The Essential Guide to Prescription Drugs

2002 Edition

The Essential Guide to Prescription Drugs

2002 Edition

James J. Rybacki, Pharm.D.

HarperResource
An Imprint of HarperCollinsPublishers

To James W. Long: More than a year now since his passing, and the wound from his loss is still bleeding. I think often of the privilege I enjoyed in working with such a brilliant man, such a kind and circumspect and selfless human being.

And to Mabis Chase: A second life now ended, a second wound that refuses to heal. Mabis, his loving family, and nurses proved that even the most complicated medication schedule can be taken right on time.

Help the people in your family, the ones living with a chronic condition and taking many medicines—the Mabises in your family—find and keep taking the right medicines. Half the people who get a prescription fail to take it correctly after a year. Make sure your loved ones, the kind and gentle persons you see every day, get the therapy they need to help keep them from running out of time.

Designed by C. Linda Dingler

ISBN 0-06-001164-5

Contents

Author's Note
for the 2002 Edition

Yet another Institute of Medicine (IOM) report (*The Quality Chasm*) took more than 300 pages to tell us that our health care system is sick. Experts from major academic and other centers found that people do not have needed access to information—and that our present health care system does NOT provide high quality care on a consistent basis. What can you do? Arm yourself with *The Essential Guide to Prescription Drugs*. Learn about your medicines, the results your doctor expects from them, how long your doctor wants to wait to reach the goals of treatment, and what changes will be made if the treatment is not successful.

Some patients take this book to office visits to get a checkup for their therapy when they get a checkup for themselves. Did YOU know that current estimates tell us that half the people who get a prescription don't take it correctly? This is called nonadherence or noncompliance. What this means is that **1.5 billion of the roughly 3 billion prescriptions filled in this country this past year were taken incorrectly. More importantly, this means that many patients DID NOT get the full benefit of those medicines and probably ended up in the hospital or may even have died. This information comes out year after year—yet we still fail to see an Adherence Assessment Form (AAF) as part of our physician office, pharmacist profile, and hospital charts. I believe it's time to make adherence to medicines the sixth vital sign (see my discussion of the AAF in Points for the Physician).**

In the US, many of us may be able to afford medicines, but medicines themselves are often used poorly. A study by Avorn looking at both Canadian and US patients found that for both groups, less than half of the patients were still taking their medicines after a year. I can't begin to count the number of patients I've seen who have been started on a new drug and left on the original medicine and dose despite less than ideal results. Current therapeutics demands that GOALS of treatment and time frames to reach them be set with any new medicine. More importantly, GOALS of treatment should be communicated to the patient as well as to his or her family. If goals are not realized, doses should be adjusted, new medicines added, and new goals and time frames created to check therapy against outcomes. Look for this strategy as a hallmark of a superb doctor. We all need to take steps to change health care. Heart disease is the leading killer of US women and men. I've become a spokesperson for the American Heart Association's new Get With The Guidelines program (www.americanheart.org/getwiththeguidelines/testimonials.html). This ambitious new program seeks to standardize treatment after a first heart attack and prevent a second one from happening. The Department of Health and Human Services has developed a Healthy People 2010 set of goals. The American Heart Association has also adopted the goals, which are to decrease coronary heart disease, stroke, and risk by 25% by January 1, 2010. While this seems distant—it is an ambitious challenge. At the time of this writing there are only about 3,000 days left. Sign up for the American Heart Association's MyHeartWatch program. We all need to lower risk of heart disease and this free Internet-based program is just the ticket to help! You'll learn more about risk factors for heart disease and get recipes, reminders, and even emails to encourage your progress. Some patients may be able to log on to this program from their pharmacy or even from their doctor's office or cardiac rehab center. Visit www.americanheart.org to find out about this and other programs. Be a part of your own solution!

In order to help YOU partner with your medicines and take care of yourself, I've included a broader and updated section in every profile that will tell you about usual goals of treatment and when they are usually reached. If a prescription is given to you—LEARN WHAT THE GOALS OF TREATMENT ARE AND WHAT THE TIME FRAME IS TO ACCOMPLISH THEM. Once again, if the goals are NOT achieved—even after you've taken the medicine exactly as prescribed—it's time for YOU to call your doctor, and see if there's a better medicine. One clear example of goals and outcomes can be seen in the new National Cholesterol Education Program Adult Treatment guidelines (ATP III). This set of guidelines calls for lower cholesterol levels, more details to be tested than just a total cholesterol, and an increased emphasis on HDL, or good cholesterol. Have you ever felt that your doctor just had to go see another patient and couldn't give you enough time? I strongly encourage you to stay in your doctor's office until you understand your disease or condition and steps you can take to prevent additional problems.

The reality from the IOM report is that in health care today—YOU MUST TAKE CARE OF YOURSELF by being part of the CENTER of the health care team. This is called patient-centered care. Amazingly—the patient historically has not been involved. That short visit in your doctor's office isn't meant to tell you all about the drugs that might be prescribed. Work with your doctor as a partner in health care, your nurse practitioner and pharmacist to keep and maintain your health, and your community pharmacist to make certain you have the right medicine in the right dose at the right time. Take steps to reduce risk factors for serious diseases. We hear more and more about shortages in health care. This means that fewer people are filling more prescriptions per hour. While intentions for not making errors may be good—time constraints often lead to problems. When you get a prescription, NEVER assume that things are correct. Read the label on your bottle and read any printed information that comes with the medicine. I'm undertaking a national demonstration project and some subsequent research this year to look at some possible systems solutions for patients and medicines. The sobering truth is that health care delivery needs a lot of work, and we are just NOT getting the most from our medicines. Use the knowledge in this book to help protect you and your family.

As noted in each previous edition, no claim is made that *all* known actions, uses, side effects, adverse effects, precautions, interactions, etc., for a drug are included in the information provided in this book. Although diligent care has been taken to ensure the accuracy of the information provided during the preparation of this revision, the continued accuracy and currentness are ever subject to change relative to the dissemination of new information derived from drug research, development, and general usage.

James Joseph Rybacki, Pharm.D.

Points for the Patient

I wish that every pharmacy, every refill required a check on how well you take your medicines (I've been trying to work on this with the American Heart Association). "I'm good about taking my pills." I can't tell you how many times I've heard this, and then checked with family members or became involved in studies looking at the same patients only to find out that a new prescription had never been filled or refills were very, very late. If we make adherence to medicines the sixth vital sign and use an uncomplicated Adherence Assessment Form to help keep us on track and remind patients every time they see their doctor, pharmacist, or other health care professional—medicines can make a fundamental difference in extending our lives.

Understanding what you are facing can be half the battle in any situation. It's important to learn as much as you can about the management of your condition. Ask your doctor and pharmacist for written information, visit reputable web sites (see Table 17), and check your local libraries and national organizations for pertinent publications. I try to help sort out information for you on my web site at www.medicineinfo.com. Never be afraid to ask your doctor and pharmacist questions—you actually make their jobs easier when you help yourself. All competent physicians and pharmacists welcome the chance to help you understand your medicines, regardless of how busy they may be. If they won't give you this critical time, find another physician or pharmacist.

We are all unique, and a critical factor in successful drug therapy is tailoring each medicine to each patient. In clothing, one size actually rarely fits all. In medicines, a "one dose fits all" approach can lead to perilous prescriptions. Once a medicine is prescribed, **share the responsibility** for safe and effective drug treatment. You can help by making sure every prescriber and pharmacist who helps provide your health care is aware of all the medicines you are taking. This sounds deceptively simple, but always include prescription, nonprescription and any herbal or nutritional support you take. Don't be afraid to take a list—I've had many patients do this and welcome the complete picture. Did you know that nonprescription medicines can blunt the benefits of your prescriptions? Millions of Americans now take herbal medicines. Do not take these products for granted. Talk to your doctor or pharmacist BEFORE combining any herbal medicine with any other medicine. REMEMBER, herbal medicines are NOT presently approved or regulated in the same way as prescription medicines. They fall under the Dietary Supplement Health and Education Act (DSHEA) of 1994. These products are more potent than ever. They can have real benefits as well as serious interactions with prescription medicines. I've updated and broadened the possible herbal/prescription medicine interactions in the drug profiles to help protect you.

Another thing I'm certain of is that decreasing risk factors for heart disease IS always a good thing. Preventing a second heart attack is absolutely critical. I've undertaken the effort of writing a testimonial and being a spokesperson for the new Get With The Guidelines program of the American Heart Association. I'm confident that this bold initiative will help consumers, pharmacists, and prescribers understand how important it is to work to reduce risk factors, develop evidence-based care, and encourage and follow physician recommendations on taking their medicines. I will also push hard to develop an Adherence Assessment Form, and the systems to make it successful. Please take your first step and find out about heart disease by calling 1-800-AHA-USA1, about strokes by calling 1-800-553-6321, and about the Get With The Guidelines Program at www.americanheart.org.

We all need to be there for our families—living in the best possible health. One way to do this is by understanding, controlling, and decreasing risk factors for heart disease. It is by far the leading killer of women and men in the United States. I've been working with some excellent people this year to once again bring important and current information to you. I'll always end my upcoming new television program (*Medicines and Your Family*) with "Take your medicines and take care of your family." I'll continue to encourage you on the radio, on television, in my audiotapes, and on my web site (www.medicineinfo.com) to ask questions and be a partner in your health care! Let's take a look at some specific ways to become involved.

When Your Doctor Prescribes a Drug for You

- ALWAYS find about specific risk factors that go along with a new diagnosis. Ask if they can be modified to lower the chance of a repeat problem or to lessen the severity of an existing problem. For example—if you have suffered a mild first heart attack, learn more about what lead to this problem, the best medicines to treat your current situation, and what to do to prevent a second heart attack. Visit the consumer side of the new Get With The Guidelines program at www.americanheart.org.

- ALWAYS ask if there is nutritional support that may be required if a new prescription is being considered. For example: HMG CoA reductase inhibitors may deplete coenzyme Q in some patients. If patients begin to feel tired after starting one of the high cholesterol medicines in that class, supplementation with co-Q may help restore quality of life. Another good example are corticosteroids such as prednisone (Deltasone, Orasone, others), which can work to weaken bones by decreasing calcium absorption. Calcium supplements and a check of bone mineral density (by DEXA or PDEXA) are advisable if prednisone or similar corticosteroids are going to be taken on an ongoing basis.
- ALWAYS ask what the goals of any existing or new treatment are, and how long it should take to reach them. Ask if there are any lifestyle changes you can try to make that might help the medicine work harder for you. Please do not wait until the last minute of an office visit to bring up the real reason you came to the office. I've seen this time after time and while it's human nature to do this, it rarely gets the best results.
- Sound-alike and look-alike errors are unfortunately not unusual. One good way to help protect yourself is to ALWAYS ask that the prescription include both the **name of the drug** and the **disorder** for which the drug is taken. For example: Fosamax for osteoporosis or Zantac for heartburn. This helps avoid "sound-alike" errors. Over the phone, a person calling in Xanax may be misunderstood as saying Zantac. Zantac is for heartburn and ulcers. Xanax is for anxiety. IF the disorder being treated is named on the label, it offers a second chance for a pharmacist or certified technician to discover a mistake.
- Ask your doctor to fill out the medication map from the back of this book while you're still in the office. This helps you fit the medicines realistically into your life. Taking this step may even show that a medicine being considered by your doctor might not really work out for you. The best medicine in the world does absolutely no good if you can't or won't be able to take it. Get the most from your health care dollars.
- Tell your doctor about any known drug allergies and of any prior drug-induced adverse effects. This will let the doctor check to see whether he or she has inadvertently prescribed a medicine from the same chemical family.
- Always honestly talk about **all other drugs** (prescription, nonprescription, herbal or nutritional) that you are taking. Include alcohol, marijuana, and others. Remember that some herbal extracts contain the same ingredients found in prescription medicines and may lead

to unforeseen toxicity, or may blunt prescription drug benefits. Interestingly, still other herbal medicines can help prescription medicines work or may even duplicate some prescription drug effects. Because of this, combining an herbal with a prescription may actually require lower doses of the prescription drug. Make certain you talk to your doctor before you combine ANY medicines.

- Many medicines **require** special precautions. Examples include avoiding certain foods, alcohol, exposure to sun, certain medicines, or even hazardous activities.
- Be sure you understand how long to take a medicine. Talk with your prescriber about this and, if applicable, when and how to stop it. A hallmark of good prescribing is that goals and time frames are set at the time a medicine is first prescribed. Unfortunately when people take several different medicines, mistakes can be made. I see many cases where patients thought they understood what to do and actually stopped the wrong medicine in a complicated regimen.
- Ask your doctor to give you a **written summary** about the drug prescribed. Few people can remember all of the information and instructions that have been talked about. A concept I have pioneered is the **medication map.** Many medicine errors are made because people forget, make incorrect combinations of medicines, mistake one pill for the other, or take medicine with food when it should not be. A medication map organizes all the medicines you are taking and tells you how much, when, and with what the medicines should be taken. Take the blank form from this book to your doctor or pharmacist and ask him or her to fill in the form with you. This will help you to clarify and verify pertinent information while taking the medicine itself in the best possible way.
- ALWAYS ask your doctor if the medicine prescribed offers the best balance of price and outcomes for you. This simple question will help a busy practitioner focus on his or her available choices. Remember to ask whether the dosing has been adjusted for any compromise in kidney or liver function or other chronic condition that you may have. Diseases can also "interact" with medicines.
- Many HMOs or health care insurers may not pay for some medicines. This can impact your doctor's prescribing authority and the pharmacist's ability to fill your prescription. Write the payer to complain. The Patient's Bill of Rights may restore your access to the medicine that will give the best results!
- Tell your doctor if new symptoms develop after you start taking the drug(s) prescribed. This can protect you from early stages of Bad Med Syndrome. Some problems caused by medicines themselves are easily reversible if they are caught early. If you are found to have had a reaction to a medicine, ask your doctor to report the problem to the FDA. This reporting is critical to maintaining safe and effective medicines.

- Keep follow-up appointments with your doctor and for laboratory tests. Many drugs must be monitored closely.
- If you go to any other health care provider, tell him or her of all medications you are taking currently—prescription and nonprescription. This is also a common source of problems: People often think that all doctors have all of their medical history simply because they are doctors. Doctors are not clairvoyant. Tell them your complete history in order to get the best possible results. Remember any herbal medicines you might be taking.
- If the prescription you got was for pain management, remember that the Joint Commission on Accreditation of Healthcare Organizations has come forth with some novel and long overdue pain management standards. From now on, when you go to the hospital, pain management will be a patient right. In time, you will see posters that help increase awareness of your basic right to effective pain management. Pain is now the fifth vital sign. In your doctor's office, you will not see the Joint Commission, but it is perfectly acceptable to demand effective pain management!
- This is controversial, but I think it is smart to ask your doctor if there is a gag rule he or she is working under that restricts him or her to a limited formulary and lower-cost medicines. There may be a conflict of interest in the advice he or she is giving you.

When You Get Your Prescription Drug(s) from Your Pharmacist

- OPEN THE BAG. Unfortunately, many people don't use the considerable education and help that their pharmacist can provide. Many prescription bags are stapled shut, with the brief patient information sheet or even a Med Guide inside. You'll be glad if you open the bag! This gives you a chance (on a refill prescription) to see if the pills look the same as before. It is also a chance to look over the dose and make sure you know how often to take it. Make sure you understand this. A few minutes reading the information about the medicine **can actually save your life.**
- READ THE LABEL carefully! It's time well spent. Check that both the **name of the drug** and the **disorder** are specified. If these are missing, ask your pharmacist to call your doctor for permission to add them.
- Many managed-care organizations require pill splitting. Check with your pharmacist to see if this is something you will be expected to do. If so, ask if they will split the pills for you, or if they have a pill splitter for sale. This will help ensure that you will get an accurate dose of medicine.
- If this is a refill, check to see that the drug in the bottle is the same as the drug in your original supply. If it is not the same, ask your

pharmacist to explain the difference. (Generic drug products from different manufacturers often vary in size, shape, color, etc.)

- There are more than 1,000 drug names that "look alike" in print or "sound alike" in speech. Examples: Celebrex—Celexa, cyclosporine—cycloserine, Prilosec—Prozac, Xanax—Zantac. Mistaking one drug for the other can lead to serious problems. "Sound-alikes" cause problems when a prescription is given by telephone. Listing the **disorder** on the prescription will help the pharmacist realize the mistake. Also, many of the most-often prescribed drugs are pictured in the Color Chart insert in this book.
- Ask your pharmacist to give you **printed information sheets** about the drug(s) prescribed for you. Say YES if you are asked if you want counseling on your medicine! Make use of your pharmacist's training. Also ask this expert to fill out the **medication map** from the back of this book for you.
- Read the label. (I'm writing this again because it is so important.) I've seen people pay more attention to a peanut butter label than they do to their prescription label. These labels are a great opportunity to learn how to get the most from your medicines. They also tell about dosage forms that should not be altered (opened, crushed, or chewed) and about effects food may have.
- Use the same pharmacy for all of your medicines. Most pharmacies have a computer system. This can help prevent serious allergic reactions and significant drug interactions. Tell your pharmacist of all drugs (remember to include herbal remedies, megavitamins, alcohol and nonprescription agents) you are currently taking.

Your Responsibilities—to Yourself—as a Patient

- Know what the goals are for any medicine you take and how long it should take to reach those goals. If time goes by and the medicine does not help as it should, there are often many other options.
- Know both the generic and brand name of all drugs prescribed for you.
- If you are taking more than one drug, be sure that the label of **each container** includes the **name of the drug** and the **condition it treats.**
- Remember that foods can react with medicines. Something as simple as grapefruit juice is now known to interact with some high blood pressure medicines. The best liquid to take with most medicines is water. Be aware.
- Take a moment to make sure you understand the directions for using a drug. Ask if you're not sure.
- Many nonprescription medicines were once available only by prescription. Talk with your pharmacist or physician **BEFORE** combining any two drugs.

- Follow medicine instructions carefully and completely. **DO NOT** stop an antibiotic seven days into a 10-day prescription because you feel better. This can lead to serious illness. If you have trouble remembering to take your medications on time, ask for a dosing calendar or a weekly medication box.
- If you take medicines prescribed by more than one doctor, check the **generic names** for duplicate drugs with different brand names. This could cause serious overdoses.
- Ask your doctor and pharmacist if they offer "brown-bag sessions" for your medicines. Put all the medicines you currently take into a bag and have your pharmacist review them for potency, appropriateness, and dating.
- If you are looking at a new insurance plan or HMO, ask if there is a formulary. Find out if a mail-order pharmacy must be used. If so, ask who will regularly review your medicines and how you will be able to contact a pharmacist for questions.
- If you will be using an Internet pharmacy, look at the Guidelines for Safe and Effective Drug Use in Section One of this book. Expect pharmaceutical care, not just delivery of medicine.
- Be certain all drugs you take are "in date" (have not expired).
- Effective and timely control of pain is a basic right to which you are entitled. The Agency for Health Care Policy and Research has released *Clinical Practice Guidelines*, which outline management of cancer pain but also apply to management of pain in general. Demand that your pain be respected as much as a high fever. The American Pain Society has long asked that pain become the fifth vital sign and this is finally a reality! The Joint Commission on Accreditation of Healthcare Organizations has developed an elaborate set of guidelines on pain management. You'll see more any time you go to a hospital.
- If you are facing a terminal illness, ask whether the hospital you are considering has a palliative care program as well as a hospice program.

Suggestions for Containing the Costs of Drug Therapy

- TAKE YOUR MEDICINE IN THE RIGHT AMOUNT AT THE RIGHT TIME AND IN THE RIGHT WAY. This sounds so very basic, but is a fundamental point where we fail time and time again. Unfortunately, if you skip doses, you may lose much of the possible benefit from many medicines. Additionally, your doctor could decide to add more medicine to the ones he thinks are not helping enough, further increasing your bill as well as chances for drug interactions.
- Cooperate fully with your doctor to ensure an accurate diagnosis. Many signs or symptoms can be embarrassing to talk about, but

may be a critical part of the puzzle that could lead your doctor to an incorrect decision. An accurate and complete history helps ensure that any medicines needed will be as safe and effective as possible.

- Ask your doctor to prescribe the drug that is most appropriate for you, selecting the product that offers the best balance of price and outcomes. If you have several chronic diseases at the same time, what appears to be a more expensive antibiotic may have a better **outcome** for you than a less costly one.
- Ask your doctor or pharmacist if an acceptable generic product is available.
- If your HMO or managed care organization requires you to split pills (a present controversy), ask if they will pay for a pill splitter so that you can accomplish this accurately. If they refuse to pay for a splitter, I strongly advise you to get one yourself. Please also write to your congressperson about the managed care organization's refusal.
- Ask your doctor if there are any vitamins or minerals that you should be taking based on family history (such as folic acid to help prevent some heart attacks or calcium for osteoporosis), or even because of the medicines themselves.
- Follow your doctor's and pharmacist's advice about your prescriptions. A medicine won't do you ANY GOOD AT ALL if it stays in the bottle.
- Many HMOs and physician groups use a concept called dual-product substitution. This is a measure that I agree with. For example, some prescription products are merely different names for the same medicine (Vanceril or Beclovent; Normodyne or Trandate). It makes perfect sense that the lowest-priced brand be freely substituted for a particular prescription. Ask your doctor about this idea when he or she is writing a prescription for you.
- Ask how the HMO or physician group measures up against other groups in your area. Remember, many groups are benchmarked or measured by groups such as the National Committee on Quality Assurance (on the Web at www.ncqa.org or call them at 202-955-5697).

Points for the Pharmacist

Adherence, adherence, adherence. I could probably end this section on this critical note. Half the people who get a prescription fail to take it correctly. WHY DO I HAVE TO SAY THIS YEAR AFTER YEAR? You can make a real difference by making sure that people understand how much to take, when to take it, and what to take it with. I've been working with the American Heart Association to involve pharmacists and pharmacies in more actively encouraging adherence and getting people quality information. A pilot program with AHA and APHA actually put a kiosk in a pharmacy to give Internet access to an AHA Web-based adherence and risk factor/behavior change program. Some other pharmacist-oriented programs increased adherence rates by two to four times what had been found in some conventional health care delivery systems! Do you encourage compliance at every initial prescription and refill? Do you call or email the doctor if your patients are early or late for refills? Consider starting a compliance clinic. Start making a difference today. If you are a hospital pharmacist, find out about the American Heart Association's new Get With The Guidelines program. It's a hospital-based program designed to identify champions in hospitals, identify patients who have had a first heart attack, and then help them get the best medicines in order to prevent a second heart attack. Learn more at www.americanheart.org.

Current estimates tell us that adverse drug events or Bad Med Syndrome costs **60–100 billion dollars a year**. Failure to individualize drug therapy is widespread and is something that you can help correct. Learn the current goals and time frames to achieve those goals in current objective guidelines (such as the American Heart Association's). Don't be afraid to keep your prescribers informed about goals and guidelines. Point of care testing such as blood sugar and cholesterol checks (now available in the same machine) can be a valuable and compensated service. Many pharmacists are being paid for their expertise in medicines (cognitive services). There are many initiatives where you can help manage diabetes, compliance, asthma, and cholesterol problems and be reimbursed for the great help that you can give. I myself take appointments and help answer questions about medicines! I've also put a framework in this book for a wonderful new cognitive service: **medication mapping.** Use this form to make sure that new prescriptions your patients present to you actually work with their lives!

Many states have given pharmacists the opportunity to provide vaccinations, and large numbers of you are starting to offer them. In a setting where the pressure of time is less restrictive, you can make a great difference in helping prevent some common illnesses. It's always better to prevent a disease or condition than to have to treat it. Influenza is a great example. Pain management is another important problem. Hospital pharmacists will now see extensive Joint Commission on Accreditation of Healthcare Organizations (JCAHCO) guidelines relating to effective pain management. Pain is now the fifth vital sign! This is a near-ideal opportunity to collaborate with your physician colleagues to make a real difference.

The American Heart Association has a Compliance Action Program underway. This bold initiative intends to help consumers, pharmacists, and prescribers understand how critical it is to work to reduce risk factors, develop evidence-based care, encourage and follow physician recommendations, and improve access to emergency care for people who have heart disease or have suffered a stroke. You can find out more by calling 1-800-242-8721. I've helped them create a new tool kit. Please use it. At the time of this writing I'll be working with the American Pharmaceutical Association Foundation and the American Heart Association on a demonstration project with community pharmacists. Visit my web site for more info at www.medicineinfo.com.

Be a leader! Create a file of your prescribers who have office email. Next, talk to your customers about the importance of your new adherence program. Explain that your pharmacy works closely with physicians to get the best results from medicines. Consider a patient adherence contract, and offer a small discount for great adherence. Talk to your patients and tell them that your pharmacy actually emails your doctor when prescriptions are filled so that they know that the new medicine is being put to work! Talk to your prescribers about this new system and explain how they can be emailed right at the office if their patients never fill or are early or late with their prescription refills.

Some pharmacists have made great inroads in clinical service by helping manage medicines for asthmatics, providing vaccines (where state law allows), offering smoking cessation groups, and helping monitor anticoagulation, asthma, blood sugar, and cholesterol. Call your state board of pharmacy for more information. It's okay to accept appointments and charge a fee for cognitive services. Many stores are getting high rates of reimbursement. No one wants to contract Bad Med Syndrome, and you can be there to help prevent it. Make your systems seamless. For example, work with your hospital pharmacy colleagues to create a seamless loop with Get With The Guidelines and follow-up care. An Adherence Assessment Form (AAF) can take 90 seconds to fill out and will keep your patients taking their medicines. Consider tracking existing medicines, start dates and dosing, and adherence via a form that follows your customers from the community to the hospital to the doctor's office and back again. Also, I've created a **medication map** in this book that offers a perfect new service to help patients realistically fit medicines into their lives!

I advise consumers to take the fullest advantage of their pharmacist's training and experience. Get copies of the latest clinical guidelines for any disease state management services you are offering and keep your prescribers in the loop! The Agency for Health Care Policy and Research is advocating effective and timely control of pain as a basic human right. The American Pain Society and JCAHCO have made pain the fifth vital sign. This is another clear opportunity for you to help in offering effective therapeutic options and superb pharmaceutical care. Call 1-800-422-6237 for more information.

When You Fill a Prescription

- Clarify with the prescriber any prescription information that is illegible, uncertain, or a potential source for erroneous interpretation—by you or the patient. Remember the Institute of Medicine data—help your customers stay alive.
- Be alert to "look-alike" and "sound-alike" drug names. This is a significant cause of dispensing errors. In accepting prescriptions by telephone, confirm the brand with the generic name as a double check. If there is still some doubt, ask the caller to spell the name of the drug.
- Include both the **name of the drug** and the **disorder** on the label (for example, Fosamax for osteoporosis) if the patient does not object, and consult with the prescribing physician when necessary. This will help (1) reduce dispensing errors caused by "look-alike" and "sound-alike" drug names and (2) prevent confusion during concurrent use of multiple drugs: mistaken identity of drug and purpose, mistakenly altered dosing schedules, etc.
- Encourage your patients to look at the prescription label **with you**. Paper clip the patient drug information to the bag. Take the lead in opening the bottle, showing the patient the medicine and making sure he or she understands how much and when to take the medicine. This also gives you a final chance to earn your place as the most trusted professional.
- Check the stock bottle for accurate identification and appropriate dating. If a technician fills the prescription, be certain you open the

dispensing container as well as the completed prescription and check the drug personally.

When You Counsel the Patient as You Dispense the Filled Prescription

- Always follow up on existing medicines with an adherence or compliance check. Document this in the patient record. Ask patients to tell you how they are to take or give any new medicine. Hearing THEM tell YOU about their medicines is a great way to make sure they really understand. Clarify any points of confusion or misunderstanding. **Every refill is an opportunity to assess and encourage adherence. Don't fail your patients by forgetting to check the medicine itself. For those patients who have Internet access and who are at risk for heart disease—encourage them to sign up for American Heart Association programs to help patients (via email reminders, risk factor identification, and other measures) decrease their risk of heart attack and stroke. Tell them to visit www.americanheart.org!**
- Make sure that the patient recognizes the **name of the drug** and the **disorder being treated**. A simple way to start this important dialogue is to ask, "What did your doctor tell you this medicine was going to do for you?" Explain what the drug is supposed to do and when the expected therapeutic benefits are usually realized.
- Review the details of dosing instructions: how much to take, when to take it, and for how long. It doesn't do them any good if it stays in the bottle. A good question to ask is, "Tell me a little bit about how your doctor told you to take this medicine." See if your computer vendor has a module for medication maps. If not, ask the publisher for permission to use the map provided in this book. This can be a valuable cognitive service.
- If the medicine you are counseling patients about is for pain, encourage patients to view effective pain control as a basic right. If they were given a pain medicine in the hospital, they will have already seen signs posted in the hospital that address this issue, and will probably have had a visit from a pain management team.
- Talk about possible side effects or adverse effects that may occur. An easy way to broach this subject is to ask, "Did your doctor tell you about any possible side effects from this medicine?" Tell patients what to do if any of these occur. Encourage them to call their doctor if new signs or symptoms develop.
- Precautions are critical. This includes possible interactions with foods, beverages, drugs, or restricted activities.
- Provide **written information** about the drug(s) dispensed and the patient's **disorder** (if available).

- Clarify how best to store the medicine. Tell patients about refrigeration and avoiding the humidity of a medicine chest. If a non-childproof lid is dispensed, remind them to keep the drug out of reach whenever children are visiting.
- Remind patients that nonprescription (over-the-counter) drugs can interact with prescription drugs. Encourage them to call your pharmacy or their physician before combining any medicines.
- Always take a good medication history and repeat this at least every six months. On every visit, be certain to ask about new medicines and any herbal medicines or vitamins the patient may have added or may be considering.
- Encourage the patient to ask questions—at the time of dispensing and later—whenever the need arises. A good way to start this conversation is, "Now that we've talked, do you have any questions for me?" Encourage patients to call if they think of something later. This is often the case.
- Explain that drugs may not work in practice exactly as expected. Tell the patient to be alert to the possibility that a new symptom or sign *may* be drug related. If one of your patients does experience a novel adverse drug reaction, it is critical that you (or your technician/designate) call the FDA MedWatch at 1-800-332-1088.

Suggestions for Containing the Costs of Drug Therapy

- Assess and encourage compliance or adherence to medicines with every initial prescription and refill. The expense of nonadherence can be huge.
- As judgment dictates, fill the prescription with the most reasonably priced drug available—within legally possible and appropriate guidelines. Consult with the prescribing physician regarding generic substitution when feasible.
- If the patient is taking other drugs (prescribed by other physicians), look for drug duplications. Offer "brown-bag sessions" where patients can bring in all their medicines and get your expert help regarding possible problems.

Points for the Physician

Outcomes, goals, guidelines, seamless systems, benchmarking, and managed care: simple phrases that have significantly changed the way physicians practice medicine today. If you also add closed formularies and critical paths, in some senses clinical decision-making has become more focused. I believe that a renewed focus on outcomes simply creates an atmosphere of continuous improvement and is just good medicine. One of the best colleagues to have in attaining the best results from any medicine is a fully informed patient. Find out more about the new American Heart Association Get With The Guidelines program (GWTG). Visit www.americanheart.org. GWTG is a hospital-based initiative that seeks to increase evidence-based therapy for secondary prevention of cardiovascular disease. If your patients are cared for by hospitalists if they suffer a heart attack—you may well find them returning to you with a form outlining new medicines. Another great way to help ensure desirable outcomes is to encourage patients with Internet access to sign up for MyHeartWatch. This novel program from the American Heart Association uses repeat emails and other messages to help patients take control of risk factors for cardiovascular disease. Send them to the web at www.americanheart.org. One novel program placed a kiosk giving One of A Kind access in the waiting area of a pharmacy. Think what such a kiosk might do in your office. Patients could have something valuable to do while they wait!

Michael Weintraub, M.D., recognized this in 1991, when in his introduction to the *Yearbook of Drug Therapy* he stated, "In looking for trends in the medical literature, it is apparent that the need for the physician to be an educator of patients and their families is becoming greater and greater." In addition, citing an increased need for patient education, he summarized with the following opinion: "Treatment principles correctly applied by patients educated about their condition and involved in its management seem to be the wave of the future." More than ever before, the volume and characteristics of the drugs in use today require deliberate individualization of treatment. The overall effectiveness of any drug therapy depends on how carefully the drug is selected, dispensed, and administered. Responsible communication between physician, pharmacist, nurse, and patient must be achieved to the greatest extent possible. This process begins with you, the physician. It is absolutely unacceptable that current estimates of the expense of adverse drug events and medical errors cost **more than 100 billion dollars a year**, more than is spent on diabetes in the United States.

Your office is most probably computerized. I've been doing work to help create a seamless patient flow sheet, which I call an Adherence Assessment Form (AAF). Create your own that lists current medicines, when they were started, and their dose and interval. Send this with the patient to the hospital and insist that it is updated on discharge. Many physicians delegate care to hospitalists and you can get the best results from them by having your UPMCAF document augment continuity of care. I wish that patients could or would use the same pharmacy, but the reality is they will shop. Make sure that your patients take or send the AAF to every pharmacy that fills prescriptions for them.

I've also told patients to "learn more about their medicines" on TV programs (*The Edge of the Envelope*), in my audiotapes and on my web site (www.medicineinfo.com). Rest assured that I will continue to encourage people to ask questions and to be partners in their health care. Don't be offended if patients bring Internet information to your office. I've tried to help patients by creating Table 17—a listing of balanced and objective sites. It may be prudent to have your office staff search the net for info on the ten most common diagnoses that you make and provide that for those under your care. The good sites will tell patients that information is only to be used in conjunction with their doctor. I know that a six- to 10-minute patient visit can never explain all of the nuances of drug therapy; hopefully, this book can help patients partner with you and decrease some of the calls that you get!

When You Evaluate a Patient for Drug Therapy

- Because patients tend to save the real reason they came to see you for the end of an office visit, ask again why they scheduled an appointment before you start to review their medication history. "Tell me again about any other questions or problems that brought you to my office today." This kind of open-ended question may help circumvent derailing bombshells left for the end of the visit. Next, be certain to review the patient's drug history for known drug allergies and prior drug-induced adverse reactions.
- Ask if the patient is currently under treatment by other health care providers or if the patient has actually gotten any prescription medicines without a prescription on the Internet.

- Ask about all drugs used currently—prescription and over-the-counter. Remember that many over-the-counter agents were once prescription medicines. Herbal medicines are now widely used and can have beneficial as well as deleterious or augmentative interactions. Rules about structure/function claims can be found at http://vm.cfsan.gov/~llrd/fr000106.html. Make certain that you do not gloss over medicines they can take without ever obtaining your guidance.
- Remember the prevalence of nutriceutical use. Include these substances in your questions. Complementary care can be valuable.
- Consider a patient's history and lifestyle. Think about diseases or conditions for which the patient is at risk, and vitamins (such as folic acid for heart disease) or minerals (calcium to prevent osteoporosis and possibly reduce risk of some colon cancers) that may be used to prevent a disease or process. Rybacki's first recommendation: It is always better to prevent a disease or condition than to have to treat it. Don't forget that some prescription medicines can negatively impact quality of life unless you recommend the appropriate nutritional support.
- Make certain that you are absolutely current. Many daily fax services are available that can be individualized to your practice and can easily be read after your morning rounds.
- Establish the nature and severity of the disorder under consideration for drug treatment.
- Elicit significant coexisting disorders—possible absolute contraindications for certain drugs.
- Evaluate any suspected or obvious organ dysfunction—possible relative contraindications for certain drugs. When creatinine values are available, take the time to calculate creatinine clearance. Many drugs have breakpoints for adjustment of dosage at various levels of renal impairment. Even though an older patient's creatinine is within the "normal limits," his or her clearance will not be. For example, a 72-year-old, 70-kg man with a 1.4 creatinine will have a creatinine clearance of about 48.6 ml/min. This is **below the level where doses or intervals of kidney (renally) eliminated medicines must be adjusted**. Hepatic disease will also impact doses or intervals for many drugs, particularly those that are highly protein-bound or heavily metabolized.
- Assess the patient's potential for adherence or nonadherence with drug therapy. Remember the expense that a given prescription presents. The most brilliant prescription choice is totally ineffective if financial considerations prevent adherence with the medicine you choose. Once-a-day dosing is much easier to remember and, combined with a dosing calendar, gets excellent results. If a complicated regimen is required, there are also pager-based systems that can give patients a "beep" with the name of the medicine and instructions for using it. Find out where your patients get their prescriptions filled and part-

ner with the pharmacy to have adherence checked on EVERY refill. If you have an email service, ask to be emailed if they are early or late or if they miss a refill. See if the patient's pharmacist offers a medication mapping service. If not, map your patient's medicines yourself.

When Selecting Drugs for Therapy

- Try to match the drug's power to the patient's problem. Avoid over-prescribing—medicinal "overkill." For example, mild to moderate stress reactions (situational anxiety-tension states) respond well to antianxiety drugs; they do not require antipsychotic medication. An uncomplicated urinary tract infection with a broadly sensitive single organism does not require a broad spectrum anti-infective drug.
- Get a copy of the *Agency for Health Care Policy and Research Clinical Practice Guidelines Number 9*. The AHCPR is advocating effective and timely pain control as a basic human right. Increase your awareness of the World Health Organization Pain Ladder and the use of the agents that are primary analgesics and adjuvants. AHCPR publications are great tools to help your patients understand their medicine and their disease. Thanks to JCAHO, pain is now the fifth vital sign in your hospital.
- Always check for drug–drug, drug–food, and drug–disease interactions. Remember to take a "new" drug history periodically.
- Many new oral anti-infectives are effective against pathogens that historically required intravenous therapy. Although this allows you to avoid hospitalization, it makes the patient's adherence more critical.
- Consider the desired onset of drug action (immediate versus delayed) and the consequences or benefits of that effect.
- Choose the drug with the most favorable benefit-to-risk ratio: the best clinical effects with the fewest possible adverse reactions.
- When you prescribe narrow-therapeutic-window drugs that require periodic blood levels, be certain that blood sampling is done after the drug has reached its steady state (usually five half-lives). Understand which level is preferable to measure: "peak" level (as for theophylline), "trough" level (as for digoxin), and "peak and trough" for aminoglycosides (such as tobramycin). Many clinical pharmacists (the author included) will willingly calculate the best dose and interval for you and make a consultative recommendation. Remember that the peak to trough ratio can be a great indicator for true once-a-day dosing with oral medicines.
- Give due consideration to the patient's prior experience with other medicines similar to the one you are considering and prescribe accordingly. Prescribing a second drug from the same drug class to which a patient already has had an allergic reaction or adverse drug effect that required discontinuation of therapy or provided no therapeutic benefit is not prudent.

- Remember individual patient factors such as age, education, and cultural factors (including genetic effects on medication elimination).
- Think about the desired extent of effect (systemic or local). Some possible adverse effects can be limited by choosing an inhaled versus "pill" form.
- Set goals and time frames when you start any new medicine. Talk these over with your patient. It's amazing how many patients I see who really have no idea what their medicine is for. Frequently, dosing issues also arise, and of course, an underdose can be just as dangerous as an overdose. If drug treatment fails after a reasonable trial with good adherence, change to a drug of another chemical class, or consider combination therapy with two medicines with different mechanisms of action. For example, if viral load decreases for a time and then increases in an AIDS patient, you MUST change treatment.
- Select the drugs you prescribe critically, utilizing independent, objective reviews of available information. The "most frequently prescribed" drug is not necessarily the best drug within its class. Slick, glossy detail pieces should always be confirmed by primary literature. Some clinical pharmacists (the author included) will provide a balanced overview of the current literature.
- Even "drugs of choice" in objective reviews can be poor choices when you consider the characteristics of individual patients. A renally compromised patient may better tolerate an "alternate drug" with dual elimination (hepatic and renal) than a "drug of choice" that is limited to renal elimination.
- Remember that possible pharmacokinetic and pharmacodynamic changes in those over 65 can lead to accumulation and excessive responses to "normal" doses and dosing intervals. In general, the possibility of side effects increases with increasing dose. Many medicines have "ceiling effects," above which dose increases act only to decrease quality of life and fail to add to therapeutic benefits.
- Be objective and discerning as you review the claims made for a newly released drug within a sizable class of drugs already available. Only a small percentage of newly approved drugs each year are classified by the FDA as truly innovative or more advantageous than similar drugs in current use. The remaining medicines are largely "me too" drugs with a limited history of use and a potential for "surprises" after a period of general use. It is best to select drugs with established records that show them to be the best in their class.

When You Issue Prescriptions in Writing or by Telephone

- When prescribing for outpatient use, slow down a little and give the pharmacist time to write. ALWAYS give both the brand and generic name as this makes sense and can help YOU avoid a lawsuit arising from a sound-alike error. Consider the advantage of including both the **name of the drug** and the **therapeutic indication** (the patient's disorder) on the prescription label—for example, Vioxx (rofecoxib) for arthritis. Putting the disorder on the label will help (1) reduce dispensing errors caused by "look-alike" and "sound-alike" drug names and (2) prevent confusion that often occurs during concurrent use of multiple drugs, especially among the elderly: mistaken identity of drug and purpose, mistakenly altered dosing schedules, etc. Pain is now the fifth vital sign and a focus of new JCAHCO guidelines. If you work in a system where inpatient care is provided by hospitalists, be aware that they will in essence be charting the outcomes of YOUR outpatient pain management.

- Respect your patients' wishes as to whether they *want* the name of the disorder written on the prescription label. If they prefer you not include it, recommend that they write it on the label themselves *after* the prescription is filled.
- Keep dosing schedules as simple as possible. Once-a-day dosing improves adherence.
- Alert the pharmacist to "look-alike" and "sound-alike" drug names. Print the drug name and generic on written prescriptions. Spell the drug name and include the generic when prescribing by telephone.

When Counseling Patients About Drug Therapy

- ALWAYS stress the critical nature of adherence. If your patients are adherence-challenged, talk about pill boxes, bottle reminders, and even pager-based systems to make sure that they will take their medicines. Briefly explain the nature of the patient's disorder and its treatment. Use language that is readily understood by the average person. I've often found clinicians using language that is barely understood by the average doctor. If you use words that are on a sixth-grade level, you'll often have a patient colleague working to achieve the goals of treatment. The MyHeartWatch component of the American Heart Association web site offers patients balanced information, repeat email messages, and a real chance at continuing risk-lowering behaviors. Consider encouraging your office patients as a chance to get objective information and behavior reinforcement while they are in your office.
- Provide written information or references for educational material about the disorder. If the disorder is chronic in nature (diabetes, hypertension), explain the need to continue drug therapy indefinitely, possibly for life. It's no surprise that patients are visiting the Internet. Provide helpful web sites (see Table 17) that give balanced information. Explain that some pharmaceutical company–provided sites may not give complete information, or may skew data to favor their products.

- Briefly explain the name and nature of the drugs you are prescribing. Again, stress the importance of strict adherence with the medicine. It is wise to tell the patient—in advance—about potential adverse effects. The patient who has such effects is more likely to be understanding and forgiving if they do not come as a surprise. Talk about possible options available if the goals of therapy are not achieved in the expected time frames.
- To supplement your discussion, **provide a printed document** that summarizes the essential information the patient needs to use the drug(s) safely and effectively. This is comforting and will save you an amazing number of telephone calls and pages. Be sure the patient knows what to do if a dose is missed. Look at an add-on program to your office-management program that prints out relevant information for your patients to take home. Such services can provide detailed descriptions of drugs, general guidelines for drug use, and personalized instructions. Unfortunately, your patient may run into a pill-splitting reality with many medicines. Be aware of what managed care organizations expect your patient to do. A pill splitter can be an important assurance of correct doses.
- Explain the need for follow-up visits to monitor the effects of drug treatment and the course of the disorder. If possible, empower the patient by self-testing. For example, a fructosamine finger stick test can augment the glycosylated hemoglobins (hemoglobin A1C) that you order and also give your diabetics better results from their medicines.
- Explain that drugs may not work in practice exactly as expected. Tell the patient to be alert to the possibility that a new symptom or sign *may* be drug related. Certainly tell the patient about probable effects and what to do about them. If one of your patients does experience a novel adverse drug reaction, it is CRITICAL that you (or your designate) call the FDA MedWatch at 1-800-332-1088.
- It is virtually impossible for the FDA to test new medicines against all possible multiple pill regimens. Calling MedWatch (1-800-332-1088) fulfills your voluntary obligation to Phase Four reporting and makes medication use safer for everyone. I admit that I am the one advocating mandatory reporting. Encourage the patient to call as needed regarding any aspect of drug treatment. Some of this call volume can be successfully shifted to pharmacists trained in specific disease management. Locate these pharmacy centers of excellence and work together to get the best results for your patients. Recognize the need to adjust drug selection and/or dosage regimens to accommodate individual variability.
- Give special attention to the older patient on drug therapy. The elderly (1) generally use multiple drugs concurrently and (2) are more prone to experience adverse drug effects.
- If you refer any of your patients to a specialist, be certain to take a

repeat medication history when they are returned to your care. Check for duplications in medicines by cross-referencing brand or generic names.

- Every six months, ask your patients to bring in all the prescription, nonprescription, and herbal medicines that they routinely take. This kind of "brown bag session" can help you best understand all of the potential or actual interactions of therapies your patient is or will be taking. Remember: An informed patient can be your greatest ally in optimal therapeutics and the outcomes that will be benchmarked!

Suggestions for Containing the Costs of Drug Therapy

- When you have selected the most appropriate drug, consider its cost. If the patient requests an available generic product, direct the pharmacist to dispense one with certified bioequivalence. Because of generic product variability, caution the patient to have the prescription refilled with the identical generic (same manufacturer) each time.
- Avoid polypharmacy whenever possible. Limit the number of drugs that the patient is taking concurrently to the fewest required. Do not let the cure become the disease. Medicate serious, significant disorders; discourage the use of drugs for minor, transient complaints.
- Consider carefully any requests from patients for a prescription drug they have learned about through direct-to-consumer advertising. Explain to your patients the profit motive of the producer and assure them that you will prescribe the drug that, in your judgment, is the most appropriate for them.
- When circumstances permit, use home intravenous drug therapy in preference to hospitalization. If hospitalization is required, explore IV to PO switches and medication streamlining to help appropriately decrease length of stay.
- The move toward managed care and other health care reform initiatives brings increased scrutiny to the outcomes of your therapeutic and clinical decisions. Become more familiar with the expense of various medicinal options, as well as the specific patient populations where the benefit-to-risk and cost-to-outcome ratios make the most sense. Pharmacoeconomic and disease management approaches will bring the best balance of cost and outcome.
- Work with the pharmacy your patients use to create seamless systems. They have a lot of data, and you want to give the best care. If you have office email, ask the pharmacy to email if patients never fill or are early or late with their prescriptions. This gets you the information you need, and can prompt a quick follow-up phone call from your office staff to your compliance-challenged patients. Finding out about nonadherence or noncompliance early can help prevent catastrophic events such as stroke or MI.

The Essential Guide to Prescription Drugs

2002 Edition

1

HOW TO USE THIS BOOK

2

GUIDELINES FOR SAFE AND EFFECTIVE DRUG USE OR HOW TO PREVENT BAD MED SYNDROME

3

TRUE BREAKTHROUGHS IN MEDICINES

1

How to Use This Book

When you're sick, and finally make that decision to see your doctor—it's probably one of the worst times for you to think about the medicines you take now or even that new prescription. A visit to your physician's office can be a disconcerting experience. The reality of "managed care" is that time has been contracted, patients may only be considered covered lives, and health care providers face severe time constraints. I think that the Institute of Medicine (IOM) report on medical errors will serve to increase awareness of systems problems in health care, but the reality will still remain that most patients will have the sense of their doctor needing—not wanting—to hurry out of the exam room to see the next patient. You may be left with a prescription for yourself or a loved one that no one told you anything—and certainly not everything—about.

I've rewritten this book to help cure Bad Med Syndrome (BMS; see Glossary) and to bring you current and important information to protect yourself and your family. I can help you become a partner in your health care and will always try to supplement the direction and guidance your doctor will offer about your medicines. This principle is also ascribed to on my web site (www.medicineinfo.com) via the Health On the Net Principles. Just like the site, this Guide seeks to augment, NOT to replace, the role of your doctor.

Your new book is arranged into six sections. The first section offers insight into modern drug therapy and gives you helpful tips on preventing BMS. "True Breakthroughs in Medicines" will help identify new medicines that have gained FDA approval or that are the first new agents to treat an existing disease or condition. Section Two gives you detailed Drug Profiles covering more than 2,000 brand-name prescription drugs and nearly 400 widely used generic medicines. Selection of each drug is based on three criteria: the extent of its use, the urgency of the conditions it treats, and the volume and complexity of information essential to its proper use. You'll find that profiles are arranged alphabetically by generic name. Read carefully to be sure you have the correct medicine.

Each profile is presented in the same way and once you become familiar with the format, you'll be able to quickly find specific information on any drug. Unlike other imitators, each Essential Drug Profile contains up to 45 helpful categories of information. Let me introduce you to the other parts of your new book:

Herbal Medicines or Minerals

Because herbal medicines are so widely used, I developed a new section last year that included (where appropriate) important possible interactions between herbal and prescription medicines. Please remember that herbal products **are not regulated by the FDA as medicines. They fall under the Dietary Supplement Health and Education Act (DSHEA) of 1994.** This may mean that specific products have not been well-studied—others rely on borrowed science—and certainly that these products can interact with prescription medicines. Accordingly, I've broadened the data in your new Guide. You'll find that I'll tell you where combinations between herbs and prescription drugs may make sense, where they do not, and of course how to talk to your doctor before you move forward. This is a very dynamic area, and I'll update this section every year! There may also be information at www.medicineinfo.com that can help.

Year Introduced

At first glance, this may seem trivial, but remember, the longer the drug has been in general use, the more likely all of its actions are known and the less likely ongoing use will produce new problems. This will help you identify those medicines that are more likely to be more fully understood both because they have been used for a longer time period and because they have also been widely used.

Drug Class

Drug classes are like families—in fact, some of the profiles giving information about medicines from the same class have been arranged into Medication Family Profiles. Many actions, reactions, and interactions with other drugs are often shared by drugs of the same class. For example, *if you are allergic to one member of the cephalosporin family, you most likely will be allergic to a second cephalosporin. By the same logic, if a medicine in a certain class has not helped you, it is likely that a second one from the same class will do you little good.* Pay close attention to this aspect of medicines, since this is an area that often leads to problems or lack of results.

Prescription Required

Just because a medicine does not require a prescription (over-the-counter) does not mean the medicine is weak or is free from possible drug interactions. Remember, over the last 15 years there has been a great shift in medicines from prescription to nonprescription. Current examples include medicines for yeast infections, patches and gum to help you stop smoking, as well as ulcer medicines (histamine H2 blockers) that can also be used to prevent or treat heartburn. Virtually all of these medicines were previously available only by prescription. Always mention nonprescription medicine use when asked about the "medicines" you take.

Controlled Drug

The Controlled Substances Act of 1970 assigned medicines with a potential for abuse to a specific schedule in the United States. A Canadian schedule is also given when applicable. A description of the schedules of controlled drugs is found at the back of your Guide.

Available for Purchase by Generic Name

In general, costs can be reduced by buying a generic equivalent of a brand-name product. The key word is "equivalent." It is important to make sure that "bioavailability and bioequivalence"—the comparative composition, quality, and effectiveness of the generic versus the brand-name drug product—are the same if a substitution is made. Further discussion of bioavailability and bioequivalence may be found in Section Five, the Glossary of Drug-Related Terms.

Brand Names

I realize that generic or chemical names of medicines can be complicated, so brand names are given to help. Brand names are listed for the United States and for Canada (✤). A combination drug (one with more than one active ingredient) is identified by [CD] following the brand name. Be careful! In some cases THE SAME NAME used in both the United States and Canada will represent entirely different generic drugs (in a single drug product) or a significantly different mixture of generic medicines. If you travel between the two countries, make sure that the brand-name drug contains the same generic medicine(s).

Benefits versus Risks

The possible pros and cons for each drug are summarized. Capital letters emphasize the drug's principal benefits and risks, while lowercase letters are used for less critical benefits and risks. One look reveals the "comparative weights" of the two columns and gives a first impression about how a drug's benefits relate to its potential risks. This is meant to help you become more circumspect in your use of medicines—but is not to be the sole basis for deciding whether to use a drug. I find that the triad **failure to individualize drug selection and dose, failure to communicate goals of treatment, and lack of an effective system to repeatedly check, encourage, and follow up on how well people take their medicines (adherence) is the greatest weakness in current drug therapy and health care.**

Principal Uses

A drug may be available as a single drug product or in combination with other drugs. The "As a Single Drug Product" section tells you the primary use(s) of the drug when it is used alone in a particular product. The "As a Combination Drug Product [CD]" section tells about the primary use(s) when an active medicine is combined with other drugs in the same pill. The uses are a consensus of the medical community and reflect current research. Where appropriate, the logic for combining certain drugs is explained.

How This Drug Works

This section tells what a drug does to work. If a specific method of action has not been established, I will tell you about the current theory. This can be important in the sense that if you are taking two medicines that work in the same way or act on the same system, better combination therapy may be available.

Available Dosage Forms and Strengths

This gives you available manufacturers' dosage forms (tablets, capsules, elixirs, etc.) and strengths, without company identification. Dosage forms limited to hospital use are often not included. The section Dosage Forms and Strengths in the Glossary can help with those few abbreviations used to describe strengths of each dosage form.

Usual Adult Dosage Ranges

Dosing information represents a consensus by appropriate authorities and is the currently recommended standard. It is a guide showing how much of the drug can reasonably be expected to be both effective and safe. Under certain circumstances, your doctor may decide to modify the "standard" dose. Some dosage forms not covered (for example, extemporaneously made suppositories) may require different doses than those listed because of absorption at different routes.

Conditions Requiring Dosing Adjustments

Medical conditions can actually change the effect a medicine has on your body (technically called a drug-disease interaction). This is a fact that is **often missed** in choosing a dose or in deciding how often a medicine should be taken (dosing interval)—and can lead to BMS. For example, people over age 60 usually have an expected or "normal" age-related decline in kidney function. Throughout this book I refer to this as kidney compromise. What this means is that medicines removed by the kidneys may stay in the body longer than expected (increased half life)—not because the kidneys are diseased—but because they simply do not work as well as they used to. The real possible effect of this increased half life is that a typically prescribed dose could in reality amount to an overdose. **While the exact age when this decline starts may vary—it is critical for people at or near 60 to ask their doctor if any prescribed medicine is removed by the kidneys—and if the dose or dosing interval has been adjusted for this kidney compromise.** I also include information on liver compromise (where appropriate) as well as information on other prevalent diseases or conditions that may impact dosing.

Dosing Instructions

Food and medicines can fight. Foods can actually change how much medicine gets into your body (increasing or decreasing absorption)—and this section tells you about them. Medicines can also irritate the lining of the stomach or intestines and food can help ease this irritation. The dosing instruction section will also tell you about advisability of changing the form of the medicine itself. For example—sometimes, when medicine is urgently needed, you may have to crush the tablet or open the capsule and mix the contents with a food or beverage. On the other hand, many medicines should **NEVER** be crushed or altered to be taken. This information category identifies those forms of each drug that may be changed and those that should not be. A new feature of this section provides information on what to do if you forget your pill. If you are still uncertain— call your doctor. Another caveat on this: if you find yourself forgetting often, talk to your doctor and see if there is a medicine that might give the same benefits but not require so many doses! A good example is in the management of high blood pressure. Many patients may get great results from a newer medicine taken once or twice a day instead of one that has to be taken more frequently. There are also many reminder systems—even beeper-based ways to help you take control of your disease or condition by taking your medicine right on time.

Usual Duration of Use

Many factors determine how long a medicine must be taken. This is often an area of great controversy and patient confusion. Factors such as the nature and severity of symptoms, drug form and strength, ability of the patient to respond, use of other drugs, etc. come into play here. Some situations such as increased cholesterol or hyperlipidemia will need to be treated on an ongoing basis. It is always prudent to check results as well as problems on a regular basis. The main idea is for you and your clinician to give the medicine an appropriate amount of time to reach the goals of therapy, and to adjust the dose or even add or change the medicine if goals are not reached within the expected period of time. Where important, limitations in how long a medicine should be taken are outlined in this section.

Typical Treatment Goals and Measurements (Outcomes and Markers)

This is the second year of this NEW SECTION that you can use to get the results you deserve! One of the hallmarks of a good clinician lies in how well he or she sets and communicates, and then prescribes or adjusts, medicines to realize the goals of therapy. Unfortunately, I've often found this aspect of care to be sorely lacking. In order to help you understand what some reasonable expectations from treatment are, I've included typical goals, measurements, and results in ALL of this year's profiles. For example, the entries below pertain to blood sugar and cholesterol lowering medicines that are taken by mouth.

- Blood Sugar: The general goal for blood sugar is to return it to the usual "normal" range (generally 80–120 mg/dl), while avoiding risks of excessively low blood sugar. One study (UKPDS) used a fasting plasma sugar (glucose) of less than 108 mg/dl.
- Cholesterol: The National Institutes of Health (NIH) has released ATP III—a new set of guidelines for treating people at risk for heart disease. This National Cholesterol Education Program (NCEP) effort has some changes versus the last edition. Importantly, diabetes was added to the list of conditions that lead to increased heart disease risk. Total cholesterol targets remain at less than 200 mg/dl, but the guidelines recommend testing for the various components of total cholesterol such as low density lipoproteins (LDL) and high density lipoproteins (HDL). New designations list 100 mg/dl of LDL to be optimal, 130–159 as borderline high, 160 mg as high, and 190 mg/dl as very high. A new focus has been placed on HDL, making the "too low" reading as 40 mg/dl for this "good" cholesterol.

I hope that this new feature will let you be more involved in your health care, and will also encourage you to ask questions if the goals of your medicines are not achieved. At the time of this writing, a great new section of the American Heart Association web site is called MyHeartWatch. This can help you with some specific heart disease (cardiovascular) risk factor goals. Visit them at www.americanheart.org.

This Drug Should Not Be Taken If

These entries are the absolute contraindications to the use of the drug (see Contraindication in the Glossary). By consensus, these are circumstances where the medicine should NEVER be taken. Tell your doctor **immediately** if any information in this category applies to you.

Inform Your Physician Before Taking This Drug If

These entries tell you relative contraindications to a medicine. One way to think of this is as a relative benefit-to-risk decision. Again, tell your physician or other prescriber if these factors apply to you.

Possible Side Effects

Here you can learn about natural, expected, and usually unavoidable medicine actions—the normal and anticipated consequences of taking it. This gives a realistic perspective balancing side effects with goals of treatment. I emphasize that these are POSSIBLE side effects.

Possible Adverse Effects

These are unusual, unexpected, and infrequent drug effects that are often called adverse drug reactions or effects. These range from mild to serious. In order to more accurately define how frequently these effects happen, I've developed the following approach:

- Possible: An effect that has been documented for other drugs in the same family but not the profiled drug. Also assigned when the effect occurs in some limited patient populations and not in others.
- Case Reports: An effect that has been documented to happen, but has been seen only in isolated cases.
- Rare: An effect that is seen in less than 2 percent of patients. Another way to look at this is that 98 percent of people will take the medicine and NOT have the effect.
- Infrequent: An effect that is seen in 2 to 10 percent of patients.
- Frequent: Effects that happen in more than 10 percent of patients.

Tell your doctor if you suspect you may be having an adverse drug effect. **Serious adverse reactions may start with mild, unthreatening symptoms, and serious problems may be avoided if you call right away.** It's also possible to have an adverse reaction that has not yet been reported. Don't discount an adverse effect just because it's not listed. *A properly selected drug usually has a comparatively small chance of producing serious harm.* Knowing that a drug can cause a serious adverse reaction should not deter you from using it when it has been properly selected and its use will be carefully supervised.

If you have had a reaction to a medicine, make sure to remember to ask that your doctor REPORT THIS REACTION. One problem with our system of medicine surveillance is that reporting of adverse effect of medicines is VOLUNTARY for health care professionals. Less than 3% of serious adverse reactions are reported, and this can leave the next family vulnerable to the same undesirable experience. Your doctor (or his staff) can call 1-800-FDA-1088 (1-800-332-1088).

Possible Effects on Sexual Function

This information is often NOT something people want to discuss, or something that patients are told about. Currently available information (often inadequate and vague) from all reliable sources is presented. Both physician and patient are well advised to discuss frankly any potential effect that drug therapy could have on sexual expression.

Adverse Effects That May Appear Similar to Natural Diseases or Disorders

Medicines can actually cause effects similar to widely diagnosed diseases or disorders. Quite often this inadvertent error is compounded by prescribing another drug to relieve the "symptoms" of the first. My father was prescribed a medicine for his "arthritis" when he was actually having an adverse effect from a medicine for his heart rhythm. For milder symptoms (e.g., nasal congestion or diarrhea from reserpine), the oversight may not be too serious. But in the case of my father, the mistake was devastating. This section tells you about this common flaw.

Natural Diseases or Disorders That May Be Activated by This Drug

Many drugs can "activate" latent disorders that may not be recognized as drug induced. If a new and seemingly unrelated disorder starts during treatment with any new medicine, ask your doctor if it may be drug related.

Possible Effects on Laboratory Tests

Most drugs have significant effects on body chemistry and organ systems. Some effects are intended and beneficial (therapeutic); others are unintended, unavoidable, and potentially harmful. Timely use of laboratory tests lets us check how well a drug is working, detect early drug toxicity, assign some lab test changes to drug and lab test interactions, and also check the course of the condition being treated.

Caution

This category gives you information on aspects of drug actions and/or drug uses that require special emphasis. Occasionally, this section may actually relate to information provided in other categories. Once again, this is an important feature this Guide offers to help you take care of your family.

Precautions for Use: Infants and Children

Doses often MUST be changed for infants and children under 12 years of age, and some drugs and/or treatment situations call for special precautions. When administering any prescription or over-the-counter drug, it is best to ask your doctor or pharmacist about needed precautions. New FDA regulations will now require study of medicines in children where the drugs are specifically used in children.

Precautions for Use: Those Over 60 Years of Age

Our bodies do not remain the same over time, and people age at different rates and in different ways. Assessment of "age" must be based upon individual mental and physical condition, and never on years alone. Changes that accompany aging may affect the actions of the body on the drug, actions of the drug on the body—and even how well the medicine is removed. Appropriate precautions are outlined in this category.

Advisability of Use During Pregnancy: Pregnancy Category

Information about safe use of a particular drug during pregnancy was one of the most forceful concerns that led to the formal petitioning of the Food and Drug Administration in 1975 to make sure that information was disclosed to the public. The FDA definitions of the five pregnancy categories are listed at the back of this book. The FDA does not make the initial category assignment; this is the responsibility of the manufacturer that markets the drug. The initial designation is then subject to review and modification by the FDA. The "Pregnancy Category" designations presented in each profile were determined after thorough review of pertinent literature and consultation with appropriate authorities. They are offered at this time for initial guidance only. They may not be "official" and may not have the endorsement of either the manufacturer or the FDA. If controversy exists among researchers or manufacturers, you may find more than one pregnancy category for the same medicine.

Advisability of Use If Breast-Feeding

This section tells you about effects of the drug on milk production. You will also learn if the drug goes into human milk, and the possible effects of the drug on the nursing infant. Prudent recommendations are given where appropriate. Also included are impacts of disease where appropriate.

Suggested Periodic Examinations While Taking This Drug

Getting the best results from your medicines often means that your doctor may ask you to get tests while you take the drug(s) he or she has prescribed. Which exams and when they are made depend on your past and present medical history, the nature of the condition being treated, the dose and duration of drug use, and your doctor's observations of your response. For example, checking finger stick blood sugar and fructosamine or hemoglobin A1C while taking an oral glucose-lowering (oral hypoglycemic) medicine is critical. On the other hand, there may be many occasions when your doctor decides no examinations are necessary. Always tell your doctor about all developments you think may be drug related.

While Taking This Drug, Observe the Following: Herbal Medicines or Minerals

Since many millions of people are taking herbal medicines as well as minerals, I think it is critical to tell you about herbs and prescription or nonprescription medicines. I've tried to bring you timely data that tells about possible harmful combinations as well as situations where herbal medicines can actually increase beneficial effects of some prescription drugs. Complementary and beneficial use of herbal medicines may allow for lower prescription drug doses (this may be very beneficial since it may also help you avoid side effects). Data have been difficult to come by, and you may find that not all profiles carry this kind of interaction or the same depth of coverage.

I have broadened the information since last year's groundbreaking inclusion of such information, and will continue to update this important aspect of care. DO NOT ASSUME that because it's herbal, it's natural and will not interact with your medicines. Because new prescription drug–herbal medicine interactions are always being discovered, NEVER combine any herbal or prescription or nonprescription drug without first talking to your pharmacist and doctor. I've also included the URLs of some helpful web sites in the tables near the end of this book.

While Taking This Drug, Observe the Following: Marijuana Smoking

The widespread "social" use of marijuana by virtually all age groups and the approval of medicinal smoking of marijuana in two states have led to inquiries about interactions between the active chemicals in marijuana smoke and medicines in common use. Currently available literature on the health aspects of marijuana use contains very little practical information concerning the potential for drug interactions. The limited information presented in this category of selected Drug Profiles represents those possible interactions considered likely to occur in view of the known pharmacological effects of the principal components of marijuana and of the medicine reviewed in the profile. In most instances, the interaction statements are not based on documented evidence, since very little is available. The conclusions stated—derived by logical inductive reasoning—represent the concurrence of authorities with expertise in this field. There is a well-designed study of medical marijuana use underway at the time of this writing.

While Taking This Drug, Observe the Following: Other Drugs

This confusing and often controversial area of drug information is divided into five subcategories of possible interactions between drugs. Look carefully at the wording of each subcategory heading (see also Interaction in Glossary). Some of the drugs listed do not have a representative profile. If you are using one of these drugs, ask your doctor or pharmacist for help about potential interactions. A brand name (or names) that follows the generic name of an interacting drug is given as an example only. It is not intended to mean that the particular brand(s) named has interactions that are different from other brands of the same generic drug. If you are taking the generic drug, all brand names under which it is marketed MUST be considered as possible interactants. Medicines in the same or similar families may also interact.

Driving, Hazardous Activities

Clearly, medicines can change coordination and alertness. The information in this category applies not just to driving motor vehicles, but to any activity of a dangerous nature, such as operating machinery, working on ladders, using power tools, and handling weapons. Your individual response and degree of reaction may vary from others'. Talk with your doctor or pharmacist if you take a medicine that may impair your abilities.

Aviation

Military pilots enjoy the expert guidance and surveillance provided by the flight surgeon, but no tightly structured control system exists for their civilian counterparts. The need for practical information regarding the possible effects of medicinal drugs on flight performance, however, is the same for pilots in all settings. This section can tell civilian pilots how a particular drug may affect their eligibility to fly and when it is advisable or necessary to consult a designated Aviation Medical Examiner or an FAA medical officer.

Occurrence of Unrelated Illness

Some medicines—for instance, "oral hypoglycemics" such as glipizide—require careful regulation of doses to maintain a constant drug effect within critical limits. In this section of your book, emphasis is given to those illnesses that might affect drug use. For example, if a body-wide infection were to occur, the oral hypoglycemic dose may not work and insulin injections may be temporarily required in order to maintain blood sugar in an appropriate range.

Discontinuation

How and when to stop a medicine are often as important as starting a medicine in the first place. Unfortunately, this aspect of drug use is often overlooked when a medicine is first discussed. Your doctor should always approach treatment with medicines with specific goals and time frames to reach those goals when the medicine is FIRST started, for example, reducing a blood pressure of 159/93 to 120/75 in two months using a particular medicine. Additionally, it is often mandatory that patients be fully informed on when to discontinue, when not to discontinue, and precisely how to stop use of the drug. In some cases, when one medicine is stopped, other drugs being taken at the same time may also need to be adjusted. The doctor who is primarily responsible for your overall medicine management must be kept informed of all the drugs you are taking at a given time and if and when any of them are stopped.

I believe that the remaining information categories in the Drug Profiles are self-explanatory, but I always welcome your letters and questions. I have also started a web site called **Medicine Information** and can be reached at www.medicineinfo.com.

Section Three is called "The Leading Edge" and offers what are, in my opinion, medicines that show great promise and are just over the horizon from FDA approval. Some of these medicines may not actually be approved, but they give such significant hope that they're worth consideration. The information may let patients facing serious diseases ask to be included in scientific studies and get the medicine prior to actual approval.

Section Four is a presentation of Drug Classes arranged alphabetically by their chemical or therapeutic (generic) class. Because of chemical composition and biological activities, some drugs appear in two or more classes. For example, the drug product with the brand name Diuril will be represented by its generic name, chlorothiazide, in three drug classes: the Thiazide Diuretics (a chemical classification), the Diuretics (a drug action classification), and the Antihypertensives (a disease-oriented classification). Please use the Drug Classes to your advantage. I can't count the number of times I've seen busy physicians discover an allergy or problem with a particular medicine, only to turn right around and prescribe a medicine **from the same class.** This section can protect you from this kind of error.

Frequently in the Drug Profiles in Section Two you are advised to "see (a particular) Drug Class." This alerts you to a possible drug contraindication, or to possible interactions with certain foods, alcohol, or other drugs. In each case, you can find the more readily recognized brand names for each drug listed generically within a drug class by looking at the appropriate Drug Profile. Timely use of these references can help you avoid many possible hazards of medication.

Section Five is a Glossary of Drug-Related Terms used throughout the book. The preferred use of each term is explained. Frequent references to the Glossary are made in the Drug Profiles. Use of the Glossary will help you understand how to recognize and interpret significant drug effects.

Section Six offers tables of drug information. The title and introductory description explain the content and purpose of each table. The tables give you another source of ready reference. I've included a Medication Map as Table 15 because it is a way for you to use your doctor's or pharmacist's expertise to arrange all of the medicines you take into a reasonable schedule. It is also something I strongly advocate that you take to the hospital with you. If a new prescription or medicine is to be given, make sure that the prescriber knows about all of the "pills" you presently take. When it's time to go home from the hospital or to leave your doctor's office, take the time to have them help you get the most from your medicines.

Table 16 identifies medicines that have been removed from the market. This may help protect you from medicines that may still be available in other countries (or on the Internet) and not available on US shelves. Please use the index of brand and generic names in the back of the book. It is a single alphabetical listing that provides page references to the appropriate Drug Profile(s) for all drugs found in this book. Read the introductory explanation of the special features of this combined index.

Because of the explosion of information on the Internet, I've also created a new table that tells you the URLs of a number of web sites that I have found to be objective and valuable (Table 17). I've updated and broadened this part of the book for this edition. Regard the Internet cautiously. If you decide to buy medicines from the Net—make sure you have a prescription from your doctor and are then buying from a reputable company. Much has been heard this year about counterfeit medicines. You can actually call the National Association of Boards of Pharmacy at 847-698-6227 or visit them on the Web at www.nabp.net and find out if a site really does belong to a licensed pharmacy.

2

Guidelines for Safe and Effective Drug Use or How to Prevent Bad Med Syndrome

MEDICINES AND PHARMACY ON THE INTERNET

There has been an explosion of emails, advertisements, health claims, prescription-less drug ordering, and even pharmacies on the Internet. While I cover some aspects in the Do and Do Not sections, I think this subject is important enough to break it out into a separate section. Mergers and changes in scope of service have occurred in pharmacy, as they have in other businesses. Amidst the change, there are still some common characteristics of appropriate pharmacies and medicines on the Internet. At a minimum these include:

- The pharmacy site requires a prescription for a prescription medicine and provides a way for you to prove that you have one. Given the present state of the Internet, it appears prudent to stick with "known" companies. The largest current online pharmacies are walgreens.com and cvs.com.
- The site requires a medication history. This history should include allergies, current weight and height, and illnesses as well as ALL prescription and nonprescription medications and herbal or nutritional supplements you are currently taking. This ensures that you will be getting appropriate pharmaceutical care (checking your medicines for interactions, errors, appropriate doses, etc.).
- Information on the site is referenced. This is critical; much of the Internet is unregulated. You should look for footnotes, endnotes, or

parenthetical references or organization references placed appropriately relative to the information you have read. If such notes are not present, the information may be untrue, opinion, or inappropriately slanted. Make sure to talk to the person who prescribed any medicines for you BEFORE you make any changes based on information not provided by that prescriber—even from a well-referenced source.

- A statement disclosing how, with which references, and by whom your current prescription and any existing prescriptions will be checked for accuracy, possible drug interactions, and appropriate disease-, age-, or condition-related dosing changes. The site will also provide a way to talk to a human about questions about your medicines and possible adverse effects.
- Medicines arrive in an appropriate, labeled container that has any needed auxiliary labels on it as well. Please make sure to ask that the disease or condition being treated by the medicine is included on the label
- Medicines can be obtained by anyone and can be shipped from anywhere. Unfortunately, not everyone has your best interests at heart. There have been a lot of news stories about counterfeit medicines—fake drugs or water substituted for expensive treatments. A real pharmacy with a board to inspect it and help ensure quality is a great idea. You can call the National Association of Boards of Pharmacy at 847-698-6227 or visit them on the Web at www.nabp.net and find out if a site really does belong to a licensed pharmacy.
- Information is a powerful ally when you are taking any medicine. When you look for information on a site, check to be sure that site has a date and date revised section. This tells you that information is being reviewed and kept current.

DO NOT

- order a prescription medicine without a prescription from the Internet. Even if you can get the medicine, you will not have the benefit of your doctor's, pharmacist's or nurse practitioner's training to help protect you. This can be a prescription for disaster. You also often have no way of knowing that what is supposed to be in the pill is actually what is there.
- automatically trust information that you get over the Internet. Appropriate information has references and at least a byline of a reputable person. If you find information that is troubling to you, talk to your doctor or pharmacist before you act on that information.
- pressure your doctor to prescribe drugs that, in his or her judgment, you do not need. A pill is not always the answer.
- blindly accept care from any provider. Ask your HMO or medical group how their results or outcomes compare to other groups in the area and the country.

- assume that all doctors know all the drugs you take. Always ask your doctor or pharmacist BEFORE combining any other medicine with medicines already prescribed.
- accept a stapled prescription bag. ALWAYS OPEN a stapled bag, check the brief patient information that may be inside the bag, and make sure you understand it. If there is a Med Guide with the prescription, read that carefully as well. While you are in the pharmacy, read the prescription label and make sure it makes sense. Look at the pills, and (especially on refill drugs) check to see that they look the same as they did before. On new prescriptions, ask that the prescription be checked to make sure it is the correct medicine.
- take prescription drugs on your own or on the advice of friends and neighbors because your symptoms are "just like theirs"—ESPECIALLY NOT FROM THE INTERNET WITHOUT A PRESCRIPTION. Drug therapy must be individualized, based on liver and/or kidney function, medicines you currently take, and many other factors.
- offer drugs prescribed for YOU to anyone else without a physician's guidance.
- change the dose or timing of any drug without the advice of your physician (except when the drug appears to be causing adverse effects).
- leave it to a guess that you've taken your medicine. ALWAYS get a dosing calendar or make one so that you can check off **each dose** as you take it.
- continue to take a drug that you feel is causing problems, until you are able to talk with your doctor.
- store your medicines in a bathroom medicine cabinet. This is often an area of high humidity, which can (even though the bottle is closed) enter the medicine and degrade the active drug. Select a lockable kitchen cabinet out of reach of children.
- take any drug (prescription or nonprescription) while pregnant or nursing an infant until you talk to your doctor or pharmacist. Many herbal combinations may have active ingredients similar to those found in prescription medicines.
- take any more medicines than are absolutely necessary. (The greater the number of drugs taken at the same time, the greater the likelihood of adverse effects.)
- withhold from your doctor information about previous prescription or nonprescription drug use. He or she will want to know what has helped and what has caused problems.
- take any drug in the dark. Identify every dose of medicine carefully in adequate light to be certain you are taking the intended drug.
- in general store drugs on a bedside table. In the dark and in a sleepy state, it's easy to get confused. Drugs for emergency use, such as nitroglycerin, are an exception. It is best to have only one such drug at the bedside for use during the night.

DO

- visit the FDA web site at www.fda.gov on a regular basis to check medicines removed from the market and other press releases. Many parts of this site are now consumer friendly. Checking your medicines to make sure you are not continuing to take a medicine that has been removed from the market (see Table 16) is prudent.
- talk with your doctor about the results or outcomes expected from any medicine being considered. Understand that taking the medicine EXACTLY as it is prescribed is critical. Missing one pill in a three-times-a-day regimen may cause you to lose the benefits of all of the medicine.
- talk with your HMO or medical group every year about how their results or outcomes compare to other providers of health care in the area and in the country. This is especially important for businesses, because the preferred provider they choose impacts the health of many people.
- ask your HMO or medical group or pharmacy what their disease management programs are and how any specific disease or condition that you may have is addressed within the scope of their disease management plan. Find out how the results or outcomes of the program compare with other programs in the area or the country.
- know the name (and correct spelling) of the drug(s) you are taking. It is best to know both the brand name and the generic name.
- understand that finding information on the Internet is often only a starting point. Make sure you openly talk to your doctor before you take any action regarding medicines because you saw something on the Net.
- open the prescription bag and the bottle WHILE YOU ARE STILL IN THE PHARMACY. This will give you a chance to best use the training and experience of your pharmacist and will also let you make sure you understand how to best take your medicine. If the prescription is a refill, make sure the pills are the same as the ones originally prescribed. If they are not, ask why.
- read the package labels of all nonprescription drugs so that you know what is in them. This is especially critical when you realize that many of these medicines have names that do not reflect all of the active compounds that are in them.
- take the medicine exactly as prescribed. If you think there will be a change in your ability to take the medicine, call your doctor before you make any change. For example, taking one dose of a medicine that should be taken three times a day often will NOT give one third of the desired effect. I've been asked this kind of question often. Taking a medicine less frequently than prescribed will often give no beneficial effects, especially for those medicines that require a relatively constant blood level to work.

- put a dosing calendar or a reminder note on the refrigerator or near your car keys. Get a watch with an alarm and set it for the times when you need to take your medicine.
- thoroughly shake all liquid suspensions of drugs to ensure uniform distribution of ingredients.
- use a standardized measuring device for giving liquid medicines by mouth. The household "teaspoon" varies greatly in size.
- follow your doctor's advice on dietary or other measures designed to help the prescribed drugs work their best. For example, decreasing or eliminating salt when taking high blood pressure medicines may help you achieve desired drug effects with smaller doses.
- tell your anesthesiologist, surgeon, and dentist of *all* drugs you are taking, before any surgery.
- tell your doctor if you become pregnant while you are taking any drugs from any source.
- keep a written record of *all* drugs (prescription and nonprescription), vaccines, and herbal remedies you take during your entire pregnancy—name, dose, dates taken, and reasons for use.
- keep a written record of *all* drugs (and vaccines) to which you become allergic or have an adverse reaction to. This should be done for each member of the family, especially the elderly or infirm.
- keep a written record of *all* drugs (and vaccines) to which your children become allergic or experience an adverse reaction to.
- fill out "Your Personal Drug Profile" (Table 14). Get the number of your Poison Control Center **today** and post it by your telephone. The worst time to try to find an emergency number is while there is a dire need for it. Fill in the Medication Map (Table 15), and ask your doctor if the times selected and combinations of medicines are appropriate.
- tell your doctor of all known or suspected allergies, especially allergies to drugs. Be sure that allergies are a part of your medical record. People with allergies are four times more prone to drug reactions.
- call your doctor immediately if you think you are having an overdose, side effect, or adverse effect from a drug.
- ask if it is safe to drive a car, operate machinery, or engage in other hazardous activities while taking the drug(s) prescribed.
- ask if it is safe to drink alcoholic beverages while taking the drug(s) prescribed. We often forget that alcohol is a drug with its own pharmacology and drug-drug interactions.
- find out if any particular foods, beverages, or other prescription or nonprescription medicines should be avoided while taking the drug(s) prescribed.
- keep all appointments for follow-up examinations or laboratory tests.
- ask for help to understand any point that confuses you. If you are concerned about remembering information or instructions for use, ask for written materials.
- throw away all outdated drugs.

- ask your doctor if a prescribed medicine offers the best balance of cost and outcomes for you.
- store all drugs for intermittent use out of the reach of children. This is critical for those of you with grandchildren who visit infrequently.

PREVENTING ADVERSE DRUG REACTIONS

It is always better to prevent a condition or disease than to have to treat it. This is especially true in the case of adverse drug reactions where the cure can become the disease. As our understanding of drug actions and reactions has expanded, we have learned that many adverse effects are, to some extent, predictable and preventable. Eleven contributing factors are now well recognized:

Previous Adverse Reaction to a Drug

People who have had an adverse drug reaction in the past are more likely to have adverse reactions to other drugs, even though the drugs are unrelated. This suggests that some people may have a genetic (inborn) predisposition to unusual or abnormal drug responses. *Always tell your doctor about any history of prior adverse drug experiences*.

Allergies

Some people are allergic by nature (have hay fever, asthma, eczema, hives) and are more likely to develop allergies to drugs. The allergic patient must be watched very closely when medicines are used. Known drug allergies must be written in the medical record. The patient must tell every health care provider that he or she is allergic by nature and is allergic to specific drugs. *Provide this information without waiting to be asked*. Your doctor will then be able to avoid prescribing those drugs that could provoke an allergic reaction, as well as related (cross-sensitivity) drugs.

Contraindications

Both patient and physician must strictly observe contraindications to any drug under consideration. *Absolute contraindications* include those conditions and situations that prohibit the use of the drug for any reason. *Relative contraindications* are those conditions that, in the judgment of the physician, do not preclude the use of the drug but make it essential that special care be given to its use. Often dosing adjustments, additional supportive measures, and close supervision are needed.

Precautions in Use

Patients should know any special precautions needed while taking a drug. This includes advisability of use during pregnancy or while nursing; precautions on sun exposure (or ultraviolet lamps); avoidance of extreme heat or cold, heavy physical exertion (such as with fluoroquinolone antibiotics), etc.

Dose

It is important to take any medicine exactly as prescribed. *This is most important with drugs that have narrow margins of safety*. Even once-a-day medications should be taken at the same time of day or night to ensure the most constant blood levels. Call your doctor if nausea, vomiting, diarrhea, or other problems interfere with taking your medicine as prescribed.

Interactions

Some drugs can interact with foods (including vitamins and some herbal remedies), alcohol, and other drugs (prescription and nonprescription) to cause serious adverse effects. *The patient must be told about all likely interactants*. If, during the course of treatment, you feel you have discovered a new interaction, tell your doctor so that its full significance can be determined.

Warning Symptoms

Many drugs will cause symptoms that are early warnings of a developing adverse effect: for example, severe headaches or visual disturbances *before* a stroke in a woman taking oral contraceptives. *It is imperative that you know symptoms and signs that could be early warnings of adverse reactions*. The patient is then empowered to act in his or her own behalf by calling the doctor before taking another dose of the medicine. Adverse reactions should be reported to the FDA following its current guidelines.

Examinations to Monitor Drug Effects

Many drugs in common use can damage vital body tissues (such as bone marrow, liver, kidney, eye structures, etc.)—especially when these drugs are used for a long time or in high doses. Sometimes these adverse effects are not discovered until a newly approved drug has been in wide use for a long time. This damage may be reversible if found quickly. *Cooperate fully with your doctor when he or she asks for periodic exams to check for adverse drug effects.*

Advanced Age and Debility

When we age or as some disease processes progress, vital organs may not work as well and can greatly influence the body's response to drugs. These patients often poorly tolerate drugs with inherent toxic potential and frequently need smaller doses at longer intervals. *The effects of drugs on the elderly and severely ill are often unpredictable*. Great care must be taken to prevent or minimize adverse effects.

Appropriate Drug Choice

The use of any medicine is always a benefit-to-risk decision. The medication used should offer the best balance of overall cost (including lab tests) and outcomes (including quality of life). Many adverse reactions can be prevented if both physician and patient exercise good judgment and restraint.

Polypharmacy

Unfortunately, the cure can become the disease. Patients who are cared for by several physicians may end up with several drugs prescribed separately by more than one physician for different disorders—often without appropriate communication between patient and prescriber. This frequent practice can lead to serious drug-drug interactions. **Every patient should routinely talk to *each* health care provider about all the drugs—prescription and nonprescription—that he or she may be taking**. It is **mandatory** that each prescriber has this information before prescribing additional drugs.

DRUGS AND THE ELDERLY

Advancing age brings changes that can alter how you react to medicines. An impaired digestive system may interfere with drug absorption. Declines in liver and kidney ability to metabolize and remove drugs may lead to toxic drug levels. We slowly lose the ability to maintain "steady state" (or homeostasis) and face increased sensitivity of many tissues to the actions of drugs, even in "normal" drug doses. If aging causes a decline in understanding, memory, vision, or coordination, these patients may not always use drugs safely and effectively. Adverse reactions to drugs occur three times more frequently in the older population. An unwanted drug response can change an independent older person into a confused or helpless patient. For these reasons, drug treatment in the elderly must **always** be accompanied by the most careful consideration of the individual's health and tolerances. Once-daily dosing may be the only viable option.

Guidelines for the Use of Drugs by the Elderly

- Make sure that drug treatment is needed. Many health problems of the elderly can be managed **without** the use of drugs.
- Avoid (if possible) the use of many drugs at one time.
- Dosing schedules should be as simple as possible. Once a medicine is selected, ask your doctor if a once- or twice-a-day formulation is available and appropriate.
- Treatment with most drugs is often best started by using less-than-standard doses. Maintenance doses should be individualized and are often smaller for those over 60 years of age.

- Avoid large tablets and capsules if other dosage forms are available. Liquid forms are easier for the elderly or debilitated to swallow.
- Have all drug containers labeled with the drug name and directions for use in large, easy-to-read letters.
- Ask the pharmacist to package drugs in easy-to-open containers. Avoid childproof caps and stoppers.
- Do not take any drug in the dark. Identify each dose of medicine carefully in adequate light to be certain you are taking the intended drug.
- To avoid taking the wrong drug or an extra dose, do not routinely leave medicines on a bedside table. Drugs for emergency use, such as nitroglycerin, are an exception. It is best to have only one such drug at the bedside for use during the night.
- Drug use by older people may require supervision; watch constantly to ensure safe and effective use.
- Remember the adage: "Start low, go slow, and (when appropriate) learn to say no."

Drugs Best Avoided by the Elderly Because of Increased Possibility of Adverse Reactions

antacids (high sodium)*	diethylstilbestrol	oxyphenbutazone
barbiturates*	estrogens	phenacetin
benzodiazepines	indomethacin	phenylbutazone
(long-acting)	monoamine oxidase	tetracyclines*
cyclophosphamide	(MAO) inhibitors*	

Drugs That Should Be Used by the Elderly in Reduced Dosages Until Full Effect Has Been Determined

anticoagulants (oral)*	cortisone-like drugs*	prazosin
antidepressants*	cimetidine	pseudoephedrine
antidiabetic drugs*	digitalis preparations*	quinidine
antihistamines*	diuretics* (all types)	sildenafil (Viagra)
antihypertensives*	ephedrine	sleep inducers
anti-inflammatory drugs*	epinephrine	(hypnotics)*
barbiturates*	haloperidol	terbutaline
beta-blockers*	isoetharine	thyroid preparations
carvedilol (Coreg)	nalidixic acid	
colchicine	narcotic drugs	

Drugs That May Cause Confusion and Behavioral Disturbances in the Elderly

acyclovir	bromocriptine	pentazocine
albuterol	carbamazepine	phenytoin
amantadine	cimetidine	primidone
anticholinergics*	digitalis preparations*	quinidine
antidepressants*	diuretics*	ranitidine

*See Drug Classes, Section Four.

antidiabetic drugs*
antihistamines*
anti-inflammatory drugs*
asparaginase
atropine* (and drugs
  containing belladonna)
barbiturates*
benzodiazepines*
beta-blockers*

ergoloid mesylates
famotidine
haloperidol
levodopa
meprobamate
methocarbamol
methyldopa
narcotic drugs
nizatidine

reserpine
sedatives
sleep inducers
  (hypnotics)*
thiothixene
tranquilizers (mild)*
trihexyphenidyl

Drugs That May Cause Orthostatic Hypotension in the Elderly

antidepressants*
antihypertensives*
diuretics* (all types)

neuroleptics*
sedatives
tranquilizers (mild)*

phenothiazines*
selegiline
vasodilators*

Drugs That May Cause Sluggishness, Unsteadiness, and Falling in the Elderly

barbiturates*
beta-blockers*
chlordiazepoxide
clorazepate

diazepam
diphenhydramine
flurazepam
halazepam

methyldopa
prazepam
sleep inducers
  (hypnotics)*

Drugs That May Cause Constipation and/or Retention of Urine in the Elderly

acebutolol
amantadine
amiodarone
androgens
anticholinergics*
antidepressants*
anti-parkinsonism
  drugs*

atropinelike drugs*
calcium
cholestyramine
epinephrine
ergoloid mesylates
famotidine
iron (some forms)
isoetharine

ketorolac
metoclopramide
narcotic drugs
phenothiazines*
ranitidine
sucralfate
terbutaline

Drugs That May Cause Loss of Bladder Control (Urinary Incontinence) in the Elderly

diuretics* (all types)
sedatives
sleep inducers
  (hypnotics)*

tacrine
thioridazine

tranquilizers (mild)**

MEASURING DRUG LEVELS IN BLOOD
(THERAPEUTIC DRUG MONITORING)

People vary greatly in the nature and degree of their responses to medicines, and often, blood levels can help find the best dose. Frequently, the clinical response to a medicine shows that the drug is working as intended. For some drugs, however, especially those with narrow safety

*See Drug Classes, Section Four.

margins, toxic reactions may closely resemble the symptoms being treated. In many cases, the patient's expected response is not in keeping with his or her clinical condition.

By measuring blood levels at appropriate times, your doctor or clinical pharmacist can adjust dosing schedules, reduce the risk of toxicity, and achieve the best results or outcomes. These levels also tell the clinician if you've been taking your medicines as prescribed. Some medications require both a peak and trough level to ensure best results, and timing of blood sampling is critical.

In general, sampling should be avoided during the two hours after an oral dose, because during this absorption period, blood levels do not represent tissue levels of the drug, and the tissue is where many medicines actually work. The peak, or highest, level of the drug can measure several things: toxic levels within the body or how effectively bacteria are killed, for instance. The trough, or lowest, level tells how effectively a medicine is cleared from the body between doses. This can also be important, because if too much drug remains, toxicity can result, and if too little stays, it may not work well. Your doctor may also use peak-to-trough ratios to understand how often a particular medicine should be taken.

The following drugs are those most suitable for therapeutic drug monitoring. If you are using any of these on a regular basis, ask your doctor about checking blood levels. Let me remind you that these numbers are ranges where effects are usually seen, but people react differently. Therapeutic ranges listed are not absolute fixed levels where lack of effect or toxicity definitely occur. One patient may have a therapeutic response at a level lower than the low end of the range while another won't react at all. A blood level higher than the high end of the range is not always toxic but is a level higher than desirable, and dosing changes should be made. Fortunately, most clinicians "treat the patient, not the level."

Generic Name/Brand Name	*Blood Level Range*
acetaminophen/Tylenol, etc.	10–20 mcg/ml
amikacin/Amikin	12–25 mcg/ml (peak)
	5–10 mcg/ml (trough)
amiodarone/Cordarone	0.8–2.8 mcg/ml
	(controversial)
amitriptyline/Elavil, etc.	
(combined with nortriptyline)	120–250 ng/ml
amoxapine/Asendin	200–500 ng/ml
aspirin (other salicylates)	100–250 mcg/ml
carbamazepine/Tegretol	5–10 mcg/ml
chloramphenicol/Chloromycetin	10–25 mcg/ml
chlorpromazine/Thorazine	50–300 ng/ml
ciprofloxacin/Cipro	0.94–3.4 mcg/ml
clonazepam/Klonopin	10–50 mg/ml
cyclosporine/Sandimmune	100–150 ng/ml

desipramine/Norpramin, Pertofrane	150–300 ng/ml
digitoxin/Crystodigin	15–30 ng/ml
digoxin/Lanoxin	0.5–2.0 ng/ml
diltiazem/Cardizem	0.1–0.4 mcg/ml
disopyramide/Norpace	2.0–4.5 mcg/ml
doxepin/Adapin, Sinequan	100–275 mg/ml
ethosuximide/Zarontin	40–100 mcg/ml
flecainide/Tambocor	0.2–1.0 mcg/ml
flucytosine/Ancobon	50–100 mcg/ml
gentamicin/Garamycin	4.0–10 mcg/ml (peak)
	less than 2 mcg/ml (trough)
gold salts/Auranofin, etc.	1.0–2.0 mcg/ml
imipramine/Janimine, Tofranil, etc.	150–300 ng/ml
kanamycin/Kantrex	25–35 mcg/ml
lidocaine/Xylocaine, etc.	1.4–6.0 mcg/ml
lithium/Lithobid, Lithotabs, etc.	0.3–1.3 MEq/L
mephobarbital/Mebaral	1–7 mcg/ml
methotrexate/Mexate	up to 0.1 mcmol/L
methsuximide/Celontin	up to 1.0 mcg/ml
metoprolol/Lopressor	20–200 ng/ml
mexiletine/Mexitil	0.75–2.0 mcg/ml
nifedipine/Procardia	25–100 ng/ml
nortriptyline/Aventyl, Pamelor	50–150 ng/ml
combined with amitriptyline	125–250 ng/ml
phenobarbital/Luminal, etc.	10–25 mcg/ml
phenytoin/Dilantin	10–18 mcg/ml
primidone/Mysoline	6–12 mcg/ml
procainamide/Pronestyl	4–10 mcg/ml
(NAPA metabolite)	4–10 mcg/ml
propafenone	0.06–1 mcg/ml
propranolol/Inderal	50–100 ng/ml
protriptyline/Vivactil	70–250 ng/ml
quinidine/Quinaglute, etc.	1.0–4.0 mcg/ml
(specific to quinidine test method)	
sulfadiazine/Microsulfon	100–120 mcg/ml
sulfamethoxazole/Gantanol	90–100 mcg/ml
theophylline/Aminophylline, etc.	10–20 mcg/ml
thioridazine/Mellaril	50–300 ng/ml
tobramycin/Nebcin	4.0–10 mcg/ml (peak)
	less than 2 mcg/ml (trough)
tocainide/Tonocard	5–12 mcg/ml
trimethadione/Tridione	10–30 mcg/ml
trimethoprim/Proloprim	1–3 mcg/ml
valproic acid/Depakene	50–100 mcg/ml
vancomycin/Vancocin	30–40 mcg/ml (peak)
	5–10 mcg/ml (trough)
verapamil/Calan	0.06–0.2 mcg/ml

3

True Breakthroughs in Medicines

Happily, every year we gain some great advances in medicines—this section tells you about some of the best, identifies novel treatment approaches, and gives truly new uses of existing medicines. I distinguish between "me too" products (that may simply be an existing drug with minor chemical changes) and forward-looking advances. I believe that this section can help you make sure you are getting the very latest treatment. This data changes on a regular basis. One way to follow up on medicines themselves is to visit the FDA web site at www.fda.gov and look at the type of approval the medicine was given. A "chemical type one" designation is a new molecular entity—something that has never existed before. "Chemical type four" designations are new combinations of medicines. These two categories coupled with the latest research can help you find the latest in therapy. I also have an Update on New Medicines report on my web site at www.medicineinfo.com.

ACUTE CORONARY SYNDROMES AND THE CURE TRIAL

The CURE trial (Clopidogrel in Unstable Angina to prevent Recurrent Events) was reported at the American College of Cardiology meeting and was immediately termed "a blockbuster" clinical result by clinicians and researchers. One of the lead researchers estimated that widespread use of clopidogrel (Plavix) combined with aspirin in patients with acute coronary syndromes (such as unstable angina or non-Q-wave MI) could prevent 50,000 to 100,000 heart attacks, strokes, or deaths EACH YEAR in North America. I think of the great possible benefit this combination could have for my father had it only been available. Talk to your doctor to see if it makes sense for you.

ADHERENCE (COMPLIANCE) PROGRAMS (MyHeartWatch)

I've been the pharmacist representative to the Compliance Action Program (CAP) of the American Heart Association and have been working to get pharmacists and pharmacies more involved in helping people get great quality information and reminders to keep taking their medicines. You may have seen me talking on television about this. The focus is how well people take their medicines—in fact, the best medicine in the world will not do you any good at all if it stays in the bottle. I have had many consults asking me why a given medicine failed to work, only to talk to the patient and find out that the medicine itself was either not being taken or was being taken as needed (when the patient felt bad). A new patient program called MyHeartWatch is a web-based program that can help you identify your risks for heart disease and make some changes. Take a look at www.americanheart.org. This is a prescription for success! You can also call the AHA at 1-800-242-8721 or fax at 1-214-706-5233. I strongly encourage you to make a donation just like me.

ASPIRIN

I include aspirin once again in this section, because it can be one of the easiest ways to help limit the damage from a heart attack. The current American Heart Association recommendation for persons who appear to be suffering a heart attack is to (if they do not have any contraindications) give them a non-enteric full-dose aspirin. This measure can help limit the size of the heart attack and possible heart muscle damage. Ongoing low-dose aspirin use may help prevent a first heart attack in people who are at risk. Talk to your doctor to see if regular use of aspirin makes sense for you.

FUSION INHIBITOR

Historically, all of the available HIV treatments fell into the nucleoside reverse transcriptase inhibitor, non-nucleoside reverse transcriptase inhibitor, and protease inhibitor classes. A novel way to attack the AIDS virus was clearly needed, and was discovered by Trimeris pharmaceutical. The new approach is called a fusion inhibitor—helping to keep HIV from entering cells and killing them. The experimental drugs are known as T-20 and T-1249 and continue to move toward approval. The T-20 compound is expected to be available no later than 2003! I believe that fusion inhibitors will become an integral part of combination HIV therapy.

HUMAN GENOME

There are some 3 billion base pairs, and an estimated 40,000 genes estimated in the human genome. Some 20 diseases cause more than 80% of deaths around the world. About 200–300 genes are responsible for these diseases. Amazingly, the human genome is now mostly known. Considering that about every three weeks we in essence get a new heart from the same set of genes, if controlling the genes becomes a reality—we can possibly knock out heart disease by knocking out the bad gene of a pair. Watch closely!

GET WITH THE GUIDELINES

You'd think that prescribing medicines and having patients take them after they've suffered a first heart attack would be well-standardized and followed. Unfortunately—this is NOT the case! The situation is called secondary prevention (secondary prevention of cardiovascular disease). One data set found that only 37% of patients with increased cholesterol actually got a statin (HMG-CoA reductase inhibitor). The American Heart Association has launched a new program called Get With The Guidelines (GWTG) to address this problem. GWTG is a hospital-based initiative seeking to help patients and their families understand the goals of treatment and get the best medicines started. You can find out more by visiting www.americanheart.org/getwiththeguidelines.html. I am a spokesperson for this program. You can read my testimonial by visiting www.americanheart.org/getwiththeguidelines/testimonials.html.

INSTITUTE OF MEDICINE REPORT

Prior editions have detailed the Institute of Medicine (IOM) report that showed that medical errors kill up to 98,000 Americans every year. That report (*To Err Is Human*) was a true breakthrough because it worked to focus attention on errors and how they can be prevented. A newer report released in 2001 titled *The Quality Chasm* exceeded 300 pages and found that our health care system does not consistently deliver high quality care. Like the previous report, this new one took a hard look at health care and will serve to challenge the system and government to improve.

ISLET CELL TRANSPLANT

Islet cells are the cells in the pancreas that make insulin to help your body control blood sugar. Researchers at the University of Alberta in Canada recently transplanted these cells from one person to another. The result (in conjunction with a new medicine to suppress rejection called sirolimus or Rapamune) was astounding. The eight diabetics previously took as many as 15 insulin shots a day, but after the transplant no longer required the shots.

LEUKEMIA PILL (STI-571, IMATINIB OR GLEEVEC)

Historically, treatments for leukemias have required an intravenous approach. The first tests of a new treatment started in 1999 and lead to STI-571 (signal transduction inhibitor). Research has shown that patient responses to STI are more rapid and also more frequent than standard therapy. This medicine works to turn off a biological switch (gene output) that leads to a kind of leukemia called chronic myelogenous leukemia (CML). The early research by Novartis showed that 30 of 31 patients tested had normal blood counts after a month of treatment. Subsequently, the FDA fast-tracked the medicine (see Glossary), approving it in record time for CML. This medicine also starts a new field called pharmacogenomics. The initial success of STI-571 (imatinib or Gleevec) has also lead to trials in a rare kind of GI tumor called GIST or gastrointestinal stromal tumor. This tumor is found in some 5,000 people in the US. The drug appears to work in those tumors by turning off a gene called C-kit which causes cells relying on that gene to grow relentlessly. I'll update you via www.medicineinfo.com as things progress. The company clinical trials hotline is 1-800-340-6843.

NIH CHOLESTEROL GUIDELINES

The National Institutes of Health has released ATP III as part of the update to the National Cholesterol Education Program or NCEP. It is projected that when widely followed, these guidelines will save many many lives. Key points in these new guidelines include acknowledging diabetes as one of the conditions that increases risk of heart disease, modifying risk factors, and recommending routine testing for all of the cholesterol fractions (lipoprotein profile) versus total cholesterol alone. These new guidelines also recommend a desirable total cholesterol of 200 mg/dl as before, but change LDL to 100 mg/dl as optimal, 130–159 mg/dl as borderline high, 160 mg/dl as high, and 190 mg/dl as very high. One other noteworthy change is that "good cholesterol" or HDL has been made more important. The "too low" measure for HDL has been increased to 40 mg/dl. I think that all of these changes combined will work to get more people the treatment they need earlier in what becomes a fatal disease process. Congratulations to NIH for this bold initiative.

DRUG PROFILES

Drugs Reviewed in This Section

Included are detailed and annually updated Drug Profiles of **more than 2,000 brands** and nearly 400 drugs of major importance. The criteria are that the medicine:

1. Is used to treat or prevent a prevalent, relatively serious significant disease or disorder.

2. Is recognized by experts to be among the "best choices" in its class.

3. Has a current benefit-to-risk ratio that compares favorably with those in its class or is the only available alternative therapy for those who cannot tolerate the first-line medicine.

4. May require special information and guidance for both the health care practitioner (physician, dentist, pharmacist, nurse) and the consumer (patient and family) for safe and effective use.

5. Is suitable (safe and practical) for use in an outpatient setting (home, work site, school, etc.). It can be self-administered or may require dosing by trained medical personnel (as with home intravenous therapy or free-standing cancer, emergency or pain centers).

ACARBOSE (A KAR BOZ)

Introduced: 1996   **Class:** Alpha glucosidase inhibitor; antidiabetes agent, oral   **Prescription:** USA: Yes   **Controlled Drug:** USA: No; Canada: No
Available as Generic: No
Brand Names: Glucobay, Precose, ♣Prandase

BENEFITS versus RISKS	
Possible Benefits	*Possible Risks*
EFFECTIVE LOWERING OF BLOOD SUGAR	Gas (flatulence) and abdominal pain (often decreases over time)
DECREASED RISK OF HIGH BLOOD PRESSURE, BLINDNESS, HEART DISEASE OR OTHER LONG-TERM DAMAGE OF UNCONTROLLED DIABETES (WITH BETTER OR TIGHTER CONTROL OF BLOOD SUGAR)	Increased liver function tests Combination use poses a risk of excessively low blood sugar (hypoglycemia) like other agents
MAY BE USED IN COMBINED TREATMENT WITH METFORMIN, INSULIN OR A SULFONYLUREA IF NEEDED TO REACH BLOOD SUGAR CONTROL GOALS	

▷ **Principal Uses**

As a Single Drug Product: Uses currently included in FDA-approved labeling: (1) Used with diet in diabetics who don't require insulin, yet don't have good (tight control of 80–120 mg/dl or as defined as acceptable by their doctor) blood sugar control with diet alone; (2) can be combined with a sulfonylurea (see Drug Classes) if diet plus acarbose or diet and sulfonylurea do not control blood sugar as well as needed; (3) can be combined with metformin or insulin if diet plus acarbose or diet plus sulfonylurea do not achieve blood sugar control goals.

Other (unlabeled) generally accepted uses: (1) Combination treatment of diabetics (type one) who require insulin.

How This Drug Works: By blocking the chemicals (enzymes) intestinal alpha glucosidase and pancreatic alpha amylase, this medicine impairs starch and sucrose digestion and actually keeps sugar low after meals.

Available Dosage Forms and Strengths

Tablets — 25 mg, 50 mg, 100 mg

▷ **Recommended Dosage Ranges** (Actual dose and schedule must be determined individually for each patient.)

Infants and Children: Safety and effectiveness not established in those less than 18 years old.

18 to 65 Years of Age: To start, 25 mg three times daily, taken at the start of each meal (after first bite). Dose increases are made at 4- to 8-week intervals to achieve blood sugar control while minimizing intestinal side effects (using 50 mg three times daily at the start of each meal). If response is not acceptable, patients weighing more than 132 pounds (60 kg) may be given doses up to 100 mg three times daily. Those weighing less than 60 kg should NOT be given more than 50 mg three times daily. If a dose increase doesn't give better sugar control, consider dose decrease.

Over 65 Years of Age: No specific recommendations unless kidney function is very limited, in which case a kidney specialist may be prudent.

Conditions Requiring Dosing Adjustments

Liver Function: Specific dosing changes do not appear to be needed. The intestinal wall and bacteria extensively contribute to removal of this medicine.

Kidney Function: Increases in drug levels may occur and dose decreases may be needed. Specific guidelines not available. Only about 2% is usually removed by the kidneys.

▷ **Dosing Instructions:** Take this pill after starting to eat breakfast, lunch and dinner—after the first bite of a meal has been eaten. Dosing must be individualized. Gas (flatulence) or diarrhea is a common side effect, but often decreases over time. Limiting sucrose (read the food label) can also help.

If dose changes are made at 4- to 8-week intervals, the best sugar response and the least potential gas (flatulence) or diarrhea are realized. Often blood sugar is checked one hour after a meal (1 hr postprandial) and the dose adjusted to get the best balance of blood sugar and side effects (also avoiding too low a blood sugar). If you forget a dose but remember it while you are still eating, take it immediately. If you remember the dose just after finishing your meal, take the dose now (if you remember later than this, take your next dose with your next meal). Do not double doses or take acarbose between meals. Check your blood sugar as your doctor has instructed.

Usual Duration of Use: Use will be ongoing. Regular use is required for good blood sugar (glucose) control. DO NOT MISS DOSES. Keeping the sugar close to normal can minimize diabetic problems.

Typical Treatment Goals and Measurements (Outcomes and Markers)

Blood Sugar: The general goal for blood sugar is to return it to the usual "normal" range (generally 80–120 mg/dl), while avoiding risks of excessively low blood sugar. One study (UKPDS) used a fasting plasma sugar (glucose) of less than 108 mg/dl. Keeping blood sugar in the normal range helps avoid complications of diabetes.

Fructosamine and Glycosylated Hemoglobin: Fructosamine levels (a measure of the past two to three weeks of blood sugar control) should be less than or equal to 310 micromoles per liter. Glycosylated hemoglobin or hemoglobin A1C (a measure of the past 2–3 months of blood sugar control) should be less than or equal to 7.0%. The American Heart Association also recognizes glycosylated hemoglobin control in their new primary and secondary cardiovascular disease prevention guidelines.

Possible Advantages of This Drug

May be used in combination with oral hypoglycemics (such as sulfonylureas, insulin or metformin (see Drug Classes) to get the best control of blood sugar. Uses a different (novel) mechanism than other oral hypoglycemic drugs.

▷ **This Drug Should Not Be Taken If**
- you have had an allergic reaction to it previously.
- you are in diabetic ketoacidosis.

- your history includes intestinal obstruction or you have a partial obstruction of the intestine.
- you have inflammatory bowel disease or colon ulceration.
- serum creatinine is over 2 mg/dl (talk to your doctor).
- you have cirrhosis of the liver, or if your liver function tests (LFTs) have become known to you and they are increased.
- you have an intestinal condition that may worsen (such as a megacolon or bowel obstruction) if increased gas (flatus) forms.
- you have a long-standing (chronic) intestinal disease altering digestion or your ability to absorb materials from the intestine.
- you are pregnant or are breast-feeding your infant (no data exist on use in pregnancy or breast-feeding).
- you are less than 18 years old.

▷ **Inform Your Physician Before Taking This Drug If**
- you have an infection (insulin may be required).
- you do not know what the symptoms of hypoglycemia are.
- you have a history of kidney or liver disease.
- you will have surgery with general anesthesia.
- you forgot to tell your doctor about all the drugs you take.
- you are also taking a sulfonylurea.
- you are unsure of how much or how often to take acarbose.

Possible Side Effects (natural, expected and unavoidable drug actions)
　　Gas (flatulence) or diarrhea (results from bacterial action on sugars) and tends to decrease over time.

▷ **Possible Adverse Effects** (unusual, unexpected and infrequent reactions)
　　If any of the following develop, consult your physician promptly for guidance.
　　Mild Adverse Effects
　　Allergic reactions: skin redness (erythema), itching (urticaria).
　　Sleepiness, headache, dizziness—of questionable cause (may be blood sugar control signs or symptoms).
　　Pain or swelling of the belly (abdomen)—frequent.
　　Gas (flatulence) or diarrhea—frequent (often eases over time).
　　Serious Adverse Effects
　　Low blood sugar if combined with sulfonylureas or other medicines such as insulin—possible.
　　Anemia—rare in clinical approval trials, but not seen in later studies.
　　Increased liver enzymes—case reports (62 developing this problem in 2–8 months—with an unclear relationship to the drug). May be more common in women than in men.
　　Ileus—case reports and in those with prior bowel blockage history.

▷ **Possible Effects on Sexual Function:** None reported.

Possible Effects on Laboratory Tests
　　Glycated protein (fructosamine): trending toward normal (good effect).
　　Hemoglobin A1C: trending more toward normal (good effect).
　　Blood sugar one hour after eating (postprandial): decreased.
　　Serum lipids: variable effect.
　　Liver enzymes: may be increased.

CAUTION
1. This medicine itself does not cause hypoglycemia. Low sugar may result if combined with metformin, insulin or sulfonylureas.
2. Infections may cause loss of sugar control and require temporary insulin use.
3. This medicine is part of the total management of diabetes. A properly prescribed diet and regular exercise are still required for best control of blood sugar.
4. If your kidneys fail or worsen, tell your doctor. This drug should not be used if serum creatinine is greater than 2 mg/dl.

Precautions for Use

By Infants and Children: Safety and effectiveness for those under 18 not established.

By Those Over 60 Years of Age: Specific changes are not made at this time.

▷ **Advisability of Use During Pregnancy**

Pregnancy Category: B. See Pregnancy Risk Categories at the back of this book.

Animal studies: No significant increase in birth defects in rats or rabbits.

Human studies: Adequate studies of pregnant women are not available. Insulin is often the drug of first choice for blood sugar control in pregnancy. Ask your doctor for help.

Advisability of Use If Breast-Feeding

Presence of this drug in breast milk: Yes, in rats. No human data available. Avoid drug or refrain from nursing.

Habit-Forming Potential: None.

Effects of Overdose: Temporary gas (flatus), abdominal discomfort and diarrhea.

Possible Effects of Long-Term Use: Beneficial effects on blood sugar, lowered risk of cardiovascular disease and of high blood pressure with better sugar control.

Suggested Periodic Examinations While Taking This Drug (at physician's discretion)

Periodic blood sugar one hour after eating.

Glycated protein (fructosamine).

Hemoglobin A1C levels.

Liver function tests (transaminases)—checked every three months during the first year, then periodically thereafter. Patients taking other medicines that can be toxic to the liver should be tested more frequently.

Serum iron or iron-binding capacity prudent if anemia develops.

▷ **While Taking This Drug, Observe the Following**

Foods: Closely follow the diet your doctor has prescribed. Blood sugar control can help avoid or delay diabetes problems! Vitamin C in high dose may worsen blood sugar control.

Herbal Medicines or Minerals: Using chromium may change the way your body is able to use sugar. Some health food stores advocate vanadium as mimicking the actions of insulin, but possible toxicity and need for rigorous studies presently preclude recommending it. DHEA may change sensitivity to insulin or insulin resistance. Hawthorn, ginger, garlic, ginseng and licorice, nettle and yohimbe may change blood sugar. Because these products can have an effect—talk to your doctor BEFORE combining any of these herbal medicines with acarbose. Echinacea purpurea (injectable) and blonde psyllium seed or husk should NOT be taken by people living with diabetes.

Beverages: No restrictions. May be taken with milk—mindful of the limits of the diet that your doctor has recommended.

▷ *Alcohol:* No interaction with acarbose. If you also take a sulfonylurea (see Drug Classes), alcohol can exaggerate lowering of blood sugar or cause a disulfiramlike (see Glossary) reaction.

Tobacco Smoking: No interactions expected, but I advise everyone to stop smoking.

▷ *Other Drugs*

Acarbose may increase the effects of
- insulins (see Drug Classes), further lowering blood sugar for patients who do not respond to acarbose alone (a beneficial effect when blood sugar is closely watched).
- metformin (Glucophage) may further lower blood sugar for patients who are not controlled by diet or acarbose alone (beneficial effect as above).
- sulfonylureas (see Drug Classes), causing further lowering of blood sugars (not an acarbose effect). This may be used for therapeutic benefit.
- warfarin (Coumadin)—INR testing more often is advisable.

Acarbose *taken concurrently* with
- activated charcoal (various) may blunt the benefits of acarbose.
- amylase (pancreatin) may blunt the benefits of acarbose.
- clofibrate (Atromid-S) may result in hypoglycemia.
- digestive enzyme products that contain amylase or lipase may result in loss of blood sugar control.
- digoxin (Lanoxin) may cause lower (subtherapeutic) blood levels of digoxin and loss of benefits (three case reports).
- disopyramide (Norpace) may result in hypoglycemia.
- high-dose aspirin or other salicylates and some NSAIDs (see Drug Classes) may result in hypoglycemia.
- monoamine oxidase (MAO) inhibitors (see Drug Classes) may increase glucose tolerance, leading to excessively low blood sugar.
- sulfonamide antibiotics (see Drug Classes) may pose an increased risk for low blood sugar (hypoglycemia).

The following drugs may *decrease* the effects of acarbose:
- adrenocorticosteroids (see Drug Classes).
- beta-blockers (see Drug Classes).
- calcium channel blockers (see Drug Classes).
- furosemide (Lasix) and bumetanide (Bumex).
- isoniazid (INH).
- nicotinic acid.
- pancreatin (or any medicines containing carbohydrate dividing enzymes such as amylase or pancreatin).
- phenytoin (Dilantin).
- rifampin (Rifadin, others).
- theophylline (Theo-Dur, others).
- thiazide diuretics (see Drug Classes).
- thyroid hormones (see Drug Classes).

▷ *Driving, Hazardous Activities:* Use caution until degree of drowsiness you may
       see is known.
   Aviation Note: Diabetes *is a disqualification* for piloting. Consult a designated
       Aviation Medical Examiner.
   Exposure to Sun: No restrictions.
   Heavy Exercise or Exertion: Caution advised because this drug lowers peak in
       blood sugar after meals. Discuss dosing changes with your doctor.
   Occurrence of Unrelated Illness: Illness can change blood sugar control and
       beneficial results from this medicine. Temporary use of insulin may be
       required if you are sick such as in the case of infection.
   Discontinuation: **Never** stop acarbose before calling your doctor.

ACEBUTOLOL (a se BYU toh lohl)

Introduced: 1973   **Class:** Antihypertensive, beta-adrenergic blocker, heart
rhythm regulator   **Prescription:** USA: Yes   **Controlled Drug:** USA: No;
Canada: No   **Available as Generic:** Yes
Brand Names: ❀Apo-Acebutolol, ❀Gen-Acebutolol, ❀Med-Acebutolol,
❀Monitan, ❀Rhotral, Sectral

BENEFITS versus RISKS	
Possible Benefits	*Possible Risks*
EFFECTIVE ANTIHYPERTENSIVE (MILD–MODERATE HIGH PRESSURE) MAY BE USED ALONE OR IN COMBINATION WITH OTHER ANTIHYPERTENSIVES, ESPECIALLY DIURETICS	CONGESTIVE HEART FAILURE IN ADVANCED HEART DISEASE
	Masking of low blood sugar (hypoglycemia) in diabetics
MAY DECREASE DEATHS OCCURRING AFTER HEART ATTACK	Rare lupus erythematosus syndrome
LONG-TERM USE CAN DECREASE DEATH AND HEART PROBLEMS	
HELPS PREVENT ABNORMAL HEART RHYTHMS	
Because this drug also has intrinsic sympathomimetic activity it may help in patients with high cholesterol (dyslipidemia) because it avoids increases in serum triglycerides	
May be particularly useful in people with asthma or diabetes (because of heart or cardioselectivity)	

▷ **Principal Uses**
   As a Single Drug Product: Uses currently included in FDA-approved labeling:
       (1) Treats mild to moderate high blood pressure alone or in combination;

(2) used to prevent premature ventricular heartbeats and ventricular arrhythmias; (3) treats diuretic resistant high blood pressure.

Other (unlabeled) generally accepted uses: (1) Stabilizes angina pectoris; (2) used after a heart attack to help prolong life; (3) may have a role in easing the symptoms of panic attacks (antidepressants may actually PREVENT panic attack occurrence).

How This Drug Works: It blocks sympathetic nervous system effects and slows the rate and force of the heart, reducing the extent of blood vessel contraction, expanding the walls and lowering blood pressure. Also slows nerve impulse speed through the heart, which helps ease some heart rhythm disorders.

Available Dosage Forms and Strengths

Capsules — 100 mg (in Canada), 200 mg, 400 mg

Tablets — 100 mg, 200 mg and 400 mg (in Canada)

▷ **Recommended Dosage Ranges** (Actual dose and schedule must be determined for each patient individually.)

Infants and Children: Not indicated.

18 to 65 Years of Age: High blood pressure: 200 mg a day works for some, but most patients require 400–800 mg a day, rarely 1,200 (given as 600 mg twice a day). Heart selectivity decreases as doses increase.

Arrhythmias: 400 mg daily, as 200 mg taken morning and evening (12 hours apart). Increased as needed and tolerated. 600–1,200 mg a day is a typical effective dose. Total dose should not exceed 1,200 mg every 24 hours (600 mg twice a day).

Angina: 600 to 1,600 mg are divided into two or three equal doses given 8 to 12 hours apart.

Over 65 Years of Age: Bioavailability (amount taken into your body) doubles. Lower ongoing doses are needed, 800 mg a day **maximum.**

Conditions Requiring Dosing Adjustments

Liver Function: Used with caution in compromised liver function.

Kidney Function: Dose must be decreased by up to 75% in severe kidney failure.

▷ **Dosing Instructions:** May be taken without regard to eating. Capsule may be opened when taken. NEVER stop this drug abruptly. If you forget a dose: take it right away unless it's within 4 hours of your next regular dose. If it IS within 4 hours of the next dose, just take the scheduled dose. Do NOT double doses.

Usual Duration of Use: Use on a regular schedule for 5 to 14 days may be required to see peak benefits in lowering blood pressure or stopping premature heartbeats. Long-term use determined by sustained benefit and response to a combined program (weight decrease, salt restriction, smoking cessation, etc.) in high blood pressure and response of abnormal heart rhythm. Do NOT skip doses.

Typical Treatment Goals and Measurements (Outcomes and Markers)

Blood Pressure: The most recent treatment guidelines (JNC VI) actually define optimal blood pressure (BP) as less than 120/80 and high normal as 139/89. The American Diabetes Association recommends that clinicians try to reach a goal of 130/80. Most clinicians try to achieve a BP that achieves the best balance of lower cardiovascular risk while avoiding the problem of too low a blood pressure. The goal and time frame (see peak benefits above) should be discussed with you when the prescription is written. Combination therapy is common if blood pressure goals are not reached.

Abnormal Heartbeats: The general goal is to return the heart to a normal rhythm or at least to markedly reduce the occurrence of abnormal heartbeats. In life-threatening arrhythmias, the goal is to abort the abnormal beats and return the pattern to normal. Success at ongoing suppression may involve ambulatory checks of heart rate and rhythm for a day (such as in Holter monitoring). This kind of testing involves placement of adhesive-backed temporary electrodes on the skin in several positions around the heart. A small heart rate and rhythm (EKG or ECG) recording device is carried around via a shoulder strap and records what the heart is doing over 24 hours. Once the recording is made, a scanning machine reviews the record, tallies abnormal heartbeats or rhythms and gives a close and extended look at how the heart is reacting or benefiting from the medicines that the patient is taking. Repeat measurements can be made if doses are changed to check the success at keeping the heart in normal sinus rhythm!

Possible Advantages of This Drug: Slows the heart less than most other beta-blocker drugs, and low doses are less likely to cause asthma attacks in asthmatics. May cause less frequent problems with blood vessels in the legs (peripheral vascular insufficiency) than non-selective beta blockers such as propranolol.

▷ **This Drug Should Not Be Taken If**
- you have had an allergic reaction to it previously.
- you are in heart failure (overt).
- you have a severely slow (bradycardia) heart rate or serious heart block (second or third degree AV).
- you are taking, or took in the past 14 days, any monoamine oxidase (MAO) type A inhibitor drug (see Drug Classes).

▷ **Inform Your Physician Before Taking This Drug If**
- you have had an adverse reaction to any beta-blocker (see Drug Classes).
- you have serious heart disease or episodes of heart failure (this drug may aggravate it).
- you have disease of the mitral valve or aorta.
- you have hay fever (allergic rhinitis), asthma, chronic bronchitis or emphysema.
- you have an overactive thyroid function (hyperthyroidism).
- you have problems with circulation to your arms and legs (peripheral vascular disease or intermittent claudication).
- you have a history of low blood sugar (hypoglycemia).
- you have impaired liver or kidney function.
- you have diabetes or myasthenia gravis.
- you take digitalis, quinidine or reserpine, or any calcium blocker (see Drug Classes).
- you will have surgery with general anesthesia.
- you do not know how much or how often to take acebutolol.
- you have not asked if the dose was adjusted for age-related kidney decline or kidney disease.

Possible Side Effects (natural, expected and unavoidable drug actions)

Lethargy and fatigability, cold extremities—rare; slow heart rate, light-headedness in upright position (see Orthostatic Hypotension in Glossary) possible.

▷ **Possible Adverse Effects** (unusual, unexpected and infrequent reactions)

If any of the following develop, consult your physician promptly for guidance.

Mild Adverse Effects

Allergic reactions: skin rash, itching—rare.

Fatigue—frequent.

Headache, dizziness, insomnia, fatigue or abnormal dreams—infrequent.

Indigestion, nausea, constipation, diarrhea—infrequent.

Decreased tearing with long-term use—case reports.

Increased frequency and painful or nighttime urination—infrequent.

Joint and muscle discomfort, fluid retention (edema)—infrequent.

Serious Adverse Effects

Allergic reactions may be more severe or less responsive to epinephrine.

Mental depression or low blood sugar—rare.

Liver toxicity—case reports (may be a hypersensitivity reaction).

Chest pain, shortness of breath, precipitation of congestive heart failure—rare.

Rebound or withdrawal chest pain (angina) if this medicine is suddenly stopped—possible.

Bronchial asthma attack (in people with asthma)—possible.

Positive ANA and lupus erythematosus—infrequent to frequent, up to 33%.

▷ **Possible Effects on Sexual Function:** Impotence, decreased libido, Peyronie's disease (see Glossary)—case reports to 2%.

Possible Effects on Laboratory Tests

Antinuclear antibodies (ANA) and LE cells: often positive after 3 to 6 months.

Free fatty acids (FFA): decreased.

Glucose tolerance test (GTT): decreased; abnormal tests at 60 and 120 minutes—possible.

Potassium: mild increases.

CAUTION

1. *Do not stop this drug suddenly* without the knowledge and help of your physician. Carry a note that says that you take this drug.
2. Nasal decongestants may cause sudden and SEVERE increases in blood pressure. Call your physician or pharmacist before using nasal decongestants and ask if they should ever be used.
3. Report any tendency to emotional depression.
4. This medicine may worsen preexisting kidney insufficiency.

Precautions for Use

By Infants and Children: Safety and effectiveness for those under 12 years not established. If this drug is used, watch for fainting as a sign of low blood sugar (hypoglycemia) if a meal is skipped.

By Those Over 60 Years of Age: All antihypertensive drugs used cautiously. High blood pressure should be lowered slowly, avoiding risks (such as stroke or heart attack) of excessively low blood pressure. Small doses and frequent blood pressure checks needed. Total daily dose should not exceed 800 mg.

Watch for dizziness, falling, confusion, hallucinations, depression or frequent urination.

▷ **Advisability of Use During Pregnancy**
Pregnancy Category: B. See Pregnancy Risk Categories at the back of this book.
Animal studies: No significant increase in birth defects in rats or rabbits.
Human studies: Adequate studies of pregnant women are not available.
Use this drug only if clearly needed. Ask your doctor for help.

Advisability of Use If Breast-Feeding
Presence of this drug in breast milk: Yes, and concentrated.
Avoid drug or refrain from nursing.

Habit-Forming Potential: None.

Effects of Overdose: Weakness, slow pulse, low blood pressure, fainting, cold and sweaty skin, congestive heart failure, possible coma and convulsions.

Possible Effects of Long-Term Use: Decreased heart reserve and heart failure in some people with advanced heart disease.

Suggested Periodic Examinations While Taking This Drug (at physician's discretion)
Blood pressure checks (treated to attain goals).
Heart and liver function tests.
ANA titer.

▷ **While Taking This Drug, Observe the Following**
Foods: Follow a sensible low-cardiovascular-risk diet. Avoid excessive salt intake.
Herbal Medicines or Minerals: Ginseng may increase blood pressure, blunting the benefits of this medicine. Hawthorn, saw palmetto, ma huang, goldenseal, yohimbe and licorice may also cause increased blood pressure. Calcium and garlic may help lower blood pressure. Indian snakeroot has a German Commission E monograph indication for hypertension—talk to your doctor. Eleuthero root and ephedra should be avoided by people living with hypertension.
Beverages: No restrictions. May be taken with milk.
▷ *Alcohol:* Alcohol may exaggerate lowering of blood pressure and may increase its mild sedative effect.
Tobacco Smoking: Nicotine may reduce this drug's effectiveness and can worsen closing of bronchial tubes seen in regular smokers. I advise everyone to quit smoking.
Marijuana Smoking: Marijuana may increase blood pressure and reduce this drug's effectiveness. DO NOT COMBINE.
▷ *Other Drugs*
Acebutolol may ***increase*** the effects of
• other antihypertensive drugs, excessively lowering the blood pressure. Dose adjustments may be necessary.
• reserpine (Ser-Ap-Es, etc.), causing sedation, depression, slow heart rate and low blood pressure.
Acebutolol ***taken concurrently*** with
• alfentanil (Alfenta) or fentanyl may result in severe slowing of the heart leading to sinus arrest. Use with great caution.

- alpha-one-adrenergic blockers (such as prazosin) may result in a severe drop in blood pressure (especially when patients stand) in response to a first dose of this medicine. Use with great caution.
- amiodarone (Cordarone) may result in severe slowing of the heart leading to sinus arrest. Use with great caution.
- calcium channel blockers such as mibefradil (Posicor) or verapamil (Calan) may lead to increased risk of abnormal heart rate or rhythm.
- clonidine (Catapres) may cause rebound high blood pressure if clonidine is withdrawn while acebutolol is still being taken.
- digoxin (Lanoxin) may change heart conduction.
- diltiazem (Cardizem) may result in increased acebutolol effects.
- fluoxetine (Prozac), fluvoxamine (Luvox), paroxetine (Paxil) or venlafaxine (Effexor) may decrease removal of acebutolol from the body (not reported as yet). Caution is advised.
- insulin may cause low blood sugar (hypoglycemia).
- methyldopa (Aldomet) may lead to unexpected increases in blood pressure.
- NSAIDs (see Drug Classes) may result in decreased acebutolol benefits.
- oral antidiabetic drugs (see Drug Classes) may result in slow recovery from low blood sugar.
- ritonavir (Norvir) and perhaps other protease inhibitors may increase the metabolism of this medicine and blunt therapeutic benefits of acebutolol.

The following drugs may *decrease* the effects of acebutolol:
- indomethacin (Indocin) and some other "aspirin substitutes" (NSAIDs) can blunt acebutolol's antihypertensive effect.
- rifabutin (Mycobutin) and other drugs that may increase (induce) cytochrome P450 enzymes in the liver (the ones that help the body remove medicines like acebutolol) may result in loss of benefits of acebutolol even if every dose of acebutolol is being taken.

▷ *Driving, Hazardous Activities:* Use caution—may cause drowsiness.

Aviation Note: The use of this drug *is a disqualification* for piloting. Consult a designated Aviation Medical Examiner.

Exposure to Sun: No restrictions.

Exposure to Heat: Hot environments can exaggerate the effects of this drug.

Exposure to Cold: Elderly need to prevent hypothermia (see Glossary).

Heavy Exercise or Exertion: This drug can intensify increased blood pressure (hypertensive) response to isometric exercise. Talk to your doctor about how much and how to exercise.

Occurrence of Unrelated Illness: Fevers can lower blood pressure and require decreased doses. Nausea or vomiting may interrupt the dosing schedule. Ask your doctor for help.

Discontinuation: **DO NOT** stop the drug suddenly. Gradual dose decreases over 2–3 weeks (tapering) is recommended. Ask your doctor for help.

ACETAZOLAMIDE (a set a ZOHL a mide)

Introduced: 1953 **Class:** Anticonvulsant, antiglaucoma, diuretic, sulfonamides
Brand Names: ♣Acetazolam, Diamox, Diamox Sequels, Diamox Sustained Release

BENEFITS versus RISKS	
Possible Benefits	*Possible Risks*
REDUCTION OF INTERNAL EYE PRESSURE in some glaucoma cases	Rare bone marrow, liver or kidney injury
	Acidosis with long-term use—possible
CONTROL OF ABSENCE (PETIT MAL) SEIZURES	Increased risk of kidney stones
TREATMENT OF PERIODIC PARALYSIS	Tingling in the arms and legs (paresthesia)
	Paralysis—rare
REDUCES FLUID IN CONGESTIVE HEART FAILURE	Bone weakening (with long-term use)—possible
PREVENTION OR LESSENING OF SYMPTOMS OF ACUTE MOUNTAIN SICKNESS	

Author's Note: This profile has been further shortened to make room for more widely used medicines.

ACETIC ACIDS

(Nonsteroidal Anti-Inflammatory Drug Family)

Diclofenac (di KLOH fen ak)   **Etodolac** (e TOE doh lak)   **Indomethacin** (in doh METH a sin)   **Ketorolac** (KEY tor o lak)   **Nabumetone** (na BYU me tohn)   **Sulindac** (sul IN dak)   **Tolmetin** (TOHL met in)

Introduced: 1976, 1986, 1963, 1991, 1984, 1976, 1976, respectively   **Class:** Mild analgesic, NSAID   **Prescription:** USA: Yes   **Controlled Drug:** USA: No;   Canada: No   **Available as Generic:** USA: Yes, all except nabumetone; Canada: No

Brand Names: Diclofenac, ✤Apo-Diclo, Arthrotec [CD], Cataflam, ✤Novo-Difenac, ✤Nu-Diclo, Voltaren, Voltaren Ophthalmic, Voltaren SR, Voltaren Timed Release; Etodolac, Lodine, Lodine XL; Indomethacin, ✤Apo-Indomethacin, Indameth, ✤Indocid, ✤Indocid-SR, ✤Indocid PDA, Indocin, Indocin-SR, ✤Novo-methacin, ✤Nu-Indo, Zendole; Ketorolac, Acular (ketorolac ophthalmic), Toradol; Nabumetone, ✤Apo-Nabumetone, ✤Novo-Nabumetone ✤Nu-Nabumetone ✤PMS-Nabumetone, Relafen, Sulindac, ✤Apo-Sulin, Clinoril, ✤Novo-Sundac; Tolmetin, Tolectin, Tolectin DS, Tolectin 600

BENEFITS versus RISKS	
Possible Benefits	*Possible Risks*
EFFECTIVE RELIEF OF MILD TO MODERATE PAIN AND INFLAMMATION	Gastrointestinal pain, ulceration, bleeding
	Liver or kidney damage
Decreased stomach (GI) problems (etodolac and Arthrotec CD form)	Fluid retention
	Bone marrow depression
	Pneumonitis (sulindac)
	Aseptic meningitis (diclofenac)
	Possible severe skin reactions (diclofenac, etodolac and sulindac)

▷ **Principal Uses**

As a Single Drug Product: Uses currently included in FDA-approved labeling:
(1) All of the drugs in this class except ketorolac are approved to treat
osteoarthritis; (2) all of the drugs in this class except ketorolac and
etodolac are approved to relieve rheumatoid arthritis; (3) etodolac is used
to treat mild to moderate pain; (4) indomethacin, diclofenac and sulindac
are useful in ankylosing spondylitis; (5) sustained-release form of
indomethacin as well as the immediate-release form of sulindac help
symptoms of tendonitis, bursitis and acute painful shoulder; (6) tolmetin
eases symptoms of juvenile rheumatoid arthritis; (7) sulindac therapy is
useful in acute gout; (8) ophthalmic form of diclofenac is useful after
cataract surgery and refractive surgery of the cornea (decreasing pain and
sensitivity to light); (9) ketorolac is approved (ophthalmic form) for use in
decreasing pain and sensitivity to light (photophobia) after refractive surgery; (10) Arthrotec is used in patients with osteo or rheumatoid arthritis
who are at high risk for damage to the stomach or intestine (gastric or
duodenal ulcer risk); (11) diclofenac is used to help dysmenorrhea.

**Author's Note: Because of the approval and more widespread use of
other medicines in this family (acetic acid NSAIDs) that can be taken
by mouth (PO) and that have a more favorable benefit to risk profile,
information on ketorolac intravenous and oral has been deleted from
this profile. Ophthalmic ketorolac information remains.**

Other (unlabeled) generally accepted uses: (1) Diclofenac used intramuscu-
larly is effective in acute migraine headache and kidney colic; (2)
indomethacin helps reduce systemic reactions in kidney transplants and
addresses low-grade neonatal intraventricular hemorrhage; (3) ketorolac
has been helpful in reducing swelling after cataract surgery; (4) sulindac is
effective in treating colon polyps and easing diabetic neuropathic pain; (5)
NSAIDs have shown conflicting results in preventing colon cancer; (6)
sulindac may be useful in lowering amounts of amniotic fluid (amniore-
duction); (7) one study of 2,765 patients found NSAIDs of use in preventing decline of thinking ability in older patients; (8) indomethacin was
compared to ibuprofen in infants with patent ductus arteriosus. Results of
the 148-infant study found that ibuprofen offered similar benefits while
causing fewer cases of decreased urine output (oliguria).

How These Drugs Work: These drugs reduce prostaglandins (and related compounds), chemicals that cause inflammation and pain.

Available Dosage Forms and Strengths

Diclofenac sodium:

Suppositories — 50 mg, 100 mg (Canada)

Tablets — 25 mg, 50 mg

Tablets (timed release),

prolonged action — 50 mg, 75 mg, 100 mg (Canada)

Ophthalmic solution — 1 mg/1 ml

Etodolac:

Capsules — 200 mg, 300 mg

Tablets, extended-release form— 400 mg, 600 mg

Indomethacin:

Capsules — 25 mg, 50 mg, 75 mg

Gelatin capsule (Canada) — 25 mg, 50 mg

Capsules, SR (prolonged action) — 75 mg
Oral suspension — 25 mg/5 ml
Suppositories — 50 mg, 100 mg

Ketorolac:

Tablets — 10 mg
Ophthalmic solution — 3 ml, 5 ml, 10 ml (0.5%)
Injection — 15 mg, 30 mg

Nabumetone:

Tablets — 500 mg, 750 mg

Sulindac:

Tablets — 150 mg, 200 mg

Tolmetin:

Capsules — 400 mg, 492 mg
Gelatin capsules — 400 mg (Canada)
Tablets — 200 mg, 600 mg

▷ **Usual Adult Dosage Ranges**

Diclofenac potassium: Maximum daily dose is 200 mg.

Diclofenac sodium: 100 to 200 mg daily to start in two to five divided doses. Reduction to the minimum effective dose is advisable. Maximum daily dose is 225 mg.

Diclofenac ophthalmic: 1 drop of 1 mg per milliliter in the eye that underwent cataract surgery, four times a day, starting 24 hours AFTER surgery and continuing for 2 weeks.

Etodolac: For osteoarthritis: A starting dose of 800 to 1,200 mg is given in divided doses. The lowest effective dose is advisable, and effective treatment has been accomplished with 200 to 400 mg daily.

Etodolac extended-release form (Lodine XL): Allows once-a-day dosing for many patients. Dosing range is 400 to 1,000 mg daily. Maximum dose is 1,000 mg daily.

Indomethacin: For arthritis and related conditions: 25 to 50 mg two to four times daily. If needed and tolerated, dose may be increased by 25 or 50 mg per day at intervals of 1 week. For acute gout: 100 mg initially; then 50 mg three times per day until pain is relieved. Maximum daily dose is 200 mg.

Indomethacin SR form: 75 mg daily for ankylosing spondylitis or rheumatoid arthritis.

Ketorolac ophthalmic: One drop four times daily for allergic conjunctivitis.

Nabumetone: 1,000 mg daily as a single dose is given. Dose is increased as needed and tolerated to 1,500 mg daily. The lowest effective daily dose is advisable. Maximum daily dose is 2,000 mg. Some clinicians divide dosing into two equal daily doses.

Sulindac: Therapy is started with 150 to 200 mg twice daily taken 12 hours apart for ankylosing spondylitis. Maximum daily dose is 400 mg.

Tolmetin: 400 mg three times daily is started, with usual ongoing doses of 600 to 1,600 mg as needed and tolerated. Total daily dose should not exceed 1,600 mg for osteoarthritis or 2,000 mg for rheumatoid arthritis. Children 2 years of age or older may be given 20 mg per kg of body mass orally, divided into three or four doses daily. The dose may be increased as needed and tolerated to a maximum daily dose of 30 mg per kg of body mass.

Note: Actual dose and dosing schedule must be determined for each patient individually.

Conditions Requiring Dosing Adjustments

Liver Function: These drugs are extensively metabolized in the liver. They should be used with caution in patients with liver compromise.

Kidney Function: All nonsteroidal anti-inflammatory drugs may inhibit prostaglandins and alter kidney blood flow in patients with kidney (renal) compromise. Use with caution or not at all in patients with kidney compromise.

▷ **Dosing Instructions:** Take with or following food to prevent stomach irritation. Take with a full glass of water and remain upright (do not lie down) for 30 minutes. Regular-release tablets may be crushed, but not extended-release forms. The regular capsules may be opened, but not the prolonged-action capsules. Food actually increases absorption of nabumetone. Ketorolac ophthalmic should NOT be used while soft contacts are worn. If you forget a dose: Take the missed dose right away. If it is almost time to take the next dose, skip the missed dose and continue the medicine on your regular schedule. DO NOT double doses.

Usual Duration of Use: Continual use on a regular schedule for 1 to 2 weeks is usually necessary to determine drug benefit in relieving arthritic discomfort. The usual length of treatment for bursitis or tendonitis for indomethacin or sulindac is 7 to 14 days. Ketorolac oral or IV when used is only for short-term pain treatment (a MAXIMUM of 5 days regardless of the way [route] that it is taken). Ophthalmic ketorolac dosing is open-ended. Long-term use of the other agents in this class requires physician supervision.

Typical Treatment Goals and Measurements (Outcomes and Markers)

Pain: Most clinicians treating pain use a device called an algometer to check your pain. This looks like a small ruler, but lets the clinician better understand your pain. The goals of treatment then relate to where the level of pain started (for example, a rating of 7 on a zero to ten scale) and what the cause of the pain was. Pain medicines may also be used together (in combination) in order to get the best result or outcome. If your pain control is not acceptable to YOU (remember, in hospitals and outpatient settings, etc., pain control is a patient right) and if after a week of arthritis pain treatment results are not acceptable, be sure to call your doctor as you may need a different medicine or combination.

Arthritis: Control of arthritis symptoms (pain, loss of mobility, decreased ability to accomplish activities of daily living) is paramount in returning patient quality of life and to checking the results (beneficial outcomes) from these medicines. Some arthritis specialists use WOMAC (see Glossary) to measure results.

▷ **These Drugs Should Not Be Taken If**
- you have had an allergic reaction to them previously.
- you are subject to asthma or nasal polyps caused by aspirin.
- you are pregnant (all NSAIDs during the last 3 months of pregnancy) or you are breast-feeding.
- you have active peptic ulcer disease or any form of gastrointestinal ulceration or bleeding.
- you have active liver disease.
- you wear soft contact lenses (diclofenac).

- you have a bleeding disorder or a blood cell disorder.
- you have severe impairment of kidney function.
- you have severe aortic narrowing (coarctation).
- you have a history of rectal bleeding or proctitis (indomethacin suppositories).
- you have porphyria (diclofenac, indomethacin).

▷ **Inform Your Physician Before Taking This Drug If**
- you are allergic to aspirin or to other aspirin substitutes.
- you have an infection.
- you have a history of peptic ulcer disease, Crohn's disease, ulcerative colitis or any type of bleeding disorder.
- you have a history of epilepsy, Parkinson's disease or mental illness (psychosis).
- you have impaired liver or kidney function.
- you have high blood pressure or a history of heart failure.
- you are taking acetaminophen, aspirin or other aspirin substitutes or anticoagulants.

Possible Side Effects (natural, expected and unavoidable drug actions)
Drowsiness, ringing in ears, fluid retention.

▷ **Possible Adverse Effects** (unusual, unexpected and infrequent reactions)
If any of the following develop, consult your physician promptly for guidance.

Mild Adverse Effects
Allergic reactions: skin rash, hives, itching, localized swellings of face and/or extremities.
Headache—infrequent (diclofenac and nabumetone) to frequent (indomethacin).
Dizziness, feelings of detachment—infrequent.
Mouth sores, indigestion, nausea, vomiting, diarrhea—infrequent.
Ringing in the ears—possible.
Temporary loss of hair (indomethacin)—case reports.

Serious Adverse Effects
Allergic reactions: worsening of asthma, difficult breathing, mouth irritation.
Angioneurotic edema (nabumetone)—rare.
Blurred vision, confusion, depression—rare.
Active peptic ulcer, with or without bleeding—possible.
Liver damage with jaundice (see Glossary)—case reports.
Kidney damage with painful urination, bloody urine, reduced urine formation—rare.
Porphyria (nabumetone)—case report.
Bone marrow depression (see Glossary): fatigue, fever, sore throat, bleeding or bruising—case reports.
Thrombophlebitis—frequent (intravenous diclofenac use).
Severe skin rash (Stevens-Johnson syndrome—diclofenac, etodolac, sulindac)—case reports.
Fluid retention, increased blood pressure or edema—possible with all.
Congestive heart failure worsening—possible.
Peripheral neuritis (see Glossary): numbness, pain in extremities (indomethacin)—rare.
Lung fibrosis (nabumetone)—case reports.
Pancreatitis (sulindac)—rare; (indomethacin)—case reports.

Pneumonitis (sulindac)—rare; (diclofenac)—case report.

Aseptic meningitis (diclofenac)—rare.

Seizures (indomethacin only)—case reports.

▷ **Possible Effects on Sexual Function:** Enlargement and tenderness of both male and female breasts (indomethacin, sulindac)—rare.

Nonmenstrual vaginal bleeding (indomethacin)—rare.

Impotence (indomethacin, diclofenac, nabumetone)—rare.

Decreased libido (indomethacin)—rare.

Uterine bleeding (etodolac, sulindac)—rare.

Possible Delayed Adverse Effects: Mild anemia due to "silent" blood loss from the stomach.

Adverse Effects That May Mimic Natural Diseases or Disorders

Liver reactions may suggest viral hepatitis. Pancreatitis has occurred with sulindac.

Natural Diseases or Disorders That May Be Activated by These Drugs

Peptic ulcer disease, ulcerative colitis. Borderline clotting problems. Kidney disease.

Possible Effects on Laboratory Tests

Complete blood cell counts: decreased red cells, hemoglobin, white cells and platelets—rare.

INR (prothrombin time): increased.

Blood lithium level: increased.

Liver function tests: increased liver enzymes (ALT/GPT, AST/GOT and alkaline phosphatase), increased bilirubin.

Blood sugar (glucose): increased (indomethacin only)—rare.

Kidney function tests: increased blood creatinine and urea nitrogen (BUN) levels (kidney damage).

Fecal occult blood test: positive.

Urine protein (tolmetin only): may be falsely positive.

CAUTION

1. The FDA now requires a warning label on all nonprescription pain (analgesic) and fever (antipyretic) products that have aspirin or other salicylates, ibuprofen, naproxen sodium, ketoprofen or acetaminophen in them (NSAIDs) that says: ALCOHOL WARNING: IF YOU CONSUME 3 OR MORE ALCOHOLIC DRINKS EVERY DAY, ASK YOUR DOCTOR WHETHER YOU SHOULD TAKE [THE MEDICINE IN QUESTION] OR OTHER PAIN RELIEVERS/FEVER REDUCERS. [THE INGREDIENT] MAY CAUSE STOMACH BLEEDING.

    This is a new warning intended to help protect patients from possible stomach or liver damage.

2. Dose should be limited to the smallest amount that produces reasonable improvement.

3. These drugs may mask early signs of infection. Tell your doctor if you think you are developing an infection of any kind.

4. Congestive heart failure in elderly patients may be unmasked or worsened. Risk appears to increase with use of higher doses.

Precautions for Use

By Infants and Children:

Diclofenac, etodolac, nabumetone, sulindac: Safety and efficacy for those under 12 years of age not established.

Indomethacin: This drug frequently impairs kidney function in infants. Fatal liver reactions are possible in children between 6 and 12 years of age; avoid the use of this drug in this age group. Note: This medicine is used in infants (patent ductus arteriosus intravenously).

Tolmetin: Safety and efficacy for those under 2 years of age not established.

By Those Over 60 Years of Age: Small doses are advisable until tolerance is determined. Watch for any signs of liver or kidney toxicity, fluid retention, dizziness, confusion, impaired memory, depression, peptic ulcer or diarrhea, often with rectal bleeding.

▷ **Advisability of Use During Pregnancy**

Pregnancy Category: Indomethacin, diclofenac, tolmetin: B. Sulindac: B in first two trimesters. Nabumetone: C in first two trimesters. Not recommended in last trimester. Indomethacin, etodolac, nabumetone and sulindac (D in last trimester): D. (Indomethacin is also category D if used after 34 weeks or for more than 48 hours.) See Pregnancy Risk Categories at the back of this book.

Animal studies:

Indomethacin: significant toxicity and birth defects reported in mice and rats.

Diclofenac: Mouse, rat and rabbit studies reveal toxic effects on the embryo but no birth defects.

Nabumetone, tolmetin: Rat and rabbit studies revealed no defects.

Human studies:

Indomethacin: Adequate studies of pregnant women are not available. However, birth defects have been attributed to the use of this drug during pregnancy. The manufacturer recommends that indomethacin not be taken during pregnancy.

Diclofenac, nabumetone, sulindac, tolmetin: Adequate studies of pregnant women are not available. Avoid this drug completely during the last 3 months of pregnancy. Use it during the first 6 months only if clearly needed. Ask your doctor for guidance.

Etodolac: Adequate studies of pregnant women not available. The manufacturer advises that this drug be avoided during pregnancy.

Nabumetone: Fetal cardiovascular system adversely affected if used in the last trimester, so not recommended for last 3 months.

Advisability of Use If Breast-Feeding

Presence of these drugs in breast milk: Yes (all).

Avoid drugs or refrain from nursing (may have bad effects on infant's nervous system).

Habit-Forming Potential: None.

Effects of Overdose: Drowsiness, agitation, confusion, nausea, vomiting, diarrhea, disorientation, seizures, coma.

Possible Effects of Long-Term Use: Indomethacin and tolmetin: eye changes— deposits in the cornea, alterations in the retina. Irritation of the stomach and intestine.

Suggested Periodic Examinations While Taking These Drugs (at physician's discretion)

Complete blood cell counts.

Liver and kidney function tests.

Complete eye examinations if vision is altered in any way.

Stool for hidden (occult) blood (may actually be positive from these drugs).

▷ **While Taking These Drugs, Observe the Following**

Foods: No restrictions. These medicines are taken with food to decrease stomach irritation.

Herbal Medicines or Minerals: Ginseng, ginkgo, alfalfa, clove oil, feverfew, cinchona bark and garlic may also change clotting, so combining those herbals with these medicines is not recommended. Talk to your doctor BEFORE combining any medicines. NSAIDs may decrease feverfew effects. Since St. John's wort and some of these medicines may increase sensitivity to the sun, CAUTION IS ADVISED. Hay flower, mistletoe herb and white mustard seed carry German Commission E monograph indications for arthritis.

Nutritional Support: Indomethacin: Take 50 mg of vitamin C (ascorbic acid) daily.

Beverages: No restrictions. May be taken with milk.

▷ *Alcohol:* Used with caution: see FDA warning above. Alcohol can irritate the lining of the stomach. If excessive alcohol use is combined with the irritating effect of these medicines, risk of stomach and intestinal problems such as ulceration or bleeding can be increased.

Tobacco Smoking: No interactions expected. I advise everyone to quit smoking.

▷ *Other Drugs*

Medicines in this family may ***increase*** the effects of

- aminoglycoside antibiotics (amikacin, others—see Drug Classes) by increasing blood levels.
- anticoagulants such as warfarin (Coumadin) and increase the risk of bleeding; monitor INR (prothrombin time), adjust dose accordingly.
- cyclosporine (Sandimmune) and cause toxicity.
- digoxin (Lanoxin)—indomethacin only.
- lithium and cause lithium toxicity (except sulindac, which may decrease lithium levels).
- methotrexate (Mexate, others) and cause toxic levels.
- phenytoin (Dilantin) because of increased drug levels.
- tacrolimus (Prograf) and increase risk of decreased kidney function.
- thrombolytics such as streptokinase or TPA.
- zidovudine (AZT) and lead to toxicity of either medicine (indomethacin).

Medications in this class may ***decrease*** the effects of

- ACE inhibitors (see Drug Classes).
- beta-blocker drugs (see Drug Classes) and reduce their antihypertensive effectiveness.
- bumetanide (Bumex).
- captopril (Capoten).
- ethacrynic acid (Edecrin).
- furosemide (Lasix) and other loop diuretics.
- thiazide diuretics (see Drug Classes).

Medications in this class ***taken concurrently*** with the following drugs may increase the risk of bleeding or serious side effects; avoid these combinations or use with great caution:

- aspirin or other NSAIDs (EVEN NONPRESCRIPTION FORMS).
- dicumarol.
- diflunisal (Dolobid).
- dipyridamole (Persantine).

- low-molecular-weight heparins (Lovenox, others).
- ofloxacin (Floxin) can increase risk of seizures.
- probenecid (Pro-Biosan, others).
- sulfinpyrazone (Anturane).
- valproic acid (Depakene).
- warfarin (Coumadin).

Medications in this class *taken concurrently* with:
- alendronate (Fosamax) may increase risk of stomach or intestinal irritation.
- colestipol and cholestyramine will reduce beneficial effects of the NSAIDs (diclofenac and sulindac).
- ritonavir (Norvir) and other medicines that affect the cytochrome P-450 system in the liver will lead to altered blood levels of these medicines.

▷ *Driving, Hazardous Activities:* These drugs may cause drowsiness, dizziness or impaired vision. Restrict activities as necessary.

Aviation Note: The use of these drugs *may be a disqualification* for piloting. Consult a designated Aviation Medical Examiner.

Exposure to Sun: Caution: Several medicines in this class have caused increased sensitivity (photosensitivity—see Glossary).

ALBUTEROL (al BYU ter ohl)

Other Name: Salbutamol   **Introduced:** 1968   **Class:** Antiasthmatic, bronchodilator   **Prescription:** USA: Yes   **Controlled Drug:** USA: No; Canada: No   **Available as Generic:** Yes

Brand Names: Airet, ✦Alti-Salbutamol, ✦Apo-Salvent, Combivent [CD], Diskhaler, ✦Novo-Salmol, Proventil HFA, Proventil Inhaler, Proventil Repetabs, Proventil Tablets, Rotahaler, ✦Salbutamol, ✦Ventodisk Rotacaps, Ventolin Inhaler, Ventolin Nebules, Ventolin Rotacaps, Ventolin Syrup, Ventolin Tablets, Volmax Sustained-Release Tablets, Volmax Timed-Release Tablets

BENEFITS versus RISKS	
Possible Benefits	*Possible Risks*
VERY EFFECTIVE RELIEF OF BRONCHOSPASM	Increased blood pressure or heart rate
	Fine hand tremor
	Potential hyperactivity in children under twelve
	Angina in patients with coronary artery disease
	Irregular heart rhythm and fatalities— possible, with excessive use
	Paradoxical spasm of the bronchi

▷ **Principal Uses**

As a Single Drug Product: Uses currently included in FDA-approved labeling: (1) Relieves acute bronchial asthma and reduces frequency and severity of chronic, recurrent asthmatic attacks; (2) helps prevent exercise-induced bronchospasm.

Other (unlabeled) generally accepted uses: (1) May have a role (nebulized)

where blood potassium is too high; (2) limited use in patients with premature labor—especially if the cervix is dilated less than 3 centimeters.

How This Drug Works: By acting on adenyl cyclase, a chemical called cyclic AMP is increased. In response to increased cyclic AMP, this drug relaxes muscle (smooth) that is found in the uterus, skeletal muscle blood vessels (vascular bed) and the bronchi. In some lung disease, albuterol also works to help the lungs move mucus and decreases chemical release from mast cells.

Available Dosage Forms and Strengths

Aerosol —	90 mcg per press (actuation)
—	100 mcg per press (Canada)
—	120 mcg per press
Capsules for inhalation (technique is important) (Canada) —	200 mcg, 400 mcg
Nasal inhaler (Canada) —	100 mcg/dose
Solution for inhalation —	0.83% and 0.5%
Rotacaps —	200 mcg
Syrup —	2 mg/5 ml
—	2.4 mg/5 ml
Tablets —	2 mg, 4 mg
Tablets, sustained release —	4 mg, 4.8 mg, 8 mg, 9.6 mg
Tablets, timed release —	4 mg, 8 mg
Ventodisk (Canada) —	200 mcg and 400 mcg per disk

▷ **Recommended Dosage Ranges** (Actual dose and schedule must be determined for each patient individually.)

Capsules for inhalation (Rotahaler): Dose for children more than 4 years old and for adults is to use the contents of one capsule (200 mcg) via the Rotahaler device every 4 to 6 hours.

Metered dose inhaler—Adults and children 12 or older: Two inhalations (180 mcg) repeated every 4 to 6 hours. For some patients, one inhalation every 4 hours may be enough. Taking a larger number of inhalations is not recommended. If the dose that previously worked does not provide relief, call your doctor immediately. The status of your asthma must be examined.

Author's Note: Proventil Repetabs and Volmax are FDA-approved to treat bronchospasm in patients 6 years old or older.

Preventing exercise-caused asthma: Two inhalations (180 mcg of Ventolin form) 15 minutes BEFORE exercise.

Tablets (immediate release)—2 to 4 mg three to four times daily (every 8 to 6 hours).

Tablets (sustained release)—One or two tablets every 12 hours.

Do not exceed eight inhalations (720 mcg) or 32 mg (tablet form) every 24 hours. Some manufacturers limit tablets to 16 mg every 24 hours.

Conditions Requiring Dosing Adjustments

Liver Function: Low doses and caution needed in liver disease.

Kidney Function: No specific changes in dosing are available.

Heart (Coronary Artery) Disease: A maximum starting dose should be 1 mg in order to avoid chest pain (angina).

Thyroid Disease: People with low (hypoactive) thyroids may require increased doses.

▷ **Dosing Instructions:** May be taken on empty stomach or with food or milk. Nonsustained-release tablets may be crushed. Sustained-release forms should NEVER be crushed. For inhaler, follow the written instructions carefully. Do not use excessively. If you forget a dose: Use the inhaler as soon as possible. Do not double doses.

Usual Duration of Use: Do not use beyond the time necessary to stop episodes of asthma.

Typical Treatment Goals and Measurements (Outcomes and Markers)

Asthma: Short-acting beta agonists like albuterol are used to prevent or treat reversible spasms of the bronchial tubes. The peak effect happens 1 to 2 hours after dosing. Many clinicians use FEV1 to check benefits as well as decreased need for hospitalizations. One center in London used measurement of peak flow (patients were asked to blow three times in quick succession into a special measuring meter) to help decide how long patients should remain in the hospital. Calculations between the first and last breath measurements were made. Patients who had a ratio of less than one were said to have a decreased peak flow (indicating inflammation) and were kept in the hospital for an additional 3 days. Patients with a ratio of more than one (acceptable peak flow and relative absence of inflammation) were successfully sent home from the hospital. In any patient, if the usual therapeutic response to this medicine is not seen, call your doctor right away.

▷ **This Drug Should Not Be Taken If**
- you have had an allergic reaction to any form of it.
- you have an irregular heart rhythm or a fast heartbeat (tachycardia—Volmax).
- you have a specific problem with the aorta (idiopathic hypertrophic subvalvular stenosis—Volmax form).
- you have an overactive thyroid (hyperthyroid).
- you are taking, or took in the past 2 weeks, any monoamine oxidase (MAO) type A inhibitor (see Drug Classes).

▷ **Inform Your Physician Before Taking This Drug If**
- you have a heart or circulatory disorder, especially high blood pressure, coronary heart disease or aneurysms.
- you have diabetes.
- you have pheochromocytoma.
- you take any form of digitalis or any stimulant drug.
- you take other prescription or nonprescription medications that weren't discussed when albuterol was prescribed.
- you are going to have a baby (this medicine may alter contractions).
- you are unsure how much or how often to take albuterol.

Possible Side Effects (natural, expected and unavoidable drug actions)

Aerosol: dryness or irritation of mouth/throat, altered taste.

Tablet: nervousness, palpitation, fast heart rate (tachycardia)—infrequent. Heart effect may not be seen with nebulized albuterol.

▷ **Possible Adverse Effects** (unusual, unexpected and infrequent reactions)
If any of the following develop, consult your physician promptly for guidance.

Mild Adverse Effects
Itching—rare.
Headache, dizziness, restlessness, insomnia—infrequent.
Fine hand tremor—frequent.
Nausea—rare.
Leg cramps, flushing of skin—rare.
Difficulty urinating—rare.
Rapid heart rate—infrequent.
Decreased platelets—possible, but not clinically significant.

Serious Adverse Effects
Hypersensitivity reaction—case report.
Heart attack—case reports after intravenous or excessive inhalation use.
Abnormal heartbeats—possible.
Chest pain (angina)—possible with higher doses in patients with coronary artery disease.
Hallucinations or convulsions (with excessive dosing)—possible.
Decreased blood potassium (hypokalemia)—possible and dose related.
High blood sugar (hyperglycemia)—possible and more likely with intravenous use.

▷ **Possible Effects on Sexual Function:** None reported.

Natural Diseases or Disorders That May Be Activated by This Drug
Latent coronary artery disease, diabetes, or high blood pressure.

Possible Effects on Laboratory Tests
Blood aldosterone: increased.
Blood HDL cholesterol level: may be slightly increased.
Blood glucose level: increased.
Blood potassium: decreased.
Blood platelets: decreased (with high doses).
Blood magnesium: one study showed doses greater than 500 mcg lowered magnesium.

CAUTION
1. This drug may be dangerous if patients increase dose and/or frequency, as it may result in rapid or irregular heart rhythm and fatalities with overuse. A July 2001 report from the Dutch Centre for Human Drug Research found that when possible, high-dose inhaled albuterol may be best given with oxygen.
2. Use of this drug by inhalation with beclomethasone aerosol (Beclovent, Vanceril) may increase the risk of fluorocarbon propellant toxicity (fluorocarbons are being phased out). Use albuterol aerosol 20 to 30 minutes before beclomethasone aerosol to reduce toxicity and enhance the penetration of beclomethasone.
3. Serious heart rhythm problems or cardiac arrest can result from excessive or prolonged inhalation.
4. In general, women have been found to have higher peak blood levels (Cmax) after oral doses than men. Therefore, women may have an

increased risk of adverse effects (like lowered potassium or tremor) even with "therapeutic or usual" doses.

5. Call your doctor if you begin to increase the number of times you use this drug on a daily basis. Tolerance to the effects of this drug has been reported.

Precautions for Use

By Infants and Children: Dosing in children is often calculated on a mg per kg basis.

By Those Over 60 Years of Age: Avoid excessive and continual use. If asthma is not relieved promptly, other drugs will have to be tried. Watch for nervousness, palpitations, irregular heart rhythm and muscle tremors. Doses of 2 mg by mouth three or four times daily are prudent.

▷ Advisability of Use During Pregnancy

Pregnancy Category: C. See Pregnancy Risk Categories at the back of this book.
Animal studies: Cleft palate reported in mice.
Human studies: Adequate studies of pregnant women are not available.
Avoid use during first 3 months if possible.

Advisability of Use If Breast-Feeding

Presence of this drug in breast milk: Yes.
Avoid drug or refrain from nursing.

Habit-Forming Potential: A few cases of dependency and abuse have been described. These may be cases of use for the effect of the propellants (propellants are changing) or the drug itself.

Effects of Overdose: Nervousness, palpitation, rapid heart rate, life-threatening arrhythmias, sweating, headache, tremor, vomiting, chest pain.

Possible Effects of Long-Term Use: Loss of effectiveness.

Suggested Periodic Examinations While Taking This Drug (at physician's discretion)

Blood pressure measurements, evaluation of heart status, frequency of bronchospasms.

▷ While Taking This Drug, Observe the Following

Foods: No restrictions. Because this medicine may lead to minor lowering of potassium, talk to your doctor about possible need to increase potassium in your diet (see Table 13).

Herbal Medicines or Minerals: Using St. John's wort, ma huang, ephedrine-like compounds or kola while taking this medicine may result in unacceptable central nervous system stimulation. Talk to your doctor and pharmacist BEFORE making any combinations. Fir or pine needle oil should NOT be used by asthmatics. Ephedra alone does carry a German Commission E monograph indication for asthma treatment. If you are allergic to plants in the Asteraceae family (aster, chrysanthemum, daisy or ragweed), you may also be allergic to echinacea, chamomile, feverfew and St. John's wort.

Beverages: Avoid excessive caffeine as found in coffee, tea, cola and chocolate.

▷ *Alcohol:* No interactions expected.

Tobacco Smoking: Smoking constricts airways. I advise everyone to quit.

▷ *Other Drugs*

Albuterol *taken concurrently* with

- amphetamines may worsen cardiovascular side effects.
- bendroflumethiazide (Corzide, Naturetin) and other thiazide and loop diuretics (see Drug Classes) may result in additive lowering of blood potassium.
- beta-blockers such as propranolol (Inderal) results in loss of effect of both medications.
- dopamine (Intropin) may worsen adverse effects on the heart. Avoid this combination.
- ephedrine (Bronkaid, Tedrigen) may result in excessive heart effects.
- ipratropium (Atrovent) can result in better (longer time) opening of the bronchi (beneficial interaction).
- isoproterenol (Isuprel) may result in worsening of heart (cardiac) side effects.
- monoamine oxidase (MAO) type A inhibitor drugs can cause very high blood pressure and undesirable heart stimulation.
- pancuronium (Pavulon) or vecuronium (Norcuron) may lead to bronchospasm and delayed recovery of neuromuscular function.
- phenylephrine (Dimetapp, Dristan, others) may worsen bad effects on the heart (adverse reaction), and the combination is not recommended.
- phenylpropanolamine (Acutrim, Alka-Seltzer Plus, Contac, others) may worsen bad effects on the heart (adverse reaction). Do not combine.
- pseudoephedrine (Sudafed, others) may worsen adverse heart effects. DO NOT COMBINE.
- theophylline (Theo-Dur, others) may result in rapid removal of theophylline and loss of therapeutic theophylline effect.
- tricyclic antidepressants (see Drug Classes) may cause a severe increase in blood pressure.

▷ *Driving, Hazardous Activities:* Use caution if excessive nervousness or dizziness occurs.

Aviation Note: The use of this drug *is a disqualification* for piloting. Consult a designated Aviation Medical Examiner.

Exposure to Sun: No restrictions.

Heavy Exercise or Exertion: Use caution. Excessive exercise can cause (induce) asthma in some asthmatics.

ALENDRONATE (a LEN druh nate)

Introduced: 1996   **Class:** Second-generation bisphosphonate   **Prescription:** USA: Yes   **Controlled Drug:** USA: No   **Available as Generic:** No   **Brand Name:** Fosamax

```
┌─────────────────────────────────────────────────────────────┐
│                    BENEFITS versus RISKS                     │
│       Possible Benefits              Possible Risks          │
│  EFFECTIVE TREATMENT OF MALE    Esophageal irritation        │
│    AND FEMALE OSTEOPOROSIS      Minor muscle pain            │
│  INCREASE IN BONE MASS                                       │
│  PREVENTION OF OSTEOPOROSIS                                  │
│  ONCE-WEEKLY TREATMENT AND/                                  │
│    OR PREVENTION OF                                          │
│    OSTEOPOROSIS                                              │
│  DECREASED RISK OF BONE                                      │
│    FRACTURES                                                 │
│  SYMPTOM RELIEF IN PAGET'S                                   │
│    DISEASE                                                   │
│  PREVENTION OF POST-                                         │
│    MENOPAUSAL OSTEOPOROSIS                                   │
│  PREVENTION OF OSTEOPOROSIS                                  │
│    IN THOSE TAKING                                           │
│    CORTICOSTEROID-TYPE                                       │
│    (STEROID) MEDICINES                                       │
└─────────────────────────────────────────────────────────────┘
```

▷ **Principal Uses**

As a Single Drug Product: Uses currently included in FDA-approved labeling: (1) Treatment of postmenopausal osteoporosis; (2) treatment of Paget's disease; (3) prevention of postmenopausal osteoporosis; (4) prevention of osteoporosis in people who take corticosteroid-type medicines; (5) once weekly prevention or treatment of osteoporosis.

Other (unlabeled) generally accepted uses: (1) approved in Canada in combination with hormone replacement therapy (estrogen or estrogen plus progesterone) to increase positive outcomes on increased bone mass; (2) expected to work in the prevention and treatment of male osteoporosis.

How This Drug Works: This medicine works at the brush border of the osteoclast cell (inhibiting enzymes in the mevalonate pathway). This prevents the cell from resorbing (gobbling up) bone while the osteoblast (bone-building cell) continues to work. The end result is bone-building and decreased fracture risk.

Available Dosage Forms and Strengths

Tablets — 5 mg, 10 mg, 35 mg, 40 mg, 70 mg

▷ **Recommended Dosage Ranges** (Actual dose and schedule must be determined for each patient individually.)

Infants and Children: Efficacy and safety are not established.

18 to 65 Years of Age: Treatment of osteoporosis in women after menopause: 70 mg once a week OR 10 mg taken once daily.

Osteoporosis prevention in women after menopause: 35 mg once a week OR 5 mg once daily. I strongly recommend an appropriate amount of dietary calcium and/or calcium supplementation to ensure adequate calcium every day. Discuss the need for vitamin D with your doctor. Calcium and vitamin D are critical in osteoporosis prevention and treatment.

Prevention of glucocorticoid-induced osteoporosis: 5 mg daily in one study.

Treatment of glucocorticoid-induced osteoporosis: 5 mg once daily. In postmenopausal women who are NOT taking estrogen, the dose for this indication is 10 mg once daily.

Paget's disease: 40 mg once daily for 6 months.

Over 65 Years of Age: Same as in those 18 to 65 years old.

Conditions Requiring Dosing Adjustments

Liver Function: No changes needed.

Kidney Function: Lower doses for patients with kidney compromise. Patients with creatinine clearances (see Glossary) less than 35 ml/min **should not** be given this medicine.

▷ **Dosing Instructions:** TAKE THIS MEDICINE WITH 6 TO 8 OUNCES OF TAP WATER TO GET THE BEST RESULTS. DO NOT take this drug with food or other drugs. The therapeutic benefit will be decreased. Take it at least half an hour before the first food or liquids (other than plain tap water) of the day. Avoiding food or drink for more than 30 minutes lets more medicine get into your body to go to work. **DO NOT** lie down for 30 minutes (preferably an hour) after taking this drug (decreases risk of irritation of the esophagus). If you forget a dose: Take the medicine right away, unless it is nearly time for your next dose. If you are taking it once weekly, call your doctor. DO NOT double doses.

Usual Duration of Use: In Paget's disease, this medicine is used once daily for 6 months, with recheck after that. In treating osteoporosis after menopause, many doctors get a bone mineral density test (DEXA or PDEXA presently most widely used) to help decide to start therapy and then get a second test 2 years later or order certain laboratory tests to check results or outcome of therapy. Further study is needed to find the best dosing strategies in long-term (greater than 5 years) use of alendronate (cyclic or ongoing).

Typical Treatment Goals and Measurements (Outcomes and Markers)

Fracture of bone is a critical issue when bones weaken and become osteoporotic. The World Health Organization has generated guidelines that establish weak bone (osteopenia) and osteoporosis based on certain patient populations. If this medicine is being used to prevent osteoporosis, a typical strategy would be to obtain a measure of bone mineral density such as a DEXA scan. The medicine would be started based on risk factors, medicines (such as glucocorticoids) that are being taken and the results of the DEXA scan itself. Laboratory tests (such as N-telopeptides) may be tested to augment treatment decisions. Once the medicine is started, a DEXA is often rechecked in 2 years to assess the beneficial effects of this medicine. Some clinicians will also recommend check of height (height loss) as well as an earlier repeat DEXA, PDEXA, ultrasound and/or laboratory test in patients with a family history of rapid perimenopausal bone loss. In Paget's disease, this medicine is used once daily for 6 months, with recheck after that.

Possible Advantages of This Drug

This drug increases bone mass more than other available (anti-resorptive) drugs, which then decreases the risk of fractures. This medicine also helps form normal bone (microarchitecture). Alendronate also offers the adherence (taking the medicine as prescribed) benefits of once-weekly dosing.

▷ **This Drug Should Not Be Taken If**
- you are allergic to the drug or its components.
- you have a low blood calcium (hypocalcemia). Talk to your doctor.
- you have a significant kidney disease (medicine should NOT be taken if creatinine clearance less than 35 ml/min—no data).
- you are unable to sit or stand for 30 minutes after taking this medicine (increased risk of esophageal problems).
- you are pregnant or are nursing your infant.
- you have esophageal disease (abnormal esophagus) or difficulty emptying the esophagus.

▷ **Inform Your Physician Before Taking This Drug If**
- you have ulcers or inflammation of the duodenum.
- you have difficulty swallowing.
- you have a vitamin D deficiency.
- you have a diet poor in calcium (low calcium diet).

Possible Side Effects (natural, expected and unavoidable drug actions)

Irritation of the esophagus and potential ulceration—rare. This effect is worsened if patients lie down soon after taking drug.

▷ **Possible Adverse Effects** (unusual, unexpected and infrequent reactions)

If any of the following develop, consult your physician promptly for guidance.

Mild Adverse Effects

Allergic reactions: rare skin rash or redness.

Headache—infrequent.

Gas (flatulence), diarrhea or constipation—infrequent.

Pain in the muscles or skeleton (musculoskeletal)—infrequent.

Mild calcium decrease—2% decrease (some patients at 10 mg daily).

Mild decrease in phosphorus—up to 6%.

Mild muscle pain—infrequent with the 10-mg dose.

Fever (drug fever) with intravenous use—rare.

Serious Adverse Effects

Allergic reactions: none reported.

Esophageal ulceration—rare. (Increased risk if you lie down after taking this drug. Best NOT to lie down for at least half an hour after taking this medicine.) One case report of a patient with a history of peptic ulcer disease who had stomach surgery and was also taking aspirin who developed an ulcer (anastamotic) and had mild hemorrhaging.

Inflammation of the sclera (scleritis)—rare (probably idiosyncratic).

Drug fever (intravenous form)—frequent.

▷ **Possible Effects on Sexual Function:** None reported.

Possible Effects on Laboratory Tests

Serum calcium or phosphorus: lowered—infrequent.

Liver function tests: increased—rare (with intravenous form) (asymptomatic and transient).

CAUTION

1. A "dear doctor" letter was sent out by the FDA warning of increased occurrence of esophageal ulceration. This may have been caused by patients taking the medicine with less water than directed and by patients who took the medicine and went back to bed. Take this medi-

cine with a full glass of tap water and DO NOT LIE DOWN for 30 minutes after taking this drug.

2. Patients who take more than 10 mg of alendronate a day may need to avoid aspirin and aspirin-containing compounds because upper gastrointestinal adverse effects may be increased in this situation if the medicines are combined (at any alendronate dose).

3. Other causes of osteoporosis besides estrogen or aging (secondary osteoporosis) must be ruled out.

4. Depression (long-standing) may be a risk factor for osteoporosis (probably diet related). Talk with your doctor about an osteoporosis test if depression is a problem for you.

5. Talk to your doctor if you develop eye symptoms while taking this medicine.

Precautions for Use

By Infants and Children: Safety and efficacy in this age group have not been established.

By Those Over 65 Years of Age: The amount that goes into the body (bioavailability) and the places alendronate goes (disposition) are similar to those less than 65. No specific dosing changes needed. Increased sensitivity to this drug is possible.

▷ **Advisability of Use During Pregnancy**

Pregnancy Category: C. See Pregnancy Risk Categories at the back of this book.

Animal studies: Studies in rats have shown toxicity to the mother as well as neonatal death following dosing of alendronate during pregnancy.

Human studies: Adequate studies of pregnant women are not available.

Avoid this medicine during pregnancy.

Advisability of Use If Breast-Feeding

Presence of this drug in breast milk: Yes in rats; unknown in humans.

Avoid drug or refrain from nursing.

Habit-Forming Potential: None.

Effects of Overdose: Nausea, vomiting, hypocalcemia and hypophosphatemia. Heartburn, ulceration of the upper gastrointestinal tract.

Possible Effects of Long-Term Use: Increased bone density and decreased fracture risk (beneficial).

Suggested Periodic Examinations While Taking This Drug (at physician's discretion)

Tests of bone mineral density (DEXA, PDEXA, ultrasound or QCT), check of lab tests of bone loss or formation.

Blood calcium.

Measurement of height.

▷ **While Taking This Drug, Observe the Following**

Foods: DO NOT TAKE THIS DRUG WITH FOOD.

Herbal Medicines or Minerals: Soy or other plant-derived phytoestrogens may work to complement alendronate, but have not been studied. Ipriflavone is a synthetic flavonoid currently investigational for osteoporosis (which both inhibits bone resorption by reducing osteoclast recruitment and encourages osteoblast function). Combined use with alendronate has not been studied.

Adequate elemental calcium and vitamin D are needed. Calcium supplements should be taken at least half an hour after taking alendronate. Effervescent calcium (resulting in a solution) may be absorbed more rapidly and help avoid problems.

Beverages: ANY liquid other than water will DECREASE the amount of alendronate that gets into your body to help you. It is critical that this medicine only be taken with 6 to 8 ounces of water.

▷ *Alcohol:* Alcohol (especially in high doses) may act as a bone-forming cell (osteoblast) poison, and excessive use is a risk factor for osteoporosis. Alcohol may also irritate the stomach lining.

Tobacco Smoking: Smoking is a risk factor for osteoporosis. STOP SMOKING.

▷ *Other Drugs*

Alendronate *taken concurrently* with

- antacids may decrease the total absorption of alendronate and decrease its therapeutic benefit.
- aspirin or aspirin-containing products or salicylates may pose an increased risk of upper gastrointestinal adverse effects if more than 10 mg of alendronate is taken daily. Although other NSAIDs (see Drug Classes) were not presented as potential problems with alendronate doses greater than 10 mg, caution is advised for this benefit to risk decision.
- calcium products (various) will blunt absorption of alendronate. Wait at least half an hour after taking alendronate to take any other medicine including a calcium supplement. Effervescent calcium forms may offer an advantage considering their speed of absorption.
- estrogens (various) taken by a few women in clinical trials did not present problems. This combination was recently (both estrogen and/or estrogen plus a progestin) approved in Canada.
- foscarnet (Foscavir) may result in an additive decrease in calcium.
- magnesium (various) may increase stomach/intestine upset.
- medicines in general should NOT be taken at the same time as alendronate. Separate any dose of alendronate and any other medicine by at least half an hour.
- mesalamine or olsalazine may increase stomach/intestine upset.
- ranitidine (Zantac) (intravenous form and perhaps oral form) may double how much alendronate gets into your body. The clinical importance of this is not yet known.

The following drugs may *decrease* the effects of alendronate:

- Because a small amount of alendronate gets into the body under the best conditions, take alendronate with a full 6 to 8 ounces of water. Take any other drugs at least half an hour after alendronate.

▷ *Driving, Hazardous Activities:* No specific limitations.

Aviation Note: The use of this drug is ***probably not a disqualification*** for piloting. Consult a designated Aviation Medical Examiner.

Exposure to Sun: No restrictions.

Heavy Exercise or Exertion: If your bone density is low, heavy aerobic exercise may not be a good idea. Discuss this with your doctor. In general, weight-bearing exercise stimulates receptors (mechanoreceptors) to release factors that result in increased bone strength.

Discontinuation: Talk with your doctor **before** stopping this medicine.

ALLOPURINOL (al oh PURE i nohl)

Introduced: 1963   **Class:** Antigout, xanthine oxidase inhibitor   **Prescription:** USA: Yes   **Controlled Drug:** USA: No; Canada: No   **Available as Generic:**   USA: Yes; Canada: No

Brand Names: ✿Alloprin, ✿Apo-Allopurinol, Lopurin, ✿Novo-Purol, ✿Purinol, ✿Riva-Purinol, Zurinol, Zyloprim

BENEFITS versus RISKS	
Possible Benefits	*Possible Risks*
EFFECTIVE CONTROL OF GOUT	Increased frequency of acute gout
CONTROL OF HIGH BLOOD URIC	initially
ACID DUE TO POLYCYTHEMIA,	Peripheral neuritis
LEUKEMIA, CANCER AND	Allergic reactions in skin, lung, blood
CHEMOTHERAPY	vessels and liver
More beneficial in patients who	Bone marrow depression
remove more than one gram of	Kidney toxicity
uric acid in a day	
May have a role in restoring blood	
vessel lining cells (endothelial cell)	
function in people with diabetes	
and mild high blood pressure	

▷ **Principal Uses**

As a Single Drug Product: Uses currently included in FDA-approved labeling: (1) Long-term gout therapy to prevent acute gout (does not relieve sudden gout attacks); (2) helps prevent high blood levels of uric acid in people who have recurrent uric acid or calcium oxalate kidney stones, people getting chemotherapy or radiation for cancer or who take thiazide diuretics (see Drug Classes).

Other (unlabeled) generally accepted uses: (1) May decrease pain and occurrence of mouth sores in people receiving 5-fluorouracil chemotherapy; (2) may help prostate swelling (nonbacterial prostatitis) not caused by bacteria; (3) early data show benefits in blood circulation damage (ischemic tissue damage); (4) may help Chagas' disease; (5) appears to ease refractive epilepsy in children; (6) effective in combination with quinine in treating malaria; (7) may have a role in helping restore how well the cells lining blood vessels (endothelial cells) work in people with diabetes and mild high blood pressure (300 mg a day in a 1-month study).

How This Drug Works: Works to change chemicals called purines' removal (metabolism) by the body. This medicine does this without changing the ability of the body to make purines that are important to the body. Allopurinol blocks the enzyme xanthine oxidase, thereby decreasing uric acid formation that is the root cause of gout. It also uses a feedback mechanism to block purine synthesis (requires hypoxanthine guanine phosphoribosyltransferase).

Available Dosage Forms and Strengths

Tablets — 100 mg, 200 mg, 300 mg

▷ **Usual Adult Dosage Ranges:** Starts as 100 mg every 24 hours, then increased by 100 mg every 24 hours (1 week apart) until uric acid level is normal (6 mg/dl or less). Usual dose is 200–300 mg every 24 hours for mild gout, and 400 to 600 mg every 24 hours for moderate to severe gout. Daily doses of 300 mg or less may be taken as a single dose. Doses exceeding 300 mg daily should be divided into two or three equal portions. For high uric acid levels associated with cancer (to prevent uric acid nephropathy): 600–800 mg every 24 hours, divided into three equal portions (with high water intake). Kidney stone (calcium oxalate) recurrence prevention: 200–300 mg per day. Extemporaneously made mouthwash: 5–6 mg/ml suspension has been used several times a day to prevent 5-FU stomatitis.

Note: Actual dosage and schedule must be determined for each patient individually.

Conditions Requiring Dosing Adjustments

Liver Function: Dose adjustment in liver compromise is not documented.

Kidney Function: Dosing must be adjusted in kidney compromise.

Malnutrition: Malnourished or low-protein-diet patients will not remove this drug normally and are at risk for toxicity. Doses must be decreased.

▷ **Dosing Instructions:** Best taken with food or milk (or a meal) to reduce stomach irritation. Tablet may be crushed. Drink 2 to 3 quarts (10 to 12 glasses) of liquids daily if your doctor says it's ok (not contraindicated). If you forget a dose: Take the medicine as soon as you remember it, unless it is close to the time for the next dose—simply take the dose at the next scheduled time. Do NOT double doses.

Usual Duration of Use: Regular use for several months may be needed to prevent acute gout attacks. Ongoing use for years often needed for adequate control.

Typical Treatment Goals and Measurements (Outcomes and Markers)

Uric Acid: Blood uric acid levels often decrease in 48 to 72 hours and may reach normal range in 1 to 3 weeks. Attacks of gout should become shorter and lessen in severity over time.

▷ **This Drug Should Not Be Taken If**
- you have had an allergic reaction to it previously.
- you are having an acute gout attack.

▷ **Inform Your Physician Before Taking This Drug If**
- you have a family history of hemochromatosis.
- you have a history of liver or kidney disease.
- you have had a blood cell or bone marrow disorder.
- you have a seizure or convulsive disorder (epilepsy—a slow withdrawal from this treatment is needed).
- you take other prescription or nonprescription medications not discussed when allopurinol was prescribed.
- you are unsure how much or how often to take allopurinol.
- you are on a low-protein diet.
- you do not drink very much water—talk to your doctor about this.
- you are pregnant.

Possible Side Effects (natural, expected and unavoidable drug actions)

Acute gout may still occur during the first several weeks of therapy. Ask your doctor about using other drugs during this period.

▷ **Possible Adverse Effects** (unusual, unexpected and infrequent reactions)

If any of the following develop, consult your physician promptly for guidance.

Mild Adverse Effects

Allergic reactions: skin rash, hives, itching—frequent; drug fever.

Confusion, agitation, headache, dizziness, drowsiness—rare.

Nausea, vomiting, diarrhea, stomach cramps—rare.

Taste disturbance—possible.

Loss of scalp hair—rare.

Serious Adverse Effects

Allergic reactions: severe skin reactions—infrequent.

High fever, chills, joint pains, swollen glands, kidney or liver damage—rare.

Idiosyncratic reaction: catatonia, paresthesia, agitation.

Hepatitis with or without jaundice (see Glossary): yellow eyes and skin, dark-colored urine, light-colored stools (may be part of allergy)—rare.

Kidney damage (acute tubular necrosis or interstitial nephritis)—case reports—rare.

Bone marrow depression (see Glossary)—rare.

Blood vessel inflammation/damage—rare (risk increased in kidney failure and thiazide diuretic use at the same time).

Peripheral neuritis—rare.

Bronchospasm (part of hypersensitivity)—rare.

Eye damage (macular), cataract formation—rare

▷ **Possible Effects on Sexual Function:** Rare cases of bladder inflammation have been reported.

Adverse Effects That May Mimic Natural Diseases or Disorders

Toxic liver reaction may suggest viral hepatitis.

Severe skin reactions may resemble the Stevens-Johnson syndrome (erythema multiforme). One case report of Stevens-Johnson with combined allopurinol and captopril has been made.

Possible Effects on Laboratory Tests

Complete blood cell counts: decreased red cells, hemoglobin and platelets; increased eosinophils.

Liver function tests: increased ALT/GPT, AST/GOT and alkaline phosphatase.

CAUTION

1. Call your doctor immediately if you develop a rash. This can be the first sign of an allergic reaction. Prompt action may avoid a more serious reaction.
2. A patient with an allopurinol allergy had cross-allergenicity and allergic reaction to acyclovir (Zovirax).
3. In the first few weeks of therapy, frequency of gout attacks may increase. These subside with ongoing therapy.
4. Drug should not be started in acute gout. It does not help.
5. Vitamin C in doses of 2 g or more daily can increase the risk of kidney stone formation during the use of allopurinol.
6. Patients with kidney function decline are more likely to have allergic reactions to this drug.
7. Frequency of rash may be increased in patients also taking a penicillin.
8. Allergic-type kidney damage can result if thiazide diuretics (see Drug Classes) are taken with allopurinol. Avoid this combination.

9. Patients on low-protein diets will not eliminate allopurinol normally. Doses must be decreased.
10. Dosing MUST be adjusted to kidney function. If you are 60 or older, "normal" declines in kidney function may require decreased doses. Talk to your doctor.

Precautions for Use

By Infants and Children: Not used in children except for increased uric acid caused by malignant growths. Watch closely for allergic skin reactions and blood cell disorders. The toxicity of azathioprine (Imuran) or mercaptopurine (Purinethol) may be increased in children receiving chemotherapy. For this kind of secondary hyperuricemia: 150 mg per day in children less than 6. Response is checked in 2 days and the dose is adjusted to response. Those 6–10 years old receive 300 mg a day with the same response check and dose changes as required.

By Those Over 60 Years of Age: Smaller starting and ongoing doses of this drug must be used (age-related decrease in kidney function).

▷ **Advisability of Use During Pregnancy**

Pregnancy Category: C. See Pregnancy Risk Categories at the back of this book.
Animal studies: Results are conflicting and inconclusive.
Human studies: Adequate studies of pregnant women are not available.
   Avoid use of drug during the first 3 months. Use during the last 6 months only if clearly needed.

Advisability of Use If Breast-Feeding

Presence of this drug in breast milk: Yes.
Avoid drug or refrain from nursing.

Habit-Forming Potential: None.

Effects of Overdose: Nausea, vomiting or diarrhea. Hypersensitivity reactions, kidney and liver function decline.

Possible Effects of Long-Term Use: Beneficial decreases in uric acid.

Suggested Periodic Examinations While Taking This Drug (at physician's discretion)

Blood uric acid levels.
Complete blood cell counts.
Liver and kidney function tests.
Eye examinations (possible cataract formation or macular damage).

▷ **While Taking This Drug, Observe the Following**

Foods: Talk to your doctor about a low-purine diet (such as avoiding liver, lentils, anchovies, etc.). A low-protein diet may increase toxicity risk if dose isn't decreased.
Herbal Medicines or Minerals: Acerola is high in vitamin C. Inosine, like acerola, may increase uric acid levels. Aspen should be avoided in gout. Lipase may worsen gout (read the labels on all neutraceuticals). Goutweed (*Aegopodium podagraria*) does not have enough data to assess effectiveness.
Beverages: No restrictions. May be taken with milk.
▷ *Alcohol:* Alcohol can worsen gout. Best to avoid it.
Tobacco Smoking: No interactions expected. I advise everyone to quit smoking.

▷   *Other Drugs*

Allopurinol may *increase* the effects of
- azathioprine (Imuran) and mercaptopurine (Purinethol), making dose decreases necessary.
- didanosine (Videx) which was noted in a case report of two patients with impaired kidneys.
- oral anticoagulants (see Drug Classes) such as warfarin (Coumadin). INR should be checked more often.
- theophylline (aminophylline, Elixophyllin, Theo-Dur, etc.).

Allopurinol *taken concurrently* with
- ampicillin, amoxicillin (and perhaps other penicillins) may increase the incidence of skin rash.
- antacids containing aluminum will decrease the therapeutic effect of allopurinol.
- captopril (Capoten) or other ACE inhibitors (see Drug Classes) can increase the likelihood of allergic reactions. CAUTION.
- chlorpropamide (Diabinese)) can cause hypoglycemia.
- cyclophosphamide (Cytoxan, Neosar) may result in cyclophosphamide toxicity.
- cyclosporine (Sandimmune) can cause cyclosporine toxicity.
- iron salts may lead to excess liver iron. Avoid combining.
- mercaptopurine (Purinethol) increases toxicity risk.
- probenecid (Benemid, others) may increase probenecid levels.
- tamoxifen (Nolvadex) may result in increased allopurinol levels and increased risk of liver toxicity.
- thiazide diuretics (see Drug Classes) may decrease kidney function.
- theophylline (Theo-Dur, etc.) may cause toxic theophylline levels.
- vidarabine (Vira-A) may increase risk of neurotoxicity.

▷   *Driving, Hazardous Activities:* Drowsiness may occur in some people. Use caution.
Aviation Note: The use of this drug *may be a disqualification* for piloting. Consult a designated Aviation Medical Examiner.
Exposure to Sun: No restrictions.
Discontinuation: If you have a seizure disorder, this medicine dose should be slowly decreased and then stopped.

ALPRAZOLAM (al PRAY zoh lam)

Introduced: 1973   **Class:** Antianxiety drug, benzodiazepines   **Prescription:** USA: Yes   **Controlled Drug:** USA: C-IV*; Canada: No   **Available as Generic:** Yes

Brand Names: Alprazolam Intensol, ♣Apo-Alpraz, ♣Med-Alprazolam, ♣Novo-Alprazol, ♣Nu-Alpraz, Xanax

Warning: The brand names Xanax and Zantac are similar and can lead to serious medication errors. Xanax is alprazolam. Zantac is ranitidine, which treats peptic ulcers and heartburn. Make sure your prescription was filled correctly.

*See Schedules of Controlled Drugs at the back of this book.

BENEFITS versus RISKS	
Possible Benefits	*Possible Risks*
RELIEF OF ANXIETY AND NERVOUS TENSION	Habit-forming potential with prolonged use
EFFECTIVE TREATMENT OF PANIC DISORDER	Minor impairment of mental functions with therapeutic doses
Wide margin of safety with therapeutic doses	Tachycardia and palpitations
May have some action as an antidepressant	

▷ **Principal Uses**

As a Single Drug Product: Uses currently included in FDA-approved labeling: (1) Used for short-term relief of mild to moderate anxiety and nervous tension; (2) helps relieve anxiety associated with neurosis; (3) decreases frequency and severity of panic disorder.

Other (unlabeled) generally accepted uses: (1) Can help control extreme PMS symptoms; (2) lessens a variety of types of cancer pain when given with various narcotics; (3) eases agoraphobia; (4) decreases symptoms in essential tremor; (5) decreases loudness of ear ringing in tinnitus; (6) can be helpful in alcohol withdrawal; (7) eases irritable bowel syndrome; (8) eases anxiety sometimes seen with depression; (9) helpful in reducing anticipatory vomiting from chemotherapy.

How This Drug Works: Calms by enhancing the action of the nerve transmitter gamma-aminobutyric acid (GABA), which in turn blocks higher brain centers.

Available Dosage Forms and Strengths

     Tablets — 0.25 mg, 0.5 mg, 1 mg, 2 mg

Oral solution — 0.25 mg, 0.5 mg, 1 mg/5 ml

            — 0.25 mg/2.5 ml

▷ **Usual Adult Dosage Ranges:** *For anxiety and nervous tension:* 0.25–0.5 mg three times daily. Maximum dose is 4 mg every 24 hours, taken in divided doses—but the lowest effective dose should be used.

For panic disorder: Initially 0.5 mg three times daily; increase dose by 1 mg every 3 to 4 days as needed and tolerated. Some patients stopped having panic attacks with 6 mg a day. Maximum daily dose is 10 mg.

For treatment of alcohol withdrawal: Dosing is variable—one source reported a mean oral daily dose to be 2.2 mg.

Note: Actual dosage and schedule must be determined for each patient individually.

Conditions Requiring Dosing Adjustments

Liver Function: A starting dose of 0.25 mg is prudent in patients with advanced liver disease. Slow increase in dose only if needed.

Kidney Function: The manufacturer does not define specific dose reductions.

Obesity: Takes a longer time to reach final concentrations in obese people. Doses should be calculated based on ideal rather than actual body weight.

Alcoholism: Because of some of the physiological and liver changes in alcoholism, removal of drug from the body may be delayed. Lower doses/longer times (intervals) between doses are needed.

▷ **Dosing Instructions:** May be taken on empty stomach or with food or milk. Tablet may be crushed. Do not stop this drug abruptly if taken for more than 4 weeks (stop slowly by decreasing 0.5 mg every 3 days or longer). If you forget a dose, but have missed by less than an hour, take the missed dose. If it is almost time for your next scheduled dose, skip the missed dose. Do NOT double doses.

Usual Duration of Use: Several days to several weeks. Continual use should not exceed 8 weeks without evaluation by your doctor.

Author's Note: The National Institute of Mental Health has a new information page on anxiety. It can be found on the World Wide Web (www.nimh.nih.gov/anxiety).

Typical Treatment Goals and Measurements (Outcomes and Markers)

Anxiety or panic: Goals for anxiety and panic tend to be more vague and subjective than hypertension or cholesterol. Frequently, the patient (in conjunction with physician assessment) will largely decide if anxiety has been modified to a successful extent. The Hamilton depression scale is widely used to assess depression. In the case of panic attacks, decreased number of trips to the hospital or ER visits may be a useful measure. In both cases, the ability of the patient to return to normal activities is a hallmark of successful treatment.

▷ **This Drug Should Not Be Taken If**
* you have had an allergic reaction to it previously.
* you are pregnant (first 3 months).
* you have acute narrow-angle glaucoma.
* you have myasthenia gravis.

▷ **Inform Your Physician Before Taking This Drug If**
* your history includes palpitations or tachycardia (may be worsened).
* you are allergic to benzodiazepines (see Drug Classes).
* you are pregnant or planning pregnancy.
* you are breast-feeding your infant.
* you have a history of depression or serious mental illness (psychosis).
* you have a history of alcoholism or drug abuse.
* you have impaired liver or kidney function.
* you have open-angle glaucoma.
* you have a seizure disorder (epilepsy).
* you have severe chronic lung disease.
* you take other prescription or nonprescription medications that were not discussed when alprazolam was prescribed for you.
* you are unsure how much or how often to take alprazolam.

Possible Side Effects (natural, expected and unavoidable drug actions)
Drowsiness, light-headedness—frequent.

▷ **Possible Adverse Effects** (unusual, unexpected and infrequent reactions)
If any of the following develop, consult your physician promptly for guidance.

Mild Adverse Effects
Allergic reactions: skin rash, hives.
Headache, dizziness, fatigue, blurred vision, dry mouth—infrequent.
Drowsiness—frequent, up to 50%.
Nausea, vomiting, constipation—infrequent.
Increased salivation—infrequent.

Serious Adverse Effects

Confusion, hallucinations, depression, excitement, agitation (paradoxical reaction)—case reports to rare.

Tachycardia and palpitations—infrequent.

Increased liver enzymes—rare.

Increased white blood cells (leukocytosis) or decreased blood cells (pancytopenia)—case reports and of questionable causation.

Low blood pressure (hypotension)—case report.

▷ **Possible Effects on Sexual Function:** Rare but documented: inhibited female orgasm (5 mg/day); impaired ejaculation (3.5 mg/day); decreased libido, impaired erection (4.5 mg/day); altered timing and pattern of menstruation (0.75–4 mg/day).

Possible Effects on Laboratory Tests

Liver function tests: increased ALT/GPT, AST/GOT—rare and insignificant.

Urine screening tests for drug abuse: may be positive (depends upon amount of drug taken and testing method).

CAUTION

1. Do not stop taking this drug abruptly if it has been taken continually for more than 4 weeks.
2. Some nonprescription drugs with antihistamines (allergy and cold medicines, sleep aids) can cause excessive sedation.
3. This medicine is removed from the body by some liver enzymes called cytochrome P450 3A4. Medicines that block this enzyme system will tend to increase alprazolam levels. Medicines that induce or increase P450 activity will tend to lower alprazolam levels and blunt effectiveness.
4. People with ongoing severe conditions such as cancer may not tolerate "typical" starting doses; 0.25 mg twice or three times a day as a starting dose is prudent. The dose may be increased as needed and tolerated.

Precautions for Use

By Infants and Children: Safety and effectiveness for those under 18 not established.

By Those Over 60 Years of Age: Starting dose should be 0.25 mg two or three times daily. Watch for excessive drowsiness, dizziness, unsteadiness and incoordination (possible low blood pressure).

▷ **Advisability of Use During Pregnancy**

Pregnancy Category: D. See Pregnancy Risk Categories at the back of this book.

Animal studies: Diazepam (a closely related benzodiazepine) can cause cleft palate in mice and skeletal defects in rats. No data on alprazolam.

Human studies: Some studies suggest an association between diazepam use and cleft lip and heart deformities. Adequate studies in pregnant women are not available.

Avoid use during entire pregnancy if possible.

Advisability of Use If Breast-Feeding

Presence of this drug in breast milk: Yes.

Avoid drug or refrain from nursing.

Habit-Forming Potential: This drug can cause psychological and/or physical dependence (see Glossary), especially if used in large doses for an extended period of time.

Effects of Overdose: Marked drowsiness, weakness, feeling of drunkenness, staggering gait, tremor, stupor progressing to deep sleep or coma.

Possible Effects of Long-Term Use: Psychological and/or physical dependence.

Suggested Periodic Examinations While Taking This Drug (at physician's discretion)

None required for short-term use.

▷ **While Taking This Drug, Observe the Following**

Foods: No restrictions.

Herbal Medicines or Minerals: Kava and valerian may exacerbate central nervous system depression (avoid this combination). Kola nut, Siberian ginseng, mate, ephedra and ma huang may blunt the benefits of this medicine. While St. John's wort is indicated for anxiety, it is also thought to increase (induce) cytochrome P450 enzymes and will tend to blunt alprazolam effectiveness if combined with alprazolam. St. John's wort may also worsen sun sensitivity caused by alprazolam.

Beverages: Avoid excessive caffeine-containing beverages: coffee, tea, cola (counteracts effects). This drug may be taken with milk.

▷ *Alcohol:* Use with extreme caution. Alcohol may increase the sedative effects of alprazolam. Alprazolam may increase the intoxicating effects of alcohol. Avoid alcohol completely—throughout the day and night—if you find it necessary to drive or engage in any hazardous activity.

Tobacco Smoking: Heavy smoking may reduce calming. I advise quitting smoking.

Marijuana Smoking: Occasional (once or twice weekly): Increased sedative effect.

Daily: Marked increase in sedative effect.

▷ *Other Drugs*

Alprazolam may *increase* the effects of
- digoxin (Lanoxin) and cause digoxin toxicity.

Alprazolam may *decrease* the effects of
- levodopa (Sinemet, etc.) and reduce its effect in treating Parkinson's disease.

The following drugs may *increase* the effects of alprazolam:
- amprenavir (Agenerase).
- itraconazole or ketoconazole (azole antifungals).
- birth control pills (oral contraceptives—various kinds).
- cimetidine (Tagamet).
- delavirdine (Rescriptor).
- disulfiram (Antabuse).
- fluconazole (Diflucan).
- fluoxetine (Prozac).
- fluvoxamine (Luvox).
- isoniazid (INH, Rifamate, etc.).
- macrolide antibiotics (such as erythromycin, clarithromycin or azithromycin—see Drug Classes).
- medicines that inhibit a liver enzyme (CYP3A4) will increase alprazolam levels (talk to your pharmacist).
- omeprazole (Prilosec).
- paroxetine (Paxil).

- propoxyphene (Darvon, etc.).
- ritonavir (Norvir) and perhaps other protease inhibitors (see Drug Classes).
- sertraline (Zoloft).
- valproic acid (Depakene).

The following drugs may **decrease** the effects of alprazolam:

- carbamazepine (Tegretol).
- rifampin (Rimactane, etc.).
- theophylline (aminophylline, Theo-Dur, etc.).

Alprazolam **taken concurrently** with

- alcohol (ethanol) will worsen coordination and mental abilities.
- benzodiazepines (see Drug Classes) can cause increased central nervous system (CNS) depression.
- buspirone (Buspar) can result in additive CNS depression.
- central nervous system active agents (see Antihistamine and Antipsychotic Drug Classes) can cause increased CNS depression.
- narcotics (morphine, etc.) cause additive CNS depression.
- nefazodone (Serzone) may double the blood level.
- tricyclic and other kinds of antidepressants (see Drug Classes) results in additional CNS depression.

▷ *Driving, Hazardous Activities:* This drug can impair mental alertness, judgment, physical coordination and reaction time. Avoid hazardous activities accordingly.

Aviation Note: The use of this drug **is a disqualification** for piloting. Consult a designated Aviation Medical Examiner.

Exposure to Sun: Use caution; rare photosensitivity reports (see Glossary).

Discontinuation: If this drug has been taken for an extended period of time, do not stop it abruptly. Slowly reduce dose by 1 mg per week until a total daily dose of 4 mg is reached; by 0.5 mg per week until a total daily dose of 2 mg is reached; and then by 0.25 mg per week thereafter. Ask your doctor for help.

AMANTADINE (a MAN ta deen)

Introduced: 1966　**Class:** Anti-parkinsonism, antiviral　**Prescription:** USA: Yes　**Controlled Drug:** USA: No; Canada: No　**Available as Generic:** USA: Yes; Canada: Yes

Brand Names: Antadine, Symadine, Symmetrel

BENEFITS versus RISKS	
Possible Benefits	*Possible Risks*
Partial relief of rigidity, tremor and impaired motion in all forms of parkinsonism	Skin rashes, mild to severe
	Confusion, hallucinations
	Congestive heart failure
Prevention and treatment of respiratory infections caused by influenza type A viruses*	Increased prostatism (see Glossary)
	Abnormally low white blood cell counts

*Does **NOT** prevent or treat viral infections other than those caused by influenza type A viruses.

▷ **Principal Uses**

As a Single Drug Product: Uses currently included in FDA-approved labeling: (1) Treats all forms of parkinsonism; (2) prevents or treats respiratory tract infections caused by influenza type A virus (rimantadine is the drug of first choice because of amantadine's more frequent CNS side effects); (3) eases drug-induced extrapyramidal symptoms.

Other (unlabeled) generally accepted uses: (1) Role in managing behavioral problems in brain injuries, autism, others; (2) some success reversing symptoms of mild dementia; (3) eases some resistant myoclonic or absence seizures; (4) may help bedwetting (enuresis) in children; (5) may ease fatigue in multiple sclerosis (MS) patients; (6) may give increased (short-term) responses as part of combination therapy of hepatitis C.

How This Drug Works: It increases a nerve transmitter (dopamine) in some nerve centers and reduces muscular rigidity, tremor and impaired movement associated with parkinsonism. May help some dyskinesias by blocking glutamate transmission in the globus pallidus. Helps wearing off or dyskinesia with advancing disease. By keeping the influenza from entering cells, it prevents the flu.

Available Dosage Forms and Strengths

Capsules (gelatin and softgel) — 100 mg

Syrup — 50 mg/5 ml

▷ **Usual Adult Dosage Ranges**

Anti-parkinsonism: 100 mg once or twice daily. Some patients may benefit from up to 400 mg daily. In general, many clinicians keep the total daily dose at 300 mg.

Antiviral: 200 mg once daily or 100 mg every 12 hours.

Children 1 to 9 years old: Treatment of type A flu: The CDC recommends 5 mg per kg per day up to 150 mg per day in order to prevent the flu, but decrease amantadine toxicity risk. The manufacturer gives a dosing range of: 4.4 to 8.8 mg per kg of body mass per day, up to a maximum of 150 mg once daily.

Children 10 and older: for those less than 40 kg, the CDC recommends 5 mg per kg per day (regardless of age). For those more than 40 kg, 100 mg twice daily is recommended.

Fatigue in multiple sclerosis: 100 mg two times a day for adults.

Note: Actual dose and schedule must be determined for each patient individually.

Conditions Requiring Dosing Adjustments

Liver Function: No dosing changes currently thought to be needed.

Kidney Function: Must be carefully adjusted to blood levels in people with kidney problems. Those with creatinine clearances of 30–50 ml/min should receive 100 mg daily. Those with 15–29 clearance should receive 100 mg every other day. Those with clearances less than 15 should receive 200 mg once a week.

Epilepsy: Doses of 200 mg/day should be avoided, as seizure risk may increase.

▷ **Dosing Instructions:** May be taken with or following meals. Can open the capsule to take it. If you forget a dose: Take the missed dose right away. If it is almost time to take the next dose, skip the missed dose and continue the medicine on your regular schedule. DO NOT double doses. If effectiveness is lost, the medicine can be gradually reduced (tapered) to zero and then restarted.

Usual Duration of Use: Use on a regular schedule for up to 2 weeks usually needed to see best effect in relieving Parkinson's symptoms. Long-term use (months to years) requires periodic check of response and dose changes. May allow for some levodopa decreases, but benefits may only last 6 months. See your doctor on a regular basis. Following exposure to influenza type A, protection requires continual daily doses for at least 10 days. During influenza epidemics, this drug may be given for 6 to 8 weeks.

Typical Treatment Goals and Measurements (Outcomes and Markers)

Parkinson's: The general goal is to ease movement problems and to allow for lowering of the levodopa dose. Benefits may be limited to about 6 months and therapy will then need to be adjusted.

Influenza (flu): Lessens the severity and length of time for the flu. PLEASE NOTE that a flu shot (or the new nasal spray "shot") is still the best way to deal with (PREVENT) the flu.

▷ **This Drug Should Not Be Taken If**
  • you have had an allergic reaction to it previously.

▷ **Inform Your Physician Before Taking This Drug If**
  • you have any type of seizure disorder.
  • you have a history of a serious emotional or mental disorder.
  • you have a history of heart disease, especially previous heart failure.
  • you have impaired liver or kidney function.
  • you have a history of lowering of blood pressure when you stand (orthostatic hypotension).
  • you have a history of peptic ulcer disease.
  • you have eczema or recurring eczemalike skin rashes.
  • you are taking any drugs for emotional or mental disorders.
  • you take other prescription or nonprescription medicines not discussed when amantadine was prescribed for you.
  • you have a history of low white blood cell counts.
  • you are unsure how much or how often to take this medicine.

Possible Side Effects (natural, expected and unavoidable drug actions)

Light-headedness, dizziness, weakness, feeling faint (see Orthostatic Hypotension in Glossary). Dry mouth, constipation. Reddish-blue pattern or patchy skin discoloration on your legs or feet (livedo reticularis—transient and unimportant).

▷ **Possible Adverse Effects** (unusual, unexpected and infrequent reactions)
  If any of the following develop, consult your physician promptly for guidance.

Mild Adverse Effects

Allergic reaction: skin rash.

Headache, nervousness, irritability, inability to concentrate, insomnia, nightmares—rare to infrequent.

Unsteadiness, visual disturbances, slurred speech—infrequent.

Swelling (fluid retention) (arms, feet or ankles)—case report.

Difficulty breathing—possible.

Urine retention—rare.

Loss of appetite, nausea, vomiting—infrequent.

Serious Adverse Effects
Allergic reaction: severe eczemalike skin rashes.
Idiosyncratic reactions: confusion, depression, hallucinations, aggression—case reports to rare.
Increased seizure activity in epileptics—possible.
Congestive heart failure—rare.
Aggravation of prostatism (see Glossary)—possible.
Elevated liver function tests—rare.
Low white blood cell counts: fever, sore throat, infection—rare.
Catatonia or seizures (if abruptly stopped).
Myasthenia gravis—case reports.

▷ **Possible Effects on Sexual Function:** None reported.

Adverse Effects That May Mimic Natural Diseases or Disorders
Mood changes, confusion or hallucinations may suggest a psychotic disorder.
Swelling of the legs and feet may suggest (but not necessarily indicate) heart, liver or kidney disorder.

Natural Diseases or Disorders That May Be Activated by This Drug
Latent epilepsy, incipient congestive heart failure.

Possible Effects on Laboratory Tests
Liver function tests: increased (AST/GOT, alkaline phosphatase).
Kidney function tests: brief increase—blood urea nitrogen (BUN).

CAUTION
1. NARROW margin of safety. Maximum dose is 400 mg in 24 hours. Watch for adverse effects with doses over 200 mg a day.
2. Initial anti-parkinsonism benefit may last 3 to 6 months. If this happens, ask your doctor if a new drug or dose is needed.
3. May increase susceptibility to German measles. Avoid exposure to anyone with active German measles.
4. Watch for early signs of congestive heart failure: shortness of breath on exertion or during the night, mild cough, swelling of feet or ankles. Report these promptly to your doctor.
5. May increase risk of seizures in people with epilepsy.
6. If you have been taking this medicine to help Parkinson's disease—do not stop it abruptly. Abruptly stopping this medicine may lead to Parkinsonian type crisis.

Precautions for Use
By Infants and Children: Safety and effectiveness for those under 18 not established.
By Those Over 60 Years of Age: Confusion, delirium, hallucinations and disorderly conduct may develop. Prostatism may be aggravated.

▷ **Advisability of Use During Pregnancy**
Pregnancy Category: C. See Pregnancy Risk Categories at the back of this book.
Animal studies: Birth defects reported in rat studies; no defects reported in rabbit studies.
Human studies: Adequate studies of pregnant women are not available. Single case of heart lesions. Ask your doctor for help.

Advisability of Use If Breast-Feeding

Presence of this drug in breast milk: Yes.

Nursing infant may develop skin rash, vomiting or urine retention. Avoid drug or refrain from nursing.

Habit-Forming Potential: This drug has a potential for abuse because of its ability to cause euphoria, hallucinations and feelings of detachment.

Effects of Overdose: Hyperactivity, disorientation, confusion, visual hallucinations, aggressive behavior, severe toxic psychosis, seizures, heart rhythm disturbances, drop in blood pressure.

Possible Effects of Long-Term Use: Livedo reticularis (see "Possible Side Effects" above). Congestive heart failure in predisposed people.

Suggested Periodic Examinations While Taking This Drug (at physician's discretion)

White blood cell counts.

Liver and kidney function tests.

Evaluation of heart function.

▷ **While Taking This Drug, Observe the Following**

Foods: No restrictions.

Herbal Medicines or Minerals: Calabar bean (chop nut, Fabia, ordeal nut, others) is unsafe when taken by mouth (physostigmine is the active ingredient) and should never be taken by people with Parkinson's disease. Echinacea purpurea should be avoided by those with multiple sclerosis.

Beverages: No restrictions. May be taken with milk.

▷ *Alcohol:* May impair mental function, lower blood pressure excessively.

Tobacco Smoking: No interactions expected. I advise everyone to quit smoking.

Marijuana Smoking: Added drowsiness.

▷ *Other Drugs*

Amantadine may increase the effects of

- atropinelike drugs used to treat parkinsonism, especially benztropine (Cogentin), orphenadrine (Disipal) and trihexyphenidyl (Artane). Amantadine can increase results, but if doses are too large, these drugs (taken with amantadine) may cause confusion, delirium, hallucinations and nightmares.
- levodopa (Dopar, Larodopa, Sinemet, etc.) and enhance results. Combination may cause acute mental disturbances.

The following drugs may increase the effects of amantadine:

- amphetamine and amphetaminelike stimulant drugs may cause excessive stimulation and adverse behavioral effects.
- hydrochlorothiazide with triamterene may increase the blood level of amantadine and cause toxicity.

Amantadine taken *concurrently* with

- cotrimoxazole may increase risk of CNS stimulation or arrhythmias.
- hydrochlorothiazide (Dyazide, Esidrix, others) may increase risk of amantadine toxicity.
- sulfamethoxazole may increase risk of CNS stimulation or arrhythmia.
- triamterene may increase risk of CNS toxicity.
- trimethoprim may increase risk of CNS toxicity.
- zotepine (Nipolept) may decrease amantadine benefits.

▷ *Driving, Hazardous Activities:* May cause drowsiness, dizziness, blurred vision or confusion. If these drug effects occur, avoid hazardous activities.

Aviation Note: The use of this drug *may be a disqualification* for piloting. Consult a designated Aviation Medical Examiner.

Exposure to Sun: No restrictions.

Exposure to Cold: Use caution. Excessive chilling may enhance the development of livedo reticularis (see "Possible Side Effects" above).

Discontinuation: When used to treat parkinsonism, this drug should not be stopped abruptly (slowly tapering is prudent). Sudden discontinuation may cause an acute Parkinsonian crisis. When treating influenza A infections, drug is continued for 48 hours after symptoms stop.

AMILORIDE (a MIL oh ride)

Introduced: 1967 **Class:** Diuretic **Prescription:** USA: Yes **Controlled Drug:** USA: No; Canada: No **Available as Generic:** Yes

Brand Names: ❦Apo-Amilzide, Midamor, ❦Moduret [CD], Moduretic [CD], ❦Novamilor [CD], ❦Nu-Amilzide [CD]

BENEFITS versus RISKS	
Possible Benefits	*Possible Risks*
EFFECTIVE DIURETIC WITH DECREASED POTASSIUM LOSS	ABNORMALLY HIGH BLOOD POTASSIUM WITH EXCESSIVE USE
	Rare heart arrhythmias
	Rare kidney toxicity
	Rare liver toxicity

▷ **Principal Uses**

As a Single Drug Product: Uses currently included in FDA-approved labeling: (1) Eliminates excessive fluid (edema) seen in congestive heart failure; (2) treats high blood pressure, especially those prone to low potassium; (3) thiazide-caused low blood potassium.

As a Combination Drug Product [CD]: Combined with other thiazide diuretics to prevent excess potassium loss.

Other (unlabeled) generally accepted uses: (1) May be able to help dissolve kidney stones in patients unable to tolerate surgery; (2) can help correct increased urination that occurs in patients taking lithium; (3) can help prevent lowered magnesium and potassium seen in patients who are given amphotericin B for serious fungal infections.

How This Drug Works: This drug promotes loss of sodium and water from the body and potassium retention by altering kidney enzymes that control urine formation.

Available Dosage Forms and Strengths

Tablets — 5 mg

▷ **Usual Adult Dosage Ranges:** One 5-mg dose a day, preferably in the morning. May increase up to 15 mg daily as needed and tolerated. Should not exceed 20 mg every 24 hours. **Note: Actual dose and schedule must be determined for each patient individually.**

Conditions Requiring Dosing Adjustments

Liver Function: Extreme caution in patients with severe liver disease.

Kidney Function: Should NOT be used in patients who can't make urine or who have acute kidney failure or creatinine clearance less than 50 ml/min.

▷ **Dosing Instructions:** Best taken when you wake up, with food. Tablet may be crushed for administration. If you forget a dose: Take the medicine right away, unless it is nearly time for your next dose, then omit the missed dose and take the medicine when it was next scheduled. DO NOT double doses. Once excess fluid is removed, use may be intermittent in some patients.

Usual Duration of Use: Ongoing long-term use to treat high blood pressure. Some clinicians use this medicine as needed (PRN) to remove abnormal fluid accumulation. Use every other day also minimizes imbalance of sodium and potassium.

Typical Treatment Goals and Measurements (Outcomes and Markers)

Blood Pressure: The most recent treatment guidelines (JNC VI) actually define optimal blood pressure (BP) as less than 120/80 and high normal as 139/89. The American Diabetes Association has chosen 130/80 as a new target. Most clinicians try to achieve a BP that achieves the best balance of lower cardiovascular risk while avoiding the problem of too low a blood pressure. The goals and time frame should be discussed with you when the prescription is written.

▷ **This Drug Should Not Be Taken If**
- you have had an allergic reaction to it before.
- your blood potassium level is greater than 5.5 mEq per liter and/or your serum creatinine is more than 1.5 mg/dl and your blood urea nitrogen (BUN) is more than 30 mg/dl (talk to your doctor about this).
- you have diabetic nerve damage (diabetic nephropathy).
- your kidneys are not making urine (anuria).

▷ **Inform Your Physician Before Taking This Drug If**
- you are allergic to any similar drug.
- you have diabetes or glaucoma.
- you have reason to believe that minerals such as potassium or chloride (electrolytes) are out of balance in your body.
- you have kidney disease or impaired kidney function.
- you take a different diuretic, blood pressure drug, digitalis or lithium.
- you don't know how much to take or how often to take it.

Possible Side Effects (natural, expected and unavoidable drug actions)

Abnormally high blood potassium level—infrequent.

Abnormally low blood sodium level, dehydration, decreased blood magnesium, constipation—possible.

Dizziness on standing (orthostatic hypotension)—possible.

▷ **Possible Adverse Effects** (unusual, unexpected and infrequent reactions)

If any of the following develop, consult your physician promptly for guidance.

Mild Adverse Effects

Allergic reactions: skin rash, itching—rare-infrequent.

Headache—infrequent.

Dizziness, weakness, fatigue, numbness and tingling—case reports (related to electrolyte problems).

Dry mouth, nausea, vomiting, stomach pains, diarrhea—infrequent.
Decreased ability to taste salt—possible.
Loss of scalp hair—rare.

Serious Adverse Effects
Idiosyncratic reactions: joint and muscle pains.
Liver or kidney toxicity—rare.
Abnormally low sodium or high potassium—possible.
Increased internal eye pressure (of concern in glaucoma)—rare.
Depression, visual disturbances, ringing in ears, tremors—infrequent.
Bone marrow depression—rare (questionable cause).
Palpitations and arrhythmias—rare.
Decreased circulation to the legs (with combination furosemide use)—case
reports.

▷ **Possible Effects on Sexual Function:** Does not appear to be a present side
effect.

Adverse Effects That May Mimic Natural Diseases or Disorders
Nervousness, confusion or depression may mimic spontaneous mental disorder.

Natural Diseases or Disorders That May Be Activated by This Drug
Preexisting peptic ulcer, latent glaucoma.

Possible Effects on Laboratory Tests
Blood cholesterol level: decreased.
Blood creatinine level: increased with long-term use.
Blood potassium level: possibly increased.
Blood uric acid level: decreased with long-term use.
Blood sodium level: possibly decreased.

CAUTION
1. Do **NOT** take potassium supplements or eat more high-potassium foods.
2. More frequent potassium levels are needed if you take digitalis compounds.
3. Do not stop this drug abruptly unless your doctor says you must.

Precautions for Use
By Infants and Children: Oral dosing with 0.625 mg per kg of body mass daily
has been used to promote water loss (diuresis) in young patients weighing
from 6 to 20 kg.
By Those Over 60 Years of Age: Declines in kidney function may make it likely
that you will retain potassium. Limit use of this drug to periods of 2 to 3
weeks if possible. The dose MUST be reduced. May cause too much water
loss, possible increased tendency of the blood to clot and increased risk of
clots (thrombosis, heart attack, stroke).

▷ **Advisability of Use During Pregnancy**
Pregnancy Category: B. See Pregnancy Risk Categories at the back of this book.
Animal studies: No birth defects reported.
Human studies: Adequate studies of pregnant women are not available.
Use only if clearly needed.

Advisability of Use If Breast-Feeding
Presence of this drug in breast milk: Unknown, but probably present.
This drug may suppress milk production. Avoid drug if possible. If use is nec-

essary, watch nursing infant closely and stop drug or nursing if adverse effects develop.

Habit-Forming Potential: None.

Effects of Overdose: Thirst, drowsiness, fatigue, weakness, nausea, vomiting, confusion, numbness and tingling of face and extremities, irregular heart rhythm, shortness of breath.

Suggested Periodic Examinations While Taking This Drug (at physician's discretion)

Complete blood counts.
Blood levels of sodium, potassium, magnesium and chloride.
Kidney function tests.
Easing of edema.

▷ **While Taking This Drug, Observe the Following**

Foods: Avoid excessive salt restriction and high-potassium foods. Taking this drug with food may help nausea and stomach upset.

Herbal Medicines or Minerals: Ginseng may increase blood pressure, blunting the benefits of this medicine. Arginine (a medicine used to treat metabolic alkalosis but also found as supplements has led to severe increases in potassium in some patients who had previously (and recently) been given spironolactone. Eleuthero root, hawthorn, saw palmetto, ma huang, goldenseal and licorice may cause increased blood pressure—blunting the beneficial effects of this medicine. Couch grass may worsen edema due to heart or kidney problems. Indian snakeroot, calcium and garlic may help lower blood pressure. Talk to your doctor and pharmacist BEFORE adding any herbal medicines.

Beverages: No restrictions. May be taken with milk.

▷ *Alcohol:* Use caution. Alcohol can exaggerate the blood-pressure-lowering effect of this drug and cause orthostatic hypotension (see Glossary).

Tobacco Smoking: No interactions expected. I advise everyone to quit smoking.

▷ *Other Drugs*

Amiloride may ***increase*** the effects of
• other blood-pressure-lowering drugs. Dose decreases may be needed.

Amiloride may ***decrease*** the effects of
• digoxin (Lanoxin, etc.) and reduce its effect in treating heart failure.

Amiloride ***taken concurrently*** with
• ACE inhibitors (see Drug Classes) such as benazepril or angiotensin II antagonists (valsartan [Diovan], etc.) may result in abnormally high blood potassium.
• arginine (various) may cause extreme and life-threatening potassium increases.
• chlorpropamide (Diabinese) may lead to excessively low blood sodium.
• cyclosporine (Sandimmune, others) may cause excessively high potassium levels.
• digoxin (Lanoxin) may decrease benefits (positive inotropic effect) of digoxin.
• dofetilide (Tikosyn) may cause serious irregular heartbeats. Combine only with great caution and careful patient monitoring.
• lithium (Lithobid) may cause lithium toxicity.

- metformin (Glucophage) may increase Glucophage levels and increase lactic acidosis or excessively lowered blood sugar (hypoglycemia) risk.
- NSAIDs (see Drug Classes) may decrease therapeutic effect.
- potassium supplements may result in extremely elevated blood potassium levels.
- quinidine (Quinaglute, others) may prolong the QRS interval and increase risk of abnormal heartbeats.
- spironolactone (Aldactone, Aldactazide) or triamterene (Dyrenium, Dyazide) may cause dangerous potassium levels. Avoid combining.
- tacrolimus (Prograf) may cause excessive potassium levels. Increased potassium checks are prudent.
- triamterene (Dyazide) may cause excessively high potassium levels and should not be combined.

▷ *Driving, Hazardous Activities:* May cause drowsiness, dizziness and orthostatic hypotension. If these drug effects occur, avoid hazardous activities.

Aviation Note: The use of this drug *may be a disqualification* for piloting. Consult a designated Aviation Medical Examiner.

Exposure to Sun: No restrictions.

Exposure to Heat: Caution is advised. Excessive sweating can cause water, sodium and potassium imbalance. Hot environments can cause lowering of blood pressure.

Occurrence of Unrelated Illness: Call your doctor if you contract an illness causing vomiting or diarrhea.

Discontinuation: With high doses or prolonged use, withdraw this drug gradually. Excessive potassium loss may occur with sudden withdrawal.

AMINOPHYLLINE (am in OFF i lin)

Other Name: Theophylline ethylenediamine

Introduced: 1910   **Class:** Antiasthmatic, bronchodilator, xanthines   **Prescription:** USA: Yes   **Controlled Drug:** USA: No; Canada: No   **Available as Generic:** Yes

Brand Names: Aminophyllin, Mudrane [CD], Mudrane GG [CD], ♣Palaron, Phyllocontin, Somophyllin, ♣Somophyllin-12, Truphylline

Author's Note: This drug is actually (79%) theophylline. See the theophylline profile for further details.

AMIODARONE (AM EE oh dur ohn)

Introduced: 1986   **Class:** Antiarrhythmic, Class III agent   **Prescription:** USA: Yes   **Controlled Drug:** USA: No; Canada: No   **Available as Generic:** Yes

Brand Names: Cordarone, ♣Alti-Amiodarone, Braxan, ♣Gen-Amiodarone, ♣Med-Amiodarone, ♣ Novo-Amiodarone, Pacerone

BENEFITS versus RISKS

Possible Benefits	*Possible Risks*
EFFECTIVE TREATMENT OF SELECTED LIFE-THREATENING HEART RHYTHM DISORDERS	SIGNIFICANT LIVER ENZYME (CYP3A) DRUG INTERACTIONS
TREATMENT OF ATRIAL FIBRILLATION (LOW MEDICINE DOSE)	LUNG (PULMONARY) TOXICITY
	SLOWED HEART RATE (BRADYCARDIA)
PREVENTION OF ATRIAL FIBRILLATION RECURRENCE (LOW DOSE)	Some isolated cases of arrhythmia worsening
	Tingling in the extremities (peripheral neuropathy)
BENEFICIAL EFFECTS ON HEART FAILURE	Liver toxicity
INTRAVENOUS USE OF GREAT BENEFIT (NEWER DATA) IN CARDIAC ARREST AND IN ADVANCED CARDIAC LIFE SUPPORT (ACLS) WHEN CARDIAC ARREST HAS RESULTED FROM (SECONDARY TO) VENTRICULAR ARRHYTHMIA	Changes in thyroid gland function (hypo or hyper)
	Heart conduction or rhythm abnormalities
	Microdeposits in the eye (cornea)
	Very long half-life
EFFECTIVE IN TREATING VENTRICULAR ARRHYTHMIAS AND FAST HEART RATE (TACHYCARDIA) THAT HAS FAILED TO RESPOND TO (REFRACTORY) TO OTHER AGENTS	
Very long half-life	

▷ **Principal Uses**

As a Single Drug Product: Uses currently included in FDA-approved labeling: (1) Treats abnormal rhythms in the heart ventricles (life-threatening ventricular arrhythmias such as recurrent hemodynamically unstable ventricular tachycardia).

Other (unlabeled) generally accepted uses: (1) Chest pain (angina pectoris); (2) suppression of abnormal heart rhythms in severe congestive heart failure (CHF) and may ease CHF itself; (3) effective in treating ventricular arrhythmias seen in heart inflammation patients (myocarditis) caused by Chagas' disease; (4) supraventricular arrhythmias (such as atrial fibrillation); (5) treats drug-induced (sotalol) torsade de pointes; (6) survivors of sudden heart attack (acute myocardial infarction) who have frequent or repetitive premature ventricular depolarizations (VPDs) may benefit from amiodarone therapy; (7) prevented repeat (recurrent) atrial fibrillation better than propafenone or sotalol in the Canadian CTAF study.

How This Drug Works: Originally classified as a class three antiarrhythmic. Appears to work on the complete spectrum (blocks the sodium channel, slows heart rate and impedes the AV node by blocking beta-adrenergic receptors as well as calcium channels) of classes. It also lengthens ventricular and atrial repolarization time by inhibiting the potassium channel. These effects help restore normal heart rate and rhythm. Amiodarone also decreases cytokines (such as tumor necrosis factor or TNF and interleukin 6 or IL-6), which may explain its benefits in heart failure.

Available Dosage Forms and Strengths
> Injection — 50 mg/ml
> Tablet — 200 mg

▷ **Usual Adult Dosage Ranges:** *Supraventricular arrhythmias:* Oral dosing has been started at 600–1,200 mg daily for one to two weeks, and then lowered (tapered) to 400–600 mg daily for one to three weeks and then lowered further to the lowest possible ongoing (maintenance) dose. The typical blood (scrum) level in patients who have been successfully treated was 1.9 micrograms per milliliter and the median dose was 200 mg a day in one study. Some elderly patients have gained control of their atrial fibrillation using 100 mg a day.

Ventricular arrhythmias: Oral doses are 800–1,600 mg per day as a loading dose for one to three weeks or longer (based on how well the heart rhythm problem responds), and then doses are gradually lowered to no more than 400 mg a day. Some European clinicians use generally lower ongoing doses.

Note: Actual dose and schedule must be determined for each patient individually.

Conditions Requiring Dosing Adjustments

Liver Function: Dosing hasn't been studied in liver failure, but since there is extensive liver metabolism, decreased doses and use of blood levels to guide dosing appear prudent in liver compromise. The medicine is also removed in the bile. Talk to your doctor if you have a block or periodic block in your bile duct (such as a gallstone) and this medicine is being considered.

Kidney Function: Dosing changes do NOT appear to be needed.

▷ **Dosing Instructions:** Tablets should be swallowed whole and may be taken with or following food to reduce stomach irritation. If you forget to take a dose: omit that dose and continue with the next scheduled dose. If you forget to take it for two or more days—call your doctor.

Usual Duration of Use: Regular use for 10 days may be required (with oral dosing) to begin to help ventricular tachycardia, but may take three to six weeks. Several months may be required to see the peak benefits. Long-term use requires supervision and ongoing evaluation by your doctor.

Typical Treatment Goals and Measurements (Outcomes and Markers)

Abnormal heartbeats: The general goal is to return the heart to a normal rhythm or at least to markedly reduce the occurrence of abnormal heartbeats. In life-threatening arrhythmias, the goal is to abort the abnormal beats and return the pattern to normal. Success at ongoing suppression may involve ambulatory checks of heart rate and rhythm for a day (such as in Holter monitoring). This kind of testing involves placement of adhesive-backed temporary electrodes on the skin in several positions around the heart. A small heart rate and rhythm (EKG or ECG) recording device is carried around via a shoulder strap and records what the heart is doing over 24 hours. Once the recording is made, a scanning machine reviews the record, tallies abnormal heartbeats or rhythms and gives a close and extended look at how the heart is reacting or benefiting from the medicines that the patient is taking. Repeat measurements can be made if doses are changed to check the success at keeping the heart in normal sinus rhythm!

Possible Advantages of This Drug: Other antiarrhythmics such as quinidine and procainamide can be associated with development of antinuclear antibodies (ANA). One study showed that amiodarone does NOT induce ANA. Because of its broad mechanism of action, may be effective where other antiarrhythmics fail. Has additional direct beneficial effects on heart failure that other heart rhythm modifiers do not have.

▷ **This Drug Should Not Be Taken If**
- you had an allergic reaction to amiodarone or similar drugs.
- you have second-degree, third-degree AV block (and do not have a pacemaker).
- you have "sick sinus" syndrome or severe heart slowing (sinus bradycardia—talk with your doctor).
- you are in heart (cardiogenic) shock.

▷ **Inform Your Physician Before Taking This Drug If**
- you have had unfavorable reactions to antiarrhythmic drugs.
- you have heart disease, especially "heart block."
- you have a history of heart attack, heart muscle changes (cardiomegaly), slow heartbeat or low blood pressure (especially with intravenous dosing).
- you have had a heart attack.
- you have impaired liver function.
- you have low blood platelets.
- your vision is impaired (this drug may cause microdeposits on the cornea).
- your blood electrolytes (such as potassium or magnesium) are not in balance.
- you have lung disease (pulmonary dysfunction).
- you live or will travel to a place where your heart rhythm cannot be checked (this medicine can help abnormal heartbeats, but may also worsen them and this must be checked when treatment is started).
- the left ventricle of your heart does not work correctly (left ventricular dysfunction).
- you have thyroid problems (hypo or hyper thyroidism).
- your job requires you to work outside in the sun or you already take other medicines that can increase sun sensitivity.

Possible Side Effects (natural, expected and unavoidable drug actions)
Inflammation of the vein (with intravenous use)—possible.
Microdeposits in the cornea—frequent with long-term (more than six months) use.

▷ **Possible Adverse Effects** (unusual, unexpected and infrequent reactions)
If any of the following develop, consult your physician promptly for guidance.
Mild Adverse Effects
Allergic reactions: skin rash, itching—case reports.
Blue-gray skin discoloration—rare to frequent (also sun sensitivity—see below).

Headache, tiredness or sleep disturbances—rare-infrequent.

Movement problems (incoordination-ataxia), fatigue, dizziness—infrequent.

Lowered blood pressure (more common with the intravenous form)—up to frequent.

Swelling of the epididymis (epididymitis)—infrequent.

Increased serum creatinine—possible.

Cholesterol changes (increased in one study and lowered in another)—possible.

Increased liver function tests—infrequent to frequent (should be clinically monitored and dose lowered or medicine stopped if persistent).

Loss of appetite, indigestion, nausea, vomiting—infrequent to frequent (usually responds to dosing adjustment or dividing).

Increased creatinine—case reports (usually happens during first six months of treatment).

Serious Adverse Effects

Allergic reaction—toxic epidermal necrolysis (TEN)—case report.

Neuropathy—frequent.

Abnormal thyroid function (hypo or hyper)—rare to frequent (may happen within one to 73 months).

Abnormal heart rhythm (such as excessive heart slowing)—infrequent.

Torsade de pointes—rare.

Lung toxicity (pulmonary)—rare to frequent (includes fatal cases).

High blood sugar (glucose)—rare (not seen in a small later study).

Jaundice (see Glossary) or liver toxicity—infrequent.

Optic neuritis—rare.

Abnormally low blood platelets—rare.

▷ **Possible Effects on Sexual Function:** Impotence or loss of libido—case reports. Swelling and tenderness of male breast tissue (gynecomastia)—case report.

Adverse Effects That May Mimic Natural Diseases or Disorders

Reversible jaundice may suggest viral hepatitis. Abnormal heart rhythms may mimic slow (brady) arrhythmias from other causes.

Natural Diseases or Disorders That May Be Activated by This Drug

Abnormal heart rhythms, abnormal thyroid function, epididymal swelling may mimic infectious epididymitis.

Possible Effects on Laboratory Tests

Blood platelets: rarely decreased.

Liver function tests: increased liver enzymes (ALT/GPT, AST/GOT, and alkaline phosphatase), increased bilirubin.

Blood urea nitrogen (BUN)—increased.

Increased or decreased thyroid function.

CAUTION

1. Thorough heart exam (including electrocardiogram) is critical prior to using this drug.
2. Periodic heart exams are needed to follow drug responses. Some people may have heart rhythm or function declines. Close monitoring of heart rate, rhythm and overall performance is essential.
3. Dose must be individualized. Do not change your dose without your doctor's supervision.

4. Talk with your doctor about signs and symptoms of thyroid function changes. This medicine contains iodine; consequently protein-bound iodine (PBI) testing will NOT detect thyroid problems.
5. Do not take any other antiarrhythmic drug while taking this drug unless directed to do so by your doctor.

Precautions for Use

By Infants and Children: In pediatric patients, amiodarone is given on a mg-per-kg-of-body-mass basis. Dose is then divided into equal doses, given at times determined by patient response. Some patients from one to four years old will receive 10 to 20 mg per kg of body mass per day, divided into equal doses and given every six hours. Initial use of this drug requires hospitalization and supervision by a qualified pediatrician.

By Those Over 60 Years of Age: Watch closely for light-headedness, dizziness, unsteadiness and tendency to fall. Older patients may be more susceptible to problems from heart slowing and should be closely followed once this medicine is started.

▷ Advisability of Use During Pregnancy

Pregnancy Category: D. See Pregnancy Risk Categories at the back of this book.
Animal studies: Can cause thyroid changes, maternal and embryo death in rabbits given 10 mg per kg or greater.
Human studies: Adequate studies of pregnant women are not available. This medicine should be used only if the potential benefit outweighs fetal risk.

Advisability of Use If Breast-Feeding

Presence of this drug in breast milk: Yes.
Refrain from nursing.

Habit-Forming Potential: None.

Effects of Overdose: Extremely slow heart rate (bradycardia), excessively low blood pressure, heart block (AV) and possibly cardiogenic shock as well as liver toxicity.

Possible Effects of Long-Term Use: Microdeposits in the cornea of the eye.

Suggested Periodic Examinations While Taking This Drug (at physician's discretion)

Liver function tests BEFORE starting treatment and every six months thereafter.
Electrocardiograms.
Complete blood counts.
Blood levels.

▷ While Taking This Drug, Observe the Following

Foods: No restrictions. Food may actually help avoid upset stomach.
Herbal Medicines or Minerals: Using St. John's wort, ma huang, ephedra or kola while taking this medicine may result in unacceptable heart stimulation. Belladonna, henbane, *Scopolia*, pheasant's eye extract or lily-of-the-valley or squill powdered extracts should NOT be taken if you have abnormal heart rhythms. Since St. John's wort and amiodarone may increase sun sensitivity, the combination is NOT advised. Pyridoxine may increase risk of phototoxicity.
Beverages: Your doctor may ask you to restrict caffeine intake. May be taken with milk.

▷   *Alcohol:* Use caution. Alcohol can increase the blood-pressure-lowering effects and may have an undesirable effect on heart rhythm in high doses.

Tobacco Smoking: Nicotine can irritate the heart, reducing effectiveness. I advise everyone to quit smoking.

▷   *Other Drugs*

Amiodarone may ***increase*** the effects of

- antihypertensive drugs and cause excessive lowering of blood pressure.
- atropinelike drugs (see Drug Classes).
- cyclosporine (Sandimmune, others) and lead to cyclosporine toxicity if cyclosporine doses are not lowered.
- digoxin (Lanoxin) by increasing blood level.
- procainamide (Procan SR, others) and NAPA.
- warfarin (Coumadin, etc.); check INR (prothrombin times) more often, and adjust dosing.

Amiodarone ***taken concurrently*** with

- amprenavir (Agenerase), indinavir (Crixivan), ritonavir (Norvir) and perhaps other protease inhibitors (see Drug Classes) may increase amiodarone blood levels and lead to toxicity.
- beta blockers (see Drug Classes) may result in abnormally low heart rates or sinus arrest. Extreme caution is advised.
- calcium channel blockers (see Drug Classes) should be avoided in patients with partial block (AV) or sick sinus syndrome.
- cimetidine (Tagamet) can increase amiodarone levels.
- cisapride (Propulsid) may lead to serious heart rhythm problems. DO NOT COMBINE.
- clonazepam (Klonopin) caused clonazepam toxicity in one case report. Caution is advised.
- digoxin (Lanoxin) can cause digoxin toxicity.
- disopyramide (Norpace) can prolong QT interval and lead to abnormal heart rhythms.
- dofetilide (Tikosyn) can lead to heart toxicity.
- dolasetron (Anzemet) can lead to heart toxicity.
- fentanyl (Actiq, Duragesic) may lead to low blood pressure, slow heart rate and lowered ability of the heart to work (cardiac output).
- flecainide (Tambocor) may allow lower flecainide dose to get the same effect.
- gatifloxacin (Tequin) may result in abnormal QT intervals and lead to abnormal heart rhythms. DO NOT COMBINE.
- halofantrine (Halfan) can lead to heart toxicity.
- insulin or oral antidiabetic drugs (see Drug Classes) may result in blunted blood sugar benefits.
- lidocaine (various) may lead to lidocaine toxicity. Extreme caution is advised.
- methotrexate (Rheumatrex, others) increases risk of methotrexate toxicity. Extreme caution is advised.
- mexiletine (Mexitil) may result in abnormal heart beats. Caution is advised.
- moxifloxacin (Avelox) may result in abnormal heart beats. DO NOT COMBINE.
- nelfinavir (Viracept) may result in amiodarone toxicity. DO NOT COMBINE.
- phenytoin (Dilantin) or fosphenytoin (Cerebyx) can result in phenytoin, phosphenytoin and amiodarone toxicity.

- propafenone (Rythmol) may lead to propafenone toxicity. Reduced propafenone doses may be needed.
- quinidine can cause increases in quinidine levels.
- ritonavir (Norvir) may increase amiodarone levels and could result in abnormal heart beats. DO NOT COMBINE.
- sotalol (Betapace) may result in increased risk of abnormal heart rhythms because of prolongation of the QT interval. This combination is NOT recommended.
- sparfloxacin (Zagam) may result in increased risk of abnormal heart rhythms. DO NOT COMBINE.
- verapamil (Calan, others) can precipitate or worsen congestive heart failure.

The following drugs may *decrease* the effects of amiodarone:

- cholestyramine (Questran, others) by increasing removal (enterohepatic elimination) of amiodarone.
- rifabutin (Mycobutin).
- rifampin (Rimactane, Rifadin).

▷ *Driving, Hazardous Activities:* May cause dizziness or blurred vision. Limit activities as needed.

Aviation Note: The use of this drug may be a disqualification for piloting. Consult a designated Aviation Medical Examiner.

Exposure to Sun: Use caution. This drug causes photosensitization (see Glossary).

Exposure to Heat: Use caution. The use of this drug in hot environments may increase the risk of heatstroke.

Occurrence of Unrelated Illness: Vomiting, diarrhea or dehydration can affect this drug's action adversely. Report such developments promptly.

Discontinuation: This drug should not be stopped abruptly after long-term use. Ask your doctor for help regarding gradual dose reduction.

AMITRIPTYLINE (a mee TRIP ti leen)

Introduced: 1961   **Class:** Antidepressant   **Prescription:** USA: Yes
Controlled Drug: USA: No; Canada: No   **Available as Generic:** Yes
Brand Names: Amitid, Amitril, ♣Apo-Amitriptyline, ♣Elatrol, Elavil, ♣Elavil Plus [CD], Emitrip, Endep, Enovil, Etrafon [CD], ♣Etrafon-A [CD], ♣Etrafon-D [CD], Etrafon-Forte [CD], ♣Levate, ♣Novo-Triptyn, PMS-Levazine [CD], SK-Amitriptyline, ♣Triavil [CD]

BENEFITS versus RISKS	
Possible Benefits	*Possible Risks*
EFFECTIVE RELIEF OF ENDOGENOUS DEPRESSION	ADVERSE BEHAVIORAL EFFECTS: Confusion, disorientation, hallucinations
Additive (adjunctive) therapy in some pain syndromes (such as peripheral neuropathic pain or pain after herpes infections—post-herpetic neuralgia)	CONVERSION OF DEPRESSION TO MANIA in manic-depressive disorders
	Irregular heart rhythms—possible
	Blood cell abnormalities—rare

▷ **Principal Uses**

As a Single Drug Product: Uses currently included in FDA-approved labeling: (1) Eases symptoms of spontaneous (endogenous) depression; (2) helps depression resistant (refractory) to a single medicine.

Other (unlabeled) generally accepted uses: (1) Additive (adjuvant) therapy in chronic pain/pain syndromes (such as peripheral neuropathic pain); (2) eases agitation; (3) helps diabetic nerve (neuropathy) pain; (4) is an alternative in intractable hiccups; (5) combined with other medicines to ease the pain of postherpetic neuralgia; (6) some benefit easing pain of chronic vulvar burning (vulvodynia); (7) used in fish (ciguatera) poisoning.

As a Combination Drug Product [CD]: Combined with chlordiazepoxide to relieve anxiety and depression. Also available in combination with perphenazine, a phenothiazine, to relieve severe agitation that may occur with depression.

How This Drug Works: Eases depression by restoring normal levels of two nerve impulse chemicals (norepinephrine and serotonin).

Available Dosage Forms and Strengths

Injection — 10 mg/ml

Oral suspension — 10 mg/5 ml

Tablets — 10 mg, 25 mg, 50 mg, 75 mg, 100 mg, 150 mg

▷ **Usual Adult Dosage Ranges:** Intramuscular injection is given as 80 to 120 mg per day divided into four doses. Switch to oral form made as soon as possible. Oral dosing starts with 25 mg two to four times daily. May be increased cautiously as needed/tolerated by 10 to 25 mg daily at intervals of 1 week with dose increases usually made later in the day or at bedtime. Usual ongoing dose is 50 to 100 mg daily. Total dose should not exceed 150 mg daily. Once the best dose is found, it may be taken at bedtime as one dose. Some clinicians start with 50 mg at bedtime. **Note: Actual dose and schedule must be determined for each patient individually.**

Conditions Requiring Dosing Adjustments

Liver Function: Specific guidelines not available; however, low doses and a check of blood levels are prudent.

Kidney Function: Lower doses and blood level checks are needed with kidney failure (18% of drug is removed this way).

▷ **Dosing Instructions:** May be taken without regard to meals. Immediate-release form tablets may be crushed to take it. DO NOT CRUSH SUSTAINED-RELEASE form (available in Great Britain). If you forget a dose: Take the medicine right away, unless it is nearly time for your next dose. If you only take one dose at bedtime, don't take the missed dose in the morning, skip the missed dose and take the next dose right on schedule. DO NOT double doses.

Usual Duration of Use: Some benefit in 1 to 2 weeks, but peak benefit may take 30 days or longer. Long-term use should not exceed 6 months without follow-up evaluation. In a set of guidelines issued by the American College of Physicians, older and newer antidepressants were found to give equal results in treating depression. Older medicines were found to generally have more frequent constipation, dizziness, dry mouth, blurred vision and tremors while newer medicines caused more diarrhea, headache and nausea. The importance here is that many options are available and possible side effects can be somewhat tailored to try to avoid overlap.

Typical Treatment Goals and Measurements (Outcomes and Markers)

Depression: The general goal: to lessen the degree and severity of depression, letting patients return to their daily lives. Specific measures of depression involve testing or inventories (such as the Hamilton Depression Inventory) and can be valuable in helping check benefits from this medicine.

Pain syndromes: The general goal: to decrease pain to a manageable level. Pain should be appropriately checked (assessed), and progress defined based on lowering of overall pain level and improved quality of life.

▷ **This Drug Should Not Be Taken If**
- you are allergic to any of the brand names listed above.
- you are taking, or have taken within the past 14 days, any monoamine oxidase (MAO) type A inhibitor drug (see Drug Classes).
- you are recovering from a recent heart attack.
- you are pregnant.

▷ **Inform Your Physician Before Taking This Drug If**
- you have a history of diabetes, epilepsy (or other seizure disorder), glaucoma, heart disease, prostate gland enlargement or overactive thyroid function.
- you will have surgery with general anesthesia.
- you have heart-induced chest pain (angina pectoris).
- you have a rapid heart rate that occurs spontaneously (paroxysmal tachycardia).
- you have narrow-angle glaucoma.
- you are unsure how much or how often to take this drug.
- you have a history of schizophrenia—this drug may worsen any paranoia.
- you have a history of prostate or sexual problems.
- you have a liver or kidney disorder.
- you have a blood cell disorder.
- you have a history of intestinal block (ileus).

Possible Side Effects (natural, expected and unavoidable drug actions)

Drowsiness, blurred vision, dry mouth, constipation, impaired urination

▷ **Possible Adverse Effects** (unusual, unexpected and infrequent reactions)

If any of the following develop, consult your physician promptly for guidance.

Mild Adverse Effects

Allergic reactions: skin rash, hives, swelling of face or tongue, drug fever (see Glossary).

Headache, dizziness, weakness, fainting, unsteady gait, tremors—infrequent.

Peculiar taste, irritation of tongue or mouth, nausea, indigestion—rare to infrequent.

Fluctuation of blood sugar levels—possible.

Increased dental cavities (caries)—increased risk.

Restlessness, nightmares—rare.

Change in the ability to perceive tones—case report.

Serious Adverse Effects

Allergic reactions: hepatitis (see Glossary).

Idiosyncratic reactions: neuroleptic malignant syndrome (see Glossary).

Confusion or hallucinations—may be more likely in older patients and with higher doses.

Bowel obstruction (ileus)—rare.

SIADH (see Glossary)—rare.

Excessively low blood pressure (hypotension)—possible.

Seizures—rare.

Severe eye or other movement problems—case reports.

Heart palpitation and irregular rhythm—rare and more likely with increasing doses or overdose.

Bone marrow depression (see Glossary): fatigue, weakness, fever, sore throat, abnormal bleeding or bruising—rare.

A lupus erythematosus–like syndrome has been reported—questionable causality.

Peripheral neuritis (see Glossary): numbness, tingling, pain, loss of arm or leg strength—possible.

Parkinson-like disorders (see Glossary): often mild and infrequent—more likely in the elderly.

Liver toxicity—rare.

Serotonin syndrome—possible.

Worsening of paranoid psychosis in schizophrenic patients—possible.

▷ **Possible Effects on Sexual Function:** Decreased libido—rare.

Increased libido (possible antidepressant effect), inhibited female orgasm, inhibited ejaculation—case reports.

Male and female breast enlargement, milk production, swelling of testicles, impotence—case reports.

These effects usually disappear within 2 to 10 days after discontinuation of the drug.

Adverse Effects That May Mimic Natural Diseases or Disorders

Liver toxicity may suggest viral hepatitis.

Natural Diseases or Disorders That May Be Activated by This Drug

Latent diabetes, epilepsy, glaucoma, impaired urination due to prostate.

Possible Effects on Laboratory Tests

Complete blood counts: decreased white cells and platelets; increased eosinophils.

Liver function tests: increased ALT/GPT, AST/GOT, alkaline phosphatase, increased bilirubin.

Blood glucose levels: increased or decreased (fluctuations).

CAUTION

1. Make sure you make follow-up visits to your doctor.
2. Best to withhold this drug if electroconvulsive therapy (ECT, "shock" treatment) is to be used.

Precautions for Use

By Infants and Children: Safety and effectiveness for those under 12 years old not established.

By Those Over 60 Years of Age: During the first 2 weeks watch for confusion, agitation, forgetfulness, delusions, and hallucinations. Decreased dose or stopping the drug may be needed. Unsteadiness may predispose to falling and injury. May worsen impaired urination seen with prostate gland enlargement (prostatism).

▷ **Advisability of Use During Pregnancy**

Pregnancy Category: C. See Pregnancy Risk Categories at the back of this book.

Animal studies: Skull deformities reported in rabbits.

Human studies: There have been reports of developmental delays, limb deformities, and central nervous system (CNS) problems in infants whose mothers had taken amitriptyline during pregnancy. Adequate studies of pregnant women are not available.

Use during pregnancy is a benefit-to-risk decision.

Advisability of Use If Breast-Feeding

Presence of this drug in breast milk: Yes.

One source says this medicine is NOT compatible with breast-feeding. Do not breast-feed or discontinue the medicine (talk to your doctor first).

Habit-Forming Potential: If prolonged therapy has been given, stopping this medicine suddenly can lead to headache, nausea, and weakness (malaise). Rare reports of hypomania or mania have been made 2 to 7 days after stopping therapy with tricyclic antidepressants.

Effects of Overdose: Confusion, hallucinations, marked drowsiness, heart palpitations, dilated pupils, tremors, stupor, deep sleep, coma, convulsions.

Suggested Periodic Examinations While Taking This Drug (at physician's discretion)

Complete blood cell counts.

Liver function tests.

Serial blood pressure readings and electrocardiograms.

▷ **While Taking This Drug, Observe the Following**

Foods: Excessive vitamin C can blunt therapeutic benefit of this drug. May also increase appetite and cause excessive weight gain.

Herbal Medicines or Minerals: Since amitriptyline and St. John's wort may act to increase serotonin, the combination is not advised. St. John's wort also increases sun sensitivity. Since part of the way ginseng works may be as a MAO inhibitor, do not combine with amitriptyline. Indian snakeroot, kava kava and yohimbe are also best avoided while taking this medicine.

Beverages: No restrictions. May be taken with milk.

▷ *Alcohol:* Even modest amounts of alcohol can lead to blackouts. Discuss any alcohol use with your doctor as this combination can markedly increase the intoxicating effects of alcohol and brain function depression.

Tobacco Smoking: May hasten the removal of this drug from your body. I advise you to quit smoking.

▷ *Other Drugs*

Amitriptyline may *increase* the effects of

- albuterol or other direct sympathomimetic drugs (amphetamines, epinephrine).
- antihistamines (such as diphenhydramine—Benadryl, others), which can increase the risk of urinary retention, chronic glaucoma and bowel obstruction (ileus). This is especially problematic in the elderly.
- atropinelike drugs (see Drug Classes).
- cimetidine (Tagamet).
- disulfiram (Antabuse), which can worsen the disulfiram effect if alcohol is consumed.

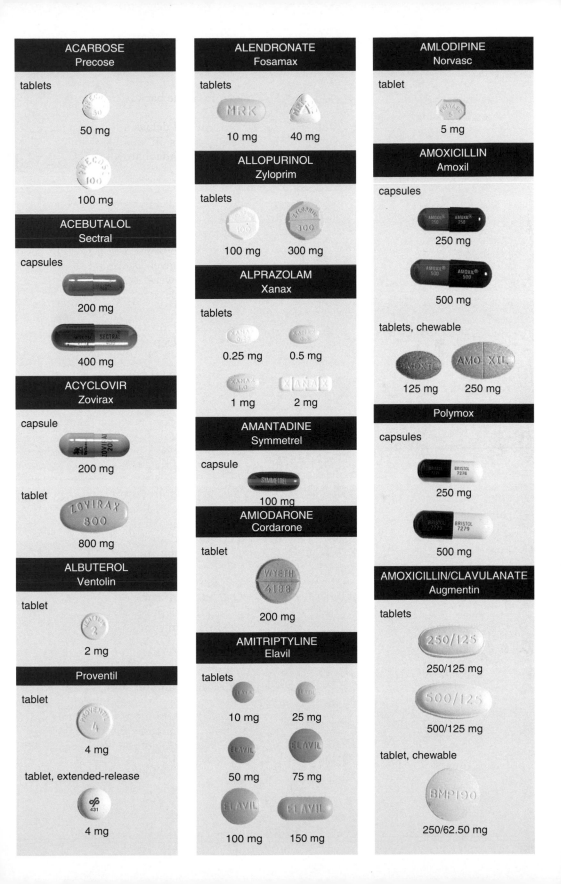

ACARBOSE
Precose

tablets

50 mg

100 mg

ACEBUTALOL
Sectral

capsules

200 mg

400 mg

ACYCLOVIR
Zovirax

capsule

200 mg

tablet

800 mg

ALBUTEROL
Ventolin

tablet

2 mg

Proventil

tablet

4 mg

tablet, extended-release

4 mg

ALENDRONATE
Fosamax

tablets

10 mg   40 mg

ALLOPURINOL
Zyloprim

tablets

100 mg   300 mg

ALPRAZOLAM
Xanax

tablets

0.25 mg   0.5 mg

1 mg   2 mg

AMANTADINE
Symmetrel

capsule

100 mg

AMIODARONE
Cordarone

tablet

200 mg

AMITRIPTYLINE
Elavil

tablets

10 mg   25 mg

50 mg   75 mg

100 mg   150 mg

AMLODIPINE
Norvasc

tablet

5 mg

AMOXICILLIN
Amoxil

capsules

250 mg

500 mg

tablets, chewable

125 mg   250 mg

Polymox

capsules

250 mg

500 mg

AMOXICILLIN/CLAVULANATE
Augmentin

tablets

250/125 mg

500/125 mg

tablet, chewable

250/62.50 mg

AMPICILLIN
Omnipen

capsule

500 mg

Polycillin

capsules

250 mg

500 mg

ATENOLOL
Tenormin

tablets

25 mg 50 mg 100 mg

ATORVASTATIN
Lipitor

tablet

10 mg

AZATHIOPRINE
Imuran

tablet

50 mg

AZITHROMYCIN
Zithromax

capsule

250 mg

BECLOMETHASONE
Beclovent

inhaler

Vanceril

inhaler

BENAZEPRIL
Lotensin

tablets

5   10   20

5 mg 10 mg 20 mg

BENZTROPINE
Cogentin

tablets

0.5 mg 1 mg 2 mg

BETAXOLOL
Kerlone

tablets

10 mg 20 mg

BITOLTEROL
Tornalate

inhaler

BUDESONIDE
Rhinocort

nasal inhaler

BUMETANIDE
Bumex

tablets

0.5 mg   1 mg

2 mg

BUPROPION
Wellbutrin

tablets

75 mg   100 mg

BUSPIRONE
BuSpar

tablets

5 mg   10 mg

CAPTOPRIL
Capoten

tablets

12.5 mg 25 mg 50 mg

CARBAMAZEPINE
Tegretol

tablet

200 mg

tablet, chewable

100 mg

CARTEOLOL
Cartrol

tablet

2.5 mg

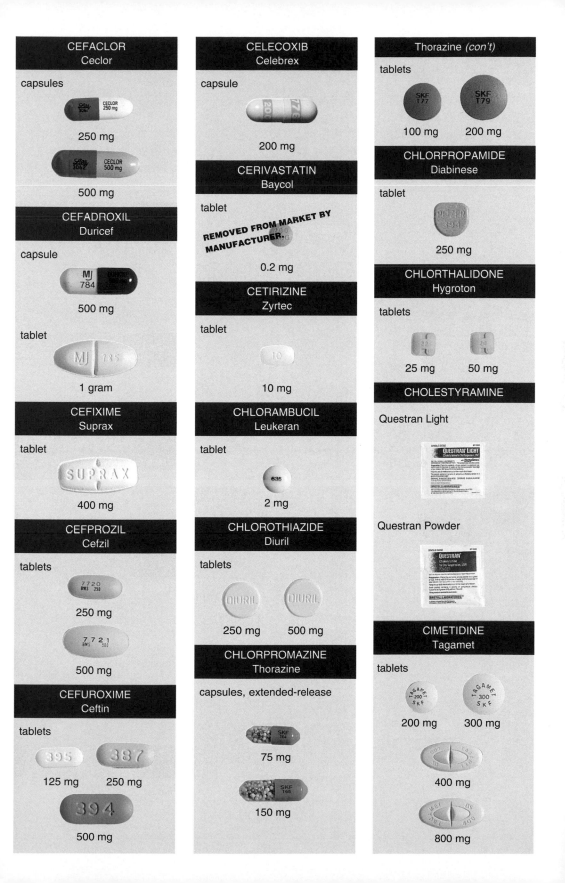

CEFACLOR
Ceclor

capsules

250 mg

500 mg

CEFADROXIL
Duricef

capsule

500 mg

tablet

1 gram

CEFIXIME
Suprax

tablet

400 mg

CEFPROZIL
Cefzil

tablets

250 mg

500 mg

CEFUROXIME
Ceftin

tablets

125 mg   250 mg

500 mg

CELECOXIB
Celebrex

capsule

200 mg

CERIVASTATIN
Baycol

tablet

REMOVED FROM MARKET BY MANUFACTURER.

0.2 mg

CETIRIZINE
Zyrtec

tablet

10 mg

CHLORAMBUCIL
Leukeran

tablet

2 mg

CHLOROTHIAZIDE
Diuril

tablets

250 mg   500 mg

CHLORPROMAZINE
Thorazine

capsules, extended-release

75 mg

150 mg

Thorazine *(con't)*

tablets

100 mg   200 mg

CHLORPROPAMIDE
Diabinese

tablet

250 mg

CHLORTHALIDONE
Hygroton

tablets

25 mg   50 mg

CHOLESTYRAMINE

Questran Light

Questran Powder

CIMETIDINE
Tagamet

tablets

200 mg   300 mg

400 mg

800 mg

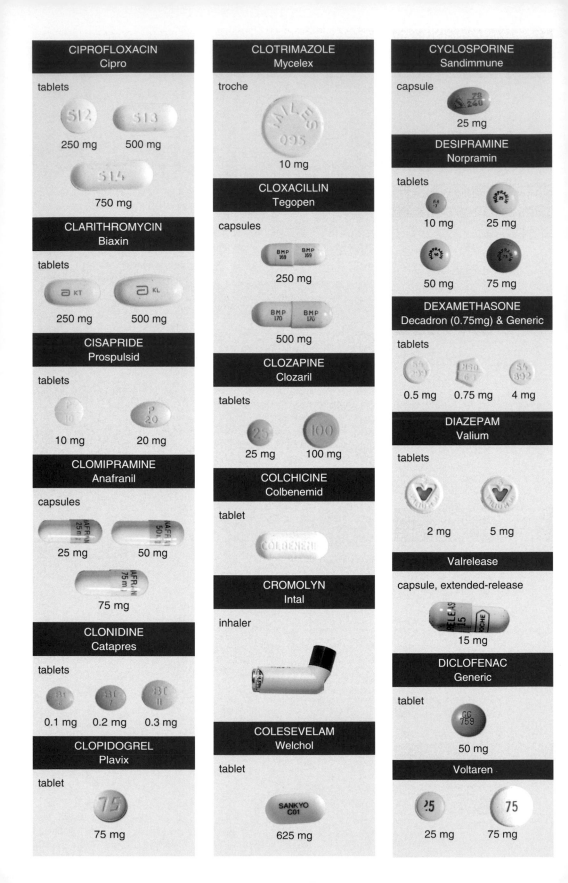

CIPROFLOXACIN
Cipro
tablets

250 mg 500 mg

750 mg

CLARITHROMYCIN
Biaxin
tablets

250 mg 500 mg

CISAPRIDE
Prospulsid
tablets

10 mg 20 mg

CLOMIPRAMINE
Anafranil
capsules

25 mg 50 mg

75 mg

CLONIDINE
Catapres
tablets

0.1 mg 0.2 mg 0.3 mg

CLOPIDOGREL
Plavix
tablet

75 mg

CLOTRIMAZOLE
Mycelex
troche

10 mg

CLOXACILLIN
Tegopen
capsules

250 mg

500 mg

CLOZAPINE
Clozaril
tablets

25 mg 100 mg

COLCHICINE
Colbenemid
tablet

CROMOLYN
Intal
inhaler

COLESEVELAM
Welchol
tablet

625 mg

CYCLOSPORINE
Sandimmune
capsule

25 mg

DESIPRAMINE
Norpramin
tablets

10 mg 25 mg

50 mg 75 mg

DEXAMETHASONE
Decadron (0.75mg) & Generic
tablets

0.5 mg 0.75 mg 4 mg

DIAZEPAM
Valium
tablets

2 mg 5 mg

Valrelease
capsule, extended-release

15 mg

DICLOFENAC
Generic
tablet

50 mg

Voltaren

25 mg 75 mg

DIDANOSINE
Videx

tablet

25 mg

DIFLUNISAL
Dolobid

tablets

250 mg   500 mg

DIGOXIN
Lanoxicaps

capsules

0.1 mg   0.2 mg

Lanoxin

tablets

0.125 mg   0.25 mg   0.5 mg

DILTIAZEM
Cardizem

tablets

30 mg   60 mg

90 mg

120 mg

Cardizem CD

capsules

180 mg

Cardizem CD

capsules *(cont.)*

240 mg

300 mg

Cardizem SR

capsules

60 mg   90 mg

120 mg

DIPHENHYDRAMINE
Benadryl

capsules

25 mg   50 mg

DISOPYRAMIDE
Norpace

capsules

100 mg   150 mg

Norpace CR

capsules, extended-release

100 mg

150 mg

DISULFIRAM
Antabuse

tablets

250 mg   500 mg

DONEPEZIL
Aricept

tablet

5 mg

DOXAZOSIN
Cardura

tablets

1 mg   2 mg

4 mg   8 mg

DOXEPIN
Sinequan

capsules

10 mg   25 mg

50 mg

DOXYCYCLINE
Zenith generic

tablet

100 mg

ENALAPRIL
Vasotec

tablet

2.5 mg

ERGOTAMINE
Ergostat

tablet

2 mg

ERYTHROMYCIN
Ery-Tab

tablet, delayed-release

333 mg

E-Mycin

tablets, delayed-release

250 mg   333 mg

Eryc

capsule, delayed-release

250 mg

Erythrocin

tablets

250 mg   500 mg

ESTROGENS
Estrace

tablets

1 mg   2 mg

Ogen

tablets

0.625 mg   1.5 mg

Premarin

tablets

0.3 mg   0.625 mg

0.9 mg   1.25 mg

2.5 mg

ETANERCEPT
Enbrel

single use vial

25 mg

ETHAMBUTOL
Myambutol

tablet

400 mg

ETHOSUXIMIDE
Zarontin

capsule

250 mg

FAMOTIDINE
Pepcid

tablets

20 mg   40 mg

FELODIPINE
Plendil

tablets

5 mg   10 mg

FENOPROFEN
Nalfon

capsule

200 mg

FEXOFENADINE
Allegra

capsule

6 mg

FINASTERIDE
Proscar

tablet

5 mg

FLUCONAZOLE
Diflucan

tablets

50 mg   100 mg

FLUCYTOSINE
Ancobon

capsule

500 mg

FLUOXETINE
Prozac

capsule

20 mg

Sarafem

pulvule

20 mg

FLURAZEPAM
Dalmane

capsules

15 mg   30 mg

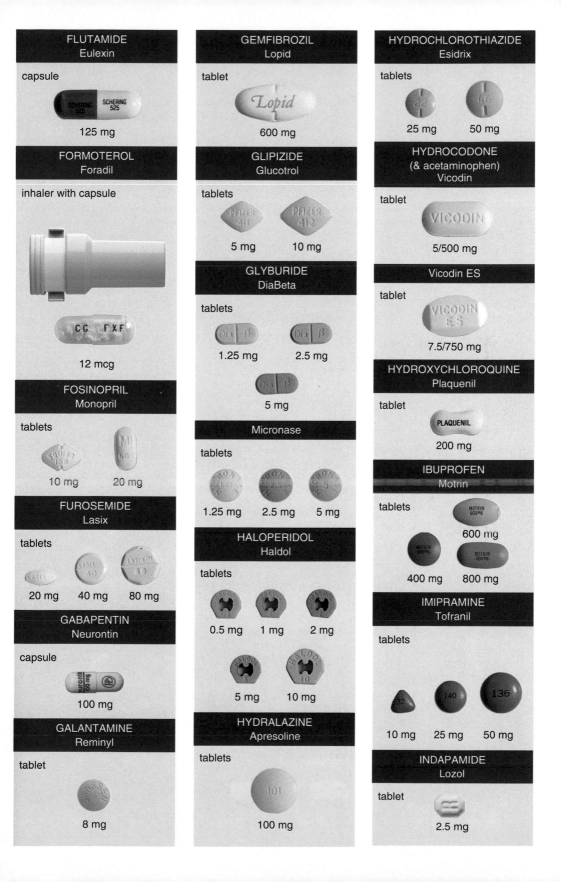

FLUTAMIDE
Eulexin

capsule

125 mg

FORMOTEROL
Foradil

inhaler with capsule

12 mcg

FOSINOPRIL
Monopril

tablets

10 mg   20 mg

FUROSEMIDE
Lasix

tablets

20 mg   40 mg   80 mg

GABAPENTIN
Neurontin

capsule

100 mg

GALANTAMINE
Reminyl

tablet

8 mg

GEMFIBROZIL
Lopid

tablet

600 mg

GLIPIZIDE
Glucotrol

tablets

5 mg   10 mg

GLYBURIDE
DiaBeta

tablets

1.25 mg   2.5 mg

5 mg

Micronase

tablets

1.25 mg   2.5 mg   5 mg

HALOPERIDOL
Haldol

tablets

0.5 mg   1 mg   2 mg

5 mg   10 mg

HYDRALAZINE
Apresoline

tablets

100 mg

HYDROCHLOROTHIAZIDE
Esidrix

tablets

25 mg   50 mg

HYDROCODONE
(& acetaminophen)
Vicodin

tablet

5/500 mg

Vicodin ES

tablet

7.5/750 mg

HYDROXYCHLOROQUINE
Plaquenil

tablet

200 mg

IBUPROFEN
Motrin

tablets

600 mg

400 mg   800 mg

IMIPRAMINE
Tofranil

tablets

10 mg   25 mg   50 mg

INDAPAMIDE
Lozol

tablet

2.5 mg

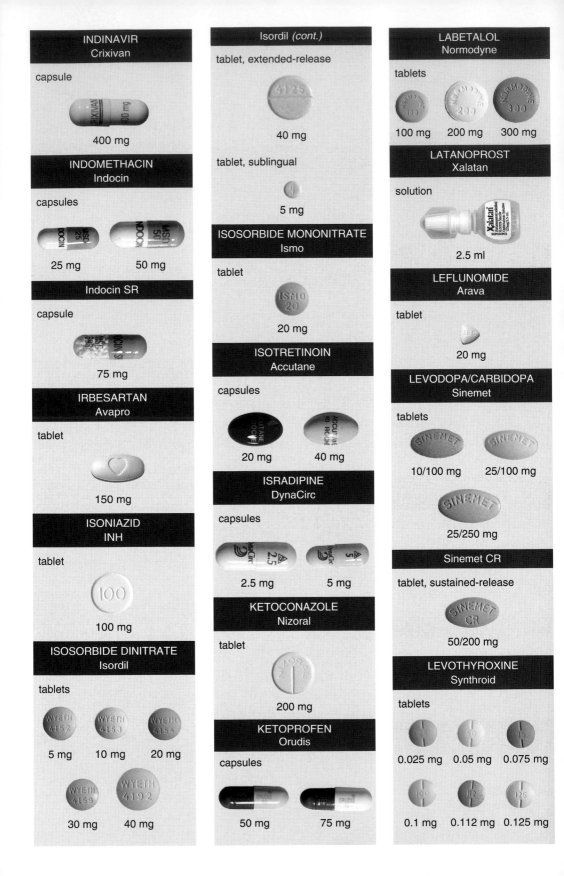

INDINAVIR
Crixivan

capsule

400 mg

INDOMETHACIN
Indocin

capsules

25 mg   50 mg

Indocin SR

capsule

75 mg

IRBESARTAN
Avapro

tablet

150 mg

ISONIAZID
INH

tablet

100 mg

ISOSORBIDE DINITRATE
Isordil

tablets

5 mg   10 mg   20 mg

30 mg   40 mg

Isordil *(cont.)*

tablet, extended-release

40 mg

tablet, sublingual

5 mg

ISOSORBIDE MONONITRATE
Ismo

tablet

20 mg

ISOTRETINOIN
Accutane

capsules

20 mg   40 mg

ISRADIPINE
DynaCirc

capsules

2.5 mg   5 mg

KETOCONAZOLE
Nizoral

tablet

200 mg

KETOPROFEN
Orudis

capsules

50 mg   75 mg

LABETALOL
Normodyne

tablets

100 mg   200 mg   300 mg

LATANOPROST
Xalatan

solution

2.5 ml

LEFLUNOMIDE
Arava

tablet

20 mg

LEVODOPA/CARBIDOPA
Sinemet

tablets

10/100 mg   25/100 mg

25/250 mg

Sinemet CR

tablet, sustained-release

50/200 mg

LEVOTHYROXINE
Synthroid

tablets

0.025 mg   0.05 mg   0.075 mg

0.1 mg   0.112 mg   0.125 mg

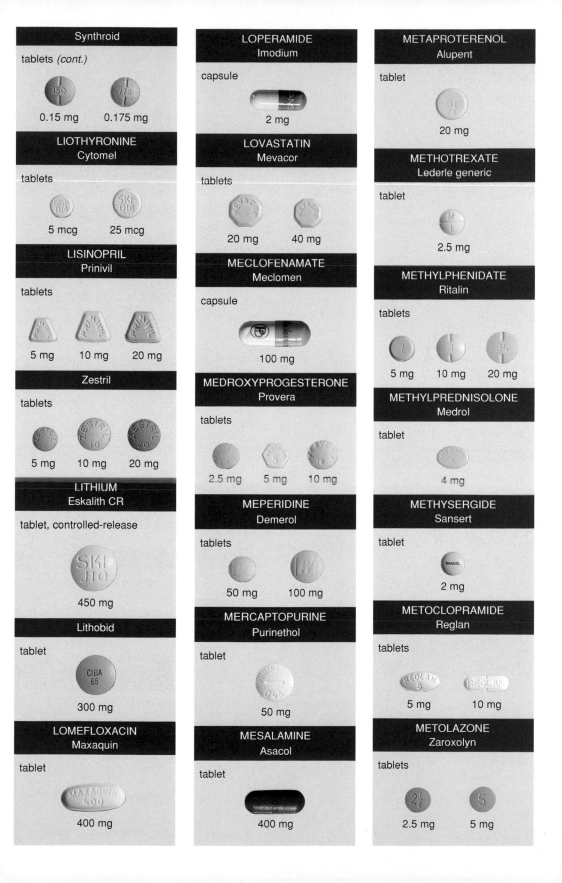

Synthroid
tablets *(cont.)*

0.15 mg   0.175 mg

LIOTHYRONINE
Cytomel

tablets

5 mcg   25 mcg

LISINOPRIL
Prinivil

tablets

5 mg   10 mg   20 mg

Zestril

tablets

5 mg   10 mg   20 mg

LITHIUM
Eskalith CR

tablet, controlled-release

450 mg

Lithobid

tablet

300 mg

LOMEFLOXACIN
Maxaquin

tablet

400 mg

LOPERAMIDE
Imodium

capsule

2 mg

LOVASTATIN
Mevacor

tablets

20 mg   40 mg

MECLOFENAMATE
Meclomen

capsule

100 mg

MEDROXYPROGESTERONE
Provera

tablets

2.5 mg   5 mg   10 mg

MEPERIDINE
Demerol

tablets

50 mg   100 mg

MERCAPTOPURINE
Purinethol

tablet

50 mg

MESALAMINE
Asacol

tablet

400 mg

METAPROTERENOL
Alupent

tablet

20 mg

METHOTREXATE
Lederle generic

tablet

2.5 mg

METHYLPHENIDATE
Ritalin

tablets

5 mg   10 mg   20 mg

METHYLPREDNISOLONE
Medrol

tablet

4 mg

METHYSERGIDE
Sansert

tablet

2 mg

METOCLOPRAMIDE
Reglan

tablets

5 mg   10 mg

METOLAZONE
Zaroxolyn

tablets

2.5 mg   5 mg

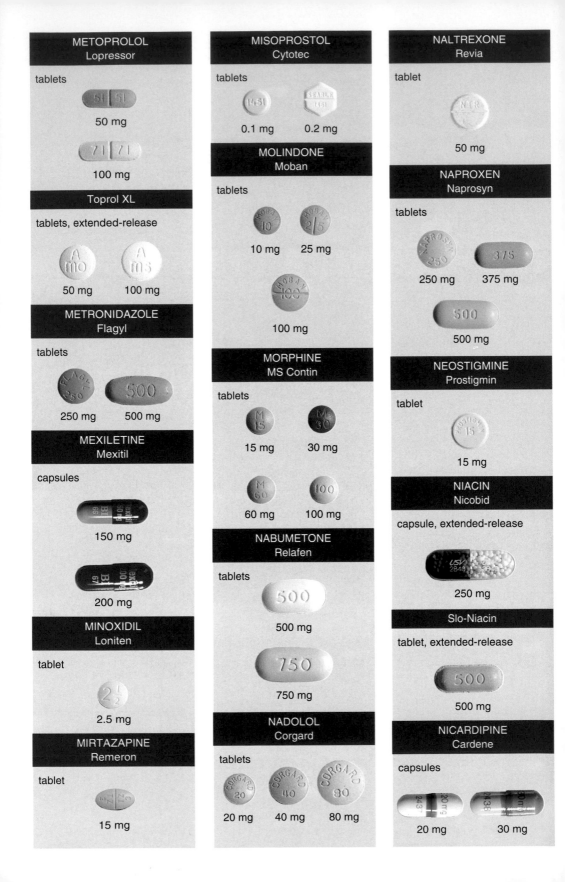

METOPROLOL
Lopressor

tablets

50 mg

100 mg

Toprol XL

tablets, extended-release

50 mg   100 mg

METRONIDAZOLE
Flagyl

tablets

250 mg   500 mg

MEXILETINE
Mexitil

capsules

150 mg

200 mg

MINOXIDIL
Loniten

tablet

2.5 mg

MIRTAZAPINE
Remeron

tablet

15 mg

MISOPROSTOL
Cytotec

tablets

0.1 mg   0.2 mg

MOLINDONE
Moban

tablets

10 mg   25 mg

100 mg

MORPHINE
MS Contin

tablets

15 mg   30 mg

60 mg   100 mg

NABUMETONE
Relafen

tablets

500 mg

750 mg

NADOLOL
Corgard

tablets

20 mg   40 mg   80 mg

NALTREXONE
Revia

tablet

50 mg

NAPROXEN
Naprosyn

tablets

250 mg   375 mg

500 mg

NEOSTIGMINE
Prostigmin

tablet

15 mg

NIACIN
Nicobid

capsule, extended-release

250 mg

Slo-Niacin

tablet, extended-release

500 mg

NICARDIPINE
Cardene

capsules

20 mg   30 mg

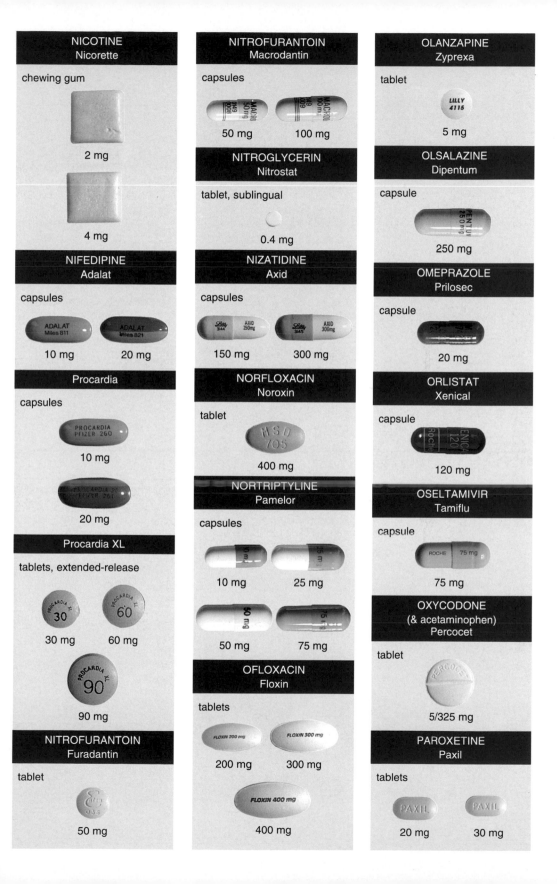

NICOTINE
Nicorette

chewing gum

2 mg

4 mg

NIFEDIPINE
Adalat

capsules

ADALAT Miles 811 · 10 mg

ADALAT Miles 821 · 20 mg

Procardia

capsules

PROCARDIA PFIZER 260 · 10 mg

PROCARDIA 20 PFIZER 261 · 20 mg

Procardia XL

tablets, extended-release

PROCARDIA XL 30 · 30 mg

PROCARDIA XL 60 · 60 mg

PROCARDIA XL 90 · 90 mg

NITROFURANTOIN
Furadantin

tablet

50 mg

NITROFURANTOIN
Macrodantin

capsules

MACRO 50 mg · 50 mg

MACRO 100 m.l · 100 mg

NITROGLYCERIN
Nitrostat

tablet, sublingual

0.4 mg

NIZATIDINE
Axid

capsules

Lilly 3144 · AXID 150mg · 150 mg

Lilly 3145 · AXID 300mg · 300 mg

NORFLOXACIN
Noroxin

tablet

MSD 705 · 400 mg

NORTRIPTYLINE
Pamelor

capsules

10 mg

25 mg

50 mg

75 mg

OFLOXACIN
Floxin

tablets

FLOXIN 200 mg · 200 mg

FLOXIN 300 mg · 300 mg

FLOXIN 400 mg · 400 mg

OLANZAPINE
Zyprexa

tablet

LILLY 4115 · 5 mg

OLSALAZINE
Dipentum

capsule

PENTUM 250 mg · 250 mg

OMEPRAZOLE
Prilosec

capsule

20 mg

ORLISTAT
Xenical

capsule

Roche · XENICAL 120 · 120 mg

OSELTAMIVIR
Tamiflu

capsule

ROCHE 75 mg · 75 mg

OXYCODONE
(& acetaminophen)
Percocet

tablet

PERCOCET · 5/325 mg

PAROXETINE
Paxil

tablets

PAXIL · 20 mg

PAXIL · 30 mg

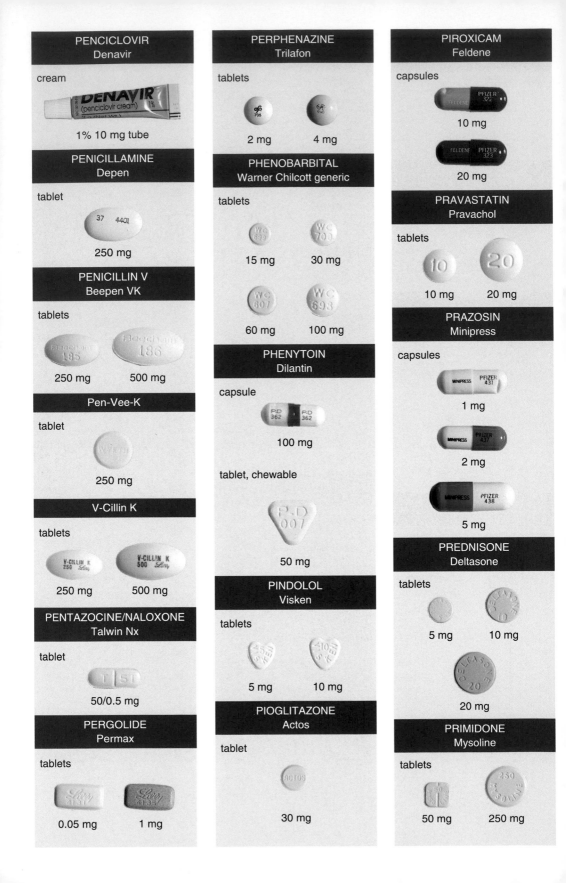

PENCICLOVIR
Denavir

cream

1% 10 mg tube

PENICILLAMINE
Depen

tablet

250 mg

PENICILLIN V
Beepen VK

tablets

250 mg   500 mg

Pen-Vee-K

tablet

250 mg

V-Cillin K

tablets

250 mg   500 mg

PENTAZOCINE/NALOXONE
Talwin Nx

tablet

50/0.5 mg

PERGOLIDE
Permax

tablets

0.05 mg   1 mg

PERPHENAZINE
Trilafon

tablets

2 mg   4 mg

PHENOBARBITAL
Warner Chilcott generic

tablets

15 mg   30 mg

60 mg   100 mg

PHENYTOIN
Dilantin

capsule

100 mg

tablet, chewable

50 mg

PINDOLOL
Visken

tablets

5 mg   10 mg

PIOGLITAZONE
Actos

tablet

30 mg

PIROXICAM
Feldene

capsules

10 mg

20 mg

PRAVASTATIN
Pravachol

tablets

10 mg   20 mg

PRAZOSIN
Minipress

capsules

1 mg

2 mg

5 mg

PREDNISONE
Deltasone

tablets

5 mg   10 mg

20 mg

PRIMIDONE
Mysoline

tablets

50 mg   250 mg

PROBENECID
Benemid

tablet

500 mg

PROCAINAMIDE
Pronestyl

capsule

500 mg

Procan-SR

tablets, extended-release

500 mg

750mg

PROCHLORPERAZINE
Compazine

capsules

10 mg   15 mg

tablet

5 mg

PROPAFENONE
Rythmol

tablet

150 mg

PROPRANOLOL
Inderal

tablets

10 mg   20 mg   40 mg

60 mg   80 mg

Inderal LA

capsules, extended-release

60 mg   80 mg

120 mg

160 mg

PYRAZINAMIDE
Lederle generic

tablet

500 mg

PYRIDOSTIGMINE
Mestinon

tablet

60 mg

PYRIMETHAMINE
Daraprim

tablet

25 mg

QUINAPRIL
Accupril

tablets

5 mg   10 mg

20 mg   40 mg

QUINIDINE
Quinaglute

tablet

324 mg

RALOXIFENE
Evista

tablet

60 mg

RAMIPRIL
Altace

capsules

2.5 mg   5 mg

10 mg

RANITIDINE
Zantac

tablets

150 mg   300 mg

REPAGLINIDE
Prandin

tablets

0.5 mg   1 mg   2 mg

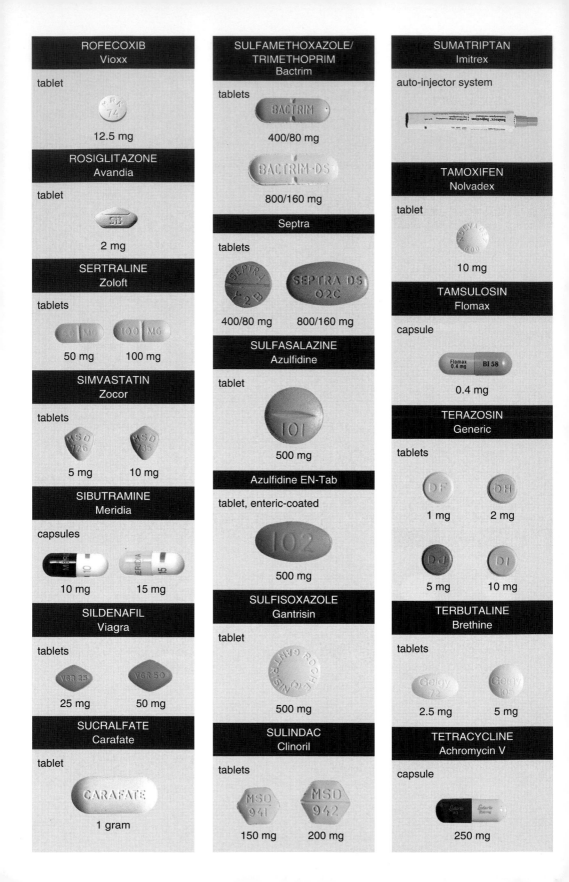

ROFECOXIB
Vioxx

tablet

12.5 mg

ROSIGLITAZONE
Avandia

tablet

2 mg

SERTRALINE
Zoloft

tablets

50 mg   100 mg

SIMVASTATIN
Zocor

tablets

5 mg   10 mg

SIBUTRAMINE
Meridia

capsules

10 mg   15 mg

SILDENAFIL
Viagra

tablets

25 mg   50 mg

SUCRALFATE
Carafate

tablet

1 gram

**SULFAMETHOXAZOLE/
TRIMETHOPRIM**
Bactrim

tablets

400/80 mg

800/160 mg

Septra

tablets

400/80 mg   800/160 mg

SULFASALAZINE
Azulfidine

tablet

500 mg

Azulfidine EN-Tab

tablet, enteric-coated

500 mg

SULFISOXAZOLE
Gantrisin

tablet

500 mg

SULINDAC
Clinoril

tablets

150 mg   200 mg

SUMATRIPTAN
Imitrex

auto-injector system

TAMOXIFEN
Nolvadex

tablet

10 mg

TAMSULOSIN
Flomax

capsule

0.4 mg

TERAZOSIN
Generic

tablets

1 mg   2 mg

5 mg   10 mg

TERBUTALINE
Brethine

tablets

2.5 mg   5 mg

TETRACYCLINE
Achromycin V

capsule

250 mg

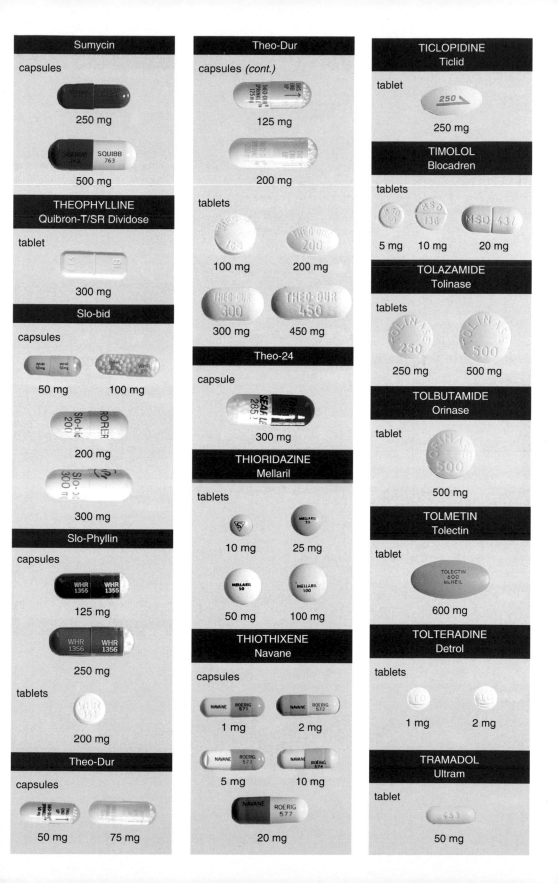

Sumycin

capsules

250 mg

500 mg

THEOPHYLLINE
Quibron-T/SR Dividose

tablet

300 mg

Slo-bid

capsules

50 mg   100 mg

200 mg

300 mg

Slo-Phyllin

capsules

125 mg

250 mg

tablets

200 mg

Theo-Dur

capsules

50 mg   75 mg

Theo-Dur

capsules *(cont.)*

125 mg

200 mg

tablets

100 mg   200 mg

300 mg   450 mg

Theo-24

capsule

300 mg

THIORIDAZINE
Mellaril

tablets

10 mg   25 mg

50 mg   100 mg

THIOTHIXENE
Navane

capsules

1 mg   2 mg

5 mg   10 mg

20 mg

TICLOPIDINE
Ticlid

tablet

250 mg

TIMOLOL
Blocadren

tablets

5 mg   10 mg   20 mg

TOLAZAMIDE
Tolinase

tablets

250 mg   500 mg

TOLBUTAMIDE
Orinase

tablet

500 mg

TOLMETIN
Tolectin

tablet

600 mg

TOLTERADINE
Detrol

tablets

1 mg   2 mg

TRAMADOL
Ultram

tablet

50 mg

TRAZODONE
Desyrel

tablets

50 mg   100 mg

150 mg

**TRIAMTERENE/
HYDROCHLOROTHIAZIDE**
Dyazide

capsule

50/25 mg

Maxzide

tablets

37.5/25 mg   75/50 mg

TRIFLUOPERAZINE
Stelazine

tablets

1 mg   2 mg   5 mg

TRIMETHOPRIM
Trimpex

tablet

100 mg

VALACYCLOVIR
Valtrex

tablet

500 mg

VALPROIC ACID
Depakote Sprinkle

capsule

125 mg

Depakote

tablets

125 mg   250 mg

500 mg

VENLAFAXINE
Effexor

tablet

25 mg

VERAPAMIL
Calan

tablets

80 mg   120 mg

Calan SR

tablets, extended-release

120 mg   180 mg

240 mg

Verelan

capsules, extended-release

120 mg

Verelan

capsules, extended-release
(*cont.*)

180 mg

Verelan

capsules, extended-release
(*cont.*)

240 mg

WARFARIN
Coumadin

tablets

1 mg   2 mg   2.5 mg

5 mg   7.5 mg   10 mg

ZAFIRLUKAST
Accolate

tablet

20 mg

ZALEPLON
Sonata

capsule

10 mg

ZILEUTON
Zyflo

tablet

600 mg

ZIPRAZIDONE
Geodon

capsule

20 mg

Amitriptyline may *decrease* the effects of
- clonidine (Catapres).
- guanethidine (Ismelin).
- guanfacine (Tenex).
- methyldopa, which can result in reduced amitriptyline and/or methyldopa benefits.

Amitriptyline *taken concurrently* with
- amphetamines can cause excessive amitriptyline responses.
- amprenavir (Agenerase), ritonavir (Norvir) and perhaps other protease inhibitors (see Drug Classes) can lead to amitriptyline toxicity.
- anticoagulants such as warfarin (Coumadin) may cause an increased risk of bleeding.
- baclofen (Lioresal) may lead to muscle weakness and memory loss.
- bepridil (Vascor) can lead to heart rhythm problems. DO NOT COMBINE.
- carbamazepine (Tegretol) may decrease the blood level of amitriptyline.
- cisapride (Propulsid) can lead to heart rhythm problems. DO NOT COMBINE.
- diazepam (Valium) and perhaps other benzodiazepines (see Drug Classes) can result in additive loss of psychomotor skills.
- dofetilide (Tikosyn) can lead to heart rhythm problems. DO NOT COMBINE.
- enflurane (various) may increase seizure risk. DO NOT COMBINE.
- epinephrine may cause an increased risk of rapid heart rate and high blood pressure.
- estrogens (see Drug Classes) may increase amitriptyline drug levels.
- ethanol (alcohol) may give additive central nervous system toxicity.
- fluconazole (Diflucan) can result in very high levels of amitriptyline.
- fluoxetine (Prozac) can result in very high levels of amitriptyline.
- fluvoxamine (Luvox) can result in very high levels of amitriptyline.
- gatifloxacin (Tequin), grepafloxacin (Raxar), moxifloxacin (Avelox) or sparfloxacin (Zagam) may result in heart toxicity—DO NOT COMBINE.
- meperidine (Demerol) worsens breathing (respiratory) depression risk.
- monoamine oxidase (MAO) type A inhibitor drugs may cause high fever, delirium and convulsions (see Drug Classes).
- phenytoin (Dilantin) or fosphenytoin (Cerebyx) can lead to amitriptyline toxicity.
- potassium (various) may lead to ulceration from potassium as amitriptyline may slow the intestine.
- quinidine (Quinaglute, etc.) can result in increased antidepressant blood levels.
- salmeterol (Serevent) should be used with great care because of increased cardiovascular risk (changes in blood pressure, pulse and electrocardiograms or EKGs).
- sertraline (Zoloft) can lead to heart rhythm problems. DO NOT COMBINE.
- thyroid preparations may impair heart rhythm and function. Ask your doctor for help with adjustment of thyroid dose.
- tramadol (Ultram) may increase risk of seizures. This combination is not advised.
- venlafaxine (Effexor) can result in very high levels of amitriptyline.
- verapamil (Calan, others) can result in very high levels of amitriptyline.
- warfarin (Coumadin) may lead to increased bleeding risk. More frequent INRs are prudent.

▷ *Driving, Hazardous Activities:* This drug may impair mental alertness, judgment, physical coordination and reaction time. Avoid hazardous activities.

Aviation Note: The use of this drug **is a disqualification** for piloting. Consult a designated Aviation Medical Examiner.

Exposure to Sun: This drug may cause photosensitivity (see Glossary).

Exposure to Heat: May inhibit sweating and impair the body's adaptation to hot environments, increasing risk of heatstroke. Avoid saunas.

Exposure to Cold: Older patients should avoid prolonged cold exposure (conducive to hypothermia—see Glossary).

Discontinuation: It is best to stop this drug gradually. Abrupt withdrawal after long-term use can cause headache, malaise and nausea.

AMLODIPINE (am LOH di peen)

Introduced: 1986   **Class:** Anti-anginal, antihypertensive, calcium channel blocker   **Prescription:** USA: Yes   **Controlled Drug:** USA: No; Canada: No   **Available as Generic:** No

Brand Names: Lotrel [CD], Norvasc

Controversies in Medicine: Medicines in this class have had many conflicting reports. The FDA has held hearings on the calcium channel blocker (CCB) class. Amlodipine got the first FDA approval to treat high blood pressure or angina in those with congestive heart failure. Some data appear to show that amlodipine lowers the risk of stroke or heart attack in people with coronary artery disease. Some research at New York University found that nifedipine is a cause of reversible male infertility. CCBs are currently second-line agents for high blood pressure according to the JNC VI (see Glossary).

BENEFITS versus RISKS	
Possible Benefits	*Possible Risks*
EFFECTIVE PREVENTION OF BOTH MAJOR TYPES OF ANGINA	DOSE-RELATED CHANGES IN HEART RHYTHM
EFFECTIVE TREATMENT OF HYPERTENSION	Peripheral edema (fluid retention in feet and ankles)
	Dose-related palpitations
	Other medicines in the same family have rare concern about depression, memory loss or malignancy

▷ **Principal Uses**

As a Single Drug Product: Uses currently included in FDA-approved labeling: (1) Treats angina pectoris due to spontaneous coronary artery spasm (Prinzmetal's variant angina) that is not associated with exertion; (2) classical angina-of-effort (caused by "hardening" or atherosclerosis of coronary arteries) in people who don't respond or can't tolerate nitrates or beta-blockers; (3) mild to moderate hypertension; (4) hypertension or angina in people who also have congestive heart failure.

Other (unlabeled) generally accepted uses: (1) May keep early atherosclerotic lesions from getting worse; (2) can help stop premature labor; (3) helps some symptoms in cases of lung (pulmonary) hypertension; (4) can work to lower blood pressure and decrease the amount of protein in the urine (microalbuminuria) of diabetics; (5) may ease silent myocardial ischemia in combination with a beta blocker; (6) some limited use in preventing migraines.

As a Combination Drug Product [CD]: In combination with benazepril offers the benefits of an ACE inhibitor and a calcium channel blocker.

How This Drug Works: This drug blocks normal passage of calcium through cell walls, inhibiting coronary artery and peripheral arteriole narrowing. As a result, this drug

- prevents spontaneous coronary artery spasm (Prinzmetal's angina).
- decreases heart rate and contraction force in exertion, making effort-induced angina less likely.
- opens contracted peripheral arterial walls, lowering blood pressure. (Also lessens heart work and helps prevent angina.)

The combination form (Lotrel) adds the benefits of inhibiting angiotensin converting enzyme (ACE) via the active benazeprilat form.

Available Dosage Forms and Strengths

Lotrel tablets — 2.5/10 mg, 5/10 mg and 5/20 mg
Tablets — 2.5 mg, 5 mg, 10 mg

▷ **Recommended Dosage Ranges** (Actual dose and schedule must be determined for each patient individually.)

Infants and Children: Dosage not established.

12 to 65 Years of Age: High blood pressure: 2.5 to 10 mg daily, in a single dose. The fixed combination (Lotrel form) is usually given as one to two capsules a day. In older (or frail patients) some clinicians limit the dose of the amlodipine component to 2.5 mg a day.

Chronic angina: 5 to 10 mg daily; 10 mg may improve exercise ability in stable angina patients.

Congestive heart failure: 5 mg once daily for 2 weeks with increase to 10 mg as needed and tolerated.

Over 65 Years of Age: Lower doses (2.5 mg for high blood pressure and 5 mg for angina) are prudent and effective.

Conditions Requiring Dosing Adjustments

Liver Function: Patients with damaged livers started on a daily 2.5-mg dose for high blood pressure, 5 mg for angina. Then dosing may be slowly increased as needed or tolerated.

Kidney Function: No adjustment in dosing is needed.

Low Protein or Starvation: This drug is moved around the body by a protein called albumin. If protein is low, in liver failure or starvation, increased effect may be seen with "normal" doses. Start therapy with low doses. Increase only if needed or tolerated.

▷ **Dosing Instructions:** May be taken with or following food to reduce stomach irritation. The tablet may be crushed. If you forget a dose: Take the medicine right away, unless it is nearly time for your next dose, then omit the missed dose and take the medicine when it was next scheduled. DO NOT double doses.

Usual Duration of Use: Regular use for 2 to 4 weeks often needed to see benefit in reducing angina frequency or severity of angina and in high blood pressure control. Best to use the lowest dose that works for long-term use (months to years). Periodic evaluation by your doctor is needed.

Typical Treatment Goals and Measurements (Outcomes and Markers)

Blood Pressure: The most recent treatment guidelines (JNC VI) define optimal blood pressure (BP) as less than 120/80 and high normal as 139/89. Most clinicians try to achieve a BP that confers the best balance of lower cardiovascular risk and avoids the problem of too low a blood pressure. The goals and time frame should be discussed with you when the prescription is written.

Possible Advantages of This Drug

Slow onset and prolonged effect, allowing effective once-a-day treatment for both angina and high blood pressure.

▷ **This Drug Should Not Be Taken If**
- you have had an allergic reaction to it previously.
- you have active liver disease.
- you have low blood pressure—systolic below 90 mm Hg.
- you have atrioventricular block or sick sinus syndrome (talk to your doctor).
- your left heart ventricle doesn't work well (dysfunctional).

▷ **Inform Your Physician Before Taking This Drug If**
- you have had a bad reaction to any calcium blocker.
- you take digitalis or a beta-blocker (see Drug Classes).
- you are taking any drugs that lower blood pressure.
- you have had congestive heart failure, heart attack or stroke.
- you have a contracted or narrowed (stenosed) aorta.
- you are subject to disturbances of heart rhythm.
- you have a history of drug-induced liver damage.
- you develop a rash or other skin reaction while taking this medicine.
- you are unsure how much or how often to take this drug.
- you have circulation problems in your hands.
- you have muscular dystrophy.

Possible Side Effects (natural, expected and unavoidable drug actions)

Swelling of feet and ankles, flushing (4.5% in women and 1.5% in men) and sensation of warmth.

Impaired sense of smell.

▷ **Possible Adverse Effects** (unusual, unexpected and infrequent reactions)

If any of the following develop, consult your physician promptly for guidance.

Mild Adverse Effects

Allergic reactions: skin rash (call your doctor, as persistent rashes may become serious).

Headache (up to 12%), dizziness (dose related)—infrequent.

Fatigue, nausea or constipation—infrequent.

Dose-related palpitations, low dose—rare; 10 mg—infrequent.

Overgrowth of the gums (gingival hyperplasia)—up to 40% with drugs in the same class.

Increased urge to urinate at night—rare.

Visual changes (eye pain, double vision)—rare.

Ringing in the ears (tinnitus)—rare.

Cough, muscle pain—infrequent.

Dose-related flushing (4.5% in women and 1.5% in men)—infrequent.

Elevated liver enzymes (may be a hypersensitivity, usually resolves)—rare.

Serious Adverse Effects

Allergic reactions: exfoliative dermatitis (very rare).

Idiosyncratic reactions: Parkinson-like symptoms—case report.

Dose-dependent edema (up to 6.2% in those over 65)—infrequent.

Exfoliative dermatitis or erythema multiforme—rare.

Agranulocytosis (only other medicines in this class)—case reports.

Rebound angina—if drug is abruptly stopped—possible.

Difficulty breathing (dyspnea)—infrequent (up to 15% in the PRAISE trial as pulmonary edema).

▷ **Possible Effects on Sexual Function:** Sexual dysfunction (both men and women)—1–2%.

Swelling and tenderness of male breast tissue (gynecomastia)—case report.

Adverse Effects That May Mimic Natural Diseases or Disorders

An allergic rash and swelling of the legs may resemble erysipelas.

Possible Effects on Laboratory Tests

Liver function tests: transient increases in liver enzymes.

CAUTION

1. Make sure all your health care providers know you take this drug. List this drug on a card in your purse or wallet.
2. Nitroglycerin or other nitrate drugs can be used as needed to ease acute angina pain. If your attacks become more frequent or intense, call your doctor promptly.

Precautions for Use

By Infants and Children: Safety and effectiveness for use by those under 12 not established.

By Those Over 60 Years of Age: May be more likely to be weak, dizzy or faint or fall. Be careful to prevent injury. Low starting doses are prudent.

▷ **Advisability of Use During Pregnancy**

Pregnancy Category: C. See Pregnancy Risk Categories at the back of this book.

Animal studies: No information available.

Human studies: Adequate studies of pregnant women are not available.

Avoid this drug during the first 3 months. Use during the last 6 months only if clearly needed. Ask your physician for guidance.

Advisability of Use If Breast-Feeding

Presence of this drug in breast milk: Unknown.

Avoid drug or refrain from nursing.

Habit-Forming Potential: None.

Effects of Overdose: Weakness, fainting, fast pulse, low blood pressure, slow heartbeat, metabolic acidosis, low potassium and calcium, sinus arrest, heart attack, seizures.

Possible Effects of Long-Term Use: Possible overgrowth of the gums.

Suggested Periodic Examinations While Taking This Drug (at physician's discretion)

Heart function tests: electrocardiograms; blood pressure check while supine, sitting and standing.

▷ **While Taking This Drug, Observe the Following**

Foods: This medicine is increased by grapefruit or grapefruit juice. Avoid eating grapefruit for an hour after taking this medicine. Avoid excessive salt intake.

Herbal Medicines or Minerals: Ginseng may increase blood pressure, blunting the benefits of this medicine. Eleuthero root, hawthorn, saw palmetto, ma huang, goldenseal and licorice may also cause increased blood pressure. Indian snakeroot, calcium and garlic may help lower blood pressure. Ask your doctor if calcium and/or garlic makes sense for you. Talk to your doctor BEFORE adding any herbal medicines.

Beverages: See foods above. May be taken with milk.

▷ *Alcohol:* Use caution. Alcohol may exaggerate the drop in blood pressure.

Tobacco Smoking: Nicotine may reduce the effectiveness of this drug. I advise everyone to quit smoking.

Marijuana Smoking: Possible reduced effectiveness of this drug; mild to moderate increase in angina; possible changes in electrocardiogram, confusing interpretation.

▷ *Other Drugs*

Amlodipine *taken concurrently* with

- adenosine (Adenocard) may cause extended problems with slow heart rate.
- amiodarone (Cordarone) may worsen AV block or cause further slowing of the heart in partial atrioventricular (AV) block or sick sinus syndrome.
- azole antifungals (such as fluconazole [Diflucan] or itraconazole [Sporanox]) and imidazoles (see Drug Classes) such as ketoconazole (Nizoral) may lead to toxic amlodipine blood levels.
- beta-blocker drugs or digitalis preparations (see Drug Classes) may cause heart rate and rhythm problems.
- cyclosporine (Sandimmune) causes increased cyclosporine blood levels and increased risk of toxicity.
- delavirdine (Rescriptor) may cause increased amlodipine levels and toxicity.
- dofetilide (Tikosyn) may cause dofetilide toxicity.
- medicines that inhibit cytochrome P450 3A4 will increase amlodipine blood levels and those that induce 3A4 will decrease amlodipine blood levels.
- NSAIDs or oral anticoagulants such as Coumadin (warfarin—see Drug Classes) may lead to increased risk of bleeding in the gastrointestinal (GI) tract.
- quinupristin/dalfopristin (Synercid) may cause extended amlodipine effects or toxicity.
- rifampin (Rifater, others) may result in decreased therapeutic benefit of amlodipine.
- ritonavir (Norvir) and probably other protease inhibitors (see Drug Classes) may lead to amlodipine toxicity.

The following drug may *increase* the effects of amlodipine

- cimetidine (Tagamet).

▷ *Driving, Hazardous Activities:* This drug may cause dizziness. Restrict activities as necessary.

Aviation Note: Coronary artery disease *is a disqualification* for piloting. Consult a designated Aviation Medical Examiner.

Exposure to Sun: Four case reports of phototoxicity have been made. Caution is advised.

Exposure to Heat: Caution is advised. Hot environments can exaggerate the blood-pressure-lowering effects of this drug. Observe for light-headedness or weakness.

Heavy Exercise or Exertion: This drug may improve your ability to be more active without resulting angina pain. Use caution.

Discontinuation: Do not stop this drug abruptly—gradual withdrawal is often prudent. Watch for development of rebound angina.

AMOXAPINE (a MOX a peen)

Introduced: 1970   **Class:** Antidepressant   **Prescription:** USA: Yes
Controlled Drug: USA: No; Canada: No   **Available as Generic:** Yes
Brand Name: Asendin

BENEFITS versus RISKS	
Possible Benefits	*Possible Risks*
EFFECTIVE RELIEF OF PRIMARY DEPRESSIONS: ENDOGENOUS, NEUROTIC, REACTIVE	ADVERSE BEHAVIORAL EFFECTS: CONFUSION, DELUSIONS, DISORIENTATION, HALLUCINATIONS
	CONVERSION OF DEPRESSION TO MANIA IN MANIC-DEPRESSIVE DISORDERS
	Rare blood cell abnormalities
	Rare movement disorders
	Rare seizures
	Rare liver toxicity

Author's Note: Since use of this medicine has declined in favor of newer medicines, the information in this profile has been shortened.

AMOXICILLIN (a mox i SIL in)

AMOXICILLIN/CLAVULANATE (a mox i SIL in/KLAV yu lan ayt)

AMPICILLIN (am pi SIL in)

Please see the penicillin family profile for further information.

ANGIOTENSIN CONVERTING ENZYME (ACE) INHIBITOR FAMILY

Benazepril (ben AY ze pril)   **Captopril** (KAP toh pril)   **Enalapril** (e NAL a pril)   **Fosinopril** (Foh SIN oh pril)   **Lisinopril** (li SIN oh pril)

Quinapril   (KWIN a pril)   **Ramipril**   (RAH mi pril)

Introduced: 1985, 1979, 1981, 1986, 1988, 1984, 1985, respectively   **Class:** ACE inhibitor, antihypertensive   **Prescription:** USA: Yes   **Controlled Drug:** USA: No; Canada: No   **Available as Generic:** Yes (captopril and enalapril)

Brand Names: Benazepril: Lotensin, Lotensin HCT [CD], Lotrel [CD], Captopril: ✹Apo-Capto, Capoten, Capozide [CD], ✹Novo-Captopril, ✹Nu-Capto, ✹Syn-Captopril, Enalapril: Lexxel [CD], ✹Vaseretic (also in U.S.) [CD], Vasotec, Fosinopril: Monopril, Lisinopril: Prinivil, Prinzide [CD], Zestoretic [CD], Zestril, Quinapril: Accupril, Accuretic, Ramipril: Altace

Author's Note: Ramipril (Altace) plus felodipine is available as a combination product in Canada only. Perindopril (Aceon), moexipril (Univasc), moexipril/hydrochlorothiazide (Uniretic), trandolapril (Mavik) and trandolapril/verapamil (Tarka) information will be added to this profile in future editions if differential benefits emerge from clinical studies.

BENEFITS versus RISKS

Possible Benefits	*Possible Risks*
RAMIPRIL HAS DATA SHOWING THAT IT CAN DECREASE THE RISK OF HEART ATTACK AND STROKE (lowered cardiovascular events by 22% in the HOPE trial; it is unknown if this is a class effect or not)	Impaired white blood cell production—rare (not for ramipril)
	Bone marrow depression—rare (not for ramipril)
EFFECTIVE CONTROL OF MILD TO SEVERE HIGH BLOOD PRESSURE	Allergic swelling of face, tongue, throat, vocal cords—possible
USEFUL ADJUNCTIVE TREATMENT FOR CONGESTIVE HEART FAILURE	Kidney damage—rare (enalapril, lisinopril, quinapril and ramipril lower risk)
MAY DECREASE RISK OF KIDNEY PROBLEMS IN DIABETICS TAKING INSULIN (CAPTOPRIL)	Liver damage—rare (not for ramipril)
MAY REDUCE RISK OF DEATH AND/OR CONGESTIVE HEART FAILURE AFTER HEART ATTACK (RAMIPRIL, CAPTOPRIL AND LISINOPRIL ARE FDA-APPROVED FOR THIS)	
MAY BE DRUGS OF FIRST CHOICE FOR PATIENTS WITH HIGH BLOOD PRESSURE WHO EXERCISE	
COMBINATION USE OF PERINDOPRIL WITH INDAPAMIDE REDUCED RISK OF RECURRENT STROKE BY NEARLY HALF IN ONE STUDY	
Quinapril has been shown to stimulate growth of new blood vessels in laboratory animals	

▷ **Principal Uses**

As Single Drug Products: Uses currently included in FDA-approved labeling: (1) Treats all degrees of high blood pressure; (2) may help prevent death after heart attacks; (3) used in advanced heart failure; (4) used in diabetics who have kidney problems; (5) helps people live longer (improves survival) in cases of congestive heart failure; (6) ramipril approved to lower risk of heart and blood vessel disease (cardiovascular) in people with coronary artery disease, stroke, diabetes or peripheral vascular disease who have one or more risk factors (for example—high cholesterol or blood pressure).

Author's Note: Enalapril was studied in the ABCD trial and was found to control blood pressure and also decrease risk of heart attack in people living with diabetes. Follow-up research is pending.

Other (unlabeled) generally accepted uses: (1) Helps relieve symptoms of cystinuria (captopril); (2) may ease rheumatoid arthritis symptoms (captopril or enalapril); (3) can help Raynaud's phenomenon symptoms (captopril); (4) lisinopril may help prevent migraines; (5) enalapril and quinapril may be helpful in aortic regurgitation; (6) helps treat increased blood pressure resulting from blood vessel problems in the kidneys (renovascular hypertension) in people who can't have angioplasty or surgery; (7) combination use of indapamide with perindopril (Aceon) reduced risk of repeat stroke by nearly 50% in one study.

Author's Note: One large study found that patients using captopril had similar low rates of nonfatal and fatal heart (cardiovascular) events to patients taking beta-blockers or diuretics. Another study showed that fosinopril cut the risk of heart attack or stroke by 51% in people who have high blood pressure and diabetes.

As Combination Drug Products [CD]: In combination with hydrochlorothiazide, captopril, enalapril, lisinopril and benazepril offer the benefits of an ACE inhibitor and a diuretic. Benazepril has also been combined with amlodipine, a calcium channel blocker.

How These Drugs Work: By blocking an enzyme system (angiotensin converting enzyme or ACE), these drugs relax arterial walls and lower pressure. This decreases the work a heart has to do and improves performance. Benefits after heart attack come from blunting reaction to catecholamines, scavenging free-radicals and increasing prostacyclin or bradykinin. Some members of this class must be converted by the liver to the active drug form. Combined therapy with diuretics helps ease fluid load. Combination with a calcium channel blocker works by blocking calcium channels and acts primarily on peripheral circulation to lower blood pressure. Amlodipine offers the further advantage of getting into the body well (bioavailability) and increased binding when blood flow is compromised (ischemic conditions and low pH).

Available Dosage Forms and Strengths

Benazepril:

Capsules — 2.5 mg of amlodipine with 10 mg of benazepril, 5 mg of amlodipine with 10 mg of benazepril and 5 mg of amlodipine with 20 mg of benazepril (Lotrel form)

Tablets — 5 mg, 10 mg, 20 mg, 40 mg (Lotensin)

Captopril:

> Tablets — 12.5 mg, 25 mg, 50 mg, 100 mg
> Tablet, combination (Capozide) — 25 or 50 mg captopril with
> 15 or 25 mg of
> hydrochlorothiazide

Enalapril:

> Injection — 1.25 mg/ml
> Tablets — 2.5 mg, 5 mg, 10 mg, 20 mg
> Tablets (Vaseretic) — 10 mg enalapril and 25 mg of
> hydrochlorothiazide

Fosinopril:

> Tablets — 10 mg, 20 mg, 40 mg

Lisinopril:

> Tablets — 2.5 mg, 5 mg, 10 mg, 20 mg,
> 30 mg, 40 mg
> Tablet, combination (Prinzide, Zestoretic) — 20 mg lisinopril with 12.5 or
> 25 mg of hydrochlorothiazide

Quinapril:

> Tablets — 5 mg, 10 mg, 20 mg, 40 mg
> Tablet, combination (Accuretic) — 10 or 20 mg of quinapril with
> 12.5 or 25 mg of
> hydrochlorothiazide

Ramipril:

> Capsules (gelcaps in Canada) — 1.25 mg, 2.5 mg, 5 mg, 10 mg

▷ **Usual Dosage Ranges for Infants and Children**

Captopril: One study used a starting dose of 0.01 to 0.25 mg per kg of body mass every 12 hours in infants; 0.05 to 0.5 mg per kg of body mass three times daily has been used in older children. Maximum dose is 2 mg/kg per dose up to three times a day.

Enalapril: Malignant Hypertension: 0.625–1.25 mg per dose, given every 6 hours. Maximum dose is 5 mg every 6 hours intravenously. In hypertension (while not recommended by the manufacturer): 0.04 mg per kg of body weight daily.

Quinapril, benazepril, ramipril, fosinopril and lisinopril: Dosage not established in infants and children.

▷ **Usual Adult Dosage Ranges**

For high blood pressure:

Captopril: 25 mg two or three times daily for 1–2 weeks. If pressure goals are not met—dose may be increased to 50 mg three times daily if needed. If blood pressure still not acceptable, a diuretic (low dose similar to 25 mg of hydrochlorothiazide) or change to a combination form may be needed. Maximum daily dose is 450 mg.

Enalapril (if not also taking a diuretic): 5 mg once daily starting dose. Usual ongoing dose is 10 to 40 mg daily in a single dose or divided into two equal doses. Total daily dose should not exceed 40 mg if kidney function is impaired. If pressure goals are not met by enalapril alone, a diuretic can be added (pill burden is decreased by fixed dose combinations).

Fosinopril (18 to 60 years of age): For hypertension, initially 10 mg once daily. Usual maintenance dose is 20 to 40 mg daily taken in a single dose. Total daily dosage should not exceed 80 mg.

Quinapril, benazepril, lisinopril (12 to 60 years of age): 10 mg once daily for those not taking a diuretic; 5 mg once daily if taking a diuretic. Usual ongoing dose is 20 to 40 mg daily, taken in a single dose. If once-a-day dosing does not give stable blood pressure control over the day, divide the dose equally into morning and evening doses. Total daily dose is 80 mg.

Ramipril: Initially 2.5 mg once daily for 2 to 4 weeks. Usual ongoing dose is 2.5 to 20 mg daily in a single dose or two divided doses. If taking diuretics, either stop diuretic for 3 days before starting this drug or begin treatment with 1.25 mg of this drug.

For congestive heart failure (CHF):

Captopril: Doses of 25 mg three times daily are suggested. Lower doses (6.25 to 12.5 mg) three times daily reduce risk of excessively low blood pressure.

Enalapril: 2.5 to 10 mg once or twice daily. Usually combined with other medications. Maximum is 40 mg daily.

Fosinopril: Starting doses of 5 mg (especially for dehydrated patients or those who have kidney failure) to 10 mg have been recommended. Some studies have used once-daily dosing. Dosing must be individualized.

Ramipril: Test dose of 1.25 mg, then a dose of 2.5 to 5 mg twice a day.

To decrease cardiovascular risk:

Ramipril: Starting dose 2.5 mg a day, followed by 5 to 10 mg daily.

After a heart attack:

Captopril: A test dose of 6.25 mg is given to see if excessive lowering of the blood pressure occurs. Test usually delayed until 3 days after heart attack. If the test is tolerated, 12.5 mg is given three times a day. This dose is then increased toward a goal of 50 mg three times a day.

Enalapril: Test dose of 2.5 mg (24 hours after a heart attack), followed by 2.5 mg twice a day, with increase (titration) to 20 mg as quickly as tolerated (in the EDEN study).

Lisinopril (when hemodynamically stable): 5 mg may be given within 24 hours after symptoms started. If this dose is tolerated, a repeat dose is given 24 hours later and then increased to 10 mg a day. Therapy continues for at least 6 weeks.

Ramipril: 10 mg a day started within 24 hours has been used. Protocol driven systems have used 1.25 mg to start, then 2.5 mg given 12 hours later, followed by daily interval increases to 10 mg once a day.

Diabetic kidney problems (nephropathy) and eye problems (retinopathy):

Captopril: Success has been achieved with 50 mg twice daily in two large studies. The manufacturer suggests a starting dose of 25 mg three times a day.

Over 60 Years of Age:

Captopril: Dosing interval is adjusted to any age-related decrease in creatinine clearance or glomerular filtration rate. The initial change (cut point) is from 75 to 35 ml/minute: dose every 12 to 24 hours. Dosing is started once a day and increased as needed and tolerated.

Enalapril: Same as in younger patients, with dosing corrected for age-related decline in kidney function.

Benazepril: Same as 12 to 60 years of age, if kidney function is normal. If kidney function is significantly impaired, reduce dose by 50%. Total daily maximum is 40 mg in those with impaired kidneys.

Fosinopril: Same as 18 to 60 years of age, but these patients may be more sensitive to fosinopril. Smaller and more gradual dose increases are prudent as needed and tolerated.

Lisinopril: Exercise tolerance was improved by 2.5 to 20 mg daily. Any needed dose increases should be made at longer intervals between adjustments.

Quinapril: Same as 12 to 60 years of age, if kidney function is normal. If kidney function is significantly impaired, reduce dose by 50%. The total daily dose should not exceed 40 mg.

Ramipril: Small doses are advisable until tolerance has been determined. Sudden and excessive lowering of blood pressure can predispose to stroke or heart attack in those with impaired brain circulation or coronary artery heart disease.

Note: Actual dose and schedule must be determined for each patient individually.

Conditions Requiring Dosing Adjustments

Liver Function:

Captopril: Must be used with extreme caution and started at a lower dose in liver failure.

Enalapril: In patients with liver compromise, the dose may need to be **increased** because less of the drug is activated.

Fosinopril: Is a prodrug and is changed into fosinoprilat (the active form) by the liver. Use with caution and in lower doses by patients with liver compromise.

Quinapril, benazepril and lisinopril: The liver is minimally involved in removing these drugs.

Ramipril: Close monitoring for adverse effects is prudent.

Kidney Function:

Benazepril: For people with creatinine clearances of less than 30 ml/min, or serum creatinine greater than 3 mg/dl (ask your doctor), the starting dose should be 5 mg once daily.

Captopril: Increased blood level and risk of adverse effects (low blood counts and protein in the urine) if used in kidney failure. **Must** decrease dose according to decreases in creatinine clearance. The lowest effective dose must be used.

Enalapril: Patients with mild to moderate kidney failure can be given 5 mg/day. In severe kidney failure, maximum dose is 2.5 mg/day.

Fosinopril: This drug undergoes liver and bile (dual hepatobiliary) and kidney (renal) elimination. Patients with renal compromise (especially those with renal artery stenosis) should start on a decreased dose, with slow dose increases if needed.

Lisinopril: Patients with moderate kidney failure should be started on 5 mg daily. In severe kidney failure, the patient can take 2.5 mg of lisinopril daily. This drug is contraindicated in kidney blood flow problems (renal artery stenosis). Combination (with hydrochlorothiazide) drugs (fixed dose products) should NOT be used in kidney failure as loop (see Drug Classes) diuretics are more effective.

Quinapril: Patients with mild kidney failure can take 10 mg daily. Those with moderate kidney failure should take 5 mg daily. In severe kidney failure, 2.5 mg per day may be taken. If needed and tolerated, dose increases should only be made every 2 weeks.

Ramipril: For patients with moderate kidney failure or creatinine values of greater than 2.5 mg/dl, 1.25 mg of ramipril can be taken daily.

Diabetes:

Enalapril: Patients with diabetes with decreased creatinine clearance and protein in the urine (proteinuria) should be given decreased doses.

▷ **Dosing Instructions**

Captopril: Best taken on empty stomach, 1 hour before meals.

Enalapril, quinapril, benazepril, ramipril, fosinopril and lisinopril: May be taken without regard to food. All ACE drugs should be taken at the same time each day, and all ACE tablets at the time of this writing may be crushed if needed to make them easier to take. If extended-release forms are present when you read this profile—talk to your doctor and pharmacist before crushing any dosage form. If you forget a dose: Take the medicine right away, unless it is nearly time for your next dose, then skip or omit the missed dose and take the medicine when it was next scheduled. DO NOT double doses.

Usual Duration of Use: Several weeks of use on a regular schedule may be required to see best benefits in lowering high blood pressure and for other uses. Use may be a partnership for life for taking control of high blood pressure and when used in kidney disease. Periodic evaluation by your doctor is needed.

Typical Treatment Goals and Measurements (Outcomes and Markers)

Blood Pressure: The most recent treatment guidelines (JNC VI) define optimal blood pressure (BP) as less than 120/80 and high normal as 139/89. The American Diabetes Association recommends 130/80 as the target for people living with diabetes. Most clinicians try to achieve a BP that confers the best balance of lower cardiovascular risk and avoids the problem of too low a blood pressure. Blood pressure duration is generally increased with beneficial restriction of sodium. The goals and time frame should be discussed with you when the prescription is written. If goals are not met, it is not unusual to increase doses or add on medicines.

Possible Advantages of These Drugs

Quinapril, benazepril, ramipril, fosinopril and lisinopril control blood pressure effectively with one daily dose with relatively low incidence of adverse effects (ramipril at present has the most favorable data). No adverse influence on asthma, cholesterol blood levels or diabetes. Sudden withdrawal does not result in a rapid increase in blood pressure.

Captopril has a special chemical (sulfhydryl group) at its active site. This may help it ease intolerance to nitrates. Lisinopril and captopril DO NOT require activation by the liver to work. They may be drugs of choice in situations where an ACE inhibitor is desirable and liver compromise is also present. Quinapril goes into tissues well and may have a future role in treating or preventing problems (dysfunction) of the lining (endothelium) of blood vessels. Quinapril also has some laboratory data showing it to be able to stimulate growth of new blood vessels in laboratory animals. The Joint National Committee number six (see JNC VI in Glossary) advocates ACE inhibitors as preferred medicines in diabetics with high blood pressure who have protein in their urine.

Ramipril has important and robust data to show it decreases risk of heart attack and stroke! The HOPE trial showed ramipril to decrease risk of death from any heart (cardiovascular) event by 25%, nonfatal heart attack by 20% and nonfatal stroke by 32%. This is remarkable by itself, yet dramatic when coupled with a 30% lowering of development of diabetes and kidney disease in people living with diabetes.

ACE inhibitors in general are drugs of first choice in African Americans who are at risk for or who have kidney (renal) problems (dysfunction). The African American Study of Kidney Disease and Hypertension research showed that African Americans with nephrosclerosis and hypertension who took ramipril (Altace) were found to have a 41% lower risk of end-stage kidney disease and death than those taking amlodipine (a calcium channel blocker).

▷ **These Drugs Should Not Be Taken If**
- you have had an allergic reaction to them.
- you develop swelling of the tongue, face or throat while taking this drug or with a previous ACE inhibitor. Call your doctor immediately if this effect starts while taking this medicine.
- you are pregnant (last 6 months).
- you currently have a blood cell or bone marrow disorder.
- you have an abnormally high level of blood potassium.

▷ **Inform Your Physician Before Taking These Drugs If**
- you develop swelling of the tongue, face or throat while taking this drug. Call your doctor immediately.
- you are planning pregnancy or to breast-feed your child.
- you have kidney disease or impaired kidney function.
- you have had an allergic reaction while undergoing desensitization for bee stings (ask your doctor).
- you have scleroderma or systemic lupus erythematosus.
- you have any form of heart or liver disease.
- you have diabetes.
- you have an elevated potassium level.
- you have a blood cell disorder.
- you take other antihypertensives, diuretics, nitrates, allopurinol (Zyloprim), Indocin or potassium supplements.
- you will have surgery with general anesthesia.
- you have renal artery stenosis (ask your doctor).
- you are taking medicines that suppress the immune system.
- you are unsure how much to take or how often to take it.

Possible Side Effects (natural, expected and unavoidable drug actions)
Dizziness, light-headedness, fainting (excessive drop in blood pressure). Increased heart rate on standing (captopril).
Scalded mouth sensation for some class members.
Impaired sense of smell—case reports for enalapril.
Nausea or constipation, increased blood potassium—all rare.
Cough—rare to infrequent.

▷ **Possible Adverse Effects** (unusual, unexpected and infrequent reactions)
If any of the following develop, consult your physician promptly for guidance.
Mild Adverse Effects
Allergic reactions: skin rash, psoriasis—rare to infrequent.
Swelling of face, hands or feet; fever—rare.

Ringing in the ears (tinnitus)—lisinopril—rare.

Lost or altered (metallic or salty) taste, mouth or tongue sores—case reports.

Hair loss—captopril—possible.

Headache—infrequent.

Nightmares, joint pain—rare.

Increased temperature (hyperthermia)—case reports (captopril).

Low blood sugar—case reports (idiosyncratic?—and limited clinical effect)—captopril and enalapril.

Rapid heart rate on standing—case reports.

Vulvovaginal itching—case reports (enalapril).

Serious Adverse Effects

Allergic reactions: swelling (angioedema) of face, tongue and/or vocal cords—rare; can be life-threatening—case reports.

Bone marrow depression (neutropenia, anemia, aplastic anemia): weakness, fever, sore throat, bleeding or bruising—rare (infrequent in kidney failure and collagen vascular disease)(not reported for ramipril).

Hemolytic or aplastic anemia—case reports (not for ramipril).

Kidney damage: water retention (edema)—case reports for some (first 8 months usually for captopril).

Elevated blood potassium (hyperkalemia)—case reports.

Rare fluid formation around the heart (pericarditis)—case reports (captopril).

Hallucinations—rare (captopril, quinapril and enalapril).

Stevens-Johnson syndrome, lupus erythematosus or other serious skin conditions (some members of this class)—rare.

Pancreatitis—case reports with some members of this class.

Liver damage (with or without jaundice)—rare.

▷ **Possible Effects on Sexual Function:** Decreased male libido—rare. Impotence. Swelling and tenderness of male breast tissue (gynecomastia)—rare.

Possible Effects on Laboratory Tests

Complete blood counts: decreased red cells, hemoglobin, white cells and platelets; increased eosinophils.

Blood antinuclear antibodies (ANA): increased (captopril, lisinopril).

Blood cholesterol and triglycerides: decreased (benazepril) (7.6–13.1%).

Blood sodium level: decreased.

Blood urea nitrogen level (BUN): increased.

Blood uric acid level: may be increased (ramipril).

Insulin sensitivity: increased—captopril.

Blood potassium level: may be increased.

Liver function tests: increased liver enzymes (alkaline phosphatase, AST/GOT, LDH), increased bilirubin—possible.

Urine ketone tests: false positive results with Keto-Diastix and Chemstrip-6 (captopril).

Blood sugar (glucose): decreased—case reports (captopril).

Venereal Disease Research Laboratory (VDRL): rare false-positive results (captopril).

Digoxin blood level: may read falsely low with fosinopril.

CAUTION

1. If possible, may be best to stop all other antihypertensive drugs (especially diuretics) for 1 week before starting.

2. **Tell your doctor immediately if you become pregnant.** These drugs should not be taken after the first 3 months of pregnancy.
3. **Report promptly** any signs of infection (fever, sore throat) and any indications of water retention (weight gain, swollen feet or ankles).
4. Many salt substitutes contain potassium; ask your doctor before using.
5. Blood counts and urine analyses are needed **before taking these medicines.**
6. The FDA has started to evaluate blood levels of ACE inhibitors (trough to peak ratios—T/P—see Glossary) to check how these medicines should be dosed best. Talk to your doctor about this concept.
7. One observational epidemiologic study found that ACE inhibitors were often prescribed in lower than recommended doses and were also underused. Check your ACE inhibitor dose, and ask if an ACE inhibitor is appropriate if you are NOT currently taking one.
8. High blood pressure rarely has symptoms. If this medicine is controlling your blood pressure, STAY ON IT—even if you never felt sick from your prior high blood pressure.

Precautions for Use
By Infants and Children: Benazepril, enalapril, fosinopril, lisinopril, quinapril and ramipril: Safety and effectiveness not established.
By Those Over 60 Years of Age: Small starting doses advisable. Sudden or excessive lowering of blood pressure can cause stroke or heart attack.

▷ **Advisability of Use During Pregnancy**
Pregnancy Category: C during the first 3 months; **D during the last 6 months** (last two trimesters). See Pregnancy Risk Categories at the back of this book.
Animal studies: Birth defects found in some animals for some ACE inhibitors.
Human studies: The use of ACE inhibitor drugs during the last 6 months of pregnancy is known to possibly cause very serious injury and possible death to the fetus; skull and limb malformations, lung defects and kidney failure have been reported in over 50 cases (captopril) worldwide.
Avoid these drugs completely during the last 6 months. During the first 3 months of pregnancy, use this drug only if clearly needed. Ask your doctor for guidance.

Advisability of Use If Breast-Feeding
Presence of this drug in breast milk: Yes, in small amounts (captopril, enalapril and ramipril); benazepril—in very small amounts; lisinopril, quinapril, fosinopril—unknown.
Monitor nursing infant closely, and discontinue drug or nursing if adverse effects develop. Breast-feeding while taking ramipril is not recommended.

Habit-Forming Potential: None.

Effects of Overdose: Excessive drop in blood pressure—light-headedness, dizziness, fainting.

Possible Effects of Long-Term Use: Gradual increase in blood potassium level, cough.

Suggested Periodic Examinations While Taking These Drugs (at physician's discretion)
Before drug is started: complete blood cell count, urine analysis and blood potassium level.

Once started: Blood counts during the first 3 months, then periodically. Urine protein every month for the first 9 months, then periodically. Periodic blood potassium tests. ANA titer.

▷ **While Taking This Drug, Observe the Following**

Foods: Talk to your doctor about salt intake.

Herbal Medicines or Minerals: Ginseng may increase blood pressure, blunting the benefits of this medicine. Hawthorn, saw palmetto, ma huang, goldenseal and licorice may also cause increased blood pressure. Calcium and garlic may help lower blood pressure. One case report of excessively low zinc in a kidney (polycystic kidney) patient for captopril. Talk with your doctor before combining any herbal medicine with your current prescriptions.

Nutritional Support: **Do not** take potassium supplements unless directed by your doctor. Case reports of zinc deficiency have been made (captopril). Large amounts of garlic, soy and calcium may lower blood pressure. A small study by Hong at Sungkyukwan University in Seoul found that use of 256 mg of iron daily over a 4-week treatment period found all of the treatment group to have their cough improved with three patients nearly stopping this adverse effect. Further research is needed. Talk to your doctor to find out if additional research has been done, if this iron benefit only applies to patients with low iron or if a consensus has developed that rational use of iron while avoiding iron side effects makes sense for you.

Beverages: No restrictions. May be taken with milk.

▷ *Alcohol:* Alcohol can further lower blood pressure. Use with caution.

Tobacco Smoking: Smoking can certainly irritate the airways and since these medicines can also lead to cough, smoking is not advisable. I advise everyone to quit smoking.

▷ *Other Drugs*

These medicines *taken concurrently* with

- allopurinol (Zyloprim) may increase risk of serious skin reactions.
- azathioprine (Imuran) may result in severe anemia.
- clomipramine (Anafranil, others) may result in clomipramine toxicity and confusion, mood changes and irritability. Lower doses may be required if these medicines are combined.
- cyclosporine (Sandimmune) may result in kidney failure that takes a while to appear (delayed acute renal dysfunction).
- erythropoietin (various) may result in lowered erythropoietin benefits.
- iron (various) may result in decreased ACE inhibitor absorption and blunted benefits. Separate dosing by 1 to 2 hours.
- interferons (alpha and beta) may greatly increase risk of blood problems with some members of this class. DO NOT combine (lisinopril, quinapril, benazepril—case reports).
- lithium (Lithobid, others) may result in toxic blood lithium levels and **toxicity.**
- loop diuretics (such as Lasix or Bumex; see Drug Classes) may cause excessively low blood pressure on standing (postural hypotension) but may also be therapeutically needed.
- metformin (Glucophage) lead to high potassium levels and lactic acidosis in a diabetic patient with kidney compromise who combined metformin and enalapril.

- oral hypoglycemic agents (glyburide—Glynase, others) may result in decreased insulin resistance and the need to decrease the dose of the oral hypoglycemic agent (enalapril only).
- phenothiazines (see Drug Classes) may result in postural hypotension.
- potassium preparations (K-Lyte, Slow-K, etc.) will increase blood potassium with risk of serious heart rhythm disturbances.
- potassium-sparing diuretics—amiloride (Moduretic), spironolactone (Aldactazide), triamterene (Dyazide)—may increase blood levels of potassium with risk of serious heart rhythm disturbances.
- rifampin (Rifadin) or rifabutin (Mycobutin) may cause decreased therapeutic benefit from enalapril.
- thiazide diuretics (hydrochlorothiazide, others) may result (especially in older people) in increased levels of enalaprilat (the active medicine) and increased reduction in blood pressure. May be used to therapeutic benefit.
- cotrimoxazole (trimethoprim component; Bactrim, Trimpex, others) may increase blood potassium (risk of serious heart rhythm disturbances).

The following drugs may *decrease* the effects of these medicines:
- antacids—by decreasing captopril (and perhaps other ACEs) absorption. Separate doses by 2 hours.
- COX-II inhibitors.
- ibuprofen (Motrin), indomethacin (Indocin) or other NSAIDs (see Drug Classes).
- naloxone (Narcan).
- salicylates (aspirin, etc.) or other NSAIDs (see Drug Classes).

▷ *Driving, Hazardous Activities:* Usually no restrictions. Be aware of possible drops in blood pressure with resultant dizziness or faintness.

Aviation Note: The use of these drugs *may be a disqualification* for piloting. Consult a designated Aviation Medical Examiner.

Exposure to Sun: Caution is advised. Some drugs in this class can cause photosensitivity (captopril, ramipril).

Exposure to Heat: Caution is advised. Excessive perspiring may drop blood pressure.

Occurrence of Unrelated Illness: Call your doctor to report any disorder causing vomiting or diarrhea. Fluid and chemical imbalances must be corrected as soon as possible.

Discontinuation: Captopril, lisinopril, quinapril, fosinopril and benazepril have been stopped abruptly without causing a sudden increase in blood pressure (though not recommended). Ask your doctor before stopping any drug for any reason.

ANGIOTENSIN II RECEPTOR ANTAGONIST FAMILY

Candesartan (KAN da sar tan)   **Eprosartan** (Eh PRO sar tan)   **Irbesartan** (Ir BAH sar tan)   **Losartan** (LOW sar tan)   **Telmisartan** (TELL mih sar tan)   **Valsartan** (VAL sar tan)

Introduced: 1998, 1999, 1997, 1995, 1998, 1997, respectively   **Class:** Angiotensin II antagonists (ARBs)   **Prescription:** USA: Yes   **Controlled Drug** USA: No; Canada: No   **Available as Generic:** USA: No; Canada: No

Brand Names: *Candesartan:* Atacand, Atacand HCT [CD]; *Eprosartan:* Teveten; *Irbesartan:* Avapro, Avalide [CD]; *Losartan:* Cozaar, Hyzaar [CD]; *Telmisartan:* Micardis; *Valsartan:* Diovan, Diovan HCT [CD]

Author's Note: Information in this profile will be broadened in subsequent editions to include data on eprosartan and telmisartan if the data warrant inclusion. Early information showed that using eprosartan WITH an ACE inhibitor reduced blood pressure (diastolic—the bottom blood pressure number) in people with chronic heart failure—yet did NOT increase heart rate as an undesirable effect.

BENEFITS versus RISKS	
Possible Benefits	*Possible Risks*
EFFECTIVE CONTROL OF HIGH BLOOD PRESSURE	Increased liver function tests (all except irbesartan)
DECREASED NUMBER OF DEATHS FROM CONGESTIVE HEART FAILURE (LOSARTAN)	
Decreased cough side effect versus ACE inhibitors	
Candesartan increases insulin sensitivity	

▷ **Principal Uses**

As a Single Drug Product: Uses currently included in FDA-approved labeling: (1) Treatment of high blood pressure; (2) decreases abnormal size of the left ventricle (left ventricular hypertrophy)(losartan); (3) candesartan works to increase insulin sensitivity.

Author's Note: The JNC VI (see Glossary) report placed use of these medicines as appropriate in patients who have indications for ACE therapy but do not tolerate those medicines (such as intolerable ACE inhibitor–induced cough). The International Society for Hypertension recommended this class of medicines as first-line treatment in patients with heart failure. Some early data show some reversal of fibrosis in animals treated with losartan.

Other (unlabeled) generally accepted uses: The ELITE study compared losartan to an ACE inhibitor (in patients over 65 with ejection fraction mean of 30%) and found a significant decrease in deaths for any reason (all-cause death) in treating congestive heart failure. (1) Congestive heart failure; (2) excessive protein excretion in diabetic patients (nephropathy).

As Combination Drug Products [CD]: These medicines have been combined with hydrochlorothiazide in fixed-dose forms. These drugs complement each other, making the combination a more effective antihypertensive.

How These Drugs Work: They block the effects of angiotensin II by binding to a specific site (the AT1 receptor). This helps the blood vessels stay open and lowers blood pressure. These drugs and some of their metabolites also block aldosterone, something of benefit in congestive heart failure. When combined with hydrochlorothiazide, these medicines have the added benefit of removing excessive accumulation of body water.

Available Dosage Forms and Strengths

Candesartan:

Tablet — 4 mg, 8 mg, 16 mg and 32 mg

Tablet (*Atacand HCT*) — candesartan 16mg or 32 mg and hydrochlorothiazide (HCTZ) 12.5 mg

Irbesartan:

Tablet — 75 mg, 150 mg, 300 mg

Tablet (*Avalide* irbesartan and HCTZ) — irbesartan 150 or 300 mg and HCTZ 12.5 mg

Losartan:

Tablet — 25 mg, 50 mg

Tablet (*Hyzaar*) — losartan 50 mg and HCTZ 12.5 mg

Valsartan:

Tablet — 80 mg and 160 mg

Tablet (*Diovan HCT*) — valsartan 80 mg and HCTZ 12.5 mg

— valsartan 160 mg and HCTZ 12.5 mg

▷ **Recommended Dosage Ranges** (Actual dose and schedule must be determined for each patient individually.)

Infants and Children: Not recommended for use in this age group.

18 to 60 Years of Age:

Candesartan: Starting dose of 16 mg a day in patients who have normal blood volume (normovolemic). Hypovolemic patients are given lower starting doses. Some European countries use lower starting doses in all patients and a maximum of 8 mg. Doses may be increased as needed and tolerated to 32 mg once daily.

Irbesartan: Starting dose of 150 mg daily. This dose may be increased as needed and tolerated to 300 mg daily. A starting dose of 75 mg daily is used in people also taking hydrochlorothiazide.

Losartan: A starting dose of 50 mg daily is used. If the blood pressure response is not sufficient, the same dose may be divided into two equal doses and given twice daily. The dose may also be increased as needed and tolerated and taken in two divided doses daily. Peak effects may not be seen for 3 to 6 weeks before dosing changes are made. The maximum daily dose is 100 mg.

Valsartan: Starting dose is 80 mg daily. Dosing may be increased to a maximum of 320 mg once daily as needed and tolerated. Many clinicians will change to a combination HCTZ form if goals are not met with a 160-mg dose of the single-ingredient product.

Over 60 Years of Age:

Candesartan: No initial dose change needed, but some older patients may be more sensitive than younger ones.

Irbesartan: No age-related changes needed.

Losartan: Patients who are dehydrated or have a decreased intravascular volume should take 25 mg once daily as a starting dose.

Valsartan: No clinically relevant changes.

Author's Note: Some clinicians start combination forms containing hydrochlorothiazide (HCTZ) only after target goals for blood pressure are not met with the ARB alone. Dosing is then usually started with the lowest available combination dose and increased as needed

and tolerated. Hydrochlorothiazide (HCTZ) side effects may be a mixture of rare dose-independent (such as pancreatitis) and dose-dependent problems (such as excessive lowering of potassium, which is largely avoided using this low-HCTZ form).

Conditions Requiring Dosing Adjustments

Liver Function:

Candesartan: No changes in mild liver compromise. Some European clinicians start at 2 mg daily.

Irbesartan: No changes needed.

Losartan: This drug is extensively changed (metabolized) in the liver to an active metabolite. The starting dose should be 25 mg. Dosing is then increased as needed and tolerated at weekly intervals. The fixed-dose drug Hyzaar should not be used by patients with liver failure.

Valsartan: Maximum starting dose is 80 mg in mild to moderate liver failure. Drug has not been used in severe liver failure.

Kidney Function:

Candesartan: No change in starting dose in mild kidney compromise.

Irbesartan: No changes needed.

Losartan: No dosing changes appear to be needed. The fixed-dose combination Hyzaar should not be used by patients with creatinine clearances (see Glossary) less than 30 ml/min.

Valsartan: Some clinical trials started dosing at 40 mg daily with increase to 80 mg after 28 days as needed and tolerated.

▷ **Dosing Instructions:** Food slows the absorption of losartan and valsartan but does not decrease the total absorption. Irbesartan and candesartan can be taken with or without food. If you forget a dose: take it right away unless it's nearly time for your next regular dose. If it is nearly dosing time, just take the scheduled dose. DO NOT double doses.

Usual Duration of Use: Regular use for 3 to 4 weeks is usually needed to determine peak effectiveness in controlling high blood pressure. Long-term use (months to years) requires periodic evaluation of response and dose adjustment. See your doctor on a regular basis.

Typical Treatment Goals and Measurements (Outcomes and Markers)

Blood Pressure: The most recent treatment guidelines (JNC VI) actually define optimal blood pressure (BP) as less than 120/80 and high normal as 139/89. The American Diabetes Association has chosen a new target of 130/80. Most clinicians try to achieve a BP that achieves the best balance of lower cardiovascular risk while avoiding the problem of too low a blood pressure. It is certainly critical to reach the goal blood pressure and maintain it over time! The goal and time frame (see peak benefits above) should be discussed with you when the prescription is written.

Possible Advantages of These Drugs

A completely new mechanism of action in treating high blood pressure. Lower rate of cough side effect than ACE inhibitors. Candesartan has NOT been associated with dry cough in any clinical trial. Once-daily dosing can improve patient compliance. Irbesartan: dosing changes NOT needed in those over 60 or in people with kidney or liver disease. Candesartan: The cytochrome P-450 system is NOT involved in removal of the medicine. Candesartan appears to avoid dry cough side effect and also works to increase sensitivity to insulin, making it a preferred agent for patients with high blood pressure who also have insulin resistance. Irbesartan offers the advantage of avoiding dosing adjustments in patients over 60. Irbesartan also appears to avoid potential of liver damage.

▷ **These Drugs Should Not Be Taken If**
- you had an allergic reaction to them previously (note: HCTZ combinations should also be avoided by people with sulfonamide allergies).
- you have stenosis of the kidney arteries on both sides (bilateral) renal artery stenosis (candesartan).
- you have primary hyperaldosteronism (candesartan).
- you are pregnant.

▷ **Inform Your Physician Before Taking These Drugs If**
- you have a history of liver or kidney disease.
- you have a history of circulation problems in the brain.
- you are breast-feeding your infant.
- you have a history of lupus erythematosus (losartan).
- you have a history of aspirin or penicillin allergy (losartan).
- you have a history of disease in the blood vessels that supply the heart (coronary artery disease) or aortic or mitral valve stenosis or stenosis of one kidney artery.
- you have abnormal heart rhythms (cardiac).
- you are taking a diuretic (doses may need to be lowered).
- you are uncertain how much to take or how often to take it.

Possible Side Effects (natural, expected and unavoidable drug actions) Taste disorders.
Candesartan may cause flushing and/or excessive sweating in some patients.
Headache is possible with any of these medicines—though less than placebo for some.
First-dose excessive lowering of blood pressure is probably possible with all of these medicines (reported first for losartan).

▷ **Possible Adverse Effects** (unusual, unexpected and infrequent reactions)
If any of the following develop, consult your physician promptly for guidance.
Mild Adverse Effects
Allergic reactions: skin rash.
Dizziness, headache or sleep disturbances—infrequent.
Fatigue or muscle cramps—infrequent.
Nose bleed—case reports for candesartan and valsartan.
Cough—possible for some members (up to 3.4% losartan, 2.8% irbesartan, 0.8% valsartan and not reported with candesartan in clinical trials).
Diarrhea—infrequent.
Serious Adverse Effects
Allergic reactions: not defined.
Swelling of the face and lips (angioedema)—case reports for losartan and irbesartan.
Migraine headaches—rare.
Gout—rare and of questionable cause (losartan).
Liver toxicity—case reports (irbesartan, losartan, valsartan).

Kidney toxicity—possible with irbesartan.

Dose-related increase in blood potassium (hyperkalemia) (losartan).

Anemia—case reports, minimal clinical significance (candesartan, losartan, valsartan).

Neutropenia—rare (valsartan).

Movement problem (ataxia)—rare (valsartan).

▷ **Possible Effects on Sexual Function:** Decreased libido, impotence—both rare (losartan and valsartan).

Possible Delayed Adverse Effects: None reported.

▷ **Adverse Effects That May Mimic Natural Diseases or Disorders**

Increases in liver function tests may mimic infectious hepatitis (irbesartan, losartan and valsartan).

Natural Diseases or Disorders That May Be Activated by This Drug: None reported.

Possible Effects on Laboratory Tests

Losartan, irbesartan, candesartan and valsartan: Liver function tests: increased. Potassium level: may be increased.

Increased kidney function tests: creatinine possible with irbesartan.

CAUTION

1. Goals are set in the current approach to antihypertensive therapy. If the blood pressure lowering goals are not met in a reasonable amount of time, dosing changes and/or new medicines must be started.

2. Patients with low renin levels (often the case in African American patients) may get a lessened benefit from some of these medicines.

3. These drugs should not be taken during pregnancy.

Precautions for Use

By Infants and Children: Safety and effectiveness for use by those under 18 years of age have not been established.

By Those Over 60 Years of Age: People in this age group may be more sensitive to the effects of medicines that lower blood pressure. Lower starting doses are indicated for patients who are dehydrated.

▷ **Advisability of Use During Pregnancy**

Pregnancy Category: C in the first 3 months, D in the fourth month through birth. See Pregnancy Risk Categories at the back of this book.

Animal studies: Rat studies have produced kidney toxicity and death in fetuses.

Human studies: Information from adequate studies of pregnant women is not available.

If pregnancy is detected, these medicines should be stopped as soon as possible.

Advisability of Use If Breast-Feeding

Presence of this drug in breast milk: Unknown, but expected (losartan), yes in rats (candesartan and irbesartan).

Avoid drug or refrain from nursing.

Habit-Forming Potential: None.

Effects of Overdose: Severe decreases in blood pressure and dizziness. Possible increased or decreased heart rate.

Possible Effects of Long-Term Use: Not defined.

Suggested Periodic Examinations While Taking This Drug (at physician's discretion)

Periodic checks of blood pressure (high blood pressure is treated to a target lowering of blood pressure and should be kept there).

Liver function tests (irbesartan, losartan, and valsartan). May be prudent for all these medicines as they are structurally similar.

Kidney function tests when starting and at two and four weeks into treatment. Some clinicians also check kidney function after any dose increases as well (irbesartan).

▷ **While Taking This Drug, Observe the Following**

Foods: Follow the diet that your doctor has prescribed.

Herbal Medicines or Minerals: Ginseng may increase blood pressure, blunting the benefits of these medicines. Hawthorn, saw palmetto, ma huang, goldenseal, yohimbe and licorice may also increase blood pressure. Calcium and garlic may help lower blood pressure and could be part of complementary care. Indian snakeroot has a German Commission E monograph indication for hypertension—talk to your doctor. Eleuthero root and ephedra should be avoided by people living with hypertension. St. John's wort can cause sun sensitivity. Since some of these medicines can cause sun sensitivity also—-caution is advised.

Nutritional Support: Specific measures are not indicated.

Beverages: Avoid excessive caffeine intake.

▷ *Alcohol:* Alcohol may intensify the blood pressure lowering effects of this medicine. Ask your doctor for guidance.

Tobacco Smoking: No interactions expected. I advise everyone to quit smoking.

Marijuana Smoking: May increase the blood pressure lowering effects of this drug.

▷ *Other Drugs*

These medicines *taken concurrently* with

- ACE inhibitors (see Drug Classes) when combined with CD HCTZ forms may lead to severe first-dose lowering of blood pressure (hypotension). Low-dose ACE and caution are critical—yet the combination is also therapeutically useful.
- corticosteroids (methylprednisolone, others—see Drug Classes) may lead to excessive loss of potassium when used with the HCTZ combination forms of these medicines. Caution is advised.
- fluconazole (Diflucan) may blunt clinical benefits of losartan by blocking conversion to an active chemical. If these medicines are combined—watch for changes in therapeutic benefits.
- hydrochlorothiazide (various) may increase clinical benefits (redundant with CD forms unless extra fluid loss desired and HCTZ dose less than maximum).
- lithium (Lithobid, others) (case reports for some HCTZ combinations) resulted in lithium toxicity. Caution is advised.
- moxonidine (Cynt, available in Germany) may result in additive lowering of blood pressure.
- ritonavir (Norvir) may change losartan blood levels.

Losartan and valsartan *taken concurrently* with

- amiloride, spironolactone and triamterene (potassium-sparing diuretics) may lead to undesirable increases in potassium.

Candesartan *taken concurrently* with

- insulin and perhaps other oral hypoglycemic agents may increase response to insulin or oral agents because of increased insulin sensitivity. This may be used to clinical advantage.

▷   *Driving, Hazardous Activities:* These drugs may cause confusion or dizziness. Restrict activities as necessary.

Aviation Note: The use of these drugs *may be a disqualification* for piloting. Consult a designated Aviation Medical Examiner.

Exposure to Sun: Caution is advised. Isolated cases of photosensitivity have been reported.

Exposure to Heat: Caution: Excessive sweating (perspiration) may lead to dehydration and an excessive blood pressure lowering effect of these drugs.

Discontinuation: Talk with your doctor before stopping these medicines for any reason.

ANTI-ALZHEIMER'S DRUG FAMILY

Donepezil (DON ep a zill)   **Rivastigmine** (REEVA stig meen)   **Tacrine** (TA kreen)   **Galantamine** (GAH lan tah meen)

Introduced: 1993, 2000, 1996, 2001   **Class:** Acetylcholinesterase inhibitor, anti-Alzheimer's drug, nicotinic acid receptor blocker (galantamine only) **Prescription:** USA: Yes   **Controlled Drug:** USA: No; Canada: No **Available as Generic:** USA: No

Brand Names: *Donepezil:* Aricept; *Rivastigmine:* Exelon; *Tacrine:* Cognex; *Galantamine:* Reminyl

Author's Note: Information on rivastigmine will not be broadened in this edition as a Dear Health Care Provider letter has been issued regarding severe vomiting. Information on galantamine will be broadened in subsequent editions if clinical data warrant. CAUTION: in Canada felodipine, a calcium channel blocker, carries the brand name Renedil. Because this is so similar sounding a name, errors may occur during a telephone prescription.

BENEFITS versus RISKS	
Possible Benefits	*Possible Risks*
IMPROVEMENT OF MEMORY IN MILD TO MODERATE ALZHEIMER'S DISEASE	LIVER TOXICITY (TACRINE) Nausea Dizziness
IMPROVEMENT OF SYMPTOMS IN MILD TO MODERATE ALZHEIMER'S DISEASE	
MILD TO MODERATE ALZHEIMER'S PATIENTS CONTINUED TO BENEFIT FROM SUSTAINED TREATMENT FOR MORE THAN ONE YEAR (DONEPEZIL)	
WORKS ON ACETYLCHOLINESTERASE AND ALLOSTERIC NICOTINIC RECEPTORS (GALANTAMINE ONLY)	
Once-daily dosing	

▷ **Principal Uses**

As a Single Drug Product: Uses currently included in FDA-approved labeling: Treats mild to moderate Alzheimer's disease symptoms (both medicines).

Author's Note: Guidelines from the American Psychiatric Association (APA) recommend use of vitamin E alone or in combination with donepezil as first-line therapy for delaying symptoms of patients with mild to moderate Alzheimer's. An early study of the herbal medicine called ginkgo biloba has also shown benefits, but the two medicines have not been studied together. Galantamine may need to undergo comparative trials to further define its place in therapy.

Other (unlabeled) generally accepted uses: (1) Donepezil may have a role in people who have memory problems after brain injuries.

How These Drugs Work: Alzheimer's disease is thought to be caused by a loss of nerve cells that make a nerve transmitter (acetylcholine). Donepezil and tacrine act to increase levels of a neurotransmitter (acetylcholine) in the brain. Galantamine also works to increase levels of acetylcholine and has been found to have activity at nicotinic acid receptors.

Available Dosage Forms and Strengths

Donepezil:
Tablets — 5 mg, 10 mg
Galantamine:
Tablets — 4 mg, 8 mg and 12 mg
Tacrine:
Capsules — 10 mg, 20 mg, 30 mg, 40 mg

▷ **Recommended Dosage Ranges** (Actual dosage and schedule must be determined for each patient individually.)

Infants and Children: No data are available on use of these drugs in infants and children.

18 to 60 Years of Age:

Donepezil: Start with 5 mg once daily at bedtime, and keep at this dose for 6 weeks. As needed and tolerated increase to 10 mg. The 10-mg dose has had increased GI side effects.

Tacrine: Start at 10 mg four times a day (between meals). This can be increased at 6-week intervals if needed. Maximum daily dose is 160 mg.

Galantamine: Dosing was started at either 32 or 24 mg a day in one early study at Baylor. Patients could then continue galantamine for an additional 2 years at a dose of 24 mg a day. Current labeling calls for a starting dose of 4 mg twice a day (with meals). This dose is then continued for 4 weeks and is increased to 8 mg twice a day, and then increased to 16 mg twice a day if needed and tolerated.

Over 60 Years of Age: Same as 18 to 60 years of age.

Conditions Requiring Dosing Adjustments

Liver Function:

Donepezil: Lower doses and blood levels prudent in liver disease.

Tacrine: Not used at all with previous liver toxicity (bilirubin more than 3 mg per dl) and used with caution in liver compromise.

Galantamine: Not used at all in severe liver disease and used with caution and with more time between dose increases in liver compromise.

Kidney Function: Dose decreases in kidney compromise not now indicated for donepezil or tacrine. Galantamine should NOT be used in people with creatinine clearance (see Glossary) less than or equal to 9 ml /min. In mild kidney compromise (renal function decline), dose increases should be made slowly and with great care.

▷ **Dosing Instructions:** The donepezil tablet may be crushed and is not affected by food. The tacrine capsule may be opened and best taken 1 hour before meals. Food decreases tacrine body levels by 30 to 40%. If you forget a dose: take it right away unless it's nearly time for your next regular dose. If it IS nearly time, just take the scheduled dose. DO NOT double doses.

Usual Duration of Use: Regular use for 3 to 4 weeks may be needed to see improvement from either medicine. Dose increases are made at 4- to 6-week intervals. Long-term use (months to years) requires periodic evaluation of response and dose. If benefits do not occur within 6 weeks, patients or family members should talk with the prescriber about stopping these drugs. Research shows that donepezil benefits continue for more than a year with regular use.

Typical Treatment Goals and Measurements (Outcomes and Markers)

Thinking and cognition: Improvement in the Mini-Mental State examination, Alzheimer's Disease Assessment Scale (ADAS-cog) and/or global function using the Clinician Interview Based Assessment of Change. Assessments should be made periodically as benefits from these medicines will decay over time.

Possible Advantages of These Drugs

Improvement of memory and other symptoms of mild to moderate Alzheimer's with fewer side effects than other agents. Donepezil has a more favorable side effect profile than tacrine, offers once-a-day dosing and also avoids liver damage. Donepezil benefits continue for more than 140 weeks with regular use.

Currently a "Drug of Choice"

Donepezil is preferred for treatment of symptoms in mild to moderate Alzheimer's disease.

▷ **These Drugs Should Not Be Taken If**

Donepezil:
• you have had an allergic reaction to it previously.
Tacrine:
• you have had an allergic reaction to it previously.
• you have bronchial asthma.
• you had tacrine liver toxicity and bilirubin levels greater than 3 mg/dl.
• you have an overly active thyroid (hyperthyroidism).
• you have peptic ulcer disease.
• you have an intestinal or urinary tract obstruction.

▷ **Inform Your Physician Before Taking These Drugs If**

• you have a history of seizure disorder.
• you have had liver disease.
• you have a history of peptic ulcer disease.
• you have a slow heartbeat (bradycardia), abnormal electrical conduction in your heart (AV conduction defect) or excessively low blood pressure.

- you take an NSAID (see Drug Classes).
- you take muscle relaxants.
- you have glaucoma (angle closure).
- you have asthma.
- you are anemic or have low blood platelets.
- you will be having surgery (donepezil may enhance some muscle relaxants).

Possible Side Effects (natural, expected and unavoidable drug actions)

Symptoms of cholinergic excess (abdominal upset, agitation).

▷ **Possible Adverse Effects** (unusual, unexpected and infrequent reactions)

If any of the following develop, consult your physician promptly for guidance.

Mild Adverse Effects

Allergic reactions: skin rash.

Increased sweating—rare.

Increased urination—infrequent.

Muscle aches—infrequent.

Lowered blood pressure—possible.

Nausea/vomiting, diarrhea, decreased appetite—infrequent to frequent.

Dizziness, confusion, insomnia—infrequent.

Serious Adverse Effects

Allergic reactions: anaphylactoid reactions.

Dose-related increase in liver function tests (starts 6 to 8 weeks after therapy begins)—frequent (tacrine only).

Hallucinations—case report (tacrine).

Inner ear problems—rare (tacrine).

Purpura—infrequent (tacrine).

Severe decrease in white blood cells—one tacrine case report.

Anemia or low blood platelets—infrequent (donepezil).

Slow heart rate (bradycardia) or abnormal rhythm—possible to rare.

Seizures—case reports (tacrine).

▷ **Possible Effects on Sexual Function:** Very rare effect of causing lactation (tacrine). Donepezil has had case reports of increased libido.

Possible Delayed Adverse Effects: Liver toxicity (tacrine only), rash, low white blood cell count (tacrine only).

Adverse Effects That May Mimic Natural Diseases or Disorders

Liver toxicity of tacrine may mimic acute hepatitis.

Natural Diseases or Disorders That May Be Activated by These Drugs

May worsen bronchial asthma and precipitate seizures. May exacerbate peptic ulcer disease.

Possible Effects on Laboratory Tests

Tacrine:

Liver function tests: increased SGOT, SGPT and CPK.

Complete blood count: decreased white blood cells.

Donepezil: decreased hematocrit or platelets.

CAUTION

1. These drugs should **NOT** be stopped abruptly. Sudden decline in thinking may happen (acute deterioration of cognitive abilities).
2. Changes in color of stools (light or very black—tacrine) should be promptly reported to your doctor.

3. These drugs do **NOT** alter the course of Alzheimer's disease. Over time, benefits may be lost.
4. The dose of tacrine **must** be lowered by 40 mg per day if liver function tests (transaminases) rise three to five times the upper normal value.
5. Females achieve 50% higher tacrine blood levels than men. Dose-related side effects may occur sooner (with lower doses) in women than in men. Beneficial doses may be lower for women than men.
6. Donepezil shows benefits for more than 140 weeks with regular ongoing use. Interruption of therapy is NOT appropriate for that time span.
7. Galantamine is removed by two widely used liver enzymes (cytochrome P-450 2D6 and 3A4). Medicines that inhibit these enzymes will increase blood levels of galantamine, which may lead to toxic effects—requiring galantamine dosing decreases while or if the medicines are combined.

Precautions for Use

By Infants and Children: Safety and effectiveness for those under 18 years of age not established.

By Those Over 60 Years of Age: No specific changes are presently indicated.

▷ **Advisability of Use During Pregnancy**

Pregnancy Category: B for galantamine, C for donepezil and tacrine. See Pregnancy Risk Categories at the back of this book.

Animal studies: Data not available.

Human studies: Adequate studies of pregnant women are not available. Consult your doctor.

Advisability of Use If Breast-Feeding

Presence of these drugs in breast milk: Unknown.

Monitor nursing infant closely, and discontinue drug or nursing if adverse effects develop.

Habit-Forming Potential: None.

Effects of Overdose: May precipitate a cholinergic crisis—severe nausea and vomiting, slow heartbeat, low blood pressure, extreme muscle weakness, collapse and convulsions.

Suggested Periodic Examinations While Taking These Drugs (at physician's discretion)

Assessment of mental status: periodically—check benefits or loss of benefits as Alzheimer's progresses.

For tacrine, liver function tests should be checked every 2 weeks for the first 16 weeks of therapy, then monthly for 2 months, and then every 3 months ongoing if the same dose is used. If dose is increased, liver tests are checked weekly for 7 weeks and then on the above schedule.

Tacrine and donepezil patients need complete blood counts periodically or if symptoms of low blood count occur.

▷ **While Taking These Drugs, Observe the Following**

Foods: Tacrine is best NOT taken with food. Donepezil is not affected by food.

Herbal Medicines or Minerals: Data from appropriate scientific studies about combination of these medicines with ginkgo biloba is not available and cannot be recommended. A well-designed study of ginkgo biloba DID show it to be effective in mild to moderate Alzheimer's.

Beverages: No restrictions.

▷ *Alcohol:* Occasional small amounts of alcohol are okay. Frequent use may worsen memory problems and affect the liver.

Tobacco Smoking: No interactions expected. I advise everyone to quit smoking.

Marijuana Smoking: Additive dizziness may occur.

▷ *Other Drugs*

These medicines may ***increase*** the effects of
- bethanechol (Duvoid, others).
- theophylline (Theo-Dur, others) by doubling the drug level (reported for tacrine).
- succinylcholine (Anectine, others).

These medicines may ***decrease*** the effects of
- anticholinergic medications (see Drug Classes).

The following drug may ***increase*** the effects of tacrine:
- cimetidine (Tagamet).

These medicines ***taken concurrently*** with
- carbamazepine (Tegretol), dexamethasone, phenobarbital, fosphenytoin (Cerebyx), phenytoin (Dilantin) or rifampin (Rifater, others) may decrease therapeutic benefits of the anti-Alzheimer drugs.
- dexamethasone (various) may blunt donepezil benefits.
- ibuprofen (Motrin, others) was associated with delirium in one case report on tacrine.
- ketoconazole, quinidine and perhaps ritonavir (Norvir) or other protease inhibitors (see Drug Classes) may lead to increased risk of donepezil or tacrine toxicity.
- medicines removed by cytochrome P-450 enzymes (2D6 and 3A4) or that inhibit those enzymes may lead to toxic levels of all of these medicines. Caution is advised.
- NSAIDs (see Drug Classes) may cause additive stomach upset.

▷ *Driving, Hazardous Activities:* These drugs may cause confusion or dizziness. Restrict activities as necessary.

Aviation Note: The use of these drugs may be a disqualification for piloting. See a designated Aviation Medical Examiner.

Exposure to Sun: No restrictions.

Exposure to Heat: Increased sweating may occur rarely with tacrine. The combination of increased sweating and hot environments may lead to more rapid dehydration.

Discontinuation: These drugs should NOT be abruptly stopped. Some adverse effects are dose related and may abate if the dose is decreased. Slow withdrawal of the drug is indicated if it is not tolerated.

ANTI-LEUKOTRIENE FAMILY

Montelukast: (mon TELL oo cast)   **Zafirlukast** (zah FUR lew kast)
Zileuton (ZEYE loo ton)

Introduced: 1998, 1996, 1997   **Class:** Antiasthmatic, anti-leukotriene, 5-lipoxygenase inhibitor (zileuton)   **Prescription:** USA: Yes   **Controlled Drug:** USA: No; Canada: No   **Available as Generic:** No

Brand Names: *Montelukast:* Singulair; *Zafirlukast:* Accolate; *Zileuton:* Zyflo

---

BENEFITS versus RISKS

Possible Benefits	*Possible Risks*
EFFECTIVE PREVENTION AND CHRONIC TREATMENT OF BRONCHIAL ASTHMA	Headache Nausea Liver enzyme increase
May have a role in treating bronchospasm caused by exercise (montelukast, zafirlukast)	
May have a role in treating hay fever (zafirlukast)	
May have a role in preventing or treating allergies to cats (zafirlukast)	

▷ **Principal Uses**

As a Single Drug Product: Uses currently included in FDA-approved labeling: (1) Prevent recurrence of asthmatic episodes; (2) chronically treat asthmatic episodes; (3) zafirlukast is approved to prevent and for long-term treatment of asthma in patients 5 years old or older; (4) montelukast is approved to prevent and for long-term treatment of asthma in adults and in pediatric patients who are 2 years old or older as well as for use in preventing asthma induced by exercise.

Author's Note: These medicines are indicated as Step Two medicines (alternatives to low-dose inhaled steroids, cromolyn or nedocromil in mild persistent asthma) in the National Institutes of Health's (NIH, NHLBI) "Guidelines for Diagnosis and Management of Asthma."

Other (unlabeled) generally accepted uses: (1) montelukast and zafirlukast may have a role in preventing spasm of the bronchi caused by exercise; (2) zileuton may have a role in preventing allergic rhinitis or aspirin-sensitive asthma; (3) zafirlukast combined with loratadine yielded superb results in treating hay fever symptoms in a study of 458 patients; (4) zafirlukast may help prevent allergic reactions to cats.

How These Drugs Work: Zafirlukast and montelukast work by blocking (leukotriene receptor antagonist) action of chemicals called leukotrienes (slow-reacting substances of anaphylaxis). Zileuton works by blocking creation of (leukotriene pathway inhibitor) leukotrienes themselves. By inhibiting action or formation of leukotrienes, all medicines help keep the airways open.

Available Dosage Forms and Strengths

Montelukast:
    Chewable tablets — 4 mg and 5 mg
        Tablet — 10 mg

Zafirlukast:
        Tablet — 10 mg and 20 mg

Zileuton:
        Tablet — 600 mg

▷ **Recommended Dosage Ranges** (Actual dosage and schedule must be determined for each patient individually.)

Children 2 to 5:
    Montelukast only: One 4-mg chewable tablet in the evening.

Children 5 or older:
   Zafirlukast: FDA approved June of 2001.
Children 6 to 14:
   Montelukast only: One 5-mg chewable tablet in the evening.
12 to 60 Years of Age:
   Montelukast (15 to 60 years of age): 10 mg once a day, taken in the evening.
   Zafirlukast: 20 mg twice daily 7 years of age.
   Zileuton: 600 mg four times a day.
Over 60 Years of Age:
   Montelukast: No difference in safety or efficacy, but increased sensitivity to the drug can't yet be ruled out.
   Zafirlukast: Maximum blood level can be twice that of younger patients. Prudent to lower doses, but specific guidelines have not been developed. Package insert notes that using typical dose did not result in adverse effects in clinical trials.
   Zileuton: Same as those for 12 to 60 years old.
   Author's Note: These medicines may be continued during an acute worsening (exacerbation) of asthma, but are not to be used to treat a sudden (acute) asthma attack.

Conditions Requiring Dosing Adjustments
Liver Function:
   Montelukast has NOT been studied in liver compromise, but is removed by liver (CYP450 3A4, 2C9 and 2A6) so lower doses may be prudent.
   Zafirlukast stays in the body up to 60% longer in patients with alcoholic cirrhosis. Lower doses and blood levels appear prudent.
   Zileuton should not be given if active liver disease is present.
Kidney Function: Dosage changes not needed for the medicines in this class.

▷ **Dosing Instructions:** Montelukast should be taken in the evening. Zafirlukast should be taken on an empty stomach, 1 hour before or 2 hours after a meal. Zileuton may be given with or without food. These medicines are NOT to be used to stop a sudden (acute) asthma attack. If you forget a dose: take it right away unless it's nearly time for your next regular dose. If it IS nearly time, just take the scheduled dose. DO NOT double doses.

Usual Duration of Use: Both zafirlukast and zileuton start to work in half an hour. Montelukast peaks and also starts to work in 3–4 hours. It lasts for 24 hours. Zafirlukast significantly relaxes bronchi in 30 minutes, and lasts for 12 hours after a typical dose. Zileuton peaks in 2–4 hours, and with multiple doses may last up to 7 days. Ongoing use requires periodic follow-up with your doctor.

Typical Treatment Goals and Measurements (Outcomes and Markers)
Asthma: The frequency of asthma attacks as well as the severity of asthma attacks that occur (such as those requiring an emergency department visit) are a benchmark of effectiveness. Pulmonary function tests such as FEV1 are valuable measures to assess response. Some clinicians also use the number of times a rescue inhaler must be used as well as daily and night (nocturnal) symptom scores as clinical fine points. Goals should be communicated and checked.

Possible Advantages of These Drugs
   A completely new mechanism of action in preventing asthma and some allergic reactions. Once-daily dosing can improve patient compliance.

▷ **These Drugs Should Not Be Taken If**
- you have had an allergic reaction to them.
- you have active liver disease or increased liver enzymes (transaminases) greater than three times the upper normal limit (zileuton).

▷ **Inform Your Physician Before Taking These Drugs If**
- you have a liver disease (montelukast or zafirlukast).
- you are having a sudden (acute) asthma attack.
- you are a child less than 12 years old (zafirlukast).
- you are taking warfarin (zafirlukast).
- you have impaired kidney function (zafirlukast or zileuton).
- you drink large amounts of alcohol (zileuton).
- you develop a rash, tingling of the arms or legs, flu-like symptoms or sinusitis.
- you are pregnant or are breast-feeding your baby.

Possible Side Effects (natural, expected and unavoidable drug actions)
Not defined at present.

▷ **Possible Adverse Effects** (unusual, unexpected and infrequent reactions)
If any of the following develop, consult your physician promptly for guidance.
Mild Adverse Effects
Allergic reactions: skin rash, hives.
Headache—frequent (montelukast, zafirlukast).
Fatigue, weakness—infrequent.
Dizziness—rare for zafirlukast, infrequent for zileuton.
Nausea or abdominal pain—infrequent.
Muscle pain—rare for zafirlukast, infrequent for zileuton.
Serious Adverse Effects
Allergic reactions: possible.
Idiosyncratic reactions: drug-induced lupus erythematosus—case reports.
Liver toxicity (increased enzyme tests)—rare for zafirlukast, less frequent for montelukast, infrequent for zileuton.
Decreases in steroid doses may be followed by onset of Churg-Strauss syndrome (montelukast and zafirlukast, possibly zileuton)—rare.

▷ **Possible Effects on Sexual Function:** None reported.

Natural Diseases or Disorders That May Be Activated by These Drugs Since all three medicines may increase liver enzymes, hidden (subclinical) liver problems may be activated.

Possible Effects on Laboratory Tests
Liver function tests (SGPT, SGOT, LDH): may be increased.

CAUTION
1. The chewable montelukast tablet has phenylalanine (0.842 mg per 5-mg tablet). People with PKU must be advised.
2. Talk with your doctor about continuing other asthma drugs once you start one of these medicines.
3. Since these medicines can affect the liver, it is critical that you have lab tests of liver function as your doctor orders them.
4. One case report of drug fever for zafirlukast.
5. All these medicines may be rare causes of Churg-Strauss syndrome. Call your doctor if you develop a rash, tingling of the arms or legs, flu-like symptoms or sinusitis.

Precautions for Use

By Children: Make certain that these medicines are taken in the amount and for the number of times they are ordered.

By Those Over 65 Years of Age: Zafirlukast goes to higher peak blood levels and remains in the body longer in those over 65, so smaller starting doses are indicated. Montelukast and zileuton are not changed by age.

▷ **Advisability of Use During Pregnancy**

Pregnancy Category: Montelukast and zafirlukast: B; zileuton: C. See Pregnancy Risk Categories at the back of this book.

Animal studies: Montelukast—no teratogenicity at 320 times the maximum human dose in rats. Zafirlukast—no teratogenicity up to 160 times maximum recommended human dose given to mice. Zileuton—adverse effects were seen in rats given 18 times the typical human dose.

Human studies: Adequate studies of pregnant women are not available.

Ask your doctor for guidance.

Advisability of Use If Breast-Feeding

Presence of this drug in breast milk: Yes (zafirlukast); unknown (montelukast [but yes in rats], zileuton).

Avoid drug or refrain from nursing.

Habit-Forming Potential: None.

Effects of Overdose: No overdose experience in humans for montelukast (900 mg a day was given for a week in one study without any adverse effects) or zafirlukast. Zileuton overdose experience is limited. One patient received 6.6 to 9.0 g of zileuton, which caused vomiting, but recovered without ill effects.

Possible Effects of Long-Term Use: Possible increased liver enzymes.

Suggested Periodic Examinations While Taking This Drug (at physician's discretion)

Periodic liver function tests.

▷ **While Taking This Drug, Observe the Following**

Foods: Zafirlukast should be taken on an empty stomach; no restrictions for montelukast or zileuton.

Herbal Medicines or Minerals: Using St. John's wort with zafirlukast may cause a problem as St. John's wort has known interactions with CYP 3A4 and 2C9—the enzymes that remove zafirlukast. Fir or pine needle oil should NOT be used by asthmatics. Ephedra alone does carry a German Commission E monograph indication for asthma treatment. Talk to your doctor as this has not been studied with leukotriene inhibitors. If you are allergic to plants in the Asteraceae family (aster, chrysanthemum, daisy or ragweed), you may also be allergic to echinacea, chamomile, feverfew and St. John's wort.

Beverages: No restrictions.

▷ *Alcohol:* May worsen drowsiness.

Tobacco Smoking: Smoking may lower levels of zileuton and is NOT advisable for anyone, least of all people living with asthma. I advise everyone to quit smoking.

Marijuana Smoking: May cause additive drowsiness.

▷ *Other Drugs*

These medicines *taken concurrently* with

• aspirin (various brands) may cause zafirlukast toxicity.

• astemizole (Hismanal) may lead to heart toxicity with zileuton.

- beta-blocker drugs (see Drug Classes) may cause beta-blocker toxicity if combined with zileuton.
- dofetilide (Tikosyn) may increase dofetilide blood levels.
- erythromycin (E-Mycin, etc.) may decrease zafirlukast's benefits.
- phenobarbital (various) may lower montelukast blood levels.
- propranolol (Inderal) and perhaps other beta-blockers (see Drug Classes) cause excessive/undesirable beta blockage.
- rifampin (Rifater) may lower montelukast blood levels.
- terfenadine (Seldane) may decrease zafirlukast blood levels and its therapeutic benefits. Zileuton may decrease terfenadine (and perhaps other similarly structured minimally sedating antihistamine levels) and lead to toxicity. DO NOT combine.
- theophylline (Theo-Dur, others) may decrease zafirlukast blood levels and its therapeutic benefits. Zileuton may result in doubling of theophylline levels and require reduced theophylline doses.
- warfarin (Coumadin) may lead to increased risk of bleeding (zafirlukast and zileuton). More frequent INRs are needed.

▷ *Driving, Hazardous Activities:* These drugs may cause dizziness. Restrict activities as necessary.

Aviation Note: The use of these drugs *may be a disqualification* for piloting. Consult a designated Aviation Medical Examiner.

Exposure to Sun: No restrictions.

Discontinuation: Do not stop these medicines without first talking with your doctor.

ASPIRIN* (AS pir in)

Other Names: acetylsalicylic acid, ASA

Introduced: 1899   **Class:** Analgesics, mild; antiplatelet, antipyretic, NSAIDs, salicylates   **Prescription:** USA: No   **Controlled Drug:** USA: No; Canada: No   **Available as Generic:** Yes

Brand Names: Added Strength Analgesic Pain Reliever, Adult Strength Pain Reliever [CD], Aggrenox [CD], Alka-Seltzer Effervescent Pain Reliever and Antacid [CD], Alka-Seltzer Night Time [CD], Alka-Seltzer Plus [CD], Alka-Seltzer Plus Cold [CD], Anacin [CD], Anacin Maximum Strength [CD], ✤Anacin w/Codeine [CD], ✤Ancasal, APC [CD], APC w/Codeine [CD], ✤APO-ASA, Arthritis Pain Formula [CD], Arthritis Strength Bufferin, A.S.A. Enseals, ✤Asasantine [CD], Ascriptin [CD], Ascriptin A/D [CD], Aspergum, ✤Aspirin,* Asprimox, ✤Astrin, Axotal [CD], Azdone [CD], Bayer Aspirin, Bayer Children's Chewable Aspirin, Bayer Enteric Aspirin, Bayer Plus, BC Powder, Buffaprin, Bufferin [CD], Bufferin Arthritis Strength [CD], Bufferin Extra Strength [CD], Bufferin w/Codeine [CD], Cama Arthritis Pain Reliever [CD], Cardioprin, Carisoprodol Compound [CD], Cope [CD], Coricidin [CD], ✤Coryphen, ✤Coryphen-Codeine [CD], ✤C2 Buffered [CD], Darvon Compound [CD], Direct Formulary Aspirin, ✤Dristan [CD], Easprin, Ecotrin, 8-Hour Bayer, Empirin, Empirin w/Codeine No. 2, 4 [CD], ✤Entrophen, Excedrin

---

*In the United States, aspirin is an official generic designation. In Canada, Aspirin is the Registered Mark of Bayer Company Division of Sterling Drug Limited.

[CD], Excedrin Extra Strength Geltabs [CD], Excedrin Migraine* [CD], Fiori-nal [CD], ❧Fiorinal-C [Q],-C [h] [CD], Fiorinal w/Codeine [CD], Genacote, Genprin, Goody's Headache Powder [CD], Halprin, Hepto [CD], Lortab ASA [CD], Low Dose Adult Chewable Aspirin, Marnal [CD], Maximum Bayer Aspirin, Measurin, Midol Caplets [CD], Momentum [CD], Norgesic [CD], Nor-gesic Forte [CD], Norwich Aspirin, ❧Novasen, Orphenadrine [CD], PAP w/Codeine [CD], Percodan [CD], Percodan-Demi [CD], ❧Phenaphen [CD], ❧ Phenaphen No. 2, 3, 4 [CD], Propoxyphene Compound [CD], ❧Riphen-10, Robaxisal [CD], ❧Robaxisal-C [CD], Roxiprin [CD], ❧692 [CD], SK-65 Com-pound [CD], Soma Compound [CD], St. Joseph Children's Aspirin, ❧Supasa, Synalgos [CD], Synalgos-DC [CD], Talwin Compound [CD], Talwin Com-pound-50 [CD], ❧Tecnal Tablet [CD], ❧Triaphen-10, ❧217 [CD], ❧217 Strong [CD], ❧292 [CD], Vanquish [CD], Verin, Wesprin, Zorprin

BENEFITS versus RISKS	
Possible Benefits	*Possible Risks*
EFFECTIVE RELIEF OF MILD TO MODERATE PAIN AND INFLAMMATION	Stomach irritation, bleeding and/or ulceration
REDUCTION OF FEVER	Decreased numbers of white blood cells and platelets
PREVENTION OF BLOOD CLOTS	Hemolytic anemia—rare
PREVENTION OF HEART ATTACK (a benefit when satisfactory blood pressure control has been achieved prior to starting aspirin)	Liver toxicity—rare
	Bronchospasm in asthmatics—possible
	Hemorrhagic strokes—case reports/increased risk
PREVENTION OF STROKE	Full-dose use (not low-dose) carries an
PREVENTION OF COLON CANCER	increased risk of hospitalization for
MAY ACT TO LIMIT THE SIZE AND SEVERITY OF HEART ATTACK ONCE IT HAS STARTED	congestive heart failure in the elderly (NSAIDs as a class effect)
TREATMENT OF MIGRAINE HEAD-ACHES (EXCEDRIN MIGRAINE ONLY)	

▷ **Principal Uses**

As a Single Drug Product: Uses currently included in FDA-approved labeling: (1) Relieves mild to moderate pain and eases symptoms in conditions causing inflammation or high fever. Treats musculoskeletal disorders, especially acute and chronic arthritis, as well as painful menstruation (dysmenorrhea). Used selectively to: (2) reduce risk of first heart attack; (3) reduce the risk of repeat heart attack; (4) prevent platelet embolism to the brain (in men); (5) reduce risk of clots (thromboembolism) after heart attack and in people with artifi-cial heart valves and after hip surgery (see Blood Platelets in Glossary); (6) help prevent a second stroke in people who have had a stroke; (7) help prevent strokes in people with transient ischemic attack (TIA) history; (8) help prevent migraine headaches (Excedrin Migraine only); (9) treat TIA in women and men; (10) treat sudden heart attack (acute myocardial infarction or AMI) in men and women; (11) decrease risk of heart attack in patients with unstable angina; (12) treat pleurisy associated with systemic lupus erythematosus.

***Author's Note: Excedrin Migraine is the first nonprescription medicine to be FDA-approved to treat mild to moderate migraine headaches.**

Other (unlabeled) generally accepted uses: (1) Long-term use may decrease the risk of colon polyps or colon cancer in women (may apply to men as well); (2) may limit size and severity of a heart attack if aspirin is taken immediately after symptoms are recognized and is continued for at least 30 days after the heart attack; (3) can help reduce flushing caused by niacin; (4) used after carotid artery surgery (endarterectomy) to prevent TIA or stroke; (5) general data supporting NSAID use and decreased Alzheimer's risk; (6) one 1999 study found that low dose (100 mg) of aspirin given 8 hours after waking or at bedtime worked to decrease blood pressure in women at risk for gestational hypertension or preeclampsia.

As a Combination Drug Product [CD]: Frequently combined with other mild or strong analgesic drugs to enhance pain relief. Also combined with antihistamines and decongestants in many cold preparations to relieve headache and general discomfort. Aggrenox combines 200 mg of dipyridamole with 25 mg of aspirin.

How This Drug Works: Reduces prostaglandins, chemicals involved in the production of inflammation and pain. By modifying the temperature-regulating center in the brain, dilating blood vessels and increasing sweating, aspirin reduces fever. Works on blood clotting elements called platelets to inactivate prostaglandin G/H synthase. This inactivation leads to almost complete suppression of platelet ability to make thromboxanes. By preventing the production of thromboxane in blood platelets, aspirin inhibits formation of blood clots.

Available Dosage Forms and Strengths

Capsules, enteric coated — 500 mg

Capsules, enteric-coated granules — 325 mg

Gum tablets — 227.5 mg

Suppositories — 60 mg, 120 mg, 125 mg, 130 mg, 195 mg, 200 mg, 300 mg, 325 mg, 600 mg, 650 mg, 1.2 g

Tablets — 65 mg, 81 mg, 165 mg, 325 mg, 496 mg, 500 mg

Tablets, chewable — 81 mg

Tablets, enteric coated — 81 mg, 165 mg, 325 mg, 500 mg, 650 mg, 975 mg

Tablets, prolonged action — 80 mg (Canada), 650 mg, 800 mg, 975 mg

▷ **Usual Adult Dosage Ranges:** *In men or women having a heart attack:* One (325 mg) nonenteric-coated aspirin (then call 911). If only enteric-coated aspirin is available, it should be chewed in order to make it enter the body faster. Aspirin is then continued for 30 days after the heart attack. Some studies have continued it for up to 2 years.

In stroke: 50–325 mg showed a benefit in the CAST study.

In preventing transient ischemic attacks (TIA): 325–900 mg a day has been used. Low-dose treatment of TIA has used 50–325 mg. For the Aggrenox combination form: Prevention of stroke in people who have had transient brain blood flow problems (ischemia) or those who have suffered an ischemic stroke from a clot (thrombosis)—one capsule in the morning and in the evening has been used.

For pain or fever: 325 to 650 mg every 4 hours and as needed for fever (ongoing pain or fever use should be medically supervised).

Arthritis (and related conditions): 3,600 to 5,400 mg daily in divided doses.

Prevention of blood clots: 80–162 mg daily or every other day. Low-dose, long-term daily aspirin may also decrease risk of colon cancer or heart attacks. **Note: For long-term use, actual dosage and schedule must be determined for each patient individually.** FDA advocates 75–325 mg daily for unstable angina or a previous heart attack to reduce risk of death or another heart attack. The US Preventive Services Task Force recommends clinicians consider low-dose aspirin use in patients who are 40 or older who have significantly increased risk of heart attack (myocardial infarction or MI) and who are not contraindicated low-dose aspirin.

Conditions Requiring Dosing Adjustments

Liver Function: This medication should be avoided in severe liver disease.

Kidney Function: Avoided or used with caution in patients with kidney problems. NOT to be used in severe (creatinine clearance less than 10 ml/min) kidney failure.

Glucose-6-Phosphate Dehydrogenase (G6PD) Deficiency: May cause destruction of red blood cells in patients with G6PD deficiency.

▷ **Dosing Instructions:** Take with food, milk or a full glass of water to reduce stomach upset. Regular tablets may be crushed and capsules opened for administration. Enteric-coated tablets, prolonged-action tablets, A.S.A. Enseals, Cama tablets and Ecotrin tablets should not be crushed. If you forget a dose: take it right away unless it's nearly time for your next regular dose. Aggrenox capsules SHOULD NOT be chewed. If it IS nearly time, just take the scheduled dose. DO NOT double dose.

Usual Duration of Use: Short-term use is recommended—3 to 5 days for fever or cold symptoms. Daily use should not exceed 10 days without physician supervision. Use on a regular schedule for 1 week usually needed to see benefit in relieving chronic arthritis symptoms. Response must be evaluated and dose adjusted in long-term use. Ongoing use for prevention of heart attack, colon cancer or stroke REQUIRES ongoing supervision by your doctor, even though aspirin is not a prescription drug.

Typical Treatment Goals and Measurements (Outcomes and Markers)

Pain: Most clinicians treating pain use a device called an algometer to check your pain. This looks like a small ruler, but lets the clinician better understand your pain. The goals of treatment then relate to where the level of pain started (for example, a rating of 7 on a zero to ten scale) and what the cause of the pain was. Pain medicines may also be used together (in combination) in order to get the best result or outcome. If your pain control is not acceptable to YOU after a week of arthritis pain treatment, be sure to call your doctor as you may need a different medicine or combination.

Cardiovascular disorders (strokes and heart attacks): The clear marker here is prevention of a first or second stroke or heart attack.

Possible Advantages of This Drug: Inexpensive medicine that treats a wide variety of conditions and can also help prevent heart attacks, colon cancer and strokes.

▷ **This Drug Should Not Be Taken If**
- you have had an allergic reaction to any form of aspirin.
- you have a history of urticaria/angioedema or spasm of the bronchi with rhinoconjunctivitis with aspirin, other NSAID or selective COX II inhibitor

(adults who developed nasal polyps, asthma, chronic rhinitis or ongoing angioedema or urticaria make these reactions more likely).
- you have any type of bleeding disorder (such as hemophilia).
- you have active peptic ulcer disease.
- you are in the last 3 months of pregnancy.
- it smells like vinegar. This indicates decomposition of aspirin.

▷ **Inform Your Physician Before Taking This Drug If**
- you are taking any anticoagulant drug.
- you are taking a COX II inhibitor and this medicine is prescribed.
- you are taking oral antidiabetic drugs.
- you have a history of peptic ulcer disease or gout.
- you have lupus erythematosus.
- you are pregnant or planning pregnancy.
- you have asthma, carditis or nasal polyps.
- you plan to have surgery of any kind (used in different doses before some kinds of surgery and not at all before others).
- you take prescription or nonprescription medications not discussed when aspirin was recommended for you.
- you are unsure how much to take or how often to take it.
- you have a history of liver or kidney problems.
- you have low glucose-6-phosphate dehydrogenase (G6PD).
- you have a history of vasospastic (Prinzmetal's) angina (may be worsened by this drug).
- you drink three or more alcoholic drinks a day (see cautions).

Possible Side Effects (natural, expected and unavoidable drug actions)

Mild drowsiness in sensitive patients.

Interference with usual blood clotting.

▷ **Possible Adverse Effects** (unusual, unexpected and infrequent reactions)

If any of the following develop, consult your physician promptly for guidance.

Mild Adverse Effects

Allergic reactions: skin rash, hives, nasal discharge (resembling hay fever), nasal polyps.

Stomach irritation, heartburn, nausea, vomiting, constipation—infrequent to frequent.

Lowering of the blood sugar—rare.

Serious Adverse Effects

Allergic reactions: acute anaphylactic reaction (see Glossary), allergic destruction of blood platelets (see Glossary) and bruising—rare.

Idiosyncratic reactions: hemolytic anemia (see Glossary)—rare.

Stevens-Johnson syndrome—possible.

Hemorrhagic stroke in some populations—case reports.

Erosion of stomach lining, with silent bleeding—may be dose and frequency related.

Activation of peptic ulcer, with or without hemorrhage—frequent with long-term non-enteric-coated use.

Bone marrow depression (see Glossary): fatigue, weakness, fever, sore throat, abnormal bleeding or bruising—possible.

Hepatitis with jaundice (see Glossary): yellow skin and eyes, dark-colored urine, light-colored stool—possible, especially with daily use of more than 2 grams (2,000 mg).

Hearing toxicity (ototoxicity)—more common with higher doses and long-term use.

Kidney function decline—possible in kidney failure patients who depend on prostaglandins for their kidneys to work.

Bronchospasm when used in patients with nasal polyps, asthma—possible.

May worsen angina attacks and increase their frequency—possible.

Reye's syndrome if used during viral illness—DO NOT USE.

▷ **Possible Effects on Sexual Function:** None reported.

Adverse Effects That May Mimic Natural Diseases or Disorders Liver damage may suggest viral hepatitis or reveal (unmask) low-level (subclinical) liver disease. May lead to decline in kidney function in people with borderline kidney disease.

Possible Effects on Laboratory Tests

Complete blood counts: decreased red cells, hemoglobin, white cells and platelets.

Bleeding time: prolonged.

INR (prothrombin time): increased by large doses; decreased by small doses.

Blood glucose level: decreased.

Blood uric acid level: increased by small doses; decreased by large doses.

Liver function tests: increased ALT/GPT, AST/GOT, alkaline phosphatase.

Thyroid function tests: increased T3 uptake, free T3 and free T4; decreased TSH, T3, T4 and free thyroxine index (FTI).

Urine sugar tests: false positive with Clinitest or Benedict's solution.

Fecal occult blood test: positive with large doses of aspirin.

CAUTION

1. The FDA now requires a warning noting that people who have three or more alcoholic drinks a day may have increased risk of stomach bleeding if they also use aspirin (problems may also occur with lower alcohol use).
2. **Aspirin is a drug.** We tend to have an unrealistic sense of its safety and its potential for adverse effects. TALK TO YOUR DOCTOR TO SEE IF BENEFITS OUTWEIGH RISKS OF REGULAR ASPIRIN USE. A meta-analysis of 55,462 patients and 16 clinical trials found an increased risk of stroke (12 strokes for every 10,000 patients). The study concluded that benefits may outweigh risks for many populations.
3. Do NOT take more than three tablets (975 mg) at one time; allow at least 4 hours between doses; and do not take more than 10 tablets (3,250 mg) in 24 hours without physician supervision.
4. An outcome study of 5,499 men found that the risk of stroke with aspirin treatment related to blood pressure. One conclusion is that blood pressure should be satisfactorily controlled BEFORE aspirin therapy for prevention of CHD is started.
5. Remember that aspirin can
   • cause new illnesses.
   • complicate existing illnesses.
   • complicate pregnancy.
   • complicate surgery.
   • interact unfavorably with other drugs.

- When a health care professional asks, "Are you taking any drugs?" the answer is yes if you are taking aspirin. This also applies to *any* non-prescription drug you may be taking (see Over-the-Counter Drugs in the Glossary).
- **Controversies in medicine:** Some clinicians think that aspirin will remove some of the benefits of ACE inhibitors (see Drug Classes) if these two medicines are taken together.
- Aspirin tends to be underused in people with diabetes and in patients with coronary artery disease (one study found only 26% use). If you are living with diabetes, or have coronary artery disease, ask your doctor if aspirin makes sense for you.

Precautions for Use

By Infants and Children: Reye's syndrome (brain and liver damage in children, often fatal) can follow flu or chickenpox in children and teenagers. Some reports suggest that the use of aspirin by children with flu or chickenpox can increase the risk of developing this complication. Consult your physician before giving aspirin to a child or teenager with chickenpox, flu or similar infection.

Usual dosage schedule for children (Up to 2 years of age—consult physician):

2 to 4 years of age — 160 mg/4 hours, up to 5 doses/24 hours.
4 to 6 years of age — 240 mg/4 hours, up to 5 doses/24 hours.
6 to 9 years of age — 320 mg/4 hours, up to 5 doses/24 hours.
9 to 11 years of age — 400 mg/4 hours, up to 5 doses/24 hours.
11 to 12 years of age — 480 mg/4 hours, up to 5 doses/24 hours.

Do not exceed 5 days of continual use without talking to your doctor. Give all doses with food, milk or a full glass of water.

By Those Over 60 Years of Age: Watch for signs of high blood level: irritability, ringing in the ears, deafness, confusion, nausea or stomach upset. Aspirin can cause serious stomach bleeding. This can occur as "silent" bleeding of small amounts over a long time. Sudden hemorrhage can occur, even without a history of stomach ulcer. Watch for gray- to black-colored stools, an indication of stomach bleeding.

▷ **Advisability of Use During Pregnancy**

Pregnancy Category: C/D. See Pregnancy Risk Categories at the back of this book.

Animal studies: Significant birth defects due to this drug have been reported.

Human studies: Information from studies of pregnant women indicates no increased risk of birth defects in 32,164 pregnancies exposed to aspirin. Studies show, however, that the regular use of aspirin during pregnancy is often detrimental to the health of the mother and the welfare of the fetus. Anemia, hemorrhage before and after delivery and an increased incidence of stillbirths and newborn deaths have been reported. There are data that support use of aspirin in low doses to prevent toxemia of pregnancy in some women with a history of this problem.

Ask your doctor for help. Avoid aspirin altogether during the last 3 months unless your doctor prescribes it.

Advisability of Use If Breast-Feeding

Presence of this drug in breast milk: Yes.
Avoid drug or refrain from nursing.

Habit-Forming Potential: Extended high-dose use may cause a psychological dependence (see Glossary).

Effects of Overdose: Stomach distress, nausea, vomiting, ringing in the ears, dizziness, impaired hearing, blood chemistry imbalance, stupor, fever, deep and rapid breathing, twitching, delirium, shock, hallucinations, convulsions.

Possible Effects of Long-Term Use

A form of psychological dependence (see Glossary). Anemia due to chronic blood loss from erosion of stomach lining. The development of stomach ulcer. The development of "aspirin allergy"—nasal discharge, nasal polyps, asthma. Kidney damage. Prolonged bleeding time, critical in the event of injury or surgery.

Suggested Periodic Examinations While Taking This Drug (at physician's discretion)

Complete blood cell counts.

Kidney function tests and urine analyses.

Liver function tests.

▷ **While Taking This Drug, Observe the Following**

Foods: May decrease the total amount of aspirin per dose that is absorbed.

Herbal Medicines or Minerals: Many herbal medicines may interact with aspirin. Examples include ginkgo, garlic, ginger, ginseng and feverfew. St. John's wort may increase sensitivity to the sun, and caution is advised as additive sensitivity may develop.

Nutritional Support: Do not take large doses of vitamin C while taking aspirin regularly.

Beverages: No restrictions. May be taken with milk.

▷ *Alcohol:* Use of alcohol and aspirin at the same time may increase risk of stomach damage and may prolong bleeding time (see cautions).

Tobacco Smoking: No interactions expected. I advise everyone to quit smoking.

▷ *Other Drugs*

Aspirin may ***increase*** the effects of

• adrenocortical steroids (see Drug Classes), leading to additive stomach irritation and possible bleeding.

• insulin (various brands including insulin lispro) and require dosage adjustment when more than 650 mg of aspirin is taken daily.

• heparin and cause abnormal bleeding.

• methotrexate and increase its toxic effects.

• oral anticoagulants (see Drug Classes) such as low-molecular-weight heparins (see Drug Classes) and warfarin (Coumadin) and cause abnormal bleeding.

• oral antidiabetic drugs (see Drug Classes) and cause hypoglycemia. Dosage adjustments are often necessary—particularly with first-generation agents.

• tiludronate (Skelid) by increasing blood levels by 50%.

• thrombolytics such as TPA and reteplase (Retavase). Careful monitoring is advised if these medicines are combined.

• valproic acid (Depakene).

Aspirin may ***decrease*** the effects of

• ACE inhibitors—since vein opening or vasodilator prostaglandins may account for some of the ACE beneficial effects and aspirin inhibits prostaglandins, aspirin may blunt ACE inhibitor benefits. Still, many clinicians feel that the benefits of aspirin and ACE use after a heart attack outweigh any blunting effect.

- beta-adrenergic-blocking drugs (see Drug Classes).
- captopril (Capoten).
- enalapril (Vasotec) by decreasing enalapril's beneficial increase in heart (cardiac) output.
- furosemide (Lasix).
- other NSAIDs (see Drug Classes).
- phenytoin (Dilantin) and fosphenytoin (Cerebyx) by decreasing phenytoin or fosphenytoin blood levels (high aspirin doses).
- probenecid (Benemid) and reduce its effectiveness in the treatment of gout—with aspirin doses of less than 2 g every 24 hours.
- spironolactone (Aldactazide, Aldactone, others) and reduce its diuretic effect.
- sulfinpyrazone (Anturane) and reduce its effectiveness in the treatment of gout—with aspirin doses of less than 2 g every 24 hours.
- tiludronate (Skelid) by decreasing the amount getting into the body.

Aspirin *taken concurrently* with
- alendronate (Fosamax) or other bisphosphonates (tiludronate or Skelid or risedronate or Actonel) may result in increased risk of stomach upset/diarrhea and decreases bisphosphonate.
- celecoxib (Celebrex) or rofecoxib (Vioxx) (see Drug Classes) increases risk of stomach ulcers.
- clopidogrel (Plavix) is a benefit-to-risk decision because increased risk of bleeding. Talk to your doctor to see if the benefits (see CURE trial above) of combining aspirin and clopidogrel outweigh any increased bleeding risk.
- cortisonelike drugs (see Drug Classes) increases risk of stomach ulcers.
- diltiazem (Cardizem) may result in increased risk of bleeding.
- high blood pressure (antihypertensive) medicines may blunt their therapeutic benefit, especially those that are diuretics such as furosemide (Lasix), spironolactone or thiazides (see Drug Classes).
- intrauterine devices (IUDs) may result in decreased IUD effectiveness.
- lithium (Lithobid) may increase lithium blood levels.
- low-molecular-weight heparins (Lovenox, Fragmin, others) increases the risk of bleeding.
- methotrexate (Mexate) may cause toxicity.
- niacin (various) may BENEFICIALLY decrease flushing from niacin.
- quinidine (Quinaglute, others) may increase risk of bleeding.
- valproic acid (Depakote) may cause toxic blood levels.
- varicella vaccine (Varivax) may result in Reye's syndrome. **Avoid aspirin and other salicylates for 6 weeks following Varivax inoculation**.
- verapamil (Calan, others) may cause increased bleeding risk.
- zafirlukast (Accolate) may increase zafirlukast blood levels and increase adverse effects.

The following drugs may *increase* the effects of aspirin:
- acetazolamide (Diamox).
- cimetidine (Tagamet).
- para-aminobenzoic acid (Pabalate).

The following drugs may *decrease* the effects of aspirin:
- antacids, with regular continual use.
- cholestyramine (Questran, others)—will decrease the amount of aspirin that goes to work; separate doses by 30 minutes.

- cortisonelike drugs (see Drug Classes).
- urinary alkalinizers (sodium bicarbonate, sodium citrate).

▷ *Driving, Hazardous Activities:* No restrictions or precautions.

Aviation Note: It is advisable to watch for mild drowsiness and restrict activities accordingly.

Exposure to Sun: Use caution, may cause photosensitivity.

Discontinuation: Aspirin should be stopped 1 week before some kinds of surgery. There are some data for use of low-dose aspirin in some cases (such as in carotid endarterectomy).

ATENOLOL (a TEN oh lohl)

Introduced: 1973   **Class:** Anti-anginal, antihypertensive, beta-adrenergic blocker   **Prescription:** USA: Yes   **Controlled Drug:** USA: No; Canada: No   **Available as Generic:** Yes

Brand Names: ♣Apo-Atenolol, ♣Novo-Atenolol, ♣Nu-Atenolol, ♣PMS-Atenolol, Tenoretic [CD], Tenormin

BENEFITS versus RISKS	
Possible Benefits	*Possible Risks*
EFFECTIVE ANTI-ANGINAL DRUG in the management of effort-induced angina	CONGESTIVE HEART FAILURE in advanced heart disease
EFFECTIVE, WELL-TOLERATED ANTIHYPERTENSIVE in mild to moderate high blood pressure	Worsening of angina in coronary heart disease (abrupt withdrawal)
DECREASES DEATH AFTER HEART ATTACK	May lead to low blood sugar in type one diabetics
DECREASES MORBIDITY AFTER HEART ATTACK	Masking of low blood sugar (hypoglycemia) in drug-treated diabetes
HELPS PREVENT MIGRAINE HEADACHES	Provocation of bronchial asthma (with high doses)

▷ **Principal Uses**

As a Single Drug Product: Uses currently included in FDA-approved labeling: (1) Treats classical, effort-induced angina pectoris; (2) used for mild to moderately severe high blood pressure (may be used alone or in combination with other antihypertensive drugs, such as diuretics); (3) used following heart attacks to prolong life, help decrease risk of a second heart attack, decrease the size of the heart attack and reduce risk of abnormal heartbeats.

Other (unlabeled) generally accepted uses: (1) Can help people with stage fright; (2) may have a role in preventing migraine headaches; (3) can have an adjunctive role in alcohol withdrawal; (4) helps congestive heart failure when used with fosinopril (Monopril); (5) taken before and after surgery, this drug can help maintain blood flow to the heart and decrease death.

As a Combination Drug Product [CD]: Used in combination with a thiazide diuretic (chlorthalidone) to combine the benefits of a beta-blocker with the excess-fluid-losing properties of a thiazide. This attacks high blood pressure using two different mechanisms.

How This Drug Works: It blocks some actions of the sympathetic nervous system, reducing heart rate and contraction force and reducing oxygen needs as the heart works, and it reduces blood vessel contraction, resulting in opening and lowering of blood pressure.

Available Dosage Forms and Strengths

Injection — 5 mg/10 ml

Tablets — 25 mg, 50 mg, 100 mg

Tablets, combination — 50 mg, 100 mg of atenolol with 25 mg of chlorthalidone

▷ **Usual Adult Dosage Ranges**

Hypertension: Initially 50 mg once daily. Dose may be increased gradually at intervals of 7 to 10 days as needed and tolerated up to 100 mg every 24 hours. The usual maintenance dose is 50 to 100 mg every 24 hours. The total dose should not exceed 100 mg every 24 hours.

Angina: Starting dose is 50 mg once daily. May be gradually increased at 7- to 10-day intervals as needed and tolerated up to 100 mg every 24 hours. Usual ongoing dose is 50 to 100 mg every 24 hours. Some patients require 200 mg daily.

After a heart attack (post-MI): Within 12 hours after the attack, 5 mg of this drug is given intravenously. This is followed by a second 5-mg intravenous dose 10 minutes later. Twelve hours after the second intravenous dose, 50 mg is given orally, followed by a second 50 mg 12 hours later. Oral dosing is continued at 100 mg orally for the next 10 days. **Note: Actual dose and schedule must be determined for each patient individually**.

Conditions Requiring Dosing Adjustments

Liver Function: No decreases needed (liver has a small removal role).

Kidney Function: The dose must be decreased, with 25 mg a day as a maximum dose in some people.

▷ **Dosing Instructions:** Food decreases the amount of drug that gets into your body by up to 20%. Better taken on an empty stomach. Tablet may be crushed to take it. **DO NOT** stop this drug abruptly. If you forget a dose: take it right away unless it's within 8 hours of your next regular dose. If it IS within 8 hours of the next dose, just take the scheduled dose. DO NOT double doses.

Usual Duration of Use: Regular use for 3 to 7 days usually needed to see this drug's benefits in lowering blood pressure. Peak benefits may take two weeks. Meeting blood pressure goals will decide long-term use. Medicines are often coupled to an overall program of weight reduction, salt restriction, smoking cessation, etc. May take 3 months for peak chest pain benefits. See your doctor regularly.

Typical Treatment Goals and Measurements (Outcomes and Markers)

Blood Pressure: The most recent treatment guidelines (JNC VI) actually define optimal blood pressure (BP) as less than 120/80 and high normal as 139/89. The American Diabetes Association (ADA) defines a target goal in diabetics of 130/80. Most clinicians try to achieve a BP that achieves the best balance of lower cardiovascular risk while avoiding the problem of too low a blood pressure. The goal and time frame (see peak benefits above) should be discussed with you when the prescription is written.

Possible Advantages of This Drug: Least likely of all beta-blocker drugs to cause central nervous system adverse effects: confusion, hallucinations, nervousness, nightmares.

▷ **This Drug Should Not Be Taken If**
- you have had an allergic reaction to it previously.
- you are in heart failure (overt).
- you have an abnormally slow heart rate or a serious form of heart block.
- you are taking, or have taken within the past 14 days, any monoamine oxidase (MAO) type A inhibitor drug (see Drug Classes).
- you are in cardiogenic shock.

▷ **Inform Your Physician Before Taking This Drug If**
- you've had beta-blocker adverse reactions (see Drug Classes).
- you have a history of serious heart disease, with or without episodes of heart failure.
- you have a history of hay fever (allergic rhinitis), asthma, chronic bronchitis, chronic obstructive pulmonary disease (COPD) or emphysema.
- you have been taking clonidine.
- you have a history of overactive thyroid function (hyperthyroidism).
- you have low blood sugar (hypoglycemia)—may hide some symptoms of hypoglycemia.
- you have impaired liver or kidney function.
- you have diabetes or myasthenia gravis.
- you take digitalis, quinidine, reserpine or any calcium blocker (see Drug Classes).
- you take clonidine (atenolol should be stopped a few days before stopping clonidine).
- you will have surgery with general anesthesia.
- you take prescription or nonprescription drugs not discussed when atenolol was prescribed.
- you are unsure how much or how often to take this drug.

Possible Side Effects (natural, expected and unavoidable drug actions)

Lethargy, fatigability, cold extremities, slow heart rate, light-headedness in upright position (see Orthostatic Hypotension in Glossary)—all reported during treatment.

▷ **Possible Adverse Effects** (unusual, unexpected and infrequent reactions)
If any of the following develop, consult your physician promptly for guidance.

Mild Adverse Effects

Allergic reactions: skin rash, itching.

Headache, abnormal dreams—infrequent.

Dizziness, tiredness or depression—frequent.

Indigestion, nausea, diarrhea—infrequent.

Joint and muscle discomfort, fluid retention (edema)—possible.

Serious Adverse Effects

Allergic reactions: may contribute to seriousness and refractory allergic reactions.

Chest pain, shortness of breath, can lead to congestive heart failure—rare.

May lead to an asthma attack (in asthmatic people)—possible.

Angina or rebound hypertension—if abruptly stopped.

Difficulty walking (intermittent claudication)—controversial.

Psychosis—case reports.

Systemic lupus erythematosus—case reports.

▷ **Possible Effects on Sexual Function:** Decreased libido and impaired potency (50 to 100 mg per day). This drug is less likely to cause lowered ability to achieve a completely firm penis (reduced erectile capacity) than most drugs of its class. Impotence—rare.

Possible Effects on Laboratory Tests

Blood cholesterol, LDL and VLDL cholesterol levels: no effect with doses of 50 mg/day; increased with doses of 100 mg/day.

Blood triglyceride levels: no effect with doses of 50 mg/day; increased with doses of 100 mg/day.

Blood HDL cholesterol levels: no effect with doses of 50 mg/day; decreased with doses of 100 mg/day.

CAUTION

1. Control your high blood pressure for life! Even though it usually does not have any signs or symptoms, high blood pressure does damage. Control your pressure and take your medicine. Visit www.americanheart.org for information on MyHeartWatch—a new Web-based program to help you decrease heart disease risk factors.
2. *DO NOT stop this drug suddenly* without the guidance of your doctor. Carry a note in your purse or wallet that says you take this drug.
3. Talk to your doctor or pharmacist BEFORE using nasal spray or pill decongestants. These may cause sudden increases in blood pressure when combined with beta-blocker drugs.
4. Report any tendency to emotional depression to your doctor.

Precautions for Use

By Infants and Children: Safety and effectiveness by those under 12 years of age not established. However, if this drug is used, watch for development of low blood sugar (hypoglycemia), especially if meals are skipped.

By Those Over 60 Years of Age: Proceed *cautiously* with all antihypertensive drugs. High blood pressure should be reduced slowly, avoiding excessively low blood pressure. Small doses and frequent blood pressure checks are needed. Sudden and excessive decrease in blood pressure can predispose to stroke or heart attack. Maximum daily dosage is 100 mg. Watch for dizziness, unsteadiness, tendency to fall, confusion, hallucinations, depression or urinary frequency.

▷ **Advisability of Use During Pregnancy**

Pregnancy Category: D. See Pregnancy Risk Categories at the back of this book.

Animal studies: Increased resorptions of embryo and fetus reported in rats, but no birth defects.

Human studies: Adequate studies of pregnant women are not available, but the drug has caused fetal harm. This drug has been used during the last 3 months of pregnancy; however, fetal growth may be slowed and the child may be born with low blood pressure and temperature.

Ask your doctor for guidance.

Advisability of Use If Breast-Feeding

Presence of this drug in breast milk: Yes.

Avoid drug if possible. If drug is necessary, observe nursing infant for slow heart rate and indications of low blood sugar.

Habit-Forming Potential: None.

Effects of Overdose: Weakness, slow pulse, low blood pressure, fainting, cold sweaty skin, congestive heart failure, coma and convulsions.

Possible Effects of Long-Term Use: Reduced heart reserve or heart failure in some people with advanced heart disease.

Suggested Periodic Examinations While Taking This Drug (at physician's discretion)
Measurements of blood pressure.
Valuation of heart function.

▷ **While Taking This Drug, Observe the Following**
Foods: Can decrease total atenolol absorption by 20%. Best to avoid excessive salt intake.
Herbal Medicines or Minerals: Ginseng may increase blood pressure, blunting the benefits of this medicine. Hawthorn, saw palmetto, ma huang, goldenseal, yohimbe and licorice may also cause increased blood pressure. Calcium and garlic may help lower blood pressure. Indian snakeroot has a German Commission E monograph indication for hypertension—talk to your doctor. Eleuthero root and ephedra should be avoided by people living with hypertension.
Beverages: No restrictions. May be taken with milk.
▷ *Alcohol:* Use caution. Alcohol may exaggerate this drug's ability to lower blood pressure and may increase its mild sedative effect.
Tobacco Smoking: Nicotine may reduce this drug's effectiveness. I advise everyone to quit smoking.
▷ *Other Drugs*
Atenolol may *increase* the effects of
• other antihypertensive drugs and cause excessive lowering of blood pressure. Dosage adjustments may be necessary.
• reserpine (Ser-Ap-Es, etc.) and cause sedation, depression, slowing of heart rate and lowering of blood pressure.
Atenolol *taken concurrently* with
• amiodarone (Cordarone) may result in cardiac arrest.
• ampicillin or bacampicillin may result in lower blood levels of atenolol.
• calcium (various) may result in **large decreases** in atenolol blood levels.
• calcium channel blockers (dihydropyridine forms—various) may result in heart impairment or severe lowering of blood pressure. Caution is advised with this combination, but it may have good therapeutic use.
• clonidine (Catapres) requires close monitoring for rebound high blood pressure if clonidine is stopped while atenolol is still being taken.
• digoxin (Lanoxin) may result in very slow heart rates.
• insulin requires close monitoring to avoid undetected hypoglycemia (see Glossary).
• oral antidiabetic drugs (see Drug Classes) may result in prolonged low blood sugar.
• phenothiazines (see Drug Classes) may increase the effects of both agents and result in phenothiazine toxicity or excessively low blood pressure.
• quinidine (Quinaglute) may cause additive lowering of the blood pressure.
• ritodrine (Yutopar) may blunt ritodrine benefits.
• verapamil can result in undesirable slowing of the heart rate and excessively low blood pressure.

The following drugs may *decrease* the effects of atenolol:
- antacids—decrease atenolol absorption.
- aspirin (various).
- indomethacin (Indocin), and possibly other "aspirin substitutes," or NSAIDs, which may impair atenolol's blood pressure lowering (antihypertensive) effect.

▷ *Driving, Hazardous Activities:* Use caution until the full extent of drowsiness, lethargy and blood pressure change has been determined.

Aviation Note: The use of this drug is *a disqualification* for piloting. Consult a designated Aviation Medical Examiner.

Exposure to Sun: No restrictions.

Exposure to Heat: Caution is advised. Hot environments can lower blood pressure and exaggerate the effects of this drug.

Exposure to Cold: Caution is advised. Can enhance the circulatory deficiency that may occur with this drug. The elderly should be careful to prevent hypothermia (see Glossary).

Heavy Exercise or Exertion: Avoid exertion that causes light-headedness, excessive fatigue or muscle cramping. This drug may worsen the blood pressure response to isometric exercise.

Occurrence of Unrelated Illness: Fever can lower blood pressure and require a decreased dose. Nausea or vomiting may interrupt the dosing schedule. Ask your physician for help.

Discontinuation: Avoid stopping this drug suddenly. If possible, gradual reduction of dose over a period of 2 to 3 weeks is recommended. During such reduction, physical activity is best kept to a minimum. Ask your doctor for help.

ATORVASTATIN (a TOR va stat in)

Introduced: 1996   **Class:** Cholesterol-lowering agent, HMG-CoA reductase inhibitor   **Prescription:** USA: Yes   **Controlled Drug:** USA: No; Canada: No   **Available as Generic:** No
Brand Name: Lipitor

BENEFITS versus RISKS	
Possible Benefits	*Possible Risks*
REDUCTION OF TOTAL AND LDL CHOLESTEROL	Drug-induced hepatitis (without jaundice)—rare
DECREASED TRIGLYCERIDES	Drug-induced myositis (muscle inflammation)—rare
INCREASES HDL-C (GOOD CHOLESTEROL) IN PEOPLE WITH PRIMARY HYPER-CHOLESTEROLEMIA AND MIXED DYSLIPIDEMIA	Decreased coenzyme Q10
May help prevent bone loss in type two diabetics	

▷ **Principal Uses**

As a Single Drug Product: Uses currently included in FDA-approved labeling:
   (1) Treats high blood cholesterol (in people with Types IIa and IIb hyper-

cholesterolemia) due to increased fractions of low-density lipoprotein (LDL) cholesterol; (2) also works in primary dysbetalipoproteinemia (Fredrickson Type III) and in patients with elevated serum triglycerides (Fredrickson Type IV). Used in conjunction with a cholesterol-lowering diet. Should not be used until an adequate trial of nondrug methods has proved to be ineffective; (3) also helps familial hypercholesterolemia; (4) approved to increase HDL-C (good cholesterol) in people with primary hypercholesterolemia and mixed dyslipidemia.

Other (unlabeled) generally accepted uses: (1) A *New England Journal of Medicine* study found that atorvastatin was as effective as getting an angioplasty when it was used to treat stable heart (coronary) artery disease; (2) prevention of coronary heart disease; (3) treats abnormal fat (lipid) changes caused by protease inhibitors; (4) may help prevent bone loss (osteoporosis) in type two diabetics; (5) may help prevent clogging (restenosis) of tubes (stents) placed in coronary arteries.

How This Drug Works: Blocks a liver enzyme that starts making cholesterol. Lowers low-density lipoproteins (LDL), the cholesterol fraction thought to increase risk of coronary heart disease. Since the amount of cholesterol is reduced in the liver, the VLDL fraction may also be decreased.

Available Dosage Forms and Strengths
Tablets — 10 mg, 20 mg, 40 mg

▷ **Recommended Dosage Ranges** (Actual dosage and schedule must be determined for each patient individually.)
Infants and Children: Data are not available.
18 to 65 Years of Age: Start with 10 mg once daily. Increase as needed and tolerated to a maximum of 80 mg daily. Lipid levels best rechecked within 2 to 4 weeks of starting or changing the dose.
Over 65 Years of Age: Some research shows that usual doses may result in higher levels than seen in younger patients. It appears prudent that the lowest dose (10 mg) be used and LDL-C levels be checked to guide any dose increases. Dose increases must be made after weighing the benefits and risks, mindful that any given dose may result in a higher than expected blood level.

Conditions Requiring Dosing Adjustments
Liver Function: Caution should be used in patients with liver compromise. In those with liver damage caused by alcohol, removal from the body has been prolonged. A 10-mg dose appears prudent. Like other HMG-CoA medicines, atorvastatin should not be given during active liver disease.
Kidney Function: The manufacturer does not recommend dosing changes.

▷ **Dosing Instructions:** The tablet may be crushed or split. Better taken on an empty stomach. Since cholesterol is made at the fastest rate between midnight and 5 a.m., clinicians advise patients to take such medicines at bedtime. If you forget a dose, take it immediately unless it is almost time for your next dose. If your next dose is shortly due, skip the missed dose and just take the next scheduled dose. DO NOT double doses.

Usual Duration of Use: Use on a regular schedule for 2 to 4 weeks usually determines the effectiveness of this drug in reducing blood levels of total and LDL-C cholesterol. Increases in HDL may take longer. Use is usually ongoing. Long-term use (months to years) requires periodic physician evaluation and follow-up.

Typical Treatment Goals and Measurements (Outcomes and Markers)

Cholesterol: The National Institutes of Health has released ATP III as part of the update to the National Cholesterol Education Program or NCEP. Key points in these new guidelines include acknowledging diabetes as one of the conditions that increases risk of heart disease, modifying risk factors and recommending routine testing for all of the cholesterol fractions (lipoprotein profile) versus total cholesterol alone. These new guidelines also recommend a desirable total cholesterol of 200 mg/dl as before, but change optimal LDL to 100 mg/dl, 130–159 mg/dl as borderline high, 160 mg/dl as high and 190 mg/dl as very high. One other noteworthy change is that "good cholesterol" or HDL has been made more important. The "too low" measure for HDL has been increased to 40 mg/dl. Take your medicine and reach these new targets! Electron beam computed tomography (EBCT) is an important tool to use in conjunction with these laboratory studies. Findings show that even patients who meet cholesterol goals (particularly females over 55) can still be at significant cardiovascular risk. EBCT then defines that risk by giving a calcium score and a "virtual tour" of the coronary arteries.

Possible Advantages of This Drug: Recent studies indicate that drugs of this class (HMG-CoA reductase inhibitors) are more effective and better tolerated than other drugs currently available for reducing total and LDL-C cholesterol. Atorvastatin decreased LDL by up to 51% in one study (the most of any medicine in this family). Another study showed this medicine to be as effective as angioplasty when used to treat coronary artery disease that is stable. This medicine is easily split. At the time of this writing, the price is the same for a 20 or 80 mg tablet. Splitting tablets (get a pill splitter for accuracy) can lower costs a lot. One short-term outcome study of changing other statins to this medicine (therapeutic interchange of atorvastatin for simvastatin or pravastatin) found that both significant lowering of LDL and cost savings occurred.

This Drug Should Not Be Taken If
- you have had an allergic reaction to it previously.
- you have active liver disease or increased liver function tests that are unexplained.
- you are pregnant or are breast-feeding your infant.

Inform Your Physician Before Taking This Drug If
- you have previously taken any other drugs in this class: lovastatin (Mevacor), simvastatin (Zocor).
- you have liver disease or impaired liver function.
- you have kidney disease.
- you are not using any method of birth control or you are planning pregnancy.
- you regularly consume substantial amounts of alcohol.
- you develop unexplained muscle weakness, pain or tenderness.
- you have any type of chronic muscular disorder.
- goals were set by another doctor and have not been met using this medicine.

Possible Side Effects (natural, expected and unavoidable drug actions)
None with usual doses.

Possible Adverse Effects (unusual, unexpected and infrequent reactions)
  If any of the following develop, consult your physician promptly for guidance.
  Mild Adverse Effects
    Allergic reactions: skin rash—infrequent.
    Headache—infrequent to frequent, rare drowsiness.
    Flu-like syndrome—infrequent.
    Diarrhea, constipation or gas (flatulence)—infrequent.
    Muscle pain (myalgia)—infrequent with 20-mg dose (tell your doctor right away if this happens).
  Serious Adverse Effects
    Allergic reactions: not reported as yet.
    Marked and persistent abnormal liver function tests (without jaundice)—case reports to rare.
    Acute myositis (muscle pain and tenderness)—rare to infrequent with 10- to 80-mg doses.
    Rhabdomyolysis with sudden kidney failure—rarely reported with other HMG-CoA medicines.
    One case report of euphoria, confusion and short-term memory problems.
Possible Effects on Sexual Function: Decreased libido or impotence (2%).
Possible Delayed Adverse Effects: Increased liver enzymes. Decreased coenzyme Q10 (co-Q10 or ubiquinone).
Natural Diseases or Disorders That May Be Activated by This Drug
  Latent liver disease.
Possible Effects on Laboratory Tests
  Blood total cholesterol, LDL cholesterol and triglyceride levels: decreased.
  HDL: increased.
CAUTION
  1. If pregnancy occurs while taking this drug, stop drug immediately and call your doctor.
  2. Report promptly any development of muscle pain or tenderness, especially if accompanied by fever or malaise.
  3. Report promptly the development of altered or impaired vision so that appropriate evaluation can be made (visual changes have been reported with some other HMG-CoA medicines).
  4. If CPK levels become markedly elevated, this medicine should be stopped.
Precautions for Use
  By Infants and Children: Safety and effectiveness for those under 18 years of age not established.
  By Those Over 60 Years of Age: Blood levels for those over 65 may be higher than those reached by the same dose in younger people.
  Advisability of Use During Pregnancy
  Pregnancy Category: X. See Pregnancy Risk Categories at the back of this book.
  Animal studies: Rat studies reveal decreased pup survival and maturity with high-dose studies.
  Human studies: Adequate studies of pregnant women are not available.
    This drug should be avoided during entire pregnancy.

Advisability of Use If Breast-Feeding
Presence of this drug in breast milk: Yes, in rats; expected in humans.
Avoid drug or refrain from nursing.

Habit-Forming Potential: None.

Effects of Overdose: Increased indigestion, stomach distress, nausea, diarrhea with other HMG-CoA medicines.

Possible Effects of Long-Term Use: Abnormal liver function tests. Decreased coenzyme Q10 (co-Q10 or ubiquinone).

Suggested Periodic Examinations While Taking This Drug (at physician's discretion)
Blood cholesterol studies: total cholesterol, HDL and LDL fractions.
Liver function tests before treatment, at 6 and 12 weeks (the same for any dose increases) and then semiannually (every 6 months) thereafter. Ask your physician for guidance.

Author's Note: A related medicine called cerivastatin (Baycol) was removed from the market because of liver changes. It is unknown at the time of this writing if the FDA will review similar medicines and ask for more frequent checks of liver function.

Electron beam computed tomography (EBCT) can help predict silent ischemia and other problems with blood vessels that supply the heart itself. This also may help define the results (outcomes) you are getting from this medicine.

▷ **While Taking This Drug, Observe the Following**
Foods: Follow a standard low-cholesterol diet.
Herbal Medicines or Minerals: No data exist from well-designed clinical studies about garlic and atorvastatin combinations and cannot presently be recommended. Additionally, garlic may inhibit blood clotting (platelet) aggregation—something to consider if you are already taking a platelet inhibitor. The FDA has allowed one dietary supplement called Cholestin to continue to be sold. This preparation actually contains lovastatin. Since use of two HMG-CoA inhibitors may increase risk of rhabdomyolysis or myopathy, the combination is NOT advised. Some products containing plant sterols (Benecol) may be useful as complementary care. Soy (milk, tofu, etc.) contains phytoestrogens that have led to an FDA-approved health claim for reducing risk of heart disease (if they have at least 6.25 grams of soy protein per serving). Substituting soy for some of the meat in your diet can help avoid cardiovascular problems. Lastly, because atorvastatin can deplete coenzyme Q10, supplementation may be needed.
Beverages: DO NOT take this medicine with grapefruit juice. Excessive blood levels and increased risk of muscle damage may occur. May be taken with water or milk.
▷ *Alcohol:* Excessive alcohol not recommended.
Tobacco Smoking: No interactions expected. I advise everyone to quit smoking.
▷ *Other Drugs*
Atorvastatin may ***increase*** the effects of
• clofibrate (Atromid-S) and other fibric acid derivatives—has been associated with increased risk of muscle damage (rhabdomyolysis).

Atorvastatin *taken concurrently* with

- amprenavir (Agenerase) and ritonavir (Norvir) and perhaps other protease inhibitors may increase atorvastatin levels and the risk of muscle damage (myopathy).
- antacids decreases the amount of atorvastatin that gets into your body.
- azole antifungals (such as itraconazole or Sporanox) may increase the risk for muscle damage (myopathy).
- birth control pills (oral contraceptives) may increase the levels of the contraceptives (certain kinds) and may increase risk of adverse effects.
- colesevelam (Welchol) results in better lowering of LDL-C.
- colestipol (Colestid) results in lowered atorvastatin blood levels, but better lowering of LDL-C.
- cyclosporine (Sandimmune) may increase the risk for myopathy.
- digoxin (Lanoxin, others) can increase digoxin levels (and possibly lead to toxic effects).
- erythromycin (and perhaps other macrolide antibiotics) may increase the risk for myopathy.
- fluconazole (Diflucan) or itraconazole (Sporanox) or ketoconazole (Nizoral) will increase risk of myopathy. Extreme caution is advised.
- fosphenytoin (Cerebyx) and phenytoin (Dilantin) may blunt atorvastatin therapeutic effects.
- gemfibrozil (Lopid) may increase the risk of muscle damage (myopathy).
- medicines that change cytochrome P450 3A4 (inhibitors will increase atorvastatin levels and inducers will blunt atorvastatin therapeutic effects).
- nefazodone (Serzone) may lead to atorvastatin toxicity.
- niacin (various) may increase the risk for myopathy. Niacin may also increase homocysteine levels—a risk factor for heart disease.
- oral contraceptive (norethindrone and ethinyl estradiol) level increases are likely. Increased monitoring for adverse effects is prudent.
- quinupristin/dalfopristin (Synercid) may increase the risk for myopathy by increasing atorvastatin blood levels.

▷ *Driving, Hazardous Activities:* This drug may cause drowsiness. Restrict activities as necessary.

Aviation Note: The use of this drug *may be a disqualification* for piloting. Consult a designated Aviation Medical Examiner.

Exposure to Sun: No restrictions.

Occurrence of Unrelated Illness: Call your doctor if another physician (such as a specialist) diagnoses a sudden liver problem.

Discontinuation: Do not stop this drug without your doctor's knowledge and help. There may be a significant increase in blood cholesterol levels if this medicine is stopped.

AURANOFIN (aw RAY noh fin)

Introduced: 1976   **Class:**   Antiarthritic   **Prescription:** USA: Yes
Controlled Drug: USA: No; Canada: No   **Available as Generic:** Yes
Brand Name: Ridaura

BENEFITS versus RISKS	
Possible Benefits	*Possible Risks*
REDUCTION OF JOINT PAIN, TENDERNESS AND SWELLING IN ACTIVE, SEVERE RHEUMATOID ARTHRITIS	SIGNIFICANTLY REDUCED LEVELS OF RED AND WHITE BLOOD CELLS AND BLOOD PLATELETS
Effective when taken by mouth	LIVER DAMAGE WITH JAUNDICE
	Diarrhea
	Ulcerative colitis
	Skin rash
	Mouth sores
	Kidney toxicity (protein in the urine)
	Lung damage

Author's Note: Given the FDA approval of DMARDS (see Glossary), this profile has been shortened to make room for more widely used medicines.

AZATHIOPRINE (ay za THI oh preen)

Introduced: 1965   **Class:** Antiarthritic, immunosuppressive   **Prescription:** USA: Yes   **Controlled Drug:** USA: No; Canada: No   **Available as Generic:** Yes

Brand Name: Imuran, ✦Med-azathioprine, ✦Riva-azathioprine

BENEFITS versus RISKS	
Possible Benefits	*Possible Risks*
REDUCTION OF JOINT PAIN, TENDERNESS AND SWELLING in active, severe, resistant rheumatoid arthritis	UNACCEPTABLE ADVERSE EFFECTS IN 15% OF USERS
	REDUCED LEVELS OF WHITE BLOOD CELLS
PREVENTION OF REJECTION IN ORGAN TRANSPLANTATION	REDUCED LEVELS OF RED BLOOD CELLS AND PLATELETS
	LIVER DAMAGE WITH JAUNDICE
	POSSIBLE INCREASED RISK OF MALIGNANCY

Principal Uses

As a Single Drug Product: Uses currently included in FDA-approved labeling: (1) Helps prevent transplanted organ rejection (mainly kidneys); (2) also used in active, severe rheumatoid arthritis (in adults) failing conventional treatment. Other (unlabeled) generally accepted uses: (1) Used to treat lupus erythematosus, ulcerative colitis, chronic active hepatitis and other "autoimmune" disorders; (2) decreases rejection rates (combination therapy) preventing heart transplant failures; (3) very useful in actinic dermatitis.

How This Drug Works: It impairs metabolism of purines, DNA and RNA. This blunts the immune reaction responsible for rheumatoid arthritis, lupus erythematosus, etc.

Available Dosage Forms and Strengths
 Injection — 100 mg per 20-ml vial
 Tablets — 50 mg

▷ **Usual Adult Dosage Ranges:** *As immunosuppressant:* 3–5 mg per kg of body mass daily, 1 to 3 days before transplantation surgery; for ongoing postoperative use—1–2 mg per kg of body mass daily.

 In rheumatoid arthritis (RA): 1 mg per kg of body mass daily for 6 to 8 weeks; increased by 0.5 mg per kg of body mass every 4 weeks as needed. Maximal daily dose is 2.5 mg per kg of body mass. Total dose may be taken once daily or divided into equal doses taken 12 hours apart. Ongoing dose should be the lowest effective dose (optimal is often 1–3 mg/kg/day). **Note: Actual dose schedule must be determined for each patient individually.**

Conditions Requiring Dosing Adjustments
 Liver Function: The drug may need to be stopped if jaundice occurs. Liver function must be closely watched.
 Kidney Function: The dose must be decreased by up to 50% in kidney failure.

▷ **Dosing Instructions:** Take with or following food to reduce stomach upset. Tablet may be crushed. If you forget a dose: and you just take one dose a day, take the next scheduled dose. DO NOT double doses. If you take more than one dose a day, take the missed dose as soon as possible. If it is nearly time for your next dose, take the two doses at the same time. If you miss more than one dose, please call your doctor.

Usual Duration of Use: Use on a regular schedule for 12 weeks is usually needed to determine this drug's effectiveness in helping rheumatoid arthritis. Patients who do not respond within 12 weeks may be considered refractory. Successful use for more than a decade has been reported. See your physician regularly.

Typical Treatment Goals and Measurements (Outcomes and Markers)
 Organ Transplantation: The balance here is a difficult range between prevention of organ rejection and toxicity (bone marrow suppression and gastrointestinal problems). Doses are generally lowered to 1–3 mg/kg/day. Complete blood cell counts and gastrointestinal disturbance are balanced with organ function (such as creatinine and BUN in kidney transplantation).

▷ **This Drug Should Not Be Taken If**
- you have had an allergic reaction to it previously.
- you are pregnant and this drug is prescribed to treat rheumatoid arthritis.
- you have an active blood cell or bone marrow disorder.
- you are taking, or have recently taken, any form of chlorambucil (Leukeran), cyclophosphamide (Cytoxan) or melphalan (Alkeran) (alkylating agents).

▷ **Inform Your Physician Before Taking This Drug If**
- you have any kind of active infection.
- you have any form of cancer.
- you have gout or are taking allopurinol (Zyloprim).
- you have a history of blood cell or bone marrow disorders.
- you have impaired liver or kidney function.
- you are taking an ACE inhibitor (see Drug Classes). Use of azathioprine with these medicines has severely lowered white blood cell counts.
- you are taking any form of gold, penicillamine or an antimalarial drug for arthritis.

- you develop an infection or have had unusual bleeding or easy bruising.
- you plan pregnancy in the near future.
- you take other prescription or nonprescription medicines not discussed when azathioprine was prescribed.
- you are unsure how much to take or how often to take it.

Possible Side Effects (natural, expected and unavoidable drug actions) Development of infection.

▷ **Possible Adverse Effects** (unusual, unexpected and infrequent reactions)
If any of the following develop, consult your physician promptly for guidance.

Mild Adverse Effects
Allergic reaction: skin rash—rare.
Loss of appetite, nausea, vomiting, diarrhea—infrequent to frequent.
Sores on lips and in mouth—possible.
Muscle aches—infrequent.

Serious Adverse Effects
Allergic reactions: drug fever (see Glossary), joint and muscle pain—rare.
Pancreatitis: severe stomach pain with nausea and vomiting—rare.
Pericarditis—case reports.
Bone marrow depression (see Glossary): fatigue, weakness, fever, sore throat, abnormal bleeding or bruising—dose dependent.
Liver damage: yellow eyes, dark urine (see Hepatitis and Jaundice in Glossary)—rare.
Drug-induced lung damage (pneumonitis): cough, shortness of breath—possible.
Development of cancer: skin cancer, reticulum-cell sarcoma, lymphoma, leukemia—possible.

▷ **Possible Effects on Sexual Function:** Reversal of male infertility due to sperm antibodies; this drug suppresses autoantibodies and permits the normal accumulation of sperm. May also decrease sperm counts.

Possible Delayed Adverse Effects: Bone marrow depression may occur after stopping this drug.

Adverse Effects That May Mimic Natural Diseases or Disorders
Liver damage may suggest viral hepatitis.

Possible Effects on Laboratory Tests
Complete blood cell counts: decreased red cells, hemoglobin, white cells and platelets.
Blood amylase and lipase levels: increased.
Blood uric acid levels: increased; decreased in gout patients.
Liver function tests: increased liver enzymes (ALT/GPT, AST/GOT and alkaline phosphatase); increased bilirubin.
Sperm counts: decreased.

CAUTION
1. Promptly report infection—fever, chills, lip sores, etc.
2. Inform your physician promptly if you become pregnant.
3. Periodic blood counts are mandatory.
4. Talk to your doctor BEFORE you get any shots (vaccines).

Precautions for Use
By Infants and Children: Safety and effectiveness in those under 12 years of age are not established.

By Those Over 60 Years of Age: The smallest effective dose should be used, as this reduces the risk of toxic reactions.

▷ **Advisability of Use During Pregnancy**

Pregnancy Category: D. See Pregnancy Risk Categories at the back of this book.

Animal studies: Birth defects reported in rodent studies.

Human studies: This drug exhibits teratogenic effects and also poses a risk of suppression of the immune system of the newborn. Adequate studies of pregnant women are not available. **Avoid completely** during entire pregnancy if possible.

Advisability of Use If Breast-Feeding

Presence of this drug in breast milk: Yes.

Avoid drug or refrain from nursing.

Habit-Forming Potential: None.

Effects of Overdose: Immediate—nausea, vomiting, diarrhea. Delayed—lowered white blood cell and platelet counts, liver and kidney toxicity.

Possible Effects of Long-Term Use: Susceptibility to infection, bone marrow depression, development of malignancies.

Suggested Periodic Examinations While Taking This Drug (at physician's discretion)

Complete blood cell counts.

Liver function tests.

▷ **While Taking This Drug, Observe the Following**

Foods: No restrictions and may help stomach upset.

Herbal Medicines or Minerals: Some patients use echinacea to attempt to boost their immune systems. Unfortunately, use of echinacea is not recommended in people with damaged immune systems. This herb may also actually weaken any immune system if it is used too often or for too long a time.

Beverages: No restrictions. May be taken with milk.

▷ *Alcohol:* No interactions expected.

Tobacco Smoking: No interactions expected. I advise everyone to quit smoking.

▷ *Other Drugs*

Azathioprine may *decrease* the effects of

- certain muscle relaxants (gallamine, pancuronium, tubocurarine) and make it necessary to increase their dosage.
- oral anticoagulants (warfarin, etc.) and requires increased doses.

The following drug may *increase* the effects of azathioprine:

- allopurinol (Zyloprim)—may increase its activity and toxicity and make it necessary to reduce its dosage.

Azathioprine *taken concurrently* with

- ACE inhibitors (see Drug Classes) such as captopril or enalapril may cause severe white blood cell count lowering or anemia.
- cotrimoxazole (Bactrim, others) can cause severe lowering of white blood cell counts.
- cyclosporine (Sandimmune, others) may lead to decreased cyclosporine levels, requiring more frequent blood level checks and dosing adjustments.
- prednisolone will result in lower prednisolone blood levels and risk of decreased therapeutic benefit.

- vaccines (live—various) may result in abnormal patient responses to the vaccines and risk of infection by the live vaccine itself.
- warfarin (Coumadin) may result in decreased anticoagulant effectiveness.

▷ *Driving, Hazardous Activities:* No restrictions.

Aviation Note: The use of this drug *may be a disqualification* for piloting. Consult a designated Aviation Medical Examiner.

Exposure to Sun: No restrictions.

Discontinuation: A gradual reduction in dosage is preferable. Consult your physician for a withdrawal schedule.

AZITHROMYCIN (a zith roh MY sin)

See the macrolide antibiotics profile for further information.

BACAMPICILLIN (bak am pi SIL in)

See the new penicillins profile for further information.

BECLOMETHASONE (be kloh METH a sohn)

Introduced: 1976 **Class:** Antiasthmatic, cortisonelike drugs **Prescription:** USA: Yes **Controlled Drug:** USA: No; Canada: No **Available as Generic:** No

Brand Names: ✤Apo-Beclomethasone-AQ, ✤Beclodisk, ✤Becloforte, Beclovent, ✤Beclovent Rotacaps, ✤Beclovent Rotahaler, Beconase AQ Nasal Spray, Beconase Nasal Inhaler, ✤Med-Beclomethasone-AQ, ✤Nu-Beclomethasone, ✤Propaderm, ✤Propaderm-C, QVAR, Vancenase AQ Nasal Spray, Vancenase Nasal Inhaler, Vanceril

BENEFITS versus RISKS	
Possible Benefits	*Possible Risks*
EFFECTIVE RELIEF OF ALLERGIC RHINITIS	FUNGUS INFECTIONS OF THE MOUTH AND THROAT
EFFECTIVE CONTROL OF SEVERE, CHRONIC ASTHMA	Localized areas of "allergic" pneumonia
HELPS PREVENT NASAL POYLPS	Changes in lining of the nose (nasal mucosa)
	Increased cataract risk
	Possible osteoporosis

▷ **Principal Uses**

As a Single Drug Product: Uses currently included in FDA-approved labeling: (1) Bronchial asthma in people who don't have sufficient response to bronchodilators and need cortisonelike drugs for asthma control; (2) prevents nasal polyp return after surgical removal; (3) treats seasonal and perennial rhinitis in children and adults (AQ nasal forms).

Other (unlabeled) generally accepted uses: (1) Helps lung disease (bronchopulmonary dysplasia) allowing smaller daily prednisone doses; (2) helps hoarseness seen in LE and juvenile rheumatoid arthritis.

How This Drug Works: It increases cyclic AMP, thus increasing epinephrine, which opens bronchial tubes and fights asthma. Also reduces local lung inflammation in the respiratory tract.

Available Dosage Forms and Strengths

Inhalant — 17 g (50 mcg)

Nasal inhaler — 16.8 g (42 or 82 mcg each)

Nasal spray — 0.042%, 42 mcg and 84 mcg per spray (52 mcg in Canada)

Oral inhaler — 16.8 g (200 doses of 42 mcg each, 50 mcg in Canada)

Rotacaps (Canada) — 100- and 200-mcg capsules

Topical lotion (Canada) — 0.025%

▷ **Usual Adult Dosage Ranges**

Infants and Children: Data are not available for infants. Children 6–12 years old may receive: Nasal inhaler—one inhalation (42 mcg) in each nostril three times a day. Oral inhalation (42 mcg)—One to two inhalations, three or four times a day depending on the response. Some clinicians use 4 inhalations twice daily. Oral inhalation (double strength—84 mcg)—2 inhalations twice a day. Maximum is 5 inhalations (420 mcg for Vanceril Double Strength).

18 to 65 Years of Age: Nasal inhaler—one to two inhalations (42–84 mcg) in each nostril twice daily. Oral inhaler (double strength)—two inhalations (of 84 mcg) twice daily. For severe asthma—6 to 8 inhalations daily. Nasal polyp prevention after surgery: 42 or 84 mcg in each nostril twice daily (Beconase AQ form). Maximum daily dose should not exceed 10 inhalations.

Those Over 65 Years of Age: Doses similar to those used in younger patients have been effective and safe. In some cases, oral-steroid-dependent patients have been able to slowly taper and then stop oral steroids while taking beclomethasone.

Note: Actual dose and schedule must be determined for each patient individually.

Conditions Requiring Dosing Adjustments

Liver Function: Use with caution in patients with liver compromise.

Kidney Function: No adjustments in dosing expected to be needed.

▷ **Dosing Instructions:** May be used without regard to eating. Shake the inhaler well before you use it. Make sure you understand how to use any dosage form. Rinse the mouth and throat (gargle) with water thoroughly after each inhalation. If you forget a dose: Use the inhaler as soon as possible. DO NOT double doses.

Usual Duration of Use: Regular use for 1 to 4 weeks is usually needed to see this drug's effectiveness in relieving severe, chronic allergic rhinitis and in controlling severe, chronic asthma. Up to 2 weeks may be needed to relieve rhinitis by nasal inhalation. Long-term use must be physician-supervised. See your doctor regularly.

Typical Treatment Goals and Measurements (Outcomes and Markers)

Asthma: This medicine is NOT useful in a sudden asthma attack, but is used to decrease the severity and frequency of attacks. Some clinicians also use the number of times a rescue inhaler is used as another clinical benchmark. FEV1 is widely used to check results when this test is available to the patient. During the course of using this medicine—if it becomes less beneficial (helps less than it used to), call your doctor immediately.

▷ **This Drug Should Not Be Taken If**
- you have had an allergic reaction to any form of this drug.
- you are having severe acute asthma or status asthmaticus that requires more intense treatment for prompt relief.
- other antiasthmatic drugs can control your asthma that are not related to cortisone.
- your asthma requires cortisonelike drugs infrequently for control.
- you have a form of nonallergic bronchitis with asthmatic features.

▷ **Inform Your Physician Before Taking This Drug If**
- you take or recently took any cortisone-related drug (including ACTH by injection) for any reason (see Drug Classes).
- you have a history of tuberculosis of the lungs.
- you have chronic bronchitis or bronchiectasis.
- you think you have an active infection of any kind, especially a respiratory infection.
- you have recently been exposed to chickenpox or other viral illnesses.
- you are prone to nosebleeds (epistaxis) (nasal forms).
- you are unsure how much to take or how often to take this drug.

Possible Side Effects (natural, expected and unavoidable drug actions)
Fungus infections (thrush) of the mouth and throat.

▷ **Possible Adverse Effects** (unusual, unexpected and infrequent reactions)
If any of the following develop, consult your physician promptly for guidance.
Mild Adverse Effects
Allergic reaction: skin rash—rare.
Dryness of mouth, hoarseness, sore throat, cough—possible.
Nosebleeds (epistaxis)—infrequent.
May decrease growth rate in children—possible.
Serious Adverse Effects
Allergic reaction: localized areas of "allergic" pneumonitis (lung inflammation).
Bronchospasm, asthmatic wheezing—rare.
Shrinking of the nasal tissues (nasal atrophy)—possible.
Yeast infections (up to 41%)—frequent.
Increased risk of cataracts with long-term (chronic) use.
Osteoporosis (any corticosteroid can cause this)—possible.

▷ **Possible Effects on Sexual Function:** None reported.

Natural Diseases or Disorders That May Be Activated by This Drug
Cortisone-related drugs having systemic effects impair immunity and lead to reactivation of "healed" or dormant tuberculosis. People with a history of tuberculosis must be watched closely while using this drug.

Possible Effects on Laboratory Tests
Blood cortisol levels: decreased.
Bone mineral density: decreased with chronic use.

CAUTION

1. This drug should not be relied upon for immediate relief of acute asthma.
2. If you required cortisonelike drugs *before* starting this inhaler, you may again require a cortisonelike drug if you are injured, have an infection or need surgery.
3. If severe asthma returns while using this drug, call your doctor immediately. Cortisonelike drugs may be required.
4. Carry a personal ID card saying that you have used (if true) cortisone-related drugs in the past year.
5. Wait 5 to 10 minutes after using a bronchodilator inhaler such as epinephrine, isoetharine or isoproterenol (which should be used first) before this drug. This permits greater penetration of beclomethasone into the lung. The time between inhalations also reduces risk of adverse propellant effects.
6. This drug does NOT replace systemic steroids, but may allow dosage decreases in some patients.
7. If this medicine is to be used long-term, a bone mineral density test before treatment and every two years is prudent.

Precautions for Use

By Infants and Children: Safety and effectiveness for use of the nasal inhaler or oral inhaler by those under 6 years of age has not been established. Maximum daily dose in children 6 to 12 years of age varies with the product being used.

By Those Over 60 Years of Age: People with bronchiectasis should be watched closely for the development of lung infections.

▷ **Advisability of Use During Pregnancy**

Pregnancy Category: C. See Pregnancy Risk Categories at the back of this book.

Animal studies: Mouse, rat and rabbit studies reveal significant birth defects due to this drug.

Human studies: Adequate studies of pregnant women are not available.

Avoid drug during the first 3 months. Use infrequently and only as clearly needed during the last 6 months.

Advisability of Use If Breast-Feeding

Presence of this drug in breast milk: Probably yes.

Avoid drug or refrain from nursing.

Habit-Forming Potential: With recommended dosage, a state of functional dependence (see Glossary) is not likely to develop. There have been a small number of cases reported where the aerosol was abused for the fluorocarbon propellants.

Effects of Overdose: Indications of cortisone excess (due to systemic absorption)—fluid retention, flushing of the face, stomach irritation, nervousness.

Suggested Periodic Examinations While Taking This Drug (at physician's discretion)

Inspection of nose, mouth and throat for fungus infection.

Inspection of the nose tissues for nasal atrophy.

Assessment of adrenal function in people using cortisone-related drugs for an extended time prior to this drug.

Lung X-ray if a prior history of tuberculosis.

Measures of bone mineral density (DEXA or PDEXA) and cataract check.

▷ **While Taking This Drug, Observe the Following**

Foods: No specific restrictions beyond those advised by your physician.

Herbal Medicines or Minerals: Fir or pine needle oil should NOT be used by asthmatics. Ephedra alone does carry a German Commission E monograph indication for asthma treatment. If you are allergic to plants in the Asteraceae family (aster, chrysanthemum, daisy or ragweed), you may also be allergic to echinacea, chamomile, feverfew and St. John's wort. Talk to your doctor BEFORE adding it to any medicines that you already take.

Beverages: No specific restrictions.

▷ *Alcohol:* No interactions expected.

Tobacco Smoking: Smoking can reduce the benefits of this drug. I advise everyone to quit smoking.

▷ *Other Drugs*

The following drugs may ***increase*** the effects of beclomethasone:

- some antiepileptic medicines such as phenytoin (Dilantin)—may increase risk of osteoporosis.
- flunisolide (Nasalide).
- inhalant bronchodilators—epinephrine, isoetharine, isoproterenol.
- oral bronchodilators—aminophylline, ephedrine, terbutaline, theophylline, etc.

Beclomethasone ***taken concurrently*** with

- alendronate (Fosamax) helps prevent steroid-induced osteoporosis.

▷ *Driving, Hazardous Activities:* No restrictions.

Aviation Note: The use of this drug and the disorder for which this drug is prescribed ***may be disqualifications*** for piloting. Consult a designated Aviation Medical Examiner.

Exposure to Sun: No restrictions.

Occurrence of Unrelated Illness: Acute infections, serious injuries and surgery can create an urgent need for cortisone-related drugs. Call your doctor immediately in the event of new illness or injury.

Discontinuation: If this drug has made it possible to reduce or stop ongoing cortisonelike drugs, do not stop this drug abruptly. If you must stop this drug, call your doctor. You may need to resume cortisone medicines.

Special Storage Instructions: Store at room temperature. Avoid exposure to temperatures above 120 degrees F (49 degrees C). Do not store or use this inhaler near heat or open flame. Protect from light.

BENAZEPRIL (ben AY ze pril)

Class: ACE inhibitor, antihypertensive

Please see the new angiotensin converting enzyme (ACE) inhibitor family profile for more information.

BENZTROPINE (BENZ troh peen)

Introduced: 1954   **Class:** Anti-parkinsonism, atropinelike drugs   **Prescription:** USA: Yes   **Controlled Drug:** USA: No; Canada: No   **Available as Generic:** USA: Yes; Canada: Yes

Brand Names: ❦Apo-Benztropine, ❦Bensylate, Cogentin ❦PMS Benztropine

```
┌─────────────────────────────────────────────────────────────────┐
│                     BENEFITS versus RISKS                         │
│      Possible Benefits                    Possible Risks          │
│  PARTIAL RELIEF OF SYMPTOMS      Atropinelike side effects: blurred│
│     OF PARKINSON'S DISEASE          vision, dry mouth, constipation,│
│  RELIEF OF DRUG-INDUCED             impaired urination             │
│     EXTRAPYRAMIDAL REACTIONS     Toxic psychosis—rare             │
│                                  Tardive dyskinesia—rare          │
└─────────────────────────────────────────────────────────────────┘
```

▷ **Principal Uses**

> *As a Single Drug Product:* Uses currently included in FDA-approved labeling: (1) Used with other drugs to treat all types of parkinsonism (if relief is inadequate, more potent drugs—levodopa or bromocriptine—may supplement Cogentin); (2) controls parkinsonian reactions from some antipsychotic drugs (such as phenothiazines); (3) eases parkinsonian symptoms after encephalitis.
>
> Other (unlabeled) generally accepted uses: (1) helps sweaty palms (combined with psychotherapy); (2) can help drooling in developmentally disabled patients.
>
> **Author's Note: Many clinicians are obtaining excellent results with higher-dose vitamin E for decreasing parkinsonian symptoms seen with some antipsychotic medicines. Some use it in combination with benztropine.**

How This Drug Works: Restores a more normal balance of two brain chemicals (acetylcholine and dopamine), thereby decreasing parkinsonism symptoms.

Available Dosage Forms and Strengths

> Injection — 1 mg/ml, 2 mg/ml
> Tablets — 0.5 mg, 1 mg, 2 mg

▷ **Usual Adult Dosage Ranges:** *For Parkinson's disease:* 0.5 to 2 mg daily, taken in a single dose by mouth at bedtime. *For drug-induced parkinsonian reactions:* 1 to 4 mg daily, either in a single dose or in two to three divided doses. The total daily dose should not exceed 6 mg. For Parkinson's symptoms after encephalitis: Starting doses of 2 mg/day are used. May then be increased as needed or tolerated to 4 to 6 mg per day. **Note: Actual dosage and schedule must be determined for each patient individually.**

Conditions Requiring Dosing Adjustments

> *Liver Function:* Use with **Caution:** in patients with impaired liver function.
> *Kidney Function:* Caution: Decreased kidney function may lead to an increased blood level and an increased risk of adverse effects.

▷ **Dosing Instructions:** May be taken with or following food to reduce stomach irritation. Tablet may be crushed. If you forget a dose, take the missed dose as soon as possible. If it is nearly time for your next dose, skip the missed dose and continue benztropine on its regular schedule. DO NOT double doses.

Usual Duration of Use: Regular use for 2 to 4 weeks usually needed to see peak benefit relieving symptoms of parkinsonism. Long-term use (months to years) requires physician supervision.

Typical Treatment Goals and Measurements (Outcomes and Markers)

> *Parkinson's:* This medicine helps treat symptoms of Parkinson's disease, but does NOT halt its progression and combination therapy is often required. Usual

goals are to decrease symptom severity and improve quality of life. Regular physician assessment is required as symptoms change or exacerbate.

▷ **This Drug Should Not Be Taken If**
- you have had an allergic reaction to it.
- you are a child under 3 years of age.
- you have tardive dyskinesia.
- you have narrow-angle glaucoma (untreated).

▷ **Inform Your Physician Before Taking This Drug If**
- you have had an unfavorable reaction to atropine or atropinelike drugs.
- you have glaucoma or myasthenia gravis.
- you have heart disease or high blood pressure.
- you have a history of liver or kidney disease.
- you have difficulty emptying the urinary bladder, especially if due to an enlarged prostate gland.
- you are taking, or took in the past 2 weeks, any monoamine oxidase (MAO) type A inhibitor (see Drug Classes).
- you take prescription or nonprescription medicines not discussed when benztropine was prescribed for you.
- you are unsure how much to take or how often to take it.
- you will be exposed to extreme heat for extended periods, such as some iron smelters or tropical climates.
- you have a history of bowel obstructions.

Possible Side Effects (natural, expected and unavoidable drug actions)
Nervousness, blurring of vision, dryness of mouth, constipation, impaired urination. (These often subside as drug use continues.)

▷ **Possible Adverse Effects** (unusual, unexpected and infrequent reactions)
If any of the following develop, consult your physician promptly for guidance.

Mild Adverse Effects
Allergic reaction: skin rashes—rare.
Headache, dizziness, drowsiness, muscle cramps—possible.
Indigestion, nausea, vomiting—reported.
Fast heart rate (tachycardia)—infrequent.
Memory problems—possible.

Serious Adverse Effects
Idiosyncratic reactions: abnormal behavior, confusion, delusions, hallucinations, toxic psychosis—case reports.
Tardive dyskinesia—case reports.
Dystonia—rare.
Bowel obstruction—case reports.
Abnormal temperature (hyperthermia)—case reports.

▷ **Possible Effects on Sexual Function** Reversal of male impotence due to the use of fluphenazine (a phenothiazine antipsychotic drug).
Male infertility (0.5 to 6 mg per day).
May help treat priapism.

Natural Diseases or Disorders That May Be Activated by This Drug
Latent glaucoma, latent myasthenia gravis.

Possible Effects on Laboratory Tests
Prolactin: may be increased (especially if taken with haloperidol).

CAUTION

1. Many over-the-counter (OTC) drugs for allergies, colds and coughs should NOT be combined with benztropine. Ask your doctor or pharmacist for help.
2. This drug may aggravate tardive dyskinesia (see Glossary). Ask your physician for guidance.

Precautions for Use

By Infants and Children: Safety and effectiveness for those under 3 years of age not established. Children are especially susceptible to the atropinelike effects.

By Those Over 60 Years of Age: Small starting doses are prudent. Increased risk of confusion, nightmares, hallucinations, increased internal eye pressure (glaucoma) and impaired urination associated with prostate gland enlargement (prostatism).

▷ **Advisability of Use During Pregnancy**

Pregnancy Category: C. See Pregnancy Risk Categories at the back of this book.
Animal studies: No data available.
Human studies: Adequate studies of pregnant women are not available.
Avoid use if possible, especially close to delivery. This drug can impair the infant's intestinal tract following birth.

Advisability of Use If Breast-Feeding

Presence of this drug in breast milk: Unknown.
Ask your doctor for help.

Habit-Forming Potential: Occasional reports of anti-Parkinsonian drug abuse have been made. Sudden withdrawal of benztropine may lead to craving, restlessness, nervousness and depression. Propranolol (20–80 mg three times daily) or diazepam (Valium) has been used to ease these symptoms.

Effects of Overdose: Weakness, drowsiness, stupor, impaired vision, rapid pulse, excitement, confusion, hallucinations, dry, hot skin, skin rash, dilated pupils.

Possible Effects of Long-Term Use: Increased internal eye pressure—possible glaucoma, especially in the elderly.

Suggested Periodic Examinations While Taking This Drug (at physician's discretion)
Measurement of internal eye pressure at regular intervals. Check of continued effectiveness of the drug itself.

▷ **While Taking This Drug, Observe the Following**

Foods: No restrictions.

Herbal Medicines or Minerals: See marijuana below. Additionally, talk to your doctor BEFORE adding any herbs to any medicines that you already take. Phenylalanine (200–500 mg daily) has been used by some clinicians to ease Parkinson's. Calabar bean (chop nut or ordeal bean) and octacosanol should be AVOIDED by people living with Parkinson's.

Beverages: No restrictions.

▷ *Alcohol:* Use caution. Alcohol may increase the sedative effects.

Tobacco Smoking: No interactions expected, but I advise everyone to quit smoking.

Marijuana Smoking: May increase heart rate to unacceptable levels. Avoid completely if this increased heart rate will be a problem for you.

▷ *Other Drugs*

Benztropine may *decrease* the effects of
- cisapride (Propulsid).
- haloperidol (Haldol).
- phenothiazines (Thorazine, others).

The following drugs may *increase* the effects of benztropine:
- antihistamines may add to the dryness of mouth and throat.
- monoamine oxidase (MAO) type A inhibitor drugs may intensify all effects of this drug (see Drug Classes).
- tricyclic antidepressants (Elavil, etc.) may add to eye effects and further increase internal eye pressure (dangerous in glaucoma).

Benztropine *taken concurrently* with
- amantadine (Symmetrel) may cause increased confusion and possible hallucinations.
- clozapine (Clozaril) can cause increased risk of elevated temperatures, neurological adverse effects and bowel obstruction (ileus).
- procainamide (Procanbid, etc.) may increase risk of heart conduction problems.

▷ *Driving, Hazardous Activities:* Drowsiness and dizziness may occur. Avoid hazardous activities until full effects and tolerance have been determined.

Aviation Note: The use of this drug *is a disqualification* for piloting. Consult a designated Aviation Medical Examiner.

Exposure to Sun: No restrictions.

Exposure to Heat: Use caution. This drug may reduce sweating, cause an increase in body temperature and increase risk of heatstroke.

Heavy Exercise or Exertion: Use caution. Avoid in hot environments.

Discontinuation: Do not stop this drug abruptly. Ask your doctor how to reduce the dose gradually.

BETAXOLOL (be TAX oh lohl)

Introduced: 1983   **Class:** Antihypertensive, beta-adrenergic blocker
Prescription: USA: Yes   **Controlled Drug:** USA: No; Canada: No
Available as Generic: No

Brand Names: Betoptic, Betoptic-Pilo [CD], Betoptic-S, Kerlone, ✤Novo-Betaxolol

BENEFITS versus RISKS	
Possible Benefits	*Possible Risks*
EFFECTIVE, WELL-TOLERATED ANTIHYPERTENSIVE IN MILD TO MODERATE HIGH BLOOD PRESSURE	CONGESTIVE HEART FAILURE in advanced heart disease
EFFECTIVE TREATMENT OF CHRONIC, OPEN-ANGLE GLAUCOMA	Worsening of angina in coronary heart disease (abrupt withdrawal)
PROLONGATION OF LIFE AFTER HEART ATTACK	Masking of low blood sugar (hypoglycemia) in diabetes
Treatment of ocular hypertension	Provocation of bronchial asthma (with high doses)
	Rare anemia and low blood platelets

▷ **Principal Uses**

As a Single Drug Product: Uses currently included in FDA-approved labeling: Used to treat (1) mild to moderate high blood pressure (alone or combined with other antihypertensive drugs, such as diuretics); (2) chronic open-angle glaucoma (eyedrops); (3) ocular hypertension; (4) Betoptic-Pilo—reduces elevated eye pressure in primary open-angle glaucoma who have failed Betoptic-S therapy.

Other (unlabeled) generally accepted uses: (1) The oral form may help decrease death (mortality) from a heart attack; (2) helps decrease incidence and severity of chest pain (angina); (3) can ease aggressive behavior in selected psychiatric patients; (4) can treat selected cases of stuttering.

How This Drug Works: By blocking some sympathetic nervous system actions, it reduces heart rate and contraction force, lowers blood ejection pressure and reduces oxygen needed by the heart. Relaxes blood vessel walls, resulting in expansion and lower blood pressure. Reduces internal eye pressure.

Available Dosage Forms and Strengths

Eyedrops (solution) — 2.8 mg/ml, 5.6 mg/ml
Eyedrops (suspension) — 0.25%
— 0.25%/1.75% (Betoptic Pilo)
Tablets — 10 mg, 20 mg

▷ **Usual Adult Dosage Ranges:** *Hypertension:* Initially 10 mg once daily. Dose may be increased at intervals of 7 to 14 days as needed and tolerated up to 20 mg every 24 hours. Usual ongoing dose is 10 to 15 mg daily. Some patients have tolerated 40 mg daily well, but had no benefit in reduced blood pressure. Total maximum is 20 mg daily.

For use in glaucoma: One or two drops of the 2.8 mg/ml solution or one drop of the 5.6 mg/ml twice daily.

Betoptic-Pilo (reducing intraocular pressure in primary open-angle glaucoma failing Betoptic-S therapy): Follow label instructions. **Note: Actual dose and schedule must be determined for each patient individually.**

Conditions Requiring Dosing Adjustments

Liver Function: Use with caution; this drug is metabolized in the liver. Dose decreases not routinely needed.

Kidney Function: Starting dose is 5 mg. The dose is increased as needed and tolerated by 5 mg every 2 weeks for a maximum of 20 mg daily.

▷ **Dosing Instructions:** May be taken without regard to eating. The tablet may be crushed. Do not stop this drug abruptly. If you forget a dose: take it right away unless it's within 8 hours of your next regular dose. If it IS within 8 hours of the next dose, just take the scheduled dose. DO NOT double doses.

Usual Duration of Use: Regular use for 10 to 14 days usually needed to see this drug's effectiveness in lowering blood pressure. Long-term use determined by success in lowering blood pressure and response to overall treatment program (weight reduction, salt restriction, smoking cessation, etc.). See your doctor regularly. Use for glaucoma will be ongoing.

Typical Treatment Goals and Measurements (Outcomes and Markers)

Blood Pressure: The most recent treatment guidelines (JNC VI) actually define optimal blood pressure (BP) as less than 120/80 and high normal as 139/89. The American Diabetes Association (ADA) has chosen a target of 130/80 for people living with diabetes. Most clinicians try to achieve a BP that achieves the best balance of lower cardiovascular risk while avoiding the problem of too low a blood pressure. The goal and time frame (see peak benefits above) should be discussed with you when the prescription is written.

Glaucoma: Return of eye pressure (intraocular pressure) to normal and avoidance of consequences of increased pressure. If this medicine does not work well enough by itself, combination treatment is typical.

Possible Advantages of This Drug: Usually effective and well-tolerated with a single dose daily, which is easier to remember to take. Twice-daily dosing for glaucoma also enhances compliance. Suspension form may be better tolerated than the solution form.

▷ **This Drug Should Not Be Taken If**
- you have had an allergic reaction to it previously.
- you have heart (overt) failure or cardiogenic shock.
- you have an abnormally slow heart rate (bradycardia) or a serious heart block (second or third degree).
- you are taking, or took in the past 14 days, any monoamine oxidase (MAO) type A inhibitor (see Drug Classes).

▷ **Inform Your Physician Before Taking This Drug If**
- you have had an adverse reaction to any beta-blocker (see Drug Classes).
- you have serious heart disease or episodes of heart failure.
- you have a history of hay fever (allergic rhinitis), asthma, chronic bronchitis or emphysema. Some drugs in this class are contraindicated in asthmatics.
- you have overactive thyroid function (hyperthyroidism).
- you have a history of low blood sugar (hypoglycemia) or diabetes.
- you have impaired liver or kidney function.
- you have narrowing of the vessels in your legs or arms (peripheral vascular disease). Discuss this with your doctor.
- you have myasthenia gravis.
- you take digitalis, quinidine or reserpine, or any calcium blocker drug (see Drug Classes).
- you will have surgery with general anesthesia.
- you take prescription or nonprescription medications not discussed when betaxolol was prescribed for you.
- you are unsure how much to take or how often to take it.

Possible Side Effects (natural, expected and unavoidable drug actions)
Lethargy, fatigue (up to 10%), cold extremities—rare; slow heart rate, light-headedness in upright position (see Orthostatic Hypotension in Glossary).

Possible Adverse Effects (unusual, unexpected and infrequent reactions)
If any of the following develop, consult your physician promptly for guidance.
Mild Adverse Effects
Allergic reactions: skin rash, itching—rare.
Hair loss—rare.
Headache (up to 15%)—frequent.
Dizziness, fatigue—infrequent.
Insomnia or abnormal dreams—infrequent.
Indigestion, nausea, diarrhea—infrequent.
Joint and muscle discomfort—infrequent.

Fluid retention (edema)—rare.

Difficulty breathing—infrequent.

Serious Adverse Effects

Allergic reactions: may make allergic reactions more difficult to treat (refractory).

Mental depression or anxiety—rare.

Increased blood sugar (hyperglycemia) in non-insulin-dependent diabetics—possible.

Chest pain, shortness of breath, congestive heart failure—rare.

Induction of bronchial asthma (in asthmatic individuals)—possible.

Low blood platelets and anemia—rare.

Congestive heart failure—rare.

Angina (if pill form abruptly stopped).

Intermittent problems walking (intermittent claudication)—possible.

Heart attack (myocardial infarction)—rare.

Author's Note: Adverse effects from eye drops happen rarely versus pill form.

▷ **Possible Effects on Sexual Function:** Decreased libido, impotence—rare and less frequent than other medicines in this class.

Altered menstrual patterns (reported rarely with other medicines in this class)—possible.

Adverse Effects That May Mimic Natural Diseases or Disorders

Reduced blood flow to extremities may mimic Raynaud's disease (see Glossary).

Possible Effects on Laboratory Tests

Glaucoma-screening test (measurement of internal eye pressure): pressure is decreased (false low or normal value).

Antinuclear antibodies (ANA) test: positive in 5.3% of users.

Blood potassium: slightly increased.

Blood platelet counts and hemoglobin: decreased—rare.

Blood glucose: increased in non-insulin-dependent diabetics.

CAUTION

1. Do not stop this drug suddenly without calling your doctor. Always carry a note with you that says you are taking this drug.
2. Ask your physician or pharmacist before using nasal decongestants. These can cause sudden increases in blood pressure when combined with beta-blocker drugs.
3. Levobetaxolol (Betaxon) is NOT the same medicine as betaxolol.
4. Report any tendency to emotional depression.
5. Eye (ophthalmic) form may cause additive effects on blood pressure if taken with the pill form.

Precautions for Use

By Infants and Children: Safety and effectiveness for those under 12 years of age not established.

By Those Over 60 Years of Age: Caution: High blood pressure should be slowly reduced, avoiding risks associated with excessively low blood pressure. Treatment should be started with 5 mg daily and blood pressure checked often. Sudden, rapid and excessive reduction of blood pressure can cause stroke or heart attack. Total daily dosage should not exceed 10 to 15 mg. Watch for dizziness, unsteadiness, tendency to fall, confusion, hallucinations, depression or urinary frequency. This age group is more prone to develop excessively slow heart rates and hypothermia.

▷ **Advisability of Use During Pregnancy**

Pregnancy Category: C. See Pregnancy Risk Categories at the back of this book.

Animal studies: Rat studies reveal increased resorptions of embryo and fetus, retarded growth and development of newborn, and mild skeletal defects.

Human studies: Adequate studies of pregnant women are not available.

Avoid use of drug during the first 3 months if possible. Avoid use during labor and delivery because of the possible effects on the newborn infant.

Advisability of Use If Breast-Feeding

Presence of this drug in breast milk: Yes.

Avoid drug if possible. If drug is necessary, observe nursing infant for slow heart rate and indications of low blood sugar.

Habit-Forming Potential: None.

Effects of Overdose: Weakness, slow pulse, low blood pressure, fainting, cold and sweaty skin, congestive heart failure, possible coma and convulsions.

Possible Effects of Long-Term Use: Reduced heart reserve and eventual heart failure in susceptible individuals with advanced heart disease.

Suggested Periodic Examinations While Taking This Drug (at physician's discretion)

Measurements of blood pressure.

Evaluation of heart function.

▷ **While Taking This Drug, Observe the Following**

Foods: No restrictions. Avoid excessive salt intake.

Herbal Medicines or Minerals: Ginseng may increase blood pressure, blunting the benefits of this medicine. Hawthorn, saw palmetto, ma huang, goldenseal, yohimbe and licorice may also increase blood pressure. Calcium and garlic may help lower blood pressure. Indian snakeroot has a German Commission E monograph indication for hypertension—talk to your doctor. Eleuthero root and ephedra should be avoided by people living with hypertension. Belladonna, ephedra, henbane leaf and scopolia root should be avoided by people living with glaucoma.

Beverages: No restrictions. May be taken with milk.

▷ *Alcohol:* Use with caution. Alcohol may exaggerate oral form lowering of blood pressure and may increase its mild sedative effect.

Tobacco Smoking: Nicotine may reduce this drug's effectiveness. High drug doses worsen bronchial constriction caused by regular smoking. I advise everyone to quit smoking.

▷ *Other Drugs*

Betaxolol may ***increase*** the effects of

- other antihypertensive drugs and cause excessive lowering of blood pressure. Dosage decreases may be necessary.
- reserpine (Ser-Ap-Es, etc.) and cause sedation, depression, slowing of heart rate and lowering of blood pressure (light-headedness, fainting).
- verapamil and cause additive risk of congestive heart failure and slow heart rate (bradycardia).

Betaxolol *taken concurrently* with
- amiodarone (Cordarone) may result in extremely slow heart rate and arrest.
- calcium channel blockers (Diltiazem, etc. or other dihydropyridine forms) may severely lower blood pressure.
- clonidine (Catapres) requires close monitoring for rebound high blood pressure if clonidine is stopped while betaxolol is still being taken.
- digoxin (Lanoxin) may prolong AV conduction time and digoxin toxicity.
- fluoroquinolone (see Drug Classes) antibiotics may cause an increase in betaxolol blood levels and lead to toxicity.
- fluvoxamine (Luvox) may cause excessive slowing of the heart and very low blood pressure.
- insulin requires close supervision to avoid hypoglycemia (see Glossary).
- methyldopa (various) may lead to an exaggerated hypertensive response to stress.
- oral antidiabetic drugs (see Drug Classes) may prolong recovery from low blood sugars.
- phenothiazines (see Drug Classes) may result in additive blood pressure lowering effects.
- rifabutin (Mycobutin) may decrease betaxolol benefits.
- ritonavir (Norvir) and perhaps other protease inhibitors (see Drug Classes) may decrease betaxolol benefits.
- venlafaxine (Effexor) may cause excessive slowing of the heart and very low blood pressure.
- zileuton (Zyflo) may cause excessive blood pressure lowering.

The following drugs may *decrease* the effects of betaxolol:
- indomethacin (Indocin) and possibly other "aspirin substitutes," or NSAIDs, may impair betaxolol's antihypertensive effect.

▷ *Driving, Hazardous Activities:* Use caution until the full extent of drowsiness, lethargy and blood pressure change has been determined.

Aviation Note: The use of this drug *is a disqualification* for piloting. Consult a designated Aviation Medical Examiner.

Exposure to Sun: No restrictions.

Exposure to Heat: Caution is advised. Hot environments can lower blood pressure and exaggerate the effects of this drug.

Exposure to Cold: Caution is advised. Cold environments can enhance the circulatory deficiency in the extremities that may occur with this drug. The elderly should be careful to prevent hypothermia (see Glossary).

Heavy Exercise or Exertion: Talk with your doctor about an exercise program that is right for you, mindful of this medicine and your physical condition.

Occurrence of Unrelated Illness: Fever can lower blood pressure and require dosing changes. Nausea or vomiting may interrupt dosing. Ask your doctor for help.

Discontinuation: DO NOT stop this drug suddenly. Gradual physician-supervised dose reduction over 2 to 3 weeks is recommended.

BITOLTEROL (bi TOHL ter ohl)

Introduced: 1985   **Class:** Antiasthmatic, bronchodilator   **Prescription:** Yes   **Controlled Drug:** No   **Available as Generic:** No
Brand Name: Tornalate

> ┌───┐
> **BENEFITS versus RISKS**
> *Possible Benefits*   *Possible Risks*
> EFFECTIVE PREVENTION AND   Fine hand tremor
>   RELIEF OF ASTHMA   Nervousness
>   Throat irritation
>   Irregular heart rhythm (with
>   excessive use)
> └───┘

▷ **Principal Uses**

As a Single Drug Product: Uses currently included in FDA-approved labeling: (1) Relieves sudden (acute) asthma and frequency and severity of ongoing, recurrent asthmatic attacks; (2) helps asthmatics dependent on steroids.

Other (unlabeled) generally accepted uses: (1) May be more useful than other agents opening bronchi in chronic obstructive pulmonary disease (COPD); (2) helps prevent exercise-induced asthma in adults.

How This Drug Works: By increasing cyclic AMP, this drug relaxes bronchial muscles and relieves asthmatic wheezing.

Available Dosage Forms and Strengths

Aerosol inhaler — 15 ml (300 inhalations of 0.37 mg each)
Inhalation solution — 0.2 percent

▷ **Usual Adult Dosage Ranges:** *For acute bronchospasm:* Two inhalations separated by 1 to 3 minutes, followed by a third inhalation in 3 to 4 minutes if needed. Preventing bronchospasm: Two inhalations every 8 hours. Maximum inhalation dose is two inhalations every 4 hours.

For children over 12: Same as adult bronchospasm dose. **Note: Actual dose and schedule must be determined for each patient individually.**

Conditions Requiring Dosing Adjustments

Liver Function: Use with caution in severe liver compromise.
Kidney Function: Significant kidney removal; however, specific dosage guidelines are unavailable.

▷ **Dosing Instructions:** May be used without regard to eating. Follow the written directions for use carefully. The American Thoracic Society advocates use of the open mouth technique (ask your doctor or pharmacist) for metered dose inhalers. This appears to help the medicine work better (improved distribution). Do not overuse this drug. If you forget a dose: Use the inhaler as soon as possible. Do not double doses.

Usual Duration of Use: Do not use beyond the time necessary to stop episodes of asthma. Ask your doctor for help regarding prevention of asthma attacks.

Typical Treatment Goals and Measurements (Outcomes and Markers)

Breathing: Short-acting beta agonists like albuterol are used to prevent or treat reversible spasms of the bronchial tubes. The peak effect happens 1 to 2 hours after dosing. Many clinicians use the FEV1 results as a marker of benefits. If the usual benefit in restoring ease of breathing is not realized, call your doctor.

▷ **Possible Advantages of This Drug:** Selective for beta-2 receptors and therefore usually avoids significant heart (cardiovascular) effects.

▷ **This Drug Should Not Be Taken If**
- you have had an allergic reaction to it previously.
- you are taking, or took, a monoamine oxidase (MAO) type A inhibitor (see Drug Classes) in the past 2 weeks.

▷ **Inform Your Physician Before Taking This Drug If**
- you have any type of heart or circulatory disorder, especially high blood pressure or coronary heart disease.
- you currently have an irregular heart rhythm.
- you have diabetes, epilepsy or an overactive thyroid gland.
- you are taking any form of digitalis or any stimulant drug.
- you are unsure how much to take or how often to take it.
- you are pregnant and are nearing the time of delivery of your baby (may complicate labor and delivery).

Possible Side Effects (natural, expected and unavoidable drug actions)

Dryness or irritation of mouth or throat.

▷ **Possible Adverse Effects** (unusual, unexpected and infrequent reactions)
   If any of the following develop, consult your physician promptly for guidance.

Mild Adverse Effects

Headache, dizziness, nervousness, insomnia—infrequent.

Fine tremor of hands—frequent.

Nausea, indigestion—infrequent.

Coughing—infrequent.

Fast heart rate (tachycardia)—rare.

Serious Adverse Effects

Excessive use can cause irregular heart rate or rhythm or increased blood pressure.

Paradoxical bronchospasm—rare.

▷ **Possible Effects on Sexual Function:** None reported.

Natural Diseases or Disorders That May Be Activated by This Drug

Latent coronary artery disease, diabetes or high blood pressure.

Possible Effects on Laboratory Tests

None reported.

CAUTION
1. Combination use of this drug by inhalation with beclomethasone aerosol (Beclovent, Vanceril) may increase the risk of toxicity due to fluorocarbon propellants. Use bitolterol aerosol 20 to 30 minutes before beclomethasone aerosol. This reduces toxicity risk and enhances penetration of beclomethasone.
2. Excessive or prolonged inhalation use can reduce benefits and cause serious heart rhythm disturbances.

Precautions for Use

By Infants and Children: Safety and effectiveness for children under 12 years of age not established.

By Those Over 60 Years of Age: Avoid excessive and continual use. If acute asthma is not relieved promptly, other drugs will be needed. Watch for nervousness, palpitations, irregular heart rhythm and muscle tremors.

▷ **Advisability of Use During Pregnancy**
Pregnancy Category: C. See Pregnancy Risk Categories at the back of this book.
Animal studies: Cleft palate reported in mice.
Human studies: Adequate studies of pregnant women are not available.
Avoid use during first 3 months if possible.

Advisability of Use If Breast-Feeding
Presence of this drug in breast milk: Unknown.
Avoid drug or refrain from nursing.

Habit-Forming Potential: None.

Effects of Overdose: Nervousness, palpitation, rapid heart rate, sweating, headache, tremor, vomiting, abnormal heart rhythms, chest pain.

Possible Effects of Long-Term Use: Loss of effectiveness.

Suggested Periodic Examinations While Taking This Drug (at physician's discretion)
Blood pressure measurements.
Evaluation of heart status.
FEV1 (improvement marker).

▷ **While Taking This Drug, Observe the Following**
Foods: No restrictions.
Herbal Medicines or Minerals: Using St. John's wort, ma huang, ephedrine-like compounds or kola while taking this medicine may result in unacceptable central nervous system stimulation (tremor, nervousness). If you are allergic to plants in the Asteraceae family (aster, chrysanthemum, daisy or ragweed), you may also be allergic to echinacea, chamomile, feverfew and St. John's wort. Fir or pine needle oil should NOT be used by asthmatics. Ephedra alone does carry a German Commission E monograph indication for asthma treatment.
Beverages: Avoid excessive caffeine—coffee, tea, cola, chocolate—as xanthines in these foods and beverages may lead to added nervousness.
▷ *Alcohol:* No interactions expected.
Tobacco Smoking: No interactions expected, but the smoke itself can irritate airways. I advise everyone to quit smoking.
▷ *Other Drugs*
Bitolterol *taken concurrently* with
• entacapone (Comtan) may cause large increases in blood pressure and undesirable heart stimulation.
• monoamine oxidase (MAO) type A inhibitors (see Drug Classes) may cause large increases in blood pressure and undesirable heart stimulation.
▷ *Driving, Hazardous Activities:* Use caution if excessive nervousness or dizziness occurs.
Aviation Note: The use of this drug *is a disqualification* for piloting. Consult a designated Aviation Medical Examiner.
Exposure to Sun: No restrictions.
Heavy Exercise or Exertion: Use caution. Excessive exercise can induce an asthma attack.

BROMOCRIPTINE (broh moh KRIP teen)

Introduced: 1975   **Class:** Anti-parkinsonism, ergot derivative   **Prescription:** USA: Yes   **Controlled Drug:** USA: No; Canada: No   **Available as Generic:** No

Brand Names: Normatine, Parlodel

Author's Note: This profile has been shortened to make room for more widely used medicines.

BUDESONIDE (byou DES oh nyde)

Introduced: 1994 (Rhinocort), 1997 (Turbuhaler)   **Class:** Antiasthmatic, cortisonelike drugs   **Prescription:** USA: Yes   **Controlled Drug:** USA: No; Canada: No   **Available as Generic:** No

Brand Names: ✷Entocort, ✷Gen-Budesonide-AQ, Pulmicort, ✷Pulmicort Nebuamp, Pulmicort Respules and Turbuhaler, Rhinocort Aqua, Rhinocort Turbuhaler

BENEFITS versus RISKS	
Possible Benefits	*Possible Risks*
EFFECTIVE RELIEF OF ALLERGIC RHINITIS	FUNGUS INFECTIONS OF THE MOUTH AND THROAT
EFFECTIVE CONTROL OF ASTHMA	Changes in lining of the nose (nasal mucosa)
TENDS TO HAVE MORE LOCAL THAN SYSTEMIC EFFECTS (HIGH RATIO)	Increased cataract risk
	Osteoporosis risk

▷ **Principal Uses**

As a Single Drug Product: Uses currently included in FDA-approved labeling: (1) Ongoing treatment of bronchial asthma in people who don't have sufficient response to bronchodilators and need cortisonelike drugs for asthma control; (2) treats seasonal and perennial rhinitis in children and adults (nasal form).

Other (unlabeled) generally accepted uses: (1) May help bring and maintain remission in Crohn's disease; (2) eases nasal polyps (nasal polyposis).

How This Drug Works: It reduces inflammation (arachidonic acid pathway) and decreases response to immediate and delayed hypersensitivity. Also reduces local lung inflammation in the respiratory tract.

Available Dosage Forms and Strengths

Nasal inhaler — 7 g (32 mcg per press)
    Nasal spray — 200-dose canister (50 mcg per dose) (Canada)
    Oral inhaler — 200 doses of 1 or 4 mg per ml
    Spacer form — same as above (200 doses of 1 or 4 mg per ml)
    Turbuhaler — 200 mcg (100 and 400 mcg in Canada)

▷ **Recommended Dosage Ranges**

Infants and Children:

Seasonal rhinitis (children 6 or older): Pressurized nasal inhaler—two inhalations in each nostril twice a day, morning and evening, or 4 inhalations in each nostril in the morning (256 mcg maximum).

Perennial allergic rhinitis: Same dose, but see cautions section.

Seasonal and perennial rhinitis (for those 12 or older): Nonaerosol pump spray—one puff (50 mcg) in each nostril twice daily. This may be increased to 2 puffs twice daily if required (256 mcg maximum).

Asthma: oral inhalation form (in those more than 6 and based on prior treatment): (a) Bronchodilators alone—200 mcg twice a day; (b) inhaled corticosteroids—200 mcg twice daily; (c) oral corticosteroids—400 mcg twice daily. Children under 12 years old are given one puff or 0.2 mg twice a day with a maximum of 2 puffs a day (0.8 mg). Some clinicians use 400 mcg per square meter.

Author's Note: Use in pediatrics may slow a child's rate of growth.

Adults:

Seasonal rhinitis: Nasal inhaler—256 mcg a day, given as 2 inhalations in each nostril twice daily (morning and evening) or 4 inhalations once a day in the morning. The effect should be checked in 3 to 7 days and the medicine stopped in 3 weeks if an adequate response isn't achieved.

Perennial rhinitis: Same dose as seasonal rhinitis, but see cautions section. Once adequate benefits have been seen, the dose is then slowly decreased to the lowest dose that works. If symptoms return while doses are being lowered, the dose may be increased back to the starting dose (briefly) and then decreased back to the dose that worked before the symptoms returned.

Asthma (use in is based on prior treatment): Oral inhaler—people receiving (a) bronchodilators alone—200–400 mcg twice a day; (b) inhaled corticosteroids—200–400 mcg twice daily; (c) oral corticosteroids—400–800 mcg twice daily. If asthma has been controlled by corticosteroids taken by mouth, the budesonide inhaler must be used at the same time as the oral corticosteroids for about 1 week. After a week, the oral corticosteroid can be SLOWLY tapered. The patient should be closely watched for the return of asthma or other effects (see cautions).

Those Over 65 Years of Age: Doses similar to those used in younger patients have been effective and safe.

Note: Actual dose and schedule must be determined for each patient individually.

Conditions Requiring Dosing Adjustments

Liver Function: Use with caution in patients with liver compromise. This drug may stay in the body longer in people with liver damage, and lower doses appear prudent.

Kidney Function: No adjustments in dosing appear to be required.

▷ **Dosing Instructions:** May be used without regard to eating. Rinse the mouth and throat (gargle) with water thoroughly after each inhalation. If you forget a dose: Use the inhaler or spray as soon as possible. DO NOT double doses.

Usual Duration of Use: Regular use for 1 to 2 weeks is often needed to see the best response from the oral inhalation form in asthma, but Pulmicort form may work in a day in some patients. The nasal inhalation form may go to work in 3–7 days. This is why results are checked after 3–7 days and at 3 weeks. If acceptable relief isn't seen in 3 weeks, the drug should be stopped. Once relief is achieved, the dose should be decreased at 2- to 4-week intervals to the minimum effective dose. Long-term use must be physician-supervised. See your doctor regularly.

Typical Treatment Goals and Measurements (Outcomes and Markers)

Asthma: Frequency and severity of asthma attacks should ease. Some clinicians also use decreased frequency of rescue inhaler use as a further clinical indicator. It is critical that this medicine is used regularly to get the best results. An additional goal of therapy is to use the lowest effective dose. Some people keep their improvements when doses are lowered, while others relapse. Those with a less than 2-fold improvement in airway response and people who stay in the moderate to severe asthma range despite high budesonide doses may be more likely to relapse. If the usual benefit is not realized, call your doctor.

Allergic rhinitis: Symptoms such as itchy, runny nose, sore throat and post-nasal drip should all ease once this medicine begins to work. Because there may be some seasonality to the pollen or molds that can cause rhinitis, talk to your doctor about exactly how you should use this medicine.

Possible Advantages of This Drug

Turbuhaler form avoids pressurized metered dose inhaler CFCs as well as increased amount of drug in the lung. Intranasal form causes less depression of free cortisol. Inhaled forms cause less of a systemic effect than the same medicine taken by mouth. Medicines in this class are considered first-line treatment by many clinicians in allergic rhinitis because they slow (attenuate) early-phase reactions and suppress late-phase allergic reactions (they may also cost less). In asthma, inhaled steroids have been recommended in revised guidelines for those with more than infrequent or mild asthma.

▷ **This Drug Should Not Be Taken If**
- you have had an allergic reaction to any form of this drug.
- you are having severe acute asthma or status asthmaticus that requires more intense treatment for prompt relief.
- other antiasthmatic drugs can control your asthma that are not related to cortisone.
- your asthma requires cortisonelike drugs infrequently for control.

▷ **Inform Your Physician Before Taking This Drug If**
- you take or recently took any cortisone-related drug (including ACTH by injection) for any reason (see Drug Classes).
- you have a history of tuberculosis of the lungs.
- you have chronic bronchitis or bronchiectasis.
- you think you have an active infection of any kind, especially a respiratory infection or herpes of the eye.
- you have recently been exposed to chickenpox or other viral illnesses.
- you are prone to nosebleeds (epistaxis) or have nose ulcers or have had nose surgery (nasal forms).
- you are unsure how much to take or how often to take this drug.
- you are a child and your growth rate has not been checked.

Possible Side Effects (natural, expected and unavoidable drug actions)

Fungus infections (thrush) of the mouth and throat.

Suppression of the adrenal glands—possible.

Stinging of nasal tissues (nasal form)—possible.

▷ **Possible Adverse Effects** (unusual, unexpected and infrequent reactions)

If any of the following develop, consult your physician promptly for guidance.

Mild Adverse Effects

Allergic reaction: skin rash—infrequent.

Headache—frequent (oral inhalation).

Dryness of mouth, hoarseness, sore throat, cough—possible.

Nosebleeds (epistaxis)—infrequent.

Weight gain—infrequent.

Serious Adverse Effects

Allergic reaction: localized areas of "allergic" pneumonitis (lung inflammation).

Bronchospasm, asthmatic wheezing—rare.

Behavioral changes—case reports.

Nose perforation (septal)—rare.

Increased susceptibility to chickenpox—possible.

Growth slowing (growth retardation)—possible.

Increased risk of cataracts with long-term (chronic) use.

Osteoporosis (any corticosteroid can cause this)—possible.

▷ **Possible Effects on Sexual Function:** None reported.

Natural Diseases or Disorders That May Be Activated by This Drug

Cortisone-related drugs having systemic effects impair immunity and lead to reactivation of "healed" or dormant tuberculosis. People with a history of tuberculosis must be watched closely while using this drug.

Possible Effects on Laboratory Tests

Blood cortisol levels: decreased.

HDL may increase.

Bone mineral density: may be decreased with chronic use.

CAUTION

1. The substance (sorbitan trioleate) that this medicine is delivered in (vehicle) may cause symptoms that are like rhinitis. Doses early in treatment may suppress these symptoms, and they may slowly come back once the dose is lowered. If this occurs and the dose can't be lowered, other treatment may be needed.

2. The maker of the pressurized nasal inhaler uses the amount of drug released from the nasal adapter (32 mcg) to determine the dose. The nasal inhaler actually releases 50 mcg.

3. Use in people with asthma REQUIRES regular use in order to get the best results. Please do not skip doses.

4. This drug should not be relied upon for immediate relief of acute asthma.

5. The inhaled powder form does not prevent asthma precipitated by exercise.

6. If you required cortisonelike drugs before starting this inhaler, you may again require a cortisonelike drug if you are injured, have an infection or need surgery. Extreme care must be taken if you are being changed from corticosteroids that work in the whole body (systemically active) to this medicine.

7. If severe asthma returns while using this drug, call your doctor immediately. Cortisonelike drugs may be required.

8. Carry a personal ID card saying that you have used (if true) cortisone-related drugs in the past year.

9. This drug may allow dosage decreases in some patients.

10. If this medicine is to be used long-term, a bone mineral density test before treatment and every 2 years is prudent.

Precautions for Use

By Infants and Children: Safety and effectiveness as described above. Children may be more susceptible to adverse effects of this drug and should be watched closely.

By Those Over 60 Years of Age: People with bronchiectasis should be watched closely for the development of lung infections.

▷ **Advisability of Use During Pregnancy**

Pregnancy Category: C. See Pregnancy Risk Categories at the back of this book.

Animal studies: Mouse, rat and rabbit studies reveal significant birth defects due to this drug.

Human studies: Adequate studies of pregnant women are not available.

Talk with your doctor.

Advisability of Use If Breast-Feeding

Presence of this drug in breast milk: Unknown.

Avoid drug or refrain from nursing.

Habit-Forming Potential: With recommended dosage, a state of functional dependence (see Glossary) is not likely to develop.

Effects of Overdose: Indications of cortisone excess (due to systemic absorption)—fluid retention, flushing of the face, stomach irritation, nervousness.

Suggested Periodic Examinations While Taking This Drug (at physician's discretion)

Inspection of nose, mouth and throat for fungus infection.

Inspection of the nose tissues for damage.

Assessment of adrenal function in people using cortisone-related drugs for an extended time prior to this drug.

Lung X-ray if a prior history of tuberculosis.

Measures of bone mineral density (DEXA, ultrasound or PDEXA) and cataract check.

▷ **While Taking This Drug, Observe the Following**

Foods: No specific restrictions beyond those advised by your physician.

Herbal Medicines or Minerals: Fir or pine needle oil should NOT be used by asthmatics. Ephedra alone does carry a German Commission E monograph indication for asthma treatment. If you are allergic to plants in the Asteraceae family (aster, chrysanthemum, daisy or ragweed), you may also be allergic to echinacea, chamomile, feverfew and St. John's wort. Taking added calcium and vitamin D while taking this medicine is prudent. Talk to your doctor BEFORE adding any herbals to this medicine.

Beverages: No specific restrictions.

▷ *Alcohol:* No interactions expected.

Tobacco Smoking: Smoking can reduce the benefits of this drug. I advise everyone to quit smoking.

▷ *Other Drugs*

The following drugs may *increase* the effects of budesonide:

- some antiepileptic medicines such as phenytoin (Dilantin) may increase risk of osteoporosis.
- inhalant bronchodilators—epinephrine, isoetharine, isoproterenol.
- methylphenidate (Ritalin) may cause increased growth suppression.
- oral bronchodilators—aminophylline, ephedrine, terbutaline, theophylline, etc.

Budesonide *taken concurrently* with:
- amiodarone (Cordarone) may cause increased risk of Cushing's syndrome (because of liver enzyme-CYP450 3A4 inhibition) Careful clinical follow-up is needed.
- ketoconazole (Nizoral) and other inhibitors of CYP450 3A4 may cause increased budesonide levels. Caution is advised.

▷ *Driving, Hazardous Activities:* No restrictions.
Aviation Note: The use of this drug and the disorder for which this drug is prescribed *may be disqualifications* for piloting. Consult a designated Aviation Medical Examiner.
Exposure to Sun: No restrictions.
Occurrence of Unrelated Illness: Acute infections, serious injuries and surgery can create an urgent need for cortisone-related drugs. Call your doctor immediately in the event of new illness or injury.
Discontinuation: If this drug has made it possible to reduce or stop ongoing cortisonelike drugs, *do not* stop this drug abruptly. If you must stop this drug, call your doctor. You may need to resume cortisone medicines.

BUMETANIDE (byu MET a nide)

Introduced: 1983   **Class:** Diuretic   **Prescription:** USA: Yes; Canada: No   **Controlled Drug:** USA: No   **Available as Generic:** Yes
Brand Name: Bumex, Burinex

BENEFITS versus RISKS	
Possible Benefits	*Possible Risks*
POTENT, EFFECTIVE DIURETIC BY MOUTH OR INJECTION	ABNORMALLY LOW BLOOD POTASSIUM with excessive use
TREATS CONGESTIVE HEART FAILURE, HIGH BLOOD PRESSURE AND FLUID BUILDUP IN KIDNEY FAILURE	Decreased magnesium with chronic therapy Blood disorders—rare

▷ **Principal Uses**
▷ *As a Single Drug Product:* Uses currently included in FDA-approved labeling: (1) Removes fluid excess in patients with congestive heart failure, kidney or liver disease; (2) eases edema in people who fail to respond to or will not tolerate furosemide (Lasix).
Other (unlabeled) generally accepted uses: (1) Used as an adjunct to other therapy in high blood pressure (hypertension); (2) can help older people decrease the number of times they must get up at night to urinate (nocturia); (3) eases the amount of fluid that can build up in the lungs (pulmonary edema).
How This Drug Works: Increases removal of salt and water from the body (through increased urine production). Reduces sodium and amount of fluid in the blood.
Available Dosage Forms and Strengths
Injection — 0.25 mg/ml (2-ml ampules)
Tablets — 0.5 mg, 1 mg, 2 mg

▷ **Usual Adult Dosage Ranges:** 0.5 to 2 mg daily, usually taken in the morning as a single dose. If needed, an additional second or third dose may be taken later in the day at 4- to 5-hour intervals. The total daily dose should not exceed 10 mg. Alternate-day dosage (every other day) may work for some people, and this approach is recommended as the safest way to control edema. **Note: Actual dose and schedule must be determined for each patient individually.**

Conditions Requiring Dosing Adjustments

Liver Function: Rapid body fluid removal can cause a coma in liver failure patients. Use of loop diuretics only done under close medical supervision (hospital or outpatient care center).

Kidney Function: NOT recommended for use in progressive renal failure.

▷ **Dosing Instructions:** May be crushed when taken and given with or following food to reduce stomach irritation. If you forget a dose: take it right away unless it's nearly time for your next regular dose. If it IS nearly time for the next dose, just take the scheduled dose. DO NOT double doses.

Usual Duration of Use: Two to three days of regular use often needed to see peak effect relieving fluid buildup (edema). Once peak benefit is realized, intermittent use reduces risk of sodium, potassium, magnesium and water imbalance. Long-term use requires supervision by your doctor.

Typical Treatment Goals and Measurements (Outcomes and Markers)

Blood pressure: The most recent treatment guidelines (JNC VI) actually define optimal blood pressure (BP) as less than 120/80 and high normal as 139/89. The American Diabetes Association has chosen a target of 130/80 as the blood pressure goal for people living with diabetes. Most clinicians try to achieve a BP that achieves the best balance of lower cardiovascular risk while avoiding the problem of too low a blood pressure. Because this medicine works to remove excess fluid, additional markers of response include increased urination (intake and output may be checked) as well as decreased swelling (edema) of the ankles. The goals and time frame should be discussed with you when the prescription is written. In high blood pressure patients, this medicine is usually reserved as additional (adjunctive) treatment in patients with kidney problems.

Congestive heart failure: Used to remove excessive fluid which builds up in the body. Typical treatment markers include resolution of ankle swelling and increased output of fluid (diuresis).

Possible Advantages of This Drug

Diuretic effect is usually complete in 4 hours; diuretic effect of furosemide usually lasts from 6 to 8 hours.

▷ **This Drug Should Not Be Taken If**
- you have had an allergic reaction to it or to sulfonamides.
- coma caused by liver failure is present.
- severe electrolyte or fluid imbalance.
- you have developed a marked increase in creatinine or blood urea nitrogen (BUN) while taking this drug.
- your kidneys are unable to produce adequate urine (oliguria).

▷ **Inform Your Physician Before Taking This Drug If**
- you are allergic to any form of "sulfa" drug.
- you are pregnant or planning pregnancy.

- you have a blood disorder.
- you have impaired liver or kidney function.
- you have diabetes, a diabetic tendency or a history of gout.
- you have impaired hearing or develop hearing loss during therapy.
- you have low blood platelets.
- you are taking: cortisone, digitalis, oral antidiabetic drugs, insulin, probenecid (Benemid), indomethacin (Indocin), lithium or drugs for high blood pressure.
- you will have surgery with general anesthesia.
- you are unsure how much to take or how often to take it.

Possible Side Effects (natural, expected and unavoidable drug actions)
Light-headedness on arising from sitting or lying position (see Orthostatic Hypotension in Glossary).
Increase in level of blood sugar, affecting control of diabetes.
Increase in level of blood uric acid, affecting control of gout.
Decreased blood potassium and sodium with muscle weakness and cramping.
Decreased blood magnesium.

▷ **Possible Adverse Effects** (unusual, unexpected and infrequent reactions)
If any of the following develop, consult your physician promptly for guidance.
Mild Adverse Effects
Allergic reactions: skin rashes, hives, itching.
Headache, dizziness, vertigo, fatigue, weakness, sweating, earache—rare.
Nausea, vomiting, stomach pain, diarrhea—infrequent.
Breast nipple tenderness, joint and muscle pains or cramps—rare.
Serious Adverse Effects
Serious skin rash (Stevens-Johnson syndrome)—case reports.
Liver coma (in preexisting liver disease)—possible.
Abnormally low magnesium, potassium and sodium (electrolytes): possible with long-term or high-dose use—rare to frequent.
Low white blood cells and platelets (leukopenia and thrombocytopenia)—rare.
Kidney failure—rare.
Pseudoporphyuria—case report.
Pancreatitis—case reports.
Elevated blood glucose—infrequent.
Lung fibrosis—case reports.
Hearing toxicity (ototoxicity)—rare.

▷ **Possible Effects on Sexual Function:** Difficulty maintaining an erection; premature ejaculation (0.5 to 2 mg daily)—rare.
Male breast enlargement and tenderness (gynecomastia)—case reports.

Natural Diseases or Disorders That May Be Activated by This Drug
Latent diabetes, gout.

Possible Effects on Laboratory Tests
White blood cell counts: increased—usual; decreased—rare.
Blood platelets: decreased.
Blood sugar (glucose): increased.
Blood lithium or uric acid levels: increased.
Blood potassium, magnesium or chloride: decreased.

CAUTION

1. High doses can cause excessive excretion of water, sodium and potassium, with loss of appetite, nausea, weakness, confusion and profound drop in blood pressure (circulatory collapse).
2. May cause digitalis toxicity by depleting potassium. If you are taking a digitalis preparation (digitoxin, digoxin), ensure an adequate intake of high-potassium foods.
3. People with cirrhosis of the liver must never increase their dose unless told to do so by their doctor. Excess dosing can cause liver coma.
4. People who take lithium may experience lithium toxicity.

Precautions for Use

By Infants and Children: Safety and effectiveness for those under 6 months of age not established. If 6 months or older, 0.015 mg per kg is used. If ongoing doses are needed, an intermittent schedule such as every other day or every 2–4 days is used.

By Those Over 60 Years of Age: Small starting doses are advisable. You may be more susceptible to the development of impaired thinking, orthostatic hypotension, potassium loss and elevation of blood sugar. Overdose and prolonged use can cause excessive loss of body water, thickening of the blood and an increased risk of blood clots, stroke, heart attack or thrombophlebitis.

▷ **Advisability of Use During Pregnancy**

Pregnancy Category: C, D by one researcher. See Pregnancy Risk Categories at the back of this book.

Animal studies: Ten times the maximum therapeutic human dose caused bone defects in rabbits.

Human studies: Adequate studies of pregnant women are not available.

Only used in pregnancy if a very serious complication of pregnancy occurs for which this drug is significantly beneficial.

Advisability of Use If Breast-Feeding

Presence of this drug in breast milk: Unknown.

Avoid drug or refrain from nursing.

Habit-Forming Potential: None.

Effects of Overdose: Weakness, lethargy, dizziness, confusion, nausea, vomiting, muscle cramps, thirst, electrolyte disturbances, drowsiness progressing to deep sleep or coma, weak and rapid pulse.

Possible Effects of Long-Term Use: Impaired balance of water, salt and potassium in blood and body tissues. Dehydration with possible increased blood viscosity and potential for abnormal clotting. Increased blood sugar in some patients.

Suggested Periodic Examinations While Taking This Drug (at physician's discretion)

Complete blood counts.

Blood levels of sodium, potassium, magnesium, chloride, sugar, uric acid.

Liver and kidney function tests.

▷ **While Taking This Drug, Observe the Following**

Foods: Salt restriction and a high-potassium diet may be needed. Ask your doctor. See Table 13, "High-Potassium Foods."

Herbal Medicines or Minerals: Ginseng may increase blood pressure, blunting the benefits of this medicine. Hawthorn, saw palmetto, ma huang, goldenseal and licorice may also cause increased blood pressure. Calcium and garlic may help lower blood pressure. Dandelion root has diuretic properties. Talk to your doctor BEFORE combining any herbals with this medicine.

Beverages: No restrictions unless directed by your doctor. May be taken with milk.

▷ *Alcohol:* Alcohol can exaggerate the blood pressure lowering effect of this drug and cause orthostatic hypotension (see Glossary).

Tobacco Smoking: No interactions expected. I advise everyone to quit smoking.

▷ *Other Drugs*

Bumetanide may **increase** the effects of
- antihypertensive drugs. Careful decreases in dose are needed to prevent excessive lowering of the blood pressure.

Bumetanide *taken concurrently* with
- ACE inhibitors (see Drug Classes) may result in severe lowering of blood pressure on standing (postural or orthostatic hypotension).
- aminoglycoside antibiotics (amikacin, gentamicin, kanamycin, neomycin, streptomycin, tobramycin, viomycin) increases the risk of hearing loss.
- cephalosporins (see Drug Classes) may increase risk of kidney toxicity.
- cortisone-related drugs may cause excessive potassium loss and also blunted therapeutic benefits.
- digitalis-related drugs (see Drug Classes) requires very careful monitoring to prevent serious disturbances of heart rhythm.
- lithium (Lithobid, others) may increase lithium toxicity risk.

The following drugs may *decrease* the effects of bumetanide:
- indomethacin (Indocin) or other NSAIDs (see Drug Classes) may reduce its diuretic effect.

▷ *Driving, Hazardous Activities:* Caution: Varying degrees of dizziness, weakness or orthostatic hypotension (see Glossary) may occur.

Aviation Note: The use of this drug *may be a disqualification* for piloting. Consult a designated Aviation Medical Examiner.

Exposure to Sun: No restrictions.

Occurrence of Unrelated Illness: Report vomiting or diarrhea promptly to your doctor.

Discontinuation: It may be advisable to stop this drug 5 to 7 days before major surgery. Ask your doctor for help.

BUPROPION (byu PROH pee on)

Other Name: Amfebutamone **Introduced:** 1986 **Class:** Antidepressant **Prescription:** USA: Yes **Controlled Drug:** USA: No; Canada: No **Available as Generic:** USA: Yes
Brand Names: Wellbutrin, Wellbutrin SR, Zyban

BENEFITS versus RISKS

Possible Benefits | *Possible Risks*

EFFECTIVE IN SMOKING
  CESSATION (ZYBAN)
EFFECTIVE TREATMENT OF
  MAJOR DEPRESSIVE
  DISORDERS
SEXUAL DESIRE MAY BE
  INCREASED IN SOME PEOPLE
  AND USED IN TREATMENT
MAY HELP ADHD IN ADULTS
Offers a different class than tricyclic,
  MAO or SSRI antidepressants

DRUG-INDUCED SEIZURES—RARE
Excessive mental stimulation:
  excitement, anxiety, confusion,
  hallucinations, insomnia
Conversion of depression to mania in
  manic-depressive disorders

▷ **Principal Uses**

As a Single Drug Product: Uses currently included in FDA-approved labeling: (1) Helps smokers quit smoking (Zyban); (2) treatment of major depressive disorders.

Other (unlabeled) generally accepted uses: (1) May ease chronic fatigue syndrome symptoms; (2) can reduce cocaine craving when combined with psychotherapy; (3) drug of choice in people who have significant weight gain while taking tricyclic antidepressants; (4) can help some cases of low back pain not responding to other agents; (5) increased sexual desire in 77% of patients in one study; (6) an Alabama Veterans Affairs medical center study found this drug to be effective in post-traumatic stress disorder; (7) works to help people stop using smokeless tobacco; (8) is an alternative to stimulant-type medicines to treat attention deficit hyperactivity disorder (ADHD) based on one cohort study with variable dosing (both in children and in adults).

How This Drug Works: Bupropion increases levels of two nerve transmitters (norepinephrine and dopamine). It is biochemically unique and works differently from other antidepressants (may be a benefit if other medicines have failed). How it works in quitting smoking is unknown.

Available Dosage Forms and Strengths

Tablets, immediate release — 75 mg, 100 mg

Tablets, sustained release — 50 mg (Canada), 100 mg, 150 mg

Zyban Tablets, sustained release only — 150 mg

▷ **Recommended Dosage Ranges** (Actual dose and schedule must be determined for each patient individually.)

Infants and Children: Dosage not established for those under 18 years of age.

18 to 60 Years of Age:

Depression: For first 3 days, 100 mg in the morning and evening. On the fourth day, dose may be increased to 100 mg in the morning, at noon, and in the evening; total daily dose of 300 mg. This schedule of 100 mg, three times daily, 6 hours apart, is used for 3 to 4 weeks. If needed and beneficial, dose may be slowly increased to a maximum of 450 mg daily. Increases should not exceed 100 mg per day in a period of 3 days. No single dose should exceed 150 mg. If daily dose is 450 mg, take 150 mg in the morning, then 100 mg every 4 hours for three more doses. The lowest effective dose should be used. Drug should be stopped if significant improvement is not seen after a trial of 450 mg daily. Doses higher than 450 mg daily may only increase risk of seizures.

Smoking cessation: 150 mg once a day for 3 days, then 150 mg twice daily for 7 to 12 weeks. If progress has not been made in 7 weeks, talk with your doctor.

ADHD in adults: 100 to 200 mg of the SR form twice daily.

Over 60 Years of Age: Same as 18 to 60 years of age.

Conditions Requiring Dosing Adjustments

Liver Function: Lower dosages and caution in monitoring should be used.

Kidney Function: The dose must be decreased in people with damaged kidneys or who develop kidney damage while taking this drug.

Dosing Instructions: May be taken with food to reduce stomach upset. Best to swallow the tablet whole, not chewing or crushing it; this drug has a bitter taste and a local numbing effect on the lining of the mouth. Sustained-release forms should never be crushed or altered. If you forget a dose (and you take the regular-release tablets): Take the medicine right away, unless it is nearly time for your next dose. For the sustained-release forms: Don't take the missed dose, simply take the next scheduled dose. DO NOT double doses. Call your doctor if you miss more than one dose.

Usual Duration of Use: Regular use for 3–4 weeks needed to realize benefits in depression. Long-term use (months to years) requires periodic evaluation of response and dose. For use in quitting smoking: Use for 7–12 weeks. See your doctor regularly.

Typical Treatment Goals and Measurements (Outcomes and Markers)

Depression: The general goal: to help lessen the degree and severity of depression, letting patients return to their daily lives. In a set of guidelines issued by the American College of Physicians, older and newer antidepressants were found to give equal results in treating depression. Older medicines were found to generally have more frequent constipation, dizziness, dry mouth, blurred vision and tremors while newer medicines caused more diarrhea, headache and nausea. The importance here is that many options are available and possible side effects can be somewhat tailored to try to avoid overlap.

Smoking Cessation: The general goal: to stop smoking. Combination with a "quit smoking" course and/or support group can increase beneficial results.

Possible Advantages of This Drug: Causes less atropinelike side effects: blurred vision, dry mouth, constipation, impaired urination. Does not cause sedation or orthostatic hypotension (see Glossary).

▷ **This Drug Should Not Be Taken If**
- you have had an allergic reaction to it previously.
- you have a history of anorexia nervosa or bulimia (may be associated with increased seizure risk).
- you have a seizure disorder of any kind.
- you are taking, or took in the past 14 days, any monoamine oxidase (MAO) type A inhibitor (see Drug Classes).

▷ **Inform Your Physician Before Taking This Drug If**
- you have had any adverse effects from antidepressant drugs.
- you are pregnant or planning pregnancy.
- you are breast-feeding your infant.

- you have a history of mental illness, head injury or brain tumor.
- you have a history of alcoholism or drug abuse.
- you have any kind of heart disease, especially a recent heart attack.
- you have impaired liver or kidney function.
- you take prescription or nonprescription drugs not discussed when bupropion was prescribed for you.
- you take other medicines that can make seizures more likely.

Possible Side Effects (natural, expected and unavoidable drug actions)

Nervousness, anxiety, confusion, insomnia.

Weight loss of more than 5 pounds—frequent.

▷ **Possible Adverse Effects** (unusual, unexpected and infrequent reactions)

If any of the following develop, consult your physician promptly for guidance.

Mild Adverse Effects

Allergic reactions: skin rash, itching—rare to infrequent.

Headache, dizziness, tremor, agitation (9.7% more than placebo) or blurred vision (4.3% more than placebo)—infrequent.

Indigestion, nausea and vomiting, constipation—infrequent.

Dry mouth or edema—frequent.

Excessive sweating (diaphoresis)—frequent.

Ringing in the ears (tinnitus)—possible.

Palpitations—frequent.

Serious Adverse Effects

Drug-induced seizures—rare, more common with high doses.

Change of depression to mania in manic-depressive disorders—possible.

Psychosis in patients with psychotic predisposition—possible.

Decreased or increased white blood cell counts or low platelets—case reports.

Liver toxicity—case reports.

▷ **Possible Effects on Sexual Function:** A study at the University of Alabama found 77% of patients experienced increased sexual desire.

Impotence—infrequent; however, another study reported a decrease in sexual dysfunction when patients were switched from fluoxetine (Prozac) to bupropion.

Altered menstruation up to 3.6% more than placebo in clinical trials—infrequent.

Possible Delayed Adverse Effects: None reported.

Natural Diseases or Disorders That May Be Activated by This Drug

Latent epilepsy, latent psychosis, manic phase of bipolar affective disorder.

Possible Effects on Laboratory Tests

White blood cell or platelet counts: increased or decreased.

CAUTION

1. Take exactly the amount prescribed; rapid dose increases can cause seizures. Watch closely for excessive stimulation.
2. Ask your doctor or pharmacist BEFORE taking any other prescription or nonprescription drug.
3. Do not take any monoamine oxidase (MAO) type A inhibitor while taking this drug (see Drug Classes). If you have taken a MAO inhibitor, wait 2 weeks before starting bupropion.

Precautions for Use

By Infants and Children: Safety and effectiveness for those under 18 years of age not established.

By Those Over 60 Years of Age: Age-related liver or kidney function decline may require dose decreases.

▷ **Advisability of Use During Pregnancy**

Pregnancy Category: B. See Pregnancy Risk Categories at the back of this book.

Animal studies: Rat and rabbit studies reveal no significant birth defects.

Human studies: Adequate studies of pregnant women are not available.

Use this drug only if clearly needed. Ask your doctor for help. A pregnancy registry has been established at 888-825-5249. Encourage your doctor to register you if you have taken this medicine while pregnant.

Advisability of Use If Breast-Feeding

Presence of this drug in breast milk: Yes.

Avoid drug or refrain from nursing.

Habit-Forming Potential: Remote with use of recommended doses. Slight potential for abuse by those who abuse stimulant drugs.

Effects of Overdose: Headache, agitation, confusion, hallucinations, seizures, loss of consciousness.

Possible Effects of Long-Term Use: Not reported.

Suggested Periodic Examinations While Taking This Drug (at physician's discretion)

Liver and/or kidney function tests as appropriate.

▷ **While Taking This Drug, Observe the Following**

Foods: No restrictions.

Herbal Medicines or Minerals: Ginseng, ma huang, yohimbe and St. John's wort may interact with antidepressants, so combining those herbals with this medicine is not recommended.

Beverages: No restrictions. May be taken with milk.

▷ *Alcohol:* Avoid completely. Alcohol may predispose to the development of seizures.

Tobacco Smoking: No interactions expected. I advise everyone to quit smoking.

Marijuana Smoking: Avoid completely; it may lead to psychotic behavior.

▷ *Other Drugs*

The following drugs taken concurrently with bupropion may increase the risk of major seizures:

- antidepressants (tricyclic) or other bupropion-containing medicines.
- clozapine (Clozaril).
- fluoxetine (Prozac).
- haloperidol (Haldol).
- lithium (Lithobid, others).
- loxapine (Loxitane).
- maprotiline (Ludiomil).
- molindone (Moban).
- phenothiazines (see Drug Classes).
- thioxanthenes (see Xanthine Drug Class).
- trazodone (Desyrel).

Bupropion *taken concurrently* with

- carbamazepine (Tegretol) may result in lowered carbamazepine levels.
- cimetidine (Tagamet) may lead to increased bupropion levels.

- flecainide (Tambocor) may lead to increased flecainide levels (interference with P450 2D6). The manufacturer suggests that flecainide doses be used at the lower end of the dose range if these medicines are combined. Flecainide blood levels are prudent.
- levodopa results in increased nausea, restlessness and tremor.
- MAO inhibitors (see Drug Classes) can lead to sudden toxicity. Do not combine.
- metoprolol (Toprol XL, others) can lead to toxicity. Lower metoprolol doses are prudent.
- phenobarbital may result in decreased levels.
- phenytoin (Dilantin) or fosphenytoin (Cerebyx) may result in decreased phenytoin or fosphenytoin levels.
- propafenone (Rythmol) can lead to toxicity. Lower propafenone doses and blood levels are prudent.
- risperidone (Risperdal) and other medicines removed from the body by P450 2D6 may lead to increased blood levels of the medicine removed by P450 2D6. Lower doses and careful patient follow-up are prudent if these medicines are combined.
- ritonavir (Norvir) and probably other protease inhibitors may lead to increased blood levels of bupropion and toxicity—DO NOT COMBINE.
- zolpidem (Ambien) may lead to hallucinations.

▷ *Driving, Hazardous Activities:* This drug may cause dizziness, drowsiness or seizures. Restrict activities as necessary.

Aviation Note: The use of this drug *is a disqualification* for piloting. Consult a designated Aviation Medical Examiner.

Exposure to Sun: No restrictions.

Discontinuation: Do not stop this drug abruptly. Ask your doctor for help.

BUSPIRONE (byu SPI rohn)

Introduced: 1979   **Class:** Antianxiety drug   **Prescription:** USA: Yes
Controlled Drug: USA: No; Canada: No   **Available as Generic:** Yes
Brand Names: ❧Apo-buspirone, Buspar, Buspar Dividose, ❧Med-buspirone, ❧Buspirex, Censpar, Sorbon

BENEFITS versus RISKS	
Possible Benefits	*Possible Risks*
EFFECTIVE RELIEF OF MILD TO MODERATE ANXIETY	Mild dizziness, faintness or headache—uncommon
DECREASED RISK OF SEDATION OR DEPENDENCE THAN OTHER AGENTS	Tachycardia—rare
	Restlessness, depression, tremor or rigidity (with high doses)—rare

▷ **Principal Uses**

As a Single Drug Product: Uses currently included in FDA-approved labeling: (1) Relieves mild to moderate anxiety and nervous tension (useful in elderly, alcoholics and addiction-prone people because of its lack of significant sedative effects or abuse potential); (2) helps control self-injurious behaviors or aggression in developmentally disabled adults.

Other (unlabeled) generally accepted uses: (1) May reduce alcohol craving in alcoholics; (2) can help aggression or hyperactivity in autistics; (3) may decrease symptoms in obsessive-compulsive disorder; (4) can help in sexual dysfunction in people with generalized anxiety disorder; (4) may help decrease smoking urge in smokers; (5) can help prevent chronic tension headaches and migraines.

How This Drug Works: Changes brain chemicals (dopamine, norepinephrine, serotonin), resulting in a calming effect. Decreases actions of serotonin using nerve cells (neurons) in part of the brain (nuclei raphe). Also a partial agonist at serotonin reuptake sites (5HT1A).

Available Dosage Forms and Strengths
Tablets — 5 mg, 10 mg
Tablets scored (Dividose) — 15 mg

▷ **Usual Adult Dosage Ranges:** Initially 7.5 mg twice daily; if needed, dose can be increased by 5 mg/day every 2 to 3 days. Some patients respond well to total daily doses of 20–30 mg which are divided into two or three equal doses. Maximum daily dose is 60 mg. **Note: Actual dose and schedule must be determined for each patient individually.**

Conditions Requiring Dosing Adjustments
Liver Function: Use with caution in severe liver failure. Doses must be decreased.
Kidney Function: Use with caution in severe kidney problems. Dose should be decreased to 25–50% of normal dose.

▷ **Dosing Instructions:** The tablet may be crushed and taken without regard to food. If you forget a dose, but have missed by less than an hour, take the missed dose. If it is almost time for your next scheduled dose, skip the missed dose and simply take the next scheduled dose. DO NOT double doses.

Usual Duration of Use: Regular use for 7 to 14 days may be needed to see full benefit in relieving anxiety and nervous tension. Continual use should not exceed 8 weeks without evaluation by your doctor. **Author's Note: The National Institute of Mental Health has a new information page on anxiety. It can be found on the World Wide Web (www.nimh.nih.gov/anxiety).**

Typical Treatment Goals and Measurements (Outcomes and Markers)
Anxiety or panic: Goals for anxiety and panic tend to be more vague and subjective than hypertension or cholesterol. Frequently, the patient (in conjunction with physician assessment) will largely decide if anxiety has been modified to a successful extent. In the case of panic attacks, decreased number of trips to the hospital or emergency department visits may be a useful measure. In both cases, the ability of the patient to return to normal activities is a hallmark of successful treatment.

Possible Advantages of This Drug: Relieves anxiety or tension without severe sedation or impaired thinking. Low abuse potential compared to benzodiazepines. Actually appeared to improve driving-related skills in one study.

▷ **This Drug Should Not Be Taken If**
• you have had an allergic reaction to this medicine.
• you take, or took in the last 2 weeks, a MAO inhibitor (see Drug Classes). May increase blood pressure.

▷ **Inform Your Physician Before Taking This Drug If**
- you take other drugs that affect the brain or nervous system: tranquilizers, sedatives, hypnotics, analgesics, narcotics, antidepressants, antipsychotic drugs, anticonvulsants or anti-parkinsonism drugs.
- you have impaired liver or kidney function.
- you take fluoxetine (Prozac) for depression.

Possible Side Effects (natural, expected and unavoidable drug actions)
Mild drowsiness (less than with benzodiazepines) (up to 16%)—frequent; lethargy is possible. Infrequent dry mouth.

▷ **Possible Adverse Effects** (unusual, unexpected and infrequent reactions)
If any of the following develop, consult your physician promptly for guidance.

Mild Adverse Effects
Headache, faintness, paradoxical excitement—infrequent.
Dizziness—infrequent to frequent.
Tingling and touch sensation changes (paresthesias)—rare.
Insomnia and dream disturbances, depression—possible.
Increased blood pressure—case reports.
Nausea—infrequent.

Serious Adverse Effects
Tachycardia or palpitations—infrequent.
With high doses: dysphoria, restlessness, rigidity, tremors—possible.
Movement disorders—case reports.
Apnea increases (in some patients with sleep apnea)—possible.

▷ **Possible Effects on Sexual Function:** Difficult or absent orgasm—case report.
May increase prolactin; however, no cases of male breast tenderness or enlargement have been reported.

Possible Effects on Laboratory Tests
Growth hormone: Conflicting increases or lack of effect on growth hormone levels.
Blood prolactin levels: dose-related increase.

CAUTION
This drug is reported to have very mild sedative effects and no abuse potential; however, it should be used with caution and only when clearly needed. Actual dysphoria has been reported with higher doses and may preclude its recreational use.

Precautions for Use
By Infants and Children: Safety and effectiveness for those under 18 years of age not established.
By Those Over 60 Years of Age: Expected to be tolerated much better than benzodiazepines and barbiturates. Watch for increased dizziness or weakness and avoid falls.

▷ **Advisability of Use During Pregnancy**
Pregnancy Category: B. See Pregnancy Risk Categories at the back of this book.
Animal studies: No birth defects found in rat and rabbit studies.
Human studies: Adequate studies of pregnant women are not available.
Discuss any use of this drug during pregnancy with your doctor.

Advisability of Use If Breast-Feeding

Presence of this drug in breast milk: Excreted in rat milk; probably also in humans.

Avoid drug or refrain from nursing.

Habit-Forming Potential: Does not appear to cause addiction; however, more studies are needed. Higher doses result in a dysphoric reaction, which may keep it from becoming a drug involved in recreational use.

Effects of Overdose: Drowsiness, fatigue, nausea, dysphoria, tingling sensations (paresthesias) and a rare chance of seizures.

Possible Effects of Long-Term Use: None reported.

Suggested Periodic Examinations While Taking This Drug (at physician's discretion)

Periodic check of heart rate.

▷ **While Taking This Drug, Observe the Following**

Foods: No restrictions; taking with food may result in a clinically insignificant increase in absorption of this drug.

Herbal Medicines or Minerals: Hawthorn and ephedra may react antagonistically to buspirone. Avoid those medicines. Valerian may interact additively (drowsiness) and caution is advised until the full extent of the combination is seen. Hops, Indian snakeroot, passionflower herb and St. John's wort carry German Commission E monograph indications for anxiety. Indian snakeroot and kava kava are contraindicated in depression and well-designed studies in anxiety combined with this medicine are not available. Talk to your doctor BEFORE you add any herbal medicine to buspirone.

Beverages: No restrictions.

▷ *Alcohol:* Milder problems than diazepam (Valium), but avoid the combination.

Tobacco Smoking: No interactions expected. I advise everyone to quit smoking.

Marijuana Smoking: Additive increase in drowsiness.

▷ *Other Drugs:*

Buspirone taken concurrently with

- citalopram (Celexa) may result in serotonin syndrome. This combination is not advisable.
- clozapine (Clozaril) may result in serious lowering of blood sugar and stomach bleeding.
- diazepam (Valium) may increase risk of headache, dizziness and nausea.
- diltiazem (Cardizem, etc.) may increase buspirone drug concentrations. Watch for increased drowsiness—lower buspirone doses may be needed.
- dofetilide (Tikosyn) may increase blood levels of dofetilide and risk of adverse effects. If this combination must be used, low doses of dofetilide and careful patient follow-up are critical.
- erythromycin (various) may increase blood levels of buspirone and risk of adverse effects.
- fluoxetine (Prozac) may increase underlying anxiety or mental disorder such as obsessive-compulsive disorder. Combination is best avoided, but if deemed clinically necessary, patients should be closely watched for worsening of symptoms.
- fluvoxamine (Luvox) resulted in serious slowing of the heart (bradycardia) in one case report (peak buspirone level was doubled). A later trial in

healthy volunteers found elevated blood levels, but no clinical changes. Caution is advised.

- itraconazole (and perhaps other similar antifungals) may increase blood levels of buspirone and risk of adverse effects.
- MAO inhibitors (see Drug Classes) such as phenelzine (Nardil) may result in large blood pressure increases. DO NOT COMBINE.
- narcotics such as oxycodone (Percodan) may result in additive sedation and potential decreases in breathing (respiratory depression).
- nefazodone (Serzone) may increase blood levels of buspirone and risk of adverse effects. If this combination must be used, low doses of buspirone and careful patient follow-up are critical.
- paroxetine (Paxil) may increase blood levels of buspirone and risk of adverse effects. If this combination must be used, lower doses of buspirone and careful patient follow-up are critical.
- rifampin (Rifater, others) may decrease buspirone blood levels. If this combination must be used, buspirone doses may need to be increased.
- trazodone (Desyrel) may lead to liver toxicity. Liver tests should be obtained regularly if the two drugs are combined.
- venlafaxine (Effexor) may lead to decreased buspirone benefits or venlafaxine toxicity.
- verapamil (Calan, etc.) may increase blood levels of buspirone and risk of adverse effects.

▷ *Driving, Hazardous Activities:* This drug may cause dizziness, faintness or fatigue. Restrict activities as necessary.

Aviation Note: The use of this drug *may be a disqualification* for piloting. Consult a designated Aviation Medical Examiner.

Exposure to Sun: No restrictions.

CALCITONIN (kal si TOH nin)

Other Names: Salcatonin, thyrocalcitonin

Introduced: 1977, 1995 (nasal spray form)   **Class:** Anti-osteoporotic, hormone   **Prescription:** USA: Yes   **Controlled Drug:** USA: No; Canada: No   **Available as Generic:** USA: Yes (one injectable form); Canada: No

Brand Names: Calcimar, Cibacalcin, Miacalcin Injection, Miacalcin Nasal Spray

BENEFITS versus RISKS	
Possible Benefits	*Possible Risks*
PARTIAL RELIEF OF SYMPTOMS OF PAGET'S DISEASE OF BONE	Nausea (with or without vomiting)
NASAL FORM CAN INCREASE BONE MASS	Allergic reactions
Effective adjunctive treatment of postmenopausal osteoporosis	
Effective adjunctive treatment of abnormally high blood calcium levels (associated with malignant disease)	

Author's Note: Information in this profile has been shortened to make room for more widely used medicines.

CAPECITABINE (CAP eh sit ah been)

Introduced: 2001 for colon cancer Class: Antineoplastic   **Prescription:** USA: Yes   **Controlled Drug:** USA: No; Canada: No   **Available as Generic:** No

Brand Names: Xeloda

Author's Note: This medicine was first approved for treatment of breast cancer, and now has been approved for treatment of metastatic colorectal cancer. This first treatment for such cancers to be available taken by mouth (oral), capecitabine is changed (metabolized) into 5-fluorouracil in the body. Capecitabine causes fewer mouth ulcers and less diarrhea and nausea, but seems to cause pain and swelling of the hands and feet more frequently than other therapies. Information in this profile will be broadened when more specific information becomes available.

CAPTOPRIL (KAP toh pril)

Introduced: 1979   **Class:** ACE inhibitor, antihypertensive
   Please see the new angiotensin converting enzyme (ACE) inhibitor family profile for more information.

CARBAMAZEPINE (kar ba MAZ e peen)

Introduced: 1962   **Class:** Anticonvulsant, antineuralgic, pain syndrome modifier   **Prescription:** USA: Yes   **Controlled Drug:** USA: No; Canada: No   **Available as Generic:** Yes

Brand Names: ♣Apo-Carbamazepine, Carbitrol Extended Release, ♣Dom-carbamazepine-CR, Epitol, ♣Mazepine, ♣Novo-Carbamaz, ♣PMS Carba-mazepine, Taro-carbamazepine, Tegretol, Tegretol Chewable Tablet, ♣Tegretol-CR, Tegretol-XR

BENEFITS versus RISKS	
Possible Benefits	*Possible Risks*
RELIEF OF PAIN IN TRIGEMINAL NEURALGIA	BONE MARROW DEPRESSION (reduced formation of all blood cells)—RARE
EFFECTIVE CONTROL OF CERTAIN TYPES OF EPILEPTIC SEIZURES	Liver damage with jaundice—rare
Relief of pain in some rare forms of nerve pain (neuralgia)	

▷ **Principal Uses**

As a Single Drug Product: Uses currently included in FDA-approved labeling: (1) pain relief in true trigeminal neuralgia (tic douloureux) or glossopharyngeal neuralgia; (2) for control of several types of epilepsy (grand mal, tonic-clonic, psychomotor/temporal lobe, complex partial and mixed seizure patterns). Precise diagnosis and careful management are mandatory.

Other (unlabeled) generally accepted uses: Beneficial in (1) bipolar affective disorders; (2) schizoaffective disorders; (3) resistant schizophrenia; (4) post-traumatic stress disorder; (5) tabes dorsalis; (6) diabetic neuropathy; (7) hemifacial spasm; (8) cocaine withdrawal; (9) aggression in some Alzheimer's patients; (10) helping hiccups and belching associated with flutter of the diaphragm; (11) treating nerve problems from thiamine deficiency; (12) possibly having a role in pain that occurs when an arm or leg is amputated (phantom limb pain); (13) easing a perceived repetitive ear noise called clicking tinnitus.

How This Drug Works: Reduces impulses at certain nerve terminals and relieves pain (of trigeminal neuralgia). Also reduces excitability of nerve fibers in the brain, decreasing likelihood, frequency and severity of seizures.

Available Dosage Forms and Strengths

Oral suspension — 100 mg/5 ml

Tablets — 200 mg (400 mg in Canada)

Tablets, chewable — 100 mg, 200 mg

Tablets, controlled release — 200 mg

Tablets, extended release — 100 mg, 200 mg, 400 mg

▷ **Recommended Dosage Ranges:** *Epilepsy:* Initially 200 mg every 12 hours (regular or extended-release tablets). Suspension is started at 100 mg four times a day. Dose may be increased at weekly intervals by 200 mg daily as needed and tolerated and as guided by drug levels. The dose is given twice daily for the extended-release tablets (in general, extended-release forms are given in the same total daily dose—but are given less often). The regular release tablets are given three times daily. Because suspensions give higher peak blood levels in the body, they are generally given in smaller, more frequent doses. Total daily dosage should generally not exceed 1,200 mg, but rare uses of 1,600 mg have been required.

Migraine prevention (prophylaxis): 10–20 mg per kg of body weight per day separated into two equal daily doses has been used.

Infants and Children: Children under age 6 are given 10–20 mg per kg of body mass. This dose is divided into three equal doses and is given three times daily. Increased as needed or tolerated based on clinical response and blood levels. Children over 12 are given 200 mg twice daily or 100 mg of the suspension four times daily. The dose can then be increased by 200 mg a day after a week, as needed and tolerated—guided by blood levels and clinical response. The typical dose that works is in the range of 17–25 mg/kg/day. Maximum is 1,000 mg or lower.

Note: Actual dosage and schedule must be determined for each patient individually. Dosing must be guided by blood levels.

Conditions Requiring Dosing Adjustments

Liver Function: Use with extreme caution, in lower doses and closely watched. May have to be stopped in active liver disease.

Kidney Function: May be toxic to kidneys. Use with extreme caution and in smaller dose in patients with kidneys that already do not work well.

Heart Attack: Changes in blood distribution (perfusion) and protein binding may give much higher than expected blood levels. More frequent lab tests are needed to guide dosing and avoid toxicity.

▷ **Dosing Instructions:** Take at same time each day, with or following food to reduce stomach irritation. Regular-release tablet may be crushed for administration. Extended-release tablet should not be altered. The suspension SHOULD NOT be given at the same time as other medicines or diluents. If you forget a dose: Take the medicine as soon as you remember it, unless it is close to the time for the next dose—simply take the dose at the next scheduled time. DO NOT double doses. Call your doctor if you miss more than one dose.

Usual Duration of Use: Regular use for 3 months may be needed to see effect in easing of trigeminal neuralgia. Longer periods, with dose changes, may be required for control of epileptic seizures. Careful evaluation of tolerance and response should be made every 3 months during long-term treatment.

Typical Treatment Goals and Measurements (Outcomes and Markers)
Seizures: The general goal for this medicine is effective seizure control. Neurologists tend to define effective on a case-by-case basis depending on the seizure type and patient factors.

Currently a "Drug of Choice"
For patients with partial seizures (without or with secondary generalization).

▷ **This Drug Should Not Be Taken If**
- you have had an allergic reaction to it previously.
- you have active liver disease.
- you currently have a blood cell or bone marrow disorder.
- you currently take, or have taken within the past 14 days, a monoamine oxidase (MAO) type A inhibitor (see Drug Classes).

▷ **Inform Your Physician Before Taking This Drug If**
- you have had an allergic reaction to any tricyclic antidepressant drug (see Drug Classes).
- you have taken this drug in the past.
- you have had any blood or bone marrow disorder, especially drug induced.
- you have a history of liver or kidney disease.
- you have depression or other mental disorder.
- you have had thrombophlebitis.
- you have high blood pressure, heart disease or glaucoma.
- you take more than two alcoholic drinks a day.
- you take prescription or nonprescription drugs not discussed when carbamazepine was prescribed for you.
- you are unsure how much to take or how often to take it.
- you are pregnant or are breast-feeding your baby.

Possible Side Effects (natural, expected and unavoidable drug actions)
Dry mouth and throat, constipation, impaired urination.

▷ **Possible Adverse Effects (unusual, unexpected and infrequent reactions)**
If any of the following develop, consult your physician promptly for guidance.
Mild Adverse Effects
Allergic reactions: skin rash, hives, itching, drug fever—rare to infrequent.
Dizziness, drowsiness, unsteadiness—may be frequent when therapy is started (often eases).

Fatigue, blurred vision, confusion—infrequent.

Exaggerated hearing, ringing in ears—case reports.

Loss of appetite, nausea, vomiting, indigestion, diarrhea—may be frequent when starting therapy.

Acne or hair loss—case reports.

Decreased sense of taste—possible.

Aching of muscles and joints, leg cramps—case reports.

Serious Adverse Effects

Allergic reactions: severe dermatitis with peeling of skin, irritation of mouth and tongue, swelling of lymph glands—case reports.

Idiosyncratic reactions: lung inflammation (pneumonitis), cough, shortness of breath.

Agranulocytosis may also be idiosyncratic—case reports.

Lowering of white blood cells (leukopenia): may be up to 10%—infrequent.

Low thyroid hormones—rare.

Bone marrow depression (see Glossary) (agranulocytosis, hemolytic or aplastic anemia) or thrombocytopenia: fatigue, weakness, fever, sore throat, abnormal bleeding or bruising—case reports.

Pseudolymphoma or systemic lupus erythematosus—case reports.

Abnormal heartbeats (bradyarrhythmias)—case reports.

Liver damage with jaundice (see Glossary): yellow eyes or skin, dark-colored urine, light-colored stools—case reports.

Kidney damage or porphyria—case reports.

Mental depression or agitation/psychosis or paradoxical increase in seizures—case reports.

Abnormally elevated urine output (SIADH)—case reports.

Neuroleptic malignant syndrome or aseptic meningitis—case reports.

Abnormal movement and muscle contractions—case reports.

Pancreatitis—case reports.

Retinopathy, visual hallucinations, peripheral neuritis (see Glossary)—case reports.

Vitamin D deficiency (especially if other risk factors are present). This may lead to osteoporosis.

▷ **Possible Effects on Sexual Function:**

Decreased libido and/or impotence—case reports.

Possible male infertility.

This drug is used to control hypersexuality (exaggerated sexual behavior) that can result from injury to the temporal lobe of the brain.

Adverse Effects That May Mimic Natural Diseases or Disorders

Liver reactions may suggest viral hepatitis. Lung reactions may suggest interstitial pneumonitis. SLE syndrome mimics SLE.

Natural Diseases or Disorders That May Be Activated by This Drug

Latent psychosis, systemic lupus erythematosus, osteoporosis.

Possible Effects on Laboratory Tests

Complete blood cell: decreased red cells, hemoglobin, white cells and platelets; increased eosinophils, increased white cells.

Blood calcium level: decreased.

Blood sodium: may be lowered in SIADH.

INR (prothrombin time): decreased.

Thyroid hormones: falsely decreased blood levels.

Blood urea nitrogen level (BUN): increased.

Liver function tests: increased liver enzymes (ALT/GPT, AST/GOT and alkaline phosphatase), increased bilirubin.

Urine pregnancy tests: false negative or inconclusive results with Prepurex, Predictor, Gonavislide, Pregnosticon.

ANA: positive if SLE effect begins.

CAUTION

1. This drug should be used only after less toxic drugs have failed.
2. *Before* the first dose is taken, blood cell counts, liver function tests and kidney function tests should be obtained.
3. Careful periodic testing for blood cell or bone marrow toxicity is *mandatory*.
4. *This drug should not be used* to prevent recurrence of trigeminal neuralgia when it is in remission.
5. *Do not stop this drug suddenly* if it is being used to control seizures.
6. If exposed to humidity, tablet hardens, resulting in poor absorption and erratic control of seizures. Store in a cool, dry place; avoid bathrooms. Try a locking kitchen cabinet.
7. Case reports have been made about an allergic (atypical cross-sensitivity) reaction in people who are allergic to phenytoin who are given carbamazepine. Talk to your doctor if you have this allergy and carbamazepine is prescribed for you.

Precautions for Use

By Infants and Children: Careful testing of blood production and liver and kidney function must be performed regularly. This drug can reduce the effectiveness of other anticonvulsant drugs. Blood levels of all anticonvulsant drugs should be checked if this drug is added to the treatment program.

By Those Over 60 Years of Age: Can cause confusion and agitation. Watch for aggravation of glaucoma, coronary artery disease (angina) or prostatism (see Glossary).

▷ Advisability of Use During Pregnancy

Pregnancy Category: D. See Pregnancy Risk Categories at the back of this book.

Animal studies: Rat studies reveal significant birth defects.

Human studies: Adequate studies of pregnant women are not available.

Avoid completely during the first 3 months. Use during the last 6 months only if clearly needed.

Advisability of Use If Breast-Feeding

Presence of this drug in breast milk: Yes.

Avoid drug or refrain from nursing.

Habit-Forming Potential: None.

Effects of Overdose: Dizziness, drowsiness, disorientation, tremor, involuntary movements, nausea, vomiting, flushed skin, dilated pupils, stupor progressing to coma, cardiac arrest.

Possible Effects of Long-Term Use: Water retention (edema), impaired liver function, possible jaundice.

Suggested Periodic Examinations While Taking This Drug (at physician's discretion)

Complete blood counts weekly during the first 3 months and then monthly.

Liver and kidney function tests.

Eye examinations.

Bone mineral density tests (for osteoporosis).

▷ **While Taking This Drug, Observe the Following**

Foods: No restrictions. There may be a minor increase in absorption if taken with food.

Herbal Medicines or Minerals: Using kola or ma huang may result in unacceptable central nervous system stimulation. Since part of the way that ginseng may work is as an MAO inhibitor, combination with this medicine is not recommended. Valerian and kava kava may interact to increase drowsiness. St. John's wort may also cause increased sun sensitivity—caution is advised.

Beverages: No restrictions. May be taken with milk.

▷ *Alcohol:* Avoid alcohol, unless your doctor approves alcohol use.

Tobacco Smoking: No interactions expected. I advise everyone to quit smoking.

▷ *Other Drugs*

Carbamazepine may ***increase*** the effects of

- medicines that increase heart block such at adenosine (Adenocard). Where possible, carbamazepine should not be given until adenosine has cleared from the body (roughly 4.32 or 5 half-lives, which is 4 days).
- sedatives, tranquilizers, hypnotics and narcotics, and enhance their sedative effects.

Carbamazepine may ***decrease*** the effects of

- adrenocortical steroids (see Drug Classes).
- alprazolam (Xanax).
- amprenavir (Agenerase).
- antidepressants (see Drug Classes).
- bupropion (Wellbutrin, Zyban).
- corticosteroids (such as prednisone or cortisone; see Drug Classes).
- cyclosporine (Sandimmune).
- doxycycline (Doxy-II, Vibramycin, etc.).
- felodipine (Plendil).
- haloperidol (Haldol) or other phenothiazines.
- isradipine (DynaCirc).
- lamotrigine (Lamictal).
- midazolam (Versed).
- nelfinavir (Viracept).
- olanzapine (Zyprexa).
- tacrolimus (Prograf) blood levels and dosing adjusted to tacrolimus levels is prudent.
- tetracyclines (see Drug Classes).
- tramadol (Ultram) and cause loss of tramadol efficacy.
- valproic acid (Depakene, etc.).
- vincristin (Oncovin).
- warfarin (Coumadin). Increased frequency of INR testing is indicated.

Carbamazepine ***taken concurrently*** with

- acetaminophen (Tylenol, others) may increase risk of acetaminophen liver toxicity.

- birth control pills (oral contraceptives) may lower blood levels of the birth control pills and result in pregnancy.
- chlorpromazine (Thorazine) solution may form a rubbery orange precipitate that is passed in the stool. DO NOT combine.
- cisplatin (Platinol, others).
- clozapine (Clozaril) may result in serious bone marrow suppression.
- delavirdine (Rescriptor) may lower trough levels of delavirdine.
- doxorubicin (Doxil, others).
- felbamate (Felbatol) may result in decreased carbamazepine levels and seizures.
- itraconazole (Sporanox) may cause loss of itraconazole benefits.
- ketorolac (Toradol) may blunt carbamazepine benefits.
- lithium (Lithobid, others) may cause serious neurological problems: confusion, drowsiness, weakness, unsteadiness, tremors and twitching.
- monoamine oxidase (MAO) type A inhibitor drugs (see Drug Classes) may cause severe toxic reactions.
- N-acetylcysteine (various) may blunt seizure control.
- phenytoin (Dilantin, etc.) and fosphenytoin (Cerebyx) may cause unpredictable fluctuations of blood levels of both drugs and impair seizure control.
- primidone (Mysoline) may blunt carbamazepine effectiveness.
- sildenafil (Viagra) may result in changes in blood levels.
- terfenadine (Seldane), and perhaps other nonsedating antihistamines, may result in carbamazepine toxicity.
- theophylline (Theo-Dur, etc.) may reduce the effects of both drugs.
- thioridazine (Mellaril) solution may form a rubbery orange precipitate that is passed in the stool. DO NOT combine.

The following drugs may *increase* the effects of carbamazepine:

- cimetidine (Tagamet).
- danazol (Danocrine).
- diltiazem (Cardizem)—and perhaps other calcium channel blockers.
- flu shots (influenza vaccine).
- fluoxetine (Prozac); may lead to toxicity.
- fluvoxamine (Luvox); may result in toxicity.
- isoniazid (INH).
- ketoconazole (Nizoral) and fluconazole (Diflucan).
- macrolide antibiotics—erythromycins, clarithromycin or troleandomycin (not azithromycin).
- nefazodone (Serzone).
- nicotinamide (nicotinic acid amide).
- omeprazole (Prilosec).
- propoxyphene (Darvon, Darvocet, etc.).
- quinupristin/dalfopristin (Synercid) may lead to increased blood levels of carbamazepine and toxicity. Blood levels are prudent and carbamazepine dose decreases may be required.
- rifampin (rifampicin) may result in toxicity.
- ritonavir (Norvir) and perhaps other protease inhibitors such as amprenavir (Agenerase) (see Drug Classes).
- verapamil (Calan, Isoptin).

▷ *Driving, Hazardous Activities:* Can cause dizziness, drowsiness or blurred vision. Adjust activities.

Aviation Note: The use of this drug *is a disqualification* for piloting. Consult a designated Aviation Medical Examiner.

Exposure to Sun: This drug can cause photosensitivity (see Glossary). Use caution until sensitivity to sun is known.

Heavy Exercise or Exertion: Use caution if you have coronary artery disease. Can intensify angina and reduce tolerance for physical activity.

Occurrence of Unrelated Illness: You MUST tell all health care providers that you take this drug.

Discontinuation: If treating trigeminal neuralgia, attempts to reduce the maintenance dose or to stop this drug are needed every 3 months. If used to control epilepsy, this drug *must not be stopped abruptly*.

Special Storage Instructions: Store tablets in a cool, dry place. Protect from humid conditions (**DO NOT store in a bathroom medicine cabinet**) as this can decrease potency of both brand or generic forms by serious percentages.

CARTEOLOL (KAR tee oh lohl)

Introduced: 1983   **Class:** Antihypertensive, beta-adrenergic blocker
Prescription: USA: Yes   **Controlled Drug:** USA: No; Canada: No
Available as Generic: Yes (ophthalmic)
Brand Names: Cartrol, Ocupress, Occupress

BENEFITS versus RISKS	
Possible Benefits	*Possible Risks*
EFFECTIVE, WELL-TOLERATED ANTIHYPERTENSIVE	Congestive heart failure worsening (in some patients)
EFFECTIVE GLAUCOMA TREATMENT	Worsening of angina in coronary heart disease (abrupt withdrawal)
Prevention of angina	Masking of low blood sugar (hypoglycemia) in drug-treated diabetics
May help prevent complications and left ventricle damage after a heart attack	Provocation of asthma in asthmatics
May help prevent tolerance to nitrates	

▷ **Principal Uses**

As a Single Drug Product: Uses currently included in FDA-approved labeling: (1) Treats mild to moderate high blood pressure, alone or in combination with other drugs, such as diuretics; (2) helps lower eye (intraocular) pressure in people with glaucoma or ocular hypertension.

Other (unlabeled) generally accepted uses: (1) Increases amount of exercise that can be performed before angina occurs; (2) can help decrease aggressive behavior; (3) decreases risk of abnormal heart rhythms; (4) has shown benefits after heart attacks—preserving left heart ventricle function and preventing second heart attacks; (5) may help lessen panic attacks.

How This Drug Works:
- Blocks certain actions of the sympathetic nervous system.
- Reduces the heart rate and contraction force, lowering ejection pressure of blood leaving the heart.

- Reduces extent of blood vessel wall contraction, relaxing the walls and lowering blood pressure.
- Reduces elevated eye pressure (intraocular) and relieves glaucoma symptoms.

Available Dosage Forms and Strengths
Ophthalmic solution — 5 ml, 10 ml (1%)
Tablets — 2.5 mg, 5 mg

▷ **Usual Adult Dosage Ranges:** *High blood pressure (hypertension):* Starts with 2.5 mg daily (by itself or combined with a water pill or diuretic) once a day. If needed because blood pressure goals are not reached, the dose can be gradually (peak benefits from a given dose may take several days up to several weeks) increased to 5 or 10 mg a day. This medicine has a ceiling effect, and doses above 10 mg are not likely to confer added benefit.

For glaucoma or eye (ocular) hypertension: One drop in the affected eye or eyes two times a day. **Note: Actual dose and schedule must be determined for each patient individually.**

Conditions Requiring Dosing Adjustments
Liver Function: Liver does play a role in removing this medicine, but how much of a role is not defined. Decreased doses are probably needed in severe liver failure.
Kidney Function: Dosing interval **MUST** be decreased in kidney failure. In severe compromise, 5 mg is given every 48 to 72 hours.

▷ **Dosing Instructions:** Tablet may be crushed and taken without regard to eating. Do not stop this drug abruptly. If you forget a dose: take it right away unless it's nearly time for your next daily dose. If it IS within 8 hours of the regular dose, skip the missed dose and just take the scheduled dose. DO NOT double doses.

Usual Duration of Use: Regular use for up to 3 weeks may be needed to see effectiveness in lowering blood pressure. Long-term use (months to years) is determined by lowering of blood pressure and response to a overall program (weight reduction, salt restriction, smoking cessation, etc.). See your doctor on a regular basis.

Typical Treatment Goals and Measurements (Outcomes and Markers)
Blood Pressure: The most recent treatment guidelines (JNC VI) actually define optimal blood pressure (BP) as less than 120/80 and high normal as 139/89. The American Diabetes Association suggests 130/80 as the optimal target for people living with diabetes. Most clinicians try to achieve a BP that achieves the best balance of lower cardiovascular risk while avoiding the problem of too low a blood pressure. The goal and time frame (see peak benefits above) should be discussed with you when the prescription is written.

Possible Advantages of This Drug: Adequate control of blood pressure with a single daily dose helps adherence or compliance. Causes less slowing of the heart rate than most other beta-blocker drugs.

▷ **This Drug Should Not Be Taken If**
- you have bronchial asthma.
- you have had an allergic reaction to it previously.
- you have congestive heart failure.
- you have an abnormally slow heart rate or a serious heart block (second- or third-degree AV).

▷ **Inform Your Physician Before Taking This Drug If**
- you have had an adverse reaction to any beta blocker (see Drug Classes).
- you have serious heart disease or episodes of heart failure.
- you have had hay fever (allergic rhinitis), asthma, chronic bronchitis or emphysema.
- you have a history of overactive thyroid function (hyperthyroidism).
- you have a history of low blood sugar (hypoglycemia), diabetes or myasthenia gravis.
- you have impaired liver or kidney function.
- you have a circulation problem (Raynaud's phenomenon, claudication pains in legs).
- you take any form of digitalis, quinidine or reserpine, or any calcium blocker drug (see Drug Classes).
- you will have surgery with general anesthesia.

Possible Side Effects (natural, expected and unavoidable drug actions)
Lethargy and fatigability, cold extremities, slow heart rate.
Short-term itching or eye tearing with the ophthalmic drops—frequent.

▷ **Possible Adverse Effects** (unusual, unexpected and infrequent reactions)
If any of the following develop, consult your physician promptly for guidance.
Mild Adverse Effects
Allergic reactions: skin rash—rare.
Headache, dizziness, nervousness, drowsiness—infrequent to frequent.
Indigestion, nausea, vomiting, constipation, diarrhea—infrequent.
Slight increase in blood potassium—possible.
Cough, wheezing or sinusitis—rare.
Joint and muscle discomfort, numbness of fingers or toes—rare.
Carpal tunnel syndrome—case reports with other medicines in this class.
Episodic difficulty walking (intermittent claudication with peripheral vascular disease)—possible.
Tearing and irritation (with eye use)—infrequent to frequent.
Serious Adverse Effects
Mental depression—possible, but less likely than some other beta blockers.
Chest pain, irregular heartbeat, shortness of breath; can cause congestive heart failure—possible.
Induction of bronchial asthma (in asthmatic patients)—possible.
Aggravation of myasthenia gravis—possible.
May hide symptoms of low blood sugar.

▷ **Possible Effects on Sexual Function:** Decreased libido, impotence—case reports.

Adverse Effects That May Mimic Natural Diseases or Disorders
Decreased extremity blood flow may mimic Raynaud's phenomenon (see Glossary).

Natural Diseases or Disorders That May Be Activated by This Drug
Raynaud's disease, intermittent claudication, myasthenia gravis.

Possible Effects on Laboratory Tests
Blood creatine kinase level: increased.
Blood potassium: slight increase.

CAUTION
1. ***Do not stop this drug suddenly*** without the knowledge of your doctor. Carry a note that says you are taking this drug.
2. Ask your physician or pharmacist before using nasal decongestants. These can cause sudden increases in blood pressure when combined with beta-blocker drugs.
3. Report any new tendency to emotional depression.
4. Use of the eye (ophthalmic) form may lead to additive lowering of blood pressure with other beta blockers.

Precautions for Use
By Infants and Children: Safety and effectiveness by those under 12 years of age not established.

By Those Over 60 Years of Age: **Caution**: Unacceptably high blood pressure should be reduced without creating excessively low blood pressure. Small doses and frequent blood pressure checks are needed. Sudden/excessive blood pressure lowering can cause stroke or heart attack. Watch for dizziness, confusion, depression or urinary frequency.

▷ **Advisability of Use During Pregnancy**
Pregnancy Category: C. See Pregnancy Risk Categories at the back of this book.
Animal studies: No birth defects found in rat or rabbit studies.
Human studies: Adequate studies of pregnant women are not available.
Use this drug only if clearly needed. Ask your physician for guidance.

Advisability of Use If Breast-Feeding
Presence of this drug in breast milk: Unknown in humans; yes in animals.
Avoid drug or refrain from nursing.

Habit-Forming Potential: None.

Effects of Overdose: Weakness, slow pulse, low blood pressure, fainting, cold and sweaty skin, congestive heart failure, possible coma and convulsions.

Possible Effects of Long-Term Use: Reduced heart reserve and eventual heart failure in susceptible individuals with advanced heart disease.

Suggested Periodic Examinations While Taking This Drug (at physician's discretion)
Measurements of blood pressure (treated to pressure goal within a set time frame).
Evaluation of heart function.

▷ **While Taking This Drug, Observe the Following**
Foods: No specific restrictions, but losing weight can help meet blood pressure goals. Avoid excessive salt intake.
Herbal Medicines or Minerals: Ginseng may increase blood pressure, blunting the benefits of this medicine. Hawthorn, saw palmetto, ma huang, goldenseal, yohimbe and licorice may also cause increased blood pressure. Calcium and garlic may help lower blood pressure, and the dose has to be individualized with a standardized extract. Indian snakeroot has a German Commission E monograph indication for hypertension—talk to your doctor. Eleuthero root and ephedra should be avoided by people living with hypertension. Talk to your doctor BEFORE adding any herbals.
Beverages: No restrictions. May be taken with milk.

▷   *Alcohol:* Use caution. Alcohol may exaggerate blood pressure lowering and also increase its mild sedative effect.

Tobacco Smoking: Nicotine may reduce benefits in treating high blood pressure. High doses may worsen bronchial constriction caused by regular smoking. I advise everyone to quit smoking.

▷   *Other Drugs*

Carteolol may *increase* the effects of

- other antihypertensive drugs and cause excessive lowering of the blood pressure. Dosage adjustments may be necessary.
- reserpine (Ser-Ap-Es, etc.) and cause sedation, depression, slowing of the heart rate and low blood pressure. This combination is best avoided.
- theophyllines (aminophylline, dyphylline, oxtriphylline, etc.).
- verapamil (Calan, Isoptin) and cause excessive depression of heart function; monitor this combination closely.

Carteolol *taken concurrently* with

- amiodarone (Cordarone) may cause severe slowing of the heart and sinus arrest. Do not combine these agents.
- clonidine (Catapres) requires close monitoring for rebound high blood pressure if clonidine is stopped while carteolol is still being taken. Severe rebound hypertension may occur.
- digoxin (Lanoxin) may lead to abnormal heart conduction. Caution is prudent.
- diltiazem (Cardizem) and other dihydropyridine type calcium channel blockers (like verapamil) may be very helpful in patients with normal heart function, but may result in AV conduction problems.
- epinephrine (Adrenalin, etc.) may cause sudden rise in blood pressure followed by slowing of the heart rate. Avoid this combination.
- ergot preparations (ergotamine, methysergide, etc.) may enhance serious ergot-induced constriction of peripheral circulation.
- fluoxetine (Prozac) may result in dangerous slowing of the heart or dangerously low blood pressure.
- fluvoxamine (Luvox) may result in dangerous slowing of the heart or dangerously low blood pressure.
- insulin requires close monitoring to avoid hypoglycemia (see Glossary).
- nifedipine (and perhaps other dihydroperidine calcium channel blockers) may result in excessive lowering of the blood pressure.
- oral antidiabetic drugs (see Drug Classes) may cause prolonged recovery from hypoglycemia should it occur.
- phenothiazines (see Drug Classes) can cause increased effects of both drugs.
- rifabutin (Mycobutin) may reduce carteolol's effectiveness.
- ritodrine (Yutopar) may block Yutopar actions. Maker of ritodrine does NOT recommend this combination.
- sibutramine (Meridia) may lead to increases in blood pressure.
- venlafaxine (Effexor) may lead to toxicity from either drug.
- zileuton (Zyflo) may result in increased toxicity risk from carteolol. Caution is advised.

The following drugs may *decrease* the effects of carteolol:

- indomethacin (Indocin), and possibly other "aspirin substitutes" or NSAIDs, and may impair carteolol's antihypertensive effect.

▷ *Driving, Hazardous Activities:* Use caution until the full extent of fatigue, dizziness and blood pressure change have been determined.

Aviation Note: The use of this drug *is a disqualification* for piloting. Consult a designated Aviation Medical Examiner.

Exposure to Sun: No restrictions.

Exposure to Heat: Caution is advised. Hot environments can lower the blood pressure and exaggerate the effects of this drug.

Exposure to Cold: Caution is advised. The elderly should take precautions to prevent hypothermia (see Glossary).

Heavy Exercise or Exertion: Avoid exertion that produces light-headedness, excessive fatigue or muscle cramping.

Occurrence of Unrelated Illness: Fever can lower blood pressure and require decreased doses. Illnesses that cause nausea or vomiting may interrupt the regular dosage schedule. Ask your physician for guidance.

Discontinuation: **DO NOT STOP this drug suddenly**. If possible, gradual reduction of dose over a period of 2 to 3 weeks is recommended. Ask your physician for help.

CARVEDILOL (KAR vi die lohl)

Introduced: 1997   **Class:** Alpha adrenergic blocker, antihypertensive, beta-adrenergic blocker   **Prescription:** USA: Yes   **Controlled Drug:** USA: No; Canada: No   **Available as Generic:**   No
Brand Names: Coreg, ✝Dilatrend, ✝Eucardic, ✝Proreg

BENEFITS versus RISKS	
Possible Benefits	*Possible Risks*
EFFECTIVE, WELL-TOLERATED ANTIHYPERTENSIVE	Worsening of heart failure (often responds to dose changes)
IMPROVES CONGESTIVE HEART FAILURE	Slow heartbeat
CONFERS SIGNIFICANT SURVIVAL BENEFITS IN PATIENTS WITH ADVANCED CONGESTIVE HEART FAILURE	Masking of low blood sugar (hypoglycemia) in drug-treated diabetics (possible)
	Provocation of asthma in asthmatics
MAY DECREASE RISK OF HEART PROBLEMS AND DEATH (MORBIDITY AND MORTALITY)	
WORKS ON TWO KINDS OF BETA RECEPTORS (B1 AND B2 AND ALPHA [ALPHA 1]) RECEPTORS AS WELL	

▷ **Principal Uses**

As a Single Drug Product: Uses currently included in FDA-approved labeling: (1) Treats mild to moderate high blood pressure, alone or in combination with other drugs; (2) improves congestive heart failure or CHF (one of two beta blockers along with metoprolol XL form approved for CHF).

Other unlabeled, generally accepted uses: (1) Eases frequency and severity of angina; (2) may help prevent nitrate tolerance; (3) may be of help in people with increased blood pressure in the liver blood circulation that stems from liver disease (portal hypertension).

How This Drug Works: Blocks certain actions of the sympathetic nervous system and:

- reduces the heart rate and contraction force, lowering ejection pressure of blood leaving the heart.
- reduces extent of blood vessel wall contraction, relaxing the walls and lowering blood pressure.
- after a heart attack, works to prevent inappropriate changes (remodeling) in the left ventricle, prevent repeat heart attacks and also appears to help decrease the size of the heart attack (infarct size in animals).

Carvedilol also is able to open (dilate) blood vessels in the periphery because of alpha-1 receptor blockade. This medicine acts as an antioxidant and inhibits programmed cell death.

Available Dosage Forms and Strengths
Tablets — 3.125, 6.25, 12.5, 25 mg
Tablets — 25 mg, 50 mg (Dilatrend)

▷ **Usual Adult Dosage Ranges**
For high blood pressure (hypertension): Starts with 6.25 mg twice daily. Dose may be increased to 12.5 mg twice daily and then to 25 mg twice daily at intervals of 2 weeks, as needed and tolerated. This medicine should be taken with food in order to decrease the risk of postural hypotension (see Glossary).

For angina: 25 to 50 mg twice a day (benefits are dose related).

For congestive heart failure: 3.125 mg twice a day. After 2 weeks, this dose may be increased to 6.25 mg twice daily as needed and tolerated. The dose can be subsequently doubled every 14 days to a maximum of 25 mg twice daily (for those less than 85 kg) or to 50 mg twice daily for people weighing more than 85 kg. When the dose is changed, patients should be watched for dizziness (for 2 hours after the first dose at the new level). If dizziness occurs, carvedilol should be taken with food to slow the speed at which it enters the body.

Note: Actual dose and schedule must be determined for each patient individually.

Conditions Requiring Dosing Adjustments
Liver Function: Twenty percent of the usual dose is given in people with cirrhosis of the liver. Carvedilol should NOT be used in severe liver failure.

Kidney Function: No changes thought to be needed.

▷ **Dosing Instructions:** Tablet may be crushed. Doses should be taken with food in order to decrease the risk of abnormally low blood pressure when standing up. Do not stop this drug abruptly. If you forget a dose: take it right away unless it's nearly time for your next dose. If it IS nearly time, just take the scheduled dose. DO NOT double doses.

Usual Duration of Use: Regular use brings the best results in lowering blood pressure. DO NOT SKIP DOSES. This medicine may reach its peak benefit with the first dose. Long-term use (months to years) is determined by lowering of blood pressure and response to a overall program (weight reduction, salt restriction, smoking cessation, etc). See your doctor on a regular basis.

Typical Treatment Goals and Measurements (Outcomes and Markers)

Blood Pressure: The most recent treatment guidelines (JNC VI) actually define optimal blood pressure (BP) as less than 120/80 and high normal as 139/89. The American Diabetes Association suggests 130/80 as the optimal target for people living with diabetes. Most clinicians try to achieve a BP that achieves the best balance of lower cardiovascular risk while avoiding the problem of too low a blood pressure. The goal and time frame (see peak benefits above) should be discussed with you when the prescription is written.

Possible Advantages of This Drug

Works on two kinds of beta receptors and alpha receptors as well. May reach its peak benefit with the first dose. Based on the COPERNICUS (Carvedilol Prospective Randomized Cumulative Survival Study), carvedilol confers marked survival benefits in advanced heart failure. A 2001 study of 2289 patients (with severe heart failure—ejection fraction less than 25%) undertaken at Columbia University found that carvedilol reduced death by 35%. An economic evaluation of the US Carvedilol Heart Failure Trials published in August of 2001 in *Pharmacotherapy* found carvedilol to not only reduce mortality but also save costs.

▷ **This Drug Should Not Be Taken If**

- you have bronchial asthma.
- you have had an allergic reaction to it previously.
- you have sick sinus syndrome (ask your doctor).
- you have decompensated heart failure (NYHA Class four).
- you have an abnormally slow heart rate or a serious heart block (second or third degree).

▷ **Inform Your Physician Before Taking This Drug If**

- you have had an adverse reaction to any beta blocker (see Drug Classes).
- you have serious heart disease or episodes of heart failure.
- you have had hay fever (allergic rhinitis), asthma, chronic bronchitis, or emphysema.
- you have a history of overactive thyroid function (hyperthyroidism).
- you have pheochromocytoma.
- you have a history of low blood sugar (hypoglycemia), diabetes, or myasthenia gravis.
- you have impaired liver or kidney function.
- you have a circulation problem (Raynaud's phenomenon, claudication pains in legs).
- you have low blood platelets.
- you take any form of digitalis, quinidine, or reserpine, or any calcium blocker drug (see Drug Classes).
- you will have surgery with general anesthesia.

Possible Side Effects (natural, expected, and unavoidable drug actions)

Lethargy and fatigability, cold extremities, slow heart rate, light-headedness in upright position (see Orthostatic Hypotension in Glossary)—rare when treating hypertension, infrequent when treating congestive heart failure. Dizziness—frequent.

▷ **Possible Adverse Effects** (unusual, unexpected, and infrequent reactions)
   If any of the following develop, consult your physician promptly for guidance.
   Mild Adverse Effects
   Allergic reactions: skin rash—rare.
   Headache, dizziness, nervousness, drowsiness—infrequent to frequent.
   Indigestion, nausea, vomiting, constipation, diarrhea—infrequent.
   Urination at night (nocturia) or difficulty urinating—reported with other beta blockers.
   Cough, wheezing, or sinusitis—reported with other beta blockers.
   Episodic difficulty walking (intermittent claudication with peripheral vascular disease)—possible.
   Muscle aches or back pain—case reports.
   Visual changes—infrequent.
   Serious Adverse Effects
   Allergic reactions: One case report of Stevens-Johnson syndrome.
   Lowering of blood platelets—rare.
   Slow heartbeat (bradycardia), worsening of angina—possible with higher doses.
   Fainting (syncope)—possible.
   Edema (dependent and peripheral)—rare in hypertension and infrequent in CHF.
   Increased blood sugar—possible.
   May hide symptoms of low blood sugar.
   Chest pain, irregular heartbeat, shortness of breath; can cause congestive heart failure—possible.
   Induction of bronchial asthma (in asthmatic patients)—possible.
   Aggravation of myasthenia gravis—possible.
   Resistance to epinephrine in hypersensitivity or other treatment.

▷ **Possible Effects on Sexual Function:** Impotence—case reports with other beta blockers. This rare effect is less common with heart selectivity and low fat (lipid) solubility.

Adverse Effects That May Mimic Natural Diseases or Disorders
   Decreased extremity blood flow may mimic Raynaud's phenomenon (see Glossary).

Natural Diseases or Disorders That May Be Activated by This Drug
   Intermittent claudication, diabetes.

Possible Effects on Laboratory Tests
   Blood sugar: increased or decreased in diabetics.

CAUTION
   • ***Do not stop this drug suddenly*** without the knowledge of your doctor (may cause dangerous increases in blood pressure or angina). Carry a note that says you are taking this drug.
   • Ask your physician or pharmacist before using nasal decongestants. These can cause sudden increases in blood pressure when combined with beta-blocker drugs.
   • May worsen positional blood pressure lowering (postural hypotension) in the elderly.
   • Report any new tendency to emotional depression.

- Because dizziness is a common side effect, make sure you know the extent and severity of this possible effect before undertaking activities that may be hazardous.

Precautions for Use

By Infants and Children: Safety and effectiveness in children not established.

By Those Over 60 Years of Age: **Caution:** Unacceptably high blood pressure should be reduced without creating excessively low blood pressure. Small doses and frequent blood pressure checks are needed.

Sudden/excessive blood pressure lowering can cause stroke or heart attack. Watch for dizziness, confusion, depression, or urinary frequency.

▷ **Advisability of Use During Pregnancy**

Pregnancy Category: C. See Pregnancy Risk Categories at the back of this book.

Animal studies: No birth defects found in rat or rabbit studies.

Human studies: Adequate studies of pregnant women are not available.

Use this drug only if clearly needed. Ask your physician for guidance.

Advisability of Use If Breast-Feeding

Presence of this drug in breast milk: Unknown in humans, but expected.

Avoid drug or refrain from nursing.

Habit-Forming Potential: None.

Effects of Overdose: Weakness, slow pulse, low blood pressure, fainting, cold and sweaty skin, congestive heart failure, possible coma, and convulsions.

Possible Effects of Long-Term Use: Not defined.

Suggested Periodic Examinations While Taking This Drug (at physician's discretion): Measurements of blood pressure and treatment to goals within a set time frame, blood sugar, evaluation of heart and visual function.

▷ **While Taking This Drug, Observe the Following**

Foods: No restrictions. Avoid excessive salt intake.

Herbal Medicines or Minerals: Ginseng may increase blood pressure, blunting the benefits of this medicine. Hawthorn, saw palmetto, ma huang, goldenseal, yohimbe and licorice may also cause increased blood pressure. Calcium and garlic may help lower blood pressure and doses should be individualized using a standardized extract. Indian snakeroot has a German Commission E monograph indication for hypertension—talk to your doctor. Eleuthero root and ephedra should be avoided by people living with hypertension. Ginger, vanadium and nettle may also change blood sugar. Talk to your doctor BEFORE combining any herbal medicine or mineral with carvedilol.

Beverages: No restrictions. May be taken with milk.

▷ *Alcohol:* Use caution. Alcohol may exaggerate blood pressure lowering and also increase its mild sedative effect.

Tobacco Smoking: Nicotine may reduce benefits in treating high blood pressure.

High doses may worsen bronchial constriction caused by regular smoking. I advise everyone to quit smoking.

▷ *Other Drugs*

Carvedilol may *increase* the effects of

- cyclosporine (Sandimmune, others) requiring cyclosporine dose decreases.
- other antihypertensive drugs, and cause excessive lowering of the blood pressure. Dosage adjustments may be necessary.

- reserpine (Ser-Ap-Es, etc.), and cause sedation, depression, slowing of the heart rate, and low blood pressure. This combination is best avoided.
- verapamil (Calan, Isoptin), and cause excessive depression of heart function; monitor this combination closely.

Carvedilol *taken concurrently* with

- amiodarone (Cordarone) may cause severe slowing of the heart and sinus arrest. Do not combine this agent.
- cimetidine (Tagamet) may lead to excessive levels of carvedilol and possible toxic effects.
- clonidine (Catapres) requires close monitoring for rebound high blood pressure if clonidine is stopped while carvedilol is still being taken. Severe rebound hypertension may occur.
- digoxin (Lanoxin) may lead to abnormal heart conduction. Caution is prudent.
- diltiazem (Cardizem) (like verapamil) may be very helpful in patients with normal heart function, but may result in AV conduction problems.
- epinephrine (Adrenalin, etc.) may cause sudden rise in blood pressure followed by slowing of the heart rate. Avoid this combination.
- insulin requires close monitoring to avoid hypoglycemia (see Glossary).
- nifedipine (dihydroperidine) may result in excessive lowering of the blood pressure.
- oral antidiabetic drugs (see Drug Classes) may cause prolonged recovery from hypoglycemia should it occur.
- rifabutin (Mycobutin) may reduce carvedilol's effectiveness.
- ritodrine (Yutopar) may block Yutopar actions. Maker of ritodrine does NOT recommend this combination.
- sibutramine (Meridia) may lead to increases in blood pressure.
- zileuton (Zyflo) may result in increased toxicity risk from carvedilol. Caution is advised.

The following drugs may *decrease* the effects of carvedilol:

- indomethacin (Indocin), and possibly other "aspirin substitutes" or NSAIDs, may impair carvedilol's antihypertensive effect.

▷ *Driving, Hazardous Activities:* Use caution until the full extent of fatigue, dizziness, and blood pressure change has been determined.

Aviation Note: The use of this drug *is a disqualification* for piloting. Consult a designated Aviation Medical Examiner.

Exposure to Sun: No restrictions.

Exposure to Heat: Caution is advised. Hot environments can lower the blood pressure and exaggerate the effects of this drug.

Exposure to Cold: Caution is advised. The elderly should take precautions to prevent hypothermia (see Glossary).

Heavy Exercise or Exertion: Avoid exertion that produces light-headedness, excessive fatigue, or muscle cramping.

Occurrence of Unrelated Illness: Fever can lower blood pressure and require decreased doses. Illnesses that cause nausea or vomiting may interrupt the regular dosage schedule. Ask your physician for guidance.

Discontinuation: **DO NOT STOP this drug suddenly.** If possible, gradual reduction of dose over a period of 2 to 3 weeks is recommended. Ask your physician for help.

CEPHALOSPORIN ANTIBIOTIC FAMILY
(SEF a low spoar ins)

Cefaclor (SEF a klor)   **Cefadroxil** (SEF a drox il)   **Cefixime** (SE fix eem)   **Cefprozil** (SEF proh zil)   **Ceftriaxone** (SEF try ax own)   **Cefuroxime** (SEF yur ox eem)   **Cephalexin** (SEF ah lex in)   **Loracarbef** (lor ah KAR bef)

Introduced: 1979, 1977, 1986, 1991, 1984, 1974, 1969, 1992, respectively **Class:** Antibiotics, cephalosporins **Prescription:** USA: Yes **Controlled Drugs:** USA: No; Canada: No **Available as Generic:** *Cefaclor:* yes; *Cefadroxil:* yes; *Cefixime:* no; *Cefprozil:* no; *Ceftriaxone:* no; *Cefuroxime:* yes; *Cephalexin:* yes; *Loracarbef:* no

Brand Names: *Cefaclor:* Ceclor; *Cefadroxil:* Duricef, Ultracef; *Cefixime:* Suprax; *Cefprozil:* Cefzil; *Ceftriaxone:* Rocephin; *Cefuroxime:* Ceftin, Kefurox, Zinacef; *Cephalexin:* ✣Apo-Cephalex, Cefanex, ✣Ceporex, Keflet, Keflex, Keftab, ✣Novo-Lexin, ✣Nu-Cephalex; *Loracarbef:* Lorabid

BENEFITS versus RISKS	
Possible Benefits	*Possible Risks*
EFFECTIVE TREATMENT OF INFECTIONS DUE TO SUSCEPTIBLE MICRO-ORGANISMS	ALLERGIC REACTIONS, MILD TO SEVERE (MAY ALSO BE SEEN IN THOSE ALLERGIC TO PENICILLIN)
HOME INTRAVENOUS TREATMENT OF SERIOUS INFECTIONS (ceftriaxone)	Drug-induced colitis—rare
	Superinfections (see Glossary)
	Low white blood cell or platelet counts (cefixime or ceftriaxone)—rare
ONE-INJECTION TREATMENT OF SOME CHILDHOOD EAR INFECTIONS	Anemia (ceftriaxone)—rare

▷ **Principal Uses**

As a Single Drug Product: Uses currently included in FDA-approved labeling: (1) To treat some infections of the skin and skin structures, the upper and lower respiratory tract (including middle ear infections—ceftriaxone has a one-dose indication for bacterial otitis media—and "strep" throat), some urinary tract and some postoperative wound infections; (2) treatment of advanced Lyme disease (stage 2 or 3) via home intravenous (home IV) services (ceftriaxone); (3) treatment of serious bone infections (osteomyelitis) via home IV; (4) treatment of gonorrhea (cefuroxime).

Other unlabeled, generally accepted uses: (1) May have an alternative role in helping prevent rheumatic fever if the bacteria are resistant to erythromycin (cefaclor); (2) may help treat resistant cervical infections (cefixime); (3) part of combination treatment of Whipple's disease (cefixime); (4) treats sexual assault cases and chancroid (ceftriaxone); (5) used in *Shigella* infections; (6) used to change from an intravenous medicine to one taken by mouth in order to shorten hospital stays and preserve results (cefuroxime).

How These Drugs Work: These drugs destroy susceptible infecting bacteria by interfering with their ability to produce new protective cell walls as they multiply and grow.

Available Dosage Forms and Strengths
Cefaclor:
> Capsules — 250 mg, 500 mg
> Oral suspension — 125 mg, 187 mg, 250 mg, 375 mg/5 ml

Cefadroxil:
> Capsules — 500 mg, 1,000 mg
> Gelatin capsules (Canada) — 500 mg
> Oral suspension — 125 mg, 250 mg, 500 mg/5 ml
> Tablets — 1,000 mg (1 g)

Cefixime:
> Oral suspension — 100 mg/5 ml
> Tablets — 200 mg, 400 mg

Cefprozil:
> Oral suspension — 125 mg, 250 mg/5 ml
> Tablets — 250 mg, 500 mg

Ceftriaxone:
> 250 mg of Rocephin — Boxes of 1 or 10 vial(s)
> 500 mg of Rocephin — Boxes of 1 or 10 vial(s)
> 1 g of Rocephin — Boxes of 1 or 10 vial(s) or piggyback bottles of 10
> 2 g of Rocephin — Boxes of 10 vials, or piggyback bottles of 10
> 10 g of Rocephin — Box of one 1 g or 2 g ADD-Vantage packaging

Cefuroxime:
> Intravenous — 750 mg/10 ml
> — 750 mg/50 ml
> — 750 mg/100 ml
> — 1.5 g/100 ml
> — 1.5 g/50 ml
> — 1.5 g/20 ml
> — 7.5 g/127 ml
> Oral suspension — 125 mg/5 ml, 250 mg/5 ml
> Tablets — 125 mg, 250 mg, 500 mg

Cephalexin:
> Capsules — 250 mg, 500 mg
> Oral suspension — 125 mg, 250 mg/5 ml
> Pediatric oral suspension — 100 mg/ml
> Tablets — 250 mg, 500 mg, 1,000 mg (1 g)

Loracarbef:
> Capsules — 200 mg and 400 mg
> Oral suspension — 100 mg, 200 mg/5 ml

▷ Recommended Dosage Ranges
Cefaclor: For FDA labeled uses. 250 mg every 8 hours for susceptible infections, up to 500 mg every 8 hours for severe infections. Maximum daily dose is 2 g (2,000 mg).

Cefadroxil: Skin infections—500 mg every 12 hours, or 1 g daily. "Strep" throat—500 mg every 12 hours for 10 days. Urinary tract infections—500 mg to 1 g every 12 hours, or 1 to 2 g daily. Maximum daily dose 6 g (6,000 mg).

Cefixime: 400 mg daily, taken as a single dose or as 200 mg every 12 hours. For treatment of multidrug-resistant *Salmonella*—20 mg per kg of body mass per day in equal doses every 12 hours, for at least 12 days. Uncomplicated gonorrhea—400 to 800 mg as a single dose.

Cefuroxime: See general dosing below. Blood levels in pregnancy are up to 50% lower than in non-pregnant females. Dosing in pregnancy should be adjusted to achieve the usual peak to MIC ratio needed to kill the infecting organism.

Cephalexin: 250 to 500 mg every 6 hours. Total daily dose should not exceed 4 g.

Loracarbef: 200–400 mg every 12 hours for 7–14 days depending on the infection being treated.

Infants and Children:

Cefaclor: 20 to 40 mg per kg of body mass per day is given in divided doses every 8 hours. Maximum dose is 1 g (1,000 mg) daily.

Cefadroxil: 30 mg per kg of body mass per day, given in divided doses every 12 hours.

Cefixime (for children over 6 months of age): 8 mg per kg of body mass per day, all in one dose or divided into two doses.

Cefprozil: For otitis media (6 months to 12 years of age)—15 mg per kg of body mass every 12 hours, for 10 days.

Ceftriaxone: For neonates and children less than 12 for treatment of serious infections caused by susceptible organisms (other than CNS infections such as meningitis)—50–75 mg per kg of body mass per day, given in two equally divided doses 12 hours apart (not to exceed 2 g daily). Some clinicians use 50 mg per kg of body weight per day for neonates 1 week old or younger; neonates older than 1 week and weighing 2 kg or less also receive 50 mg per kg of body mass per day; neonates older than 1 week and weighing more than 2 kg receive 50–75 mg per kg of body mass per day.

For meningitis (caused by susceptible organisms)—the dose for neonates and children 12 or younger is 100 mg per kg of body mass (no more than 4 grams or 4,000 mg) daily, divided into two equal doses given every 12 hours. The American Academy of Pediatrics suggests 80–100 mg per kg of body mass be given once daily or in two equally divided doses every 12 hours for children older than 1 month. Because the once-daily regimen is relatively new, I suggest that the 12-hour regimen be used. For serious CNS disease—children can be treated with 75–100 mg per kg of body mass IV daily for 21 days.

For heart (cardiac disease)—children can be given 75–100 mg per kg of body mass per day IV. Treatment of serious Lyme arthritis, cardiac or neurologic complications of early or late (stage 2 or 3) Lyme disease: Arthritis: 75–100 mg per kg of body mass per day IV. One recent article advocated a single dose of ceftriaxone for some childhood ear infections. For otitis media: 75–100 mg per kg of body mass per day, in four divided doses.

Cefuroxime: Oral (for children over 2)—125 mg twice a day, 250 mg twice daily for treatment of otitis media. Intravenous—Those over 3 months should be given 50 to 100 mg per kg of body mass per day, divided every 6 to 8 hours. Maximum dose is 4 g.

Cephalexin: 25 to 50 mg per kg of body mass per day in two to four divided doses. Maximum dose is 4 g (4,000 mg).

Loracarbef: For ear infection (otitis media)—30 mg per kg per day given in equal doses, taken every 12 hours for 10 days (suspension only—capsules should NOT be substituted for suspension).

12 to 60 Years of Age:

Cefprozil: Pharyngitis or tonsillitis—500 mg every 24 hours (once daily), for 10 days. Acute or chronic bronchitis—500 mg every 12 hours, for 10 days.

Bacterial pneumonia—250 mg three times a day for 14 days. Skin or skin structure infections—250 to 500 mg every 12 to 24 hours, for 10 days.

Ceftriaxone: For most infections (caused by susceptible organisms)—1–2 g daily or in equally divided doses two times a day depending on the type and severity of the infection. Children over 12 are given the adult dose. Some clinicians use 4 g daily in CNS infections in adults. This is the maximum adult dosage recommended by the manufacturer. Uncomplicated gonorrhea caused by penicillinase-producing strains of *Neisseria gonorrhoeae* (PPNG) or non-penicillinase-producing strains—Single IM 250-mg dose. Disseminated gonococcal infection should be treated by 1 g of ceftriaxone IV or IM once a day for 7 days. Acute sexually transmitted epididymitis in adults—Single 250-mg IM dose, followed by 7 days of oral tetracycline or erythromycin. For treatment of acute pelvic inflammatory disease (PID)—Single 250-mg IM dose, followed by 100 mg of oral doxycycline two times a day for 10–14 days. Treatment of serious Lyme arthritis, cardiac or neurologic complications of early or late (stage 2 or 3) Lyme disease: Arthritis—2 g IV daily. Serious CNS disease—2 g IV daily for 21 days. Cardiac disease—2 g IV per day for 21 days.

Cefuroxime: Oral—250 to 500 mg every 12 hours. Total daily dosage should not exceed 4 g. Intravenous—750 mg to 1.5 g every 8 hours.

Over 60 Years of Age:

Cefprozil: No specific age-related changes. Decreased dose in kidney failure.

Ceftriaxone: No specific changes needed.

Loracarbef: Same as adult dose unless kidney function has declined.

> **Note: Actual dosage and schedule must be determined for each patient individually for ALL of these medicines**.

Conditions Requiring Dosing Adjustments

Liver Function:

Cefaclor, cefixime, cefprozil, cefuroxime, cephalexin or loracarbef: No changes in dosing needed at present.

Cefadroxil: The liver is involved to a minimal degree, and no dosing changes are anticipated in liver compromise.

Ceftriaxone: Patients with both liver and kidney problems should have blood levels checked and a maximum dose of 2 g given.

Kidney Function:

Cefaclor: 40–80% eliminated by the kidney. For creatinine clearances (CrCl) of 10–50 ml/min, 50–100% of the usual dose at the normal interval is used. For creatinine clearances of less than 10 ml/min, 50% of the usual dose at the usual time is given.

Cefadroxil: With creatinine clearances of 10–50 ml/min, use the usual doses every 12–24 hours. For CrCl less than 10 ml/min, usual doses are given every 24–48 hours.

Cefixime: Dose **must be decreased** in mild to moderate kidney problems. In severe failure, a single dose every 48 hours is often used.

Cefprozil: With severe kidney failure, **half** the dose can be given at the usual time.

Ceftriaxone: Patients with kidney compromise must be carefully followed for adverse effects.

Cefuroxime: 750 mg once daily for most kidney compromise. Dose must be repeated after dialysis, as this medicine is dialyzable.

Cephalexin: For creatinine clearances of 10–50 ml/min, usual dose every 6 hours. For creatinine clearances less than 10 ml/min, usual dose every 8–12 hours.

Loracarbef: Usual dose for CrCl 50 ml/minute or greater. If the CrCl is 10–49 ml/min half the usual dose is given at the usual time.

Phenylketonuria (PKU): Cefprozil only: The suspension has 28 mg of phenylalanine in every 5 ml. This may preclude use of this drug in these patients.

▷ **Dosing Instructions:** May be taken on an empty stomach or with food if stomach upset occurs. Loracarbef must be taken on an empty stomach. Capsule (cefaclor, cefadroxil) may be opened and tablet forms crushed. Cefuroxime tablet can give a bitter taste that lingers. Shake suspension forms well before measuring dose (use a measured dose cup or calibrated dose measure). Intravenous forms should be brought to room temperature if they are refrigerated. Take the full course prescribed. If you forget a dose: Take the missed dose as soon as you remember it, and take any remaining doses for the day at evenly spaced time periods. If you miss more than one dose, please call your doctor.

Usual Duration of Use: Regular use for 3–5 days is usually needed to see effectiveness of these drugs in controlling the infection. Response varies with the infection. Treatment time will vary from 1 week (for some minor infections) to 6 weeks (as in some bone infections). Some cases **require 10–14 consecutive days** of treatment to prevent rheumatic fever. Follow your doctor's instructions carefully. Many clinicians ask you to call them if symptoms worsen or fever persists for 24–48 hours after you start to take these medicines.

Typical Treatment Goals and Measurements (Outcomes and Markers)

Infections: The most commonly used measures of serious infections are white blood cell counts and differentials (the kind of blood cells that occur most often in your blood) and temperature. Many clinicians look for positive changes in 24–48 hours. NEVER stop an antibiotic because you start to feel better. For many infections, a full 14 days is REQUIRED to kill the bacteria. The goals and time frame (see peak benefits above) should be discussed with you when the prescription is written.

Possible Advantages of These Drugs

One-time dosing (injection) of ceftriaxone guarantees that the medicine will be taken (adherence) by children with one kind of ear infection (acute otitis media).

These Drugs Should Not Be Taken If
- you are allergic to any cephalosporin (see Drug Classes).
- you have pseudomembranous colitis.

▷ **Inform Your Physician Before Taking These Drugs If**
- you have a history of allergy to any penicillin (see Drug Classes).
- you have a history of regional enteritis or ulcerative colitis.
- you have impaired kidney function.
- you have a history of blood clotting disorders.
- you have a history of low platelets or white blood cell count (cefprozil, cefixime or ceftriaxone).

Possible Side Effects (natural, expected and unavoidable drug actions)

Superinfections (see Glossary).

▷ **Possible Adverse Effects** (unusual, unexpected and infrequent reactions)
> **If any of the following develop, consult your physician promptly for guidance.**
>
> *Mild Adverse Effects*
> Allergic reactions: skin rash, itching, hives.
> Nausea and vomiting or mild diarrhea—most common adverse effects.
> Sore mouth or tongue—possible.
> Mild and reversible decrease in white blood cells (neutrophils) (cefaclor).
> Confusion, nervousness, insomnia, dizziness—rare.
>
> *Serious Adverse Effects*
> Allergic reactions: drug fever (see Glossary), anaphylactic reaction (see Glossary), Stevens-Johnson syndrome—rare.
> Idiosyncratic reactions: lowered white blood cell counts or platelets (cefixime, ceftriaxone, cefuroxime)—rare and idiosyncratic (cephalexin).
> Extended time for blood to clot (reported with chronic use of other second- or third-generation cephalosporins in debilitated patients and for loracarbef)—case reports to rare.
> Genital itching (may represent a fungus superinfection)—possible.
> Serum sickness (itching, joint pain and irritated swellings)—rare.
> Increased blood urea nitrogen (BUN) or serum creatinine—rare.
> Gallbladder concretions (ceftriaxone)—rare.
> Severe diarrhea may be drug-induced colitis—rare.
> Increases in liver enzymes (cefadroxil and loracarbef) and jaundice (cholestatic) (cefaclor)—rare.

▷ **Possible Effects on Sexual Function:** None reported.

Adverse Effects That May Mimic Natural Diseases or Disorders
> Skin rash and fever may resemble measles.

Possible Effects on Laboratory Tests
> Blood platelet counts: decreased—rare (see above).
> INR: may be increased (cefixime, ceftriaxone)—rare.
> PTT: extended (cefprozil)—rare.
> Liver enzymes: increased (cefaclor, cefuroxime, cefprozil, ceftriaxone)—rare.
> BUN and creatinine: increased (cefaclor, cefprozil, cefuroxime, ceftriaxone)—rare.
> White blood cell counts: decreased (cefprozil, cefixime, cefuroxime, ceftriaxone, cephalexin, loracarbef)—rare.

CAUTION
- *Do not stop these drugs* without the knowledge of your doctor (may cause dangerous bacterial resistance).
- Some drugs in this class can cause a false-positive test result for urine sugar when using Clinitest tablets, Benedict's solution or Fehling's solution, but not with Tes-Tape.
- Cefuroxime suspension and tablets DO NOT get into the body to the same extent (bioavailability). They should not be substituted on a mg of ingredient to mg of ingredient basis.

Precautions for Use
> *By Infants and Children:* Not recommended for use in infants less than 1 month old (cefaclor) or 1 year old (cephalexin). The maximal dose in children should not exceed 1 g every 24 hours (cefaclor). Dosing of other medicines in this

class is based on weight. Follow the dosing instructions exactly. Safety and effectiveness for those under 6 months not established (cefixime, cefprozil).

By Those Over 60 Years of Age: Dosage must be carefully individualized and based upon evaluation of kidney function. Natural changes in the skin may predispose to severe and prolonged itching reactions in the genital and anal regions. Such reactions should be reported promptly. The natural decline in kidney function often requires a decrease in dose and achieves the same effect as a larger dose (all but ceftriaxone).

▷ **Advisability of Use During Pregnancy**

Pregnancy Category: B. See Pregnancy Risk Categories at the back of this book.

Animal studies: No birth defects reported.

Human studies: Information from adequate studies of pregnant women is not available.

Generally considered to be safe. Ask your physician for guidance. See dosing in pregnancy above for cefuroxime.

Advisability of Use If Breast-Feeding

Presence of these drugs in breast milk: Yes, in small amounts (cefaclor, cefadroxil, ceftriaxone, cefuroxime and cephalexin); unknown (cefixime, cefprozil and loracarbef).

Ask your doctor for advice.

Habit-Forming Potential: None.

Effects of Overdose: Nausea, vomiting, stomach cramps and/or diarrhea.

Possible Effects of Long-Term Use: Superinfections (see Glossary).

Suggested Periodic Examinations While Taking These Drugs (at physician's discretion)

Complete blood cell counts.

Liver enzymes.

INR or PTT (for some of these medicines).

BUN and creatinine with long-term therapy.

▷ **While Taking These Drugs, Observe the Following**

Foods: Delays the absorption of these drugs and may result in decreased antibiotic effect: cefaclor and loracarbef—take these 1 hour before or 2 hours after eating. No restrictions: cefadroxil, cefprozil, cefixime, ceftriaxone, cefuroxime or cephalexin.

Herbal Medicines or Minerals: Echinacea: Some patients use echinacea to attempt to boost their immune systems. Unfortunately, use of echinacea is not recommended in people with damaged immune systems. This herb may also actually weaken any immune system if it is used too often or for too long a time. Do NOT take mistletoe herb, oak bark or F.C. of marshmallow root and licorice.

Beverages: No restrictions. May be taken with milk.

▷ *Alcohol:* Ceftriaxone: May cause severe nausea and vomiting.

Others: No interactions expected, but large amounts of alcohol may blunt the immune system.

Tobacco Smoking: No interactions expected. I advise everyone to quit smoking.

▷ *Other Drugs*

These medicines *taken concurrently* with

• any aminoglycoside antibiotic (see Drug Classes) may result in increased kidney (renal) toxicity.

- anticoagulants (blood thinners) such as heparin or warfarin (Coumadin) may have anticoagulant effects increased by some medicines in this class.
- birth control pills (oral contraceptives) may result in **decreased effectiveness** in preventing conception and pregnancy.
- cholestyramine may decrease cephalexin (and perhaps other drugs in this class) absorption and blunt the beneficial effects in fighting infection.
- cyclosporine (Sandimmune, others) may lead to cyclosporine toxicity with some members of this family. More frequent cyclosporine levels are prudent.
- live typhoid vaccine (Vivotif Berna) may blunt the response to the vaccine if taken with some of these medicines. Separate the last dose of antibiotic and vaccination by 24 hours.
- loop diuretics such as ethacrynic acid may result in increased risk of kidney toxicity.
- nilvadipine (Escor) may increase cephalosporin blood levels.
- probenecid (Benemid) will slow the elimination of these drugs, resulting in higher blood levels and prolonged effect.

▷ *Driving, Hazardous Activities:* Usually no restrictions.

Aviation Note: The use of these drugs *may be a disqualification* for piloting. Consult a designated Aviation Medical Examiner.

Exposure to Sun: No restrictions.

Special Storage Instructions: Oral suspension should be kept at room temperature (cefixime or loracarbef). Oral suspensions should be refrigerated (cefaclor, cefadroxil, cefprozil, cephalexin, ceftriaxone IV form). Cefuroxime may be stored at room temperature or in the refrigerator.

Observe the Following Expiration Times: Do not take the oral suspension of this drug if it is older than 14 days (cefaclor, cefadroxil, cefprozil, cephalexin or loracarbef) or 10 days (cefuroxime).

CERIVASTATIN (SIR iv a sta tin)

Introduced: 1998   **Class:** Cholesterol-lowering agent, HMG-CoA reductase inhibitor   **Prescription:** USA: Yes   **Controlled Drug:** USA: No; Canada: No   **Available as Generic:** USA: No; Canada: No

Brand Name: Baycol

Author's Note: This medicine has been voluntarily removed from the market by the manufacturer because of reports of fatal muscle damage (see Table 16 for more information).

CHLORAMBUCIL (klor AM byu sil)

Introduced: 1974   **Class:** Anticancer, immunosuppressant   **Prescription:** USA: Yes   **Controlled Drug:** USA: No; Canada: No   **Available as Generic:** USA: No; Canada: No

Brand Name: Leukeran, ❧Alti-Chlorambucil

BENEFITS versus RISKS	
Possible Benefits	*Possible Risks*
EFFECTIVE PALLIATIVE TREATMENT FOR CHRONIC LYMPHOCYTIC LEUKEMIA	BONE MARROW DEPRESSION (see Glossary)
EFFECTIVE PALLIATIVE TREATMENT FOR HODGKIN'S DISEASE AND OTHER LYMPHOMAS	INCREASED SUSCEPTIBILITY TO INFECTIONS
	CENTRAL NERVOUS SYSTEM TOXICITY
	Male and female sterility
Immunosuppression of nephrotic syndrome	Drug-induced liver or lung damage
Immunosuppression of rheumatoid arthritis	Development of secondary cancers

▷ **Principal Uses**

As a Single Drug Product: Uses currently included in FDA-approved labeling: Treats (1) chronic lymphocytic leukemia; (2) Hodgkin's lymphoma and other malignant lymphomas.

Other (unlabeled) generally accepted uses: (1) Hairy cell leukemia; (2) multiple myeloma; (3) Letterer-Siwe disease; (4) nephrotic syndrome; (5) ovarian cancer; (6) may have a role in treating rheumatoid arthritis; (7) can have a short-term role in treating systemic lupus erythematosus; (8) combined with methylprednisolone in one study to stabilize kidney disease of unknown cause (idiopathic nephropathy); (9) case reports of combination treatment with corticosteroids in Sjögren's syndrome.

How This Drug Works: This drug blocks genetic activity (impairs DNA and RNA) and inhibits production of essential proteins. This kills cancerous cells.

Available Dosage Forms and Strengths

Tablets — 2 mg, 5 mg

▷ **Usual Adult Dosage Ranges:** *For leukemia and lymphoma:* Initially (induction phase) 3–4 mg per square meter of body surface daily (usually 4–10 mg daily) is given until lowering of blood cells (cytopenias) is seen and then 1–2 mg per meter squared if needed. Intermittent doses (twice a week or monthly pulse therapy) for chronic lymphocytic leukemia have used an initial dose of 0.4 mg/kg (single dose) with the next doses increased by 0.1 mg/kg until the lymphocytes are controlled or toxicity is seen. Many clinicians think that pulse dosing is safer.

Ongoing (maintenance) dose: Often not used (increased leukemia risk).

For immunosuppression: 0.1–0.2 mg/kg of body mass daily (in refractory RA cases not responding to corticosteroids), given in a single dose, then titrated based on response and toxicity. **Note: Actual dose and schedule must be determined for each patient individually.**

Conditions Requiring Dosing Adjustments

Liver Function: Can cause liver damage. Use with extreme caution in liver compromise. Extensively metabolized.

Kidney Function: Can cause bladder inflammation; caution is advised in cases of compromised urine outflow.

▷ **Dosing Instructions:** Best to swallow the tablet whole. May be taken with food; however, food may decrease absorption by up to 20%. See your doctor if vomiting prevents you from taking chlorambucil. It is best to drink 6–8 glasses of water a day while you are taking this medicine. If you forget a dose: Take the dose immediately, unless it is nearly time for your next dose—then skip the missed dose and take the next dose on schedule. DO NOT DOUBLE DOSES. If you miss more than one dose, call your doctor.

Usual Duration of Use: Regular use for 3 to 4 weeks is usually required to see benefits in controlling leukemia or lymphoma; several months are needed to assess immunosuppression.

Typical Treatment Goals and Measurements (Outcomes and Markers)
Leukemia (chronic lymphocytic): Many clinicians use lowering of lymphocyte count and easing of lymph swelling (lymphadenopathy) as markers of response to treatment. Ongoing or maintenance treatment is usually not used.

▷ **This Drug Should Not Be Taken If**
- you have had an allergic reaction to it previously.
- you had full-course radiation therapy less than 4 weeks ago.
- you have a significant degree of bone marrow depression.
- you currently have an uncontrolled infection.

▷ **Inform Your Physician Before Taking This Drug If**
- you are allergic to melphalan (Alkeran).
- you are pregnant, planning pregnancy or breast-feeding.
- you have had bone marrow depression or blood cell disorders.
- you have a history of gout or urate kidney stones.
- you develop a skin reaction while taking this drug.
- you have a seizure disorder of any kind.
- you have a history of porphyria.
- you have impaired liver or kidney function.
- you have had cancer chemotherapy or radiation therapy.
- you are taking drugs that can impair your immunity.
- you had or recently were exposed to chickenpox or herpes zoster.

Possible Side Effects (natural, expected and unavoidable drug actions)
Decreased white blood cell and platelet counts. Decreased immunity; susceptibility to infections. Increased blood levels of uric acid, formation of kidney stones.

▷ **Possible Adverse Effects (unusual, unexpected and infrequent reactions)**
If any of the following develop, consult your physician promptly for guidance.
Mild Adverse Effects
Allergic reactions: skin rash, itching, drug fever (see Glossary)—rare.
Mouth and lip sores, nausea, vomiting—infrequent.
Serious Adverse Effects
Allergic reactions: drug-induced hepatitis with jaundice—case reports.
Delayed allergic reaction.
Cataract formation with high-dose usage—case reports.
Central nervous system toxicity: agitation, confusion, hallucinations, seizures, tremors, paralysis—case reports.
Peripheral neuritis (see Glossary)—possible.

Lung damage: cough, shortness of breath—case reports.

Bone marrow damage, aplastic anemia (see Glossary)—possible (dose-related and can be dose limiting).

Leukemia (may depend on dose and length of treatment)—possible.

Liver damage (hepatotoxicity and jaundice)—case reports.

Severe skin damage (toxic epidermal necrolysis)—case reports.

▷ **Possible Effects on Sexual Function:** Can inhibit reproduction: stops sperm production (male sterility); alters menstrual patterns, blocks ovulation and menstruation (female sterility)—possible.

Possible Delayed Adverse Effects

Severe bone marrow depression (even after drug is stopped). Secondary cancers (especially leukemia) have been reported. Lung damage (pulmonary fibrosis). Delayed allergic reaction.

Adverse Effects That May Mimic Natural Diseases or Disorders

Drug-induced seizures may suggest epilepsy. Drug-induced jaundice may suggest viral hepatitis.

Natural Diseases or Disorders That May Be Activated by This Drug

Gout, urate kidney stones, porphyria, latent epilepsy.

Possible Effects on Laboratory Tests

Complete blood counts: decreased red cells, hemoglobin, white cells and platelets.

Blood uric acid level: increased.

Liver function tests: increased liver enzymes (ALT/GPT, AST/GOT), increased bilirubin, increased icterus index.

Sperm counts: decreased or absent.

CAUTION

1. Long-term use of this drug in noncancerous conditions requires extreme caution. Risks include permanent sterility, lung damage and the development of secondary cancers. It should only be used where less toxic medicines have failed.
2. Periodic check for leukemia is appropriate.
3. Four weeks should pass after a full course of radiation therapy or chemotherapy before chlorambucil is started.
4. Have dental work prior starting drug. Bone marrow depression could lead to gum infection, bleeding and delayed healing.
5. If gout develops, allopurinol is the drug of choice for chlorambucil-caused gout symptoms.
6. Both killed or live virus vaccines will not work while you take this drug. Live virus vaccines may actually cause infection. It may take 3 months to a year for the immune system to recover after stopping this or similar drugs. People in close contact with chlorambucil patients should not get oral poliovirus vaccine. This eliminates risk of accidental exposure.
7. Immediately report: Infection, unusual bruising or bleeding, excessive fatigue, tremors or muscle twitching, trouble walking, loss of appetite with nausea or vomiting.
8. It is advisable to avoid pregnancy while taking this drug. A nonhormonal method of contraception is recommended. Call your doctor promptly if you think pregnancy has occurred.
9. High-dose treatment increases risk of seizures.

Precautions for Use

By Infants and Children: Dosage schedules and treatment monitoring should be supervised by a qualified pediatrician. Children with nephrotic syndrome can be more prone to drug-induced seizures.

By Those Over 60 Years of Age: Watch for central nervous system toxicity.

▷ **Advisability of Use During Pregnancy**

Pregnancy Category: D. See Pregnancy Risk Categories at the back of this book.

Animal studies: Rat studies reveal drug-associated defects of the nervous system, palate, skeleton and urogenital system.

Human studies: Adequate studies of pregnant women are not available. There are two known cases of an infant born with an absent kidney and ureter following exposure to this drug during early pregnancy.

If possible, this drug should be avoided during pregnancy, especially the first 3 months. A nonhormonal contraceptive is generally advisable during treatment with this and similar drugs.

Advisability of Use If Breast-Feeding

Presence of this drug in breast milk: Unknown.

Avoid drug or refrain from nursing.

Habit-Forming Potential: None.

Effects of Overdose: Fatigue, weakness, fever, sore throat, bruising, agitation, unstable gait, bone marrow depression, seizures.

Possible Effects of Long-Term Use: Permanent sterility, secondary cancers (leukemia), lung damage (pulmonary fibrosis).

Suggested Periodic Examinations While Taking This Drug (at physician's discretion)

Before drug treatment and periodically during drug use: Complete blood counts, uric acid levels, liver function tests, sperm counts.

▷ **While Taking This Drug, Observe the Following**

Foods: No restrictions.

Herbal Medicines or Minerals: Echinacea: Some patients use echinacea to attempt to boost their immune systems. Unfortunately, use of echinacea is not recommended in people with damaged immune systems. This herb may also actually weaken any immune system if it is used too often or for too long a time.

Beverages: No restrictions. May be taken with milk. Drinking 2 to 3 quarts of liquids daily can reduce kidney stone risk. Ask your doctor.

▷ *Alcohol:* Use with caution. Avoid if platelet counts are low and there is a risk of stomach bleeding.

Tobacco Smoking: No interactions expected. I advise everyone to quit smoking.

Marijuana Smoking: Best avoided. Increases risk of central nervous system toxicity. Some fungal infections (toxoplasmosis) may be contracted from marijuana itself if the immune system is weak.

▷ *Other Drugs*

Chlorambucil *taken concurrently* with

• amphotericin B (Abelcet) may increase risk of bronchial spasm, low blood pressure and kidney (nephrotoxicity) toxicity.

• antidepressant or antipsychotic (neuroleptic) drugs requires careful monitoring; these drugs lower the seizure threshold and increase the risk of chlorambucil-induced seizures.

- aspirin may increase the risk of bruising or bleeding; the platelet-reduction effects of chlorambucil and the antiplatelet action of aspirin are additive. Avoid aspirin while taking chlorambucil.
- other immunosuppressant drugs can increase the risk of infection and the development of secondary cancers.
- tramadol (Ultram) may increase risk of seizures.
- live virus vaccines (such as MMWR) may result in overwhelming infections.

▷ *Driving, Hazardous Activities:* This drug may cause nervous agitation, confusion, hallucinations or seizures. Restrict activities as necessary.

Aviation Note: The use of this drug *may be a disqualification* for piloting. Consult a designated Aviation Medical Examiner.

Exposure to Sun: No restrictions.

Discontinuation: Many factors will determine when and how this drug should be stopped. Follow your doctor's advice to get the best results.

CHLORAMPHENICOL (KLOR am fen ih coll)

Introduced: 1947   **Class:** Antibiotic   **Prescription:** USA: Yes   **Controlled Drug:**   USA: No; Canada: No   **Available as Generic:**   USA: Yes; Canada: No

Brand Names: Ak-Chlor, Chloracol, Chlorofair, Chloromycetin, Chloroptic, Chloroptic SOP, Econochlor, ❦Elase-Chloromycetin, I-Chlor, ❦Isopto Fenicol, ❦Minims, ❦Nova-Phenicol, ❦Novochlorocap, ❦Ocu-Chlor, Ophthochlor, ❦Ophtho-Chloram, Ophthocort, ❦PMS-Chloramphenicol, ❦Sopamycetin, ❦Sopamycetin/HC

BENEFITS versus RISKS	
Possible Benefits	*Possible Risks*
VERY EFFECTIVE TREATMENT OF INFECTIONS DUE TO SUSCEPTIBLE MICROORGANISMS	BONE MARROW DEPRESSION APLASTIC ANEMIA (see Glossary) Peripheral neuritis (see Glossary) Liver damage, jaundice

Author's Note: Risks are largely as defined for systemic use, not for ophthalmic use.

▷ **Principal Uses**

As a Single Drug Product: Uses currently included in FDA-approved labeling: (1) Very effective in a broad spectrum of serious infections—however, because of serious toxicity (fatal aplastic anemia), it is now reserved for life-threatening infections (such as meningitis) caused by resistant organisms and for infections in people who cannot tolerate other appropriate anti-infective drugs; (2) used in eye (intraocular) infections.

Available Dosage Forms and Strengths

Previously available capsules and oral suspensions are no longer made.

Cream — 1%

Eye/ear solutions — 0.5%

Eye ointment — 1%

Injection — 100 mg/ml

Ophthalmic/otic suspension — 2 mg/ml

▷ **Usual Adult Dosage Ranges:** Ophthalmic: Chloramphenicol plus hydrocortisone suspension or solution is given as two drops to the affected eye every 3 hours day and night for 48 hours. After this, the time between doses is usually lengthened and therapy continued until 48 hours after the eye appears normal. **Note: Actual dose and schedule must be determined for each patient individually.**

Author's Note: Because use of this medicine is largely limited to ophthalmic use, this profile has been shortened to make room for more widely used medicines.

CHLOROQUINE (KLOR oh kwin)

Introduced: 1964   **Class:** Amebecide, antimalarial   **Prescription:** USA: Yes   **Controlled Drug:** USA: No; Canada: No   **Available as Generic:** USA: Yes; Canada: No

Brand Names: Aralen, Kronofed-A-JR, ♣Novo-Chloroquine

Warning: The brand names Aralen and Arlidin are similar and can be mistaken for each other; this can lead to serious medication errors. These names represent very different drugs. Verify that you are taking the correct drug.

BENEFITS versus RISKS	
Possible Benefits	*Possible Risks*
EFFECTIVE PREVENTION AND TREATMENT OF CERTAIN FORMS OF MALARIA	INFREQUENT BUT SERIOUS DAMAGE OF CORNEAL AND RETINAL EYE TISSUES
EFFECTIVE COMBINATION TREATMENT OF SOME FORMS OF AMEBIC INFECTION	RARE BUT SERIOUS BONE MARROW DEPRESSION; aplastic anemia, deficient white blood cells and platelets
Possibly effective in palindromic rheumatism	Heart muscle damage—rare
Possibly effective in short-term treatment of systemic lupus erythematosus	Ear damage; hearing loss, ringing in ears—rare
Can be of help in refractory rheumatoid arthritis	Eye damage—rare

Author's Note: Because this medicine is not as widely used as other medicines, this profile has been shortened to make room for more widely used drugs.

CHLOROTHIAZIDE (klor oh THI a zide)

Please see the thiazide diuretic family profile.

CHLORPROMAZINE (klor PROH ma zeen)

Introduced: 1952   **Class:** Antipsychotic, phenothiazines, strong tranquilizer   **Prescription:** USA: Yes   **Controlled Drug:** USA: No; Canada: No   **Available as Generic:** Yes

Brand Names: ❦Chlorpromanyl,   ❦Largactil,   ❦Novochlorpromazine, Ormazine, Thora-Dex, Thorazine, Thorazine SR

BENEFITS versus RISKS	
Possible Benefits	*Possible Risks*
EFFECTIVE CONTROL OF ACUTE MENTAL DISORDERS	Toxic effects on the brain with long-term use—rare but possible
Beneficial effects on thinking, mood and behavior	Liver damage with jaundice—rare
Moderately effective control of nausea and vomiting	Rare blood disorders: hemolytic anemia, abnormally low white blood cell count
	Eye toxicity

▷ **Principal Uses**

As a Single Drug Product: Uses currently included in FDA-approved labeling: (1) Treats acute and chronic psychotic disorders such as agitated depression, schizophrenia and mania; (2) can be used for presurgical anxiety; (3) helps reduce symptoms in porphyrias and tetanus; (4) is used to stop prolonged hiccups; (5) lessens or stops vomiting caused by toxic chemotherapy or a potent drug used to treat fungal infections (amphotericin B).

Other (unlabeled) generally accepted uses: (1) Can be of help in complicated drug withdrawal cases; (2) lessens the symptoms of Tourette's syndrome; (3) may be of help in combination therapy of tuberculosis; (4) can be used intravenously after some heart surgeries.

Author's Note: The information in this profile has been shortened to make room for more widely used medicines.

CHLORPROPAMIDE (klor PROH pa mide)

Introduced: 1958   **Class:** Antidiabetic, sulfonylureas   **Prescription:** USA: Yes   **Controlled Drug:** USA: No; Canada: No   **Available as Generic:** Yes
Brand Names: ❦Apo-Chlorpropamide, ❦Chloronase, Diabinese, Glucamide

BENEFITS versus RISKS	
Possible Benefits	*Possible Risks*
Helps in regulating blood sugar in non-insulin-dependent diabetes (adjunctive to appropriate diet and weight control)	HYPOGLYCEMIA, severe and prolonged
	Allergic skin reactions (some severe)
	Water retention
Tight blood sugar control may avoid or delay blood vessel, heart, nerve and vision damage possible with uncontrolled increase in blood sugar	Liver damage or blood cell and bone marrow disorders—rare

Author's Note: The information in this profile has been shortened to make room for more widely used medicines.

CHLORTHALIDONE (klor THAL i dohn)

Please see the thiazide diuretics family profile.

CHOLESTYRAMINE (koh LES tir a meen)

Introduced: 1959   **Class:** Anticholesterol   **Prescription:** USA: Yes
Controlled Drug: USA: No; Canada: No   **Available as Generic:** USA: No;
Canada: No
Brand Names: Questran, Questran Light, ✤Novo-Cholamine, ✤Novo-
Cholamine Light, Prevalite
**Author's Note: Questran and Questran Light were proposed to the FDA to
be changed from prescription to nonprescription status. Approval was not
granted.**

BENEFITS versus RISKS	
Possible Benefits	*Possible Risks*
EFFECTIVE REDUCTION OF TOTAL CHOLESTEROL AND LOW-DENSITY CHOLESTEROL IN TYPE IIA CHOLESTEROL DISORDERS	Constipation (may be severe)
	Reduced absorption of fat-soluble vitamins (A, D, E, K), folic acid and niacin
Reduction of total cholesterol and LDL cholesterol	May increase triglycerides
EFFECTIVE RELIEF OF ITCHING associated with biliary obstruction	Reduced formation of prothrombin with possible bleeding
Effective binding of medicines in some drug overdoses	
Helps remove leflunomide (Arava) in patients desiring pregnancy	

▷ **Principal Uses**

As a Single Drug Product: Uses currently included in FDA-approved labeling:
(1) Reduces high blood levels of total cholesterol and low-density (LDL)
cholesterol in Type IIa cholesterol disorders; (2) relieves itching due to the
deposit of bile acids in the skin associated with partial biliary obstruction;
(3) reduces risk of heart disease in type II hyperlipoproteinemia; (4)
reduces progression of disease in coronary arteries in people with type II
hyperlipoproteinemia.

Other (unlabeled) generally accepted uses: (1) Because leflunomide (Arava)
stays in the body for a very long time, cholestyramine has been used by
some clinicians to help remove the medicine in patients desiring to become
pregnant or who are having problems with the drug; (2) may help biliary
fistulas and skin irritations seen in colostomy; (3) helps lower thyroid hormone levels if too much thyroid hormone is given; (4) treats cholesterol
ester storage disease (CESD); (5) treats relapses of resistant diarrhea
(pseudomembranous colitis); (6) eases diarrhea caused by quinidine.

How This Drug Works: Binds bile acids and bile salts in the intestine, forming
complexes then removed via feces. This process stimulates change of cholesterol to bile acids to replace those removed, reducing cholesterol levels.
By lowering bile acids, this drug reduces bile acids deposited in the skin
and relieves itching.

Available Dosage Forms and Strengths
Cans — 378 g
Chewable bars — 4 g
Packets — 4 g, 5.7 g, 9 g

▷ **Usual Adult Dosage Ranges:** *Diarrhea (pseudomembranous colitis):* 2–4 g two or three times daily.

Hypercholesterolemia: 9 g of powder (equivalent to 4 g of cholestyramine) one to six times daily. Dose may be increased slowly as needed and tolerated. The total daily dose should not exceed 72 g of powder (32 g of cholestyramine).

Itching: 4 g (one packet) once or twice daily.

Note: Actual dose and schedule must be determined for each patient individually.

Conditions Requiring Dosing Adjustments
Liver Function: Removed in the feces—no liver involvement.
Kidney Function: Not absorbed into the body.

▷ **Dosing Instructions:** Always take just before or with a meal; this drug is ineffective when taken without food. Mix the powder thoroughly in 4 to 6 ounces of water, fruit juice, milk, thin soup or a soft food such as applesauce; do not use carbonated beverages. **Do not take powder in its dry form.** Chewable bar should be chewed repeatedly before swallowing. If you forget a dose: Take the missed dose as soon as you remember it, unless it is nearly time for the next dose. DO NOT DOUBLE DOSES. Call your doctor if you find yourself forgetting doses.

Usual Duration of Use: Regular use for up to 3 weeks may be needed to see benefits in lowering cholesterol. If an adequate response does not occur in 3 months, talk with your doctor about another medicine. Long-term use (months to years) requires ongoing follow-up by your doctor.

Typical Treatment Goals and Measurements (Outcomes and Markers)
The National Institutes of Health has released ATP III as part of the update to the National Cholesterol Education Program or NCEP. Key points in these new guidelines include acknowledging diabetes as one of the conditions that increases risk of heart disease, modifying risk factors and recommending routine testing for all of the cholesterol fractions (lipoprotein profile) versus total cholesterol alone. These new guidelines also recommend a desirable total cholesterol of 200 mg/dl as before, but change optimal LDL to 100 mg/dl, 130–159 mg/dl as borderline high, 160 mg/dl as high and cite 190 mg/dl as very high. One other noteworthy change is that "good cholesterol" or HDL has been made more important. The "too low" measure for HDL has been increased to 40 mg/dl. Take your medicine and reach these new targets! Electron beam computed tomography (EBCT) is an important tool to use in conjunction with these laboratory studies because even patients who meet cholesterol goals (particularly females over 55) can still be at risk.

▷ **This Drug Should Not Be Taken If**
• you have had an allergic reaction to it previously.
• you have complete obstruction of the bile duct (biliary obstruction).
• you have type III, IV or V hyperlipoproteinemia (drug does not work in these conditions). Ask your doctor.

▷ **Inform Your Physician Before Taking This Drug If**
- you are prone to constipation.
- you have peptic ulcer disease.
- you have a bleeding disorder of any kind.
- you have impaired kidney function.
- you have phenylketonuria (PKU), as Questran Light has aspartame.
- you have a bleeding disorder.

Possible Side Effects (natural, expected and unavoidable drug actions)
Constipation; interference with normal fat digestion and absorption; reduced absorption of vitamins A, D, E and K, folic acid or niacin. Vitamin K decrease may increase bleeding tendencies. Possible tooth discoloration (do not swish this product in the mouth).

▷ **Possible Adverse Effects** (unusual, unexpected and infrequent reactions)
If any of the following develop, consult your physician promptly for guidance.
Mild Adverse Effects
Allergic reactions: skin rash, hives, tongue irritation, anal itching—rare.
Loss of appetite, heartburn, abdominal discomfort, excessive gas, nausea, vomiting, diarrhea—possible.
Constipation—frequent.
Serious Adverse Effects
Allergic reaction: asthmalike wheezing.
Vitamin K lowering, increased bleeding tendency—case reports.
Impaired calcium absorption (osteoporosis risk higher)—possible.
Gallbladder colic—case reports.
Disruption of acid-base balance (acidosis, hyperchloremic)—case reports.

▷ **Possible Effects on Sexual Function:** Increased libido (questionable).

Natural Diseases or Disorders That May Be Activated by This Drug
Peptic ulcer disease; steatorrhea (excessive fat in stools) with large doses.

Possible Effects on Laboratory Tests
Blood cholesterol and triglyceride levels: decreased (therapeutic effect).
Blood hemoglobin and iron levels: decreased (drug impairs absorption of iron).
INR (prothrombin time): increased (impaired vitamin K absorption).
Liver function tests: increased liver enzymes (ALT/GPT, AST/GOT) in a few cases; not thought to be liver damage.
Urine calcium: increased (drug impairs absorption of calcium from intestine).

CAUTION
1. This medicine may increase homocysteine and triglyceride levels—risk factors for heart disease.
2. The powder should never be taken in its dry form; always mix it thoroughly with a suitable liquid.
3. Use stool softeners and laxatives as needed if constipation develops. If you are prone to constipation, it may be prudent to start a stool softener before starting this drug.
4. This drug binds other drugs. Prudent to take all other drugs 1 to 2 hours before or 4 to 6 hours after taking cholestyramine.

Precautions for Use

By Infants and Children: Safety and effectiveness for those under 6 years of age not established. Watch carefully for development of acidosis and vitamin A or folic acid deficiency. (Ask your doctor for help.)

By Those Over 60 Years of Age: Increased risk of severe constipation. Impaired kidney function may increase acidosis risk.

▷ **Advisability of Use During Pregnancy**

Pregnancy Category: C. See Pregnancy Risk Categories at the back of this book.

Animal studies: No information available.

Human studies: Adequate studies of pregnant women are not available.

Use this drug only if clearly needed. Ensure adequate intake of vitamins and minerals. Ask your doctor for guidance.

Advisability of Use If Breast-Feeding

Presence of this drug in breast milk: No.

Because this drug causes problems in absorbing fat-soluble vitamins, caution is advised.

Habit-Forming Potential: None.

Effects of Overdose: Progressive constipation.

Possible Effects of Long-Term Use:

Deficiencies of vitamins A, D, E and K and folic acid. Calcium deficiency, osteoporosis. Acidosis (excessive retention of chloride).

Suggested Periodic Examinations While Taking This Drug (at physician's discretion)

Measurements of blood levels of total cholesterol, triglycerides, low-density (LDL) cholesterol and high-density (HDL) cholesterol.

Complete blood cell count for possible anemia.

Bone mineral density test to check osteoporosis.

▷ **While Taking This Drug, Observe the Following**

Foods: Avoid foods that tend to constipate (cheeses, etc.). Follow your doctor's recommended diet.

Herbal Medicines or Minerals: Some studies show garlic to reduce cholesterol. Since it probably works by a different mechanism than cholestyramine, the combination use may be reasonable if dosing is separated. Discuss this with your doctor. Soy milk may also offer some lowering of cholesterol. Current cholesterol therapy sets a goal for treatment, and these herbs may help reach that goal when combined with this prescription medicine.

Nutritional Support: Ask your doctor about the need for supplements of vitamins A, D, E and K, folic acid, niacin and calcium.

Beverages: Avoid carbonated beverages. Ensure adequate liquid intake (up to 2 quarts daily). This drug may be taken with milk.

▷ *Alcohol:* No interactions expected.

Tobacco Smoking: No interactions expected. I advise everyone to quit smoking.

▷ *Other Drugs*

Cholestyramine may decrease the effects of

• acetaminophen; take 2 hours before cholestyramine.

• benzafibrate (various), take 2 hours before cholestyramine.

• cephalexin (Keflex), take 2 hours before cholestyramine.

• cerivastatin (Baycol), take 2 hours before cholestyramine.

- chlorothiazide (Diuril, others), take 2 hours before cholestyramine.
- diclofenac (various), take 2 hours before cholestyramine.
- digitoxin and digoxin (Lanoxin), take 2 hours before cholestyramine.
- fenofibrate (Tricor) and perhaps other fibrates (see Drug Classes), separate doses by 4 hours.
- fluvastatin (Lescol), separate doses by 4 hours.
- furosemide (Lasix).
- iron; separate from cholestyramine doses by 4 hours.
- leflunomide (Arava), take 2 hours before cholestyramine.
- levothyroxine (Euthroid, others), take 2 hours before cholestyramine.
- methotrexate (Mexate); take 3 hours before cholestyramine.
- metronidazole (Flagyl).
- NSAIDs (some acidic ones, such as piroxicam and sulindac) (see Drug Classes).
- oral antidiabetic drugs (see Drug Classes).
- penicillin G (Pentids).
- phenobarbital; take 2 hours before cholestyramine.
- raloxifene (Evista), take 2 hours before cholestyramine.
- tetracycline (various), take 1 hour before or 4–6 hours after cholestyramine.
- thiazide diuretics (see Drug Classes); take 2 hours before cholestyramine.
- thyroxin; take 5 hours before cholestyramine.
- valproic acid (Depakene, others), take 2 hours before cholestyramine.
- warfarin; take 6 hours after cholestyramine.

Cholestyramine *taken concurrently* with
- amiodarone (Cordarone) can result in lowered amiodarone blood levels and decreased effectiveness.
- entacapone (Comtan), may increase risk of adverse effects such as diarrhea and movement disorders.
- pravastatin (Pravachol) or other HMG-CoA reductase inhibitors may work well in further lowering cholesterol if pravastatin dose is taken 1 hour before or 4 hours after cholestyramine is taken.
- salicylates (aspirin, others) can result in lowered aspirin levels and decreased effectiveness. Separate doses by at least half an hour.

▷ *Driving, Hazardous Activities:* No restrictions.
Aviation Note: The use of this drug *is usually not a disqualification* for piloting. Consult a designated Aviation Medical Examiner.
Exposure to Sun: No reports of problems at present.
Discontinuation: The dose of any potentially toxic drug taken concurrently must be reduced appropriately when this drug is discontinued.

CILOSTAZOL (SIGH low stay zahl)

Introduced: 1999   **Class:** Blood flow agent, phosphodiesterase III inhibitor
Prescription: USA: Yes   **Controlled Drug:** USA: No; Canada: No   **Available as Generic:** No
Brand Name: Pletal

BENEFITS versus RISKS

Possible Benefits

IMPROVED BLOOD FLOW IN PERIPHERAL ARTERIAL DISEASE	Worsening of congestive heart failure (CHF) (never to be used in CHF)
REDUCES PAIN OF INTERMITTENT CLAUDICATION	Palpitation Diarrhea
EARLY DATA FROM A STUDY OF 1,052 PATIENTS FOUND A SIGNIFICANT RELATIVE RISK REDUCTION (41.7 %) IN RECURRENT STROKES	Headache
Some increase in force of contraction of the heart	

▷ **Principal Uses**

As a Single Drug Product: Uses currently included in FDA-approved labeling: Management of peripheral obstructive arterial disease to improve arterial blood flow and reduce frequency and severity of muscle pain due to intermittent claudication.

Other (unlabeled) generally accepted uses: (1) May be used as part of combination treatment of problems in small vessels (microangiopathic hemolytic anemia) in graft-versus-host disease; (2) could have a role in angioplasty (percutaneous transluminal coronary) in helping keep the blood vessel from having problems after the procedure (postprocedure restenosis); (3) May have a role in preventing repeat (recurrent) strokes in people who have suffered a first stroke.

How This Drug Works: Acts as a selective inhibitor (type three) of phosphodiesterase. Works to keep platelets from clumping directed by arachidonic acid, epinephrine, thromboxane A2, platelet activating factor, ADP or collagen. Works to dilate the bronchi and decreases thrombomodulin in diabetics. Works to prevent repeat blockage of coronary arteries in dogs after a clot buster (thrombolytic) has been used (unknown in humans).

Available Dosage Forms and Strengths

Tablets — 50 mg, 100 mg

▷ **Usual Adult Dosage Ranges:** *Intermittent claudication:* 100 mg twice daily, taken half an hour before or two hours after breakfast and dinner. **Note: Actual dose and schedule must be determined for each patient individually.**

Conditions Requiring Dosing Adjustments

Liver Function: No apparent changes in mild liver impairment. This drug has NOT been studied in moderate to severe liver impairment.

Kidney Function: No changes thought to be needed.

▷ **Dosing Instructions:** Take cilostazol at the same time each day, one half hour before or two hours after breakfast and dinner. It is taken this way because food (especially a high-fat meal) INCREASES the amount that gets into your body. If you forget a dose: Take it as soon as you remember it, unless it's nearly time for your next dose, then simply take the next scheduled dose. DO NOT double doses.

Usual Duration of Use: Regular use for 2–4 weeks may show benefits, but up to 12 weeks may be required to see the full benefit of cilostazol in preventing or delaying intermittent claudication pain when walking. Long-term use (months to years) requires follow-up with your doctor and checks of progression of blood vessel problems.

Typical Treatment Goals and Measurements (Outcomes and Markers)
Claudication: Many clinicians use distance a patient can walk without leg pain as a way to standardize response. Another measure is absence of leg pain.

Possible Advantages of This Drug
Works on both blood vessel (vascular) beds and on heart function. Also keeps platelets from clumping.

▷ **This Drug Should Not Be Taken If**
- you have had an allergic reaction to it previously.
- you have an active hemorrhage.
- you have congestive heart failure.

▷ **Inform Your Physician Before Taking This Drug If**
- you have impaired liver or kidney function.
- you have low blood pressure or arrhythmias.
- you get migraines.
- you are pregnant.
- you have a bleeding problem or low blood platelets.
- you smoke tobacco.
- you are taking any antihypertensive drugs, antiplatelet medicines or anti-coagulants.

Possible Side Effects (natural, expected and unavoidable drug actions)
Prolonged bleeding time.

▷ **Possible Adverse Effects** (unusual, unexpected and infrequent reactions)
If any of the following develop, consult your physician promptly for guidance.
Mild Adverse Effects
Allergic reaction: Skin rash.
Headache (mild to severe)—frequent.
Dizziness or vertigo—rare to infrequent.
Flushing of the face—infrequent.
Runny nose—infrequent to frequent.
Edema (peripheral)—infrequent.
Back pain or muscle aches—infrequent.
Nausea—infrequent.
Diarrhea—infrequent to frequent.
Palpitations or fast heart rate—possible.
Blood sugar changes—possible.
Serious Adverse Effects
Development of heart rhythm disorders—possible.
Increased bleeding risk with low blood platelets—possible.

▷ **Possible Effects on Sexual Function:** None reported.

Possible Effects on Laboratory Tests
Bleeding time: extended.
Complete blood cell counts: rarely lowers red cells.
Blood sugar: variable changes.

CAUTION
1. May worsen migraines.
2. DO NOT USE IF YOU HAVE CONGESTIVE HEART FAILURE.

Precautions for Use

By Infants and Children: Safety and effectiveness for those less than 18 years of age not established. Use by this age group is not anticipated.

By Those Over 60 Years of Age: You may be more susceptible to this medicine. Observe closely for any adverse effects and report these promptly.

▷ **Advisability of Use During Pregnancy**

Pregnancy Category: C. See Pregnancy Risk Categories at the back of this book.

Animal studies: Increased fetal cardiovascular, kidney and skeletal problems.

Human studies: Adequate studies of pregnant women are not available. Talk to your doctor.

Advisability of Use If Breast-Feeding

Presence of this drug in breast milk: Yes in rats, expected in humans. Avoid drug or refrain from nursing.

Habit-Forming Potential: None.

Effects of Overdose: Limited data: severe headache, diarrhea, low blood pressure, fast heart rate and possible abnormal heartbeats.

Possible Effects of Long-Term Use: None reported.

Suggested Periodic Examinations While Taking This Drug (at physician's discretion)

Blood pressure measurements.

Evaluation of heart and blood vessel status.

▷ **While Taking This Drug, Observe the Following**

Foods: Best taken on an empty stomach.

Herbal Medicines or Minerals: Many herbal medicines may interact with cilostazol because of its action on blood clotting. Examples include ginkgo, garlic, ginger, ginseng and feverfew. DO NOT COMBINE THESE HERBAL MEDICINES WITH CILOSTAZOL.

Beverages: DO NOT TAKE WITH GRAPEFRUIT JUICE.

▷ *Alcohol:* Alcohol may increase the blood pressure lowering effect of this drug.

Tobacco Smoking: Smoking decreases cilostazol benefits. Avoid tobacco.

▷ *Other Drugs*

Cilostazol may *increase* the effects of
- antihypertensive drugs and cause excessive lowering of blood pressure.
- aspirin on blood clotting, but clinical significance is not known.

The following drugs may *increase* the effects of cilostazol:
- any medicine that interferes with cytochrome (CYP3A4-major or 2C9-minor) will potentially increase cilostazol blood levels (such as sibutramine [Meridia] that uses CYP3A4). In some cases, I expect that cilostazol dosing will need to be adjusted, and in others, the combination should be avoided.
- cimetidine (Tagamet).
- diltiazem (Cardizem).
- erythromycins (see Drug Classes erythromycin and clarithromycin).
- fluconazole (Diflucan).
- itraconazole (Sporanox).
- ketoconazole (Nizoral).

- metronidazole (Flagyl).
- miconazole (Monistat).
- nefazodone (Serzone).
- nelfinavir (Viracept) and perhaps other protease inhibitors (see Drug Classes), which may increase cilostazol blood levels and effects.
- sertraline (Zoloft).

Cilostazol *taken concurrently* with

- CYP-3A4 (diltiazem, erythromycin). Itraconazole, others or CYP 2C19 inhibitors such as omeprazole may result in excessively high cilostazol levels and increased risk of cilostazol toxicity unless doses are lowered.
- glipizide (Glucotrol) or other medicines that lower blood sugar may result in excessively low blood sugar.
- omeprazole (Prilosec) may lead to increased adverse effects if the cilostazol dose is not reduced to 50 mg twice daily.
- warfarin (Coumadin, etc.) finds that multiple dosing effects are not known.

The following drugs may *decrease* the effects of cilostazol:

- carbamazepine (Tegretol).
- phenytoin (Dilantin).
- rifabutin (Mycobutin).
- rifampin (Rifadin, Rimactane).
- troglitazone (Rezulin)—now removed from the US market.

▷ *Driving, Hazardous Activities:* This drug may cause dizziness. Restrict activities as necessary.

Aviation Note: The use of this drug *may be a disqualification* for piloting. Consult a designated Aviation Medical Examiner.

Exposure to Sun: No restrictions.

CIMETIDINE (si MET i deen)

Please see the histamine (H2) blocking drug family profile.

CIPROFLOXACIN (sip roh FLOX a sin)

Please see the fluoroquinolone antibiotic family profile.

CISAPRIDE (SIS a pryde)

Introduced: 1993   **Class:** Gastrointestinal drug   **Prescription:** USA: Yes
Controlled Drug: USA: No; Canada: No   **Available as Generic:** USA: No; Canada: No
Brand Names: ♣Prepulsid, Propulsid

Author's Note: This medicine is only available under severely restricted medication guidelines and as such is no longer covered as a full profile— the information in this profile has been shortened.

CITALOPRAM (SIH tal oh prahm)

Introduced: 1998   **Class:** Antidepressant   **Prescription:** USA: Yes
Controlled Drug: USA: No   **Available as Generic:** USA: No
Brand Name: Celexa

BENEFITS versus RISKS	
Possible Benefits	*Possible Risks*
EFFECTIVE TREATMENT OF DEPRESSION	Headache
	Dry mouth
Rapidly reaches steady state	Sleepiness
	Constipation

▷ **Principal Uses**

As a Single Drug Product: Uses currently included in FDA-approved labeling: (1) Treats depression; (2) treats depression that may happen after a stroke. Other (unlabeled) generally accepted uses: (1) may have a role in alcohol abuse; (2) can ease the frequency and intensity of tension headaches; (3) lacks controlled studies, but may have a role in obsessive-compulsive disorder; (4) eases symptoms of premenstrual dysphoria syndrome (PDS).

How This Drug Works: It restores normal levels of a nerve transmitter (serotonin) by selectively inhibiting the reuptake of serotonin.

Available Dosage Forms and Strengths

Oral solution — 10 mg per 5 ml

Tablets — 10 mg (Canada only), 20 mg, 40 mg

▷ **Usual Adult Dosage Ranges:** *Depression:* Starts with 20 mg in the late afternoon or early evening; if no improvement after a week, dose may be increased by 20 mg/day as needed and tolerated up to a maximum of 60 mg daily.

Alcohol abuse: 40 mg once daily.

Depression or crying after a stroke: 20 mg once daily with lower doses being used in older patients.

Infants and Children: Safety and efficacy not established.

Note: Actual dose and schedule must be determined for each patient individually.

Conditions Requiring Dosing Adjustments

Liver Function: The dose should be decreased to 20 mg daily in treating depression. A German manufacturer suggests 30 mg daily as the dose in liver dysfunction.

Kidney Function: Dosing changes do not appear to be needed. Patients with mild to moderate kidney failure should be closely watched for adverse effects as less than 15% of the original (parent) drug and 20% of metabolites are removed by the kidneys. Use of this medicine in people with severe kidney failure has not been studied.

▷ **Dosing Instructions:** The capsule may be opened and the contents mixed with any convenient food. The contents may be mixed with orange juice or apple juice (NOT GRAPEFRUIT JUICE). If you forget a dose: Take the dose right away, unless it is nearly time for your next dose—then simply take the next scheduled dose. DO NOT double doses. Call your doctor if you find yourself forgetting doses.

Usual Duration of Use: Use on a regular schedule for 1 week may reveal start of benefits in depression. Up to 6 weeks may be needed for peak effects in (1) relieving depression and (2) the pattern of both favorable and unfavorable effects. Since there are active metabolites and a long half-life, it may take several weeks before the benefits of a change in dose are seen. Long-term use requires periodic physician evaluation. Some clinical guidelines suggest that 4–9 months of treatment should continue after the symptoms of depression go away. Some clinicians use lower doses to prevent depression. People who take their medicine regularly are least likely to have a recurrence.

Typical Treatment Goals and Measurements (Outcomes and Markers)

Depression: The general goal: to at least help lessen the degree and severity of depression, letting patients return to their daily lives. Specific measures of depression involve testing or inventories (such as the Hamilton Depression Scale) can be valuable in helping check benefits from this medicine.

Possible Advantages of This Drug: Does not cause weight gain, a common side effect of tricyclic antidepressants. Less likely to cause dry mouth, constipation, urinary retention, orthostatic hypotension (see Glossary) and heart rhythm disturbances than tricyclic antidepressants. Since a large National Cancer Institute study found that those who suffer depression for 6 years or more have a generally increased risk of cancer, one benefit of effective treatment of depression with this drug may be a generally reduced risk of cancer.

▷ **This Drug Should Not Be Taken If**
- you had an allergic reaction to it previously.
- you take, or took in the last 14 days, a monoamine oxidase (MAO) type A inhibitor (see Drug Classes).

▷ **Inform Your Physician Before Taking This Drug If**
- you have had any adverse effects from antidepressant drugs.
- you have impaired liver or kidney function.
- you have a seizure disorder.
- you have a history of suicide attempt.
- you are pregnant or plan pregnancy while taking this drug.

Possible Side Effects (natural, expected and unavoidable drug actions)

Increased sweating or cough—may be frequent.

Weight loss.

Case reports of orthostatic hypotension (see Glossary).

▷ **Possible Adverse Effects** (unusual, unexpected and infrequent reactions)

If any of the following develop, consult your physician promptly for guidance.

Mild Adverse Effects

Allergic reactions: skin rash, itching—may be frequent.

Headache, insomnia, drowsiness, tremor, dizziness—infrequent to frequent (these central nervous system symptoms tend to diminish over time).

Altered taste, increased saliva or nausea—frequent.

Increased appetite or gas (flatulence)—may be frequent.

Vomiting, constipation—infrequent to frequent.

Increased heart rate—frequent.

Increased urination—case reports.

Increased liver enzymes—possible.

Blurred vision—infrequent.

Excessive sweating—frequent.

Serious Adverse Effects

Allergic reactions: not reported.

Drug-induced seizures—rare and questionable cause and effect.

Suicidal preoccupation—possible.

Activation of mania/hypomania—possible.

This medicine caused some degeneration of the retina in rats. The significance of this for humans is not known.

▷ **Possible Effects on Sexual Function:** Inhibition of ejaculation or inhibited orgasm in men and women—infrequent.

Amenorrhea—frequent.

Natural Diseases or Disorders That May Be Activated by This Drug

Latent epilepsy.

Possible Effects on Laboratory Tests

Blood sodium level: possibly decreased.

CAUTION

1. If dry mouth develops and persists for more than 2 weeks, consult your dentist for help.
2. Ask your doctor or pharmacist before taking any other prescription or over-the-counter drug while taking this medicine.
3. If you must start any monoamine oxidase (MAO) type A inhibitor (see Drug Classes), allow an interval of 5–6 weeks after stopping this drug before starting the MAO inhibitor.

Precautions for Use

By Infants and Children: Safety and effectiveness are not established.

By Those Over 60 Years of Age: Lower or less frequent doses are recommended by the German manufacturer with a maximum dose of 40 mg daily. Twenty to 30 mg once daily has been used for depression in elderly patients.

▷ **Advisability of Use During Pregnancy**

Pregnancy Category: C. See Pregnancy Risk Categories at the back of this book.

Animal studies: No birth defects due to this drug found in rat or rabbit studies.

Human studies: Adequate studies of pregnant women are not available.

Use this drug in pregnancy is a benefit-to-risk decision that MUST be discussed with your doctor.

Advisability of Use If Breast-Feeding

Presence of this drug in breast milk: Yes.

Use is a benefit-to-risk decision. There have been a few reports of weight loss, excessive somnolence and decreased feeding in babies breast-fed while the mother was taking citalopram.

Habit-Forming Potential: Not systematically studied. Caution is advised.

Effects of Overdose: Post-marketing reports of drug overdoses that included citalopram include 12 fatalities. Symptoms include agitation, sweating, tremor, nausea, vomiting, seizures, ECG changes and one possible case of torsades de pointes.

Possible Effects of Long-Term Use: None reported.

Suggested Periodic Examinations While Taking This Drug (at physician's discretion)

Check of electrolytes if symptoms of SIADH begin.

▷ **While Taking This Drug, Observe the Following**

Foods: Grapefruit in small quantities is acceptable, but see the grapefruit juice warning below.

Beverages: Grapefruit juice may lead to increased blood levels. AVOID IT. May be taken with milk or water.

Herbal Medicines or Minerals: Since citalopram and St. John's wort may act to increase serotonin, the combination is not advised. St. John's wort also increases sun sensitivity. Since part of the way ginseng works may be as a MAO inhibitor, do not combine with citalopram. Ginkgo may also have some MAO activity—hence this combination cannot be recommended. Ma huang, yohimbe, Indian snakeroot and kava kava are also best avoided while taking this medicine.

▷ *Alcohol:* This combination is NOT advisable.

Tobacco Smoking: No interactions expected, but I advise everyone to quit smoking.

▷ *Other Drugs*

Citalopram may ***increase*** the effects of
- dofetilide (Tikosyn) requiring dosing decreases.
- imipramine (Tofranil).
- metoprolol (Toprol, Lopressor, others) by increasing metoprolol blood levels.
- quinidine (Quinaglute).
- sildenafil (Viagra) by competing for CYP3A4.
- warfarin (Coumadin) and related oral anticoagulants. Test INR more often.

Citalopram **taken concurrently** with
- azole antifungals (such as fluconazole, itraconazole and ketoconazole) may lead to higher than expected citalopram blood levels and increased risk of adverse effects.
- buspirone (Buspar) may lead to serotonin syndrome. Avoid the combination.
- carbamazepine (Tegretol, others) may blunt benefits of citalopram.
- cimetidine (Tagamet) may theoretically lead to increased citalopram levels.
- cisapride (Propulsid) may lead to excessive cisapride levels and risk of serotonin syndrome.
- clarithromycin (Biaxin) may lead to citalopram toxicity—avoid the combination.
- delavirdine (Rescriptor) may lead to citalopram toxicity.
- dextromethorphan (a cough suppressant in many "DM"-labeled nonprescription cough medicines) has resulted in visual hallucinations when combined with fluoxetine, a related medicine. Caution is advised if these drugs are combined.
- diltiazem (Cardizem) may lead to excessive citalopram levels and possible serotonin syndrome.
- fenfluramine (Pondimin) may lead to serotonin syndrome—DO NOT combine.
- lithium (Lithobid, others) may increase risk of enhanced effects from serotonin. Caution is advised.
- medicines that inhibit CYP3A4 or CYP2C19 may lead to higher than expected citalopram blood levels and increased citalopram toxicity risk.

- monoamine oxidase (MAO) type A inhibitor drugs (see Drug Classes) may cause confusion, agitation, high fever, seizures and dangerous elevations of blood pressure. Avoid combining these drugs.
- naratriptan (Amerge), rizatriptan (Maxalt), sumatriptan (Imitrex) or zolmitriptan (Zomig) may lead to increased risk of incoordination, weakness or excessive reflex responses.
- selegiline (Eldepryl) can result in serotonin toxicity syndrome. Avoid this combination.
- sibutramine (Meridia) may lead to serotonin syndrome—AVOID COMBINING.
- tryptophan will result in central nervous system toxicity. Avoid the combination.
- any tricyclic antidepressant (amitriptyline, nortriptyline, etc.) may result in increased antidepressant drug levels and serotonin syndrome. Extreme caution is advised.
- tramadol (Ultram) may increase seizure risk. DO NOT COMBINE.
- verapamil (Calan) may lead to excessive citalopram levels and possible serotonin syndrome.

▷ *Driving, Hazardous Activities:* This drug may cause drowsiness, dizziness, impaired judgment and delayed reaction time. Restrict activities as necessary.

Aviation Note: The use of this drug **is a disqualification** for piloting. Consult a designated Aviation Medical Examiner.

Exposure to Sun: No restrictions.

Discontinuation: Slow drug elimination makes withdrawal effects unlikely, but call your doctor if you plan to stop this drug for any reason.

Current Controversies in Drug Management: In 1990 six patients being treated with fluoxetine experienced intense and violent suicidal preoccupation. All six had severe depression that had not responded to the use of fluoxetine for 2 to 7 weeks. For most of them, suicidal mentality persisted for 2 to 3 months after stopping the drug. Adverse publicity suggested that this may be characteristic of fluoxetine in contrast to other antidepressant drugs. A review of relevant literature on this subject reveals that the development or intensification of suicidal thoughts during treatment (regardless of the severity of depression) has been documented repeatedly for many antidepressant drugs in wide use. Suicidal thinking may emerge during treatment with any antidepressant. Recent reports establish that some patients who become suicidal while taking one antidepressant can be switched to fluoxetine and experience cessation of suicidal thinking and satisfactory relief of depression. The most recent study of fluoxetine in the *American Journal of Psychiatry* in February 1999 found that in 643 Caucasians studied, treatment of affective disorders resulted in suicidal behavior that was marginally lower than in those patients who were not treated. This is another example of the marked variability of individual response to drug therapy. The choice of a drug to treat many serious disorders remains an experiment of trial and error. Successful management requires clinical judgment (based on experience), close monitoring and appropriate doses.

CLARITHROMYCIN (klar ith roh MY sin)

Please see the macrolide antibiotic family profile.

CLINDAMYCIN (klin da MY sin)

Introduced: 1973   **Class:** Antibiotic   **Prescription:** USA: Yes
Controlled Drug: USA: No; Canada: No   **Available as Generic:** USA: Yes;
Canada: No
Brand Names: Cleocin, Cleocin Pediatric, Cleocin T, Cleocin Vaginal Cream,
✤Dalacin C, ✤Dalacin T

BENEFITS versus RISKS	
Possible Benefits	*Possible Risks*
EFFECTIVE TREATMENT FOR SERIOUS INFECTIONS OF THE LOWER RESPIRATORY TRACT, ABDOMINAL CAVITY, GENITAL TRACT IN WOMEN, BLOODSTREAM (SEPTICEMIA), SKIN, AND RELATED TISSUES CAUSED BY SUSCEPTIBLE ORGANISMS	SEVERE DRUG-INDUCED COLITIS (FATALITIES REPORTED— SYSTEMIC USE) Liver injury with jaundice—rare Reduction in white blood cell and platelet counts—rare
Combination treatment of *Pneumocystis carinii* pneumonia Effective for local treatment of acne	

▷ **Principal Uses**
   As a Single Drug Product: Uses currently included in FDA-approved labeling:
      (1) Treats serious and unusual infections of the lungs and bronchial tubes,
      organs and tissues within the abdominal cavity, the genital tract and
      pelvic organs in women, the skin and soft tissue structures and general-
      ized infections involving the bloodstream; (2) used in topical form to treat
      acne.
   Other (unlabeled) generally accepted uses: (1) Treatment of resistant gum
      disease and malaria; (2) prevention of infection of the heart; (3) combina-
      tion treatment of *Pneumocystis carinii* pneumonia (PCP), an infection
      associated with AIDS; (4) may have a role in combination therapy of toxo-
      plasmosis infections of the brain in AIDS patients.
**Author's Note: This profile has been shortened to make room for more
widely used medicines.**

CLOMIPRAMINE (kloh MI pra meen)

Introduced: 1970   **Class:** Antidepressant   **Prescription:** USA: Yes
Controlled Drug: USA: No; Canada: No   **Available as Generic:** Yes
Brand Name: Anafranil, ✤Apo-Clomipramine, ✤Novo-Clopamine, Maronil

---

BENEFITS versus RISKS

Possible Benefits	*Possible Risks*
EFFECTIVE TREATMENT OF SEVERE OBSESSIVE-COMPULSIVE NEUROSIS	DRUG-INDUCED SEIZURES
	ADVERSE BEHAVIORAL EFFECTS
Effective relief of symptoms of some types of depression	Conversion of depression to mania in manic-depressive (bipolar) disorders
	Aggravation of schizophrenia
	Liver toxicity
	Bone marrow depression and blood cell disorders

▷ **Principal Uses**

As a Single Drug Product: Uses currently included in FDA-approved labeling: Relieves severe, disabling obsessive-compulsive disorder.

Other (unlabeled) generally accepted uses: (1) eases depression; (2) relieves symptoms of panic attacks; (3) helps some phobias; (4) may help repetitive symptoms in autistics; (5) could have a role in diabetic neuropathy; (6) can help premature ejaculation; (7) may relieve severity of hair-pulling, nail-biting or arm-burning in obsessive-compulsive patients; (8) can ease symptoms in severe premenstrual syndrome.

How This Drug Works: By increasing brain nerve transmitters (mostly serotonin), it reduces frequency/intensity of obsessive-compulsive behavior.

Available Dosage Forms and Strengths

Capsules — 10 mg (Canada only), 25 mg, 50 mg, 75 mg

Tablet, sustained release — 75 mg

▷ **Usual Adult Dosage Ranges:** Starts at 25 mg daily in the evening. If needed, may be increased by 25 mg daily at 3- to 4-day intervals up to 100 mg daily (reached in 2 weeks). The 100 mg should be divided and taken after meals. Usual maintenance dose is 50 mg to 150 mg daily. Maximum daily dose is 250 mg. (Once identified, the daily dose may be given at bedtime as a single dose.) **Note: Actual dose and schedule must be determined for each patient individually.**

Conditions Requiring Dosing Adjustments

Liver Function: The dose should be decreased in patients with liver compromise.

Kidney Function: Changes in dose are not usually needed.

▷ **Dosing Instructions:** May be taken without regard to meals. If needed, the capsule may be opened and may be taken with or following food to reduce stomach upset. If you forget a dose: Take the missed dose right away, unless it's nearly time for your next dose. If you only take one dose at bedtime, call your doctor. DO NOT double doses.

Usual Duration of Use: Regular use for 3 to 4 weeks often needed to see benefits in controlling obsessive-compulsive behavior. Peak effect may take 3 or more months of use. Long-term use (months to years) requires periodic evaluation.

Typical Treatment Goals and Measurements (Outcomes and Markers)

Obsessive-compulsive disorder: The general goal: to ease the severity of the OCD in order to let the patient resume his or her usual activities. There should involve less time spent with prior obsessions or compulsions.

▷ **This Drug Should Not Be Taken If**
- you have had an allergic reaction to it previously.
- you are taking, or have taken within the past 14 days, any monoamine oxidase (MAO) type A inhibitor drug (see Drug Classes).
- you have active bone marrow depression or a current blood cell disorder.
- you have had a recent heart attack (myocardial infarction).

▷ **Inform Your Physician Before Taking This Drug If**
- you have had an adverse reaction to an antidepressant drug, especially one of the tricyclic class.
- you have a history of bone marrow or blood cell disorder.
- you have any type of seizure disorder.
- you have any type of heart disease, especially coronary artery disease or a heart rhythm disorder.
- you are subject to bronchial asthma.
- you have impaired liver or kidney function.
- you have any type of thyroid disorder or are taking thyroid medication.
- you have a history of suicide attempts.
- you have an adrenaline-producing tumor.
- you have prostatism (see Glossary).
- you have a history of alcoholism.
- you will have surgery with general anesthesia.

Possible Side Effects (natural, expected and unavoidable drug actions)
Drowsiness, increased sweating, light-headedness, blurred vision, dry mouth, constipation, impaired urination.

▷ **Possible Adverse Effects** (unusual, unexpected and infrequent reactions)
If any of the following develop, consult your physician promptly for guidance.

Mild Adverse Effects
Allergic reactions: skin rash, itching, drug fever (see Glossary)—case reports.
Headache, dizziness, nervousness, impaired memory, weakness, tremors, insomnia, muscle cramps, flushing—infrequent.
Sweating—infrequent.
Increased appetite, weight gain—infrequent.
Altered taste, indigestion, nausea, vomiting, diarrhea—infrequent.

Serious Adverse Effects
Allergic reactions: drug-induced hepatitis, with or without jaundice—case reports.
Idiosyncratic reactions: neuroleptic malignant syndrome (see Glossary)—case reports.
Adverse behavioral effects: confusion, delirium, delusions, hallucinations, paranoia—case reports.
Seizures, reduced control of epilepsy—case reports to rare.
Aggravated paranoid psychoses or schizophrenia—case reports.
Heart rhythm disturbances—case report.
Bone marrow depression (see Glossary): fatigue, weakness, fever, sore throat, infections, abnormal bleeding or bruising—case reports.
SIADH and severe lowering of blood sodium—case reports.
Liver toxicity—infrequent.
Serotonin syndrome—case reports.

▷ **Possible Effects on Sexual Function:** Altered libido, impaired (delayed) ejaculation, impotence, inhibited male orgasm, inhibited female orgasm, abnormal sperm formation, female breast enlargement with milk production, absence of menstruation—case reports.

Adverse Effects That May Mimic Natural Diseases or Disorders
Liver toxicity may suggest viral hepatitis.

Natural Diseases or Disorders That May Be Activated by This Drug
Latent epilepsy, glaucoma, prostatism, schizophrenia.

Possible Effects on Laboratory Tests
Complete blood cell counts: decreased red cells, hemoglobin, white cells and platelets.
Liver function tests: increased liver enzymes (ALT/GPT, AST/GOT)—liver damage.
Thyroid function tests: decreased TT3 and FT3.
Blood sodium: severely lowered in cases of drug-induced SIADH.

CAUTION
1. Watch for toxicity: confusion, agitation, rapid heart rate, heart irregularity. Blood levels clarify the situation.
2. Use with caution in schizophrenia. Watch closely for deterioration of thinking or behavior.
3. Use with caution in epilepsy. Watch for any change in the frequency or severity of seizures.
4. Complete blood counts should be obtained in patients who develop sore throat or fever while taking this medicine.

Precautions for Use
By Infants and Children: Safety and effectiveness for those under 10 years of age not established. Dose and management should be supervised by a properly trained pediatrician. Dosing is started at 25 mg daily and is then increased over 2 weeks to 200 mg or 3 mg per kg of body mass, whichever number is smaller.
By Those Over 60 Years of Age: Started with 10 mg at bedtime. Dose is increased as needed and tolerated to 75 mg daily in divided doses. During first 2 weeks, watch for behavioral reactions: restlessness, agitation, forgetfulness, disorientation, hallucinations. Unsteadiness or instability may predispose to falling. Prostate problems may also be aggravated.

▷ **Advisability of Use During Pregnancy**
Pregnancy Category: C. See Pregnancy Risk Categories at the back of this book.
Animal studies: No drug-induced birth defects seen in mouse or rat studies.
Human studies: Adequate studies of pregnant women are not available.
Use only if clearly needed. Avoid use during the last 3 months, if possible, to prevent withdrawal symptoms in the newborn infant: irritability, tremors and seizures.

Advisability of Use If Breast-Feeding
Presence of this drug in breast milk: Yes.
Breast-feeding appears to be safe.

Habit-Forming Potential: Psychological or physical dependence is rare and unexpected. Withdrawal symptoms have been reported, and the drug should be tapered if it is to be stopped.

Effects of Overdose: Confusion, delirium, hallucinations, drowsiness, tremors, unsteadiness, heart irregularity, seizures, stupor, sweating, fever.

Possible Effects of Long-Term Use: Neuroleptic malignant syndrome (see Glossary): Fever, fast or irregular heartbeat, fast breathing, sweating, weakness, muscle stiffness, seizures, loss of bladder control.

Suggested Periodic Examinations While Taking This Drug (at physician's discretion)

Monitoring of blood drug levels as appropriate.

Complete blood cell counts.

Liver and kidney function tests.

Serial blood pressure readings and electrocardiograms.

Visual acuity checks.

▷ **While Taking This Drug, Observe the Following**

Foods: No specific restrictions. May need to limit food intake to avoid excessive weight gain.

Herbal Medicines or Minerals: Since clomipramine and St. John's wort may act to increase serotonin, the combination is not advised. St. John's wort also increases sun sensitivity. Since part of the way ginseng and ginkgo biloba works may be as a MAO inhibitor, do not combine with this medicine. Ma huang and yohimbe are best avoided while taking clomipramine. Indian snakeroot, kava kava and yohimbe are also best avoided while taking this medicine.

Beverages: No restrictions. May be taken with milk.

▷ *Alcohol:* Avoid completely. This drug can markedly increase the intoxicating effects of alcohol; the combination can depress brain function significantly.

Tobacco Smoking: May delay the elimination of this drug and require dosage adjustment. I advise everyone to quit smoking.

Marijuana Smoking: Increased drowsiness and mouth dryness; reduced effectiveness.

▷ *Other Drugs*

Clomipramine may *increase* the effects of

• all drugs with atropinelike effects (see Drug Classes).

• all sedating drugs. Watch for excessive sedation.

Clomipramine may *decrease* the effects of

• clonidine (Catapres).

• guanadrel (Hylorel).

• guanethidine (Ismelin, Esimil).

Clomipramine **taken concurrently** with

• anticonvulsants (see Drug Classes) such as carbamazepine (Tegretol) requires careful monitoring for changes in seizure patterns and the need to adjust anticonvulsant dosage.

• bepridil (Vascor) may lead to dangerous heart rhythms.

• cisapride (Propulsid) may lead to dangerous heart rhythms.

• dofetilide (Tikosyn) may lead to dangerous heart rhythms. Do not combine.

• gatifloxacin (Tequin), grepafloxacin (Raxar), moxifloxacin (Avelox) or sparfloxacin (Zagam) may lead to dangerous heart rhythms. Combination is NOT recommended.

• medicines that affect the QTc interval of the heart may worsen the QTc interval changes if combined with clomipramine.

- monoamine oxidase (MAO) type A inhibitor drugs (see Drug Classes) may cause high fever, seizures and hypertension. Avoid combining these drugs—14 days should separate doses of either.
- phenytoin (Dilantin) or fosphenytoin (Cerebyx) may lead to phenytoin or fosphenytoin toxicity.
- stimulant drugs (amphetamine, cocaine, epinephrine, phenylpropanolamine, etc.) may cause severe high blood pressure and/or high fever.
- thyroid preparations may increase risk of heart rhythm disorders.
- tramadol (Ultram) may increase seizure risk.
- venlafaxine (Effexor) may lead to venlafaxine and clomipramine toxicity.
- warfarin (Coumadin) may cause an increased warfarin effect and bleeding. More frequent INR (prothrombin time) testing is needed.

The following drugs may *increase* the effects of clomipramine:
- ACE inhibitors (see Drug Classes).
- birth control pills (oral contraceptives).
- cimetidine (Tagamet).
- enalapril (Vasotec, Vaseretic).
- estrogens (various).
- fluoxetine (Prozac).
- fluvoxamine (Luvox).
- haloperidol (Haldol).
- medicines that interfere with or inhibit cytochrome P450 3A4, a liver enzyme that is responsible for removing clomipramine from the body.
- methylphenidate (Ritalin).
- paroxetine (Paxil).
- phenothiazines (see Drug Classes).
- propafenone (Rythmol).
- quinidine (Quinaglute).
- ranitidine (Zantac).
- ritonavir (Norvir) and perhaps other protease inhibitors (see Drug Classes).
- sertraline (Zoloft).
- verapamil (Calan, others).

The following drugs may *decrease* the effects of clomipramine:
- barbiturates (see Drug Classes).
- carbamazepine (Tegretol).
- chloral hydrate (Noctec, Somnos, etc.).
- lithium (Lithobid, Lithotab, etc.).
- reserpine (Serpasil, Ser-Ap-Es, etc.).

▷ *Driving, Hazardous Activities:* This drug may cause seizures and impair alertness, judgment, physical coordination and reaction time. Restrict activities as necessary.

Aviation Note: The use of this drug **is a disqualification** for piloting. Consult a designated Aviation Medical Examiner.

Exposure to Sun: No restrictions.

Exposure to Heat: Use caution. This drug may impair the body's adaptation to hot environments, increasing the risk of heatstroke. Avoid saunas.

Exposure to Environmental Chemicals: This drug may mask the symptoms of poisoning due to handling certain insecticides (organophosphorous types). Read their labels carefully.

Discontinuation: It is best to slowly reduce the dose over 3 to 4 weeks. Abrupt withdrawal after prolonged use may cause nausea, vomiting, diarrhea, headache, dizziness, malaise, disturbed sleep and irritability. Obsessive-compulsive behavior may worsen if drug is stopped. Other drug doses may need to be changed to adjust.

CLONAZEPAM (kloh NA ze pam)

Introduced: 1977   **Class:** Anticonvulsant, benzodiazepines   **Prescription:** USA: Yes   **Controlled Drug:** USA: C-IV*; Canada: No   **Available as Generic:** Yes

Brand Names: ✤Apo-clonazepam, Klonopin, ✤Med-clonazepam, ✤Novo-clonazepam, ✤Rivotril

Warning: Klonopin and the generic clonidine have similar names and can be mistaken for each other—a serious error. Make sure you are taking the correct drug.

BENEFITS versus RISKS	
Possible Benefits	*Possible Risks*
EFFECTIVE CONTROL OF SOME TYPES OF PETIT MAL, AKINETIC AND MYOCLONIC SEIZURES	Paradoxical reactions: excitement, agitation and hallucinations
Possibly effective in the management of panic disorders	Minor impairment of mental functions
Can help restless leg syndrome	Blood cell disorders: anemia, abnormally low white blood cell and platelet counts—rare
	Increased salivation (difficult with chronic lung disease)

▷ **Principal Uses**

As a Single Drug Product: Uses currently included in FDA-approved labeling: (1) Treats several types of epilepsy: petit mal variations, akinetic, myoclonic and absence seizure patterns; (2) used in panic disorder; (3) helps control seizures from cyclosporin A.

Other (unlabeled) generally accepted uses: (1) Eases symptoms of Tourette's syndrome; (2) relieves trigeminal neuralgia; (3) helps resistant depression; (4) can ease drug-induced mania; (5) may be of help in restless leg syndrome (Ekbom syndrome); (6) may help essential tremor symptoms; (7) eases alprazolam withdrawal.

How This Drug Works: Increases the action of a nerve transmitter (gamma-aminobutyric acid or GABA), which blocks seizures.

Available Dosage Forms and Strengths

Tablets — 0.125 mg, 0.25 mg, 0.5 mg, 1 mg, 2 mg

▷ **Usual Adult Dosage Ranges**

Seizures: Starts with 0.5 mg three times daily. Increased by 0.5 mg to 1.0 mg every 3 days, as needed and tolerated. Maximum daily dose 20 mg.

Panic disorder: 0.25 mg twice daily. Some patients may require 4 mg a day.

*See Schedules of Controlled Drugs at the back of this book.

Note: **Actual dose and schedule must be determined for each patient individually**.

Conditions Requiring Dosing Adjustments

Liver Function: The dose must be decreased in liver compromise.

Kidney Function: Watch for signs and symptoms of accumulation (see "Effects of Overdose" below).

▷ **Dosing Instructions:** May be taken on empty stomach or with food or milk. The tablet may be crushed. Do not stop this drug abruptly if taken for seizure control, or if taken for more than 4 weeks to control panic attacks. If your forget a dose: take the dose as soon as you remember it, unless it's nearly time for your next dose—if that is the case, skip the missed dose and simply take the next scheduled dose. DO NOT double doses.

Usual Duration of Use: Regular use for 2 to 3 weeks may be needed to see benefit in reducing frequency or severity of seizures. Peak control requires dose adjustments over several months. Long-term use (months to years) requires evaluation by your doctor.

Typical Treatment Goals and Measurements (Outcomes and Markers)

Seizures: The general goal for this medicine is effective seizure control. Neurologists tend to define effective on a case-by-case basis depending on the seizure type and patient factors. IF goals have not been reached, combination treatment may be needed.

Panic: Goals for panic tend to be more vague and subjective than for hypertension or cholesterol. Frequently, the patient (in conjunction with physician assessment) will largely decide if panic has been successfully controlled. Additional markers include: decreased number of trips to the hospital or ER visits may be a useful measure. The ability of the patient to return to normal activities is a hallmark of successful treatment.

▷ **This Drug Should Not Be Taken If**
- you have had an allergic reaction to it previously.
- you have acute narrow-angle glaucoma.
- you have active liver disease.

▷ **Inform Your Physician Before Taking This Drug If**
- you are allergic to any benzodiazepine (see Drug Classes).
- you have a history of alcoholism or drug abuse.
- you are pregnant or planning pregnancy.
- you have palpitations, as this drug may worsen palpitations.
- you have impaired liver or kidney function.
- you have a history of serious depression or mental disorder.
- you have asthma, emphysema, chronic bronchitis or myasthenia gravis.
- you have acute intermittent porphyria or lung disease.

Possible Side Effects (natural, expected and unavoidable drug actions)

Drowsiness—frequent (may diminish with time).

Increased salivation.

▷ **Possible Adverse Effects** (unusual, unexpected and infrequent reactions)

If any of the following develop, consult your physician promptly for guidance.

Mild Adverse Effects

Allergic reactions: skin rash, hives, itching.

Ataxia—frequent.

Weight gain—frequent.

Headache, dizziness, blurred vision, double vision, slurred speech, impaired memory, confusion, depression—possible.

Muscle weakness, uncontrolled body movements—possible.

Palpitations or hair loss—rare.

Nausea, vomiting, constipation, diarrhea, impaired urination, incontinence—case reports in older patients.

Serious Adverse Effects

Idiosyncratic reactions: paradoxical responses of excitement, hyperactivity, agitation, anger, hostility—case reports.

Hallucinations, seizures—case reports.

Blood disorders: abnormally low platelet counts—benzodiazepine case reports.

Porphyria—case reports.

Increased secretions and breathing problems, especially in those with chronic lung disease—case reports.

▷ **Possible Effects on Sexual Function:** Increased libido, enlargement of male breasts. May cause abnormally early (precocious) secondary sex characteristics in children—case reports.

Possible Effects on Laboratory Tests

Complete blood cell counts: low red or white cells, hemoglobin or platelets.

Urine tests for drug abuse: may be positive. (Results depend on amount of drug taken and test method.)

Liver function tests: increased.

CAUTION

1. Drug should not be stopped abruptly if used to control seizures.
2. Some over-the-counter products containing antihistamines (allergy and cold preparations, sleep aids) can cause excessive sedation if combined with clonazepam.
3. Adverse behavioral reactions are more common in people with brain damage, mental retardation or psychiatric disorders.
4. Decreased drug response seen in about 30% of users 3 months after therapy starts. Dose increase often needed to restore seizure control.

Precautions for Use

By Infants and Children: This drug is used to treat infants and children of all ages. Careful dosage adjustment based on weight and age is mandatory. Abnormal behavioral responses are more common in children.

By Those Over 60 Years of Age: Smaller doses and longer intervals are suggested. Watch for lethargy, indifference, fatigue, unsteadiness, disturbing dreams, paradoxical excitement, agitation, anger, hostility or rage.

▷ **Advisability of Use During Pregnancy**

Pregnancy Category: C. See Pregnancy Risk Categories at the back of this book.

Animal studies: This drug causes cleft palates, open eyelids, fused rib structures and limb defects in rabbits.

Human studies: Adequate studies of pregnant women are not available.

Avoid drug during the first 3 months if possible. Frequent use in late pregnancy may cause the "floppy infant" syndrome in newborns: weakness, lethargy, unresponsiveness, low body temperature, depressed breathing.

Advisability of Use If Breast-Feeding
> Presence of this drug in breast milk: Yes.
> Avoid drug or refrain from nursing.

Habit-Forming Potential: This drug can produce psychological and/or physical dependence (see Glossary), especially with large doses for extended periods.

Effects of Overdose: Marked drowsiness, weakness, confusion, slurred speech, staggering gait, tremor, stupor progressing to deep sleep or coma.

Possible Effects of Long-Term Use: Benefits versus risks must be considered carefully during the extended use of this drug in children. Possible adverse effects on physical or mental development may not be apparent for many years.

Suggested Periodic Examinations While Taking This Drug (at physician's discretion)
> During long-term use: Complete blood cell counts; liver function tests.

▷ **While Taking This Drug, Observe the Following**
> *Foods:* No restrictions.
> *Herbal Medicines or Minerals:* Hawthorn may react antagonistically to clonazepam. Valerian and kava kava may interact additively (drowsiness). Avoid these combinations.
>> Kava and valerian may exacerbate central nervous system depression (avoid this combination). Kola nut, Siberian ginseng, mate, ephedra and ma huang may blunt the benefits of this medicine. While St. John's wort is indicated for anxiety, it is also thought to increase (induce) cytochrome P450 enzymes and will tend to blunt clonazepam effectiveness if combined with clonazepam.
> *Beverages:* No restrictions. May be taken with milk.
▷ *Alcohol:* Use with extreme caution. Alcohol may increase the depressant effects of this drug on the brain. It is advisable to avoid alcohol completely—throughout the day and night—if it is necessary to drive or to engage in any hazardous activity.
> *Tobacco Smoking:* No interactions expected. I advise everyone to quit smoking.
> *Marijuana Smoking:* Increased sedation and significant impairment of intellectual and physical performance.
▷ *Other Drugs*

> Clonazepam *taken concurrently* with
> - amiodarone (Cordarone) may decrease elimination of clonazepam and also worsen toxicity by causing low thyroid function.
> - carbamazepine (Tegretol) may decrease blood levels and hence benefits of both medications.
> - desipramine, imipramine and other tricyclic antidepressants (see Drug Classes) can decrease the tricyclic antidepressant blood level and lessen its therapeutic benefit.
> - MAO inhibitors (see Drug Classes) may result in very low blood pressure and worsening of sedation and respiratory depression.
> - phenytoin (Dilantin) or fosphenytoin (Cerebyx) may result in decreased phenytoin or fosphenytoin levels.
> - primidone (Mysoline) may lead to excessive drowsiness.
> - ritonavir (Norvir), and perhaps other protease inhibitors (see Drug Classes), may lead to clonazepam toxicity.
> - valproic acid (Depakene, etc.) may cause continuous absence seizures.

The following drugs may *increase* the effects of clonazepam:
- antifungal medicines such as itraconazole (Sporanox) and ketoconazole (Nizoral).
- cimetidine (Tagamet).
- disulfiram (Antabuse).
- macrolide antibiotics such as azithromycin, clarithromycin or erythromycin (see Drug Classes).
- omeprazole (Prilosec).
- oral contraceptives (birth control pills).

The following drugs may *decrease* the effects of clonazepam:
- rifampin (Rifater) or rifabutin (Mycobutin).
- theophylline (aminophylline, Theo-Dur, etc.).

▷ *Driving, Hazardous Activities:* This drug can impair mental alertness, judgment, physical coordination and reaction time. Avoid hazardous activities accordingly.

Aviation Note: The use of this drug *is a disqualification* for piloting. Consult a designated Aviation Medical Examiner.

Exposure to Sun: No restrictions.

Discontinuation: Do not stop clonazepam suddenly if it was controlling any type of seizure, or if it was taken for more than 4 weeks. Dosing should be slowly decreased (tapered) to prevent a withdrawal syndrome.

CLONIDINE (KLOH ni deen)

Introduced: 1969   **Class:** Antihypertensive   **Prescription:** USA: Yes
Controlled Drug: USA: No; Canada: No   **Available as Generic:** USA: Yes; Canada: No
Brand Names: ✤Apo-Clonidine, Catapres, Catapres-TTS, Combipres [CD], ✤Dixarit, Duraclon, ✤Novo-Clonidine, ✤Nu-Clonidine

BENEFITS versus RISKS	
Possible Benefits	*Possible Risks*
EFFECTIVE ANTIHYPERTENSIVE IN MILD TO MODERATE HIGH BLOOD PRESSURE	ACUTE WITHDRAWAL SYNDROME (rebound hypertension) with abrupt discontinuation
Effective control of menopausal hot flashes (in selected cases)	Raynaud's phenomenon (cold fingers or toes)
Effective help in narcotic withdrawal	
May have a role as a second-line medicine for people who are trying to quit smoking	

▷ **Principal Uses**
As a Single Drug Product: Uses currently included in FDA-approved labeling: Used in combination with other medicines to treat mild to moderate high blood pressure.

Other (unlabeled) generally accepted uses: (1) Helps prevent migraine headache; (2) helps improve outcomes in some head injuries; (3) can aid menopausal hot flashes and severe menstrual cramps; (4) lessens symptoms of alcohol or narcotic drug withdrawal; (5) helped atrial fibrillation in one study; (6) second-line drug in controlling high blood pressure in congestive heart failure patients; (7) case reports of benefits in water contact pain (aquadynia); (8) useful in some diabetic nerve damage (peripheral neuropathy); (9) may have a use protecting the kidneys (renal protective) from cyclosporine or in coronary artery bypass surgery; (10) useful in Tourette's syndrome; (11) second-line agent in quitting smoking.

As a Combination Drug Product [CD]: Available in combination with chlorthalidone. The different ways in which these drugs work complement each other, making the combination a more effective antihypertensive.

How This Drug Works: Decreases action of the brain (vasomotor center), limiting the sympathetic nervous system's constriction of blood vessels and blood pressure increases. Chlorthalidone combination helps remove excess water from the body that contributes to high blood pressure.

Available Dosage Forms and Strengths
Patches — 2.5 mg, 5.0 mg, 7.5 mg
Tablets — 0.1 mg, 0.2 mg, 0.3 mg

▷ **Usual Adult Dosage Ranges:** *Tablets:* Initially 0.1 mg twice daily. Increased by 0.1 to 0.2 mg daily as needed and tolerated. Usual range is 0.2 to 0.6 mg daily, taken in two doses. Maximum daily dose is 2.4 mg. Some clinicians set maximum of 1.2 mg daily. *Patches:* Applied once a week. Hypertension in children has been treated with 5 to 10 mcg per kg of body mass per day, divided into two or three doses.

Note: Actual dose and schedule must be determined for each patient individually.

Conditions Requiring Dosing Adjustments
Liver Function: This drug is changed into six active forms. The dose must be decreased in liver compromise.
Kidney Function: Some kidney patients may require higher ongoing doses to get the best blood pressure.

▷ **Dosing Instructions:** Tablets may be taken without regard to eating. The tablet may be crushed. Patches should not be altered. If you forget a dose: For the patch form—put the patch on as soon as you remember it. If you are more than 3 days late, call your doctor. If you forget a regular release tablet, take the missed dose right away unless it is nearly time for your next dose, then skip the missed dose and take the regularly scheduled dose. DO NOT double doses. If you have trouble remembering this medicine, talk with your doctor.

Usual Duration of Use: Use on a regular schedule for 2 to 3 weeks may be needed to see this drug's full benefit in lowering high blood pressure. If target goals are not met by the expected time frame, changes should be made. Long-term use (months to years) requires physician supervision and guidance.

Typical Treatment Goals and Measurements (Outcomes and Markers)
Blood Pressure: The most recent treatment guidelines (JNC VI) actually define optimal blood pressure (BP) as less than 120/80 and high normal as 139/89. The American Diabetes Association suggests a target of 130/80 for those living with diabetes. Most clinicians try to achieve a BP that achieves the best balance of lower cardiovascular risk while avoiding the problem

of too low a blood pressure. The goal and time frame (see peak benefits above) should be discussed with you when the prescription is written.

▷ **This Drug Should Not Be Taken If**
- you have had an allergic reaction to it previously.
- you have a problem in your heart that impacts the timing of the heartbeat or transmission of electrical impulses through the heart.

▷ **Inform Your Physician Before Taking This Drug If**
- you have a circulatory disorder of the brain.
- you have angina or coronary artery disease.
- you recently had a heart attack (MI).
- you have or have had serious emotional depression.
- you have a very slow heart rate.
- you have kidney failure.
- you have Buerger's disease or Raynaud's phenomenon.
- you are taking a tricyclic antidepressant (see Drug Classes).
- you are taking any sedative or hypnotic drugs or an antidepressant.
- you will have surgery with general anesthesia.

Possible Side Effects (natural, expected and unavoidable drug actions)
Drowsiness, dry nose and mouth, constipation—common.
Decreased heart rate, mild orthostatic hypotension (see Glossary).
Serious abnormal heartbeats possible if drug is stopped suddenly.

▷ **Possible Adverse Effects** (unusual, unexpected and infrequent reactions)
If any of the following develop, consult your physician promptly for guidance.
Mild Adverse Effects
Allergic reactions: skin rash, hives, localized swellings, itching—rare to infrequent.
Drowsiness—infrequent to frequent.
Headache, dizziness, fatigue, anxiety, sleep disorders (nightmares or vivid dreaming), dry and burning eyes—possible.
Painful parotid (salivary) gland, nausea, vomiting—case reports.
Dry mouth—frequent.
Urination at night—rare.
Increased liver function tests—case reports.
Serious Adverse Effects
Idiosyncratic reaction: Raynaud's phenomenon (see Glossary)—case reports.
Aggravation of congestive heart failure, heart rhythm disorders—case reports.
Depression, hallucinations or psychosis—case reports.

▷ **Possible Effects on Sexual Function:** Decreased libido or impotence—infrequent.
Enlargement of male breasts (gynecomastia)—rare.
Precocious puberty in females—case report.

Possible Effects on Laboratory Tests
Blood cholesterol or triglyceride levels: no consistent or significant effects.
Blood sodium level: increased.
Liver function: rare increases of enzymes (ALT/GPT, AST/GOT, alkaline phosphatase).

CAUTION
1. ***Do not stop this drug suddenly***. Sudden withdrawal can cause a severe and possibly fatal reaction.

2. Hot weather or fever can reduce blood pressure significantly. Dose adjustments may be necessary.
3. Report any tendency to depression.

Precautions for Use

By Infants and Children: Initial doses of 5–10 mcg per kg of body mass per day, divided into two or three doses, have been used. A larger evening dose and smaller morning dose can help minimize sedation during school hours when used for attention deficit hyperactivity disorder (ADHD).

By Those Over 60 Years of Age: **Proceed cautiously** with this drug. High blood pressure should be reduced slowly without the risks associated with excessively low blood pressure. Low initial doses and frequent blood pressure checks are needed. Watch for development of light-headedness, dizziness, unsteadiness, fainting and falling. Sedation and dry mouth occur in 50% of elderly users. Promptly report any changes in mood or behavior: depression, delusions, hallucinations.

▷ **Advisability of Use During Pregnancy**

Pregnancy Category: C. See Pregnancy Risk Categories at the back of this book.
Animal studies: No birth defects reported. However, this drug is toxic to the embryo in low dosage.
Human studies: Adequate studies of pregnant women are not available. The manufacturer recommends that women who are or who may become pregnant avoid this drug. Ask your doctor for help.

Advisability of Use If Breast-Feeding

Presence of this drug in breast milk: Yes.
This drug may impair milk production. Monitor nursing infant closely. Stop drug or nursing if adverse effects begin.

Habit-Forming Potential: A small number of reports regarding abuse of this drug have surfaced. It may cause extreme grogginess and lethargy when combined with diazepam (Valium).

Effects of Overdose: Marked drowsiness, weakness, dry mouth, slow pulse, low blood pressure, vomiting, stupor progressing to coma.

Possible Effects of Long-Term Use: Development of tolerance (see Glossary) with loss of drug effect; weight gain due to salt and water retention; temporary sexual impotence.

Suggested Periodic Examinations While Taking This Drug (at physician's discretion)

Blood pressure measurements.
Monitoring of body weight.

▷ **While Taking This Drug, Observe the Following**

Foods: Avoid excessive salt and ask your doctor for help with salt restriction.
Herbal Medicines or Minerals: Ginseng may increase blood pressure, blunting the benefits of this medicine. Hawthorn, saw palmetto, ma huang, goldenseal, yohimbe and licorice may also cause increased blood pressure. Calcium and garlic may help lower blood pressure and Indian snakeroot has a German Commission E monograph indication for hypertension—talk to your doctor to see if those combinations may allow some lowering of prescription medicine doses. Eleuthero root and ephedra should be avoided by people living with hypertension.
Beverages: No restrictions. May be taken with milk.

▷   *Alcohol:* Use with extreme caution. Combined effects can cause marked drowsiness and exaggerated reduction of blood pressure.

Tobacco Smoking: No expected interactions. I advise everyone to quit smoking.

▷   *Other Drugs*

Clonidine may *decrease* the effects of

- levodopa (Larodopa, Sinemet, etc.), causing an increase in parkinsonism symptoms.

Clonidine *taken concurrently* with

- beta-adrenergic blocking drugs (Inderal, Lopressor, Coreg, etc.) may increase rebound hypertension risk if clonidine is stopped first. It is best to stop the beta-blocker first and then withdraw clonidine gradually.
- cyclosporine (Sandimmune) may lead to cyclosporine toxicity.
- ephedrine (various) may dangerously increase the blood pressure raising effect of ephedrine.
- mirtazapine (Remeron) resulted in a large increase in blood pressure in one case report. Caution is advised.
- naloxone (Narcan, Talwin NX) may blunt the therapeutic effect of clonidine and result in a hypertensive response.
- niacin may decrease the facial-flushing side effect of niacin.
- nonsteroidal anti-inflammatory drugs (NSAIDs-see Drug Classes) may blunt blood pressure lowering benefits of clonidine.
- verapamil (Calan, others) may lead to problems in conduction of the heart.

The following drugs may *decrease* the effects of clonidine:

- nonsteroidal anti-inflammatory drugs (NSAIDs—see Drug Classes).
- tricyclic antidepressants (Elavil, Sinequan, etc.—see Drug Classes), possibly reducing clonidine's effectiveness in lowering blood pressure.

▷   *Driving, Hazardous Activities:* Use caution. Can cause drowsiness and impair alertness, judgment and coordination.

Aviation Note: Hypertension (high blood pressure) *is a disqualification* for piloting. Consult a designated Aviation Medical Examiner.

Exposure to Sun: No restrictions.

Exposure to Heat: Use caution. Hot environments may reduce blood pressure, making orthostatic hypotension (see Glossary) more likely.

Exposure to Cold: Use caution. May cause painful blanching and numbness of the hands and feet on exposure to cold air or water (Raynaud's phenomenon).

Heavy Exercise or Exertion: Use caution. This drug may intensify the hypertensive response to isometric exercise. Ask your doctor for help.

Occurrence of Unrelated Illness: Fever may lower blood pressure. Repeated vomiting may prevent the regular use of this drug and cause an acute withdrawal reaction. Consult your physician.

Discontinuation: **Do not stop this drug suddenly.** A severe withdrawal reaction can occur within 12 to 48 hours after the last dose. It is best to gradually decrease the dose over 3 to 4 days, and check blood pressure often.

CLOPIDOGREL (KLOW pi doh grel)

Introduced: 1998   **Class:** Antiplatelet (platelet aggregation inhibitor)   **Prescription:** USA: Yes   **Controlled Drug:** USA: No; Canada: No   **Available as Generic:** No
Brand Name: Plavix

BENEFITS versus RISKS

Possible Benefits	*Possible Risks*
PREVENTION OF DEATH IN ACUTE CORONARY SYNDROMES (ACS)	Stomach irritation, bleeding and/or ulceration (less than aspirin)
EFFECTIVE PREVENTION OF ATHEROSCLEROTIC EVENTS	Lowered white blood cells
PREVENTION OF BLOOD CLOTS	Liver toxicity
PREVENTION OF HEART ATTACK	Thrombotic thrombocytopenic purpura
PREVENTION OF STROKE	
PREVENTION OF VASCULAR DEATH	

▷ **Principal Uses**

As a Single Drug Product: Uses currently included in FDA-approved labeling: (1) Reduces atherosclerotic events (vascular death, stroke or heart attack [MI]) in people who have atherosclerosis (shown by recent MI, peripheral artery disease or stroke).

Other (unlabeled) generally accepted uses: (1) Combined use of clopidogrel with aspirin in people with unstable angina (see CURE trial below) showed that stroke, heart attack and deaths could be prevented in acute coronary syndrome patients.

How This Drug Works: Permanently (irreversibly) inhibits adenosine diphosphate (ADP)-induced platelet clumping (aggregation).

Available Dosage Forms and Strengths: Tablets — 75 mg

▷ **Usual Adult Dosage Ranges**

75 mg once a day by mouth. This approach may take 2–3 days to have a full anti-clot effect.

Conditions Requiring Dosing Adjustments

Liver Function: Dose lowering may be needed in moderate to severe liver disease.
Kidney Function: No changes thought to be needed.

▷ **Dosing Instructions:** May be taken with or without food. Talk to your doctor or pharmacist BEFORE combining this medicine with any other pill, herbal or nutritional medicine. If you forget a dose: take the missed dose as soon as you remember it, unless it is nearly time for your next dose. If this is the case, skip the missed dose and simply take the next scheduled dose. DO NOT double doses.

Usual Duration of Use: Ongoing use for prevention of atherosclerotic events MUST continue until your doctor tells you to stop this medicine. Ongoing physician supervision is required.

Typical Treatment Goals and Measurements (Outcomes and Markers)

Atherosclerotic events: Most clinicians view preventing, rather than treating an atherosclerotic event such as stroke or heart attack, as the ultimate goal of this therapy. Measurement then becomes straightforward in that fewer than expected (based on the severity of the atherosclerosis that you face) heart attack or stroke occurrences is the end point of therapy. Electron beam computed tomography (EBCT) may help define the severity of circulatory compromise.

Possible Advantages of This Drug: Significant benefit versus aspirin alone in patients with peripheral vascular disease. **Author's Note: Combined use of clopidogrel with aspirin showed dramatic results in the CURE (Clopidogrel in Unstable angina to prevent Recurrent Events) trial. One researcher estimated that 50,000 to 100,000 strokes, heart attacks or deaths in patients with acute coronary syndromes could be prevented EACH YEAR with combined aspirin and clopidogrel use.**

▷ **This Drug Should Not Be Taken If**
- you have had an allergic reaction to this drug or to any substance in the pill.
- you have any type of bleeding disorder (such as hemophilia).
- you are actively bleeding, such as from an ulcer or hemorrhage in the head.

▷ **Inform Your Physician Before Taking This Drug If**
- you are taking any anticoagulant drug.
- you are pregnant or planning pregnancy.
- you have high blood pressure.
- you plan to have surgery of any kind (drug is usually stopped 7 days BEFORE major surgery).
- you have a low white blood cell count.
- you have a history of liver problems.

Possible Side Effects (natural, expected and unavoidable drug actions)
Interference with usual blood clotting.

▷ **Possible Adverse Effects** (unusual, unexpected and infrequent reactions)
If any of the following develop, consult your physician promptly for guidance.

Mild Adverse Effects
Allergic reactions: skin rash.
Headache, fatigue, depression or dizziness—infrequent.
Flu-like symptoms—infrequent.
Loss of taste (ageusia)—case reports.
Nose bleeds—infrequent.
Sudden (acute) arthritis—case reports.
Cough—infrequent.
Increased cholesterol—infrequent.
Stomach irritation, nausea, vomiting or diarrhea—infrequent to frequent.
Increased blood pressure—infrequent.

Serious Adverse Effects
Allergic reactions: possible.
Erosion of stomach lining, with silent bleeding—possible.
Bone marrow depression (see Glossary): fatigue, weakness, fever, sore throat, abnormal bleeding or bruising—possible.
Thrombotic thrombocytopenic purpura (low blood platelets, anemia, fever, nerve and kidney changes)—20 cases reported to date (onset often within 2 weeks after treatment was started).
Hemothorax—rare.
Hemolytic uremic syndrome—case report.
Ischemic necrosis—rare.
Hepatitis with jaundice (see Glossary): yellow skin and eyes, dark-colored urine, light-colored stool—possible.
Intracranial bleeding—possible.

▷ **Possible Effects on Sexual Function:** Excessive menstrual flow (menorrhagia)—
     case reports.

Adverse Effects That May Mimic Natural Diseases or Disorders
     Liver damage may suggest viral hepatitis or reveal (unmask) low-level (sub-
     clinical) liver disease.

Possible Effects on Laboratory Tests
     Bleeding time: prolonged.
     Cholesterol: possibly increased.
     Complete blood counts: decreased white blood cells (agranulocytosis, neu-
         tropenia or granulocytopenia)—possible.
     Liver function tests: increased ALT/GPT, AST/GOT, alkaline phosphatase.

CAUTION
     1. You may take longer than usual to stop bleeding.
     2. Since this medicine is indicated for preventing problems in people with
        atherosclerosis, the atherosclerosis needs to be diagnosed by: recent
        heart attack or stroke or established peripheral artery disease.
     3. Call your doctor if you develop infections.

Precautions for Use
     By Infants and Children: Safety and efficacy not evaluated.
     By Those Over 60 Years of Age: The blood levels achieved with the standard
        dose are significantly higher than those in younger patients, but no dos-
        ing changes are presently thought to be needed. Watch for gray- to black-
        colored stools, an indication of stomach bleeding.

▷ **Advisability of Use During Pregnancy**
     Pregnancy Category: B. See Pregnancy Risk Categories at the back of this
        book.
     Animal studies: No changes in rats at up to 78 times the human dose.
     Human studies: Adequate human studies are not available.
     Talk to your doctor to see if benefit outweighs the risk.

Advisability of Use If Breast-Feeding
     Presence of this drug in breast milk: Yes in rats, unknown in humans.
     Avoid drug or refrain from nursing.

Habit-Forming Potential: None.

Effects of Overdose: One overdose (1,050 mg) resulted in no special treatment
     or adverse effects.

Possible Effects of Long-Term Use: Prolonged bleeding time, critical in the
     event of injury or surgery.

Suggested Periodic Examinations While Taking This Drug (at physician's dis-
     cretion)
     Complete blood cell counts.
     Liver function tests.

▷ **While Taking This Drug, Observe the Following**
     Foods: No effect by food on how much gets into your body.
     Herbal Medicines or Minerals: Many herbal medicines may interact with
        aspirin. Examples include ginkgo, garlic, ginger, ginseng and feverfew.
        Combining those medicines with clopidogrel is not recommended. Talk to
        your doctor BEFORE adding any herbal medicine.
     Beverages: No restrictions. May be taken with milk.

▷ *Alcohol:* Use of alcohol and clopidogrel at the same time may increase risk of stomach damage and may prolong bleeding time.

Tobacco Smoking: No interactions expected, but I advise everyone to quit smoking.

▷ *Other Drugs*

Clopidogrel may *increase* the effects of

- aspirin (various), posing an increased bleeding risk—however the CURE trial showed a dramatic benefit in ACS patients where aspirin was combined with clopidogrel.
- eptifibatide (Integrilin), leading to an increased bleeding risk.
- fluvastatin (Lescol).
- heparin, leading to increased bleeding risk.
- medicines removed by cytochrome P450 2C9 may be increased if combined with clopidogrel (an inhibitor of this enzyme).
- oral anticoagulants (see Drug Classes) such as warfarin (Coumadin) and cause abnormal bleeding.
- phenytoin (Dilantin) and fosphenytoin (Cerebyx). More frequent blood levels and dosage adjustments are prudent.
- tamoxifen (Nolvadex), leading to tamoxifen toxicity.
- tolbutamide (Orinase), leading to tolbutamide toxicity.

Clopidogrel taken concurrently with

- alendronate (Fosamax) may result in increased risk of stomach upset/diarrhea.
- cortisonelike drugs (see Drug Classes) increases risk of stomach ulcers.
- high blood pressure medicines (antihypertensives) may lessen lowering of elevated blood pressure.
- torsemide (Demadex), leading to excessive torsemide effect.
- warfarin (Coumadin), leading to increased bleeding risk. Increased frequency of INR testing is prudent.
- zafirlukast (Accolate) may cause additive inhibition of the CYP2C9 isoenzyme, possibly increasing blood levels of other medicines removed by CYP2C9.

The following drug may *decrease* the effects of clopidogrel:

- cholestyramine (Questran, others) might decrease the amount of clopidogrel that goes to work—separate doses by 30 minutes.

▷ *Driving, Hazardous Activities:* No restrictions or precautions.

Aviation Note: It is advisable to watch for dizziness and fatigue and restrict activities accordingly.

Exposure to Sun: No reports of problems.

Discontinuation: Talk to your doctor before stopping this medicine for any reason.

CLOTRIMAZOLE (kloh TRIM a zohl)

Introduced: 1976   **Class:** Antifungal   Prescription: USA: Yes, though some are nonprescription   **Controlled Drug:** USA: No; Canada: No   **Available as Generic:** USA: Yes; Canada: No

Brand Names: ❦Canesten, Clotrimaderm, Femcare, Femzol-7, Gyne-Lotrimin (1% cream and insert are nonprescription), ❦Lotriderm, Lotrimin, Lotrimin AF (nonprescription), Lotrisone, Mycelex (1% vaginal cream is nonprescription), Mycelex-G, Mycelex-7, ❦Myclo, ❦Myclo-Gyne, ❦Neo-Zol

Warning: The brand names Mycelex and Myoflex sound similar. This can lead to serious errors. Make sure you are using the correct drug.

BENEFITS versus RISKS	
Possible Benefits	*Possible Risks*
EFFECTIVE TREATMENT AND PREVENTION OF *CANDIDA* (YEAST) INFECTIONS OF THE MOUTH AND THROAT (THRUSH)	Skin and mucous membrane irritation due to sensitization (drug-induced allergy)
EFFECTIVE TREATMENT OF *CANDIDA* (YEAST) INFECTIONS OF THE SKIN	Nausea, vomiting, stomach cramping, diarrhea (when swallowed)
EFFECTIVE TREATMENT OF *CANDIDA* (YEAST) INFECTIONS OF THE VULVA AND VAGINA	
EFFECTIVE TREATMENT OF TINEA (RINGWORM) INFECTIONS OF THE SKIN	

▷ **Principal Uses**

As a Single Drug Product: Uses currently included in FDA-approved labeling: (1) Treats *Candida* (yeast) infections of skin, mouth, throat, vulva and vagina; (2) treats tinea and related infections: ringworm of the body, groin (jock itch) or feet (athlete's foot), due to susceptible fungi; (3) treats pityriasis.

Other (unlabeled) generally accepted uses: Prevention of *Candida* (yeast) infections of the mouth and throat in the management of HIV.

How This Drug Works: It damages cell walls and blocks critical enzymes, inhibiting fungal growth (with low drug levels) and kills fungus (with high drug concentrations).

Available Dosage Forms and Strengths

Cream — 1% (10 mg/g)
Lotion — 1% (10 mg/g)
Mouth lozenges — 10 mg
Topical solution — 1% (10 mg/ml)
Vaginal cream — 1% (10 mg/g), 2% (20 mg/g)
Vaginal tablets — 100 mg, 200 mg, 500 mg

▷ **Recommended Dosage Ranges** (Actual dosage and schedule must be determined for each patient individually.)

Infants and Children: Use of lozenges not recommended for children under 5 years of age; for 5 years and older, dissolve one lozenge slowly and completely in mouth five times a day for 14 days, longer if necessary.

12 to 60 Years of Age:

For Candida infections of mouth and throat: Dissolve 1 lozenge slowly and completely in mouth five times a day for 14 days; extended treatment will be necessary for people with AIDS.

For Candida and tinea infections of skin: Apply cream, lotion or solution to infected areas twice a day, morning and evening. Make certain that you use this product for the length of time specified by your doctor (if a prescription form) or by the label if you are using a nonprescription form.

For Candida infections of vulva and vagina: One applicatorful (5 g) of cream intravaginally at bedtime for 7 to 14 consecutive days; or one 100-mg tablet intravaginally at bedtime for 7 days; or two 100-mg tablets intravaginally at bedtime for 3 days; or as a single-dose treatment, one 500-mg tablet intravaginally at bedtime, one time only.

Over 60 Years of Age: Same as 12 to 60 years of age.

Conditions Requiring Dosing Adjustments

Liver Function: This drug is removed via the bile—dose should be decreased if bile duct is blocked.

Kidney Function: Dosing changes are not needed.

▷ **Dosing Instructions:** Dissolve lozenge in mouth completely, swallowing saliva as it accumulates. Do not chew the lozenge or swallow it whole. Take full course prescribed. Vaginal forms will seep out of the vagina. It's prudent to wear a minipad to protect your clothing. If symptoms persist after or worsen during a course of nonprescription forms, see your doctor. Many clinicians prefer multiple-day regimens for more complicated or severe vulvovaginal yeast infections. If you forget a dose: Take the missed dose right away, unless it is nearly time for your next dose—then skip the missed dose and just take the next scheduled dose. DO NOT double doses.

Usual Duration of Use: Regular use for 1 to 2 weeks usually needed to see benefit in controlling yeast or tinea infection. Some single-, 3- or 7-day courses are appropriate for some creams or tablets. Long-term use (as in AIDS management) requires periodic physician evaluation. Treatment failure may indicate need for new combination HIV therapy.

Typical Treatment Goals and Measurements (Outcomes and Markers)

Infections: The most commonly used measures of serious infections are white blood cell counts and differentials (the kind of blood cells that occur most often in your blood) and temperature. For uncomplicated vaginal yeast infections, many clinicians look for positive changes in 48 hours. If this is a multi-day course, NEVER stop an antifungal because you start to feel better. The goals and time frame (see peak benefits above) should be discussed with you when the prescription is written.

Possible Advantages of This Drug

Reasonably effective with minimal toxicity. More palatable than nystatin.

▷ **This Drug Should Not Be Taken If**
- you have had an allergic reaction to it previously.

▷ **Inform Your Physician Before Taking This Drug If**
- you are allergic to related antifungal drugs: fluconazole, itraconazole, ketoconazole, miconazole.
- you have liver problems and take oral clotrimazole troche.

Possible Side Effects (natural, expected and unavoidable drug actions)
None.

▷ **Possible Adverse Effects** (unusual, unexpected and infrequent reactions)
If any of the following develop, consult your physician promptly for guidance.

Mild Adverse Effects

Allergic reactions: skin rash, hives, itching, burning, swelling, blistering (not present prior to treatment)—possible.

Depression, disorientation or drowsiness—may be frequent with oral therapy.

Nausea, vomiting, stomach cramping, diarrhea (when swallowed)—frequent.

Serious Adverse Effects

Allergic reactions: sensitization of tissues (where applied locally) that will react allergically with future drug application—possible.

Liver toxicity (with oral form)—infrequent.

Author's Note: Side effects with topical forms are rare.

▷ **Possible Effects on Sexual Function:** None.

Possible Delayed Adverse Effects: Local tissue sensitization to this drug.

Possible Effects on Laboratory Tests

Liver function tests: increased liver enzyme AST/GOT in 15% of oral form users.

CAUTION

1. Avoid contact of cream, lotion and solution with the eyes.
2. Do not cover applied cream or lotion with an occlusive dressing.
3. Failure of treatment may mean resistant fungi.
4. Failure of treatment in AIDS patients may mean resistant HIV.

Precautions for Use

By Infants and Children: Use of lozenges by those under 5 years of age is not recommended.

By Those Over 60 Years of Age: No specific problems reported.

▷ **Advisability of Use During Pregnancy**

Pregnancy Category: B for vaginal or topical use. C for troches. See Pregnancy Risk Categories at the back of this book.

Animal studies: No drug-induced birth defects were found in mouse, rat or rabbit studies.

Human studies: Adequate studies of pregnant women are not available.

Ask your physician for guidance.

Advisability of Use If Breast-Feeding

Presence of this drug in breast milk: Unknown.

Watch infant closely. Stop drug or nursing if adverse effects.

Habit-Forming Potential: None.

Effects of Overdose: Excessive use of lozenges may cause nausea, vomiting or diarrhea.

Possible Effects of Long-Term Use: None reported.

Suggested Periodic Examinations While Taking This Drug (at physician's discretion)

Ongoing oral use: liver function tests.

▷ **While Taking This Drug, Observe the Following**

Foods: No restrictions.

Herbal Medicines or Minerals: Echinacea: Some patients use echinacea to attempt to boost their immune systems. Unfortunately, use of echinacea is not recommended in people with damaged immune systems. This herb may also actually weaken any immune system if it is used too often or for too long a time. Do NOT take mistletoe herb, oak bark or F.C. of marshmallow root and licorice.

Beverages: No restrictions.
▷   *Alcohol:* No interactions expected.
Tobacco Smoking: No interactions expected. I advise everyone to quit smoking.
▷   *Other Drugs:*
Clotrimazole (oral dosage forms) **taken concurrently** with
- amphotericin B lipid complex (Abelcet) may blunt benefits.
- aspirin (various) may lead to additive stomach and intestinal (GI upset, bleeding) problems.
- betamethasone (Betaderm, Diprolene, others) resulted in enhanced fungal growth (Majocchi's granulomas) in one case report.
- cyclosporine (Sandimmune) may result in cyclosporine toxicity.
- dofetilide (Tikosyn) may result in dofetilide toxicity.
- sirolimus (Rapamune) and tacrolimus (Prograf) can result in increased sirolimus or tacrolimus levels and increased risk of kidney toxicity and increased potassium and glucose.
- trimetrexate (Neutrexin) may result in trimexate toxicity.
▷   *Driving, Hazardous Activities:* No restrictions.
Aviation Note: No restrictions.
Exposure to Sun: No restrictions.
Discontinuation: As directed by your doctor.

CLOXACILLIN (klox a SIL in)

Please see the penicillin family profile.

CLOZAPINE (KLOH za peen)

Introduced: 1975   **Class:** Strong tranquilizer (antipsychotic)   **Prescription:** USA: Yes   **Controlled Drug:** USA: No   **Available as Generic:** USA: Yes
Brand Name: ✤Apo-Clozaril, Clozaril
Author's Note: In the United States, this drug is available only by special arrangement through the Clozaril National Registry. Your doctor will call 800-448-5938 to register you and then a form is filled out by the MD and pharmacy, which is faxed to 800-648-6015. The medicine can then be ordered directly from the pharmacy wholesaler. This is to make certain that required blood tests are obtained. Ask your doctor for help.

BENEFITS versus RISKS	
Possible Benefits	*Possible Risks*
EFFECTIVE CONTROL OF SEVERE SCHIZOPHRENIA THAT HAS FAILED TO RESPOND ADEQUATELY TO OTHER APPROPRIATE DRUGS	SERIOUS BLOOD CELL DISORDERS: ABNORMALLY LOW WHITE BLOOD CELL AND PLATELET COUNTS
Improvement in many refractory cases	DRUG-INDUCED SEIZURES (DEPENDING ON SIZE OF DOSE)
Useful in patients who have tardive dyskinesia	
This class of medicines may be drugs of choice in older adults	

▷ **Principal Uses**

As a Single Drug Product: Uses currently included in FDA-approved labeling: Manages severe schizophrenia that fails to respond to adequate trials of other standard antipsychotic medicines. Because of potential for serious blood cell disorders and seizures, its use is reserved for severely ill schizophrenic patients.

Other (unlabeled) generally accepted uses: (1) Severe and refractory bipolar disorder; (2) severe tardive dyskinesia (dystonic subtype)—a syndrome that can happen after some medicines are used to treat psychosis; (3) psychosis occurring after labor with lactation; (4) may help excessive urination (polydipsia) caused by other neuroleptic agents.

How This Drug Works: By blocking the place (receptor) where dopamine works, this drug corrects an imbalance of nerve impulses causing schizophrenic thought disorders.

Available Dosage Forms and Strengths

Tablets — 25 mg, 100 mg

▷ **Usual Adult Dosage Ranges:** *Resistant schizophrenia:* Starts with 12.5 mg once or two times a day; the dose is gradually increased by 25 mg to 50 mg daily, as tolerated, to reach a dose of 300 mg to 450 mg daily (divided into three doses) by the end of 2 weeks. Later increases should be limited to 100 mg one or two times a week. For ongoing (maintenance) doses, the lowest effective dose should be used. One researcher commented on dosing ranges from 50 to 900 mg daily. **Note: Actual dose and schedule must be determined for each patient individually.**

Conditions Requiring Dosing Adjustments

Liver Function: Eliminated in the liver; however, no specific dosing guidelines are available.

Kidney Function: Patients with kidney failure should be watched closely for adverse effects.

▷ **Dosing Instructions:** May be taken without regard to meals or with food if necessary to reduce stomach irritation. The tablet may be crushed. If you forget a dose: Take the missed dose as soon as you remember it, unless it is nearly time for the next scheduled dose—then skip the missed dose and take the scheduled dose on time. DO NOT double doses.

Usual Duration of Use: Benefits may be seen after 2 to 4 weeks of regular use. Peak effect may require 3 to 12 months. If no significant benefit is seen in 6 to 8 weeks, the drug should be stopped. Long-term use requires periodic evaluation by your doctor.

Typical Treatment Goals and Measurements (Outcomes and Markers)

Schizophrenia: The general goal: to ease the severity of symptoms in order to let the patient resume his or her usual activities. There should be lessened time spent with prior intrusions of abnormal thinking into more normal life.

Possible Advantages of This Drug: Rarely causes significant sexual dysfunction. Low incidence of Parkinson-like reactions (see Glossary). Only case reports of tardive dyskinesia (see Glossary). Medicines in this class are probably drugs of choice in older adults.

Currently a Drug of Choice: For treatment of severe schizophrenia in patients who have not responded to other standard antipsychotic drugs.

▷ **This Drug Should Not Be Taken If**
- you have had an allergic reaction to it previously.
- you have had severe bone marrow depression (impaired white blood cell production) with previous use of this drug.
- you have a bone marrow or blood cell disorder.
- you have epilepsy that is not controlled.
- you take any other drug that can cause bone marrow depression (see Glossary).

▷ **Inform Your Physician Before Taking This Drug If**
- you have a history of any type of seizure disorder.
- you have a history of narrow-angle glaucoma.
- you have any type of heart or circulatory disorder, especially heart rhythm abnormalities or hypertension.
- you have diabetes or glucose intolerance.
- your body is very depleted (cachectic).
- you have impaired liver or kidney function.
- you have prostatism (see Glossary).

Possible Side Effects (natural, expected and unavoidable drug actions)
Drowsiness, sedation—frequent.
Weight gain—frequent.
Dizziness, light-headedness—infrequent to frequent.
Orthostatic hypotension (see Glossary)—possible.
Blurred vision, salivation, dry mouth, impaired urination, constipation—possible.

▷ **Possible Adverse Effects** (unusual, unexpected and infrequent reactions)
If any of the following develop, consult your physician promptly for guidance.
Mild Adverse Effects
Allergic reactions: skin rash; drug fever (see Glossary), which usually occurs within the first 3 weeks of treatment and is self-limiting—rare.
Headache, tremor, fainting, sleep disorders, restlessness, confusion, depression—rare.
Increased salivation—frequent.
Rapid heartbeat, hypertension, chest pain—rare to infrequent.
Nausea, indigestion, vomiting, diarrhea—rare.

Serious Adverse Effects
Allergic reactions: asthmatic-type respiratory reaction—case reports.
Bone marrow depression: specific impairment of white blood cell production with potential for serious infection—rare.
Glucose intolerance—case reports.
Drug-induced seizures, dose-related—rare.
Tardive dyskinesia—case reports.
Abnormally low blood pressure on standing (orthostatic hypotension)—possible.
Anticholinergic syndrome—rare.
Neuroleptic malignant syndrome—case reports.

▷ **Possible Effects on Sexual Function:** Decreased libido and impotence—infrequent and dose-related (over 150 mg).
Abnormal ejaculation or priapism (see Glossary)—rare.

Adverse Effects That May Mimic Natural Diseases or Disorders

Drug-induced fever may suggest systemic infection. Because of the risk of bone marrow depression and secondary infection, any occurrence of fever must be carefully evaluated. Drug-induced seizures may suggest the possibility of epilepsy.

Natural Diseases or Disorders That May Be Activated by This Drug

Latent glaucoma, prostatism, diabetes.

Possible Effects on Laboratory Tests

White blood cell counts: decreased.

CAUTION

1. Baseline white blood cell counts must be checked before clozapine treatment is started; follow-up counts must be made every week during the entire course of treatment and for 4 weeks after discontinuation of clozapine.
2. Promptly report any signs of infection: fever, sore throat, flu-like symptoms, skin infections, painful urination, etc.
3. Report promptly light-headedness or dizziness on rising from a sitting or lying position—this could be orthostatic hypotension (see Glossary).
4. There have been case reports of glucose intolerance and diabetes mellitus with this medicine.
5. Call your doctor before taking any other medication. This includes all prescription and over-the-counter drugs.

Precautions for Use

By Infants and Children: An open label trial of 11 patients from 12 to 17 years old used 12.5 to 25 mg per day as a starting dose and increased every 4 days by one or two times the starting dose. This dosing strategy was used to treat refractory childhood-onset schizophrenia. Mean trial dose was 370 mg per day.

By Those Over 60 Years of Age: Starting doses of 6.25 to 12.5 mg are prudent with required increases not exceeding 25 mg a day. There is an increased risk of orthostatic hypotension, confusion, blood problems and prostatism. Report related symptoms promptly.

▷ **Advisability of Use During Pregnancy**

Pregnancy Category: B. See Pregnancy Risk Categories at the back of this book.
Animal studies: No birth defects due to this drug reported.
Human studies: Adequate studies of pregnant women are not available.
Use this drug only if clearly needed.

Advisability of Use If Breast-Feeding

Presence of this drug in breast milk: Yes, in animal studies.
Avoid drug or refrain from nursing.

Habit-Forming Potential: None, but a withdrawal syndrome has been reported after suddenly stopping long-term therapy.

Effects of Overdose: Marked drowsiness, delirium, hallucinations, rapid and irregular heartbeat, irregular breathing, fainting.

Possible Effects of Long-Term Use: Tardive dyskinesia—case report.

Suggested Periodic Examinations While Taking This Drug (at physician's discretion)

White blood and differential counts prior to starting therapy, every week during therapy, and for 4 weeks after stopping therapy.
Serial blood pressure measurements and electrocardiograms.

▷ **While Taking This Drug, Observe the Following**
 Foods: No restrictions.
 Herbal Medicines or Minerals: Kava and valerian may worsen drowsiness. Since part of the way that ginseng and ginkgo biloba works is as an MAO inhibitor, combination with this medicine is not advisable.
 Beverages: No restrictions. May be taken with milk.
▷ *Alcohol:* Avoid completely. Alcohol increases clozapine-induced sedation and can worsen possible undesirable side effects of clozapine on blood pressure and brain function.
 Tobacco Smoking: May accelerate the elimination of this drug and require increased dosage. I advise everyone to quit smoking.
 Marijuana Smoking: Moderate increase in drowsiness, worsening of orthostatic hypotension, increased risk of aggravating psychosis.
▷ *Other Drugs*

 Clozapine may ***increase*** the effects of
- antihypertensive drugs; observe for excessive lowering of blood pressure.
- drugs with atropinelike actions (see Drug Classes).
- drugs with sedative actions (see benzodiazepines, etc.); observe for excessive sedation.

 Clozapine ***taken concurrently*** with
- other bone marrow depressant drugs, such as carbamazepine (Tegretol), may increase the risk of impaired white blood cell production.
- buspirone (Buspar) may excessively elevate blood sugar and also lead to bleeding.
- carbamazepine (Tegretol) may increase risk of low white blood cells.
- cimetidine (Tagamet) can result in a toxic level of clozapine.
- erythromycin (E-Mycin, others) can result in increased clozapine concentrations and potential toxicity. This has been seen in a single case report, but caution is advised.
- fluoxetine (Prozac) can result in clozapine toxicity.
- fluvoxamine (Luvox) can result in clozapine toxicity.
- lithium (Lithobid, Lithotab, etc.) may increase the risk of confusional states, seizures and neuroleptic malignant syndrome (see Glossary).
- monoamine oxidase inhibitors (MAO inhibitors; see Drug Class) may cause abnormally low blood pressure and exaggerated central nervous system response.
- nefazodone (Serzone) may lead to clozapine toxicity.
- other medicines that interfere with cytochrome P450 3A4 may increase clozapine levels and increase risk of clozapine side effects or toxicity.
- paroxetine (Paxil) may lead to toxicity from either medicine.
- phenytoin (Dilantin) and fosphenytoin (Cerebyx) can cause a decreased clozapine level and result in breakthrough schizophrenia.
- risperidone (Risperdal).
- ritonavir (Norvir), and perhaps other protease inhibitors (see Drug Classes), may lead to increased risk of blood adverse effects or other adverse effects. DO NOT COMBINE.
- sertraline (Zoloft) can result in clozapine toxicity.
- tramadol (Ultram) may increase seizure risks.
- venlafaxine (Effexor) may lead to clozapine toxicity.

▷ *Driving, Hazardous Activities:* This drug may cause drowsiness, dizziness, blurred vision, confusion and seizures. Restrict activities as necessary.

Aviation Note: The use of this drug ***is a disqualification*** for piloting. Consult a designated Aviation Medical Examiner.

Exposure to Sun: No restrictions except for heat adaptation (see below).

Exposure to Heat: Use caution. This drug can cause fever and can impair the body's adaptation to heat.

Occurrence of Unrelated Illness: Infections must be vigorously treated. White blood cell response to infection must be followed closely.

Discontinuation: If possible, this drug should be discontinued gradually over a period of 1 to 2 weeks. If abrupt withdrawal is necessary, observe carefully for recurrence of psychotic symptoms.

CODEINE (KOH deen)

Introduced: 1886   **Class:** Analgesic, narcotic, opioid   **Prescription:** USA: Yes   **Controlled Drug:** USA: C-II*; Canada: No   **Available as Generic:** Yes

Brand Names: A.B.C. Compound w/Codeine [CD], AC&C [CD], Accopain, Acta-gen-C [CD], Actifed w/Codeine [CD], Afed-C [CD], Alamine-C [CD], Alamine Expectorant [CD], Ambenyl Expectorant [CD], Ambenyl Syrup [CD], Anacin 3 w/Codeine #2–4, Anacin w/Codeine [CD], APC w/Codeine [CD], Atasol-8, -15, -30 [CD], Ban-Tuiss C [CD], Benylin Syrup w/Codeine [CD], Bitex [CD], Bromanyl Cough Syrup [CD], Bromotuss, Bromphen DC [CD], Brontex [CD], Bufferin w/Codeine [CD], Butalbital Compound [CD], Chemdal Expectorant [CD], Chem-Tuss NE [CD], Cheracol [CD], Chlor-Trimeton Expectorant [CD], Coactifed [CD], Codecon-C [CD], Codehist DH, Codehist Elixir, ♣Codeine Contin (timed release), ♣Coricidin w/Codeine [CD], ♣Coryphen-Codeine [CD], ♣C2 Buffered, ♣C2 w/Codeine, Deproist [CD], Dimetane Cough Syrup-DC [CD], Dimetane Expectorant-C [CD], Dimetapp-C [CD], Dimetapp w/Codeine [CD], Empirin w/Codeine No. 2, 4 [CD], ♣Empracet-30, -60 [CD], Empracet w/Codeine No. 3, 4 [CD], ♣Emtec-30 [CD], ♣Exdol-8, -15, -30 [CD], ♣Extra Strength Acetaminophen with Codeine [CD], ♣Fiorinal-C ¼, -C ½ [CD], Fiorinal w/Codeine No. 1, 2, 3 [CD], Gecil [CD], Glydeine, Isoclor Expectorant [CD], ♣Lenoltec w/Codeine No. 1, 2, 3, 4 [CD], ♣Mersyndol, Naldecon-CX [CD], Normatane [CD], Novadyne DH [CD], ♣Novahistex C [CD], ♣Novo-Gesic, Nucochem [CD], Nucofed [CD], ♣Omni-Tuss [CD], Oridol-C [CD], Panadol w/Codeine [CD], ♣Paveral, Pedi-acof [CD], Penntuss [CD], ♣Phenaphen No. 2, 3, 4 [CD], Phenaphen w/Codeine No. 2, 3, 4 [CD], Phenergan w/Codeine [CD], Poly-Histine [CD], Promethazine CS [CD], Pyra-Phed [CD], ♣Robaxacet-8, Robaxisal-C [CD], ♣Rounox w/Codeine [CD], SK-Apap [CD], Tamine Expectorant DC [CD], ♣Tecnal C [CD], Terpin Hydrate and Codeine [CD], ♣318 AC&C [CD], Tri-afed w/Codeine [CD], Triaminic Expectorant w/Codeine [CD], ♣Triatec-8, 30 [CD], ♣Tussaminic C Forte [CD], ♣Tussaminic C Ped [CD], ♣Tussi-Organidin [CD], ♣222 [CD], ♣282 [CD], ♣292 [CD], ♣Tylenol w/Codeine [CD], Tylenol w/Codeine No. 1, 2, 3, 4 [CD], Tylenol w/Codeine Elixir [CD], ♣VC Expectorant w/Codeine, ♣Veganin [CD]

*See Schedules of Controlled Drugs at the back of this book.

BENEFITS versus RISKS	
Possible Benefits	*Possible Risks*
RELIEF OF MILD TO MODERATE PAIN	Potential for habit formation (dependence)
VERY EFFECTIVE CONTROL OF COUGH	Mild allergic reactions—infrequent
	Nausea, constipation

▷ **Principal Uses**

As a Single Drug Product: Uses currently included in FDA-approved labeling: (1) Relieves mild to moderate pain; (2) controls cough—its widest use is as an ingredient in analgesic preparations and cough remedies.

Other (unlabeled) generally accepted uses: (1) Limited role in controlling diarrhea; (2) migraine during pregnancy.

As a Combination Drug Product [CD]: Codeine is combined with other analgesics (aspirin and acetaminophen) on the World Health Organization pain ladder to increase overall pain control. It is also added to cough mixtures containing antihistamines, decongestants and expectorants.

How This Drug Works: By depressing some brain functions, this drug decreases pain perception, calms emotional responses to pain and reduces cough reflex sensitivity.

Available Dosage Forms and Strengths

Injection — 30 mg/ml, 60 mg/ml

Tablets — 15 mg, 30 mg, 60 mg

Tablets, soluble — 15 mg, 30 mg, 60 mg

▷ **Usual Adult Dosage Ranges:** *As analgesic:* 15 to 60 mg every 4 hours. **Author's Note: Current pain treatment theory calls for timed or scheduled dosing. This tends to prevent pain, rather than allowing pain to recur and then having to be treated. Some clinicians will use timed dosing immediately after surgery and then revert to as-needed dosing once the most severe period of pain has passed. Pain is now the fifth vital sign.** *For cough:* 10 to 20 mg every 4 to 6 hours as needed. Maximum daily dose 200 mg for pain, 120 mg for cough. **Note: Actual dose and schedule must be determined for each patient individually.**

Conditions Requiring Dosing Adjustments

Liver Function: The dose must be decreased in liver compromise.

Kidney Function: Dose decreased by up to 50% in moderate to severe failure.

▷ **Dosing Instructions:** Tablet may be crushed and then taken with or following food to reduce stomach irritation or nausea. If you forget a dose: take it as soon as you remember, unless it's nearly time for your next dose—then omit the dose you forgot and take the next scheduled dose. DO NOT double doses.

Usual Duration of Use: As long as it is needed to control cough (usually the shortest time required). Use for pain should not exceed 5 to 7 days without reassessment of need.

Typical Treatment Goals and Measurements (Outcomes and Markers)

Pain: Most clinicians treating pain use a device called an algometer to check your pain. This looks like a small ruler, but lets the clinician better understand your pain. The goals of treatment then relate to where the level of pain started (for example, a rating of 7 on a zero to ten scale) and what the cause of the pain was. Pain medicines may also be used together (in combination) in order to get the best result or outcome. If your pain control is not acceptable to YOU (remember, in hospitals and outpatient settings, etc., pain control is a patient right) and if after a week of pain treatment, results are not acceptable, be sure to call your doctor as you may need a different medicine or combination.

▷ **This Drug Should Not Be Taken If**
- you have had an allergic reaction to any form of it.
- you are having an acute attack of asthma.
- your breathing is depressed (respiratory depression).

▷ **Inform Your Physician Before Taking This Drug If**
- you have a history of drug abuse or alcoholism.
- you have impaired liver or kidney function.
- you have gallbladder disease, a seizure disorder or an underactive thyroid gland.
- you have chronic obstructive pulmonary disease (COPD) or other lung problems such as asthma.
- you have low blood calcium (increased sensitivity to this medicine).
- you have a history of porphyria.
- you tend to be constipated.
- you are taking any other drugs that have a sedative effect.
- you will have surgery with general anesthesia.

Possible Side Effects (natural, expected and unavoidable drug actions)
Drowsiness, light-headedness, dry mouth, urinary retention—possible.
Constipation—frequent and dose-related. (Best to start a stool softener or related medicine before codeine is started if you are prone to constipation.)

▷ **Possible Adverse Effects** (unusual, unexpected and infrequent reactions)
If any of the following develop, consult your physician promptly for guidance.
Mild Adverse Effects
Allergic reactions: skin rash, hives, itching—case reports.
Dizziness, impaired concentration, sensation of drunkenness, confusion, depression, blurred or double vision—infrequent.
Nausea, vomiting—frequent and may be dose-related.
Serious Adverse Effects
Allergic reactions: anaphylaxis, severe skin reactions—case reports.
Idiosyncratic reactions: delirium, hallucinations, excitement, increased pain sensitivity once the medicine wears off.
Seizures—rare.
Impaired breathing—dose-related.
Porphyria—case reports.
Liver toxicity—case reports.

▷ **Possible Effects on Sexual Function:** Opiates have a variety of effects on sexual response. These may range from blunting of sexual response to increased response if anxiety has been a factor inhibiting response—case reports.

Adverse Effects That May Mimic Natural Diseases or Disorders
Paradoxical behavioral disturbances may suggest psychotic disorder.

Possible Effects on Laboratory Tests

Blood platelet counts: decreased.

Blood amylase and lipase levels: increased (natural side effect).

Urine screening tests for drug abuse: may be positive. (Test results depend upon amount of drug taken and testing method used.)

CAUTION

1. If you have asthma, chronic bronchitis or emphysema, use of this drug may cause respiratory difficulty, thickening of secretions and decrease of needed cough reflex.
2. Combining this drug with atropinelike drugs can increase the risk of urinary retention and reduced intestinal function.
3. Do not take this drug following acute head injury.

Precautions for Use

By Infants and Children: Do not use this drug in children under 2 years of age (possible life-threatening respiratory depression). Children 2 to 6 years old can receive 1 mg per kg of body mass per day, divided into four equal doses. Maximum dose is 30 mg per day. Children 6 to 12 years of age can receive 5 to 10 mg per dose every 4 to 6 hours, to a maximum of 60 mg every 24 hours.

By Those Over 60 Years of Age: Small starting doses and short-term use is indicated. Expect increased risk of drowsiness, dizziness, unsteadiness, falling, urinary retention and constipation (often leading to fecal impaction).

▷ **Advisability of Use During Pregnancy**

Pregnancy Category: C; D if used in high doses or for prolonged periods near the time the baby is about to be born. See Pregnancy Risk Categories at the back of this book.

Animal studies: Skull defects reported in hamster studies.

Human studies: Adequate studies of pregnant women are not available. Some studies suggest an increase in significant birth defects when this drug is taken during the first 6 months of pregnancy. Codeine taken during the last few weeks before delivery can cause withdrawal symptoms in the newborn.

Use only if clearly needed and in small, infrequent doses.

▷ **Advisability of Use If Breast-Feeding**

Presence of this drug in breast milk: Yes, in small amounts.

Avoid drug or refrain from nursing.

▷ **Habit-Forming Potential:** Psychological and/or physical dependence can develop with use of large doses for an extended period of time. True dependence is infrequent, however, and unlikely with prudent use.

Effects of Overdose: Drowsiness, restlessness, agitation, nausea, vomiting, dry mouth, vertigo, weakness, lethargy, stupor, coma, seizures.

Possible Effects of Long-Term Use: Psychological and physical dependence, chronic constipation.

Suggested Periodic Examinations While Taking This Drug (at physician's discretion)

Periodic check for constipation, especially in older patients.

▷ **While Taking This Drug, Observe the Following**

Foods: No restrictions.

Herbal Medicines or Minerals: Valerian and kava kava may interact additively (drowsiness). Avoid these combinations. St. John's wort can change (inducing or increasing) P450 3A4 enzymes, blunting the effects of this medicine. Talk to your doctor BEFORE you combine any herbals with codeine.

Beverages: No restrictions. May be taken with milk.

▷ *Alcohol:* DO NOT COMBINE. Codeine intensifies alcohol, and alcohol intensifies codeine depressant effects on brain function, breathing and circulation.

Tobacco Smoking: Tobacco smoking may cause decreased pain tolerance and require an increased or more frequent dose of codeine. I advise everyone to quit smoking.

Marijuana Smoking: Increases drowsiness and pain relief. Mental and physical performance will be impaired.

▷ *Other Drugs*

Codeine may ***increase*** the effects of

- atropinelike drugs and increase the risk of constipation and urinary retention.
- monoamine oxidase (MAO) inhibitors and also increase central nervous system symptoms and depression.
- other drugs with sedative effects.
- tramadol (Ultram).

Codeine ***taken concurrently*** with

- quinidine may decrease codeine pain control.
- rifabutin (Mycobutin) may decrease codeine effectiveness.
- ritonavir (Norvir) may blunt codeine benefits.

▷ *Driving, Hazardous Activities:* This drug can impair mental alertness, judgment, reaction time and physical coordination. Avoid hazardous activities accordingly.

Aviation Note: The use of this drug ***is a disqualification*** for piloting. Consult a designated Aviation Medical Examiner.

Exposure to Sun: No restrictions.

Discontinuation: Best to limit use to short-term. If extended use occurs, gradual decreases in dose are prudent to minimize possible withdrawal (usually mild with codeine).

COLCHICINE (KOL chi seen)

Introduced: 1763   **Class:** Antigout **Prescription:** USA: Yes   **Controlled Drug:** USA: No; Canada: No   **Available as Generic:** Yes

Brand Names: Colbenemid [CD], Col-Probenecid [CD], Colsalide, Proben-C [CD]

BENEFITS versus RISKS	
Possible Benefits	*Possible Risks*
EFFECTIVE RELIEF OF ACUTE GOUT SYMPTOMS	Loss of hair
	Rare bone marrow depression (see Glossary)
Prevention of recurrent gout attacks	
Prevention of attacks of Mediterranean fever	Rare peripheral neuritis (see Glossary)
	Rare liver damage

▷ **Principal Uses**

As a Single Drug Product: Uses currently included in FDA-approved labeling: (1) Reduces pain, swelling and inflammation seen in acute gout attacks (many clinicians prefer NSAIDs [see Drug Classes] as drugs of first choice in acute gout); (2) also used in smaller doses to prevent recurrent gout attacks.

Other (unlabeled) generally accepted uses: (1) Prevention and control of attacks of familial Mediterranean fever; (2) may have a role in easing symptoms of Behçet's disease; (3) limited use in cirrhosis of the liver; (4) damaged disk syndrome may be helped in some patients; (5) may have a role in recurrent pericarditis; (6) can be of help in pseudogout; (7) appears to be of benefit in some lung disease (idiopathic pulmonary fibrosis); (8) treats some cases of refractory immune thrombocytopenic purpura.

As a Combination Drug Product [CD]: Colchicine combined with probenecid enhances its ability to prevent recurrent attacks of gout. Colchicine is most effective in relieving acute gout; it has some effect in preventing recurrent and chronic discomfort. Probenecid increases removal of uric acid by the kidneys and reduces risk of acute gout. This dual action is more effective than either drug used alone in long-term management of gout.

How This Drug Works: Decreasing joint tissue acid, lowering painful uric acid deposits and acute inflammation and pain. (Colchicine does not lower uric acid in the blood or increase urine removal.)

Available Dosage Forms and Strengths

Injection — 1 mg/2 ml

Tablets — 0.5 mg, 0.6 mg, 0.65 mg (also 1 mg in Canada)

▷ **Usual Adult Dosage Ranges:** *For acute attack:* 0.5 to 1.2 mg, followed by 0.5 to 0.65 mg every 1 to 2 hours until pain eases or nausea, vomiting or diarrhea occurs. Maximum total dose is 8 mg. *For preventing recurrent attacks:* 0.5 to 0.65 mg, one to three times per day. *Pericarditis:* 1 mg daily to start, followed by 0.5 mg daily. **Note: Actual dose and schedule must be determined for each patient individually.**

Conditions Requiring Dosing Adjustments

Liver Function: Caution must be used, and the dose decreased, if there is a bile obstruction. This drug should NOT be used in people with both liver and kidney compromise.

Kidney Function: For severe kidney failure, 50% of the usual dose should be given. Ongoing preventive use NOT prudent in moderate (creatinine clearance less than 50 ml/min) kidney problems. Those with creatinine clearances less than 10 ml/min should NOT be given this medicine.

▷ **Dosing Instructions:** The tablet may be crushed and then either taken on an empty stomach or with food to reduce nausea or stomach irritation. Start treatment at the first sign of an acute attack. Take the exact dose prescribed. While dosing should be individualized, once the dose needed to abort a sudden (acute) attack is identified, the patient should keep that supply on hand in order to stop an acute attack. Remember that if diarrhea or stomach and intestine (gastrointestinal) side effects happen, the drug needs to be stopped. If you forget a dose: take the dose you forgot as soon as you remember it, unless it's nearly time for your next dose. If it's nearly time for your next dose, skip the dose you missed and simply take the next scheduled dose. DO NOT double doses.

Usual Duration of Use: For acute attack, stop the drug when pain is relieved or when nausea, vomiting or diarrhea occurs; do not restart this drug for 3 days without asking your doctor. Total doses of 8 mg should not be exceeded. For prevention, use the smallest dose that works. Ask your doctor about dosing.

Typical Treatment Goals and Measurements (Outcomes and Markers)

Gout: Blood uric acid levels are not changed by this medicine (tissue deposits are), but gout pain decreases (lowered by ongoing use of this drug as in dosing section) or limiting nausea defines response or highest tolerable dose of colchicine. Call your doctor if an acute attack of gout is not stopped or if you have reached dose-limiting nausea or vomiting.

▷ **This Drug Should Not Be Taken If**
- you have had an allergic reaction to it previously.
- you have an active stomach or duodenal ulcer.
- you have active ulcerative colitis.
- you have a severe kidney or liver disorder.
- you have a serious heart disorder.
- you are pregnant.
- you have a history of blood cell disorders.

▷ **Inform Your Physician Before Taking This Drug If**
- you have peptic ulcer disease or ulcerative colitis.
- you develop diarrhea and vomiting while taking this drug.
- you have any type of heart disease.
- you have impaired liver or kidney function.
- you plan to have surgery in the near future.

Possible Side Effects (natural, expected and unavoidable drug actions)

Nausea, vomiting, abdominal cramping, diarrhea—frequent, especially with maximum doses.

▷ **Possible Adverse Effects** (unusual, unexpected and infrequent reactions)

If any of the following develop, consult your physician promptly for guidance.

Mild Adverse Effects

Allergic reactions: skin rash, hives, fever—rare.

Hair loss—reported after overdoses.

Serious Adverse Effects

Allergic reaction: anaphylactic reaction (see Glossary)—case reports.

Bone marrow depression (see Glossary): fatigue, weakness, fever, sore throat, abnormal bleeding or bruising—case reports.

Peripheral neuritis (see Glossary): numbness, tingling, pain, weakness in hands and/or feet or myopathy with nerve symptoms (facial palsy and weakness, especially with long-term use in patients with declines in kidney function)—case reports.

Rhabdomyolysis—case reports.

Porphyria—case reports.

Drooping of the eyes (ptosis)—case reports.

Inflammation of colon with bloody diarrhea—case reports.

Thrombophlebitis with intravenous use—case reports.

▷ **Possible Effects on Sexual Function:** Reversible absence of sperm (azoospermia).

Possible Delayed Adverse Effects: Impaired production of sperm, possibly resulting in birth defects.

A rare combined muscle and nerve damage syndrome.

Natural Diseases or Disorders That May Be Activated by This Drug

Peptic ulcer disease, ulcerative colitis.

Possible Effects on Laboratory Tests

Complete blood cell counts: decreased red cells, hemoglobin, white cells and platelets; increased white cells (follows initial decrease).

Prothrombin time: decreased (with concurrent use of warfarin).

Blood vitamin B_{12} level: decreased.

Liver function tests: increased liver enzymes (ALT/GPT, AST/GOT and alkaline phosphatase), increased bilirubin.

Fecal occult blood test: positive.

Sperm counts: decreased (may be marked).

CAUTION

1. If this drug causes vomiting and/or diarrhea before relief of joint pain, stop it and call your doctor.
2. Try to limit each course of treatment for acute gout to 4 to 8 mg. Do not exceed 3 mg every 24 hours or a total of 8 mg per course.
3. Omit drug for 3 days between courses to avoid toxicity.
4. Carry this drug with you while traveling if you are subject to attacks of acute gout.
5. Surgical stress can cause a gout attack. Ask your doctor how much colchicine should be taken before and after surgery to prevent gout.
6. This medicine may inhibit healing of the cornea. Talk to your doctor about this if you will have eye surgery.

Precautions for Use

By Infants and Children: Use for preventing (prophylaxis) familial Mediterranean fever in children 6 to 13 years of age was given as 0.5 mg per day and increased by 0.5 mg per day, to symptom control or a maximum of 2 mg per day. For other uses in children, dosage has not been established. Ask your physician for guidance.

By Those Over 60 Years of Age: Because the dosage needed to relieve acute gout often causes vomiting and/or diarrhea, extreme caution is advised if you have heart or circulatory disorders, reduced liver or kidney function or general debility.

▷ **Advisability of Use During Pregnancy**

Pregnancy Category: C by one manufacturer, and D by another source. See Pregnancy Risk Categories at the back of this book.

Animal studies: This drug causes significant birth defects in hamsters and rabbits.

Human studies: Adequate studies of pregnant women are not available. However, it is reported that colchicine can cause harm to the fetus.

Avoid during entire pregnancy if possible. Ask your physician for guidance.

Advisability of Use If Breast-Feeding

Presence of this drug in breast milk: Yes.

Ask your doctor for help. The American Academy of Pediatrics considers this medicine compatible with breast-feeding.

Habit-Forming Potential: None.

Effects of Overdose: Nausea, vomiting, abdominal cramping, diarrhea (may be bloody), burning sensation in throat and skin, weak and rapid pulse, progressive paralysis, inability to breathe.

Possible Effects of Long-Term Use: Hair loss, aplastic anemia (see Glossary), peripheral neuritis (see Glossary).

Suggested Periodic Examinations While Taking This Drug (at physician's discretion)

Complete blood cell counts.

Uric acid blood levels to monitor status of gout.

Sperm analysis for quantity and condition.

Liver function tests.

▷ **While Taking This Drug, Observe the Following**

Foods: Follow your doctor's advice about a low-purine diet.

Herbal Medicines or Minerals: Acerola is high in vitamin C. Inosine, like acerola, may increase uric acid levels. Aspen should be avoided in gout. Lipase may worsen gout. Goutweed (*Aegopodium podagraria*) does not have enough data to assess effectiveness. Some "herbal teas" (promoted as being beneficial for arthritis) contain phenylbutazone and other potentially toxic ingredients. Avoid herbal teas if you are not certain of their source, content and medicinal effects.

Beverages: Drink at least 3 quarts of liquids every 24 hours. This drug may be taken with milk.

▷ *Alcohol:* No interactions expected. Combination may increase the risk of gastrointestinal irritation or bleeding and raise uric acid blood levels.

Tobacco Smoking: No interactions expected. I advise everyone to quit smoking.

▷ *Other Drugs*

Colchicine *taken concurrently* with

- allopurinol (Zyloprim), probenecid (Benemid) or sulfinpyrazone (Anturane) can prevent attacks of acute gout that often occur when treatment with these drugs is first started.
- cyanocobalamin will decrease absorption of the vitamin B_{12}. Higher doses of oral cyanocobalamin may be required by patients on colchicine.
- cyclosporine (Sandimmune) may increase cyclosporine levels and result in toxicity.
- erythromycins (E.E.S., clarithromycin) can result in toxic colchicine blood levels.
- insulin may inhibit the response (biphasic) of the body to sugar.

▷ *Driving, Hazardous Activities:* Usually no restrictions when taken continually in small (preventive) doses. May cause nausea, vomiting and/or diarrhea when taken in larger (treatment) doses.

Aviation Note: The use of this drug *may be a disqualification* for piloting. Consult a designated Aviation Medical Examiner.

Exposure to Sun: No restrictions.

Exposure to Cold: This drug can lower body temperature. Use caution to prevent excessive lowering (hypothermia), especially in those over 60 years of age.

Occurrence of Unrelated Illness: Acute attacks of gout may result from injury or illness. Call your doctor for dosing adjustment if injury or new illness occurs.

COLD SORE AND GENITAL HERPES TREATMENT
FAMILY (KOLD sore)

Acyclovir (ay SI kloh veer)   **Famciclovir** (fam SEYE klo veer)   **Penci-clovir** (PEN SI kloh veer)   **Valacyclovir** (val a SY klo veer) **Docosanol cream (Abreva)** (a BREE vah):   **Author's Note: Once head-to-head trials have been conducted with prescription and this new non-prescription medicine for cold sores, information will be included in this profile. (This new medicine needs to be applied 12 hours after itching or redness and appears to work by inhibiting fusion between the skin membrane and the herpes virus envelope.)**

Other Name: *Acyclovir*: Acycloguanosine   **Other medicines:** None
Introduced: 1979, 1994, 1997, 1996   **Class:** Antiviral, cold sore medicines, anti-herpes virus   **Prescription:** USA: Yes   **Controlled Drug:** USA: No; Canada: No   **Available as Generic:** Yes acyclovir: (capsule, suspension and tablets). No for famciclovir, penciclovir, valacyclovir

Brand Names: *Ayclovir*: Zovirax; *Famciclovir*: Famvir; *Penciclovir*: Denavir; *Valacyclovir*: Valtrex

---

BENEFITS versus RISKS

Possible Benefits	*Possible Risks*
Acyclovir:	*Acyclovir systemic use*:
TREATMENT OF ENCEPHALITIS CAUSED BY HERPES SIMPLEX	Nausea, vomiting, diarrhea
	Joint and muscle pain
TREATMENT OF CHICKENPOX	Seizures or coma with IV use—rare
Acyclovir, famciclovir and valacyclovir:	*Famciclovir*:
FASTER RECOVERY FROM	Purpura
INITIAL EPISODE OF GENITAL	Paresthesias
HERPES	*Valacyclovir*:
TREATMENT OF SUDDEN (ACUTE)	Rare reports of thrombotic
SHINGLES (HERPES ZOSTER)	thrombocytopenic purpura (TTP)
PREVENTION OF RECURRENCE	in HIV and bone marrow or kidney
OF GENITAL HERPES	transplant patients
Valacyclovir:	*Acyclovir and penciclovir topical use*:
ORAL (BY MOUTH) DOSING	Skin redness or irritation
ACHIEVES BLOOD LEVELS	
SIMILAR TO THOSE OBTAINED	
FROM INTRAVENOUS DOSING	
NEWLY APPROVED 3-DAY DOSING	
FOR VALACYCLOVIR FOR	
RECURRENT GENITAL HERPES	
WILL HELP ADHERENCE	
Acyclovir, famciclovir and penciclovir:	
TREATMENT OF HERPES	
SIMPLEX OF THE LIPS (COLD	
SORES OR MUCOCUTANEOUS HERPES)	

Author's Note: Acyclovir was again rejected by the FDA for a change to non-prescription "over-the-counter" (OTC) status. This was based on fear of development of viral resistance—NOT on safety issues.

▷ **Principal Uses**

As a Single Drug Product: Uses currently included in FDA-approved labeling:

Acyclovir only: (1) Used to treat varicella (chickenpox) in children over a year old who have a chronic lung disease or skin condition, who take aspirin regularly, who are receiving short courses of corticosteroids via the lungs, or are over 13 years old and are otherwise healthy (must be started within 24 hours of symptoms); (2) used to treat brain infections caused by herpes simplex (encephalitis); (3) used to prevent herpes simplex virus infections in bone marrow transplant patients.

Acyclovir, famciclovir and valacyclovir: (1) Treats or helps prevent genital herpes; (2) treats shingles (herpes zoster).

Acyclovir and famciclovir: (1) treats skin and mucous membrane infections (mucocutaneous) caused by herpes simplex in patients with immune problems; (2) treatment of cold sores (mucocutaneous herpes) of the lips and face.

Famciclovir only: used in severe damage to the retina (retinal necrosis syndrome) in cases where acyclovir has failed to work.

Other (unlabeled) generally accepted uses: (1) Acyclovir helps treat herpes simplex infections of the eye and rectum, and pneumonia caused by the chickenpox (varicella) virus; (2) some data support its use in nonmalignant skin growths in the throat (laryngeal papillomatosis); (3) prevention of repeat episodes of herpes eye infections; (4) penciclovir may have a role in herpes infections of the genitals; (5) famciclovir may help treat hepatitis B; (6) some combination data with interferon alpha and famciclovir in treating polyarteritis nodosa are promising; (7) valacyclovir may have a role in erythema multiforme and in decreasing risk of cytomegalovirus disease in kidney transplant patients.

Author's Note: A study of 455 patients reported in JAMA found that when famciclovir was correctly taken for 1 year to suppress herpes simplex virus (HSV), nearly 75% of those patients did NOT have any HSV outbreaks during that year.

How These Drugs Work: By blocking genetic material formation of the herpes simplex virus, this drug stops viral multiplication and spread, reducing severity and duration of the herpes infection. Use at the first sign of infection (such as the "itch" of a cold sore) can prevent a full blown lesion. Famciclovir is changed in the body to penciclovir. Valacyclovir is rapidly changed into acyclovir in the body and enters the body to a much greater extent than acyclovir.

Available Dosage Forms and Strengths

Acyclovir:
Capsules — 200 mg, 400 mg, 800 mg
Intravenous — 500 mg, 1 g
Oral suspension — 200 mg/5 ml
Tablets — 200 mg, 400 mg, 500 mg, 800 mg
Ointment — 5%, 50 mg/g (Canada)

Famciclovir:
Tablets — 125 mg, 250 mg, 500 mg

Penciclovir:
Ointment — 1%

Valacyclovir:
>   Caplets — 500 mg, 1,000 mg

▷ **Recommended Dosage Ranges** (Actual dose and schedule must be determined for each patient individually.)

Infants and Children:

Acyclovir: In children less than 12 who have deficient immune systems (immunocompromised), intravenous acyclovir has been used (250 mg per square meter given over 1 hour) every 8 hours in a week-long treatment for skin and mouth herpes simplex infections. Safety and efficacy of oral use in children younger than 6 weeks of age have NOT been established.

Famciclovir, penciclovir and valacyclovir: Safety and efficacy in infants and children not established.

18 to 65 Years of Age:

Acyclovir: For first episode of genital herpes: 200 mg every 4 hours for a total of five capsules daily for 7 to 10 days (or until what your doctor describes as "clinical resolution" happens). Some clinicians use 400 mg three times a day for 7 to 10 days. Initial cases of herpes proctitis may require 400–800 mg five times daily by mouth (orally) for 10 days or until clinical resolution or 800 mg three times daily for 7–10 days until clinical resolution.

For intermittent recurrence: 200 mg every 4 hours for a total of five capsules daily for 5 consecutive days (total dose of 25 capsules) or 400 mg three times a day for 5 days. Start treatment at the earliest sign of recurrence.

For prevention of frequent recurrence: 400 mg taken twice daily for up to 12 months and then evaluation of ongoing need for this medicine.

For the ointment form: Cover all infected areas every 3 hours for a total of six times daily for 7 consecutive days. Start treatment at the earliest sign of infection (this can avoid a full-blown lesion).

In attempting to decrease the pain of herpes zoster: 800 mg five times daily (every 4 hours) for 7–10 days. Ointment use six times a day for 10 days helps the crusts form sooner.

Treatment of chickenpox: For those over 12 months old with a long-standing skin or lung condition, those being given aerosolized steroids, those taking long-term salicylates or those 13 years old (otherwise healthy): In those 2 or older: 20 mg per kg of body mass (do not exceed 800 mg) orally, four times a day for 5 days. If over 40 kg: 800 mg four times daily for 5 days. Start treatment at the first symptom or sign.

Treatment of herpes infections of the eye: 400 mg by mouth five times a day for at least 5 days.

Prevention of repeat herpes eye infections: One study used 400 mg twice a day (decreased recurrence by 45%).

Famciclovir: Shingles (herpes zoster): 500 to 750 mg is given every 8 hours for 7 days. It is important to start this medicine promptly after the diagnosis is made.

Recurrent genital herpes: 125 mg twice a day for 5 days. Once the initial infection is controlled, 250 mg twice a day has been given for up to a year.

Penciclovir: For the cream form: Cover all infected areas every 2 hours for a total of six times daily for 4 consecutive days. Start treatment at the earliest sign of infection.

Valacyclovir: Herpes zoster (shingles): Best started within 48 hours of the zoster rash; 1 g (1,000 mg) three times a day for 7 days.

Genital herpes simplex: This medicine is best started within 24 hours of the onset of symptoms and is taken as 500 mg twice daily for 10 days. It has not been established to work if it is started more than 72 hours after symptoms start.

Recurrent genital herpes simplex: 500 mg twice a day for 3 DAYS. This is new shorter dosing.

Suppression of genital herpes: 1 gram taken once a day. Some clinicians use 500 mg once a day in patients who have nine *or fewer recurrences a year. Safety and efficacy have not been established for use more than a year.*

Over 65 Years of Age (all four medicines): The dose must be adjusted if the kidneys are impaired.

Conditions Requiring Dosing Adjustments

Liver Function: All medicines: Specific adjustment in liver dysfunction is not defined. Valacyclovir is NOT recommended in people with cirrhosis.

Kidney Function:

Acyclovir: The dose MUST be adjusted in people with compromised kidney function. For example: Creatinine clearance of 25–50 ml/min gets usual dose every 12 hours; 10–25 ml/min gets usual dose once daily.

Famciclovir: In people with mild kidney compromise (creatinine clearance greater than 60 ml/min), 500 mg is given every 8 hours. Mild to moderate compromise (creatinine clearance 40 to 59 ml/min) receives 500 mg every 12 hours. Moderate to severe (creatinine clearance 20 to 39 ml/min) receives 500 mg every 24 hours.

Penciclovir: Dosing may need to be lowered in ongoing dosing cases.

Valacyclovir: Dosing changes MUST be made in patients with compromised kidneys (500 mg once a day for creatinine clearance less than 30 ml/min).

Obesity: Acyclovir: Dosing (intravenous form) should be made on ideal body weight and given as 10 mg per kg of body mass. Maximum dose is 500 mg per square meter every 8 hours.

▷ **Dosing Instructions:**

Acyclovir, famciclovir and valacyclovir: May be taken without regard to food. Acyclovir only: Capsule may be opened. The maker of this medicine recommends drinking 1 liter of water for each gram (1,000 mg) of this medicine that is taken.

All medicines: Take or apply the full course of the exact dose prescribed—interrupted therapy can lead to resistant viruses. Apply ointment forms to the lesions every 2 hours while you are awake. Start treatment at the earliest sign of infection. Use a finger cot or rubber glove to apply the ointment forms. If you forget a dose: Take or apply the missed dose as soon as you remember it, unless it is nearly time for your next dose—if that is the case, simply take the next dose right on schedule. DO NOT double doses.

Usual Duration of Use:

Acyclovir: Use on a regular schedule for 10 days is usually needed to see this drug's effect in reducing the severity and duration of the initial infection. Continual use for 6 months may be needed to prevent frequent recurrence of herpes eruptions.

Famciclovir: For herpes zoster: Regular use for 2 days determines effectiveness. Then the medicine is typically continued for 7 days. Your doctor should decide when to stop the medicine.

For recurrent genital herpes: Start at first sign of recurrence and dosing is continued for 5 days.

Penciclovir: Use on a regular schedule for 4 days usually needed to see this drug's effect in reducing the severity and duration of the infection.

Valacyclovir: Best started within 48 hours of onset of the zoster rash. Use on a regular schedule for 7 days for herpes zoster has been effective. Start therapy within 24 hours of signs of genital herpes; regular use for 10 days is appropriate for initial cases. Take the full course as prescribed. Missing doses may lead to resistance. For recurrent genital herpes, 500 mg twice a day for 3 days is a NEWLY APPROVED shorter treatment duration.

If you forget a dose: Apply the cream or ointment form as soon as you remember, but skip the missed dose if it is nearly time for your next dose. If you are taking the "pill" forms, take the missed dose as soon as you remember it, unless it is nearly time for your next dose—then skip the missed dose and continue with your next scheduled dose. DO NOT double doses.

Typical Treatment Goals and Measurements (Outcomes and Markers)

Infections: The most commonly used measures of serious infections are white blood cell counts and differentials (the kind of blood cells that occur most often in your blood) and temperature. With herpes infections, clinicians look for positive changes in the appearance of the infection (shortened time to crusting, etc.) as well as shortened time for postherpetic neuralgia. Suppressive use finds decreased frequency of outbreaks as a goal.

Possible Advantages of This Drug: Valacyclovir: Achieves blood levels similar to INTRAVENOUS acyclovir with a medicine taken by mouth (the oral route). Patients do not have to take it as many times a day as acyclovir (should help adherence). Newly approved dosing for valacyclovir in recurrent genital herpes should also help adherence.

▷ **These Drugs Should Not Be Taken If**
- you have had an allergic reaction to them previously.
- (valacyclovir) you have advanced HIV disease or have had a bone marrow or kidney transplant (increased risk of thrombotic thrombocytopenic purpura).

▷ **Inform Your Physician Before Taking These Drugs If**
Acyclovir and valacyclovir:
- you take other medicines that may cause kidney damage.
- you think you are dehydrated and can't or will not drink water.
All medicines:
- your liver, kidney or nerve function is impaired.
- you are unsure of how much or how often to take them.

Possible Side Effects (natural, expected and unavoidable drug actions)
Acyclovir and valacyclovir:
Possible increased sensitivity to light (photophobia).
With IV acyclovir—possible irritation of the vein up to 9%.
All medicines with ointment forms:
With use of ointment—mild pain or stinging at site of application.

▷ **Possible Adverse Effects** (unusual, unexpected and infrequent reactions)
If any of the following develop, consult your physician promptly for guidance.
Mild Adverse Effects: Allergic reaction: skin rash, itching.
Acyclovir: Headache (valacyclovir as well and may be frequent), dizziness, nerv-

ousness, confusion, insomnia, depression, fatigue—rare. Nausea, vomiting, diarrhea—infrequent with IV form. Joint pains, muscle cramps—rare. Acne, hair loss—rare.

Famciclovir: Nausea or diarrhea—infrequent to frequent.

Famciclovir and penciclovir: Headache—infrequent.

Valacyclovir: fast heart rate—case reports.

Serious Adverse Effects

Acyclovir: Superficial thrombophlebitis—infrequent with IV form. Seizures or coma with IV use—rare. Kidney problems—rare (especially if adequate water is taken). Low platelets or red or white blood cells—case reports rare. Colitis—case reports.

Famciclovir: Purpura or paresthesias—case reports. Rigors—rare. Increased breast cancer in male rats given extremely high doses. Does not appear to increase risk in humans.

Penciclovir: Liver enzyme abnormalities—infrequent.

Valacyclovir: Thrombotic thrombocytopenic purpura—rare and in immuno-compromised patients.

▷ **Possible Effects on Sexual Function:** None reported for these medicines.

Possible Effects on Laboratory Tests

Acyclovir and valacyclovir: Complete blood cell counts: decreased red or white cells or hemoglobin—rare.

Blood urea nitrogen (BUN)/creatinine: increased—rare (5–10% fast IV).

Liver function tests: increased—rare.

Famciclovir and penciclovir: None reported.

CAUTION

1. These drugs do not eliminate all herpes virus and are not a cure. The infection often returns. Restart treatment at the earliest sign of infection.
2. Avoid intercourse if herpes blisters and swelling are present.
3. Do not exceed the prescribed dose.
4. If severity/frequency of infections don't improve, call your doctor.
5. The manufacturer recommends drinking 1 liter (1,000 ml) of fluid for each gram (1,000 mg) of oral or intravenous form taken of acyclovir.
6. Other medicines that can form damaging crystals in the urine may lead to added kidney problem risk if combined with acyclovir.
7. Many managed care organizations require pill splitting (valacyclovir is an example). If you are required to split pills, get a pill splitter to help ensure accuracy.

Precautions for Use

By Infants and Children: Acyclovir: Specific dosing required. Fluid intake must be adequate.

Famciclovir, penciclovir and valacyclovir: Safety and efficacy not established.

By Those Over 60 Years of Age: Acyclovir and valacyclovir:

Avoid dehydration. Talk to your doctor about how much water you should take or can tolerate. Make sure dosing is adjusted for age-related decline in kidney function.

Famciclovir and penciclovir: Age-related declines in kidney function may require dosing adjustment.

▷ **Advisability of Use During Pregnancy**

Pregnancy Category:

Acyclovir: B for the oral and intravenous forms. C for the topical form. See Pregnancy Risk Categories at the back of this book.

Famciclovir and penciclovir: B. See Pregnancy Risk Categories at the back of this book.

Valacyclovir: B. See Pregnancy Risk Categories at the back of this book.

Animal studies:

Acyclovir: No birth defects found in mouse, rat or rabbit studies.

Famciclovir and penciclovir: No birth defects found in animals.

Valacyclovir: NOT teratogenic in rabbits or rats (up to 10 times the human dose).

Human studies:

Acyclovir: The pregnancy registry has followed more than 600 cases to date. Sixteen birth defects occurred, with no pattern.

Widespread (disseminated) or life-threatening herpes virus infections may warrant use of this medicine during pregnancy. Talk with your doctor about use.

Famciclovir and penciclovir: Studies not available.

Valacyclovir: Adequate studies of pregnant women are not available.

A pregnancy registry can be accessed by physicians at 1-800-722-9292, extension 39437.

Advisability of Use If Breast-Feeding

Presence of this drug in breast milk: Acyclovir: Yes. *Famciclovir*: yes in lab animals, unknown in humans. *Penciclovir*: unknown. *Valacyclovir:* Yes (documented in two women; 0.6 to 4.1 times the plasma levels).

Ask your physician for guidance: Acyclovir: often okay to breast-feed. Famciclovir: stop nursing or discontinue drug. *Valacyclovir:* Given to parents who are breast-feeding their infants with caution or not at all. Discuss benefits and risk factors with your doctor.

Habit-Forming Potential: None.

Effects of Overdose: Possible impairment of kidney function with acyclovir and valacyclovir, not defined or symptomatic management for famciclovir or penciclovir.

Possible Effects of Long-Term Use: Development of resistant strains of herpes virus. Treatment will fail if this occurs.

Suggested Periodic Examinations While Taking This Drug (at physician's discretion)

Kidney function tests for acyclovir and valacyclovir, not defined for famciclovir or penciclovir.

▷ **While Taking This Drug, Observe the Following**

Foods: No restrictions. Some claims have been made for lysine (an amino acid) but specific scientifically rigorous studies have not been made.

Herbal Medicines or Minerals: Some patients use echinacea to attempt to boost their immune systems. Unfortunately, use of echinacea is not recommended in people with damaged immune systems. This herb may also actually weaken any immune system if it is used too often or for too long a time.

Beverages: No restrictions. Acyclovir may be taken with milk. Drink 2 to 3 quarts of liquids daily (if not contraindicated for you) when you take acyclovir or valacyclovir.

▷ *Alcohol:* Acyclovir and valacyclovir: Use caution; dizziness or fatigue may be accentuated. Penciclovir and famciclovir: No restrictions.

Tobacco Smoking: No interactions expected. I advise everyone to quit smoking.

▷ *Other Drugs*

Penciclovir: No significant interactions for the cream.

The following drugs may *increase* the effects of acyclovir and valacyclovir:

- cyclosporine (Sandimmune)—use may result in increased risk of kidney toxicity.
- probenecid (Benemid)—may delay acyclovir or famciclovir elimination.

Acyclovir or valacyclovir *taken concurrently* with or by

- a patient with an allopurinol (Zyloprim) allergy may result in cross-allergenicity and allergic reaction.
- cimetidine (Tagamet) increases risk of antiviral toxicity.
- fosphenytoin (Cerebyx) or phenytoin (Dilantin) may cause loss of seizure control (lower blood levels of this seizure medicine).
- meperidine (Demerol) may result in neurologic problems.
- valproic acid (Depakote) may cause loss of seizure control (lower valproic blood levels).
- varicella vaccine (Varivax) will blunt the vaccine effectiveness.
- zidovudine (AZT) may result in severe fatigue and lethargy.

Famciclovir *taken concurrently* with

- digoxin (Lanoxin) may increase peak digoxin blood level slightly.
- probenecid (Benemid) may increase famciclovir blood levels as both medicines are removed from the body by active tubular secretion in the kidney.

▷ *Driving, Hazardous Activities:* Use caution if dizziness or fatigue occurs from acyclovir or famciclovir. Caution is advised if significant headache results from these medicines.

Aviation Note: The use of acyclovir, famciclovir or valacyclovir *may be a disqualification* for piloting. Penciclovir is probably not a disqualification. Consult a designated Aviation Medical Examiner.

Exposure to Sun: No restrictions; however, some data indicate that sun exposure may trigger release of herpes simplex from its dormant state (from the optic nerve).

COLESEVELAM (koh lee SEV eh lamb)

Introduced: 2000   **Class:** Anticholesterol   **Prescription:** USA: Yes
Controlled Drug: USA: No; Canada: No   **Available as Generic:** USA: No; Canada: No
Brand Name: Welchol

```
┌─────────────────────────────────────────────────────────────────────┐
│                      BENEFITS versus RISKS                           │
│         Possible Benefits                    Possible Risks          │
│   EFFECTIVE REDUCTION OF TOTAL      Constipation                     │
│     CHOLESTEROL AND LOW-            Reduced absorption of fat, fat-soluble │
│     DENSITY CHOLESTEROL IN            vitamins (A, D, E and K, etc.)  │
│     TYPE IIA CHOLESTEROL                                             │
│     DISORDERS                                                        │
│   ADDITIVE EFFECTS WHEN                                              │
│     COMBINED WITH HMG-CoA                                           │
│     REDUCTASE INHIBITORS                                            │
└─────────────────────────────────────────────────────────────────────┘
```

▷ **Principal Uses**

   As a Single Drug Product: Uses currently included in FDA-approved labeling: (1) Used in combination with diet changes to decrease blood cholesterol and low-density (LDL) cholesterol in Type IIa cholesterol disorders.
   Other (unlabeled) generally accepted uses: None at present.

How This Drug Works: Cross-linked hydrogel polymer that holds onto (binds) bile acids in the intestine, which prevents them from being absorbed. Because bile acids are not absorbed, more cholesterol is converted to bile acids. This effect works to lower cholesterol (upregulate the LDL receptor) by removing cholesterol from the blood (plasma).

Available Dosage Forms and Strengths
   Tablets — 625 mg

▷ **Usual Adult Dosage Ranges:** *When used alone:* this medicine is started with three tablets twice a day (with meals) or six tablets once a day with a meal. The dose can then be increased if goals are not met to seven tablets a day. This medicine should be taken with liquids.
   Combination therapy: Three tablets twice daily with meals or six tablets once daily with a meal. **Note: Actual dose and schedule must be determined for each patient individually.**

Conditions Requiring Dosing Adjustments
   Liver Function: No changes needed (zero to minimal absorption).
   Kidney Function: No changes needed (zero to minimal absorption).

▷ **Dosing Instructions:** Always take just before or with a meal and with liquids. If you forget a dose: Take the missed dose as soon as you remember it, unless it is nearly time for the next dose. DO NOT DOUBLE DOSES. Call your doctor if you find yourself forgetting doses.

Usual Duration of Use: Initial response often occurs in 2 weeks. Regular use for up to a month may be needed to see peak benefits in lowering cholesterol. If no acceptable response in 3 months with peak doses, combination therapy with an HMG-CoA is advisable. Long-term use (months to years) requires periodic follow-up with your doctor. Treat cholesterol for life!

Typical Treatment Goals and Measurements (Outcomes and Markers)
   Cholesterol: The National Institutes of Health has released ATP III as part of the update to the National Cholesterol Education Program or NCEP. Key points in these new guidelines include acknowledging diabetes as one of the conditions that increase risk of heart disease, modifying risk factors and recommending routine testing for all of the cholesterol fractions

(lipoprotein profile) versus total cholesterol alone. These new guidelines also recommend a desirable total cholesterol of 200 mg/dl as before, but change optimal LDL to 100 mg/dl, 130–159 mg/dl as borderline high, 160 mg/dl as high and cite 190 mg/dl as very high. This medicine was shown to lower LDL-C by 15–18% in clinical trials when used alone. One noteworthy change from NCEP is that "good cholesterol" or HDL has been made more important. The "too low" measure for HDL has been increased to 40 mg/dl. Take your medicine and reach these new targets! Electron beam computed tomography (EBCT) is an important tool to use in conjunction with these laboratory studies because even patients who meet cholesterol goals (particularly females over 55) can still be at risk.

▷ **This Drug Should Not Be Taken If**
- you have had an allergic reaction to it previously.
- you have a bowel block (obstruction).

▷ **Inform Your Physician Before Taking This Drug If**
- you are prone to constipation.
- you have low thyroid function (hypothyroidism).
- you have stomach or intestinal problems (gastrointestinal disorders).
- you have a bleeding disorder of any kind.

Possible Side Effects (natural, expected and unavoidable drug actions)
Constipation; interference with normal fat digestion and absorption; reduced absorption of vitamins A, D, E and K and folic acid. Binds to vitamin B_{12}-intrinsic factor complex.

▷ **Possible Adverse Effects** (unusual, unexpected and infrequent reactions)
If any of the following develop, consult your physician promptly for guidance.
Mild Adverse Effects
Allergic reactions: not reported as yet.
Joint pains—possible.
Constipation or dyspepsia—most frequent.
Loss of appetite, indigestion, heartburn, abdominal discomfort, excessive gas, nausea, vomiting, diarrhea—case reports.
Serious Adverse Effects
Fat-soluble vitamin deficiency—possible.

▷ **Possible Effects on Sexual Function:** None reported.

Natural Diseases or Disorders That May Be Activated by This Drug
Fat-soluble vitamin deficiency.

Possible Effects on Laboratory Tests
Blood cholesterol and triglyceride levels: decreased (therapeutic effect).

CAUTION
Watch carefully for constipation; use stool softeners and laxatives as needed.

Precautions for Use
By Infants and Children: Safety and effectiveness for those under 12 years of age not established.
By Those Over 60 Years of Age: Increased risk of severe constipation.

▷ **Advisability of Use During Pregnancy**
Pregnancy Category: B. See Pregnancy Risk Categories at the back of this book.
Animal studies: No information available.

Human studies: Adequate studies of pregnant women are not available. Use this drug only if clearly needed. Ensure adequate intake of vitamins and minerals to satisfy needs of mother and fetus.

Advisability of Use If Breast-Feeding

Presence of this drug in breast milk: None.

Breast-feeding is permitted.

Habit-Forming Potential: None.

Effects of Overdose: Progressive constipation.

Possible Effects of Long-Term Use: Deficiencies of vitamins A, D, E and K and folic acid. Binding of the B_{12}-intrinsic factor complex may lead to blood cell problems.

Suggested Periodic Examinations While Taking This Drug (at physician's discretion)

Measurements of blood levels of total cholesterol, low-density (LDL) cholesterol and high-density (HDL) cholesterol.

▷ **While Taking This Drug, Observe the Following**

Foods: Avoid foods that tend to constipate (cheeses, etc.). Talk to your doctor if you are considering adding soy milk or other soy products to your diet.

Herbal Medicines or Minerals: Some studies show garlic to reduce cholesterol. Since it probably works by a different mechanism than colesevelam, the combination use may be reasonable if dosing is separated. Discuss this with your doctor. Soy milk may also offer some lowering of cholesterol. Current cholesterol therapy sets a goal for treatment, and these herbs may help reach that goal when combined with this prescription medicine. Talk to your doctor before combining any herbals with colesevelam.

Nutritional Support: Ask your doctor if you need supplements of vitamins A, D, E and K, folic acid and calcium.

Beverages: Ensure adequate liquid intake (up to 2 quarts daily). This drug may be taken with milk.

▷ *Alcohol:* No interactions expected.

Tobacco Smoking: No interactions expected. I advise everyone to quit smoking.

▷ *Other Drugs*

Colesevelam may ***decrease*** the effects of

- alendronate (Fosamax); take 2 hours before colesevelam.
- fibrates (Tricor, others); take 2 hours before colestipol or 4 to 6 hours after colestipol.
- vitamin B_{12} and fat-soluble vitamins.

Colesevelam may ***increase*** the effects of

- atorvastatin (Lipitor), lovastatin (Mevacor) and simvastatin (Zocor).

▷ *Driving, Hazardous Activities:* No restrictions.

Aviation Note: The use of this drug is usually not a disqualification for piloting. Consult a designated Aviation Medical Examiner.

Exposure to Sun: No restrictions.

Discontinuation: The dose of any toxic drug combined with colesevelam must be reduced when this drug is stopped. Once colesevelam is stopped, cholesterol levels usually return to pretreatment levels in 1 month.

COLESTIPOL (koh LES ti pohl)

Introduced: 1974   **Class:** Anticholesterol   **Prescription:** USA: Yes
Controlled Drug: USA: No; Canada: No   **Available as Generic:** USA: No;
Canada: No
Brand Name: Colestid, Lestid

BENEFITS versus RISKS

Possible Benefits	*Possible Risks*
EFFECTIVE REDUCTION OF TOTAL CHOLESTEROL AND LOW-DENSITY CHOLESTEROL IN TYPE IIA CHOLESTEROL DISORDERS	Constipation (may be severe)
	Reduced absorption of fat, fat-soluble vitamins (A, D, E and K) and folic acid
EFFECTIVE RELIEF OF ITCHING associated with biliary obstruction	Reduced formation of prothrombin with possible bleeding
Treatment of some pseudomembranous colitis cases	

▷ **Principal Uses**

As a Single Drug Product: Uses currently included in FDA-approved labeling:
(1) Used in combination with diet changes to decrease blood cholesterol
and low-density (LDL) cholesterol in Type IIa cholesterol disorders; (2)
eases itching due to deposit of bile acids in skin.

Other (unlabeled) generally accepted uses: (1) Data from one study showed
that colestipol in combination with lovastatin actually caused regression
of plaque buildup (atherosclerosis) inside blood vessels; (2) some data
show that colestipol is useful in pseudomembranous colitis.

How This Drug Works: Binds bile acids and is removed in feces. Removal of bile
acids stimulates conversion of cholesterol to bile acids, which then
reduces cholesterol. By reducing levels of bile acids, this drug hastens
removal of bile acids in the skin and relieves itching.

Available Dosage Forms and Strengths

Bottles — 250 g, 500 g
Flavored Colestid Granules for oral suspension — 5 g per dose
Packets — 5 g

▷ **Usual Adult Dosage Ranges:** Starts with 5 g of powder mixed in an approved
liquid (such as orange juice, apple juice, water or grape juice) and taken
three times daily. May be increased slowly as needed and tolerated to 30 g
daily in two to four divided doses. **Note: Actual dose and schedule must
be determined for each patient individually.**

Conditions Requiring Dosing Adjustments
Liver Function: No changes needed.
Kidney Function: No changes needed.

▷ **Dosing Instructions:** Always take just before or with a meal; drug does not work if
taken without food. Mix the powder thoroughly in 4 to 6 ounces of water,
fruit juice, tomato juice, milk, thin soup or a soft food such as applesauce.
Do not take it in its dry form. If you forget a dose: Take the missed dose as

soon as you remember it, unless it is nearly time for the next dose. DO NOT DOUBLE DOSES. Call your doctor if you find yourself forgetting doses.

Usual Duration of Use: Regular use for up to a month may be needed to see peak benefits in lowering cholesterol. If no acceptable response in 3 months, combination treatment with an HMG-CoA inhibitor should be considered. Long-term use (months to years) requires periodic follow-up with your doctor.

Typical Treatment Goals and Measurements (Outcomes and Markers)

Cholesterol: The National Institutes of Health has released ATP III as part of the update to the National Cholesterol Education Program or NCEP. Key points in these new guidelines include acknowledging diabetes as one of the conditions that increases risk of heart disease, modifying risk factors and recommending routine testing for all of the cholesterol fractions (lipoprotein profile) versus total cholesterol alone. These new guidelines also recommend a desirable total cholesterol of 200 mg/dl as before, but change optimal LDL to 100 mg/dl, 130–159 mg/dl as borderline high, 160 mg/dl as high and cite 190 mg/dl as very high. One other noteworthy change is that "good cholesterol" or HDL has been made more important. The "too low" measure for HDL has been increased to 40 mg/dl. Take your medicine and reach these new targets! Electron beam computed tomography (EBCT) is an important tool to use in conjunction with these laboratory studies because even patients who meet cholesterol goals (particularly females over 55) can still be at risk.

▷ **This Drug Should Not Be Taken If**
- you have had an allergic reaction to it previously.
- you have complete biliary obstruction.

▷ **Inform Your Physician Before Taking This Drug If**
- you are prone to constipation.
- you have low thyroid function (hypothyroidism).
- you have peptic ulcer disease.
- you have a bleeding disorder of any kind.
- you have impaired kidney function.

Possible Side Effects (natural, expected and unavoidable drug actions)

Constipation; interference with normal fat digestion and absorption; reduced absorption of vitamins A, D, E and K and folic acid. Binds to vitamin B_{12}-intrinsic factor complex.

▷ **Possible Adverse Effects** (unusual, unexpected and infrequent reactions)

If any of the following develop, consult your physician promptly for guidance.

Mild Adverse Effects

Allergic reactions: skin rash—rare; hives, tongue irritation, anal itching—case reports.

Headache, dizziness, weakness, muscle and joint pains—possible.

Constipation—most frequent.

Loss of appetite, indigestion, heartburn, abdominal discomfort, excessive gas, nausea, vomiting, diarrhea—case reports.

Serious Adverse Effects

Vitamin K deficiency and increased bleeding tendency—possible.

Impaired absorption of calcium; predisposition to osteoporosis—possible.

Hypothyroidism—possible.

Disruption of normal acid-base balance of the body (metabolic acidosis)—possible with long-term use.

▷ **Possible Effects on Sexual Function:** None reported.

Natural Diseases or Disorders That May Be Activated by This Drug

Peptic ulcer disease; steatorrhea (excessive fat in stools) with large doses.

Possible Effects on Laboratory Tests

Blood cholesterol and triglyceride levels: decreased (therapeutic effect).

Blood thyroxine (T4) level: decreased when colestipol and niacin are taken concurrently (in presence of normal thyroid function).

CAUTION

1. Never take the dry powder; always mix thoroughly with a suitable liquid before swallowing.
2. Watch carefully for constipation; use stool softeners and laxatives as needed.
3. This drug may bind other drugs taken concurrently and impair their absorption. It is advisable to take all other drugs 1 to 2 hours before or 4 to 6 hours after taking this drug.

Precautions for Use

By Infants and Children: Safety and effectiveness for those under 12 years of age not established. Watch carefully for the possible development of acidosis and vitamin A or folic acid deficiency. (Ask your physician for guidance.)

By Those Over 60 Years of Age: Increased risk of severe constipation. Impaired kidney function may predispose to the development of acidosis.

▷ **Advisability of Use During Pregnancy**

Pregnancy Category: not established, B2 in Australia. See Pregnancy Risk Categories at the back of this book.

Animal studies: No information available.

Human studies: Adequate studies of pregnant women are not available.

Use this drug only if clearly needed. Ensure adequate intake of vitamins and minerals to satisfy needs of mother and fetus.

Advisability of Use If Breast-Feeding

Presence of this drug in breast milk: None.

Breast-feeding is permitted.

Habit-Forming Potential: None.

Effects of Overdose: Progressive constipation, skin changes (skin drying).

Possible Effects of Long-Term Use: Deficiencies of vitamins A, D, E and K and folic acid. Calcium deficiency, osteoporosis. Acidosis due to excessive retention of chloride. Binding of the B_{12}-intrinsic factor complex may lead to blood cell problems.

Suggested Periodic Examinations While Taking This Drug (at physician's discretion)

Measurements of blood levels of total cholesterol, low-density (LDL) cholesterol and high-density (HDL) cholesterol.

Hemoglobin and red blood cell studies for possible anemia.

Thyroid function tests.

▷ **While Taking This Drug, Observe the Following**

Foods: Avoid foods that tend to constipate (cheeses, etc.). Talk to your doctor if you are considering adding soy milk or other soy products to your diet.

Herbal Medicines or Minerals: Some studies show garlic to reduce cholesterol. Since it probably works by a different mechanism than colestipol, the combination use may be reasonable if dosing is separated. Discuss this with your doctor. Soy milk may also offer some lowering of cholesterol. Current cholesterol therapy sets a goal for treatment, and these herbs may help reach that goal when combined with this prescription medicine. Talk to your doctor before combining any herbals with colestipol.

Nutritional Support: Ask your doctor if you need supplements of vitamins A, D, E and K, folic acid and calcium.

Beverages: Ensure adequate liquid intake (up to 2 quarts daily). This drug may be taken with milk.

▷ *Alcohol:* No interactions expected.

Tobacco Smoking: No interactions expected. I advise everyone to quit smoking.

▷ *Other Drugs*

Colestipol may decrease the effects of
- acetaminophen (Tylenol); take 2 hours before colestipol.
- alendronate (Fosamax); take 2 hours before colestipol.
- aspirin; take 2 hours before colestipol.
- atorvastatin (Lipitor); take 2 hours before colestipol.
- cephalexin (Keflex); take 2 hours before colestipol.
- diclofenac (various); take 2 hours before colestipol.
- digitoxin and digoxin (Lanoxin); take 2 hours before colestipol.
- fibrates (Tricor, others); take 2 hours before colestipol or 4 to 6 hours after colestipol.
- folic acid; take 2 hours before colestipol.
- furosemide (Lasix); take 2 hours before colestipol or 4 to 6 hours after colestipol.
- hydrocortisone; take 2 hours before colestipol.
- iron preparations; take 2 to 3 hours before colestipol.
- leflunomide (Arava); take 2 hours before colestipol.
- penicillin G (Pentids); take 2 hours before colestipol.
- phenobarbital; take 2 hours before colestipol.
- pravastatin (Pravachol); take 2 hours before colestipol.
- oral antidiabetic drugs (see Drug Classes).
- raloxifene (Evista); take 2 hours before colestipol.
- tetracycline (various); take 2 hours before or 3 hours after colestipol.
- thiazide diuretics (see Drug Classes); take 2 hours before colestipol.
- thyroxine (see Thyroid Hormones Drug Class); take 5 hours before colestipol.
  - vancomycin (various oral forms); take 2 hours before colestipol or 4 to 6 hours after colestipol.
  - vitamin B_{12}.

▷ *Driving, Hazardous Activities:* No restrictions.

Aviation Note: The use of this drug is usually not a disqualification for piloting. Consult a designated Aviation Medical Examiner.

Exposure to Sun: No restrictions.

Discontinuation: The dose of any toxic drug combined with colestipol must be reduced when this drug is stopped. Once colestipol is stopped, cholesterol levels usually return to pretreatment levels in 1 month.

COX II INHIBITOR FAMILY (KOX too)

Celecoxib (SELL ah kox ib) **Rofecoxib** (ROW fah kox ib)

Introduced: 1999, 1999   **Class:** COX II Inhibitor, selective NSAID   **Prescription:** USA: Yes   **Controlled Drug:** USA: No; Canada: No   **Available as Generic:** No

Brand Names: *Celecoxib*: Celebrex; *Rofecoxib*: Vioxx

Author's Note: Some sound-alike errors have been made with Celexa and Celebrex. One drug is an antidepressant, while the other is a COX II inhibitor. Caution is advised.

BENEFITS versus RISKS	
Possible Benefits	*Possible Risks*
EFFECTIVE TREATMENT OF OSTEOARTHRITIS (both medicines)	INCREASED BLOOD PRESSURE Possible increased risk of cardiovascular event rates (see controversies in medicines note below)
EFFECTIVE RELIEF OF INFLAMMATION (both medicines)	
EFFECTIVE SHORT-TERM RELIEF OF SUDDEN (ACUTE) NONARTHRITIC PAIN (rofecoxib only)	Stomach irritation, bleeding and/or ulceration—possible but less likely than NSAIDs
TREATMENT OF PRIMARY DYSMENORRHEA (rofecoxib only)	Anemia—rare Bronchospasm in asthmatics—possible
REDUCTION OF ADENOMATOUS COLON POLYPS IN FAMILIAL ADENOMATOUS POLYPOSIS (FAP)	Allergic reactions in people allergic to sulfa drugs (celecoxib only)
TREATMENT OF RHEUMATOID ARTHRITIS (celecoxib)	
BOTH HAVE MORE FAVORABLE GASTROINTESTINAL SIDE EFFECT PROFILES THAN EXISTING NSAIDS	
May have a role in treating a kind of bladder cancer (carcinoma in situ)	
Both medicines reduce fevers	
Both may have a role in Alzheimer's	

▷ **Principal Uses**

As a Single Drug Product: Uses currently included in FDA-approved labeling: (1) Relieves sudden (acute) nonarthritic pain in adults (orthopedic and dental pain) (rofecoxib); (2) relieves signs and symptoms of osteoarthritis (both medicines); (3) treats primary dysmenorrhea (rofecoxib only); (4) relieves signs and symptoms of rheumatoid arthritis (celecoxib); (5) reduces the number of adenomatous colorectal polyps in familial adenomatous polyposis (FAP).

Other (unlabeled) generally accepted uses: (1) Rofecoxib may have a role in rheumatoid arthritis; (2) based on the way that they work, both could have a role in Alzheimer's disease; (3) may have a role in treating carcinoma in situ of the bladder.

How These Drugs Work: Inhibit cyclooxygenase (COX) II. Since COX II is the COX type (isoform) that is mostly responsible for inflammation and pain, this results in relief of pain and inflammation. COX II also causes fever in humans (along with other compounds), so these medicines work to lower fevers if they occur. Because COX I works to maintain kidney function and has a protective role in the stomach, lack of inhibition of this isoform by both medicines should result in a much more favorable side effect profile than nonselective NSAIDs.

Available Dosage Forms and Strengths
Celecoxib:
>   Capsules — 100 mg, 200 mg
Rofecoxib:
>   Oral suspension — 12.5 mg/5 ml, 25 mg/5 ml
>   Tablets — 12.5 mg, 25 mg, 50 mg

▷ **Usual Adult Dosage Ranges**
Celecoxib:
Osteoarthritis: 100 mg twice daily or 200 mg once a day.
Rheumatoid arthritis: 100 mg twice a day, increased as needed and tolerated to 200 mg twice daily.
FAP: 400 mg twice a day (taken with food).
Rofecoxib:
Osteoarthritis: Dosing is started at 12.5 mg once daily. The dose may be increased as needed and tolerated to 25 mg daily. The lowest effective dose should be used.
Sudden pain or primary dysmenorrhea: 50 mg once daily is used (use for more than 5 days for either of these conditions has NOT been studied). May have an opioid sparing effect in patients taking medicines such as morphine. **Note: Actual dosage and schedule must be determined for each patient individually.**

Conditions Requiring Dosing Adjustments
Liver Function: Celecoxib: Lower doses recommended for celecoxib in moderate liver compromise. Not recommended for use in severe liver (hepatic) problems. Rofecoxib: Use in mild (Child-Pugh score of less than 6) liver problems (dysfunction) showed that rofecoxib achieves similar blood levels as in healthy patients. A small amount of data in moderate (Child-Pugh 7–9) liver disease shows that blood levels are roughly 69% increased. Dose adjustments appear prudent. This medicine has NOT been studied in severe liver failure.
Kidney Function: Rofecoxib and celecoxib have not been studied in advanced kidney (renal) disease and are NOT recommended.

▷ **Dosing Instructions:** Celecoxib and rofecoxib: May be taken with or without food. Taking these medicines with a full glass of water is a good idea. Use of rofecoxib in treating pain or in primary dysmenorrhea has only been studied for up to 5 days. An oral rofecoxib suspension is available if you have trouble swallowing pills. For both medicines: If you forget a dose:

take the missed dose as soon as you remember it, unless its nearly time for your next scheduled dose—if this is the case, skip the missed dose and simply take the regularly scheduled dose. DO NOT double doses.

Usual Duration of Use: Celecoxib may take 1–2 weeks of regular use to work in osteoarthritis and 2 weeks in rheumatoid arthritis.

Short-term use of rofecoxib is recommended (up to 5 days) for nonarthritic pain or dysmenorrhea as longer use has NOT been studied. The medicine usually goes to work in 30 minutes but may take up to an hour. Use on a regular schedule for 1 week usually needed to see benefit in relieving osteoarthritis symptoms. Both medicines are best used in the smallest possible dose and for the shortest possible length of time (minimizes the possibility of GI adverse effects). Treatment of osteo or rheumatoid arthritis will be decided by your doctor. Follow up with your doctor on a regular basis is needed.

Typical Treatment Goals and Measurements (Outcomes and Markers)

Pain: Most clinicians treating pain use a device called an algometer to check your pain. This looks like a small ruler, but lets the clinician better understand your pain. The goals of treatment then relate to where the level of pain started (for example, a rating of seven on a zero to ten scale) and what the cause of the pain was. Pain medicines may also be used together (in combination) in order to get the best result or outcome. For example, many clinicians use acetaminophen (Tylenol, others) rescue doses to help breakthrough pain previously controlled by a COX II inhibitor. If your pain control is not acceptable to YOU (remember, in hospitals and outpatient settings, etc., pain control is a patient right and the fifth vital sign) and if after a week of arthritis pain treatment, results are not what you expect, be sure to call your doctor as you may need a different medicine or combination.

Arthritis: Control of arthritis symptoms (pain, loss of mobility, decreased ability to accomplish activities of daily living, range of motion, etc.) is paramount in returning patient quality of life and to checking the results (beneficial outcomes) from these medicines. Clinicians use the WOMAC osteoarthritis index (see Glossary) to globally assess the health status of people living with osteoarthritis. Many arthritis management or pain centers use interdisciplinary teams (physicians from several specialties, nurses, physician's assistants, physical and occupational therapists, pharmacotherapists, psychotherapists, social workers and others) to get the best results. Laboratory measures of results for rheumatoid arthritis include decreases in chemicals released by the body (acute phase reactants) such as C-reactive protein. A more general test to roughly measure inflammation is a sed rate (erythrocyte sedimentation rate).

Possible Advantages of These Drugs: Both compounds: Do NOT inhibit the COX I isoenzyme. They carry the warnings of NSAIDs but will probably be shown to have much more favorable side effect profiles. Rofecoxib: Is NOT a sulfonamide compound and avoids possible allergic sulfonamide reactions of celecoxib. Rofecoxib does not alter bleeding time, and is mainly removed by cycotosolic enzymes, versus CYP 450 2C9 removal of celecoxib. Because of rofecoxib's lack of effect on platelets, combined use of low-dose (81 mg) aspirin may be advisable for patients who have already suffered a heart attack. This issue should be discussed with your doctor as this may also increase risk of stomach/intestine (GI) problems. In a head-to-head study of 382 arthritis patients, rofecoxib was reported to relieve pain at night more effectively than celecoxib. In a head-to-head trial of 800 patients with osteoarthritis and high blood pressure, 12% of rofecoxib patients versus 6% of celecoxib patients developed higher blood pressure. Rofecoxib is extremely effective in primary dysmenorrhea.

Author's Note: At the time of this writing, controversy has erupted regarding edema in 7.7% versus 4.6% and systolic blood pressure increases of 14.9% versus 6.9% of 1,100 patients. The difference in results and hence the controversy may have resulted from larger than recommended doses of rofecoxib being used in older patients. Further study is needed using typical (usual care and age-related doses) in head-to-head trials.

▷ **These Drugs Should Not Be Taken If**
- you have had an allergic reaction to any COX II inhibitor or NSAID.
- you have active peptic ulcer disease.
- you are in the last 3 months of pregnancy.
- you have severe liver disease (not studied).
- you have a history of urticaria/angioedema or spasm of the bronchi with rhinoconjunctivitis with aspirin or other NSAID (adults who developed nasal polyps, asthma, chronic rhinitis or ongoing angioedema or urticaria make these reactions more likely).

▷ **Inform Your Physician Before Taking These Drugs If**
- you smoke, have ulcerative colitis, take corticosteroids or abuse alcohol.
- you have a bleeding disorder.
- you have a history of peptic ulcer disease.
- you have a history of heart disease or high blood pressure.
- you are pregnant or planning pregnancy.
- you have asthma, carditis or nasal polyps.
- you have a history of liver or kidney problems.
- you drink three or more alcoholic drinks a day (see cautions).

Possible Side Effects (natural, expected and unavoidable drug actions)
Not defined at present.

▷ **Possible Adverse Effects** (unusual, unexpected and infrequent reactions)
If any of the following develop, consult your physician promptly for guidance.

Mild Adverse Effects
Allergic reactions: skin rash, itching.
Dizziness—infrequent.
Auditory hallucinations (celecoxib)—case report.
Stomach irritation, heartburn—infrequent.
Increased liver enzymes—up to 15% of people who take NSAIDs. (This was a rare effect for rofecoxib in clinical trials, and 6% of people had this effect.)
Diarrhea—infrequent.
Edema/fluid accumulation—infrequent (celecoxib).

Serious Adverse Effects
Allergic reactions: acute anaphylactic reaction (see Glossary)—not reported, but possible based on NSAID experience.

Erosion of stomach lining, with silent bleeding—possible but unclear.

Gastrointestinal (GI) bleeding, ulceration or perforation—possible but unclear.

Anemia—rare

Kidney function decline—possible with other NSAIDs in kidney failure patients who depend on prostaglandins for their kidneys to work.

Bronchospasm when used in patients with nasal polyps, asthma—possible.

May worsen angina attacks and increase their frequency—possible (because of fluid retention and increased heart work).

Controversies in Medicine: At the time of this writing, an article appeared in the *Journal of the American Medical Association* that reviewed two large studies (CLASS and VIGOR trials). The authors concluded that their findings suggested a potential increase in the rate of cardiovascular events for both celecoxib and rofecoxib—the two COX II inhibitors currently available at the time of their review. They further concluded that it is mandatory for a trial specifically designed to assess cardiovascular risk and benefit of these medicines to be undertaken and that until that study is conducted, caution be used in prescribing those medicines to people at risk for cardiovascular disease (morbidity).

▷ **Possible Effects on Sexual Function:** None reported.

Adverse Effects That May Mimic Natural Diseases or Disorders

Increased liver enzymes may suggest viral hepatitis. Other NSAIDs have led to decline in kidney function in people with borderline kidney disease. Accumulation of fluid may mimic worsening of congestive heart failure.

Possible Effects on Laboratory Tests

Complete blood counts: decreased red cells or hemoglobin.

Liver function tests: increased ALT/GPT, AST/GOT, alkaline phosphatase.

Fecal occult blood test: may be positive.

CAUTION

1. The FDA requires a warning noting that people who have three or more alcoholic drinks a day may have increased risk of stomach bleeding if they also use NSAIDs (problems may also occur with lower alcohol use).

2. Since these medicines are somewhat newly approved, the full scope of possible side effects or benefits in avoidance of NSAID side effects has not been defined. Nonsteroidal drug warnings were required by the FDA to be included in the package inserts.

3. NSAIDs should be used with extreme caution in people with a previous history of gastrointestinal bleeding or ulcer disease.

4. People with asthma may have aspirin-sensitive asthma. Cross-reactivity between aspirin and these medicines may be possible.

5. When NSAIDs are taken long term, kidney damage is possible. Caution is needed if these medicines are to be used in a patient with kidney damage or in one who is dehydrated (should be rehydrated BEFORE these medicines are started).

6. Rofecoxib and celecoxib may lead to anemia. Patients should be evaluated if they are taking rofecoxib and start to show signs or symptoms of anemia.

7. Part of the removal of rofecoxib from the body happens in a way that can become full or saturated. This means a small change in dose could result in a larger than expected increase in blood level.

8. People who take NSAIDS such as these medicines can develop serious stomach or intestinal (gastrointestinal) problems. Elderly people or patients with debilitating diseases or conditions may be at increased risk for gastrointestinal problems from these medicines. While the FDA ruled that data on these medicines did not support removal of NSAID warnings from the product labels, many clinicians feel that these medicines have a more favorable adverse event profile than previously available, less selective NSAIDS.

9. These medicines may cause fluid retention, complicating high blood pressure or heart failure treatment—but this effect can generally be managed by an inexpensive and well-tolerated water pill (diuretic) such as low-dose hydrochlorothiazide.

10. See cardiovascular disease morbidity note in controversies section above.

Precautions for Use

By Infants and Children: Safety and efficacy in those less than 18 years old have NOT been established.

By Those Over 60 Years of Age: Clinical studies included many patients who were more than 75 years old. These patients showed no difference from younger patients.

▷ **Advisability of Use During Pregnancy**

Pregnancy Category: C for both medicines. See Pregnancy Risk Categories at the back of this book.

Animal studies: Slight increase in vertebral malformations in rabbits for rofecoxib. Celecoxib caused skeletal defects at two times the usual human dose.

Human studies: Adequate studies of pregnant women have NOT been performed.

These medicines should be avoided in pregnancy because of possible premature closure of the ductus arteriosus.

Advisability of Use If Breast-Feeding

Presence of this drug in breast milk: Yes for both medicines in rats, unknown in humans.

Avoid drug or refrain from nursing.

Habit-Forming Potential: None.

Effects of Overdose: No overdose data were reported in clinical trials. Supportive measures consistent with patient symptoms as well as removal of unabsorbed drug from the stomach is reasonable.

Possible Effects of Long-Term Use: Anemia due to chronic blood loss from erosion of stomach lining.

Suggested Periodic Examinations While Taking These Drugs (at physician's discretion)

Check for signs or symptoms of serious GI toxicity.

Complete blood cell counts.

Liver function tests if signs or symptoms of liver problems begin.

Increased range of motion and decreased pain in arthritis.

▷ **While Taking These Drugs, Observe the Following**

Foods: May be taken with or without food.

Herbal Medicines or Minerals: Ginseng, ginkgo, alfalfa, clove oil, feverfew, cinchona bark and garlic may also change clotting, so combining those herbals with these medicines is not recommended. NSAIDs may decrease feverfew effects. Hay flower, mistletoe herb and white mustard seed carry German Commission E monograph indications for arthritis and may be complementary. Talk to your doctor BEFORE combining any herbal medicines or prescription medicines.

Beverages: No restrictions. May be taken with milk.

▷ *Alcohol:* Use of alcohol and these medicines at the same time may increase risk of stomach irritation. See alcohol/NSAIDs warning in Cautions.

Tobacco Smoking: May increase risk of stomach irritation. I advise everyone to quit smoking.

▷ *Other Drugs*

These medicines may ***increase*** the effects of
- adrenocortical steroids (see Drug Classes), which may lead to additive stomach irritation and bleeding.
- methotrexate and increase its toxic effects.
- oral anticoagulants (see Drug Classes) such as warfarin (Coumadin) and require more frequent INR testing.

The following drugs may ***decrease*** the effects of these medicines:
- cholestyramine (Questran, others) may decrease the amount of drug that goes to work (not reported, but possible in theory). Separate doses by 30 minutes.
- rifampin (Rifater, others) by increasing liver enzymes that remove them from the body.

These medicines ***taken concurrently*** with
- ACE inhibitors—since vein-opening or vasodilator prostaglandins may account for some of the ACE beneficial effects and since data from combined use with benazepril (Lotensin) showed blunting of beneficial effects from benazepril, caution with all ACE inhibitors is prudent.
- alendronate (Fosamax) may blunt alendronate absorption and may also result in increased risk of stomach upset/diarrhea (not reported, but theoretically possible).
- cortisonelike drugs (see Drug Classes) increase risk of stomach ulcers.
- high blood pressure (antihypertensive) medicines may blunt their therapeutic benefit, especially those that are diuretics such as furosemide (Lasix) or other loop diuretics, spironolactone or thiazides (see Drug Classes).
- lithium (Lithobid) may increase lithium blood levels.
- other NSAIDs (see Drug Classes) (such as aspirin) may increase risk of stomach or intestine (GI) toxicity. The benefit-to-risk decision of combined use of aspirin with these medicines in patients who have had a heart attack (secondary prevention) may be desirable because of the lack of a needed effect on platelets or to overcome a possible effect of these medicines on clotting. Further study is needed.

The following drugs may ***increase*** the effects of celecoxib:
- amiodarone (Cordarone) by inhibiting CYP 2D6 liver enzymes that remove celecoxib from the body. This effect would also be expected for any medicine that inhibits the CYP 2D6 liver enzyme.
- fluconazole (Diflucan) by inhibiting liver enzymes that remove celecoxib from the body. Celecoxib dose decreases may be prudent if these medicines are to be combined.
- fluoxetine (Prozac) by inhibiting liver enzymes that remove celecoxib from

the body. Celecoxib dose decreases may be prudent if these medicines are to be combined.

- propafenone (Rythmol) by inhibiting liver enzymes that remove celecoxib from the body. Celecoxib dose decreases may be prudent if these medicines are to be combined.
- ritonavir (Norvir) and perhaps other protease inhibitors by inhibiting liver enzymes that remove celecoxib from the body. Celecoxib dose decreases may be prudent if these medicines are to be combined.
- sertraline (Zoloft) by inhibiting liver enzymes that remove celecoxib from the body. Celecoxib dose decreases may be prudent if these medicines are to be combined.

The following drugs may *decrease* the effects of celecoxib:

- carbamazepine (Tegretol, others) by increasing CYP 2D6 liver enzymes that remove celecoxib from the body.
- phenytoin (Dilantin) or fosphenytoin (Cerebyx) by increasing CYP 2D6 liver enzymes that remove celecoxib from the body.

▷ *Driving, Hazardous Activities:* May cause dizziness. Use caution until full effects are known.

Aviation Note: The use of these drugs *may be a disqualification* for piloting. Consult a designated Aviation Medical Examiner.

Exposure to Sun: No reported problems.

Discontinuation: May be stopped abruptly, but talk to your doctor before making any changes in your medicines.

CROMOLYN (KROH moh lin)

Other Names: Cromolyn sodium, sodium cromoglycate

Introduced: 1968   **Class:** Antiasthmatic drug, preventive   **Prescription:** USA: Yes   **Controlled Drug:** USA: No; Canada: No   **Available as Generic:** USA: Yes; Canada: Yes

Brand Names: Children's Nasalcrom, Crolom, Fisoneb [CD], Gastrocrom, Intal, ✷Intal Spincaps, ✷Intal Syncroner, ✷Nalcrom, Nasalcrom, ✷Novocromolyn, Opticrom, ✷Rynacrom

Author's Note: Cromolyn sodium (4%) as Nasalcrom is available without a prescription.

BENEFITS versus RISKS	
Possible Benefits	*Possible Risks*
LONG-TERM PREVENTION OF RECURRENT ASTHMA ATTACKS	Anaphylactic reaction (see Glossary)
Prevention of acute asthma due to allergens or exercise	Spasm of bronchial tubes, increased wheezing
Prevention and treatment of allergic rhinitis	Allergic pneumonitis (allergic reaction in lung tissue)
Prevention of bronchospasm	
RELIEF OF ALLERGIC CONJUNCTIVITIS	
Treatment of giant papillary conjunctivitis	

▷ **Principal Uses**

As a Single Drug Product: Uses currently included in FDA-approved labeling: (1) Prevents allergic reactions in the nose (allergic rhinitis, hay fever) and the bronchial tubes (bronchial asthma); (2) used to treat conjunctivitis (allergic); (3) helps prevent exercise- or environmental-induced asthma; (4) treats mastocytosis and manages several allergy-related skin disorders.

Other (unlabeled) generally accepted uses: (1) Can be used to help stop cough from ACE inhibitors (see Drug Classes); (2) helps modify the reactions in food allergies; (3) may have a small part in therapy of Bell's palsy.

How This Drug Works: Blocks the release of histamine (and other chemicals) from mast cells that worsens allergic reactions. Prevents sequence of events leading to swelling, itching and constriction of bronchial tubes (asthma).

Available Dosage Forms and Strengths

Capsules, oral — 20 mg, 100 mg

Eyedrops — 2% and 4%

Inhalation aerosol — 0.8 mg per metered spray

Inhalation capsules (powder) — 20 mg

Inhalation solution — 20 mg per ampule

Nasal insufflation (powder) — 10 mg per cartridge

Nasal solution — 40 mg/ml

▷ **Usual Adult Dosage Ranges**

Eyedrops: One to two drops four to six times daily at regular intervals.

Inhalation aerosol: 1.6 mg (two inhalations) four times daily at regular intervals for prevention of asthma, or a single dose 10 to 15 minutes before exposure to prevent allergen- or exercise-induced asthma.

Inhalation powder: 20 mg (one capsule) four times daily at regular intervals for long-term prevention of asthma; 20 mg (one capsule) as a single dose 10 to 15 minutes before exposure to prevent acute allergen- or exercise-induced asthma. Total daily maximum dosage is 160 mg (eight capsules).

Inhalation solution: Same as inhalation powder.

Nasal insufflation: Initially 10 mg in each nostril every 4 to 6 hours as needed; reduce to every 8 to 12 hours for maintenance.

Nasal solution: 2.6 mg to 5.2 mg in each nostril three to six times daily as needed.

Oral powder: ALL of the contents of capsules for oral use are poured into a half glass of hot water. This is stirred, and a half glass of cold water is added while mixing. Drink all the liquid and add more water to be sure you drink any leftover medicine. Mix cromolyn with water only, not with fruit juice, milk or foods. **Note: Actual dose and schedule must be determined for each patient individually**.

Conditions Requiring Dosing Adjustments

Liver Function: If the bile duct is damaged by liver disease, the dose must be decreased.

Kidney Function: The dose should be decreased in kidney failure.

▷ **Dosing Instructions:** Follow instructions provided with all of the dosage forms, especially inhalers and eyedrops. Do not swallow capsules intended for inhalation. (If the capsule is accidentally swallowed, drug will cause no beneficial or adverse effects.) Capsules for mouth (oral) use can be poured into 4 ounces (one half glass) of hot water as above. If you forget a dose:

take it right away unless it's nearly time for your next regular dose. If it IS nearly time, just take the scheduled dose. DO NOT double doses.

Usual Duration of Use: Regular use for 6 weeks or more is often needed for benefits in preventing asthma attacks. Onset in perennial allergic rhinitis can be 1 to 2 weeks. Eye use (ophthalmic) may work in a few days up to 6 weeks. Long-term use (months to years) requires periodic evaluation.

Typical Treatment Goals and Measurements (Outcomes and Markers)

Asthma: The frequency of asthma attacks as well as the severity of asthma attacks that occur (such as those requiring an emergency department visit) are a benchmark of effectiveness. Some clinicians also use the number of times a rescue inhaler must be used as a clinical fine point. Pulmonary function tests such as FEV1 may also be used. Goals should be communicated and checked.

Possible Advantages of This Drug

May be quite effective in the young asthmatic. Usually well tolerated. Serious adverse effects are very rare. Works against immediate responses to allergens as well as late nasal responses and isolated late nasal responses.

▷ **This Drug Should Not Be Taken If**
- you have had an allergic reaction to any dosage form of it previously.

▷ **Inform Your Physician Before Taking This Drug If**
- you are allergic to milk, milk products or lactose. (The inhalation powder contains lactose.)
- you have impaired liver or kidney function.
- you have soft contact lenses (these should not be worn while using the eyedrops).
- you have angina or a heart rhythm disorder. (The inhalation aerosol contains propellants that could be hazardous.)

Possible Side Effects (natural, expected and unavoidable drug actions)

Unpleasant taste with use of inhalation aerosol. Mild throat irritation, hoarseness, cough (minimized by a few swallows of water after each powder inhalation). Painful or difficult urination (dysuria)—rare.

▷ **Possible Adverse Effects** (unusual, unexpected and infrequent reactions)

If any of the following develop, consult your physician promptly for guidance.

Mild Adverse Effects

Allergic reactions: skin rash, hives, itching—possible.

Headache, dizziness, drowsiness—rare.

Nausea, vomiting, urinary urgency and pain (dysuria), joint pain—infrequent.

Muscle pain (myositis)—rare.

Stinging or burning of the eyes with ophthalmic use—possible.

Cough and bronchial irritation—rare.

Nosebleed or itching with nasal solution use—rare.

Serious Adverse Effects

Allergic reactions: rare anaphylactic reaction (see Glossary).

Allergic pneumonitis (allergic reaction in lung tissue)—case reports.

Propellants in the metered dose inhaler may cause problems in patients with disease of the heart arteries or a history of abnormal heart rhythms—possible.

Pericarditis—case report.

Inflammation of the arteries—case reports.

▷ **Possible Effects on Sexual Function:** None reported.

Possible Effects on Laboratory Tests

None reported.

CAUTION

1. This drug only helps **prevent** bronchial asthma—use **before** the start of acute bronchial constriction (asthmatic wheezing).
2. *Do not* use during an acute asthma attack—may worsen and prolong asthmatic wheezing.
3. This drug does not block the benefits of drugs that relieve acute asthma attacks after they start. Cromolyn is used *before and between* acute attacks to help keep them from starting; bronchodilators are used during acute attacks.
4. If you are using a bronchodilator drug by inhalation, it is best to take it about 5 minutes before inhaling cromolyn.
5. If this drug has allowed you to decrease or eliminate steroids and you are unable to tolerate cromolyn, ask your doctor about the need to start steroids once again.

Precautions for Use

By Infants and Children: Safety and effectiveness for those under 5 years of age not established for the metered dose inhaler. Inhalation capsules: For children 2 years and older—20 mg (contents of one capsule) inhaled four times a day. Young children may find a nebulized solution easier than the powder.

By Those Over 60 Years of Age: This drug does not work in the management of chronic bronchitis or emphysema.

▷ **Advisability of Use During Pregnancy**

Pregnancy Category: B. See Pregnancy Risk Categories at the back of this book.

Animal studies: Mouse, rat and rabbit studies revealed no birth defects due to this drug.

Human studies: Adequate studies of pregnant women are not available.

Use this drug only if clearly needed.

Advisability of Use If Breast-Feeding

Presence of this drug in breast milk: Unknown.

Avoid drug or refrain from nursing.

Habit-Forming Potential: None.

Effects of Overdose: No significant effects reported.

Possible Effects of Long-Term Use: Allergic reaction of lung tissue (allergic pneumonitis)—very rare.

Suggested Periodic Examinations While Taking This Drug (at physician's discretion)

Sputum analysis and X-ray if symptoms suggest allergic pneumonitis. FEV1.

▷ **While Taking This Drug, Observe the Following**

Foods: Follow physician-prescribed diet. Avoid all foods to which you are allergic.

Herbal Medicines or Minerals: If you are allergic to plants in the Asteraceae family (aster, chrysanthemum, daisy or ragweed), you may also be allergic to echinacea, chamomile, feverfew and St. John's wort. Fir or pine needle oil should NOT be used by asthmatics. Ephedra alone does carry a German Commission E monograph indication for asthma treatment. Talk to your doctor before using any herbal medicine.

Beverages: Avoid all beverages to which you may be allergic.

▷ *Alcohol:* No interactions expected.

Tobacco Smoking: No interactions with the medicine, but smoking can irritate your airways. I advise everyone to quit smoking.

▷ *Other Drugs:* Cromolyn may allow reduced dosage of cortisonelike drugs in the management of chronic asthma. Ask your doctor about dosage adjustment.

▷ *Driving, Hazardous Activities:* This drug may cause dizziness. Restrict activities as necessary.

Aviation Note: The use of this drug *may be a disqualification* for piloting. Consult a designated Aviation Medical Examiner.

Exposure to Sun: No restrictions.

Heavy Exercise or Exertion: This drug may prevent exercise-induced asthma if taken 10 to 15 minutes before exertion. It is most effective in young people.

Discontinuation: If cromolyn has made it possible to reduce or stop maintenance doses of cortisonelike drugs and you find it necessary to discontinue cromolyn, watch closely for a sudden return of asthma. A slow withdrawal (over a week) is advisable. You may have to start a cortisonelike drug as well as take other measures to control asthma.

Special Storage Instructions: Keep the powder cartridges in a dry, tightly closed container. Store in a cool place, but not in the refrigerator. Do not handle the cartridges or the inhaler when hands are wet.

CYCLOPHOSPHAMIDE (si kloh FOSS fa mide)

Introduced: 1959   **Class:** Anticancer, immunosuppressive   **Prescription:** USA: Yes   **Controlled Drug:** USA: No; Canada: No   **Available as Generic:** Yes

Brand Names: Cycloblastin, Cytoxan, Neosar, ✚Procytox

BENEFITS versus RISKS	
Possible Benefits	*Possible Risks*
CURE OR CONTROL OF CERTAIN TYPES OF CANCER	REDUCED WHITE BLOOD CELL COUNT
PREVENTION OF REJECTION IN ORGAN TRANSPLANTATION	SECONDARY INFECTION URINARY BLADDER
Possibly beneficial in rheumatoid arthritis or lupus erythematosus	BLEEDING HEART
May help selected cases of childhood nephrotic syndrome	LUNG, LIVER OR KIDNEY DAMAGE
	Loss of hair

Principal Uses

As a Single Drug Product: Uses currently included in FDA-approved labeling: (1) Treats various cancers: malignant lymphomas, multiple myeloma, sarcomas, retinoblastomas, leukemias, as well as breast and ovarian cancer; (2) also used to prevent rejection in organ transplantation and in some autoimmune disorders; (3) treats some resistant forms of nephrotic syndrome.

Other (unlabeled) generally accepted uses: (1) Used to prepare patients for autologous bone marrow transplants; (2) part of several combination chemotherapy regimens; (3) helps overall survival in combination therapy of lung or fallopian tube cancer; (4) can be part of combination therapy for Ewing's sarcoma; (5) may be of help in patients with lupus erythematosus who have interstitial lung disease or nephritis; (6) secondary role in prostate cancer; (7) high-dose therapy of anemia (aplastic anemia); (8) helps in resistant rheumatoid arthritis; (9) may have a role in drug-induced serious skin reactions (Stevens-Johnson syndrome, etc.).

How This Drug Works: Kills cancer cells during all phases of development. Suppresses primary growth and secondary spread (metastasis) of some types of cancer.

Available Dosage Forms and Strengths
Injection — vials of 100 mg, 200 mg, 500 mg, 1 g, and 2 g
Tablets — 25 mg, 50 mg

▷ **Usual Adult Dosage Ranges:** *Oral form:* 60 to 120 mg per square meter of body surface area daily or 400 mg per square meter of body surface area on days 1 to 5, every 3 to 4 weeks. As therapy continues, the dose is adjusted according to how the tumor responds or unacceptable low white blood cell counts develop. *Intravenous:* 1,000 to 1,500 mg per square meter every 3 to 4 weeks, adjusted the same as the oral form. **Note: Actual dose and schedule must be determined for each patient individually.**

Conditions Requiring Dosing Adjustments
Liver Function: Dose changes are not required in liver compromise. Toxicity may be more likely in people with liver failure.
Kidney Function: In moderate to severe kidney problems, the dose is decreased by 25–50%.

▷ **Dosing Instructions:** Tablets may be crushed and are best taken on an empty stomach. If nausea or indigestion occurs, may be taken with or following food. Liquid intake should be no less than 3 quarts every 24 hours to reduce risk of bladder irritation. If you forget a dose: take it right away unless it's nearly time for your next regular dose. If it IS nearly time, just take the scheduled dose. DO NOT double doses.

Usual Duration of Use: Use on a regular schedule is required to achieve and maintain a significant cancer remission. Initial response often happens in 1 to 3 weeks. Duration depends on response of the cancer and patient tolerance of the drug.

Typical Treatment Goals and Measurements (Outcomes and Markers)
Cancer chemotherapy: The balance here is a difficult range between killing cancer cells and toxicity (bone marrow suppression, heart and others). Complete blood cell counts, assessment of the cancer itself (as in disappearance of soft tissue bumps or masses in multiple myeloma) and resolution of increased calcium are typical markers.

▷ **This Drug Should Not Be Taken If**
• you have had an allergic reaction to it previously.
• you have an active infection of any kind.
• you have bloody urine for any reason.
• you are pregnant or are breast-feeding your infant.

▷ **Inform Your Physician Before Taking This Drug If**
- you have impaired liver, heart or kidney function.
- you have a blood cell or bone marrow disorder.
- you have had previous chemotherapy or X-ray therapy for any type of cancer.
- you take, or have taken within the past year, any cortisonelike drug (adrenal corticosteroids).
- you have diabetes.
- you will have surgery with general anesthesia.

Possible Side Effects (natural, expected and unavoidable drug actions)
Bone marrow depression (see Glossary)—low production of white blood cells and, to a lesser degree, red blood cells and blood platelets (see Glossary). Fever, chills, sore throat, fatigue, weakness, abnormal bleeding or bruising. Leukemia has been reported following cyclophosphamide therapy. Impairment of natural resistance (immunity) to infection. Weakening of the heart muscle (cardiomyopathy). Excessive urination (SIADH). Cystitis or hemorrhagic cystitis. Up to ninefold increase in bladder cancer risk.

▷ **Possible Adverse Effects** (unusual, unexpected and infrequent reactions)
If any of the following develop, consult your physician promptly for guidance.
Mild Adverse Effects
Allergic reaction: skin rash—rare.
Headache, dizziness, blurred vision—possible.
Loss of scalp hair (50% of users), darkening of skin and fingernails, transverse ridging of nails.
Nausea, vomiting (dose-related)—frequent.
Ulceration of mouth, diarrhea (may be bloody)—possible.
Serious Adverse Effects
Idiosyncratic reaction: hemolytic anemia—case reports.
Allergic reaction: anaphylaxis—possible.
Liver damage with jaundice: yellow eyes and skin, dark-colored urine, light-colored stools—rare.
Kidney damage: impaired kidney function, reduced urine volume, bloody urine—case reports.
Lowered white blood cell (granulocyte) colony formation—possible even with rheumatoid arthritis use.
Severe inflammation of bladder: painful urination, bloody urine—infrequent to frequent.
Syndrome of inappropriate antidiuretic hormone secretion (SIADH)—rare.
Intestinal or stomach bleeding (hemorrhagic colitis or GI bleed)—possible.
Drug-induced damage of heart and lung (interstitial pneumonitis) tissue—case reports.
Pancreatitis—case reports.

▷ **Possible Effects on Sexual Function:** Suppression of ovarian function—irregular menstrual pattern or cessation of menstruation (18 to 57%, depending upon dose and duration of use).
Testicular suppression—reduced or no sperm production (100% of users).

Possible Delayed Adverse Effects: Development of other types of cancer (secondary malignancies). Development of severe cystitis with bleeding from the bladder wall (may occur many months after the last dose).

Possible Effects on Laboratory Tests

Complete blood cell counts: decreased red cells, hemoglobin, white cells and platelets.

Blood sodium levels: decreased in SIADH (rare).

INR (prothrombin time): increased.

Liver function tests: increased liver enzymes (ALT/GPT, AST/GOT and alkaline phosphatase), increased bilirubin.

CAUTION

1. This drug may interfere with the normal healing of wounds.
2. This drug can cause significant changes in genetic material in both men and women (sperm and eggs or ova). Patients taking this drug must understand the potential for serious defects in children that are conceived during or following the course of medication.
3. This drug can suppress natural resistance (immunity) to infection, resulting in life-threatening illness.
4. Avoid live-virus vaccines while taking this drug (talk with your doctor about this).

Precautions for Use

By Infants and Children: This drug should not be given if the child is dehydrated. Adequate fluid intake to ensure a copious urine volume for 4 hours following each dose is needed. Prevent exposure of child to anyone with active chickenpox or shingles. This drug may cause ovarian or testicular sterility.

By Those Over 60 Years of Age: Increased risk of serious bladder problems (chemical cystitis). Patients MUST drink large amounts of water in order to keep the bladder flushed. This may increase the risk of urinary retention in men with prostatism (see Glossary).

▷ **Advisability of Use During Pregnancy**

Pregnancy Category: D. See Pregnancy Risk Categories at the back of this book.

Animal studies: Significant birth defects reported in mice, rat and rabbit studies.

Human studies: Information from studies of pregnant women indicates that this drug can cause serious birth defects or fetal death.

Avoid completely during the first 3 months. Use of this drug during the last 6 months must be carefully individualized.

Advisability of Use If Breast-Feeding

Presence of this drug in breast milk: Yes.

Avoid drug or refrain from nursing.

Habit-Forming Potential: None.

Effects of Overdose: Nausea, vomiting, diarrhea, bloody urine, water retention, weight gain, severe bone marrow depression, severe infections.

Possible Effects of Long-Term Use: Development of fibrous tissue in lungs; secondary malignancies.

Suggested Periodic Examinations While Taking This Drug (at physician's discretion)

Complete blood cell counts, every 2 to 4 days during initial treatment and then every 3 to 4 weeks during maintenance treatment.

Liver and kidney function tests.

Thyroid function tests (if symptoms warrant).

▷ **While Taking This Drug, Observe the Following**

Foods: No restrictions.

Herbal Medicines or Minerals: Echinacea: Some patients use echinacea to attempt to boost their immune systems. Unfortunately, use of echinacea is not recommended in people with damaged immune systems. This herb may also actually weaken any immune system if it is used too often or for too long a time. Talk to your doctor before taking any herbal medicine with cyclophosphamide.

Beverages: No restrictions. May be taken with milk.

▷ *Alcohol:* No interactions expected.

Tobacco Smoking: No interactions expected. I advise everyone to quit smoking.

▷ *Other Drugs*

Cyclophosphamide *taken concurrently* with

- allopurinol (Zyloprim) may increase the extent of bone marrow depression.
- amphotericin (Abelcet and others) may increase risk of kidney toxicity.
- chloramphenicol can decrease cyclophosphamide effectiveness.
- ciprofloxacin (Cipro) can result in lowered ciprofloxacin levels and the need for a larger than usual dose.
- digoxin may decrease digoxin absorption and impair digoxin's effectiveness.
- flu (influenza) vaccine, and perhaps other vaccines, may decrease the vaccine's ability to confer immunity.
- hydrochlorothiazide and other thiazide diuretics (see Drug Classes) may worsen the lowering of white blood cells (myelosuppression) caused by cyclophosphamide.
- indomethacin (Indocin) can cause fluid retention.
- live-virus vaccines should be avoided.
- ondansetron (Zofran) may blunt benefits of cyclophosphamide.
- pentostatin may cause fatal heart damage.
- ritonavir (Norvir) may lead to cyclophosphamide toxicity.
- succinylcholine can result in succinylcholine toxicity.
- tamoxifen (Nolvadex) can increase blood clot risk.
- traztuzumab (Herceptin) may increase the risk of heart problems (congestive heart failure or ventricular dysfunction).

▷ *Driving, Hazardous Activities:* Use caution if dizziness occurs.

Aviation Note: The use of this drug *may be a disqualification* for piloting. Consult a designated Aviation Medical Examiner.

Exposure to Sun: No restrictions.

Occurrence of Unrelated Illness: Any signs of infection—fever, chills, sore throat, cough or flu-like symptoms—must be promptly reported. This drug may have to be stopped until the infection is controlled. Consult your physician.

CYCLOSPORINE (SI kloh spor een)

Other Names: Ciclosporin, cyclosporin A

Introduced: 1983   **Class:** Immunosuppressant   **Prescription:** USA: Yes   **Controlled Drug:** USA: No; Canada: No   **Available as Generic:** USA: Yes; Canada: No

Brand Names: Neoral, Sandimmune, SangCya

BENEFITS versus RISKS	
Possible Benefits	*Possible Risks*
EFFECTIVE PREVENTION AND TREATMENT OF REJECTION IN ORGAN TRANSPLANTATION	MARKED KIDNEY TOXICITY DEVELOPMENT OF HYPERTENSION HIGH BLOOD PRESSURE
Some use treating severe rheumatoid arthritis, psoriasis and other inflammatory (autoimmune) conditions	Liver toxicity Low white blood cell count Development of lymphoma Excessive hair growth

▷ **Principal Uses**

As a Single Drug Product: Uses included in FDA-approved labeling: (1) Helps prevent (in conjunction with cortisonelike drugs) organ rejection in kidney, liver and heart transplantation; (2) helps treat rejection crisis; (3) the Neoral microemulsion form treats severe active rheumatoid arthritis; (4) treats refractory psoriasis.

Other (unlabeled) generally accepted uses: (1) Used in transplantation of the bone marrow; (2) used investigationally in a variety of diseases involving the immune system such as: Sjögren's, Crohn's and Grave's diseases; psoriasis; myasthenia gravis; bullous pemphigoid; pulmonary fibrosis associated with rheumatoid arthritis; rheumatoid arthritis; Sweet's syndrome; insulin-dependent diabetes; lupus erythematosus; large granular lymphocytic leukemia; and some anemias; (3) severe, steroid-dependent asthma; (4) treats severe skin reactions (toxic epidermal necrolysis) to phenytoin (Dilantin).

How This Drug Works: By inhibiting some lymphocytes (white blood cells) and their growth factors, this drug suppresses the rejection of transplanted organs.

Available Dosage Forms and Strengths

Capsules, soft gelatin — 25 mg, 100 mg

Injection, intravenous — 50 mg/ml

Oral solution — 100 mg/ml (Note: The microemulsion Neoral is NOT the same as Sandimmune)

▷ **Usual Adult Dosage Ranges:** *Transplantation:* Initially 15 mg per kg of body mass intravenously, taken 4–12 hours prior to transplantation surgery. The drug is then continued after surgery until patients can tolerate cyclosporine taken by mouth. Other immunosuppressant medicines are often used in conjunction with cyclosporine. Some clinicians have used lowest blood levels (trough) to adjust dosing; 7–14 days after surgery, the dose is usually lowered (tapered) by 5% per week to an ongoing dose taken by mouth that is equal to 5–10 mg per kg of body weight each day. Sandimmune should be given with corticosteroids.

If a conversion is made from oral Sandimmune to Neoral, Neoral dose is usually started at the same daily dose as Sandimmune, given at the same time each day in two equally divided doses. Cyclosporine trough levels should be measured twice weekly in people who were taking more than 10 mg per kg of body mass per day of Sandimmune.

Crohn's disease or severe/refractory ulcerative colitis: Therapy is started with 8–10 mg/kg/day with the medicine adjusted to response and a maximum treatment length of 6 months. **Note: Actual dose and schedule must be determined for each patient individually.**

Conditions Requiring Dosing Adjustments

Liver Function: The dose must be adjusted (based on blood levels) in liver compromise. Much of the drug is eliminated in the bile.

Kidney Function: This drug is capable of causing marked kidney toxicity. Caution is critical. Dosing usually does not change, but more frequent blood levels are indicated.

Diabetes: People who are diabetic and subsequently have kidney or pancreatic transplants will need larger than usual doses.

Hypercholesterolemia: If the blood cholesterol is 50% above normal, the dose must be decreased by 50% in order to avoid toxicity.

Obesity: Dosing **must** be based on ideal (a calculation that helps eliminate the weight that is fat) body weight.

Cystic Fibrosis: It is very difficult to appropriately dose this medication in patients who have this disease. Some patients will require as much as two times the usual dose. The dose should be adjusted to drug levels.

Multiple Organ Transplants: Patients with multiple transplants (such as pancreas and kidney) often need an increased dose of cyclosporine in order to achieve the desired effect. The dose should be determined based on blood levels.

▷ **Dosing Instructions:** Preferably taken with or immediately following food to reduce stomach irritation. The capsule should be swallowed whole; do not open, crush or chew. The oral solution should be mixed with milk, chocolate milk or orange juice (at room temperature) in a glass or ceramic cup; do not use a wax-lined or plastic container. Stir well and drink immediately. Use the same liquid to dilute the dose, because different liquids may change the amount that gets into your body and blood levels are important. DO NOT take this medicine with grapefruit juice. It is also best to take this drug at the same time each day to maintain steady blood levels.

Usual Duration of Use: Use on a regular schedule for several weeks is usually needed to prevent organ rejection or stop rejection already underway. Benefits in psoriasis or rheumatoid arthritis may take 4 to 8 weeks. Long-term use (months to years) requires follow-up by your doctor. If you forget a dose: Take the dose you missed as soon as possible, unless it's nearly time for your next dose. If that is the case, skip the missed dose and take the next scheduled dose. DO NOT double doses. If you find yourself missing doses, talk to your doctor.

▷ **This Drug Should Not Be Taken If**
- you have had an allergic reaction to it previously.
- you are getting radiation treatment.
- you have an active lymphoma or a malignancy of any type.
- you have an active, uncontrolled infection, especially chickenpox or shingles.

▷ **Inform Your Physician Before Taking This Drug If**
- you are taking any immunosuppressant drug other than cortisonelike preparations.
- you are pregnant or breast-feeding.
- you have a history of liver or kidney disease or impaired liver or kidney function.

- you have a history of hypertension or gout.
- you have a chronic gastrointestinal disorder.
- you are taking a potassium supplement or drugs that can raise the blood level of potassium.
- you have a seizure disorder.
- you have a history of a blood cell disorder.
- you take other medicines toxic to the kidney.

Possible Side Effects (natural, expected and unavoidable drug actions)
Predisposition to infections (such as pneumocystis).

▷ **Possible Adverse Effects** (unusual, unexpected and infrequent reactions)
If any of the following develop, consult your physician promptly for guidance.

Mild Adverse Effects
Allergic reactions: skin rash, itching—case reports.
Excessive hair growth—frequent in transplant patients.
Acne—rare.
Headache, confusion—infrequent.
Tremors (dose dependent)—frequent.
Mouth sores—rare.
Gum overgrowth—frequent in some reports.
Nausea/vomiting, diarrhea—infrequent.
Changes in facial features (dysmorphosis)—possible with longer-term therapy.

Serious Adverse Effects
Allergic reactions: anaphylactic reaction (see Glossary) to intravenous solution—case reports.
Kidney injury (25% kidney transplant, 37% liver and 38% heart)—frequent.
Hypertension, mild to severe (up to half of patients getting this drug)—frequent.
Blood total cholesterol: increased (while HDL decreased).
Seizures—rare to frequent (kidney, 1.8%; bone marrow, 5.5%; up to 25% of liver transplant patients).
Cortical blindness—case reports.
Liver injury—infrequent.
Pancreatitis—rare.
Low white blood cell count (leukopenia)—infrequent.
Low blood platelets (thrombocytopenia)—rare.
High blood potassium levels, blood glucose, uric acid levels (and gout), increased blood cholesterol or low blood magnesium—all possible.
Lymphoma, possibly drug-induced—rare to infrequent.
Relapse of lupus erythematosus—case reports.
Increased risk of skin cancers (risk increased by sun or UV light exposure).

▷ **Possible Effects on Sexual Function:** Enlargement and tenderness of male breast (1 to 4%)—rare to infrequent.

Adverse Effects That May Mimic Natural Diseases or Disorders
Liver toxicity may suggest viral hepatitis.

Natural Diseases or Disorders That May Be Activated by This Drug
Latent infections, hypertension, gout.

Possible Effects on Laboratory Tests
Complete blood cell counts: decreased red cells, hemoglobin and white cells.
Blood potassium level or uric acid level: increased.

Blood platelets, white cells, magnesium: decreased.

Liver function tests: increased liver enzymes (ALT/GPT, AST/GOT and alkaline phosphatase), increased bilirubin.

Kidney function tests: blood creatinine and urea nitrogen levels (BUN) increased; urine casts present.

Total cholesterol: increased. HDL: decreased.

CAUTION

1. Report promptly any indications of infection of any kind.
2. Promptly report swollen glands, sores or lumps in the skin, abnormal bleeding or bruising.
3. Call your doctor immediately if you become pregnant.
4. Periodic laboratory tests are mandatory.
5. It is best to avoid immunizations and contact with people who have recently taken oral poliovirus vaccine.

Precautions for Use

By Infants and Children: This drug has been used successfully and safely in children of all ages. Dosing is made on the adult schedule in some cases, while others require increased dosing.

By Those Over 60 Years of Age: The dose must be adjusted to any decline in kidney function.

▷ Advisability of Use During Pregnancy

Pregnancy Category: C. See Pregnancy Risk Categories at the back of this book.

Animal studies: Rat and rabbit studies reveal that this drug is toxic to the embryo and fetus. No drug-induced birth defects were found.

Human studies: Adequate studies of pregnant women are not available.

Avoid this drug during entire pregnancy unless it is clearly needed.

Advisability of Use If Breast-Feeding

Presence of this drug in breast milk: Yes.

Avoid drug or refrain from nursing.

Habit-Forming Potential: None.

Effects of Overdose: Headache, pain, facial flushing, gum soreness and bleeding, high blood pressure, atrial fibrillation, respiratory distress, seizures, coma, hallucinations, neurotoxicity, electrolyte disturbances, liver toxicity.

Possible Effects of Long-Term Use: Irreversible kidney damage, severe hypertension, abnormal growth of gums.

Suggested Periodic Examinations While Taking This Drug (at physician's discretion)

Cyclosporine blood levels.

Complete blood counts.

Liver and kidney function tests.

Magnesium, potassium and uric acid blood levels.

Cholesterol with fractions.

Blood pressure checks.

▷ While Taking This Drug, Observe the Following

Foods: Food may increase the peak blood level of cyclosporine.

Herbal Medicines or Minerals: Some patients use echinacea to attempt to boost their immune systems when they are ill. Use of echinacea is not recommended in people taking medicines to suppress their immune systems. Do

NOT take mistletoe herb, oak bark or F.C. of marshmallow root and licorice. There have been case reports of heart transplant rejection with combined use of cyclosporine and St. John's wort. DO NOT COMBINE THESE. Cyclosporine may deplete magnesium from the body. Ask your doctor if supplementation with magnesium makes sense for you. Potassium levels may be increased by cyclosporine. Avoid excessive intake of high-potassium foods. See Table 13.

Beverages: Grapefruit juice and other fruit juices increase blood levels. Milk may increase blood levels.

▷ *Alcohol:* Large amounts of alcohol may increase cyclosporine levels.

Tobacco Smoking: This interaction has not been well studied. I advise everyone to quit smoking.

▷ *Other Drugs*

Cyclosporine *taken concurrently* **with**

- ACE inhibitors (see Drug Classes) may increase the risk of kidney problems.
- acyclovir (Zovirax) may lead to increased cyclosporine levels. CAREFUL check of cyclosporine blood levels are recommended.
- aminoglycoside antibiotics (see Drug Classes) may increase kidney toxicity.
- amphotericin B (Abelcet, others) can cause serious kidney toxicity.
- aspirin substitutes (nonsteroidal anti-inflammatory drugs or NSAIDs) may increase kidney toxicity.
- azathioprine (Imuran) may increase immunosuppression.
- calcium channel blockers (see Drug Classes) may result in cyclosporine toxicity.
- clonidine (Catapres) can increase risk of kidney problems.
- ciprofloxacin (and other fluoroquinolones—see Drug Classes) may increase risk of kidney toxicity.
- cotrimoxazole (Bactrim, others) may result in decreased cyclosporine effectiveness as well as kidney toxicity.
- cyclophosphamide (Cytoxan) may increase immunosuppression.
- digoxin (Lanoxin) may result in serious digoxin toxicity.
- furosemide (Lasix) may result in increased risk of gout.
- ganciclovir (Cytovene) may result in increased kidney toxicity.
- histamine (H2) inhibitors (see Drug Classes) and ketoconazole may experience decreased cyclosporine blood levels.
- imipenem/cilastatin (Primaxin) may result in neurotoxicity.
- lovastatin (Mevacor), atorvastatin (Lipitor) and other HMG-CoA reductase inhibitors may increase risk of muscle toxicity (myopathy) or kidney failure.
- methylprednisolone (Medrol) may cause seizures.
- metronidazole (Flagyl) may result in increased cyclosporine levels and toxicity.
- nifedipine (Adalat) may worsen abnormal gum growth (gingival hyperplasia) and also cause nifedipine toxicity (low blood pressure and abnormal heartbeats).
- propafenone (Rythmol) may increase risk of cyclosporine toxicity.
- pravastatin (Pravachol) and other HMG-CoA reductase inhibitors can increase risk of muscle damage (myopathy).

- saquinavir (Fortovase, Invirase) may increase risk of cyclosporine toxicity.
- simvastatin (Zocor) may cause myopathy.
- spironolactone (various) may increase risk of excessive potassium levels.
- sulfamethoxazole and/or trimethoprim (Septra) may increase kidney toxicity.
- tacrolimus (Prograf) can cause kidney toxicity.
- thiazide diuretics (see Drug Classes) may increase adverse effects on the blood (myelosuppression).
- triamterine (various) may increase risk of excessive potassium levels.
- vaccines may blunt the benefit of the vaccine.
- valproic acid (Depakene, others) lead to liver toxicity in one patient.
- verapamil (Calan) may increase immunosuppression.

The following drugs may increase the effects of cyclosporine:

- acetazolamide.
- allopurinol (Zyloprim).
- amiodarone (Cordarone).
- ceftriaxone (Rocephin).
- cimetidine (Tagamet).
- cisapride (Propulsid).
- clarithromycin (Biaxin).
- clotrimazole (Mycelex, Gyne-Lotrimin, others).
- colchicine (Colbenemid).
- dalfopristin (Synercid).
- danazol or other anabolic steroids.
- diltiazem (Cardizem).
- econazole (Spectazole).
- erythromycin (E.E.S., others).
- fluconazole (Diflucan).
- fluvoxamine (Luvox).
- glipizide (Glucotrol) or glyburide (Diabeta).
- grepafloxacin (Raxar).
- itraconazole (Sporanox).
- ketoconazole (Nizoral).
- medicines that inhibit cytochrome P-450 3A4 liver enzymes. Caution is advised.
- methotrexate (Rheumatrex).
- methyltestosterone.
- metoclopramide (Reglan).
- miconazole (Lotrimin, Micatin).
- nonsteroidal anti-inflammatory agents (see Drug Classes).
- oral contraceptives (birth control pills).
- ritonavir (Norvir).
- tamoxifen (Nolvadex).
- terconazole (Terazol).

The following drugs may *decrease* the effects of cyclosporine:

- carbamazepine (Tegretol).
- carvedilol (Coreg).
- clindamycin (various).
- isoniazid (INH).
- nafcillin.
- octreotide (Sandostatin).

- orlistat (Xenical).
- omeprazole (Prilosec).
- phenobarbital.
- phenytoin (Dilantin) or fosphenytoin (Cerebyx).
- quinine.
- rifabutin (Mycobutin).
- rifampin (Rifadin).
- sulfadimidine, sulfadiazine and/or trimethoprim.
- ticlopidine (Ticlid).
- warfarin (Coumadin).

▷ *Driving, Hazardous Activities:* This drug may cause confusion or seizures. Restrict activities as necessary.

Aviation Note: The use of this drug *may be a disqualification* for piloting. Consult a designated Aviation Medical Examiner.

Exposure to Sun: Exposure to sunlight or other ultraviolet (UV) radiation may increase the risk of skin cancer.

Discontinuation: Do not stop this drug without your physician's guidance.

Special Storage Instructions: Keep the gelatin capsules in the blister packets until ready for use. Store below 77 degrees F (25 degrees C). Keep the oral solution in a tightly closed container. Store below 86 degrees F (30 degrees C). Do not refrigerate.

Observe the Following Expiration Times: The oral solution must be used within 2 months after opening.

DESIPRAMINE (des IP ra meen)

Introduced: 1964   **Class:** Antidepressant   **Prescription:** USA: Yes
Controlled Drug: USA: No; Canada: No   **Available as Generic:** USA: Yes; Canada: Yes
Brand Names: ✦Apo-desipramine, Deprexan, Norpramin, Pertofrane

BENEFITS versus RISKS	
Possible Benefits	*Possible Risks*
EFFECTIVE RELIEF OF ENDOGENOUS DEPRESSION	ADVERSE BEHAVIORAL EFFECTS: CONFUSION, DISORIENTATION, DELUSIONS, HALLUCINATIONS
Treats attention deficit hyperactivity disorder (ADHD) in children over 6	CONVERSION OF DEPRESSION TO MANIA IN MANIC-DEPRESSIVE (BIPOLAR) DISORDERS
Possibly beneficial in other depressive disorders	Aggravation of paranoia and schizophrenia
	Drug-induced heart rhythm disorders
	Abnormally low white blood cell and platelet counts

▷ **Principal Uses**

As a Single Drug Product: Uses currently included in FDA-approved labeling: Relieves severe depression (primary endogenous) and some secondary (exogenous) depression.

Other (unlabeled) generally accepted uses: (1) Chronic pain syndromes, including diabetic neuropathy; (2) treats attention deficit disorder (ADHD) in children over 6, adolescents and adults with hyperactivity; (3) decreases symptoms of panic disorder; (4) treats resistant malaria; (5) may help reduce binge eating in bulimia.

How This Drug Works: By increasing brain levels of nerve impulse transmitters (serotonin and norepinephrine), this drug relieves depression.

Available Dosage Forms and Strengths
Capsules — 25 mg, 50 mg
Tablets — 10 mg, 25 mg, 50 mg, 75 mg, 100 mg, 150 mg

▷ **Usual Adult Dosage Ranges:** *Depression:* Initially 25 mg two to four times daily. May be increased as needed and tolerated by 25 mg daily at intervals of 1 week. Usual ongoing dose is 100 mg to 200 mg daily. Maximum dose is 300 mg. (When determined, daily dose may be given at bedtime as a single dose.) **Note: Actual dose and schedule must be determined for each patient individually.**

Conditions Requiring Dosing Adjustments
Liver Function: Dose should be decreased in liver disease.
Kidney Function: Can cause urine retention—use with caution in kidney compromise with urine outflow problems. The hydroxy form and unconjugated amine form are increased in kidney failure. Close patient monitoring is needed.

▷ **Dosing Instructions:** May be taken without regard to meals. The capsule may be opened, and the tablet may be crushed. If you forget a dose: take the missed dose as soon as you remember it, unless it's nearly time for your next dose—then skip the missed dose and just take the next scheduled dose. If you only take this medicine once a day at bedtime, call your doctor and ask what you should do.

Usual Duration of Use: Regular use for 3 to 4 weeks is often needed to see easing of depression and peak response may require 3 months of use—be patient and give the medicine a chance to work for you. Easing of pain (when used in pain syndromes) may start sooner. Keep taking the medicine even if you feel better. DO NOT simply take the medicine when you feel depressed. People with delusions may require 7 weeks to benefit. Long-term use (months to years) requires periodic evaluation of response and dose adjustment.

Typical Treatment Goals and Measurements (Outcomes and Markers)
Depression: The general goal: to help lessen the degree and severity of depression, letting patients return to their daily lives. Some clinicians use a depression scale such as the Hamilton to check severity and results of treatment.
Pain syndromes: The general goal: to decrease pain to a manageable level. Pain should be appropriately assessed, and progress defined based on lowering of overall pain level. Pain is now the fifth vital sign according to the Joint Commission on Accreditation of Health Care Organizations (JCAHCO). Expect effective pain management as a basic right.

▷ **This Drug Should Not Be Taken If**
- you have had an allergic reaction to it previously.
- you are taking, or have taken within the past 14 days, any monoamine oxidase (MAO) type A inhibitor drug (see Drug Classes).
- you have had a recent heart attack (myocardial infarction).

▷ **Inform Your Physician Before Taking This Drug If**
- you have had an adverse reaction to another antidepressant.
- you have any type of seizure disorder.
- you have increased internal eye pressure or narrow-angle glaucoma.
- you have any type of heart disease, especially a heart rhythm disorder.
- you drink alcohol excessively.
- you have a thyroid disorder or take thyroid medication.
- you have thought about or attempted suicide.
- you have diabetes or sugar intolerance.
- you take levodopa (increased risk of heart rhythm problems with high desipramine doses).
- you have prostatism (see Glossary).
- you will have surgery with general anesthesia.

Possible Side Effects (natural, expected and unavoidable drug actions)
Mild drowsiness, light-headedness (low blood pressure), blurred vision, dry mouth, constipation, impaired urination.

▷ **Possible Adverse Effects** (unusual, unexpected and infrequent reactions)
If any of the following develop, consult your physician promptly for guidance.

Mild Adverse Effects
Allergic reactions: skin rash, hives, swelling of face or tongue, drug fever (see Glossary)—case reports.
Headache, dizziness, weakness, unsteadiness, tremors, fainting—infrequent.
Irritation of tongue or mouth, altered taste, difficulty talking—rare.
Indigestion, nausea—infrequent.
Fluctuations of blood sugar—possible.

Serious Adverse Effects
Allergic reactions: drug-induced hepatitis, with or without jaundice; anaphylactic reaction (see Glossary)—case reports.
Adverse behavioral effects: delusions, hallucinations—case reports.
Seizures; reduced control of epilepsy—case reports.
Aggravation of paranoid psychoses and schizophrenia—possible.
Heart rhythm disturbances, myocarditis—case reports.
Parkinson-like disorders, peripheral neuritis (see both terms in Glossary)—rare to infrequent.
Withdrawal symptoms—case reports of hypomania.
Abnormally low white blood cell and platelet counts: fever, sore throat, infections, abnormal bleeding or bruising—case reports.
Neuroleptic malignant syndrome—case reports.

▷ **Possible Effects on Sexual Function:** Decreased libido, increased libido (antidepressant effect), impotence, painful male orgasm, male breast enlargement (gynecomastia), female breast enlargement with milk production, swelling of testicles, decreased sperm viability—case reports.

Adverse Effects That May Mimic Natural Diseases or Disorders
Liver toxicity may suggest viral hepatitis.

Natural Diseases or Disorders That May Be Activated by This Drug
Latent diabetes, epilepsy, glaucoma, prostatism.

Possible Effects on Laboratory Tests
Complete blood cell counts: decreased red cells, hemoglobin, white cells and platelets; increased eosinophils (allergic reaction).

Blood glucose levels: unexplained fluctuations.

Liver function tests: increased liver enzymes (ALT/GPT, AST/GOT and alkaline phosphatase), increased bilirubin—all rare.

Thyroid function tests: decreased TSH and mean free thyroxin.

CAUTION

1. Watch for toxicity: confusion, agitation, fast heart rate, heart irregularity. Blood levels will be needed.

2. It is advisable to withhold this drug if electroconvulsive therapy (ECT) is to be used to treat the depression.

Precautions for Use

By Infants and Children: Safety and effectiveness for those under 6 years of age not established. This drug is being used to treat children who have attention deficit disorder, with or without hyperactivity. Dose and management must be supervised by a properly trained pediatrician.

By Those Over 60 Years of Age: Start treatment with 25 mg one or two times daily to evaluate tolerance. During the first 2 weeks of treatment, watch for confusion, restlessness, agitation, forgetfulness, disorientation, delusions or hallucinations. Also observe for unsteadiness and instability that may predispose to falling. This drug may aggravate prostatism.

▷ **Advisability of Use During Pregnancy**

Pregnancy Category: C. See Pregnancy Risk Categories at the back of this book.

Animal studies: Birth defects reported in rat and rabbit studies.

Human studies: Adequate studies of pregnant women are not available.

Use only if clearly needed. Avoid during the first 3 months if possible.

Advisability of Use If Breast-Feeding

Presence of this drug in breast milk: Yes, in small amounts.

Monitor nursing infant closely and discontinue drug or nursing if adverse effects develop.

Habit-Forming Potential: Psychological or physical dependence is rare and unexpected. Some patients may seek to abuse this medicine for its ability to create anticholinergic delirium. Case reports of hypomania on stopping the drug have been made.

Effects of Overdose: Confusion, hallucinations, drowsiness, tremors, heart irregularity, seizures, stupor, hypothermia (see Glossary).

Possible Effects of Long-Term Use: None reported.

Suggested Periodic Examinations While Taking This Drug (at physician's discretion)

Complete blood cell counts.

Liver function tests.

Serial blood pressure readings and electrocardiograms.

▷ **While Taking This Drug, Observe the Following**

Foods: No specific restrictions. Limiting food intake may avoid excess weight gain.

Herbal Medicines or Minerals: Since desipramine and St. John's wort may act to increase serotonin, the combination is not advised. St. John's wort also increases sun sensitivity. Recent data questions the results (efficacy) of St. John's wort in serious depression. Since part of the way ginseng works may be as a MAO inhibitor, do not combine with desipramine. Indian snakeroot, kava kava and yohimbe are also best avoided while taking this medicine. Talk to your doctor about herbal medicines.

Nutritional Support: High doses of vitamin C may blunt the therapeutic effects of desipramine.

Beverages: No restrictions. May be taken with milk.

▷ *Alcohol:* Avoid completely. This drug can markedly increase the intoxicating effects of alcohol; the combination can depress brain function.

Tobacco Smoking: May accelerate the elimination of this drug and require increased doses. I advise everyone to quit smoking.

Marijuana Smoking

Occasional (once or twice weekly): transient increase in drowsiness and mouth dryness as well as possible unacceptable increases in heart rate.

Daily: persistent drowsiness and mouth dryness; possible reduced effectiveness of this drug.

▷ *Other Drugs*

Desipramine may ***increase*** the effects of
- all drugs with atropinelike effects (see Drug Classes).
- all drugs with sedative effects; watch for excessive sedation.
- phenytoin (Dilantin) or fosphenytoin (Cerebyx), leading to possible toxicity.

Desipramine may ***decrease*** the effects of
- clonidine (Catapres).
- guanethidine (Ismelin, Esimil).
- guanfacine (Tenex).
- levodopa, by decreasing absorption of the levodopa.
- venlafaxine (Effexor).

Desipramine ***taken concurrently*** with
- albuterol (Ventolin) may increase the effect of albuterol on the blood vessels.
- anticonvulsants—carbamazepine (Tegretol) and phenytoin (Dilantin) are examples—require careful monitoring for changes in seizure patterns (need to adjust anticonvulsant dose).
- cisapride (Propulsid) increases risk of heart rhythm problems.
- dofetilide (Tikosyn) increases risk of heart rhythm problems. The combination should be avoided.
- ethchlorvynol (Placidyl) may cause delirium; avoid concurrent use.
- gatifloxacin (Tequin) or grepafloxacin (Raxar) may increase risk of heart rhythm problems. Combination is not recommended.
- monoamine oxidase (MAO) type A inhibitor drugs (see Drug Classes) may cause high fever, seizures and high blood pressure; avoid combining. Wait 14 days between either.
- propafenone (Rythmol) may lead to toxic desipramine levels.
- quinestrol (Estrovis) may increase or decrease desipramine levels.
- quinidine may cause desipramine toxicity.
- sparfloxacin (Zagam) may increase risk of heart rhythm problems.
- stimulant drugs (amphetamine, cocaine, epinephrine, phenylpropanolamine, etc.) may cause severe high blood pressure and/or high fever.
- thyroid preparations may increase the risk of heart rhythm disorders.
- tramadol (Ultram) may increase seizure risk.
- large doses (greater than 2 g/day) of vitamin C may lead to increased removal of desipramine and need to adjust dose.

- warfarin (Coumadin) may cause an increased risk of bleeding. Increased testing of INR is indicated.
- zolpidem (Ambien) may lead to hallucinations.

The following drugs may *increase* the effects of desipramine:
- cimetidine (Tagamet).
- fluoxetine (Prozac).
- fluvoxamine (Luvox).
- methylphenidate (Ritalin).
- nefazodone (Serzone).
- phenothiazines (see Drug Classes).
- ritonavir (Norvir) and other protease inhibitors (see Drug Classes).

The following drugs may *decrease* the effects of desipramine:
- barbiturates (see Drug Classes).
- chloral hydrate (Noctec, Somnos, etc.).
- clonazepam (Klonopin).
- estrogen (see profile for brand names).
- lithium (Lithobid, Lithotab, etc.).
- oral contraceptives (birth control pills; see profile for brand names).
- reserpine (Serpasil, Ser-Ap-Es, etc.).

▷ *Driving, Hazardous Activities:* This drug may impair mental alertness, judgment, physical coordination and reaction time. Restrict activities as necessary.

Aviation Note: The use of this drug *is a disqualification* for piloting. Consult a designated Aviation Medical Examiner.

Exposure to Sun: Use caution. This drug may cause photosensitivity (see Glossary) and changes in iris and skin pigment color with sun exposure.

Exposure to Heat: Use caution. This drug can inhibit sweating and impair adaptation to hot environments, increasing the risk of heatstroke. Avoid saunas.

Exposure to Cold: The elderly should use caution and avoid conditions conducive to hypothermia (see Glossary).

Exposure to Environmental Chemicals: This drug may mask the symptoms of poisoning due to handling certain insecticides (organophosphorous types). Read labels carefully.

Discontinuation: Best to stop this drug gradually. Abrupt withdrawal after prolonged use may cause headache, malaise and nausea. If this drug is stopped, doses of other drugs may need adjustment.

DEXAMETHASONE (dex a METH a sohn)

Introduced: 1958   **Class:** Cortisonelike drugs   **Prescription:** USA: Yes
Controlled Drug: USA: No; Canada: No   **Available as Generic:** USA: Yes; Canada: Yes

Brand Names: Aeroseb-Dex, ✤Ak-Dex, Ak-Trol [CD], Baldex, Dalalone, Dalalone DP, Dalalone LA, Decaderm, Decadron, Decadron Nasal Spray, Decadron-LA, Decadron Phosphate Ophthalmic, Decadron Phosphate Respihaler, Decadron Phosphate Turbinaire, Decadron w/Xylocaine [CD], Decadron dose pack, Decaject, Decaject LA, Decaspray, Deenar [CD], Deone-LA, ✤ Deronil, Dex-4, Dexacen-4, Dexacen LA-8, Dexacidin [CD], Dexacort, Dexameth, Dexasone, Dexasone-LA, Dexo-LA, Dexon, Dexone-E, Dexone-4,

Dexone-LA, Dexsone, Dexsone-E, Dexsone-LA, Dezone, Duo-dezone, Gammacorten, Hexadrol, Maxidex, Mymethasone, ✤Neodecadron Eye-Ear, Neodexair, Neomycin-Dex, Ocu-Trol [CD], ✤Oradexon, ✤PMS-Dexamethasone, ✤SK-Dexamethasone, ✤Sofracort, Solurex, Solurex-LA, ✤ Spersadex, Tobradex [CD], Turbinaire

BENEFITS versus RISKS	
Possible Benefits	*Possible Risks*
EFFECTIVE RELIEF OF SYMPTOMS IN A WIDE VARIETY OF INFLAMMATORY AND ALLERGIC DISORDERS	Long-term systemic use (exceeding 2 weeks) is associated with many possible adverse effects: ALTERED MOOD AND PERSONALITY,
EFFECTIVE IMMUNOSUPPRESSION IN SELECTED BENIGN AND MALIGNANT DISORDERS	CATARACTS, GLAUCOMA, HYPERTENSION, ARRHYTHMIAS, PEPTIC ULCERS, PANCREATITIS,
COMBINED WITH TOBRAMYCIN TO FIGHT BOTH INFECTION AND INFLAMMATION IN THE EYE	OSTEOPOROSIS, ASEPTIC BONE NECROSIS, INCREASED SUSCEPTIBILITY TO INFECTIONS

▷ **Principal Uses**

*As a Single Drug Product:*Uses currently included in FDA-approved labeling: (1) Used to manage serious skin disorders, asthma, allergic rhinitis, lymphoma, brain edema, shock, systemic lupus erythematosus and all types of major rheumatic disorders including bursitis, tendonitis and most forms of arthritis; (2) ulcerative disease of the colon; (3) topical cream is used to treat eczema, psoriasis, dermatitis and lichen planus; (4) used in conjunction with antibiotics in meningitis; (5) helps ease swelling in otitis media.

Other (unlabeled) generally accepted uses: (1) Adrenal insufficiency; (2) acute airway obstruction; (3) mountain sickness; (4) vomiting caused by chemotherapy; (5) cardiopulmonary bypass; (6) refractory depression; (7) relief of brain cancer symptoms; (8) combination with other drugs in multiple myeloma; (9) cases of *Pneumocystis carinii* pneumonia; (10) can help suppress male hormones (androgens) in women with acne, hirsutism or hair loss (androgenic alopecia) caused by androgens; (11) eases vomiting after cancer treatment (chemotherapy); (12) single doses may have a role in croup.

How This Drug Works: Inhibits defensive functions of certain white blood cells. It reduces the production of lymphocytes and some antibodies and acts as an immunosuppressant. When combined with tobramycin or other antibiotics in the eye, it helps relieve inflammation and pain while the antibiotic kills the infection

Available Dosage Forms and Strengths
Aerosol — 0.01% and 0.04%
Aerosol inhaler — 84 mcg per spray
Cream — 0.1%
Elixir — 0.5 mg/5 ml
Eye ointment — 0.05%
Eye solution — 0.1%
Eye suspension — 0.1% dexamethasone, 0.3% tobramycin
Gel — 0.1%
Injection — 4 mg/ml, 8 mg/ml, 10 mg/ml, 16 mg/ml, 20 mg/ml, 24 mg/ml

Oral solution — 0.5 mg/0.5 ml, 0.5 mg/5 ml
    Solution — 0.1%
Spray, topical — 10 mg/25 g
Suspension — 0.1%
    Tablets — 0.25 mg, 0.5 mg, 0.75 mg, 1 mg, 1.5 mg, 2 mg, 4 mg, 6 mg

▷ **Usual Adult Dosage Ranges**

Respihaler: For asthma, three inhalations taken three to four times a day.

Turbinaire form: Two sprays in each nostril two or three times daily. Twelve sprays is the daily maximum.

Decadron dose pack form: On the first day, 1 or 2 ml is given as an intramuscular injection (IM). On the second day, four tablets are taken—divided into two equal doses (such as two in the morning at 9 A.M. and two at 9 P.M.). The third day, the same dose is given, the fourth day two tablets are given in two equal doses, the fifth and sixth day one tablet a day is given and treatment is stopped on the seventh day.

Ophthalmic: Tobradex form is often started as one to two drops into the eye sac or sacs (conjunctival) every 2 hours during the first day or two of treatment. The dosing frequency is then gradually decreased to one or two drops every 4–6 hours depending on the severity and response of the infection to treatment.

Oral: 0.75 to 9 mg daily divided into two to four doses.

Topical (0.1% cream): Apply thin film of medicine on the affected area three or four times a day.

Oral dose for children: 0.03 to 0.15 mg per kg of body mass per day, divided into equal doses given every 6 to 12 hours, or 1–5 mg per square meter divided into equal doses and given every 6 to 12 hours. **Note: Actual dose and schedule must be determined for each patient individually.**

Conditions Requiring Dosing Adjustments

Liver Function: This drug is eliminated via the liver; however, no specific guidelines for dosing adjustments are available.

Kidney Function: Use with caution as it can cause alkalosis (a change toward a more basic condition in the body's chemistry).

Obesity: Dosing on a mg-per-kg-of-body-mass-per-day basis is recommended. It is best to measure free urinary cortisol as well.

▷ **Dosing Instructions:** Tablet may be crushed and taken with or following food to prevent stomach irritation, preferably in the morning. If you forget a dose: (suspension, solution): take the missed dose right after you remember it. If it is nearly time for your next scheduled dose, skip the missed dose and continue with the scheduled dose. DO NOT double doses. If you only take this medicine every other day, take the dose you forgot right away, unless it's late in the day. If you only remember late in the day, wait until the next morning to take the missed dose and then continue on your every other day schedule. If you forget a dose of the shot (IM injection), call your doctor for instructions.

Usual Duration of Use: For acute disorders: 4 to 10 days.

For chronic disorders: varies. Length of therapy should not exceed time needed for adequate symptomatic relief in acute self-limiting conditions or time required to stabilize a chronic condition and permit gradual withdrawal.

Typical Treatment Goals and Measurements (Outcomes and Markers)

Inflammation: The general goal is to relieve the swelling and the inflammatory response. Use in asthma should help decrease the frequency and severity of acute attacks. Some clinicians use decreased frequency of rescue inhaler use as a measure of success. Lung (pulmonary function) testing and improvement in those tests also helps define results in asthma. Lastly, clinical signs and symptoms such as wheezing, tightness in the chest and exercise tolerance should all move in favorable directions.

▷ **This Drug Should Not Be Taken If**

- you have had an allergic reaction to it previously.
- you have active peptic ulcer disease.
- you have an active herpes simplex infection of the eye.
- you have a systemic fungal infection (talk with your doctor).
- your sputum consistently grows *Candida albicans* (a yeast that may grow very quickly if steroids suppress your immune system).
- you have a psychoneurosis or psychosis.
- you have active tuberculosis.

▷ **Inform Your Physician Before Taking This Drug If**

- you have had unfavorable reactions to cortisonelike drugs.
- you have a history of peptic ulcer disease, thrombophlebitis or tuberculosis.
- you have diabetes, glaucoma, high blood pressure, deficient thyroid function or myasthenia gravis.
- you start to have restricted motion, increased pain, fever or joint swelling— may be early signs of septic arthritis.
- you have osteoporosis.
- you plan to have surgery of any kind in the near future.

▷ **Possible Side Effects** (natural, expected and unavoidable drug actions)

Increased appetite, weight gain, retention of salt and water, excretion of potassium, increased susceptibility to infection (yeast infections can be frequent in cancer patients treated with a corticosteroid). Increased facial hair. Increased white blood cell count (release from the bone marrow versus a sign of infection). **All of the possible and mild or serious adverse effects may happen with inhaled or even ophthalmic steroid use, but generally to a much reduced extent and/or severity.**

▷ **Possible Adverse Effects** (unusual, unexpected and infrequent reactions)

If any of the following develop, consult your physician promptly for guidance.

Mild Adverse Effects

Allergic reaction: skin rash—case reports.

Headache, dizziness, insomnia—possible.

Mild euphoria or depression—most common possible central nervous system (CNS) effects.

High blood pressure (may be lessened by alternate-day therapy): more likely in older patients and those who already have high blood pressure— possible.

Acid indigestion, abdominal distention—possible.

Muscle cramping and weakness—case reports.

Easy bruising (ecchymosis) or acnelike lesions—case reports.

Vaginal itching—may be frequent with intravenous dosing.

Serious Adverse Effects

Allergic reaction: anaphylaxis—case reports.

Mental and emotional disturbances of serious magnitude—infrequent.

Reactivation of latent tuberculosis—possible.

Pneumocystis carinii pneumonia—possible with immunosuppression and chronic use.

Development of peptic ulcer—rare, but risk increases with higher doses and preexisting ulcers.

Inflammation of the pancreas—rare.

Thrombophlebitis (inflammation of a vein with the formation of blood clot): pain or tenderness in thigh or leg or swelling of the foot, ankle or leg—possible with intravenous use.

Abnormal lipids (cholesterol, triglycerides, LDLs)—possible.

Abnormal heart rhythm—case reports.

Cushing's syndrome—possible with chronic use and high doses (supraphysiologic).

Suppression of the adrenal gland—possible with chronic use and more common with larger doses.

High blood sugar—risk increases with use in diabetics and with higher doses.

Excessively low blood potassium—case reports.

Abnormally slow heartbeat in infants—case reports.

Increased pressure in the eye or cataracts or glaucoma—rare to frequent.

Precipitation of porphyria—case reports.

Excessive thyroid function (questionable causality)—case reports.

Muscle changes (myopathy)—infrequent, but more likely with higher doses and some steroids.

Bone death (aseptic necrosis or avascular necrosis)—infrequent, but more likely with high initial doses.

Osteoporosis—more likely with long-term and higher-dose use.

▷ **Possible Effects on Sexual Function:** Altered timing and pattern of menstruation—case reports.

Adverse Effects That May Mimic Natural Diseases or Disorders

Pattern of symptoms and signs resembling Cushing's syndrome.

Natural Diseases or Disorders That May Be Activated by This Drug

Latent diabetes, glaucoma, peptic ulcer disease, tuberculosis.

Possible Effects on Laboratory Tests

Blood amylase level: increased (possible pancreatitis).

Blood glucose level: increased.

Digoxin testing: may falsely increase digoxin results.

Glucose tolerance test (GTT): increased.

Blood potassium level: decreased.

Thyroid function tests: decreased.

Cholesterol: increased in some studies while decreased in others.

CAUTION

1. It is best to carry a card noting that you are taking this drug, if your course of treatment is to exceed 1 week.
2. Do not stop this drug abruptly if it is used for long-term treatment.

3. If vaccination against measles, rabies, smallpox or yellow fever is required, stop this drug 72 hours before vaccination and do not resume it for at least 14 days after vaccination.
4. Children may be more sensitive to topical application because there is a larger skin surface area to body weight ratio.

Precautions for Use

By Infants and Children: Avoid prolonged use if possible. During long-term use, watch for suppression of normal growth and the possibility of increased intracranial pressure. Following long-term use, the child may be at risk for adrenal gland deficiency during stress for as long as 18 months after cessation.

By Those Over 60 Years of Age: Avoid prolonged use of this drug. Continual use (even in small doses) can increase the severity of diabetes, enhance fluid retention, raise blood pressure, weaken resistance to infection, induce stomach ulcer and accelerate the development of cataracts and osteoporosis.

▷ **Advisability of Use During Pregnancy**

Pregnancy Category: C. See Pregnancy Risk Categories at the back of this book.
Animal studies: Birth defects reported in mice, rats and rabbits.
Human studies: Adequate studies of pregnant women are not available.

Avoid completely during the first 3 months. Limit use during the last 6 months as much as possible. If used, examine infant for possible deficiency of adrenal gland function.

Advisability of Use If Breast-Feeding

Presence of this drug in breast milk: Yes.
Avoid drug or refrain from nursing.

Habit-Forming Potential: Use to suppress symptoms over an extended period of time may produce a state of functional dependence (see Glossary). In treating asthma and rheumatoid arthritis, it is best to keep the dose as small as possible and to attempt drug withdrawal after periods of reasonable improvement. Such procedures may reduce the degree of "steroid rebound"—the return of symptoms as the drug is withdrawn.

Effects of Overdose: Fatigue, muscle weakness, stomach irritation, acid indigestion, excessive sweating, facial flushing, fluid retention, swelling of extremities, increased blood pressure.

Possible Effects of Long-Term Use: Increased blood sugar (possible diabetes), increased fat deposits on the trunk of the body ("buffalo hump"), rounding of the face ("moon face"), thinning and fragility of skin, loss of texture and strength of bones (osteoporosis, aseptic necrosis), cataracts, glaucoma, increased body hair (hirsutism), retarded growth and development in children.

Suggested Periodic Examinations While Taking This Drug (at physician's discretion)

Measurements of blood pressure, blood sugar and potassium levels.
Complete eye examinations at regular intervals.
Chest X-ray if history of tuberculosis.
Determination of the rate of development of the growing child to detect retardation of normal growth.
Bone mineral density testing to assess risk of osteoporosis or thinning of bones.

▷ **While Taking This Drug, Observe the Following**

Foods: No interactions expected. Ask your physician about salt restriction or need for potassium-rich foods. During long-term use of this drug, it is advisable to eat a high-protein diet.

Herbal Medicines or Minerals: Hawthorn, ginger, garlic, ma huang, ginseng and nettle may change blood sugar. Since dexamethasone may also change blood sugar control, caution is advised.

Fir or pine needle oil should NOT be used by asthmatics. Ephedra alone does carry a German Commission E monograph indication for asthma treatment. If you are allergic to plants in the Asteraceae family (aster, chrysanthemum, daisy or ragweed), you may also be allergic to echinacea, chamomile, feverfew and St. John's wort.

During long-term use, take a vitamin D supplement and increase calcium. During wound repair, take a zinc supplement. Talk to your doctor BEFORE adding any herbal to any other medicines that you already take.

Beverages: No restrictions. Drink all forms of milk liberally.

▷ *Alcohol:* No interactions expected. Caution if you are prone to peptic ulcer disease.

Tobacco Smoking: Nicotine increases the blood levels of naturally produced cortisone and related hormones. Heavy smoking may add to the expected actions of this drug and requires close observation for excessive effects. I advise everyone to quit smoking.

Marijuana Smoking: May cause additional impairment of immunity and also is a risk factor for toxoplasmosis.

▷ *Other Drugs*

Dexamethasone may **decrease** the effects of
- indinavir (Crixivan).
- insulin (various), requiring dosing changes of insulin.
- isoniazid (INH, Niconyl, etc.).
- salicylates (aspirin, sodium salicylate, etc.), increasing ulcer risk.
- vaccines (such as flu vaccine), by blunting the immune response to them.

Dexamethasone *taken concurrently* with
- aspirin (various) and other NSAIDS (see Drug Classes) increases the risk of stomach and intestinal (gastrointestinal) ulceration.
- birth control pills (oral contraceptives) may increase dexamethasone's therapeutic effects.
- carbamazepine (Tegretol) will reduce the effectiveness of dexamethasone.
- irinotecan (Camptosar) may increase risk of low white blood cells (lymphocytopenia) and increase hyperglycemia risk.
- loop diuretics such as furosemide (Lasix) or bumetanide (Bumex) can result in additive potassium loss.
- oral anticoagulants may either increase or decrease their effectiveness; ask your doctor about increased INR testing and dose adjustment.
- oral antidiabetic drugs (see Drug Classes) will decrease their effectiveness.
- neuromuscular blocking agents (such as pancuronium [Pavulon] or vecuronium [Norcuron] may antagonize the neuromuscular blockade, increasing risk or severity of flaccid paralysis. Dose adjustments or unparalyzed periods may be advisable.

- ritonavir (Norvir), saquinavir (Fortovase) and possibly other protease inhibitors (PI—see Drug Classes) may decrease PI blood levels and increase dexamethasone blood levels.
- thiazide diuretics (see Drug Classes) will decrease their blood-pressure-lowering ability.

The following drugs may **decrease** the effects of dexamethasone:
- antacids—may reduce its absorption.
- barbiturates (Amytal, Butisol, phenobarbital, etc.).
- fosphenytoin (Cerebyx).
- phenytoin (Dilantin, etc.).
- primidone (Mysoline).
- rifabutin (Mycobutin).
- rifampin (Rifadin, Rimactane, etc.).

▷ *Driving, Hazardous Activities:* Usually no restrictions. Be alert to the rare occurrence of dizziness.

Aviation Note: The use of this drug *may be a disqualification* for piloting. Consult a designated Aviation Medical Examiner.

Exposure to Sun: No restrictions.

Occurrence of Unrelated Illness: This drug may decrease natural resistance to infection. Call your doctor if you develop an infection of any kind. It may also reduce your body's ability to respond to the stress of acute illness, injury or surgery. Keep your physician fully informed of any significant health changes.

Discontinuation: Do not stop this drug abruptly after chronic use. Ask your doctor for help about gradual withdrawal. For up to 2 years after stopping this drug, you may require it again if you have an injury, surgery or an illness.

DIAZEPAM (di AZ e pam)

Introduced: 1963   **Class:** Antianxiety drug, benzodiazepines, mild tranquilizer   **Prescription:** USA: Yes   **Controlled Drug:** USA: C-IV*; Canada: No   **Available as Generic:** Yes

Brand Names: ✤Apo-Diazepam, Diastat, ✤Diazemuls, Diazepam Intensol Oral Solution, Dizac, E-Pam, ✤Meval, ✤Novo-Dipam, Q-pam, ✤Rival, Valcaps, Valium, Valrelease, Vazepam, ✤Vivol, Zetran

BENEFITS versus RISKS	
Possible Benefits	*Possible Risks*
RELIEF OF ANXIETY AND NERVOUS TENSION	Habit-forming potential with prolonged use
Wide margin of safety with therapeutic doses	Minor impairment of mental functions
	Respiratory depression
	Jaundice—very rare

▷ **Principal Uses**

As a Single Drug Product: Uses included in FDA-approved labeling: (1) Provides short-term relief of mild to moderate anxiety; (2) relieves the symptoms of

* See Schedules of Controlled Drugs at the back of this book.

acute alcohol withdrawal: agitation, tremors, hallucinations, incipient delirium tremens; (3) eases skeletal muscle spasm; (4) provides short-term control of certain types of seizures (epilepsy, fever-induced and status epilepticus); (5) short-term relief of insomnia; (6) adjunctive use in endoscopic procedures; (7) decreases anxiety prior to electrical defibrillation of the heart (cardioversion); (8) eases severe muscle spasms; (9) rectal gel is approved as an orphan drug for intermittent sudden (acute) seizure control in some patients who fail to respond to other treatments.

Other (unlabeled) generally accepted uses: (1) Helps prevent LSD flashbacks; (2) short-term treatment of sleepwalking; (3) treatment of persistent hiccups; (4) adjunctive treatment of catatonia.

How This Drug Works: This drug calms higher brain centers by enhancing a nerve transmitter (gamma-aminobutyric acid or GABA).

Available Dosage Forms and Strengths

Capsules, prolonged action (sustained release) — 15 mg

Concentrate — 5 mg/ml

Injection — 5 mg/ml

Oral solution — 5 mg/ml, 5 mg/5 ml

Rectal gel — 2.5 mg, 5 mg, 10 mg, 15 mg, 20 mg

Tablets — 2 mg, 5 mg, 10 mg

▷ **Usual Adult Dosage Ranges:** *For anxiety:* 2 to 10 mg, two to four times daily. Dose may be increased cautiously as needed and tolerated. After 1 week of continual use, the total daily dose may be taken at bedtime. Maximum daily dose is 60 mg. Sustained-release form can be given once daily (15 mg) if it is replacing use of the immediate-release form that has been taken as a total daily dose of 15 mg divided into 5-mg doses three times a day. **Note: Actual dose and schedule must be determined for each patient individually.**

Conditions Requiring Dosing Adjustments

Liver Function: The dose must be decreased by 50% in patients with liver compromise.

Kidney Function: Caution—if 15 mg or more is given daily, diazepam metabolites may accumulate.

Obesity: Obese patients may take longer than nonobese patients to accumulate this medicine. The time that it takes to remove diazepam (elimination half-life) is prolonged in obese people. This means that obese people may take a much longer time to get the peak effect of diazepam and will also take a longer time to remove the drug from their bodies.

▷ **Dosing Instructions:** The tablet may be crushed and taken on empty stomach or with food or milk. The prolonged-action capsule should not be opened. Do not stop this drug abruptly if taken for more than 4 weeks (medicine should be slowly withdrawn or tapered). If you forget a dose: Take the dose as soon as you remember it, unless it's nearly time for your next dose. If you remember when it's nearly time for your next dose, skip the missed dose and take the next dose right on schedule. DO NOT double doses.

Usual Duration of Use: Regular use for 3 to 5 days is usually needed to see benefits in relieving moderate anxiety. Limit continual use to 1 to 3 weeks. Avoid uninterrupted and prolonged use.

Author's Note: The National Institute of Mental Health has an information page on anxiety. It can be found on the World Wide Web (www.nimh.nih.gov/anxiety).

Typical Treatment Goals and Measurements (Outcomes and Markers)

Goals for anxiety tend to be more vague and subjective than hypertension or cholesterol. Frequently, the patient (in conjunction with physician assessment) will largely decide if anxiety has been modified to a successful extent. The ability of the patient to return to normal activities is a hallmark of successful treatment.

▷ **This Drug Should Not Be Taken If**

- you have had an allergic reaction to any dosage form of it previously.
- you have acute narrow-angle glaucoma.
- it is prescribed for a child under 6 months of age.

▷ **Inform Your Physician Before Taking This Drug If**

- you are allergic to any benzodiazepine (see Drug Classes).
- you have a history of alcoholism or drug abuse.
- you are pregnant or planning pregnancy.
- you have impaired liver or kidney function.
- you have a history of serious depression or a mental disorder.
- you have asthma, emphysema, epilepsy or myasthenia gravis.

Possible Side Effects (natural, expected and unavoidable drug actions)

Drowsiness—frequent.

Lethargy, unsteadiness—rare.

"Hangover" effects on the day following bedtime use.

▷ **Possible Adverse Effects** (unusual, unexpected and infrequent reactions)

If any of the following develop, consult your physician promptly for guidance.

Mild Adverse Effects

Allergic reactions: rashes, hives—rare.

Dizziness, fainting, blurred or double vision, slurred speech, sweating, nausea—possible.

Increased liver enzymes—case report.

Ringing in the ears—case reports.

Impaired motor skills (dose-related to some extent)—frequency varies.

Serious Adverse Effects

Allergic reactions: liver damage with jaundice (see Glossary), kidney damage, abnormally low blood platelet count, anaphylaxis—case reports.

Respiratory depression—dose-related.

Bone marrow depression: low white blood cells, fever, sore throat—case reports.

Severe lowering of blood pressure, slow heart rate and cardiac arrest have been reported after rapid intravenous dosing—case reports.

Hip fracture—possible indirect effect of the medicine arising from unsteadiness.

Amnesia—dose-related.

Heart arrhythmia (intravenous form)—possible.

Obsessive-compulsive disorder following extended use and abrupt withdrawal—possible.

Paradoxical responses of excitement, agitation, anger, rage—case reports.

▷ **Possible Effects on Sexual Function:**
Altered timing and pattern of menstruation.
Small doses (2 to 5 mg/day) may help the anxiety seen in many cases of impotence in men and inhibited sexual responsiveness in women. Larger doses (10 mg/day or more) can decrease libido, impair potency in men and inhibit orgasm in women.
Swelling and tenderness of male breast tissue (gynecomastia).
Abnormally prolonged erections (priapism)—case reports.

Adverse Effects That May Mimic Natural Diseases or Disorders
Liver reaction with jaundice may suggest viral hepatitis.

Possible Effects on Laboratory Tests
White blood cell counts: decreased.
Blood thyroxine (T4) level: decreased.
Liver function tests: increased liver enzymes (ALT/GPT, AST/GOT and alkaline phosphatase), increased bilirubin—all rare.
Urine sugar tests: no drug effect with Tes-Tape; low test results with Clinistix and Diastix.
Urine screening tests for drug abuse: may be positive. (Test results depend upon amount of drug taken and testing method used.)

CAUTION
1. This drug should not be stopped abruptly if it has been taken continually for more than 4 weeks.
2. Some nonprescription (over-the-counter or OTC) drug products that contain antihistamines (allergy and cold preparations, sleep aids) can cause excessive sedation if combined with diazepam.

Precautions for Use
By Infants and Children: This drug should not be used in hyperactive or psychotic children. Watch for excessive sedation and incoordination. Usual dose in children for muscle relaxation or sedation is 0.1 to 0.8 mg per kg of body mass per day, divided into equal doses and given every 8 hours or as often as every 6 hours. The drug has been used intravenously to help seizures in neonates.
By Those Over 60 Years of Age: Small doses are indicated. Observe for lethargy, indifference, fatigue, weakness, unsteadiness, disturbing dreams, nightmares and paradoxical reactions of excitement, agitation, anger, hostility and rage.

▷ **Advisability of Use During Pregnancy**
Pregnancy Category: D. See Pregnancy Risk Categories at the back of this book.
Animal studies: Cleft palate reported in mice; skeletal defects in rats.
Human studies: Available information is conflicting and inconclusive. Some findings of increased serious birth defects. Other studies have found no significant increase in birth defects.
Frequent use in late pregnancy can cause the "floppy infant" syndrome in the newborn: weakness, lethargy, unresponsiveness, depressed breathing, low body temperature. Avoid use during entire pregnancy.

Advisability of Use If Breast-Feeding
Presence of this drug in breast milk: Yes.
Avoid drug or refrain from nursing.

Habit-Forming Potential: This drug can produce psychological and/or physical dependence (see Glossary), especially if used in large doses for an extended period of time.

Effects of Overdose: Marked drowsiness, weakness, feeling of drunkenness, staggering gait, tremor, stupor progressing to deep sleep or coma.

Possible Effects of Long-Term Use: Psychological and/or physical dependence, rare blood cell disorders.

Suggested Periodic Examinations While Taking This Drug (at physician's discretion)

Complete blood cell counts during long-term use.

▷ **While Taking This Drug, Observe the Following**

Foods: No restrictions.

Herbal Medicines or Minerals: Hawthorn may react antagonistically to diazepam. Valerian and kava kava may interact additively (drowsiness). Avoid these combinations. Kava and valerian may exacerbate central nervous system depression (avoid this combination). Kola nut, Siberian ginseng, mate, ephedra and ma huang may blunt the benefits of this medicine. While St. John's wort is indicated for anxiety, it is also thought to increase (induce) cytochrome P450 enzymes and will tend to blunt diazepam effectiveness if combined with diazepam. Do not combine any herbal medicines without talking to your doctor first.

Beverages: Avoid excessive intake of caffeine-containing beverages: coffee, tea, cola. May be taken with milk. Caffeine use may be recommended by your doctor to ease some cases of excessive diazepam-caused drowsiness.

▷ *Alcohol:* Avoid this combination. Alcohol increases the absorption of this drug and adds to its depressant effects on the brain. It is advisable to avoid alcohol completely—throughout the day and night—if it is necessary to drive or to engage in any hazardous activity.

Tobacco Smoking: Heavy smoking may reduce the calming action of this drug. I advise everyone to quit smoking.

Marijuana Smoking: Increased sedation and impairment of intellectual and physical performance.

▷ *Other Drugs*

Diazepam may *increase* the effects of
- digoxin (Lanoxin) and cause digoxin toxicity.
- phenytoin (Dilantin) or fosphenytoin (Cerebyx) and cause toxicity.

Diazepam may *decrease* the effects of
- levodopa (Sinemet, etc.) and reduce its effectiveness in treating Parkinson's disease.

Diazepam *taken concurrently* with
- fluoxetine (Prozac) may lead to diazepam toxicity.
- fluvoxamine (Luvox) can result in serious accumulation of diazepam and toxicity.
- macrolide antibiotics (see Drug Classes) may lead to toxicity.
- MAO inhibitors (see Drug Classes) may exaggerate breathing depression.
- mirtazapine (Remeron) may worsen motor skills. Avoid operating dangerous machinery or tasks requiring coordination.
- narcotics or other centrally active medicines may cause additive respiratory depression or decreased levels of consciousness.

- olanzapine (Zyprexa) may cause blood pressure lowering when you stand (orthostatic hypotension).
- propoxyphene (various) may lead to benzodiazepine (diazepam) intoxication.
- quinupristin/dalfopristin (Synercid) may lead to diazepam toxicity.

The following drugs may *increase* the effects of diazepam:
- birth control pills (oral contraceptives).
- cimetidine (Tagamet).
- cisapride (Propulsid).
- disulfiram (Antabuse).
- isoniazid (INH, Rifamate, etc.).
- itraconazole (Sporanox), ketoconazole (Nizoral) or other azole antifungals.
- macrolide antibiotics such as erythromycin or clarithromycin.
- omeprazole (Prilosec).
- ritonavir (Norvir) and other protease inhibitors (see Drug Classes).
- sertraline (Zoloft).
- valproic acid (Depakene).

The following drugs may *decrease* the effects of diazepam:
- ranitidine (Zantac).
- rifampin (Rimactane, etc.).
- rifabutin (Mycobutin).
- theophylline (aminophylline, Theo-Dur, etc.).

▷ *Driving, Hazardous Activities:* This drug can impair mental alertness, judgment, physical coordination and reaction time. Avoid hazardous activities accordingly.

Aviation Note: The use of this drug *is a disqualification* for piloting. Consult a designated Aviation Medical Examiner.

Exposure to Sun: No restrictions.

Exposure to Heat: Because of reduced urine volume, this drug may accumulate in the body and produce effects of overdose.

Discontinuation: Avoid stopping this drug suddenly if taken for over 4 weeks. Prudent to taper gradually to prevent a withdrawal syndrome (sweating, tremor, depression, hallucinations, seizures and vomiting).

DICLOFENAC (di KLOH fen ak)

Please see the acetic acid (nonsteroidal anti-inflammatory drug) family profile.

DIDANOSINE (di DAN oh seen)

Other Names: DDI, dideoxyinosine

Introduced: 1991   **Class:** Antiviral   **Prescription:** USA: Yes   **Controlled Drug:** USA: No; Canada: No   **Available as Generic:** USA: No; Canada: No

Brand Name: Videx, Videx EC

BENEFITS versus RISKS	
Possible Benefits	*Possible Risks*
DELAYED PROGRESSION OF DISEASE IN HIV-POSITIVE PATIENTS	DRUG-INDUCED PANCREATITIS DRUG-INDUCED PERIPHERAL NEURITIS
USE IN COMBINATION THERAPY OF AIDS	Drug-induced seizures
ONCE-DAILY DOSING	Liver damage—rare

▷ **Principal Uses**

As a Single Drug Product: Uses currently included in FDA-approved labeling: (1) Treats human immunodeficiency virus (HIV) infections in adults and children (6 months of age or older); (2) treatment of advanced HIV infection in those failing zidovudine. **Author's Note: Adherence or taking medicines for HIV exactly on time and in the right amount is ABSOLUTELY critical to getting the best possible results or outcomes.** The new antiretroviral therapy guidelines from NIAID take into account how easily the medicine treating HIV can fit into a patient's life. The company is actively investigating once-daily use as well as an enteric form.

Other (unlabeled) generally accepted uses: Used in combination with other antiretroviral medicines (such as protease inhibitors or hydroxyurea [Hydrea]) to treat HIV infection or AIDS.

How This Drug Works: By interfering with essential HIV enzyme systems, this drug prevents growth and reproduction of HIV particles in infected cells, limiting the severity and extent of HIV infection.

Available Dosage Forms and Strengths

Powder for oral solution (bottle) — 2 g, 4 g

Powder for oral solution (packet) — 100 mg, 167 mg, 250 mg, 375 mg

Tablets, chewable/dispersible — 25 mg, 50 mg, 100 mg, 150 mg

Tablets, extended release — 125 mg, 200 mg, 250 mg, 400 mg

▷ **Recommended Dosage Ranges** (Actual dose and schedule must be determined for each patient individually.)

Infants and Children: For those 6 months of age or older, dose is based on drug form and body surface area. Once-daily dosing HAS NOT been studied as yet in children.

Pediatric oral solution (reconstituted and mixed with buffers): 125 mg (12.5 ml) every 12 hours for body surface area of 1.1–1.4 m^2; 94 mg (9.5 ml) every 12 hours for body surface area of 0.8–1 m^2; 62 mg (6 ml) every 12 hours for body surface area of 0.5–0.7 m^2; 31 mg (3 ml) every 12 hours for body surface area of 0.4 m^2 or less. (Based on 200 mg/square meter per day.)

Chewable/dispersible tablets: 100 mg every 12 hours for body surface area of 1.1–1.4 m^2; 75 mg every 12 hours for body surface area of 0.8–1 m^2; 50 mg every 12 hours for body surface area of 0.5–0.7 m^2; 25 mg every 12 hours for body surface area of 0.4 m^2 or less. In children 1 year of age or older, each dose should be two tablets to ensure that adequate buffering is provided to prevent destruction (degradation) of the drug in stomach acid. In children younger than 1 year of age, one tablet will provide adequate buffering.

12 to 60 Years of Age: Chewable/dispersible tablets: 400 mg once a day or 200 mg every 12 hours for those weighing more than 60 kg; 250 mg once daily or 125 mg every 12 hours for those weighing less than 60 kg

EC form: 200-mg EC tablets are only part of a 400-mg once-daily regimen and dosing is based on a mg per kg of body weight basis. For example—if a patient weighs more than 60 kg, 400 mg of Videx EC should be taken daily.

Over 60 Years of Age: Same as 12 to 60 group, but the dose should be reduced if there is an age-related decline in kidney function.

Conditions Requiring Dosing Adjustments

Liver Function: Increased risk of liver toxicity if used in people with compromised liver. Doses must be decreased in liver failure.

Kidney Function: Dose must be decreased in mild to moderate kidney failure. For example: those with creatinine clearance of 30–59 ml/min who weigh 60 kg or more would receive 100 mg twice daily or 200 mg each day of the oral tablets, 100 mg twice daily of the buffered powder and 200 mg each day of Videx EC. Care must also be taken as there is an increased risk of magnesium toxicity (chewable dispersible tablets have 8.6 MEQ of magnesium each). Risk of drug-induced pancreatitis also increases in patients with kidney problems.

▷ **Dosing Instructions:** Best taken on an empty stomach, 30 minutes before or 2 hours after eating. Patients MUST take at least two of the needed tablets at each dose in order to make sure that there is adequate buffer present. This actually protects the drug itself from being destroyed by stomach acid. The Videx EC should be swallowed WHOLE.

Pediatric oral solution first reconstituted with water and then combined with equal amounts of antacid (such as Mylanta or Maalox). Shake this mixture thoroughly BEFORE you measure each dose.

Adult oral solution is made by stirring one packet into 120 ml (4 ounces) of water until the powder is dissolved; this may take up to 3 minutes. Do not mix powder with fruit juice or other acidic liquid. Swallow all of the 4-ounce solution immediately.

The chewable/dispersible buffered tablets should be thoroughly chewed, crushed or dispersed in water before swallowing. To disperse the tablet(s), stir in at least 30 ml (1 ounce) of water until all the medicine is in the water. Swallow all of preparation immediately. The mandarin orange flavor formulation of Videx disperses in water in as little as 2 minutes. These tablets are dropped whole into a glass of water and are stirred to speed dispersion in the water. If you forget a dose: take the missed dose as soon as you remember it, unless it's nearly time for your next dose—then skip the missed dose and take the next scheduled dose right on time. DO NOT double doses. Talk openly with your doctor if you are having trouble remembering doses. Some patients benefit greatly from beeper-based reminder systems.

Author's Note: Current HIV therapy involves combination use of agents from different drug classes to attack the AIDS virus from different points and delay resistance. Clinicians use viral load (see Glossary) to indicate success or failure of therapy.

Usual Duration of Use: Regular use for several months with repeat viral load and CD4 tests are needed check benefits in slowing AIDS progression. Long-term use requires follow-up with your doctor.

Typical Treatment Goals and Measurements (Outcomes and Markers)

> *HIV:* Goals for HIV treatment presently are maximum suppression of viral replication, maximum lowering of the amount of virus in your body (viral load or burden), and maximum patient survival. Markers of successful therapy include undetectable viral load, increased CD4 cells, absence of indicator or opportunistic infections (OIs) and in the case of the HIV-positive patient, delay of the infection to progress to AIDS.

Possible Advantages of This Drug

> Does not cause serious bone marrow depression (production of blood cells). Less frequent liver toxicity than some other antiretrovirals. Once-daily dosing can be a great advantage in adherence.

This Drug Should Not Be Taken If

- you have had an allergic reaction to it previously.
- you have active liver disease.
- you have had pancreatitis recently.

▷ **Inform Your Physician Before Taking This Drug If**

- you have had allergic reactions to any drugs in the past.
- you are taking any other drugs currently.
- you have a history of pancreatitis or peripheral neuritis.
- you have a history of gout or high blood uric acid level.
- you have a history of alcoholism.
- you have a history of eye problems.
- you have a history of diarrhea.
- you have had nerve damage (peripheral neuropathy) from other medicines.
- you have a history of phenylketonuria (PKU).
- you have a history of low blood platelets or blood disorder.
- you are pregnant—increased chance of metabolic problems (lactic acidosis risk).
- you have a history of low blood potassium.
- you have a history of heart failure.
- you have a seizure disorder.
- you have impaired liver or kidney function.

Possible Side Effects (natural, expected and unavoidable drug actions)

> Mild decreases in red blood cell, white blood cell and platelet counts in adults.
> Mild increases in blood uric acid levels. Increased sodium load (each buffered powder packet has 1,380 mg of sodium).
> Increased magnesium levels in patients with kidney problems.

▷ **Possible Adverse Effects** (unusual, unexpected and infrequent reactions)

> **If any of the following develop, consult your physician promptly for guidance.**

Mild Adverse Effects

> Allergic reactions: skin rash and itching—occasional in adults and common in pediatric patients.
> Headache, dizziness, insomnia, nervousness, confusion—infrequent.
> Visual disturbances—rare.
> Nausea, vomiting—may be frequent in pediatrics.
> Stomach pain and diarrhea (25% of adults and frequent in pediatric patients), dry mouth and altered taste, yeast infection of mouth—rare to infrequent.

Lowered blood pressure—rare to infrequent.

Loss of color in the retina (retinal depigmentation)—case reports.

Nose bleeds—frequent in clinical trials in children.

Increased urination—infrequent in pediatric patients.

Cough—infrequent.

Loss of hair, muscle and joint pains—rare to infrequent.

Serious Adverse Effects

Drug-induced pancreatitis, usually seen in the first 6 months—infrequent.

Drug-induced peripheral neuritis (see Glossary), usually occurring after 2 to 6 months of treatment (this effect also appears to be dose-related)—infrequent to frequent.

Muscle damage (myalgia and/or rhabdomyolysis including sudden kidney failure)—case reports.

Electrolyte imbalance (low potassium or calcium)—variable.

Increased triglycerides—frequent.

Asthma—frequent in children.

Abnormal heart rhythm—infrequent.

High blood sugar—possible.

Excessive lowering of blood pressure and passing out (syncope)—case reports to infrequent.

Serious skin rash (Stevens-Johnson syndrome)—case report.

Seizures (may be due to electrolyte problems)—rare.

Lowered white blood cell counts, lowered granulocyte (a specific white blood cell) counts and lowered blood platelets (69%) in pediatric patients—infrequent to frequent.

Lactic acidosis—case reports.

Optic neuritis and blindness—case reports.

Liver damage—rare to infrequent.

Kidney damage—rare.

▷ **Possible Effects on Sexual Function:** None reported.

Adverse Effects That May Mimic Natural Diseases or Disorders

Drug-induced liver reaction—rare at less than 0.2%—may suggest viral hepatitis.

Possible Effects on Laboratory Tests

Complete blood cell counts: decreased red cells and white cells—variable; decreased platelets—infrequent.

Blood amylase or uric acid level: increased—infrequent.

Blood electrolytes: low calcium, potassium and magnesium.

Liver function tests: increased liver enzymes (ALT/GPT, AST/GOT and alkaline phosphatase), increased bilirubin—infrequent in adults, higher in pediatric patients.

CAUTION

1. This drug **does not cure HIV infection.** Ongoing CD4 and viral load tests are prudent. The AIDS virus may still be passed to other people while you are taking this medicine.
2. Report stomach pain with nausea and vomiting to your doctor; this could indicate pancreatitis.
3. Report pain, numbness, tingling or burning in the hands or feet—could be peripheral neuritis. Drug may need to be stopped.

4. If your kidneys are damaged or your creatinine elevated, ask your doctor if accumulating magnesium will be a problem for you.
5. One current therapy approach uses STI or structured therapy interruptions to carefully attempt to evoke an immune response to HIV. This approach is presently controversial and should NOT be attempted without the supervision of your doctor.

Precautions for Use

By Infants and Children: Safety and effectiveness for those under 6 months of age not established. Children are also at risk for developing pancreatitis and peripheral neuritis. It is recommended that detailed eye examinations be performed every 6 months and at any time that visual disturbance occurs.

By Those Over 60 Years of Age: Reduced kidney function may require dose reduction.

▷ **Advisability of Use During Pregnancy**

Pregnancy Category: B. See Pregnancy Risk Categories at the back of this book.
Animal studies: Rat and rabbit studies show no birth defects.
Human studies: Adequate studies of pregnant women not available.
Consult your physician for specific guidance.

Advisability of Use If Breast-Feeding

Presence of this drug in breast milk: Unknown.
Avoid drug or refrain from nursing.
Note: HIV has been found in human breast milk. Breast-feeding may result in transmission of HIV infection to the nursing infant.

Habit-Forming Potential: None.

Effects of Overdose: Nausea, vomiting, stomach pain, diarrhea, pain in hands and feet, irritability, confusion.

Possible Effects of Long-Term Use: Peripheral neuritis (see Glossary).

Suggested Periodic Examinations While Taking This Drug (at physician's discretion)

Complete blood cell counts before starting treatment and weekly thereafter until tolerance is established.
Electrolytes.
Blood amylase levels, fractionated for salivary gland and pancreatic origin.
Liver and kidney function tests.
Viral load or viral burden in order to assess success of treatment.
CD4 counts.

▷ **While Taking This Drug, Observe the Following**

Foods: Best taken on an empty stomach.
Herbal Medicines or Minerals: Echinacea: Some patients use echinacea to attempt to boost their immune systems. Unfortunately, use of echinacea is not recommended in people with damaged immune systems. This herb may also actually weaken any immune system if it is used too often or for too long a time. Some cancer patients are looking to mistletoe (Iscador) to boost their immune systems. This HAS NOT been studied in HIV-positive patients.
Beverages: Do not take with acidic fruit juices.
▷ *Alcohol:* No interactions expected.
Tobacco Smoking: No interactions expected. I advise everyone to quit smoking.

▷   *Other Drugs*

Didanosine may ***increase*** the effects of
- zidovudine (Retrovir) and enhance its antiviral effect against HIV.

Didanosine may ***decrease*** the effects of
- ciprofloxacin (Cipro) and other fluoroquinolones (gatifloxacin [Tequin] and grepafloxacin [Raxar], levofloxacin [Levaquin] and see Drug Classes), if taken at the same time; take fluoroquinolones at least 4 hours before taking didanosine buffered solution, tablets or the oral powder.
- dapsone and render it ineffective; avoid concurrent use.
- indinavir (Crixivan) and blunt therapeutic benefits; separate dosing by 2 hours.
- itraconazole (Sporanox). Separate dosing by at least 2 hours.
- ketoconazole (Nizoral), if taken at the same time; take ketoconazole at least 2 hours before taking didanosine.
- tetracyclines (see Drug Classes), if taken at the same time; take tetracyclines at least 2 hours before taking didanosine.

Didanosine ***taken concurrently*** with
- allopurinol (various) increased didanosine absorption in two patients with damaged kidneys. Caution and blood levels are prudent if this medicine is used in patients with kidney failure.
- amprenavir (Agenerase) will probably decrease amprenavir absorption. Separate doses by at least 1 hour.
- antacids will decrease didanosine absorption and lower its therapeutic benefit.
- delavirdine (Rescriptor) may lower both drug levels. Separate doses by an hour.
- fluconazole (Diflucan) and other azole antifungals may decrease fluconazole benefits.
- histamine (H2) blocking drugs (see Drug Classes)—cimetidine, etc.—may increase didanosine toxicity.
- pentamidine or sulfamethoxazole may increase the risk of drug-induced pancreatitis; watch for significant symptoms.
- ritonavir (Norvir) will inactivate both medicines. Separate doses by 2$\frac{1}{2}$ to 3 hours.
- triazolam (Halcion) may cause confusion.
- zalcitabine (Hivid) may cause increased neurotoxicity.

▷   *Driving, Hazardous Activities:* This drug may cause dizziness and impaired vision. Restrict activities as necessary.

Aviation Note: The use of this drug ***is a disqualification*** for piloting. Consult a designated Aviation Medical Examiner.

Exposure to Sun: No restrictions.

Discontinuation: Do not stop this drug without your physician's knowledge and guidance.

DIFLUNISAL (di FLU ni sal)

Please see the acetic acid (nonsteroidal anti-inflammatory drug) family profile.

DIGITOXIN (di ji TOX in)

See the digoxin profile for further information.

DIGOXIN (di JOX in)

Introduced: 1934   **Class:** Digitalis preparations **Prescription:** USA: Yes
Controlled Drug: USA: No; Canada: No **Available as Generic:** Yes
Brand Names: ✤Digitaline Nativelle, Digitek, Lanoxicaps, Lanoxin, ✤Novodigoxin, SK-Digoxin

BENEFITS versus RISKS	
Possible Benefits	*Possible Risks*
EFFECTIVE HEART STIMULANT IN CONGESTIVE HEART FAILURE	NARROW TREATMENT RANGE Frequent and sometimes serious disturbances of heart rhythm
EFFECTIVE PREVENTION AND TREATMENT OF CERTAIN HEART RHYTHM DISORDERS	

▷ **Principal Uses**

As a Single Drug Product: Uses in current FDA-approved labeling: (1) Treats congestive heart failure; (2) restores and helps keep normal heart rate and rhythm in cases of atrial fibrillation (second-line agent behind verapamil, diltiazem or a beta-blocker), atrial flutter, PAT and atrial/supraventricular tachycardia.

Other (unlabeled) generally accepted uses: (1) Postoperative arrhythmias; (2) helps to increase left ventricular function in patients with pacemakers; (3) may have a role in treating Wolff-Parkinson-White syndrome.

How This Drug Works: Increases force of heart muscle contraction. Delays electrical transmission through the heart, helping restore normal rate and rhythm.

Available Dosage Forms and Strengths

Capsules — 0.05 mg, 0.1 mg, 0.2 mg
Elixir — 0.25 mg/5 ml, 0.125 mg/5 ml
Elixir, pediatric — 0.05 mg/ml
Injection — 0.1 mg/ml, 0.25 mg/ml
Tablets — 0.0625 mg (Canada), 0.125 mg, 0.25 mg, 0.5 mg

Author's Note: Dosing and timing of doses are critical for this medicine. The difference between toxic blood levels and therapeutic blood levels is small. Be CERTAIN you understand how and when to take this medicine.

▷ **Usual Adult Dosage Ranges:** For loading dose, 10 mcg per kilogram of lean body mass (some clinicians use ideal body weight as the math is less complicated); 10–15 mcg per kg of body mass may be needed if digoxin is being used to control abnormal heart rhythms (such as atrial fibrillation); 8–12 mcg per kg is typical if this medicine is being used for heart failure. Loading dose can be given orally or intravenously. Once decided, is often given as 50% in the first dose with remainder divided into smaller doses and given at 6- to 8-hour intervals until the desired response is achieved. Usual ongoing dose after loading is 0.125 to 0.5 mg per day, and is calculated by a specific formula. In neonatal and pediatric patients, a similar loading and ongoing strategy is used, but the amount on a mg-per-kg-of-body-mass basis is very different. **Note: Actual dose and schedule must be determined for each patient individually.**

Conditions Requiring Dosing Adjustments
Liver Function: Use with caution; blood levels should be obtained more frequently.
Kidney Function: Dose **must** be adjusted in kidney compromise. Smaller doses and some cases of dosing every other day may be needed.

▷ **Dosing Instructions:** Tablet may be crushed and is best taken at the same time each day (to help keep blood levels about the same) on an empty stomach. Can be taken with or following food; milk and dairy products may delay absorption but do not reduce the amount of drug absorbed. The capsule should be swallowed whole. If you forget a dose: Take the dose you missed as soon as you remember it, unless you are more than 12 hours late. If that is the case, skip the missed dose and simply take the next scheduled dose. DO NOT double doses. If you forget your medicine for 2 days, call your doctor for directions.

Usual Duration of Use: Regular use for 7 to 10 days needed to see benefits in relieving heart failure or controlling heart rhythm disorders. Long-term use requires physician supervision. Treatment of heart rhythm disorders and congestive heart failure will usually be ongoing.

Typical Treatment Goals and Measurements (Outcomes and Markers)
Heart failure: Because the level of this medicine in the blood must be kept in a certain range, blood levels are used to help guide dosing. When this medicine is in the correct range, it helps the heart beat more strongly, increasing the amount of work that it can do. Your doctor may use terms like cardiac output (the amount of work that your heart can do in a given amount of time), contractile force (the strength of your heart action) and edematous decrease (lowered ankle swelling) to describe how much better your heart is working. Spironolactone (Aldactone) may be combined with a water pill (diuretic) to get the best results. The goals and time frame should be discussed with you when the prescription is written.

▷ **This Drug Should Not Be Taken If**
• you have had an allergic reaction to any form of it.
• you are in ventricular fibrillation (a life-threatening heart rhythm).

▷ **Inform Your Physician Before Taking This Drug If**
• you have had an unfavorable reaction to digitalis.
• you have taken digitalis in the past 2 weeks.
• you take (or have recently taken) any diuretic drug.
• you have a history of severe lung disease.
• you have abnormal heart rhythms (such as severe slowing or bradycardia), sick sinus syndrome, rapid rate arising in the ventricles (ventricular tachycardia) or certain aortic problems.
• you have had damage to the heart muscle (myocardium), such as in a heart attack.
• you have ongoing (chronic) inflammation of part of the heart (constrictive pericarditis).

- you have a history of low blood potassium or magnesium.
- you have impaired liver or kidney function.
- you have a history of thyroid function disorder.

Possible Side Effects (natural, expected and unavoidable drug actions)

Slow heart rate.

May cause blackening of feces.

Enlargement or sensitivity of the male breast—rare.

▷ **Possible Adverse Effects** (unusual, unexpected and infrequent reactions)

If any of the following develop, consult your physician promptly for guidance.

Mild Adverse Effects

Allergic reactions: skin rash, hives.

Headache, drowsiness, lethargy, confusion, changes in vision: "halo" effect, blurring, spots, double vision, yellow-green vision—infrequent.

Changes in vaginal tissue (vaginal cornification)—case reports.

Nightmares—case reports.

Loss of appetite, nausea, vomiting, diarrhea (can be early signs of adult toxicity)—frequent.

Serious Adverse Effects

Idiosyncratic reactions: hallucinations, facial neuralgias, peripheral neuralgias, blindness—case reports.

Low blood platelets—case reports and probably an immune reaction.

Psychosis and hallucinations—associated with toxic levels.

Seizures—rare.

Serious skin rash (Stevens-Johnson syndrome)—rare.

Disorientation—most common in the elderly.

Heart rhythm disturbances—possible and dose-related.

▷ **Possible Effects on Sexual Function:**

Decreased libido and impotence in 35% of male users. Enlargement and tenderness of male breasts (gynecomastia)—case reports. Both effects are attributed to digoxin's estrogenlike action. May cause cornification of the vagina in women after menopause. Caution is advised, as this has been mistaken for cancer (endometrial).

Adverse Effects That May Mimic Natural Diseases or Disorders

Drug-induced mental changes may be mistaken for senile dementia or psychosis. May cause cornification of the vagina in women after menopause. Caution is advised as this has been mistaken for cancer (endometrial).

Possible Effects on Laboratory Tests

Blood platelet counts: rarely decreased.

Blood testosterone level: may be decreased with long-term use.

CAUTION

1. Take this medicine EXACTLY as prescribed.
2. If you take calcium supplements, ask your physician for help. Avoid large doses.
3. Prudent to carry a card that says you are taking this drug.
4. Avoid over-the-counter antacids and cold, cough or allergy remedies without first asking your doctor or pharmacist.
5. Because blood levels are so important, make sure you stay on the same brand or generic form that you are started on. If you are changed from

one form or one generic to the other, blood level checks are usually prudent.

6. May cause changes (cornification) in the vagina in women after menopause. Caution is advised, as this has been mistaken for cancer (endometrial).

Precautions for Use

By Infants and Children: Watch for indications of toxicity: slow heart rate (below 60 beats/min), irregular heart rhythms.

By Those Over 60 Years of Age: Reduced drug tolerance; smaller doses are prudent. Watch for toxicity: headache, dizziness, fatigue, weakness, lethargy, depression, confusion, nervousness, agitation, delusions, difficulty with reading. Call your doctor if these happen.

▷ **Advisability of Use During Pregnancy**

Pregnancy Category: C. See Pregnancy Risk Categories at the back of this book.

Animal studies: No birth defects reported.

Human studies: Adequate studies of pregnant women not available. However, no birth defects from the therapeutic use of this drug have been reported.

Use this drug only if clearly needed. Overdose can be harmful to the fetus.

Advisability of Use If Breast-Feeding

Presence of this drug in breast milk: Yes.

Monitor nursing infant closely and discontinue drug or nursing if adverse effects develop.

Habit-Forming Potential: None.

Effects of Overdose: Loss of appetite, excessive saliva, nausea, vomiting, diarrhea, serious disturbances of heart rate and rhythm, intestinal bleeding, drowsiness, headache, confusion, delirium, hallucinations, convulsions.

Possible Effects of Long-Term Use: May cause cornification of the vagina in women after menopause. Caution is advised, as this has been mistaken for cancer (endometrial).

Suggested Periodic Examinations While Taking This Drug (at physician's discretion)

Measurements of blood levels of digoxin, calcium, magnesium and potassium. (Time to sample blood for digoxin level: 6–8 hours after last dose or just before next dose. Recommended therapeutic range: 0.5–2.0 ng/ml.)

Electrocardiograms.

▷ **While Taking This Drug, Observe the Following**

Foods: Talk to your doctor about high-potassium foods. The peak level and rate that digoxin enters your body will decrease if taken with food.

Herbal Medicines or Minerals: Hawthorn and co-enzyme Q10 (co-Q10) can affect the way the heart works. Issues remain regarding optimum doses, monitoring strategies and possible interactions. One objective review recognized co-Q10 as adjunctive therapy for congestive heart failure. BE CERTAIN to tell your doctor that you are taking or are considering taking these herbs if you are taking digoxin or if a digoxin prescription is being considered for you or a loved one. Co-Q10 may also interact badly with aspirin. Soy (milk, tofu, etc.) contains phytoestrogens that have led to an FDA-approved health claim for reducing risk of heart disease (if they have at least 6.25 grams of soy protein per serving). It is important that potassium and magnesium levels be kept in the normal range while you are taking digoxin.

St. John's wort appears to lower digoxin levels by about 25%. This decrease may lead to loss of digoxin benefits and can be a very serious drug interaction. Couch grass or nettle should NOT be taken by patients who have increased fluid (edema) caused by heart weakness. Patients taking digoxin should NOT take lily of the valley herb, pheasant's eye or squill. Hawthorn (Crataegus variety) has been used to help heart failure, but should not be combined with heart medicines as combination use has not been studied. Use of intravenous calcium may cause a fatal interaction with digoxin. A case report of ginseng falsely elevating digoxin test levels has been made.

Beverages: Avoid excessive amounts of caffeine-containing beverages or herbs: coffee, tea, cola. May be taken with milk.

▷ *Alcohol:* No interactions expected.

Tobacco Smoking: Nicotine can cause heart muscle irritability and predispose to serious rhythm disturbances. I advise everyone to quit smoking.

Marijuana Smoking: Possible accentuation of heart failure; reduced digoxin effect; possible changes in electrocardiogram, confusing interpretation.

▷ *Other Drugs*

Digoxin **taken concurrently** with

- acarbose (Precose) may result in decreased digoxin blood levels and loss of digoxin's benefits.
- calcium (intravenously) may cause a fatal interaction.
- digoxin immune Fab (Digibind) will result in decreased blood levels. This is used to therapeutic advantage in digoxin toxicity.
- diuretics (except spironolactone or triamterene) can cause serious heart rhythm problems due to loss of potassium.
- dofetilide (Tikosyn) has been found to result in increased occurrence of an abnormal heart effect (torsades de pointes). Presently, it is unclear if this is an interaction or is a result of medicines used in sicker patients. Caution is advised.
- metformin (Glucophage) may increase metformin levels and lead to excessively low blood sugar.
- pancuronium (Pavulon) or vecuronium (Norcuron) may cause abnormal heartbeats (arrhythmia).
- propranolol or other beta-blocking medicines (see Drug Classes) may cause very slow heart rate.
- quinidine may result in decreased digoxin effectiveness and increased digoxin toxicity; careful dose adjustments are needed.
- succinylcholine may lead to abnormal heart rhythms.

The following drugs may **increase** the effects of digoxin:

- alprazolam (Xanax).
- amiloride (Midamor).
- amiodarone (Cordarone).
- amphotericin B (Abelcet, Fungizone).
- atorvastatin (Lipitor), simvastatin (Zocor) blood levels should be checked more frequently and digoxin dosing adjusted.
- benzodiazepines (Librium, Valium, etc.; see Drug Classes).
- captopril (Capoten, Capozide).
- cotrimoxazole (various).

- cyclosporine (Sandimmune).
- diltiazem (Cardizem) and other calcium channel blockers (see Drug Classes).
- disopyramide (Norpace).
- erythromycin (E.E.S., Erythrocin, etc.). May also occur with clarithromycin and azithromycin.
- ethacrynic acid.
- esomeprazole (Nexium), omeprazole (Prilosec).
- flecainide (Tambocor).
- fluoxetine (Prozac, Sarafem) and fluvoxamine (Luvox).
- gatifloxacin (Tequin).
- hydroxychloroquine.
- ibuprofen (Advil, Medipren, Motrin, Nuprin, etc.).
- indomethacin (Indocin) and other NSAIDs.
- itraconazole (Sporanox).
- methimazole (Tapazole).
- mibefradil (Posicor).
- nefazodone (Serzone).
- nifedipine (Adalat, Procardia).
- phenytoin (Dilantin).
- propafenone (Rythmol) (30–100% increased blood level).
- propylthiouracil (Propacil).
- quinine.
- quinupristin/dalfopristin (Synercid).
- ritonavir (Norvir).
- spironolactone (Aldactone).
- telmisartan (Micardis).
- tetracyclines (see Drug Classes).
- tolbutamide (Orinase).
- tramadol (Ultram).
- trazodone (Desyrel).
- trimethoprim (Septra, others).
- verapamil (Calan, Verelan, others).

The following drugs may **decrease** the effects of digoxin:
- aluminum-containing antacids (Amphojel, Maalox, etc.).
- bleomycin (Blenoxane).
- carmustine (BiCNU).
- cholestyramine (Questran).
- colestipol (Colestid).
- cyclophosphamide (Cytoxan).
- cytarabine (Cytosar).
- doxorubicin (Adriamycin).
- fluvoxamine (Luvox).
- kaolin/pectin (Donnagel, others).
- methotrexate (Mexate).
- metoclopramide (Reglan).
- miglitol (Glyset).
- neomycin.
- penicillamine (Cuprimine, Depen).
- procarbazine (Matulane).

- rifampin or rifabutin.
- St. John's wort (hypericum).
- sucralfate (Carafate).
- sulfa antibiotics or sulfasalazine.
- thyroid hormones.
- vincristine (Oncovin).

▷ *Driving, Hazardous Activities:* Usually no restrictions. This drug may cause drowsiness, vision changes and nausea. Restrict activities as necessary.

Aviation Note: Heart function disorders **are a disqualification** for piloting. Consult a designated Aviation Medical Examiner.

Exposure to Sun: No restrictions.

Occurrence of Unrelated Illness: Vomiting or diarrhea can seriously alter this drug's effectiveness. Notify your physician promptly.

Discontinuation: This drug may be continued indefinitely. Do not stop it without consulting your physician.

DILTIAZEM (dil TI a zem)

Introduced: 1977   **Class:** Anti-anginal, antihypertensive, calcium channel blocker   **Prescription:** USA: Yes   **Controlled Drug:** USA: No; Canada: No   **Available as Generic:** Yes

Brand Names: ✤Albert Diltiazem CD, ✤Apo-Diltiaz, ✤Alti-Diltiazem, Cardizem, Cardizem CD, Cardizem SR, Cartia XT, Dilacor XR, Diltia XT, Diltiazem, Diltiazem ER, Med Diltiazem SR, ✤Novo-Diltiazem, ✤Nu-Diltiaz, Pharma-Diltiaz, ✤Syn-Diltiazem, Teczem [CD], Tiamate, Tiazac

Controversies in Medicine: Medicines in this class have had many conflicting reports. The FDA has held hearings on the calcium channel blocker (CCB) class. Early research at New York University found that nifedipine is a cause of reversible male infertility. CCBs are currently second-line agents for high blood pressure according to the JNC VI (see Glossary).

BENEFITS versus RISKS	
Possible Benefits	*Possible Risks*
EFFECTIVE PREVENTION OF	Depression, confusion
BOTH MAJOR TYPES OF ANGINA	Low blood pressure
EFFECTIVE CONTROL OF MILD	Heart rhythm disturbance
TO MODERATE HYPERTENSION	Fluid retention
HELPS CONTROL ATRIAL	Liver damage—case reports
FIBRILLATION	Muscle damage—case reports
May help prevent repeat blockage of coronary arteries in heart transplant patients	

▷ **Principal Uses**

As a Single Drug Product: Uses currently included in FDA-approved labeling: Treats (1) angina pectoris (coronary artery spasm or spontaneous Prinzmetal's variant angina) or associated with exertion; (2) classical angina-of-effort (due to atherosclerotic disease); (3) mild to moderate hypertension; (4) atrial fibrillation.

Other (unlabeled) generally accepted uses: (1) Unstable angina; (2) congestive heart failure; (3) migraine prophylaxis; (4) prevention of abnormal protein excretion in the urine; (5) abnormal heart rhythms; (6) treats abnormal plaques inside blood vessels (atherosclerosis); (7) may help prevent abnormal growth of the left side of the heart (left ventricular hypertrophy) after a heart attack; (8) treats some esophageal disorders; (9) eases symptoms of an overactive thyroid gland (hyperthyroidism); (10) can ease symptoms of Raynaud's phenomenon; (11) can have a role in preserving function in kidney and heart transplant patients; (12) may protect against heart attacks or variant or unstable angina that can occur after (postoperatively) coronary artery bypass grafting; (13) could have a role in slowing the advance of low tension glaucoma; (14) may help prevent repeat blockage (restenosis) in heart transplant patients.

How This Drug Works: This drug blocks normal passage of calcium through cell walls, inhibiting coronary artery and peripheral arteriole narrowing. As a result, this drug

- prevents spontaneous coronary artery spasm (Prinzmetal's angina).
- decreases heart rate and contraction force in exertion, making effort-induced angina less likely.
- opens contracted peripheral arterial walls, lowering blood pressure (also lessens heart work and helps prevent angina).

Available Dosage Forms and Strengths

Capsules, extended release — 120 mg, 180 mg, 240 mg, 300 mg
Capsules, extended release (Tiazac only) — 120, 180, 240, 300, 360, 420 mg
Capsules, sustained release — 60 mg, 90 mg, 120 mg
Tablets, immediate release — 30 mg, 60 mg, 90 mg, 120 mg

▷ **Usual Adult Dosage Ranges:** *High blood pressure:* Sustained-release capsules are started at 60 to 120 mg twice daily or 180 to 240 mg daily. Effective dose for many patients in clinical trials was 240 to 360 mg. Daily maximum is 540 mg once a day for extended-release capsules (such as Tiazac R) and 360 mg a day for sustained-release form (such as Cardizem SR). *Angina:* Sustained release form may be started at 120 to 180 mg daily. The dose can then be increased as needed and tolerated to 480 mg over 1 to 2 weeks. Note: Actual dose and schedule must be determined for each patient individually.

Conditions Requiring Dosing Adjustments

Liver Function: Maximum daily dose in patients with liver compromise should be 90 mg. Rarely causes hepatoxicity, and a benefit-to-risk decision must be made.

Kidney Function: May be one of the best calcium channel blockers to use in kidney compromise (large liver and fecal removal). Caution must still be used. Drug can be a rare cause of kidney compromise.

▷ **Dosing Instructions:** Immediate-release form may be crushed and is best taken before meals and at bedtime. Extended-release forms should NEVER be crushed or altered. Tiazac form may be taken with or without food. If you forget a dose, take it as soon as you remember it, unless it is nearly time for your next dose—then skip the missed dose and take the next dose right on schedule. DO NOT double doses. If you find yourself forgetting doses, please talk to your doctor about possible reminder systems to help.

Usual Duration of Use: Use for 2 to 4 weeks is required to see effectiveness in decreasing angina frequency and severity and in lowering blood pressure. Smallest effective dose should be used in long-term therapy (months to years). Take control of your blood pressure for life!

Typical Treatment Goals and Measurements (Outcomes and Markers)

Blood Pressure: The most recent treatment guidelines (JNC VI) actually define optimal blood pressure (BP) as less than 120/80 and high normal as 139/89. The American Diabetes Association has chosen a target of 130/80 as the blood pressure goal for people living with diabetes. Most clinicians try to achieve a BP that achieves the best balance of lower cardiovascular risk while avoiding the problem of too low a blood pressure. The goal and time frame (see peak benefits above) should be discussed with you when the prescription is written.

Possible Advantages of This Drug

Often effective as single-drug therapy. Does not reduce blood supply to kidneys. Does not raise blood cholesterol levels. Does not induce asthma in susceptible individuals. Minimal removal by the kidneys may make this a drug of choice in people with kidney damage who require a calcium channel blocker. Beneficial in patients with high blood pressure who also have angina.

▷ **This Drug Should Not Be Taken If**
- you have had an allergic reaction to it previously.
- you have "sick sinus" syndrome (and do not have an artificial pacemaker).
- you've recently had a heart attack and your lungs are not working well (acute MI with pulmonary congestion).
- you have atrial fibrillation or flutter and an IV form is being considered.
- you have second- or third-degree heart block.
- you have a particular kind of fast heart rate (ventricular tachycardia with a wide [QRS more than 0.12 sec] complex).
- you have low blood pressure—systolic pressure below 90.
- you have heart failure (talk with your doctor).

▷ **Inform Your Physician Before Taking This Drug If**
- you had an unfavorable response to any calcium blocker drug.
- you take digitalis or a beta-blocker (see Drug Classes).
- you have a history of congestive heart failure.
- you have a narrowing or stenosis of the aorta.
- you have atrial fibrillation (talk with your doctor).
- you have impaired liver or kidney function.
- your blood pressure is excessively low.
- you have a blockage in your stomach or intestines or they are moving excessively (gastrointestinal obstruction or hypermotility).
- you develop a skin rash.
- you have a history of drug-induced liver damage.

Possible Side Effects (natural, expected and unavoidable drug actions)

Fatigue—rare.
Light-headedness, heart rate and rhythm changes in some people—rare.
Excessive growth of gum tissue (gingival hyperplasia)—possible.
Difficulty breathing or cough—possible.
Drug fever—one case report—possible.

▷ **Possible Adverse Effects** (unusual, unexpected and infrequent reactions)
    If any of the following develop, consult your physician promptly for guidance.
    Mild Adverse Effects
        Allergic reactions: skin rash, hives, itching—rare.
        Headache—may be self-limiting but frequent.
        Drowsiness, dizziness—occasional and dose-related.
        Nervousness, sleep problems, depression, confusion, hallucinations—case reports.
        Desire to be in constant motion (acathisia)—case reports.
        Overgrowth of the gums (gingival hyperplasia)—may be frequent.
        Impaired sense of smell or taste—possible.
        Increased urination—rare.
        Flushing, palpitations, fainting, slow heart rate, low blood pressure—rare.
        Nausea, indigestion, heartburn, vomiting, diarrhea, constipation—rare to infrequent.
    Serious Adverse Effects
        Serious skin rashes (Stevens-Johnson syndrome, others).
        Serious disturbances of heart rate and/or rhythm, fluid retention (edema), congestive heart failure—rare.
        Drug-induced myopathy or liver damage—rare.
        Lowering of a specific kind of white blood cell (granulocytes)—case reports with this and other calcium channel blockers.
        Lowering of blood platelets or function—case reports.
        Sudden kidney failure—case reports to rare.
        Systemic lupus erythematosus—rare.

▷ **Possible Effects on Sexual Function:** Impotence—rare.
    Swelling or tenderness of the male breast tissue (gynecomastia)—case reports.
    One reported case of heavy vaginal bleeding.

Possible Effects on Laboratory Tests
    Blood total cholesterol and triglyceride levels: no effects.
    Blood HDL cholesterol level: increased.
    Blood LDL and VLDL cholesterol levels: no effects.

CAUTION
    1. Tell health care providers that you take this drug. Carry a card in your purse or wallet saying you take diltiazem.
    2. Nitroglycerin and other nitrate drugs as needed may still be used to relieve acute angina pain. If your angina attacks become more frequent or intense, call your doctor promptly.

Precautions for Use
    By Infants and Children: Safety and effectiveness for those under 12 years of age not established.
    By Those Over 60 Years of Age: May be more likely to have weakness, dizziness, fainting and falling. Take necessary precautions to prevent injury. Report promptly any changes in your pattern of thirst and urination.

▷ **Advisability of Use During Pregnancy**
    Pregnancy Category: C. See Pregnancy Risk Categories at the back of this book.
    Animal studies: Embryo and fetal deaths and skeletal birth defects reported in mice, rats and rabbits.

Human studies: Adequate studies of pregnant women not available.
Avoid this drug during the first 3 months. Use during the last 6 months only if clearly needed. Ask your physician for help.

Advisability of Use If Breast-Feeding
Presence of this drug in breast milk: Yes.
Avoid drug or refrain from nursing.

Habit-Forming Potential: None.

Effects of Overdose: Weakness, light-headedness, fainting, slow pulse, low blood pressure, shortness of breath, congestive heart failure.

Possible Effects of Long-Term Use: None reported.

Suggested Periodic Examinations While Taking This Drug (at physician's discretion)
Evaluations of heart function, including electrocardiograms.
Liver and kidney function tests, with long-term use.

▷ **While Taking This Drug, Observe the Following**
Foods: May increase absorption and cause a 30% increase in blood levels. Avoid excessive salt intake.
Herbal Medicines or Minerals: Ginseng may increase blood pressure, blunting the benefits of this medicine. Hawthorn, saw palmetto, ma huang, goldenseal, yohimbe and licorice may also cause increased blood pressure. Garlic and calcium may work to lower blood pressure. The combination may work to require lower diltiazem doses. St. John's wort may work to lower calcium channel blocker levels (because it increases P-glycoprotein in the gut). This combination may also increase sun sensitivity. Eleuthero root and ephedra should be avoided by people living with hypertension.
Indian snakeroot has a German Commission E monograph indication for hypertension—talk to your doctor. Discuss any plans for herbal medicines or minerals with your doctor.
Beverages: No restrictions. May be taken with milk.
▷ Alcohol: Use with caution. Alcohol may exaggerate the drop in blood pressure.
Tobacco Smoking: Nicotine reduces benefits. I advise everyone to quit smoking.
Marijuana Smoking: Possible reduced effectiveness of this drug; mild to moderate increase in angina; possible changes in electrocardiogram, confusing interpretation.
▷ *Other Drugs*
Diltiazem *taken concurrently* with
• alfentanil (various) may lead to accumulation of alfentanil. Caution and lower doses of alfentanil are prudent.
• amiodarone (Cordarone) may lead to abnormal heart rhythm.
• anticoagulants (see Drug Classes) may lead to stomach or intestinal bleeding.
• aspirin can result in prolonged bleeding time or hemorrhage.
• beta-blocker drugs or digitalis preparations (see Drug Classes) may affect heart rate and rhythm. Careful patient monitoring is necessary if these drugs are combined.
• carbamazepine (Tegretol) may result in toxicity and seizures.
• cilostazol (Pletal) may result in cilostazol toxicity. Lower cilostazol doses are prudent.
• cisapride (Propulsid) may lead to heart toxicity.

- cyclosporine (Sandimmune) may result in cyclosporine toxicity and kidney failure.
- digoxin (Lanoxin) can result in digoxin toxicity.
- dofetilide (Tikosyn) may result in dofetilide toxicity. Checks of dofetilide levels and dosing adjustments to levels are prudent.
- lithium (Lithobid, others) can result in psychosis and neurotoxicity.
- lovastatin (Mevacor), simvastatin (Zocor) may increase these (and perhaps other) HMG CoA reductase inhibitor levels that rely on CYP 450 3A4 for removal, and increase risk of muscle damage. Lower HMG CoA doses and careful patient monitoring are prudent.
- midazolam (Versed) may result in midazolam toxicity. Lower doses (by 50%) and careful patient monitoring are critical.
- nifedipine (various) may result in nifedipine toxicity. Alternative medicines or nifedipine dosing adjusted to blood levels is prudent.
- nonsteroidal anti-inflammatory drugs (NSAIDs—see Drug Classes) may lead to stomach or intestinal bleeding.
- oral anticoagulants (warfarin—Coumadin, others) may result in higher than expected anticoagulation. Increased INRs and careful patient following are prudent.
- oral antidiabetic drugs (see Drug Classes) such as glipizide (Glucotrol) may result in greater than expected lowering of blood sugar and hypoglycemia.
- phenytoin (Dilantin) and fosphenytoin (Cerebyx) decreases phenytoin and fosphenytoin metabolism and may cause toxicity. Lower doses and blood level checks are prudent.
- quinidine (Quinaglute, others) may lead to quinidine toxicity.
- rifabutin (Mycobutin) may decrease diltiazem blood levels.
- rifampin (Rifadin) may result in decreased diltiazem effectiveness.
- ritonavir (Norvir) and other protease inhibitors (see Drug Profiles) may lead to diltiazem toxicity.
- tacrolimus (Prograf) may result in tacrolimus accumulation and tacrolimus toxicity.
- theophylline (Theo-Dur, others) may lead to theophylline toxicity.
- tretinoin (Vesanoid, others) may lead to tretinoin toxicity.
- triazolam (Halcion) may lead to triazolam toxicity.

The following drugs may *increase* the effects of diltiazem:
- cimetidine (Tagamet).
- fluoxetine (Prozac).
- fluvoxamine (Luvox).
- quinupristin/dalfopristin (Synercid).
- ranitidine (Zantac).
- sertraline (Zoloft).

▷ *Driving, Hazardous Activities:* Usually no restrictions. This drug may cause drowsiness or dizziness. Limit activities as necessary.

Aviation Note: Coronary artery disease *is a disqualification* for piloting. Consult a designated Aviation Medical Examiner.

Exposure to Sun: This drug may cause photosensitivity (see Glossary).

Exposure to Heat: Caution is advised. Hot environments can exaggerate the blood-pressure-lowering effects of this drug. Observe for light-headedness or weakness.

Heavy Exercise or Exertion: May improve ability to be more active without angina pain. Use caution, and avoid exercise that might be excessive and yet not result in warning pain.

Discontinuation: **Do not stop this drug abruptly.** Ask your doctor about gradual withdrawal.

DIPHENHYDRAMINE (di fen HI dra meen)

Introduced: 1946   **Class:** Antihistamines, hypnotic   **Prescription:** USA: Varies with dose   **Controlled Drug:** USA: No*; Canada: No   **Available as Generic:** Yes

Author's note: This medicine is available without a prescription and is found in many products.

Brand Names: Acetaminophen-PM, AID to Sleep, Allerdryl, Allergy Capsules, Allergy Formula, Allermax, ✤Ambenyl Expectorant [CD], Ambenyl Syrup [CD], Anacin P.M. Aspirin-Free, Banophen, Bayer Select, Beldin Syrup, Bena-D, Benadryl, Benadryl 25, Benahist, Benylin, ✤Benylin Decongestant [CD], ✤Benylin Pediatric Syrup, ✤Benylin Syrup w/Codeine [CD], ✤Caladryl [CD], Caldyphen Lotion, Children's Complete Allergy, Complete Allergy Medication, Compoz, Dermarest, Di-Delamine, Dihydrex, Diphendryl, Diphenhist, Dormarex 2, ✤Ergodryl [CD], Excedrin P.M. [CD], Extra Strength Tylenol PM, Gecil, Genahist, Gen-D-Phen, Hydramine, ✤Insomnal, Kolex, ✤Mandrax [CD], Maximum Strength Nytol, Medi-Phedryl, Midol-PM, Nervine Nighttime Sleep, Nidryl Elixir, Nighttime Cold Medicine [CD], Nite-Time, Noradryl [CD], Noradryl 25, Nytol, Pain Relief PM [CD], Pathadryl, ✤PMS-Diphenhydramine, Sinutab Maximum Strength, SK-Diphenhydramine, Sleep, ✤Sleep-Eze D, Sleep-Eze 3, Sominex, Sominex 2, Theraflu Cold Medicine (Nighttime Strength), Twilite, Tylenol PM Extra Strength, Unisom Sleepgels, Valdrene, Valu-Dryl Allergy Medicine [CD], Wal-Ben, Wal-Dryl, Wehydryl

BENEFITS versus RISKS	
Possible Benefits	*Possible Risks*
EFFECTIVE RELIEF OF ALLERGIC RHINITIS AND ALLERGIC SKIN DISORDERS	Marked sedation
	Atropinelike effects
	Accentuation of prostatism (see Glossary)
EFFECTIVE, NONADDICTIVE SEDATIVE AND HYPNOTIC	
Treatment of anaphylaxis	
Prevention and relief of motion sickness	
Partial relief of symptoms of Parkinson's disease	

▷ **Principal Uses**

As a Single Drug Product: Uses currently included in FDA-approved labeling: (1) Prevention or treatment of motion sickness (control of dizziness, nau-

*Ambenyl Syrup is C-V. See Schedules of Controlled Drugs at the back of the book.

sea and vomiting); (2) treatment of drug-induced Parkinsonian reactions, especially in children or the elderly; (3) treatment of conditions caused by histamine release (such as allergic drug reactions); (4) used as a short-term sleep aid; (5) helps hives (urticaria) that have an unknown cause (idiopathic); (6) approved to help treat symptoms of the common cold.

Other (unlabeled) generally accepted uses: (1) Cough suppression; (2) can have a role in easing the discomfort of mucositis caused by radiation therapy; (3) used in combination with metoclopramide (Reglan) to help stop vomiting caused by chemotherapy (moderately emetogenic).

As a Combination Drug Product [CD]: This drug may have a mild suppressant effect on coughing. It is combined with expectorants and codeine or dextromethorphan in some cough products.

How This Drug Works: Blocks the action of histamine. Its natural side effects are used to advantage: sedative action used to help people fall asleep; atropinelike action used in motion sickness and Parkinson-related disorders.

Available Dosage Forms and Strengths

Capsules, nonprescription — 5 mg
Capsules, prescription — 50 mg
Cream — 1%
Elixir — 12.5 mg/5 ml (14% alcohol)
Spray — 1%
Syrup — 12.5 mg/5 ml and 13.3 mg/5 ml
Tablets, nonprescription — 25 mg
Tablets, prescription — 50 mg

▷ **Usual Adult Dosage Ranges:** *Antihistamine, to prevent motion sickness, or in parkinsonism:* 25 to 50 mg every 6 to 8 hours. Maximum daily dose is 300 mg. Cough control (antitussive): 25 mg every 4 to 6 hours. Maximum daily dose is 150 mg. *As a sleep aid (hypnotic):* 50 mg at bedtime is often used. To prevent vomiting from chemotherapy: 50 mg of diphenhydramine combined with 50 mg of metoclopramide every 6 hours for 2 to 4 days. **Note: Actual dose and schedule must be determined for each patient individually.**

Conditions Requiring Dosing Adjustments

Liver Function: Caution—single doses are not expected to be a problem; however, the use of multiple doses in patients with liver compromise has not been studied.

Kidney Function: In mild kidney failure (creatinine clearance more than 50 ml/min), usual dose is given every 6 hours; every 6–12 hours in mild-moderate failure; and every 12–18 hours in severe kidney failure.

▷ **Dosing Instructions:** Tablet may be crushed and capsule may be opened and is best taken with or following food. If you forget a dose: Take the missed dose as soon as you remember unless it is almost time for your next dose—if that is the case, simply skip the missed dose and take the next dose right on schedule. DO NOT double doses.

Usual Duration of Use: Regular use for 2 to 3 days is needed to see effectiveness in easing allergic rhinitis and dermatosis symptoms. If it doesn't work after 5 days, this drug should be stopped. As a bedtime sedative (hypnotic), use only as needed. Avoid long-term use.

▷ **This Drug Should Not Be Taken If**
  • you have had an allergic reaction to it previously.
  • you are nursing your infant.
  • you are taking, or took during the past 2 weeks, any monoamine oxidase (MAO) type A inhibitor (see Drug Classes).
▷ **Inform Your Physician Before Taking This Drug If**
  • you have had an unfavorable response to any antihistamine.
  • you have narrow-angle glaucoma.
  • you have peptic ulcer disease, with any degree of pyloric obstruction.
  • you have chickenpox and are considering the topical form of this medicine.
  • you have prostatism (see Glossary).
  • you are subject to bronchial asthma or seizures (epilepsy).
  • you have difficulty urinating.
  • you have glucose-6-phosphate dehydrogenase (G6PD) deficiency.

Possible Side Effects (natural, expected and unavoidable drug actions)
  Drowsiness (diphenhydramine is the most sedating antihistamine); weakness; dryness of nose, mouth and throat; constipation; thickening of bronchial secretions.

▷ **Possible Adverse Effects** (unusual, unexpected and infrequent reactions)
  If any of the following develop, consult your physician promptly for guidance.
  Mild Adverse Effects
  Allergic reactions: skin rash, hives—rare.
  Headache, dizziness, inability to concentrate, blurred or double vision, difficult urination—infrequent.
  Reduced tolerance for contact lenses—possible.
  Nausea, vomiting, diarrhea—possible.
  Serious Adverse Effects
  Allergic reaction: anaphylactic reaction (see Glossary)—case reports.
  Idiosyncratic reactions: insomnia, excitement, confusion—case reports.
  Hemolytic anemia (see Glossary) or porphyria—case reports.
  Reduced white blood cell count: fever, sore throat, infections or blood platelet destruction (abnormal bleeding or bruising; see Glossary)—case reports.
  Movement disorders (dyskinesias)—case reports.
  Hip fractures—case reports resulting in older patients from unsteadiness from the drug versus the drug itself.

▷ **Possible Effects on Sexual Function:** Shortened menstrual cycle (early arrival of expected menstrual onset).

Natural Diseases or Disorders That May Be Activated by This Drug
  Latent epilepsy, glaucoma, prostatism.

Possible Effects on Laboratory Tests
  Red blood cell counts and hemoglobin: decreased.
  Urine screening tests for drug abuse: initial test result may be falsely **positive;** confirmatory test result will be **negative.** (Test results depend upon amount of drug taken and testing method used.)

CAUTION
  1. Stop this drug 5 days before diagnostic skin testing procedures in order to prevent false-negative test results.
  2. Do not use if you have active bronchial asthma, bronchitis or pneumonia.

3. May lead to unsteadiness in older patients (generally more sensitive to this drug), resulting in falls. Caution is advised.

Precautions for Use

By Infants and Children: This drug should not be used in premature or full-term newborn infants. Doses for children should be small, as the young child is especially sensitive to the effects of antihistamines on the brain and nervous system. For use to decrease coughing (antitussive) in children 6 to 12 years old: 12.5 mg every 4 to 6 hours. The maximum daily dose here is 75 mg/day. Avoid the use of this drug in the child with chickenpox or a flu-like infection—may lead to altered mental status and loss of coordination.

By Those Over 60 Years of Age: Increased risk of drowsiness, dizziness, unsteadiness, and impairment of thinking, judgment and memory. Can increase the degree of impaired urination associated with prostate enlargement (prostatism). Sedative effects may be misinterpreted as senility or emotional depression.

▷ **Advisability of Use During Pregnancy**

Pregnancy Category: B by the manufacturer. See Pregnancy Risk Categories at the back of this book.

Animal studies: No birth defects reported in rats or rabbits.

Human studies: Some case reports of fetal toxicity have been made. Information from studies of pregnant women is not available. A withdrawal syndrome of tremor and diarrhea was reported in a 5-day-old infant whose mother used this drug (150 mg daily) during pregnancy.

Use is a benefit-to-risk decision. Ask your doctor for help.

Advisability of Use If Breast-Feeding

Presence of this drug in breast milk: Yes.

Avoid drug or refrain from nursing.

Habit-Forming Potential: Combination use of pentazocine and diphenhydramine has become an abused intravenous drug combination. There have been rare reports of a withdrawal syndrome after use of high doses. Intravenous use has led to some rare cases of drug abuse.

Effects of Overdose: Marked drowsiness, confusion, incoordination, muscle tremors, fever, dilated pupils, stupor, coma, seizures.

Possible Effects of Long-Term Use: The development of tolerance (see Glossary) and reduced effectiveness of drug.

Suggested Periodic Examinations While Taking This Drug (at physician's discretion)

Complete blood cell counts.

▷ **While Taking This Drug, Observe the Following**

Foods: No restrictions.

Herbal Medicines or Minerals: Valerian and kava kava may interact additively (drowsiness). Avoid these combinations. Ginkgo biloba leaf extract has a German Commission E indication for vertigo, but has not been studied in combination with antihistamines and cannot presently be recommended. Talk to your doctor BEFORE adding any herbal medicines.

Beverages: No restrictions. May be taken with milk.

▷ Alcohol: Use extreme caution. The combination of alcohol and antihistamines can cause rapid and marked sedation.

Tobacco Smoking: No interactions expected. I advise everyone to quit smoking.

Marijuana Smoking: Increased drowsiness and mouth dryness; accentuation of impaired thinking.

▷ *Other Drugs*

Diphenhydramine may **increase** the effects of

- all drugs with a sedative effect such as benzodiazepines, tricyclic antidepressants and narcotics (see Drug Classes) and cause oversedation.
- amitriptyline (Elavil) and cause increased urinary retention.
- atropine and atropinelike drugs (see Drug Classes).
- metaproterenol (Alupent, others) leading to increased risk of metaproterenol toxicity.
- tramadol (Ultram), leading to increased sedation risk.

The following drugs may **increase** the effects of diphenhydramine:

- monoamine oxidase (MAO) type A inhibitor drugs (see Drug Classes); can delay elimination, exaggerating and prolonging its action.

Diphenhydramine **taken concurrently** with

- phenothiazines (see Drug Classes) may result in increased difficulty urinating, intestinal obstruction or glaucoma, especially in those over 70 years old.
- temazepam (Restoril) in pregnancy may increase risk of death of the fetus.
- tricyclic antidepressants (see Drug Classes) may cause increased risk of urinary retention.

▷ Driving, Hazardous Activities: This drug may impair alertness, judgment, coordination and reaction time. Restrict activities as necessary.

Aviation Note: The use of this drug *is a disqualification* for piloting. Consult a designated Aviation Medical Examiner.

Exposure to Sun: Caution—this drug may cause photosensitivity (see Glossary).

Exposure to Environmental Chemicals: The insecticides Aldrin, Dieldrin and Chlordane may decrease the effectiveness of this drug. Sevin may increase the sedative effects of this drug.

DISOPYRAMIDE (di so PEER a mide)

Introduced: 1969 Class: Antiarrhythmic **Prescription:** USA: Yes
Controlled Drug: USA: No; Canada: No **Available as Generic:** USA: Yes; Canada: No

Brand Names: Norpace, Norpace CR, Pisopyramide, Rythmical, ✚Rythmodan, ✚Rythmodan-LA

BENEFITS versus RISKS	
Possible Benefits	*Possible Risks*
EFFECTIVE TREATMENT OF SELECTED HEART RHYTHM DISORDERS	NARROW TREATMENT RANGE
	LOW BLOOD PRESSURE
	LOW BLOOD SUGAR (INFREQUENT)
	AGRANULOCYTOSIS—RARE
	Peripheral neuropathy
	Liver toxicity
	Heart conduction and rhythm abnormalities
	Frequent atropinelike side effects

▷ **Principal Uses**

As a Single Drug Product: Uses currently included in FDA-approved labeling: Treats abnormal rhythms in the heart ventricles (ventricular arrhythmias). It is classified as a Type 1A antiarrhythmic agent.

Other (unlabeled) generally accepted uses: (1) Abolishes and prevents recurrence of premature heartbeats in the atria (upper chambers) and ventricles (lower heart chambers); (2) treats and prevents abnormally rapid heart rates (tachycardia) beginning in the atria or the ventricles; (3) eases arrhythmias and abnormal heart pressures arising from cardiomyopathy or subaortic stenosis; (4) may have a role in easing oxygen problems in some infants (hypercyanotic attacks in tetralogy of Fallot).

How This Drug Works: Slows activity of the heart pacemaker and delays electrical impulses through the conduction system and muscle of the heart. These effects help restore normal heart rate and rhythm.

Available Dosage Forms and Strengths

Capsules — 100 mg, 150 mg

Capsules, prolonged action — 100 mg, 150 mg

Capsules, prolonged action (Canada) — 250, 322.5 mg LA

Tablet, controlled release — 100, 150 mg

Tablet, controlled release (Canada) — 250 mg

▷ **Usual Adult Dosage Ranges:** For most adults, 600 mg per day. Immediate-release form: 150 mg every 6 hours. Controlled release: 300 mg every 12 hours. If weight is less than 110 pounds (50 kg) dose is 400 milligrams/day given as 100 milligrams every 6 hours (immediate-release) or 200 milligrams every 12 hours (controlled-release); 1,600 mg every 24 hours—for refractory cases. Loading dose (if quick control is critical): For more than 50 kg, 300 mg of immediate-release form. If less than 50 kg, 200 mg (immediate-release form). **Note: Actual dose and schedule must be determined for each patient individually.**

Conditions Requiring Dosing Adjustments

Liver Function: Dose decreased in patients with liver compromise by 25 to 50%.

Kidney Function: Dosing must be adjusted in kidney compromise. In moderate to severe kidney failure: Immediate-release form is given every 12 to 24 hours. May cause urine retention and should be used with caution in patients with urinary outflow problems.

Cardiomyopathy and/or Heart Decompensation: Starting dose is limited to 100 mg of the immediate-release form every 6 to 8 hours. Care must be taken to avoid congestive heart failure or excessive lowering of blood pressure.

▷ **Dosing Instructions:** Regular capsules may be opened and are best taken on an empty stomach, 1 hour before or 2 hours after eating. May also take with or following food to reduce stomach irritation. Prolonged-action capsules should not be opened, chewed or crushed. If you forget a dose (immediate release): take the missed dose when you remember it, unless it is nearly time for your next dose—if that is the case, skip the missed dose and take the next one right on schedule. Controlled or extended release: Take the missed dose as soon as you remember it, unless it is within 4 hours of your next dose. If that is the case, skip the missed dose and take the next scheduled dose. DO NOT double doses of either form.

Usual Duration of Use: Regular use for 2 to 4 days is needed to see effectiveness in correcting or preventing rhythm disorders. Long-term use requires supervision and ongoing evaluation by your doctor.

Typical Treatment Goals and Measurements (Outcomes and Markers)

Abnormal heartbeats: The general goal is to return the heart to a normal rhythm or at least to markedly reduce the occurrence of abnormal heartbeats. In life-threatening arrhythmias, the goal is to abort the abnormal beats and return the pattern to normal. Success at ongoing suppression may involve ambulatory checks of heart rate and rhythm for a day (such as in Holter monitoring). This kind of testing involves placement of adhesive-backed temporary electrodes on the skin in several positions around the heart. A small heart rate and rhythm (EKG or ECG) recording device is carried around via a shoulder strap and records what the heart is doing over 24 hours. Once the recording is made, a scanning machine reviews the record, tallies abnormal heart beats or rhythms and gives a close and extended look at how the heart is reacting or benefiting from the medicines that the patient is taking. Repeat measurements can be made if doses are changes to check the success at keeping the heart in normal sinus rhythm!

Possible Advantages of This Drug

Both quinidine and procainamide (other medicines for abnormal heart rhythms) can be associated with development of antinuclear antibodies (ANA). One study showed that disopyramide does NOT induce ANA.

▷ **This Drug Should Not Be Taken If**

- you have had an allergic reaction to it previously.
- you have second-degree, third-degree or bifasicular heart block (and you don't have a pacemaker).
- you have "sick sinus" syndrome (talk with your doctor).
- you are in heart (cardiogenic) shock.

▷ **Inform Your Physician Before Taking This Drug If**

- you have had unfavorable reactions to antiarrhythmic drugs.
- you have heart disease, especially "heart block."
- you have a history of atrial fibrillation or flutter.
- you have a history of low blood potassium.
- you have a history of low blood pressure.
- you have a history of low white blood cells.
- you have impaired liver or kidney function.
- you have glaucoma, a family history of glaucoma or myasthenia gravis.
- you have an enlarged prostate gland.
- you are prone to low blood sugars.
- you take digitalis or any diuretic drug that can cause loss of body potassium (ask your doctor).

Possible Side Effects (natural, expected and unavoidable drug actions)

Drop in blood pressure in susceptible individuals.

Dry mouth, constipation, blurred vision, impaired urination—may be frequent.

▷ **Possible Adverse Effects** (unusual, unexpected and infrequent reactions)

If any of the following develop, consult your physician promptly for guidance.

Mild Adverse Effects
Allergic reactions: skin rash, itching—case reports.
Headache, nervousness, fatigue, muscular weakness, mild aches—infrequent.
Loss of appetite, indigestion, nausea, vomiting, diarrhea—infrequent to frequent.

Serious Adverse Effects
Idiosyncratic reaction: acute psychotic behavior—rare.
Severe drop in blood pressure, fainting—possible.
Neuropathy—case report.
Progressive heart weakness, possible congestive heart failure.
Inability to empty urinary bladder, prostatism (see Glossary).
Abnormal heart rhythms—case reports, usually within first month of use.
Low blood sugar (glucose)—infrequent.
Jaundice (see Glossary) or liver toxicity—case reports.
Porphyria—rare.
Abnormally low white blood cell count—case report.

▷ **Possible Effects on Sexual Function:** Rare impotence (300 mg/day); enlargement and tenderness of male breasts—case reports.

Adverse Effects That May Mimic Natural Diseases or Disorders
Reversible jaundice may suggest viral hepatitis. Abnormal heart rhythms such as paroxysmal tachycardia may mimic tachycardia from other causes.

Natural Diseases or Disorders That May Be Activated by This Drug
Glaucoma, myasthenia gravis.

Possible Effects on Laboratory Tests
White blood cell counts: decreased.
Liver function tests: increased liver enzymes (ALT/GPT, AST/GOT, and alkaline phosphatase), increased bilirubin.

CAUTION
1. Thorough heart exam (including electrocardiogram) is critical prior to using this drug.
2. Periodic heart exams are needed to follow drug responses. Some people may have heart rhythm or function declines. Close monitoring of heart rate, rhythm and overall performance is essential.
3. Dose must be individualized. Do not change your dose without your doctor's supervision.
4. Talk with your doctor about signs and symptoms of low blood sugar.
5. Do not take any other antiarrhythmic drug while taking this drug unless directed to do so by your doctor.

Precautions for Use
By Infants and Children: In pediatric patients, disopyramide is given on a mg-per-kg-of-body-mass basis. Dose is then divided into equal doses, given at times determined by patient response. Some patients from 1 to 4 years old will receive 10 to 20 mg per kg of body mass per day, divided into equal doses and given every 6 hours. Initial use of this drug requires hospitalization and supervision by a qualified pediatrician.
By Those Over 60 Years of Age: Reduced kidney function may require dose reductions. This drug can aggravate existing prostatism (see Glossary) and promote constipation. Watch closely for light-headedness, dizziness, unsteadiness and tendency to fall.

▷ **Advisability of Use During Pregnancy**
 Pregnancy Category: C. See Pregnancy Risk Categories at the back of this book.
 Animal studies: No birth defects reported in rats and rabbits.
 Human studies: Adequate studies of pregnant women are not available. It has been reported that this drug can cause contractions of the pregnant uterus. Use this drug only if clearly needed. Ask your physician for guidance.

Advisability of Use If Breast-Feeding
 Presence of this drug in breast milk: Yes.
 Avoid drug or refrain from nursing.

Habit-Forming Potential: None.

Effects of Overdose: Dryness of eyes, nose, mouth and throat; impaired urination; constipation; marked drop in blood pressure; abnormal heart rhythms; congestive heart failure.

Possible Effects of Long-Term Use: None reported.

Suggested Periodic Examinations While Taking This Drug (at physician's discretion)
 Electrocardiograms.
 Complete blood counts.
 Potassium blood levels.

▷ **While Taking This Drug, Observe the Following**
 Foods: No restrictions. Ask your physician regarding need for salt restriction and advisability of eating potassium-rich foods.
 Herbal Medicines or Minerals: Using St. John's wort, ma huang, ephedra or kola while taking this medicine may result in unacceptable heart stimulation. Belladonna, henbane, *Scopolia,* pheasant's eye extract or lily-of-the-valley or squill powdered extracts should NOT be taken if you have abnormal heart rhythms. Since St. John's wort and disopyramide may increase sun sensitivity, the combination is NOT advised.
 Beverages: No restrictions. May be taken with milk.
▷ *Alcohol:* Use caution. Alcohol can increase the blood-pressure-lowering effects and the blood-sugar-lowering effects of this drug.
 Tobacco Smoking: Nicotine can irritate the heart, reducing effectiveness. I advise everyone to quit smoking.
▷ *Other Drugs*
 Disopyramide may ***increase*** the effects of
 • antihypertensive drugs and cause excessive lowering of blood pressure.
 • atropinelike drugs (see Drug Classes).
 • warfarin (Coumadin, etc.); check INR (prothrombin times) more often, and adjust dosing.
 Disopyramide may ***decrease*** the effects of
 • ambenonium (Mytelase).
 • neostigmine (Prostigmin).
 • pyridostigmine (Mestinon).
 Benefits of these three drugs listed above in treating myasthenia gravis may be reduced.
 Disopyramide ***taken concurrently*** with
 • amiodarone (Cordarone) may result in an abnormal heart effect (torsade de pointes).

- beta-blockers (see Drug Classes) may result in abnormally low heart rates.
- cisapride (Propulsid) may lead to abnormal heart rhythm. DO NOT COMBINE.
- digoxin (Lanoxin) can cause digoxin toxicity.
- dofetilide (Tikosyn) may lead to heart toxicity. One source suggests waiting 3 half-lives (most conservative approach is 4.32 half-lives) before starting a dofetilide. DO NOT COMBINE.
- erythromycins (E.E.S., others) can cause increased disopyramide blood concentrations and abnormal heart effects. (Caution is advised in combining with azithromycin, clarithromycin or dirithromycin because they are structurally similar.)
- gatifloxacin (Tequin), levofloxacin (Levaquin), moxifloxacin (Avelox) or sparfloxacin (Zagam) may result in increased risk of abnormal heart rhythms. DO NOT combine.
- insulin or oral antidiabetic drugs (see Drug Classes) may result in abnormally low blood sugars.
- moxifloxacin (Avelox) may lead to abnormal heart rhythm. DO NOT COMBINE.
- phenobarbital may result in loss of disopyramide's effectiveness.
- phenytoin (Dilantin) or fosphenytoin (Cerebyx) can result in decreased disopyramide effectiveness and accumulation of a metabolite of fosphenytoin or phenytoin, which may cause a severe increase in anticholinergic effects.
- potassium supplements may result in elevated potassium levels, which can lead to disopyramide toxicity.
- quinidine can cause increases in disopyramide blood levels and decreases in quinidine levels.
- quinupristin/dalfopristin (Synercid) may lead to abnormal heart rhythm. Careful patient monitoring and possible dosing decreases of disopyramide are prudent.
- ritonavir (Norvir) and perhaps other protease inhibitors (see Drug Classes) may increase disopyramide blood levels and lead to toxicity.
- verapamil (Calan, others) can precipitate or worsen congestive heart failure.
- warfarin (Coumadin) may cause increased bleeding risk. INR must be checked more frequently.

The following drugs may **_decrease_** the effects of disopyramide:
- all diuretics that promote potassium loss.
- rifabutin (Mycobutin).
- rifampin (Rimactane, Rifadin).

▷ *Driving, Hazardous Activities:* May cause dizziness or blurred vision. Limit activities as needed.

Aviation Note: The use of this drug **_may be a disqualification_** for piloting. Consult a designated Aviation Medical Examiner.

Exposure to Sun: Use caution. This drug causes photosensitization (see Glossary).

Exposure to Heat: Use caution. The use of this drug in hot environments may increase the risk of heatstroke.

Occurrence of Unrelated Illness: Vomiting, diarrhea or dehydration can affect this drug's action adversely. Report such developments promptly.

Discontinuation: This drug should not be stopped abruptly after long-term use. Ask your doctor for help regarding gradual dose reduction.

DISULFIRAM (di SULF i ram)

Introduced: 1948   **Class:** Antialcoholism   **Prescription:** USA: Yes
Controlled Drug: USA: No; Canada: No   **Available as Generic:** USA: Yes;
Canada: No
Brand Name: Antabuse

BENEFITS versus RISKS	
Possible Benefits	*Possible Risks*
EFFECTIVE ADJUNCT IN THE TREATMENT OF CHRONIC ALCOHOLISM	DANGEROUS REACTIONS WITH ALCOHOL INGESTION
	Acute psychotic reactions
	Drug-induced liver damage
	Drug-induced optic and/or peripheral neuritis
	Low blood platelets

Principal Uses

As a Single Drug Product: Uses currently included in FDA-approved labeling: Deters abusive drinking of alcoholic beverages. It does not abolish the craving or impulse to drink.

Other (unlabeled) generally accepted uses: (1) Limited use in helping skin problems (dermatitis) caused by nickel exposure; (2) some data showing increase in infection-fighting cells (CD4) in AIDS.

How This Drug Works: This drug blocks normal liver enzyme activity after alcohol is changed to acetaldehyde. This causes accumulation of acetaldehyde and causes the disulfiram (Antabuse) reaction (see Glossary).

Available Dosage Forms and Strengths

Tablets — 250 mg, 500 mg

▷ **Usual Adult Dosage Ranges:** Once all signs of intoxication are gone and no less than 12 hours after the last alcohol drink, therapy begins with 500 mg/day for 1 to 2 weeks, followed by an ongoing dose of 250 mg/day. Range is 125 mg to 500 mg daily and is individually determined. Maximum daily dose is 500 mg. **Note: Actual dose and schedule must be determined for each patient individually.**

Conditions Requiring Dosing Adjustments

Liver Function: This drug is a benefit-to-risk decision in mild liver compromise. Disulfiram is clearly contraindicated in portal hypertension and active hepatitis.

Kidney Function: Dosing adjustments are not indicated.

Diabetes: People with diabetes who take disulfiram can be at increased risk for diabetic blood vessel (micro- and macrovascular) problems. The risk is worsened by potential adverse drug effects such as increased cholesterol levels and peripheral neuropathy.

Lung Disease: Accumulation of a metabolite may occur in severe lung problems. Drug levels or dose reduction will be needed.

▷ **Dosing Instructions:** The tablet may be crushed and taken with or following food to decrease stomach irritation. If you forget a dose: take the missed dose right away, unless it is 12 hours after you should have taken the dose—if that is the case, simply take the next scheduled dose. DO NOT double doses.

Usual Duration of Use: Use on a regular schedule for several months is needed to see effectiveness in deterring alcohol use. If tolerated well, use should continue until self-control and sobriety are ongoing.

Typical Treatment Goals and Measurements (Outcomes and Markers)

Alcoholism: This medicine does NOT cure alcoholism, but reduces the desire to drink. The goal is to stop drinking and return self-control and sobriety. Combination of this medicine with psychological help (psychotherapy) gets the best results.

▷ **This Drug Should Not Be Taken If**
- you have had a severe allergic reaction to disulfiram. (Note: The interaction of disulfiram and alcohol is not an allergic reaction.)
- you have taken any form of alcohol within the past 12 hours.
- you are pregnant.
- you have a history of psychosis.
- you are taking paraldehyde.
- you have significant exposure to ethylene dibromide where you live or work. Disulfiram inhibits the removal of this chemical and enhances the ability of ethylene dibromide to cause cancer.
- you are taking (or have taken recently) metronidazole (Flagyl).
- you have coronary heart disease or a serious heart rhythm disorder.

▷ **Inform Your Physician Before Taking This Drug If**
- you have used disulfiram in the past.
- you do not intend to avoid alcohol completely while taking this drug.
- you do not understand what will happen if you drink alcohol while taking this drug.
- you are planning pregnancy in the near future.
- you have a history of diabetes, epilepsy or kidney or liver disease.
- you take oral anticoagulants, digitalis, isoniazid, paraldehyde or phenytoin (Dilantin).
- you have a history of low thyroid function (hypothyroidism).
- you have a history of lung disease.
- you plan to have surgery under general anesthesia while taking this drug.

Possible Side Effects (natural, expected and unavoidable drug actions)

Drowsiness, lethargy during early use.

Offensive breath and body odor.

▷ **Possible Adverse Effects** (unusual, unexpected and infrequent reactions)

If any of the following develop, consult your physician promptly for guidance.

Mild Adverse Effects

Allergic reactions: skin rash, hives—case reports.

Headache, dizziness, restlessness, tremor—infrequent.

Metallic or garlic-like taste, indigestion (usually subsides in 2 weeks).

Increased cholesterol after 3–6 weeks of treatment—possible (taking 50 mg per day of pyridoxine seems to stop this).

Decreased or increased blood pressure—possible.

Serious Adverse Effects
  Allergic reactions: severe skin rashes, drug-induced hepatitis—rare.
  Idiosyncratic reaction: acute toxic effect on brain, including abnormal movements and psychotic behavior—case reports.
  Optic or peripheral neuritis (see Glossary)—case reports.
  Seizures—case reports.
  Decreased thyroid gland function—possible.
  May increase risk for blood vessel problems in people with diabetes or cause low blood platelets—case reports.
  Carpal tunnel syndrome, peripheral neuropathy—case reports.
▷ **Possible Effects on Sexual Function:** Decreased libido and/or impaired erection in users taking recommended doses of 125 to 500 mg daily—case reports.

Adverse Effects That May Mimic Natural Diseases or Disorders
  Liver reaction may suggest viral hepatitis.
  Brain toxicity may suggest spontaneous psychosis.

Possible Effects on Laboratory Tests
  Blood cholesterol level: increased.
  INR (prothrombin time): increased (taken concurrently with warfarin).
  Liver function tests: liver enzymes increased (ALT/GPT, AST/GOT and alkaline phosphatase), increased bilirubin.

CAUTION
  1. No one intoxicated with alcohol should take this drug.
  2. Patients must be fully informed about purpose and actions of this drug *before* treatment is started.
  3. Long-term use requires exam for reduced thyroid function.
  4. Carry a personal identification card noting you are taking this drug.
  5. Many herbal medicines are extracts that contain alcohol—do not combine.

Precautions for Use
  By Infants and Children: Safety and effectiveness for those under 12 years of age not established.
  By Those Over 60 Years of Age: Watch for excessive sedation when the drug is started. *Do not* perform an "alcohol trial" to see the effects of this drug.
▷ **Advisability of Use During Pregnancy**
  Pregnancy Category: C. See Pregnancy Risk Categories at the back of this book.
  Animal studies: No defects reported in rats and hamsters.
  Human studies: Two reports indicate that four of eight fetuses exposed had serious birth defects. Adequate studies of pregnant women are not available. Avoid this drug completely if possible.

Advisability of Use If Breast-Feeding
  Presence of this drug in breast milk: Unknown.
  Talk with your doctor, as this is a question of benefit of the drug versus the risk of adverse effects to the fetus.

Habit-Forming Potential: None.

Effects of Overdose: Marked lethargy, impaired memory, altered behavior, confusion, unsteadiness, weakness, stomach pain, nausea, vomiting, diarrhea.

Possible Effects of Long-Term Use: Decreased function of thyroid gland.

Suggested Periodic Examinations While Taking This Drug (at physician's discretion)

> Visual acuity.
> Liver function tests.
> Thyroid function tests.

▷ **While Taking This Drug, Observe the Following**

Foods: Avoid all foods prepared with alcohol, including sauces, marinades, vinegars, desserts, etc. Ask when dining out about use of alcohol in cooking food. Increased cholesterol after 3–6 weeks of treatment is possible. Taking 50 mg per day of pyridoxine seems to stop this side effect. Talk to your doctor!

Herbal Medicines or Minerals: Many herbal medicines such as ginseng and echinacea contain alcohol. DO NOT combine them with disulfiram. Using St. John's wort, ma huang, ephedrine-like compounds or kola while trying to stop drinking may worsen jitteriness and anxiety.

Beverages: Avoid all punches, fruit drinks, etc., that may contain alcohol. This drug may be taken with milk.

▷ *Alcohol:* ***Avoid completely in all forms*** while taking this drug and for 14 days after the last dose. Disulfiram and alcohol—even in small amounts—produces the disulfiram (Antabuse) reaction. This starts 5 to 10 minutes after alcohol: intense flushing, severe headache, shortness of breath, chest pains, nausea, repeated vomiting, sweating and weakness. If large amounts of alcohol: reaction may progress to blurred vision, vertigo, confusion, severely low blood pressure and loss of consciousness. May go on to convulsions and death. Reaction may last from 30 minutes to hours, depending upon amount of alcohol and disulfiram.

Tobacco Smoking: No interactions expected. I advise everyone to quit smoking.

Marijuana Smoking: Possible increase in drowsiness or lethargy.

▷ *Other Drugs*

Disulfiram may ***increase*** the effects of

- chlordiazepoxide (Librium) and diazepam (Valium) and cause oversedation. Other benzodiazepines such as alprazolam, clonazepam, clorazepate, flurazepam, halazepam, prazepam or triazolam may also be subject to this interaction.
- oral anticoagulants (warfarin, etc.) and increase the risk of bleeding; dose adjustments may be necessary.
- paraldehyde and cause excessive depression of brain function.
- phenytoin (Dilantin) or fosphenytoin (Cerebyx) and cause toxicity; dose must be decreased.

Disulfiram may ***decrease*** the effects of

- perphenazine (Trilafon, etc.).

Disulfiram ***taken concurrently*** with

- bacampicillin (Spectrobid) can theoretically cause a disulfiram reaction, but no cases have been reported.
- cisplatin (Platinol) can increase risk of toxicity of cisplatin.
- cyclosporine (Sandimmune) may result in a disulfiram reaction, as there is alcohol in the intravenous and oral forms of cyclosporine.
- isoniazid (INH, etc.) may cause acute mental problems and incoordination.

- metronidazole (Flagyl) may cause acute mental and behavioral disturbances, making it necessary to stop treatment.
- omeprazole (Prilosec) and possibly esomeprazole (Nexium) may result in increased disulfiram levels and toxicity.
- over-the-counter (OTC) cough syrups, tonics, etc., containing alcohol may cause a disulfiram (Antabuse) reaction; avoid concurrent use (see Over-the-Counter Drugs in Glossary).
- paraldehyde may result in a disulfiram reaction.
- theophylline (Theo-Dur, others) can lead to theophylline toxicity because the metabolism of theophylline is decreased.
- tranylcypromine (Parnate) can increase risk of hallucinations, disorientation and agitation. Monitor the patient closely if these two medicines must be used together.
- warfarin will result in an increased risk of bleeding. More frequent INR testing is recommended.

The following drugs may *increase* the effects of disulfiram:
- amitriptyline (Elavil) and perhaps other tricyclic antidepressants may enhance the disulfiram-alcohol interaction; avoid concurrent use of these drugs.

▷ *Driving, Hazardous Activities:* This drug may cause drowsiness or dizziness. Limit activities as necessary.

Aviation Note: Alcoholism *is a disqualification* for piloting. Consult a designated Aviation Medical Examiner.

Exposure to Sun: No restrictions.

Exposure to Environmental Chemicals: Thiram, a pesticide, and carbon disulfide, a pesticide and industrial solvent, can have additive toxic effects. Watch for toxic effects on the brain and nervous system.

Discontinuation: This medicine is only part of your program. Do not stop it unless you have talked with your doctor. Even if it is stopped, no alcohol should be ingested for 14 days.

DOFETILIDE (Doh FET ill eyed)

Introduced: 1999   **Class:** Antiarrhythmic   **Prescription:** USA: Yes
Controlled Drug: USA: No; Canada: No   **Available as Generic:** USA: No; Canada: No
Brand Name: Tikosyn
Author's Note: Information on this medicine will be broadened in subsequent editions as clinical use and medication benefits warrant.

DORNASE ALPHA (Door nase AL fa)

Introduced: 1994   **Class:** Anti-cystic-fibrosis   agent   **Prescription:** USA: Yes   **Controlled Drug:** USA: No; Canada: No   **Available as Generic:** USA: No; Canada: No
Brand Name: Pulmozyme

```
┌─────────────────────────────────────────────────────────────────┐
│                      BENEFITS versus RISKS                        │
│        Possible Benefits                    Possible Risks        │
│  DECREASED MUCUS                   Hoarseness                     │
│    VISCOSITY                       Antibodies to DNA              │
│  IMPROVED LUNG FUNCTION            Facial swelling (edema)        │
│  DECREASED OCCURRENCE OF                                          │
│    RESPIRATORY INFECTIONS                                        │
│  DECREASED NUMBER OF                                             │
│    HOSPITALIZATIONS                                              │
└─────────────────────────────────────────────────────────────────┘
```

▷ **Principal Uses**

As a Single Drug Product: Uses currently included in FDA-approved labeling: Eases symptoms of cystic fibrosis (used with standard therapies).

Other (unlabeled) generally accepted uses: None at present.

How This Drug Works: Large amounts of DNA are found in sputum of people with cystic fibrosis, making it thicker than normal. Dornase breaks the DNA down, making the sputum easier to remove. Other undiscovered mechanisms may also account for its benefits.

Available Dosage Forms and Strengths

Solution — 2.5-ml ampules of 1.0 mg/ml dornase alpha (2.5 mg)

▷ **Recommended Dosage Ranges** (Actual dose and schedule must be determined for each patient individually.)

Infants and Children: Now approved for patients 3 months to less than 5 years of age. Rashes, cough and runny nose (rhinitis) may happen at a higher rate in this population than in older patients.

5 to 60 Years of Age: One 2.5-mg dose administered by one of the tested nebulizers each day. Some selected patients (FVC greater than 85%) may benefit from twice-daily dosing.

Over 60 Years of Age: Same as 5 to 60 years of age.

Conditions Requiring Dosing Adjustments

Liver Function: Not defined.

Kidney Function: Not defined.

▷ **Dosing Instructions:** Solution must be refrigerated and protected from strong light. The drug should not be used if it is cloudy or discolored. Do **not** mix dornase with other medicines. Clinical trials have only been conducted with the Hudson T Up-Draft 2, Marquest Acorn II and Pulmo-Aide compressor. The reusable PARI LC Jet nebulizer and PARI PRONEB compressor were also tested. Do not use with other equipment. If you forget a dose: Administer the missed dose as soon as you remember it, unless it is almost time for your next dose—if that is the case, simply administer the next scheduled dose. DO NOT double doses.

Usual Duration of Use: Regular use for up to 8 days may be needed in cystic fibrosis. Long-term use (up to 12 months has been studied) requires periodic physician evaluation.

Typical Treatment Goals and Measurements (Outcomes and Markers)

Cystic fibrosis: Lung (pulmonary) function tests (FEV1 or FEC) are used to measure the success of treatment. Improvements in these tests may be seen in as little as 3 days. Patient clinical signs and symptoms of cystic fibrosis (such as easing of breathing difficulty or dyspnea and clearing of sputum) may also be a measure of treatment results. If the usual benefit is not realized, call your doctor.

Possible Advantages of This Drug

Reduction in number of infections, use of antibiotics and hospitalizations with minimal side effects.

▷ **This Drug Should Not Be Taken If**

- you have had an allergic reaction to it.
- you have an allergy to Chinese hamster ovary cells.

▷ **Inform Your Physician Before Taking This Drug If**

- you had a rash after the last dose was taken.
- you are uncertain how to use the nebulizer or compressor.
- you are uncertain how much to take or how often to take it.

Possible Side Effects (natural, expected and unavoidable drug actions)

Hoarseness—may be frequent.

▷ **Possible Adverse Effects** (unusual, unexpected and infrequent reactions)

If any of the following develop, consult your physician promptly for guidance.

Mild Adverse Effects

Allergic reactions: rash—infrequent to frequent (may be more likely in those 3 months to less than 5 years old).

Cough or runny nose—infrequent (may be more likely in those 3 months to less than 5 years old).

Mild pharyngitis or laryngitis—frequent.

Conjunctivitis—infrequent.

Chest pain—has been reported.

Facial swelling—rare.

Serious Adverse Effects

Allergic reactions: none defined at present.

Antibodies to DNA (2–4%).

▷ **Possible Effects on Sexual Function:** None reported.

Possible Delayed Adverse Effects: None reported.

Possible Effects on Laboratory Tests

Antibodies to DNA.

CAUTION

1. This drug should only be used with one of the studied nebulizers and compressors.
2. Do not use the drug if it is cloudy or discolored.

Precautions for Use

By Infants and Children: Rash, cough and runny nose may be more likely in those 3 months to 5 years old.

By Those Over 60 Years of Age: No changes or precautions.

▷ **Advisability of Use During Pregnancy**

Pregnancy Category: B. See Pregnancy Risk Categories at the back of this book.

Animal studies: Studies in rats and rabbits at up to 600 times the usual human dose have not revealed any harm to the fetus.

Human studies: Adequate studies of pregnant women are not available. Ask your doctor for guidance.

Advisability of Use If Breast-Feeding
Presence of this drug in breast milk: Unknown.
Avoid drug or refrain from nursing.

Habit-Forming Potential: None.

Effects of Overdose: Single doses of up to 180 times the usual human dose in rats and monkeys have been well tolerated.

Possible Effects of Long-Term Use: Not defined.

Suggested Periodic Examinations While Taking This Drug (at physician's discretion)
Periodic pulmonary function tests. Improved clearing of sputum.

▷ **While Taking This Drug, Observe the Following**
Foods: No restrictions.
Herbal Medicines or Minerals: Some herbals such as anise seed and fennel oil have German commission E monograph indications for catarrh or upper respiratory tract difficulties, but since no studies have been performed with this medicine, they cannot be recommended.
Nutritional Support: Continued enzyme and nutritional support is still needed.
Beverages: No specific restrictions.
▷ *Alcohol:* Follow your doctor's advice relative to alcohol use.
Tobacco Smoking: No interaction, but smoking irritates airways. I advise everyone to quit smoking.
▷ *Other Drugs*
Clinical studies have revealed that dornase is compatible with medicines typically used to manage cystic fibrosis. Specific drug interactions are not documented at present.
▷ *Driving, Hazardous Activities:* Specific limitations because of drug effects are not defined at present.
Aviation Note: The use of this drug *may be a disqualification* for piloting. Consult a designated Aviation Medical Examiner.
Exposure to Sun: No restrictions.
Discontinuation: This drug's benefits stop soon after its regular use is stopped. It must be continued indefinitely to maintain benefit.
Special Storage Instructions: This drug should be stored at 36–46 degrees F and should be protected from light. Unused ampules should be stored in their protective pouch in the refrigerator.

DOXAZOSIN (dox AY zoh sin)

Introduced: 1986   **Class:** Antihypertensive   **Prescription:** USA: Yes
Controlled Drug: USA: No   **Available as Generic:** Yes
Brand Names: ❧Apo-Doxazosin, Cardura, Cardura-1, Doxaloc, ❧Gen-Doxazosin, ❧Med-Doxazosin

BENEFITS versus RISKS	
Possible Benefits	*Possible Risks*
EFFECTIVE TREATMENT OF MILD TO MODERATE HYPERTENSION WHEN USED ALONE OR IN COMBINATION WITH OTHER ANTIIIYPERTENSIVE DRUGS TREATMENT OF BENIGN PROSTATIC HYPERPLASIA	"First-dose" drop in blood pressure, but without fainting Dizziness Fluid retention Rapid heart rate

Author's Note: Data from the ALLHAT trial found that alpha blockers are not drugs of first choice in high blood pressure. A recent FDA panel decided not to change the product label. Information in this profile has been truncated to make room for more widely used medicines.

DOXEPIN (DOX e pin)

Introduced: 1969 **Class:** Antidepressant **Prescription:** USA: Yes **Controlled Drug:** USA: No; Canada: No **Available as Generic:** USA: Yes; Canada: No

Brand Names: Adapin, Sinequan, ✤Triadapin, Zonalon

BENEFITS versus RISKS	
Possible Benefits	*Possible Risks*
EFFECTIVE RELIEF OF ENDOGENOUS DEPRESSION EFFECTIVE RELIEF OF ANXIETY AND NERVOUS TENSION EFFECTIVE RELIEF OF SOME KINDS OF ITCHING (TOPICAL FORM) Possibly beneficial in other depressive disorders	ADVERSE BEHAVIORAL EFFECTS: Confusion, disorientation, hallucinations, delusions CONVERSION OF DEPRESSION TO MANIA in manic-depressive (bipolar) disorders Aggravation of schizophrenia and paranoia Rare blood cell disorders Rare liver toxicity Low blood pressure on standing

Author's Note: Information in this profile has been truncated to make room for more widely used medicines.

EFAVIRENZ (e FAV i rinz)

Introduced: 1998 **Class:** Non-nucleoside reverse transcriptase inhibitor, antiretroviral, antiviral **Prescription:** USA: Yes **Controlled Drug:** USA: No; Canada: No **Available as Generic:** USA: No; Canada: No

Brand Name: Sustiva

BENEFITS versus RISKS	
Possible Benefits	*Possible Risks*
EFFECTIVE COMBINATION TREATMENT OF HIV	SIGNIFICANT CENTRAL NERVOUS SYSTEM EFFECTS
IS PART OF THE STRONGLY RECOMMENDED MEDICINES IN THE NEW NIAID GUIDELINES	Rash
May be the most effective non-nucleoside reverse transcriptase inhibitor currently available when used in combination with other antiretrovirals. Convenient once-daily dosing schedule decreases pill burden and will improve adherence.	

Author's Note: Information in this profile will be broadened or shortened as more information and outcomes become available.

ENALAPRIL (e NAL a pril)

Class: Antihypertensive, ACE inhibitor
Please see the angiotensin converting enzyme (ACE) inhibitor family profile.

EPINEPHRINE (ep i NEF rin)

Other Name: Adrenaline   **Introduced:** 1900   **Class:** Antiasthmatic, antiglaucoma, decongestant   **Prescription:** USA: Varies   **Controlled Drug:** USA: No; Canada: No   **Available as Generic:** USA: Yes; Canada: No

Brand Names: Adrenalin, Adreno-Mist, Ana-Kit, Asthmahaler, Asthmanephrine, Bronkaid Mist, ✤Bronkaid Mistometer, ✤Citanest Forte, Duranest [CD], ✤Dysne-Inhal, Epifrin, E-Pilo Preparations [CD], Epinal Ophthalmic, EpiPen, Epitrate, Marcaine, Medihaler-Epi Preparations, Micronephrine, Norocaine, Octocaine, P1E1, P2E1, P3E1, P4E1, P6E1, Primatene Mist, Propine Ophthalmic, Sensorcaine, Sus-Phrine, Thalfed [CD], Therex [CD], ✤Ultracaine, Vaponefrin, Xylocaine

BENEFITS versus RISKS	
Possible Benefits	*Possible Risks*
EFFECTIVE RELIEF OF SEVERE ALLERGIC (ANAPHYLACTIC) REACTIONS	Significant increase in blood pressure (in sensitive people)
TEMPORARY RELIEF OF ACUTE BRONCHIAL ASTHMA	Idiosyncratic reaction: Pulmonary edema (fluid formation in lungs)
Reduction of internal eye pressure (treatment of glaucoma)	Heart rhythm disorders (in sensitive people)
Relief of allergic congestion of the nose and sinuses	

▷ **Principal Uses**

As a Single Drug Product: Uses currently included in FDA-approved labeling: (1) Inhalation to relieve acute attacks of bronchial asthma; (2) as a decongestant for symptomatic relief of allergic nasal congestion and as eyedrops in the management of glaucoma; (3) treats anaphylactic shock; (4) emergency treatment of abnormal heart rhythms and in cardiopulmonary resuscitation; (5) increases beneficial effects of topical anesthetics.

Other (unlabeled) generally accepted uses: (1) Septic shock; (2) wheezing in infants; (3) croup; (4) can have a role in easing painful erections (priapism); (5) may be used in cataract surgery.

How This Drug Works: By stimulating some nerve (sympathetic) terminals, this drug:

- contracts blood vessel walls, raising blood pressure.
- inhibits histamine release into skin and internal organs.
- dilates constricted bronchial tubes, increasing the size of the airways and improving the ability to breathe.
- decreases fluid formation in the eye, increases its outflow and reduces internal eye pressure.
- decreases blood flow in the nose, shrinking swelling (decongestion) and expanding nasal airways.

Available Dosage Forms and Strengths

Aerosol — 0.2, 0.27, and 0.3 mg per spray

Eyedrops — 0.1%, 0.25%, 0.5%, 1%, 2%

Injection — 0.01, 0.1, 1, and 5 mg/ml

Nose drops — 0.1%

Solution for nebulizer — 1%, 1.25%, 2.25%

▷ **Usual Adult Dosage Ranges**

Aerosols: One inhalation, repeated in 1 to 2 minutes if needed; wait 4 hours before next inhalation.

Eyedrops: One drop every 12 hours. Dose may vary with product; follow printed instructions and label directions. **Note: Actual dose and schedule must be determined for each patient individually.**

Conditions Requiring Dosing Adjustments

Liver Function: Dose reduction is not needed in liver compromise.

Kidney Function: Dose adjustment is not defined in kidney compromise.

Diabetes: People with diabetes benefit more from standard-dose epinephrine when they are undergoing cardiopulmonary resuscitation (CPR) than they do from high dose.

▷ **Dosing Instructions:** Aerosols and inhalation solutions: After first inhalation, wait 1 to 2 minutes to see if a second inhalation is needed. If relief does not occur within 20 minutes of use, stop this drug and seek medical attention **promptly. Avoid prolonged and excessive use.** Eyedrops: During instillation of drops and for 2 minutes after, press finger against the tear sac (inner corner of eye) to prevent rapid absorption of drug into body. If you forget a dose: take (instill) the missed dose as soon as you remember it, unless it is nearly time for your next dose—then simply skip the missed dose and instill the next dose right on schedule.

Usual Duration of Use: According to individual needs. Long-term use requires physician supervision.

Typical Treatment Goals and Measurements (Outcomes and Markers)

Asthma: Short-acting sympathomimetics like epinephrine are used to prevent or treat reversible spasms of the bronchial tubes. The peak effect happens 1 to 2 hours after dosing. Goals are to return bronchial status to more acceptable status (relief of respiratory distress). If the usual benefit to your breathing is not realized, call your doctor.

▷ **This Drug Should Not Be Taken If**
- you have had an allergic reaction to it previously.
- you have narrow-angle glaucoma.
- you are in shock.
- you have organic brain damage.
- you are in labor—it may delay the second stage of labor.
- you are to undergo general anesthesia with cyclopropane or halogenated hydrocarbons.
- your heart is dilated and you have a coronary deficiency.
- you have experienced a recent stroke or heart attack.

▷ **Inform Your Physician Before Taking This Drug If**
- you have any degree of high blood pressure.
- you have any form of heart disease, especially coronary heart disease (with or without angina) or a heart rhythm disorder.
- you have diabetes or overactive thyroid function (hyperthyroidism).
- you have a history of stroke.
- you have a chronic lung disease.
- you take monoamine oxidase (MAO) type A inhibitors, phenothiazines (see Drug Classes), digitalis preparations or quinidine.

Possible Side Effects (natural, expected and unavoidable drug actions)

In some people—restlessness, anxiety, headache, tremor, palpitation, cold hands and feet, dryness of mouth and throat (with use of aerosol). Temporary increase in blood platelets. Discoloration of soft contact lenses—possible.

▷ **Possible Adverse Effects** (unusual, unexpected and infrequent reactions)

If any of the following develop, consult your physician promptly for guidance.

Mild Adverse Effects

Allergic reactions: skin rash; eyedrops may cause redness, swelling and itching of the eyelids.

Weakness, dizziness, pallor.

Serious Adverse Effects

Idiosyncratic reaction: sudden development of excessive fluid in the lungs (pulmonary edema).

In predisposed individuals—excessive rise in blood pressure with risk of stroke (cerebral hemorrhage).

Rapid heart rate and arrhythmias—case reports.

Passing out (syncope)—possible.

Seizures or porphyria—rare.

Pulmonary edema—case reports.

Pigmentation of the eye—case reports.

Kidney toxicity—rare.

▷ **Possible Effects on Sexual Function:** May ease painful and abnormally prolonged erections (priapism).

Possible Effects on Laboratory Tests

Complete blood counts: red cells and white cells increased; eosinophils decreased.

Blood glucose level: increased.

Urine sugar tests: false low or negative results with Clinistix; true positive with Benedict's or Fehling's solution.

Acidosis.

Blood platelets: temporarily increased.

CAUTION

1. Medication failure can result from frequent repeat use at short intervals. If this develops, avoid use for 12 hours, and a normal response should return.
2. Excessive use of aerosol preparations in asthmatics has been associated with sudden death.
3. May cause significant irritability of nerve pathways (conduction system) and heart muscle, predisposing to serious heart rhythm disorders. Talk with your doctor about this.
4. This drug can increase blood sugar level. If you have diabetes, test for sugar often to detect significant changes.
5. If this drug no longer works for you and you substitute isoproterenol (Isuprel), allow 4 hours between drugs.
6. Promptly throw this drug away if a pinkish-red to brown coloration or cloudiness (precipitation) occurs.

Precautions for Use

By Infants and Children: Use cautiously in small doses until tolerance is determined. Watch for weakness, light-headedness or fainting.

By Those Over 60 Years of Age: Small doses are prudent. Watch for nervousness, headache, tremor, rapid heart rate. If you have hardening of the arteries (arteriosclerosis), heart disease, high blood pressure, Parkinson's disease or prostatism (see Glossary), this drug may aggravate your disorder. Ask your doctor for help.

▷ **Advisability of Use During Pregnancy**

Pregnancy Category: C. See Pregnancy Risk Categories at the back of this book.

Animal studies: Birth defects reported in rats.

Human studies: Adequate studies of pregnant women are not available.

This drug can cause significant reduction of oxygen supply to the fetus. Use it only if clearly needed and in small, infrequent doses. Avoid during the first 3 months and during labor and delivery.

Advisability of Use If Breast-Feeding

Presence of this drug in breast milk: Yes.

Avoid drug or refrain from nursing.

Habit-Forming Potential: Tolerance to this drug (see Glossary) can develop with frequent use, but dependence does not occur.

Effects of Overdose: Nervousness, throbbing headache, dizziness, tremor, palpitation, disturbance of heart rhythm, difficult breathing, abdominal pain, vomiting of blood.

Possible Effects of Long-Term Use: "Epinephrine fastness": loss of ability to respond to this drug's bronchodilator effect. With long-term treatment of glaucoma: pigment deposits on eyeballs and eyelids, possible damage to retina, impaired vision, blockage of tear ducts.

Suggested Periodic Examinations While Taking This Drug (at physician's discretion)

Blood pressure measurements.

Blood or urine sugar measurements in diabetics.

Vision testing and measurement of internal eye pressure in glaucoma.

▷ **While Taking This Drug, Observe the Following**

Foods: No restrictions, except those that cause you to have an asthma attack.

Herbal Medicines or Minerals: Using St. John's wort, ma huang, guarana, paullinia, ephedrine-like compounds or kola while taking this medicine may result in unacceptable central nervous system stimulation. Fir or pine needle oil should NOT be used by asthmatics. Ephedra alone does carry a German Commission E monograph indication for asthma treatment, but combining it with this medicine would be like using two medicines from the same family and does not make sense. If you are allergic to plants in the Asteraceae family (aster, chrysanthemum, daisy or ragweed), you may also be allergic to echinacea, chamomile, feverfew and St. John's wort. Talk to your doctor BEFORE combining any herbal medicines with epinephrine

Beverages: No restrictions.

▷ *Alcohol:* Alcoholic beverages can increase the urinary excretion of this drug.

Tobacco Smoking: No interactions expected. I advise everyone to quit smoking.

▷ *Other Drugs*

Epinephrine *taken concurrently* with

- some beta-blockers (carvedilol, carteolol, nadolol, propranolol) may cause increased blood pressure response to epinephrine and decreased heart rate and resistance to epinephrine if it is used in anaphylaxis.
- chlorpromazine (Thorazine) or other phenothiazines (see Drug Classes) may cause decreased blood pressure and increased heart rate.
- dihydroergotamine (D.H.E.) may cause extreme increases in blood pressure.
- furazolidone (Furoxone) may cause increased blood pressure.
- guanethidine (Esimil, Ismelin) may cause increased blood pressure.
- halothane may cause abnormal heartbeats.
- monoamine oxidase (MAO) inhibitors (see Drug Classes) may lead to large and undesirable increases in blood pressure.
- pilocarpine (Ocusert) may cause increased myopia.
- tricyclic antidepressants (amitriptyline, etc.) may cause increased blood pressure and heart rhythm disturbances.
- zotepine (Nipolept) may lead to low blood pressure and reversal of epinephrine benefits.

▷ *Driving, Hazardous Activities:* This drug may cause dizziness or nervousness. Limit activities as necessary.

Aviation Note: The use of this drug *may be a disqualification* for piloting. Consult a designated Aviation Medical Examiner.

Exposure to Sun: No restrictions.

Heavy Exercise or Exertion: No interactions expected, but exercise can induce asthma in sensitive individuals.

Occurrence of Unrelated Illness: Use caution in severe burns. This drug can increase drainage from burned tissue and cause serious loss of tissue fluids and blood proteins.

Special Storage Instructions: Protect drug from exposure to air, light and heat. Keep in a cool place, preferably in the refrigerator.

Discontinuation: If this drug fails after an adequate trial, stop using it and call your doctor. It is dangerous to increase the dose or frequency.

ERGOTAMINE (er GOT a meen)

Introduced: 1926   **Class:** Antimigraine, ergot derivative   **Prescription:** USA: Yes   **Controlled Drug:**   USA: No; Canada: No   **Available as Generic:** Yes

Brand Names: Bellamine [CD], Bellaspas [CD], ✤Bellergal [CD], Bellergal-S [CD], ✤Bellergal Spacetabs [CD], Cafergot [CD], Cafergot P-B [CD], Cafetrate [CD], Drummergal [CD], Duragal-S [CD], Ercaf [CD], Ergobel [CD], Ergocaf [CD], ✤Ergodryl [CD], Ergomar, Ergostat, Genergen, ✤Gravergol [CD], ✤Gynergen, Medihaler Ergotamine, ✤Megral [CD], Oxoid, Phenerbrel-S [CD], Spastrin [CD], Wigraine [CD], ✤ Wigraine [CD], Wigrettes

BENEFITS versus RISKS	
Possible Benefits	*Possible Risks*
PREVENTION AND RELIEF OF VASCULAR HEADACHES: MIGRAINE, MIGRAINELIKE AND HISTAMINE HEADACHES	GANGRENE OF THE FINGERS, TOES OR INTESTINE AGGRAVATION OF CORONARY ARTERY DISEASE (ANGINA) INCREASED RISK OF ABORTION (if used during pregnancy)

▷ **Principal Uses**

As a Single Drug Product: Uses currently included in FDA-approved labeling: Treats vascular headaches, especially migraine and "cluster" headaches. Often effective in stopping headache if taken in the first hour following start of pain. Short-term basis use is a valid attempt to prevent or abort "cluster" headaches. The inhalation form provides rapid onset of action.

Other (unlabeled) generally accepted uses: None at present.

As a Combination Drug Product [CD]: Combined with caffeine to enhance its absorption. This makes a smaller dose of ergotamine effective and reduces risk of adverse effects with repeated use. This drug is also combined with belladonna (atropine) and barbiturates to help premenstrual tension and the menopausal syndrome—nervousness, nausea, hot flushes and sweating.

How This Drug Works: It constricts blood vessel walls in the head, preventing or relieving dilation that causes pain of migrainelike headaches.

Available Dosage Forms and Strengths

Aerosol — 9 mg/ml (0.36 mg/inhalation)

Nasal inhaler (Canada) — 9 mg/ml (360 mcg/dose)

Suppositories — 2 mg (in combination with 100 mg of caffeine)
Tablets, sublingual — 2 mg

▷ **Usual Adult Dosage Ranges:** *Inhalation:* One spray (0.36 mg) when headache starts; repeat 1 spray after 30 to 60 minutes as needed for relief, up to a maximum of 6 sprays every 24 hours. Do not exceed 15 sprays per week. *Sublingual tablets:* Dissolve 2 mg under tongue at the start of headache; repeat 2 mg in 30 to 60 minutes as needed, up to a maximum of 6 mg per attack. Do not exceed 6 mg every 24 hours or 10 mg/week. **Note: Actual dose and schedule must be determined for each patient individually.**

Conditions Requiring Dosing Adjustments
Liver Function: Should be used with caution by patients with liver compromise.
Kidney Function: This drug is a rare cause of acute renal failure and should be used with caution by patients with compromised kidneys.

▷ **Dosing Instructions:** Follow written instructions and doses **carefully.** The regular tablets (combination drug) may be crushed; sustained-release tablets should be taken whole (not crushed). Sublingual tablets should be dissolved under the tongue, not swallowed. If you forget a dose: Call your doctor as this medicine gets the best results if you take it at the first sign of migraine.

Usual Duration of Use: Regular use for several headache episodes often needed to see effectiveness in aborting or relieving vascular headache. Do not exceed recommended schedules. If headaches are not controlled after several trials of maximal doses, ask your doctor about other treatments. There are also a variety of medicines to prevent (prophylactic use) migraines.

Typical Treatment Goals and Measurements (Outcomes and Markers)
Pain: Most clinicians treating pain use a device called an algometer to check your pain. This looks like a small ruler, but lets the clinician better understand your pain. The goals of treatment then relate to where the level of pain started (for example, a rating of 7 on a zero to ten scale) and what the cause of the pain was. Pain medicines may also be used together (in combination) in order to get the best result or outcome. Specific results to migraine relate to stopping (aborting) an attack or easing the severity of an attack. Once again, the role of prophylactic medicines is clear in helping some patients avoid attacks altogether.

▷ **This Drug Should Not Be Taken If**
- you have had an allergic reaction to any dose form.
- you are pregnant or are breast-feeding your child.
- you have a severe infection (sepsis).
- you have any of the following conditions:
  angina pectoris (coronary artery disease)
  Buerger's disease
  hardening of the arteries (arteriosclerosis)
  high blood pressure (severe hypertension)
  ischemic heart disease or angina
  peptic ulcer
  malnutrition
  kidney disease or impaired kidney function
  liver disease or impaired liver function
  Raynaud's phenomenon

thrombophlebitis
glaucoma

▷ **Inform Your Physician Before Taking This Drug If**
- you are allergic or overly sensitive to any ergot preparation.
- you have a prolonged aura and migraines (aura may be further prolonged).
- you are planning to have a face-lift (rhytidectomy) or other plastic surgery. This drug may cause serious skin flap problems.

Possible Side Effects (natural, expected and unavoidable drug actions)
Usually infrequent and mild with recommended doses.
Some people may have cold hands and feet, with mild numbness and tingling.

▷ **Possible Adverse Effects** (unusual, unexpected and infrequent reactions)
If any of the following develop, consult your physician promptly for guidance.
Mild Adverse Effects
Allergic reactions: localized swellings (angioedema), itching—case reports.
Headache, drowsiness, dizziness, confusion—possible.
Chest pain, abdominal pain, numbness and tingling of fingers and toes, muscle pains in arms or legs—infrequent.
Nausea, vomiting, diarrhea—possible.
Serious Adverse Effects
Gangrene of the extremities: coldness; numbness; pain; dark discoloration; eventual loss of fingers, toes or feet—possible.
Gangrene of the intestine: severe abdominal pain and swelling; emergency surgery required—case reports.
Retroperitoneal fibrosis—case reports.
Fibrous changes in the lung (pleuropulmonary fibrosis)—case reports.
Pain syndromes (reflex sympathetic dystrophy)—possible.
Insufficient blood flow to the heart (myocardial ischemia) or arrhythmias—case reports.
Fibrous changes in the heart (myocardial fibrosis) or porphyria—case reports.
Lesions of the rectum or anus (anorectal lesions)—case reports.
Kidney failure—case reports.

▷ **Possible Effects on Sexual Function:** None reported.

Natural Diseases or Disorders That May Be Activated by This Drug
Angina pectoris (coronary artery insufficiency), Buerger's disease, Raynaud's phenomenon.

Possible Effects on Laboratory Tests: None reported.

CAUTION
1. Excessive use of this drug can actually provoke migraines and increase their frequency.
2. Do not exceed a total dose of 6 mg daily or 10 mg/week of the oral form.
3. Individual drug sensitivity varies greatly. Some may have early toxic effects while taking recommended doses. Promptly report numbness in fingers or toes, muscle cramping or chest pain.

Precautions for Use
By Infants and Children: Safety and effectiveness for those under 12 years of age are not established.

By Those Over 60 Years of Age: Natural circulation changes may make you more susceptible to adverse effects of this drug. See the preceding list of disorders that are contraindications for the use of this drug.

▷ **Advisability of Use During Pregnancy**

Pregnancy Category: X. See Pregnancy Risk Categories at the back of this book.

Animal studies: Fetal deaths reported due to this drug.

Human studies: Information from studies of pregnant women indicates that this drug can cause abortion.

This drug should be avoided during the entire pregnancy.

Advisability of Use If Breast-Feeding

Presence of this drug in breast milk: Yes.

Avoid drug or refrain from nursing. May also suppress prolactin secretion.

Habit-Forming Potential: None.

Effects of Overdose: "Ergotism": cold skin, severe muscle pain, tingling or burning pain in hands and feet, loss of blood supply to extremities resulting in tissue death (gangrene) in fingers and toes. Acute ergot poisoning: nausea, vomiting, diarrhea, cold skin, numbness of extremities, confusion, seizures, coma.

Possible Effects of Long-Term Use: A form of functional dependence (see Glossary) may develop, resulting in withdrawal headaches if the drug is stopped.

Suggested Periodic Examinations While Taking This Drug (at physician's discretion)

Evaluation of circulation (blood flow) to the extremities.

Observation for emergence of tolerance.

▷ **While Taking This Drug, Observe the Following**

Foods: No interactions expected. Avoid all foods to which you are allergic; some migraine headaches are due to food allergies. There are also often "trigger" foods. Keep a diary and try to identify, then avoid these.

Herbal Medicines or Minerals: Using ma huang or ephedrine-like compounds (ephedra) may result in additive and undesirable vasoconstriction. If you are allergic to plants in the Asteraceae family (aster, chrysanthemum, daisy or ragweed), you may also be allergic to echinacea, chamomile, feverfew and St. John's wort. St. John's wort can cause changes in the liver enzymes that help remove this medicine—talk to your doctor before combining any herbal medicine or mineral with ergotamine.

Beverages: No restrictions.

▷ *Alcohol:* Best avoided; alcohol can intensify vascular headache.

Tobacco Smoking: Best avoided; nicotine can further reduce the restricted blood flow produced by this drug.

Marijuana Smoking: Best avoided; additive effects can increase the coldness of hands and feet.

▷ *Other Drugs*

Ergotamine may **decrease** the effects of

• nitroglycerin and reduce its effectiveness in preventing or relieving angina pain.

The following drugs may **increase** the effects of ergotamine:

• amprenavir (Agenerase), indinavir (Crixivan) and ritonavir (Norvir) are removed by the same enzymes that remove ergotamine. Ritonavir actually has had reports of sudden (acute) ergotism. These combinations are to be avoided.

- beta-blockers (see Drug Classes).
- delavirdine (Rescriptor).
- dopamine (Intropin).
- erythromycins: clarithromycin (Biaxin), dirithromycin (Dynabac) or E-Mycin, ERYC, etc. Azithromycin (Zithromax) has not been reported to cause this effect.
- medicines that inhibit cytochrome P450 3A4 will lead to increased ergotamine levels, increasing toxicity risk, and those that induce P450 3A4 will blunt therapeutic effects.
- saquinavir (Fortovase).
- troleandomycin (TAO).

Ergotamine *taken concurrently* with

- triptans (naratriptan [Amerge], rizatriptan [Maxalt], sumatriptan [Imitrex] or zolmitriptan [Zomig]) may lead to prolonged vasospastic reaction. One day should pass between an ergotamine dose and triptan use.

▷ *Driving, Hazardous Activities:* This drug may cause drowsiness or dizziness. Restrict activities as necessary.

Aviation Note: Vascular headache *is a disqualification* for piloting. Consult a designated Aviation Medical Examiner.

Exposure to Sun: No restrictions.

Exposure to Cold: Avoid as much as possible. Cold further reduces restricted blood flow to the extremities.

Discontinuation: Following long-term use, it may be necessary to withdraw this drug gradually to prevent withdrawal headache. Ask your doctor for help.

ERYTHROMYCIN (er ith roh MY sin)

Please see the macrolide antibiotic family profile.

ESTROGENS (ES troh jenz)

Other Names: Chlorotrianisene, conjugated estrogens, esterified estrogens, estradiol, estriol, estrone, estropipate, quinestrol

Introduced: 1933   **Class:** Female sex hormones   **Prescription:** USA: Yes   **Controlled Drug:** USA: No; Canada: No   **Available as Generic:** USA: Yes; Canada: No

Brand Names: ✤C.E.S., Climara, ✤Climestrone, ✤Congest, Delestrogen, DV, Estinyl, Estrace, Estraderm, Estraguard, Estratab, Estrovis, Feminone, ✤Femogen, ✤Femogex, Gynetone, Gynogen LA, Menest, Menotab, Menotab-M, Menrium [CD], Milprem [CD], ✤Minestrin, ✤Neo-Pause, ✤Oestrilin, Ogen, PMB [CD], PMS-Estradiol, Premarin, Premphase [CD], Prempro [CD], (a lower dose Prempro is being studied at the time of this writing), Progynon Pellet, TACE, Valergen-10, Vivelle (transdermal), White Premarin

Author's Note: Controversy has erupted regarding estrogen replacement therapy (ERT) and hormone replacement therapy (HRT) based on results from the HERS (Heart and Estrogen/progestin Replacement Study). This trial brought into controversy the issue of benefits versus no effect versus an increased risk of problems of estrogen/progestin combination in patients where preventing a second heart attack (secondary prevention) was the goal. Controversy also resulted from higher use of statins (HMG-CoA reductase inhibitors—see Drug Classes) in the control group and high use of beta blockers and aspirin in both study and control groups. Additional ongoing studies include the Women's Health Initiative (WHI) and WISDOM. Newer data from the 2-year Women's Health, Osteoporosis, Progestin, Estrogen study (HOPE) points to the use of 1.5 mg of progestin with 0.45 or 0.3 mg of estrogen being equal in benefits to higher doses. An important new direction in research may be use of lower doses of estrogens combined with lower doses of progestins to define cardiovascular, bone health and other benefits while avoiding or lowering risks of problems. Further research is needed to define optimal doses, duration and patients who will best benefit from ERT or HRT.

BENEFITS versus RISKS	
Possible Benefits	*Possible Risks*
COMBINATION WITH SIMVASTATIN MAY REDUCE UNDESIRABLE CLOTTING FACTORS AND INFLAMMATION	INCREASED RISK OF CANCER OF THE UTERUS
RELIEF OF MENOPAUSAL HOT FLASHES AND NIGHT SWEATS	SMALL INCREASED RISK OF BREAST CANCER
PREVENTION OR RELIEF OF ATROPHIC VAGINITIS, ATROPHY OF THE VULVA AND URETHRA	Increased frequency of gallstones
PREVENTION OF POSTMENOPAUSAL HEART DISEASE (SECONDARY PREVENTION IS CONTROVERSIAL)	Accelerated growth of preexisting fibroid tumors of the uterus
PREVENTION OF POST-MENOPAUSAL OSTEOPOROSIS	Fluid retention
PATCH FORM MAY GIVE UP TO A WEEK OF ESTROGEN REPLACEMENT	Postmenopausal bleeding
EARLY DATA APPEAR TO SHOW A BENEFIT IN PREVENTING ALZHEIMER'S	Deep vein thrombophlebitis and thromboembolism (less likely with conjugated estrogens and new lower doses; more likely with synthetic unconjugated hormones)
Prevention of thinning of the skin	Increased blood pressure
Mental tonic effect	Decreased sugar tolerance
May help improve memory	
Possible lessening of the severity of age-related increases in blood pressure in some patients (further research needed)	

▷ **Principal Uses**

As a Single Drug Product: Uses currently included in FDA-approved labeling: "replacement" therapy in (1) ovarian failure or removal; (2) the menopausal syndrome; (3) postmenopausal atrophy of genital tissues; (4) postmenopausal osteoporosis; (5) selected cases of breast cancer and prostate cancer; (6) treats difficulty having sexual intercourse (dyspareunia) caused by vaginal secretion drying.

Other (unlabeled) generally accepted uses: (1) Used in combination with simvastatin (Zocor) (in one study of women averaging 57 years old) lowered LDL, increased HDL, reduced undesirable blood clotting factors and inflammation; (2) a study of 46 women (at Yale) after menopause found that estrogen increased activity in the brain in a region associated with memory; (3) may have a role in some selected cases of infertility from days 5 to 15 of a cycle to augment mucus quality (coordinated with basal body temperature).

As a Combination Drug Product [CD]: Estrogen is available in combination with chlordiazepoxide (Librium) and with meprobamate (Equanil, Miltown). These drugs provide a calming effect and ease symptoms in selected cases of menopause. See oral contraceptives profile for a discussion of estrogens and progestins.

How This Drug Works: When used to correct hormonal deficiency states, estrogens restore normal cellular activity by increasing nuclear material and protein synthesis. Frequency and intensity of menopausal symptoms are reduced when normal levels of estrogen are restored. Blood vessel effects appear to work through both nongenetic and genetic ways. Estrogen may modify inflammation that encourages buildup of plaque on vessels (atherosclerosis), relaxes the heart muscle and increases sensitivity to insulin. The precise mechanism of estrogen in protecting brain cells (neurons) from oxidative stress or amyloid protein is unknown, but the end result appears to be some protection from development of Alzheimer's disease.

Available Dosage Forms and Strengths

Capsules — 12 mg, 25 mg
Capsules (TACE) — 72 mg
Tablets — 0.02 mg, 0.05 mg, 0.1 mg, 0.3 mg,
— 0.5 mg, 0.625 mg, 0.9 mg, 1.25 mg, 2.5 mg
Transdermal patch — 0.025 mg (2 mg), 0.05 mg (4 mg),
— 0.1 mg (8 mg)
Transdermal patch — 10, 20, and 30 mg (Canada only)
Vaginal cream — 0.1, 0.625, and 1.5 mg/g

▷ **Usual Adult Dosage Ranges:** *For conjugated and esterified estrogens:* lowest doses that will control moderate to severe vasomotor symptoms that happen in menopause should be used: Starting doses of 0.625 mg with increases up to 1.25 mg daily are used. Cenestin product notes attempts to lower doses or taper the medicine should be made at 3–6 month intervals. Premarin product notes use of 1.25 mg daily for treatment of moderate to severe vasomotor symptoms. Dosing is undertaken for 21 days with 1 week off. Addition of a progestin for the last 10–13 days of the cycle is recommended to lower the occurrence of effects (endometrial hyperplasia or carcinoma) caused by estrogen alone (unopposed). Some studies suggested that combined estrogen and progestin use actually increases breast cancer risk. For other forms of estrogen: Ask your doctor. Patch form such as Climara may give a week of estrogen replacement in a small patch. **Note: Actual dose and schedule must be determined for each patient individually.**

Conditions Requiring Dosing Adjustments

Liver Function: The dose should be decreased in mild liver disease. Estrogens should not be used in acute or severe liver compromise. This drug can be lithogenic (capable of causing stones) in bile.

Kidney Function: No expected dosing changes in kidney compromise.

▷ **Dosing Instructions:** The tablets may be crushed and taken without regard to food. The capsules should be taken whole. If you forget a dose: take the dose you forgot as soon as you remember it, unless it is nearly time for your next dose—if that is the case, simply skip the missed dose and take the next dose right on schedule. DO NOT double doses. Talk to your doctor if you find yourself forgetting doses.

Usual Duration of Use: Regular use for 10 to 20 days needed to see effectiveness in easing menopausal symptoms. Long-term use requires periodic evaluation by your doctor (individualized) to see if the benefits of this medicine are being realized (depending on the use) and if it is still needed.

Typical Treatment Goals and Measurements (Outcomes and Markers)

Menopause: Most clinicians treating menopause seek goals of reduction or cessation of hot flashes, greater sense of well-being and avoidance of rapid bone loss (which can also be measured by some lab tests and DEXA testing). Longer term use of estrogen is associated with increased risk of breast cancer, so trends may be toward shorter term therapy than in the past.

▷ **This Drug Should Not Be Taken If**
- you have had an allergic reaction to it previously.
- you have a history of thrombophlebitis, embolism, heart attack or stroke.
- you have seriously impaired liver function or recent onset of liver disease.
- you have abnormal and unexplained vaginal bleeding.
- you are pregnant.
- you have sickle cell disease.
- you have or are suspected to have breast cancer (may be used to treat some kinds of breast cancer).
- you have known or suspected estrogen-dependent cancer (your doctor will determine this)—except in selected patients being treated for cancer.

▷ **Inform Your Physician Before Taking This Drug If**
- you have had an unfavorable reaction to estrogen therapy previously.
- you have a history of breast or reproductive organ cancer.
- you have fibrocystic breast changes, fibroid tumors of the uterus, endometriosis, migraine headaches, epilepsy, asthma, heart disease, high blood pressure, gallbladder disease, diabetes or porphyria.
- you retain fluid.
- you have elevated calcium and kidney disease.
- you smoke tobacco on a regular basis.
- you have a history of blood-clotting disorders.
- you plan to have surgery in the near future.

Possible Side Effects (natural, expected and unavoidable drug actions)

Fluid retention, weight gain, "breakthrough" bleeding (spotting in middle of menstrual cycle), altered menstrual pattern, resumption of menstrual flow ("periods") after natural cessation (postmenopausal bleeding), increased yeast infection susceptibility of the genitals.

▷ **Possible Adverse Effects** (unusual, unexpected and infrequent reactions)
If any of the following develop, consult your physician promptly for guidance.

Mild Adverse Effects

Allergic reactions: skin rash, hives, itching—rare.

Headache, nervous tension, irritability, depression, accentuation of migraine headaches—infrequent.

Nausea, vomiting, bloating, diarrhea—infrequent to frequent.

Tannish pigmentation of the face—possible.

Serious Adverse Effects

Allergic reactions: anaphylaxis—case reports.

Idiosyncratic reaction: cutaneous porphyria—fragility and scarring of the skin.

Can produce or worsen high blood pressure—more likely with higher doses.

Gallbladder disease, benign liver tumors, jaundice, rise in blood sugar—case reports.

Erosion of uterine cervix, enlargement of uterine fibroid tumors—possible.

Thrombophlebitis (inflammation of a vein with formation of blood clot): pain or tenderness in thigh or leg, with or without swelling of foot or leg—low dose has minimal increased risk; higher doses may carry more risk.

Pulmonary embolism (movement of blood clot to lung): sudden shortness of breath, pain in chest, coughing, bloody sputum—case reports.

Benign liver tumors (adenomas)—possible.

Systemic lupus erythematosus or porphyria—rare.

Stroke (blood clot in brain): headaches, blackout, sudden weakness or paralysis of any part of the body, severe dizziness, altered vision, slurred speech, inability to speak—case reports.

Endometrial cancer (how long increased risk continues if the drug is stopped is not clear).

Retinal thrombosis (blood clot in eye vessels): sudden impairment or loss of vision—case reports.

Heart attack (blood clot in coronary artery)—sudden pain in chest, neck, jaw or arm; weakness; sweating; nausea. Has been associated with women taking higher doses and with men using estrogen to treat prostate cancer; however, this is not clearly decided as yet. Lower progestin doses appears to provide benefits of avoiding unopposed estrogen while also avoiding some increased propensity for abnormal clots. Estrogen in lower doses appears to decrease overall risk of heart attack.

Breast cancer—increased risk possible although only a slight increase in risk. A study that followed 46,355 women after menopause found that use of estrogen with or without a progestin was associated with a slightly increased breast cancer risk. Risk appeared to increase by combination with a progestin (in contrast to earlier findings) and increased with the length of time the estrogen was taken.

▷ **Possible Effects on Sexual Function:** Swelling and tenderness of breasts, milk production.

Increased vaginal secretions.

Possible Delayed Adverse Effects: Estrogens taken during pregnancy may predispose a female child to the later development of cancer of the vagina or cervix following puberty.

▷ **Adverse Effects That May Mimic Natural Diseases or Disorders**

Liver reactions may suggest viral hepatitis.

Natural Diseases or Disorders That May Be Activated by This Drug

Latent hypertension, diabetes mellitus, acute intermittent porphyria.

Possible Effects on Laboratory Tests

Red blood cells, hemoglobin and platelets: decreased.

Blood calcium level: increased.

Blood total cholesterol level: decreased (treatment effect); increased in postmenopausal women.

Blood LDL cholesterol level: decreased in postmenopausal women.

Blood triglyceride level: no drug effect in postmenopausal women.

Blood glucose level: increased.

Glucose tolerance test (GTT): decreased.

Blood thyroid hormone (T3 and T4) levels: increased.

Blood uric acid level: decreased.

Liver function tests: increased liver enzymes (ALT/GPT, AST/GOT and alkaline phosphatase), increased bilirubin.

CAUTION

1. To avoid prolonged (uninterrupted) stimulation of breast and uterine tissues, estrogen should be taken in cycles of 3 weeks on and 1 week off of medication.
2. The estrogen in estrogen vaginal creams is absorbed systemically. It may also be absorbed through the penis during sexual intercourse and can cause enlargement and tenderness of male breast tissue.
3. Some patients may benefit from lower or may require higher than usual doses to prevent osteoporosis. Bone mineral density tests (DEXA or PDEXA) are prudent to see whether a selected dose is working.
4. Recent data found that estrogen replacement therapy was associated with a small increase in breast cancer risk. Another study found that combining estrogen with progestin increased risk of breast cancer. Risk was also found to increase the longer hormone replacement therapy (HRT) is taken. This area is now controversial, and is a benefit-to-risk decision. From recent studies, it appeared that taking HRT for 2 to 3 years for menopausal symptoms wasn't likely to increase breast cancer risk.

Precautions for Use

By Those Over 60 Years of Age: Thinking has changed on use of estrogen in older populations and benefits have been shown in the eighth decade of life. In this age group, it is advisable to attempt relief of hot flashes with nonestrogenic medicines, yet benefits have been shown in osteoporosis. During use, report promptly any indications of impaired circulation: speech disturbances, altered vision, sudden hearing loss, vertigo, sudden weakness or paralysis, angina, leg pains.

▷ **Advisability of Use During Pregnancy**

Pregnancy Category: X. See Pregnancy Risk Categories at the back of this book.

Animal studies: Genital defects reported in mice and guinea pigs; cleft palate reported in rodents.

Human studies: Information from studies of pregnant women indicates that estrogens can masculinize the female fetus. In addition, limb defects and heart malformations have been reported.

It is now known that estrogens taken during pregnancy can predispose the female child to the development of cancer of the vagina or cervix following puberty. **Avoid estrogens completely during entire pregnancy.**

Advisability of Use If Breast-Feeding

Presence of this drug in breast milk: Yes, in minute amounts.

Estrogens in large doses can suppress milk formation. Breast-feeding is considered to be safe during the use of estrogens.

Malnourished mothers may have unacceptable decreases in protein and nitrogen in their breast milk if this drug is used while breast-feeding.

Habit-Forming Potential: There has been some suggestion of estrogens having potential for psychological dependence and tolerance because of their mood-elevating properties, but clinical reports have not been presented.

Effects of Overdose: Headache, drowsiness, nausea, vomiting, fluid retention, abnormal vaginal bleeding, breast enlargement and discomfort.

Possible Effects of Long-Term Use: High blood pressure, gallbladder disease with gallstone formation, increased growth of benign fibroid tumors of the uterus. Several reports suggest possible association between the long-term use (3+ years) of estrogens and the development of cancer of the lining of the uterus as well an increasing breast cancer risk. Further studies are needed to establish a definite cause-and-effect relationship (see Glossary). Prudence dictates that women with intact uteri should use estrogens only when symptoms justify it and with proper supervision.

Suggested Periodic Examinations While Taking This Drug (at physician's discretion)

Regular (every 6 months) evaluation of the breasts and pelvic organs, including Pap smears.

Liver function tests as indicated.

▷ **While Taking This Drug, Observe the Following**

Foods: Avoid excessive use of salt if fluid retention occurs.

Herbal Medicines or Minerals: Black cohosh appears to work by: (1) suppressing luteinizing hormone; (2) binding to estrogen receptors in the pituitary; and (3) inhibiting luteinizing hormone release. The net effect is that this herb eases symptoms of menopause, but little is known about long-term use or heart and bone protective effects. This herb may interfere with the benefits of estrogen replacement therapy. Talk to your doctor before starting black cohosh if you are currently taking estrogen. Other herbal or integrative approaches to women's health are always best discussed with your doctor to develop an evidence-based approach to overall therapy and avoid possible undesirable additive or side effects.

Use of St. John's wort, echinacea or ginkgo completely blocked or lowered the ability of sperm to penetrate eggs in one study. DO NOT use these herbs if you are using a conjugated estrogen product to augment mucus quality and help infertility. Combined use of calcium and vitamin D can be a further step to help avoid osteoporosis. Talk to your doctor BEFORE adding any herbal medicines.

Beverages: No restrictions. May be taken with milk.

▷   *Alcohol:* No interactions expected.

Tobacco Smoking: Some studies show that heavy smoking (15 or more cigarettes daily) in association with use of estrogen-containing oral contraceptives significantly increases risk of heart attack (coronary thrombosis). I
advise everyone to stop smoking.

▷   *Other Drugs*

Estrogens *taken concurrently* with

* alendronate (Fosamax) have not been well studied. One small clinical
study suggested the combination was beneficial in preventing postmenopausal osteoporosis. The combination of alendronate and hormone
replacement therapy (HRT) is now approved in Canada because of excellent combination results.
* oral antidiabetic drugs (see Drug Classes) or oral blood-sugar-lowering
medicines may cause loss of glucose control and high blood sugars.
* progestins (various) may increase risk of breast cancer versus estrogen use
by itself.
* thyroid hormones may increase the bound (inactive) drug and require an
increase in thyroid dose.
* tricyclic antidepressants (Elavil, Sinequan, etc.) may enhance their adverse
effects and reduce their antidepressant effectiveness.
* vitamin C (ascorbic acid, various brands) in higher doses may result in
increased estrogen effects. A lower dose of estrogens may be indicated if
higher-dose vitamin C will be taken on an ongoing basis.
* warfarin (Coumadin) may cause alterations of prothrombin activity.
Increased doses may be needed.

The following drugs may *decrease* the effects of estrogens:

* carbamazepine (Tegretol).
* phenobarbital (Belladenal, others).
* phenytoin (Dilantin), fosphenytoin (Cerebyx).
* primidone (Mysoline).
* rifampin (Rifadin, Rimactane).

▷   *Driving, Hazardous Activities:* Usually no restrictions. Consult your physician
for assessment of individual risk and for guidance regarding specific
restrictions.

Aviation Note: Usually no restrictions, but watch for the rare occurrence of disturbed vision and restrict activities accordingly. Consult a designated Aviation Medical Examiner.

Exposure to Sun: Caution—may cause photosensitivity (see Glossary).

Discontinuation: Best to stop estrogens periodically (every 3 to 6 months) to
see if they are still needed. The dose is reduced gradually to prevent acute
withdrawal hot flashes. Avoid continual, uninterrupted use of large doses.
Stop altogether when a definite need for replacement therapy has ended.
Ask your doctor for help.

ETANERCEPT (ee TAN err sept)

Other Names: TNFR:Fc (Tumor necrosis factor receptor p75 Fc fusion protein)
Introduced: 1998   **Class:**   Disease-modifying antirheumatic drug (DMARD),

biologic response modifier   **Prescription:** USA:Yes   **Controlled Drug:**
USA: No; Canada: No   **Available as Generic:** No
Brand Name: Enbrel

<table>
<tr><td colspan="2" align="center">**BENEFITS versus RISKS**</td></tr>
<tr><td align="center">*Possible Benefits*</td><td align="center">*Possible Risks*</td></tr>
<tr><td>USEFUL IN RHEUMATOID
  ARTHRITIS
HAS A ROLE IN MANY CASES OF
  JUVENILE RHEUMATOID
  ARTHRITIS
CAN BE USED IN COMBINATION
  WITH METHOTREXATE
MAY GIVE A RESPONSE WHERE
  OTHER AGENTS HAVE FAILED
COULD HAVE A ROLE IN
  CONGESTIVE HEART FAILURE
  AND IN DECREASING RISK OF
  REPEAT HEART ATTACKS
CURRENTLY UNDER REVIEW AS
  THE FIRST PRODUCT TO BE
  CONSIDERED FOR PSORIATIC
  ARTHRITIS (either alone or in
  combination with methotrexate)</td><td align="top">INFECTIONS CAUSED BY
  IMMUNOSUPPRESSION FROM
  THE MEDICINE ITSELF
Injection site reactions
Possible development of antibodies</td></tr>
</table>

▷ **Principal Uses**

As a Single Drug Product: Uses currently included in FDA-approved labeling:
(1) Approved for INITIAL treatment of rheumatoid arthritis (RA) where previously it was used in treatment of moderate to severe rheumatoid arthritis (RA) in patients who have not responded to one or more disease-modifying antirheumatic drugs (DMARD); (2) approved for use in RA in children over 4 years old (juvenile rheumatoid arthritis).

Other (unlabeled) generally accepted uses: (1) May have a role in some kinds of wasting (cachexia) where tumor necrosis factor (TNF) is involved; (2) a small study of 18 patients showed that this drug improved the ability to walk as well as the ability of the heart to pump blood in patients with congestive heart failure (appears to be safe and efficacious); (3) data from the cholesterol and recurrent events (CARE) trial found that decreasing tumor necrosis factor (TNF) (see how this drug works, below) reduces risk of repeat heart attacks; (4) could have a role in ankylosing spondylitis; (5) currently under FDA review for approval to treat psoriatic arthritis (either alone or in combination with methotrexate).

How This Drug Works: Binds with tumor necrosis factor alpha (TNF-alpha) in the body, as well as to lymphotoxin alpha (TNF-beta), and stops their biologic actions. This drug also works to change the body's responses that are caused or regulated by TNF, such as increased levels of matrix metalloproteinase-3, serum levels of cytokines and release of substances that control white blood cell migration.

Available Dosage Forms and Strengths

Injection — 25 mg with a syringe containing 1 ml of bacteriostatic water.

▷ **Recommended Dosage Ranges** (Actual dose and schedule must be determined for each patient individually.)

Infants and Children: Not studied in children less than 4 years old. Children 4–17 years old who have moderate to severely active juvenile rheumatoid arthritis (JRA) and who did not respond to or tolerate methotrexate were given 0.4 mg/kg up to a maximum of 25 mg twice a week (subcutaneously). Twice-weekly dosing is best, given 72 to 96 hours apart.

Usual Adult Dosage Ranges: For rheumatoid arthritis (adults): 25 mg injected under the skin (subcutaneously), twice a week. (Remember to change or rotate where you inject.)

Author's Note: Demand for etanercept has been increasing and some shortages of product have occurred. A new production facility called BioNext is being developed to encompass cell culture manufacturing for etanercept. A medicine also used in rheumatoid arthritis (infliximab or Remicade) has added a black box (more stringent) warning about increased risk of infections in patients who use that medicine. The FDA will review both products in late August to decide if additional warnings are required for the products. No labeling changes were requested by the FDA for etanercept at the time of this writing.

Conditions Requiring Dosing Adjustments

Liver Function: No changes needed, as the drug is removed by the reticuloendothelial system.

Kidney Function: Dosing changes are not known to be needed in people with kidney problems.

▷ **Dosing Instructions:** It is very important that you understand how to inject this drug under the skin (subcutaneously) and NOT intravenously. Please ask your doctor or pharmacist if you do not understand the patient information on injecting. Please also remember to change (rotate) where you inject (the injection site). Talk to your doctor before injecting etanercept if you have an infection. If you forget a dose: Take the missed dose right away, unless it is nearly time for your next dose—if that is the case, skip the missed dose and take the next dose right on schedule. Call your doctor if you find yourself missing doses.

Usual Duration of Use: Use on a regular schedule determines benefit. In rheumatoid arthritis this drug usually goes to work in 1 to 4 weeks. Long-term use (months to years) requires physician supervision.

Arthritis: Control of arthritis symptoms (pain, loss of mobility, decreased ability to accomplish activities of daily living, range of motion, etc.) is paramount in returning patient quality of life and to checking the results (beneficial outcomes) from this medicine. Many arthritis management or pain centers use interdisciplinary teams (physicians from several specialties, nurses, physician's assistants, physical and occupational therapists, pharmacotherapists, psychotherapists, social workers and others) to get the best results. Specific mobility goals are often set by the physician and administered by a physical/occupational therapist. The arthritis foundation has additional information at www.arthritis.org.

Possible Advantages of This Drug Uses: A novel mechanism (against TNF) to fight arthritis as well as congestive heart failure. This may be a great advantage as the two conditions may often be found in the same person.

Works to prevent joint damage better than methotrexate and also eases symptoms faster than methotrexate. Convenient dosing schedule. A new enrollment program has been started and can be entered by patients by calling 1-888-4EN-BREL.

▷ **This Drug Should Not Be Taken If**
- you have had an allergic reaction to it previously.
- you currently have an active infection (including chronic or localized infections).
- you have an immune deficiency.

▷ **Inform Your Physician Before Taking This Drug If**
- you have poorly controlled diabetes or a suppression of the immune system or any other disease or condition that predisposes you to infections.
- you develop a new infection while taking this medicine.
- you have recently received a live virus vaccine.
- you have a history of malignancy.
- you are pregnant or planning pregnancy in the near future.
- you are breast-feeding your infant.
- you have an allergy to latex.
- you have impaired kidney function.
- you have a history of asthma or allergies to other medicines.

Possible Side Effects (natural, expected and unavoidable drug actions)
Report such developments to your physician promptly.
Discomfort at the injection site.

▷ **Possible Adverse Effects** (unusual, unexpected and infrequent reactions)
If any of the following develop, consult your physician promptly for guidance.
Mild Adverse Effects
Allergic reactions: skin rash at the injection site—possible.
Development of antinuclear antibodies—infrequent to frequent.
Cough—frequent.
Sinusitis—possible.
Upper respiratory infections—up to 29%.
Vomiting—may be frequent in some children.
Serious Adverse Effects
Allergic reactions: anaphylaxis—possible.
Central nervous system damage (demyelination)—case reports with unclear causality.
Suppression of the immune system/cells (pancytopenia/aplastic anemia)—possible.
Development of diabetes mellitus—case report.

▷ **Possible Effects on Sexual Function:** None reported.

Possible Delayed Adverse Effects: Possible development of antinuclear antibodies. Long-term effects on infections and malignancies is not fully understood.

Possible Effects on Laboratory Tests
Antinuclear antibodies (ANA): positive.

CAUTION
1. This drug must be monitored carefully by a qualified physician.
2. Make certain you understand how to inject this medicine under the skin.

3. Live-virus vaccines should be avoided during use of this drug. Live-virus vaccines could actually produce infection rather than stimulate an immune response.
4. Positive antinuclear antibodies (ANA) have been reported, but the clinical importance is not yet known.
5. The manufacturer advises against using this medicine if you have an active infection.
6. Patients should be followed closely if they develop an infection while taking etanercept, and treatment should be STOPPED in patients with serious infections or sepsis.

Precautions for Use
By Those Over 60 Years of Age: Specific changes are not indicated at present.

▷ **Advisability of Use During Pregnancy**
Pregnancy Category: B. See Pregnancy Risk Categories at the back of this book.
Human studies: Adequate studies are NOT available.
Talk to your doctor about benefits versus risks of use.

Advisability of Use If Breast-Feeding
Presence of this drug in breast milk: Unknown.
Avoid drug or refrain from nursing.

Habit-Forming Potential: None.

Effects of Overdose: One patient injected 62 mg twice a week for 3 weeks without any significant adverse effects.

Possible Effects of Long-Term Use: Positive antinuclear antibodies—significance not presently known. One case of diabetes mellitus.

Suggested Periodic Examinations While Taking This Drug (at physician's discretion)
Beneficial response to the medicine.
Sedimentation rate (ESR) and rheumatoid factor or C-reactive protein.
ANA and fasting glucose tests.
If used in congestive heart failure, tests of heart function and symptom-free walking time.

▷ **While Taking This Drug, Observe the Following**
Foods: No specific recommendations.
Herbal Medicines or Minerals: There is NO DATA on combined use of etanercept with glucosamine. There are also no data on use of etanercept with hay flower, mistletoe herb or white mustard seed. Echinacea may actually blunt the immune response if used on an ongoing basis, and therefore combination with etanercept is not advisable. Talk to your doctor before combining any herbal medicine with etanercept.
Beverages: No restrictions.
▷ *Alcohol:* No specific recommendations.
Tobacco Smoking: No interactions expected. I advise everyone to quit smoking.
Marijuana Smoking: May cause impairment of immunity.
▷ *Other Drugs*
Etanercept *taken concurrently* with
• medicines that blunt the immune system may lead to additive immune system depression if combined with etanercept.
• yellow fever, pneumococcal, smallpox or any other live vaccine may result

in decreased immune response to the vaccine as well as possible transmission of the infection BY the vaccine.

▷ *Driving, Hazardous Activities:* No restrictions.

Aviation Note: The use of this drug is ***probably not a disqualification*** for piloting, but the condition being treated may be. Consult a designated Aviation Medical Examiner.

Exposure to Sun: No restrictions.

ETHAMBUTOL (eth AM byu tohl)

Introduced: 1971 Class: Anti-infective, antituberculosis drug   **Prescription:** USA: Yes   **Controlled Drug:** USA: No; Canada: No   **Available as Generic:** USA: No; Canada: No

Brand Names: ✦Etibi, Myambutol

BENEFITS versus RISKS

Possible Benefits	*Possible Risks*
EFFECTIVE ADJUNCTIVE TREATMENT OF PULMONARY TUBERCULOSIS	RARE OPTIC NEURITIS WITH IMPAIRMENT OR LOSS OF VISION
EFFECTIVE ADJUNCTIVE TREATMENT OF AIDS-RELATED *MYCOBACTERIUM AVIUM-INTRACELLULARE* COMPLEX INFECTIONS	Rare peripheral neuritis (see Glossary) Activation of gout
Possibly effective treatment of tuberculous meningitis	

▷ **Principal Uses**

As a Single Drug Product: Uses currently included in FDA-approved labeling: Treats lung (pulmonary) tuberculosis. Used with other antitubercular drugs (currently three other medicines are added to ethambutol).

Other (unlabeled) generally accepted uses: (1) Treatment of tuberculous meningitis; (2) treatment of AIDS-related *Mycobacterium avium-intracellulare* (MAI) complex infections, in combination with other antimycobacterial drugs.

Available Dosage Forms and Strengths

Tablets — 100 mg, 400 mg

▷ **Recommended Dosage Ranges** (Actual dose and schedule must be determined for each patient individually.)

Infants and Children: Dose not established. Some authorities recommend that children under 13 years of age not be given this drug.

13 to 60 Years of Age: To start—15 mg per kg of body mass, once daily. Daily maximum is 500–1,500 mg.

For retreatment of tuberculosis—25 mg per kg of body mass, once daily for 60 days; then 15 mg per kg of body mass. Total daily dose should not exceed 900–2,500 mg.

For tuberculous meningitis or AIDS-related MAI infections—15 to 25 mg per kg of body mass, once daily.

Over 60 Years of Age: Same as 13 to 60 years of age.

▷ **This Drug Should Not Be Taken If**
- you have had an allergic reaction to it previously.
- you currently have optic neuritis or peripheral neuritis.
- you currently have active gout.
- you are not able to have visual acuity testing.

Author's Note: The information in this profile has been shortened to make room for more widely used medicines.

ETHANOL (ETH an all)

Other Names: **Prescription:** None

Nonprescription: Moonshine, alcohol, jack, white lightning, wine, beer, whiskey, vodka, others

Introduced: 1980 (prescription); 6,000 years ago (nonprescription)   **Class:** Antianxiety drug (nonprescription form)   **Prescription:** USA: Yes (IV) **Controlled Drug:** USA: No; Canada: Yes (IV)   **Available as Generic:** USA: Yes; Canada: Yes

Brand Names: **Prescription:** ❦Dilusol (38.7%), Eskaphen B, Novahistine DMX Liquid, Nyquil Nighttime Cold Medicine, Temaril (5.7%), Tuss-Ornade (5%), Vicks Formula 44D   **Nonprescription:** Robert Alison Chardonnay (12% by volume), Bud Dry, Glenlivet, Smirnoff (40% by volume), others

Warning: Clinical use is limited to intravenous treatment of methanol and antifreeze (ethylene glycol) poisoning and as a preservative. Many products contain alcohol. Ask your pharmacist for help if you must avoid alcohol. Widely used in nonprescription form as an antianxiety agent. Some data show heart (cardiac) benefit of moderate use—however, other data show increased cancer risks. Some data from the UK show that heavy drinking may actually DOUBLE the risk of strokes. Some people may not have any mental or physical changes even though a breath or blood alcohol test shows they are "legally drunk."

BENEFITS versus RISKS	
Possible Benefits	*Possible Risks*
EFFECTIVE TREATMENT OF METHANOL OR ETHYLENE GLYCOL POISONING	WITHDRAWAL SYMPTOMS SEIZURES LIVER DAMAGE (with prolonged use)
MODERATE USE MAY DECREASE HEART DISEASE/HEART ATTACK RISK	Possible increased cancer risk Heavy drinking may increase the risk of type 2 diabetes
LIGHT TO MODERATE USE (AS LITTLE AS ONE DRINK PER WEEK) MAY DECREASE RISK OF STROKE AND ISCHEMIC STROKE IN MEN	Pancreatitis Encephalopathy Low white blood cell counts and anemia Myopathy
Moderate drinking may lower the risk of type 2 diabetes	

▷ **Principal Uses**

As a *Single Drug Product:* Uses currently included in FDA-approved labeling: (1) Intravenously in very specific depletion cases as a calorie source.

Other (unlabeled) generally accepted uses: (1) Treatment of methanol or antifreeze (ethylene glycol) poisoning; (2) adjunctive treatment of cancer pain; (3) intravenous treatment of DTs (delirium tremens); (4) used to sclerose esophageal varices and stop bleeding; (5) treatment of hepatocellular cancer where severe liver problems preclude surgery; (6) used to sclerose thyroid cysts; (7) used to destroy nerve tissue (neurolytic block) in chronic pain therapy; (8) widely used in nonprescription form as an antianxiety agent; (9) one large study appears to show that use ranging up to moderate (and NO GREATER than 0.7 mg per kg of body mass for 3 days in a row) may actually help prevent coronary heart disease and heart attacks; (10) a large study of more than 22,000 men showed that light to moderate use (as little as one drink per week) appears to decrease risk of stroke and ischemic stroke in men; (11) moderate drinking (one to two drinks per day) appears to lower the risk of type 2 diabetes; (12) ethanol injection may have a role in managing benign prostatic hypertrophy (BPH).

As a *Combination Drug Product [CD]:* Uses currently included in FDA-approved labeling: Widely present in elixirs and other liquid vehicles for drugs as a preservative and partial drug action enhancer.

How This Drug Works: In antifreeze (ethylene glycol) or methanol poisoning, ethanol prevents ethylene glycol or methanol from being changed (metabolized) into toxic chemicals, letting the body remove antifreeze or methanol harmlessly. If used in nonprescription form in excess, it depresses nerve function, leading to emotional changes and disturbances of perception, coordination and intoxication. Nonprescription use of up to moderate amounts appears to decrease risk of heart and blood vessel disease, but how it works is unknown. One recent report found that beer containing vitamin B_6 helps protect against heart disease by lowering homocysteine-a risk factor for heart disease.

Available Dosage Forms and Strengths

Intravenous — 5%, 10%, 95%

Nonprescription — Each ounce of 100-proof whiskey has 15 ml of ethanol
— 6 ounces (12%) wine has 22 ml of ethanol
— 12 ounces of beer (4.9%) has 18 ml of ethanol

▷ **Recommended Dosage Ranges** (Actual dose and schedule must be determined for each patient individually.)

Infants and Children: Methanol or ethylene glycol poisoning: 40 ml per kg of body mass per day.

18 to 60 Years of Age: Methanol or ethylene glycol poisoning: A loading dose of 0.6 g per kg of body mass is given and followed by 109 to 125 mg per kg of body mass per hour to maintain a blood level of 100 mg/dl.

Coronary heart disease or heart attack prevention: It APPEARS THAT use of moderate amounts (up to 0.8 mg per kg of body mass per day or no more than 0.7 mg per kg of body mass per day for 3 days in a row) of alcohol may help in preventing risk of this kind of blood vessel disease and myocardial infarctions.

Ischemic stroke or stroke prevention: It appears that as little as one drink per week decreases risk.

Over 60 Years of Age: Same as 18 to 60 years of age for poisonings. Older people may be less able to tolerate the same amount as a younger person for the nonprescription forms. A smaller dose will generally cause an equal or greater loss of coordination or mental ability. Hypothermia risk is also increased.

Conditions Requiring Dosing Adjustments

Liver Function: Ethanol is extensively metabolized in the liver to acetaldehyde and acetyl CoA. The drug is also a clear cause of liver toxicity. The dose must be decreased in liver compromise.

Kidney Function: Kidneys are minimally involved. No changes needed.

▷ **Dosing Instructions:** If methanol or ethylene glycol poisoning is suspected: The nearest poison control center should be contacted. Oral dosing (use vodka mixed in orange juice) may be of benefit, depending on distance from a hospital or free-standing emergency center.

For nonprescription antianxiety use: Dose of this drug and the blood alcohol level varies with many factors. Critical ones are weight, metabolic activity of the liver, how much food is in the stomach, strength of alcohol in the beverage, number of "drinks" consumed over a given period of time and how well hydrated (whether there has been extreme exercise and fluid loss) you are.

Again, although a blood or breath alcohol test may be a marker for mental or physical changes, some people may not have physical or mental changes and will actually have a blood or breath alcohol level in the state-defined range of "legally drunk."

Specific levels of blood or breath alcohol do not absolutely predict impairment. Each 10 ml of ethanol increases blood ethanol of an average 150-lb (70-kg) person by 16.6 mg percent (3.6 mmol/L).

Legal definition of intoxication is a blood alcohol level of 0.10% or 100 mg/dl. "Under the influence" in Maryland is 0.07% or 70 mg/dl. Driving impairment may occur at blood levels of 0.05% (50 mg/dl) or lower.

Usual Duration of Use: Use on a regular schedule for 48 hours determines effectiveness in methanol overdose. Long-term excessive use as an antianxiety agent is NOT recommended. If you forget a dose: not applicable.

Typical Treatment Goals and Measurements (Outcomes and Markers)

Prevention of coronary heart disease: Information from big and small studies shows that taking two or fewer (see dosing above) drinks per day can help decrease the risk of coronary heart disease. Red wine appears to have the most data, but some recent information appears to show a benefit from vitamin B_6-containing beer. Goals then relate to probability of a coronary problem, and time gained without experiencing a coronary problem.

▷ **This Drug Should Not Be Taken If**
- you have had an allergic reaction to any dose form of it previously.
- you have epilepsy.
- you have a history of alcohol addiction.
- you have a urinary tract infection.
- you are pregnant.
- you are in diabetic coma.

▷ **Inform Your Physician Before Taking This Drug If**
- you have liver or kidney compromise.
- you have gout.
- you are prone to low blood sugars.
- you are a diabetic.
- you have congestive heart failure.

Possible Side Effects (natural, expected and unavoidable drug actions)
Intoxication, perception, coordination and mood changes.

▷ **Possible Adverse Effects** (unusual, unexpected and infrequent reactions)
If any of the following develop, consult your physician promptly for guidance.

Mild Adverse Effects
Allergic reactions: itching, rash, hives and flushing.
Headache, "hangover": nausea, headache, malaise—dose-related.
Sedation—dose-dependent.
Disorientation, memory loss—dose-dependent.
Color blindness or neuropathy (tingling, burning or numbness)—with chronic use.
Vitamin deficiency or muscle changes (myopathy)—with chronic use.
Stomach irritation—frequent.

Serious Adverse Effects
Allergic reactions: anaphylaxis (rash, swelling of tongue, breathing problems, flushing)—case reports.
Bronchospasm (asthmatics at increased risk)—case reports.
Respiratory depression—dose-related.
Elevated or decreased white blood cell count—possible.
Increased or decreased platelets—case reports.
Heart dysfunction (myopathy) or anemia (megaloblastic)—with chronic use.
High blood pressure—possible to frequent.
Abnormal heart rhythms (atrial and ventricular) or chest pain (angina)—increased risk.
Liver toxicity—cirrhosis possible with chronic use.
Osteoporosis—increased risk with chronic use.
Pancreatitis—increased risk with chronic higher-dose use.
Encephalopathy or cerebrovascular bleeding—increased risk with higher-dose chronic use.
Low blood sugar or ketoacidosis—especially if meals are missed or with chronic use.
Vitamin deficiency (folic acid, vitamins B_1 and B_6) or low magnesium—with chronic use.
Low potassium (especially with acute intoxication in children)—possible.
Gout (precipitated by alcohol use in those with gout)—possible.
Tolerance (with chronic use)—possible.
Withdrawal: nausea, fever, rapid heart rate, hallucinations. May progress to delirium tremens (5%): profound confusion, hallucinations, etc.—possible.

▷ **Possible Effects on Sexual Function:** Decreased libido, impotence (with excessive chronic use). Difficulty achieving an erection in males and decreased vaginal dilation in females. Chronic alcohol use may lead to tenderness and swelling of male and female breast tissue, testicular atrophy, low sperm counts, decreased menstrual blood flow and diminished capability for orgasm in females.

Possible Delayed Adverse Effects: Liver toxicity, anemia, low or high platelets, vitamin deficiency.

▷ **Adverse Effects That May Mimic Natural Diseases or Disorders**

Alcoholic cirrhosis may mimic hepatitis.

Natural Diseases or Disorders That May Be Activated by This Drug

Peptic ulcer disease.

Possible Effects on Laboratory Tests

Liver function tests: elevated ALT.

Complete blood count: decreased white blood cells, decreased hemoglobin, increased or decreased platelets.

Amylase: elevated.

Sperm count: decreased with chronic use.

Magnesium: decreased with chronic use.

CAUTION

1. The FDA now requires a warning label on all nonprescription pain (analgesic) and fever (antipyretic) products that have aspirin or other salicylates, ibuprofen, naproxen sodium, ketoprofen or acetaminophen in them (NSAIDs) that says:

   Alcohol Warning: If you consume 3 or more alcoholic drinks every day, ask your doctor whether you should take [the medicine in question] or other pain relievers/fever reducers. [The ingredient] may cause stomach bleeding. This is a new warning intended to help protect patients from possible stomach or liver damage.

2. Nonprescription form may cause FATAL increases in blood pressure if combined with cocaine.

3. With high doses (nearly pure "grain" alcohol) or many drinks (frequent dosing) over a short period of time, FATAL blood alcohol levels may be reached with the nonprescription form.

4. Some alcoholic beverages have tyramine in them. Combination of these beverages with MAO inhibitors (see Drug Classes) may lead to extreme increases in blood pressure (hypertensive crisis).

5. Data from a study of 5,766 men over more than 21 years showed that heavy drinking may DOUBLE the risk of strokes.

6. Recent data from a study of more than 22,000 men showed that light to moderate use (from one drink per week up to one drink per day) of alcohol decreased the risk of stroke or ischemic stroke. Having more than one drink per day DID NOT further decrease risk.

Precautions for Use

By Infants and Children: Safety and effectiveness for those under 12 years of age not established. Accidental and unsupervised drinking of the nonprescription form may result in severe consequences in children. Seriously low blood sugar may happen and be delayed up to 6 hours after drinking. Low potassium may also occur with high ethanol levels. Therapy is guided by blood sugar, potassium and blood alcohol (ethanol) levels. Fatality caused by low blood sugar was reported in a 4-year-old child who drank 12 ounces of a mouthwash that contained 10% ethanol.

By Those Over 60 Years of Age: Poisoning with methanol or ethylene glycol is an emergency situation, and while there may be an increased sensitivity to effects, dosing is adjusted to blood levels. The nonprescription form dosing (number of drinks) tolerated would be expected to decrease with increasing age.

▷ **Advisability of Use During Pregnancy**
Pregnancy Category: D, X if used for long periods. See Pregnancy Risk Categories at the back of this book.
Human studies: Fetal alcohol syndrome—a collection of limb, neurological and behavioral defects—occurs with excessive alcohol use.
Avoid use of this drug during your **entire** pregnancy.

Advisability of Use If Breast-Feeding
Presence of this drug in breast milk: Yes.
Avoid drug or refrain from nursing.

Habit-Forming Potential: Clearly defined alcoholism exists and occurs.

Effects of Overdose: Toxic levels result in ataxia, loss of consciousness progressing to coma, anesthesia, respiratory failure and death. Levels of 150 to 300 mg/dl may result in exaggerated emotional states, confusion and incoordination. Fatalities most often result with blood concentrations greater than 400 mg/dl. Fatal blood levels vary greatly, however, and death has been reported following levels as low as 260 mg/dl. Once again, some people will not have any mental or physical changes with an alcohol level that is in the "legally drunk" range and even with higher levels.

Possible Effects of Long-Term Use: Liver toxicity, anemia, esophageal varices, low white blood cell counts, compromised heart function, high blood pressure, depression, peripheral neuropathy, seizures, cerebrovascular accident (with acute high levels), water intoxication, vitamin and electrolyte disturbances, gastritis or ulcers, pancreatitis, muscle pain, osteoporosis, tolerance and withdrawal.

Suggested Periodic Examinations While Taking This Drug (at physician's discretion)
Blood alcohol levels and methanol or ethylene glycol levels guide therapy in poisonings.
Chronic alcohol abuse: Complete blood counts, liver function tests, amylase and lipase, electrocardiograms.

▷ **While Taking This Drug, Observe the Following**
Foods: Food may decrease the absorption of ethanol from the stomach and reduce chances of intoxication.
Nutritional Support: Vitamin support, particularly thiamin (B_1), folic acid and B_6, are needed with chronic use. Vitamin C may help eliminate ethanol.
Herbal Medicines or Minerals: Valerian and kava kava may interact additively (drowsiness). Avoid these combinations. Magnesium replacement may be needed.
Tobacco Smoking: No interactions expected. I advise everyone to quit smoking.
Marijuana Smoking: Additive central nervous system depression and possible increases in ethanol blood levels.

▷   *Other Drugs*

Ethanol may **increase** the effects of
- some antibiotics (such as doxycycline, others).
- central nervous system depressants, such as benzodiazepines, barbiturates, opioids and anesthetic agents.
- chlorpromazine (Thorazine) and will result in increased sedation.
- cocaine and result in dangerous increases in blood pressure.
- cyclosporine (Sandimmune)—with large amounts of ethanol.
- diphenhydramine (Benadryl, others) and will increase sedation.
- venlafaxine (Effexor) and may increase CNS effects of both drugs.
- warfarin (Coumadin) and require more frequent INR testing and possible dose changes.

Ethanol may **decrease** the effects of
- phenytoin (Dilantin) or fosphenytoin (Cerebyx) by reducing blood levels.
- propranolol (Inderal) by increasing propranolol elimination.

Ethanol taken concurrently with
- abacavir (Ziagen) may result in increased blood levels of abacavir and possibly an increased risk of toxicity.
- acetaminophen (Tylenol) poses an increased risk of liver damage.
- some antihistamines may increase sedation.
- amprenavir (Agenerase) solution may carry a risk of propylene glycol toxicity. Combination is NOT recommended.
- aspirin may result in increased blood loss from the stomach.
- cefamandole (Mandol), cefotetan (Cefotan), metronidazole (Flagyl), cotrimoxazole, sulfamethoxazole and cefoperazone (Cefobid) may result in disulfiramlike reaction (see Glossary).
- cimetidine (Zantac) may decrease the amount of alcohol that it takes to make you drunk (intoxicated).
- cisapride (Propulsid) may increase ethanol blood levels.
- disulfiram (Antabuse) will result in severe vomiting and intolerance.
- dronabinol (Marinol) may increase ethanol levels.
- fexofenadine (Allegra) showed NO driving performance decrease in one study of 24 healthy men.
- griseofulvin (Fulvicin) can increase the effects of alcohol.
- insulin may result in potential severe hypoglycemia.
- isoniazid may result in elevated isoniazid levels.
- ketoconazole (Nizoral) may result in disulfiramlike reactions.
- lithium (Lithobid) may result in worsened impairment of coordination and intoxication.
- metformin (Glucophage) may increase risk of lactic acidosis with ongoing or excessive ethanol use.
- methotrexate (Rheumatrex, others) may increase risk of liver damage (especially with long-term ethanol use).
- metronidazole (Flagyl) may result in a disulfiramlike reaction.
- mirtazapine (Remeron) may lead to increased risk of psychomotor impairment.
- nitroglycerin (Nitrostat, others) may result in excessive decreases in blood pressure.

- nonsteroidal anti-inflammatory drugs (NSAIDs; see Drug Classes) may lead to increased risk of stomach bleeding or liver damage.
- olanzapine (Zyprexa) may lead to excessive depression of the central nervous system.
- oral hypoglycemic agents (see Drug Classes) poses an increased risk of seriously low glucose levels.
- quetiapine (Seroquel) may worsen thinking and motor skill depression caused by ethanol.
- sibutramine (Meridia) is not recommended by the manufacturer.
- tramadol (Ultram) may lead to excessive depression of the central nervous system.
- tricyclic antidepressants (see Drug Classes) may result in increased antidepressant levels and toxicity.
- trimethoprim/sulfamethoxazole (Cotrimoxazole, Septra, Bactrim, others) may lead to a disulfiram-like reaction.
- valproic acid (Depakene, Depakote, others) may enhance central nervous depression from ethanol.
- verapamil (Calan, others) may increase the amount of time ethanol stays in the body and may pose an increased risk of intoxication.
- zaleplon (Sonata) may result in increased additive central nervous depression (impairing psychomotor functions). Combination should be avoided.
- zolpidem (Ambien) may result in increased additive central nervous depression (impairing psychomotor functions). Combination should be avoided.

▷ *Driving, Hazardous Activities:* This drug may cause drowsiness, mental impairment and coordination problems. Driving skill may be impaired at very low blood levels with the perception that capabilities are **not** reduced. Drinking and driving is not recommended. Restrict activities as necessary.

Aviation Note: The use of this drug **is a disqualification** for piloting. Consult a designated Aviation Medical Examiner.

Exposure to Sun: May result in additive dehydration.

Heavy Exercise or Exertion: May worsen the adverse effects of this drug.

Discontinuation: Abrupt discontinuation after chronic use may result in a serious withdrawal syndrome known as DT or delirium tremens.

ETHOSUXIMIDE (eth oh SUX i mide)

Introduced: 1960   **Class:** Anticonvulsant   **Prescription:** USA: Yes
Controlled Drug: USA: No; Canada: No   **Available as Generic:** Yes
Brand Name: Zarontin

BENEFITS versus RISKS	
Possible Benefits	*Possible Risks*
EFFECTIVE CONTROL OF ABSENCE SEIZURES (PETIT MAL EPILEPSY)	RARE APLASTIC ANEMIA (see Aplastic Anemia and Bone Marrow Depression in Glossary)
EFFECTIVE CONTROL OF MYOCLONIC AND AKINETIC EPILEPSY IN SOME PATIENTS	Rare decrease in white blood cells and blood platelets

▷ **Principal Uses**

As a Single Drug Product: Uses currently included in FDA-approved labeling: Used to treat petit mal epilepsy and is a drug of choice in absence seizures. Other (unlabeled) generally accepted uses: None at present.

How This Drug Works: Alters some nerve impulses, suppressing abnormal electrical activity that causes absence seizures (petit mal epilepsy).

Available Dosage Forms and Strengths

Capsules — 250 mg

Solution — 250 mg/ml

Syrup — 250 mg/5 ml

▷ **Usual Adult Dosage Ranges:** Dosing starts with 500 mg daily and can be increased by 250 mg every 4 to 7 days until acceptable control is achieved. Ending dose may be 20 to 30 mg per kg daily. Daily maximum is 1,500 mg. IMPORTANT: Blood levels increase more quickly in females than males. *For children 3 to 6 years old:* Usual starting dose is 250 mg per day. May increase by 250-mg doses every 4 to 7 days as needed. Usually 20–30 mg per kg is the once-daily dose. *More than 6 years old with absence seizures:* Same as adults.

Note: Actual dose and schedule must be determined for each patient individually.

Conditions Requiring Dosing Adjustments

Liver Function: Blood levels are recommended if the liver is damaged.

Kidney Function: No specific changes needed, but a more frequent check of blood levels may be prudent.

▷ **Dosing Instructions:** Capsule may be opened and taken with food to reduce stomach irritation. If you forget a dose: take the dose you missed as soon as you remember it, unless it is nearly time for your next dose—if that is the case, simply skip the missed dose and take the next scheduled dose right on schedule. DO NOT double doses.

Usual Duration of Use: Regular use for 1 to 2 weeks may be needed to identify the best dose and reduce frequency of absence seizures. Long-term use requires physician supervision and use is ongoing.

Typical Treatment Goals and Measurements (Outcomes and Markers)

Seizures: The general goal for this medicine is effective seizure control. Neurologists tend to define effective on a case-by-case basis depending on the seizure type and patient factors. Blood levels can help guide dosing. If this medicine is being used to treat absence seizures, EEG can be used to check clinical progress.

▷ **This Drug Should Not Be Taken If**

- you are allergic to any succinimide anticonvulsant (see Drug Classes).
- you currently have a blood cell or bone marrow disorder.

▷ **Inform Your Physician Before Taking This Drug If**

- you have a history of or active liver or kidney disease.
- you have any type of blood disorder, especially one caused by drugs.
- you have serious depression or mental illness.

Possible Side Effects (natural, expected and unavoidable drug actions)

Drowsiness, lethargy, fatigue.

▷ **Possible Adverse Effects** (unusual, unexpected and infrequent reactions)
If any of the following develop, consult your physician promptly for guidance.

Mild Adverse Effects

Allergic reactions: skin rash, hives—case reports.

Headache, unsteadiness, euphoria, impaired vision, numbness and tingling in extremities—infrequent.

Loss of appetite, nausea, vomiting, dizziness, hiccups, stomach pain, diarrhea—infrequent to frequent.

Thickening and overgrowth of gums—possible.

Serious Adverse Effects

Allergic Reaction: Swelling of tongue—case reports.

Aggravation of emotional depression and paranoid mental disorders—case reports.

Severe bone marrow depression: fatigue, fever, sore throat, abnormal bleeding or bruising—case reports.

Porphyria, myasthenia gravis or systemic lupus erythematosus—rare.

▷ **Possible Effects on Sexual Function:** Increased libido (questionable); nonmenstrual vaginal bleeding—case reports.

Natural Diseases or Disorders That May Be Activated by This Drug

Latent psychosis, systemic lupus erythematosus.

Possible Effects on Laboratory Tests

Complete blood cell counts: decreased red cells, hemoglobin, white cells and platelets; increased eosinophils.

Blood aspartate aminotransferase (AST) level: increased in 33% of users.

Blood bilirubin level: increased (rare liver damage).

Blood lupus erythematosus (LE) cells: positive—rare.

Kidney function tests: increased blood urea nitrogen (BUN) level, increased urine protein content.

CAUTION

1. May increase the frequency of grand mal seizures in people with mixed seizure disorders.
2. Periodic blood counts and other tests are mandatory.

Precautions for Use

By Infants and Children: If a single daily dose causes nausea or vomiting, give in two or three divided doses 8 to 12 hours apart. Large differences in response occur and require blood levels. Watch for a lupuslike reaction: fever, rash, arthritis.

By Those Over 60 Years of Age: Rarely used in this age group.

▷ **Advisability of Use During Pregnancy**

Pregnancy Category: C. See Pregnancy Risk Categories at the back of this book.

Animal studies: Bone defects reported in rodents.

Human studies: Three instances of birth defects have been reported. Adequate studies of pregnant women are not available.

Avoid during first 3 months. Use only if clearly needed during the final 6 months.

Advisability of Use If Breast-Feeding

Presence of this drug in breast milk: Yes, but not usually a significant level. Watch nursing infant closely and discontinue drug or nursing if adverse effects develop. If mother requires high doses, refrain from nursing. Ask your doctor for help.

Habit-Forming Potential: None.

Effects of Overdose: Drowsiness, lethargy, dizziness, nausea, vomiting, stupor progressing to coma.

Possible Effects of Long-Term Use: Systemic lupus erythematosus.

Suggested Periodic Examinations While Taking This Drug (at physician's discretion)

Complete blood counts every 2 weeks during the first months of use and then monthly thereafter.

Liver and kidney function tests.

▷ **While Taking This Drug, Observe the Following**

Foods: No restrictions.

Herbal Medicines or Minerals: Valerian and kava kava may interact additively (drowsiness). Avoid these combinations.

Beverages: No restrictions. May be taken with milk.

▷ *Alcohol:* Use caution—this drug may increase the sedative effects of alcohol. Excessive alcohol may precipitate seizures.

Tobacco Smoking: No interactions expected. I advise everyone to quit smoking.

▷ **Other Drugs**

Ethosuximide may **increase** the effects of

- phenytoin (Dilantin) and fosphenytoin (Cerebyx), by slowing elimination.

Ethosuximide *taken concurrently* with

- carbamazepine (Tegretol) may change ethosuximide blood levels.
- phenobarbital may decrease seizure control success.
- ritonavir (Norvir) and perhaps other protease inhibitors (see Drug Classes) may lead to toxicity.
- tramadol (Ultram) may increase seizure risk.
- valproic acid (Depakene) may unpredictably alter ethosuximide effects.

The following drug may *increase* the effects of ethosuximide:

- isoniazid (INH, Niconyl, etc.).

▷ *Driving, Hazardous Activities:* This drug may cause drowsiness, dizziness, unsteadiness and impaired vision. Restrict activities as necessary.

Aviation Note: Seizure disorders and the use of this drug *are disqualifications* for piloting. Consult a designated Aviation Medical Examiner.

Exposure to Sun: No restrictions.

Discontinuation: Do not stop taking this drug abruptly. Ask your physician for help with gradual dose reduction.

ETIDRONATE (e ti DROH nate)

Introduced: 1976   **Class:** Anti-osteoporotic   **Prescription:** USA: Yes
Controlled Drug: USA: No; Canada: No   **Available as Generic:** USA: No; Canada: No
Brand Name: Didronel

BENEFITS versus RISKS	
Possible Benefits	*Possible Risks*
PARTIAL RELIEF OF SYMPTOMS OF PAGET'S DISEASE OF BONE	Increased bone pain
	Bone fractures
EFFECTIVE PREVENTION AND TREATMENT OF ABNORMAL CALCIFICATION	Kidney failure
	Focal osteomalacia
Effective adjunctive treatment of abnormally high blood calcium levels (associated with malignant disease)	
Treatment of postmenopausal osteoporosis	

▷ **Principal Uses**

> *As a Single Drug Product:* Uses currently included in FDA-approved labeling: (1) Treatment of symptomatic Paget's disease of bone (excessive bone growth of skull, spine and long bones); (2) prevention and treatment of abnormal bone formation (ossification) following total hip replacement or spinal cord injury; (3) adjunctive treatment of excessively high blood calcium levels due to malignant bone disease.

> Other (unlabeled) generally accepted uses: (1) treatment of Paget's disease of bone that is not yet causing symptoms; (2) treatment of abnormal calcium levels that may result from prolonged immobilization; (3) helps hyperparathyroidism; (4) helps pulmonary alveolar microlithiasis (PAM); (5) treatment (with cyclic dosing) of postmenopausal osteoporosis.

How This Drug Works: This drug attaches to the surface of bone and slows the abnormally accelerated processes of "bone turnover" that occur in Paget's disease. In malignant bone disease, this drug slows bone destruction and reduces excessive transfer of calcium from bone to blood.

Available Dosage Forms and Strengths

> Injection — 50 mg/ml
> Tablets — 200 mg, 400 mg

▷ **Recommended Dosage Ranges** (Actual dose and schedule must be determined for each patient individually.)

Infants and Children: Dose not established.

12 to 60 Years of Age:

For Paget's disease: Initially 5 mg per kg of body mass daily, as a single dose, for up to 6 months. Discontinue for a drug-free period of 6 months. As needed, repeat, alternating 6-month courses of drug treatment and abstention. Doses above 10 mg per kg of body mass per day are only used if there is a critical need to decrease increased work output of the heart or to quickly slow down increased bone turnover.

For ossification associated with hip replacement: 20 mg per kg of body mass daily for 1 month before and 3 months after surgery.

For ossification associated with spinal cord injury: Initially 20 mg per kg of body mass daily for 2 weeks after injury; then decrease dose to 10 mg per kg of body mass daily for an additional 10 weeks.

For high blood calcium associated with malignant bone disease: 20 mg per kg of body mass daily for 30 days; if needed and tolerated, continue for a maximum of 90 days. The total daily dose should not exceed 20 mg per kg of body mass.

Over 60 Years of Age: Same as 12 to 60 years of age.

Author's Note: The information in this profile has been shortened to allow room for more widely used medicines.

ETODOLAC (e TOE do lak)

Please see the acetic acids (nonsteroidal anti-inflammatory drug) family profile.

ETRETINATE (e TRET i nayt)

Introduced: 1976   **Class:** Antipsoriasis
Brand Name: Tegison
Author's Note: The manufacturer has stopped marketing this medicine.

FAMOTIDINE (fa MOH te deen)

Please see the histamine (H2) drug family profile.

FELODIPINE (feh LOH di peen)

Introduced: 1986   **Class:** Antihypertensive, calcium channel blocker
Prescription: USA: Yes   **Controlled Drug:** USA: No   **Available as Generic:** No
Brand Names: Plendil, Altace plus felodipine [CD], Lexxel [CD], Logimax [CD], ✤Renedil
Controversies in Medicine: Medicines in this class have had many conflicting reports. The FDA has held hearings on the calcium channel blocker (CCB) class. Amlodipine got the first FDA approval to treat high blood pressure or angina in people with congestive heart failure. Early research at NYU found that nifedipine is a cause of reversible male infertility. CCBs are currently second-line agents for high blood pressure according to the JNC VI (see Glossary).

BENEFITS versus RISKS	
Possible Benefits	*Possible Risks*
EFFECTIVE TREATMENT OF MILD TO MODERATE HYPERTENSION	Peripheral edema (fluid retention in feet and ankles)

▷ **Principal Uses**
As a Single Drug Product: Uses currently included in FDA-approved labeling: Treats mild to moderate hypertension.

Other (unlabeled) generally accepted uses: (1) Treats angina; (2) arrhythmias; (3) may inhibit progression of atherosclerosis; (4) can be used in some cases of premature labor; (5) may have a role in kidney disease in diabetes (diabetic nephropathy); (6) helps kidney toxicity caused by cyclosporine (nephropathy).

As a Combination Drug Product [CD]: Available combined with enalapril (an ACE inhibitor) as the brand name Lexxel. The combination puts two different actions to work to lower blood pressure. Logimax combines felodipine with metoprolol, and Altace plus felodipine combines ramipril (an ACE inhibitor) with felodipine.

How This Drug Works: Blocks normal passage of calcium through some cell walls. This slows spread of electrical activity and reduces contraction of peripheral arterial walls, lowering blood pressure. Combination form adds the benefits of an ACE inhibitor to this calcium blocker.

Available Dosage Forms and Strengths
Tablets, sustained release — 5 mg, 10 mg
Coated tablet (Lexxel) — 5 mg enalapril and 5 mg felodipine

▷ **Recommended Dosage Ranges** (Actual dose and schedule must be determined for each patient individually.)

Infants and Children: 0.18 to 0.56 mg/kg daily have controlled blood pressure after kidney transplants.

12 to 60 Years of Age: High blood pressure: Initially 5 mg, once daily. Increased as needed and tolerated (at 2-week intervals). Usual dose range is 5–10 mg, once daily. Total daily maximum is 10 mg.

Lexxel: One tablet daily. Increased to two daily if needed.

Over 60 Years of Age: Starting dose is 2.5 mg daily. Daily maximum is 10 mg.

Conditions Requiring Dosing Adjustments
Liver Function: Starting dose is 2.5 mg daily, with a 10-mg maximum.
Kidney Function: No changes needed.

▷ **Dosing Instructions:** May take with or following food to reduce stomach upset. Tablet should be swallowed whole; do not crush or chew it. If you forget a dose: Take the missed dose as soon as you remember it, unless it is nearly time for your next dose—if that is the case, skip the missed dose and take the next dose right on schedule. As with other medicines for high blood pressure, please remember to take it. Keeping your blood pressure under control will help avoid dangerous long-term complications. Do not take this medicine with grapefruit juice.

Usual Duration of Use: Regular use for 2 to 4 weeks has shown benefits in controlling hypertension. Smallest effective dose should be used in long-term (months to years) therapy. Physician visits are essential.

Typical Treatment Goals and Measurements (Outcomes and Markers)
Blood Pressure: The most recent treatment guidelines (JNC VI) define optimal blood pressure (BP) as less than 120/80 and high normal as 139/89. The American Diabetes Association has chosen a target of 130/80 as the blood pressure goal for people living with diabetes. Most clinicians try to achieve a BP that confers the best balance of lower cardiovascular risk and avoids the problem of too low a blood pressure. The goals and time frame should be discussed with you when the prescription is written.

Possible Advantages of This Drug: Gradual onset and prolonged duration of action, permitting effective once-a-day treatment.

▷ **This Drug Should Not Be Taken If**
- you had an allergic reaction to it or similar medicines.
- you have active liver disease.
- you have severe lowering of the blood pressure.
- you have severe problems (dysfunction) in the left side of your heart.
- you have atrioventricular blockade or "sick sinus" syndrome (talk with your doctor).
- you have uncorrected congestive heart failure.

▷ **Inform Your Physician Before Taking This Drug If**
- you have had an unfavorable response to any calcium-channel-blocker drug.
- you take digitalis or a beta-blocker (see Drug Classes).
- you are taking any other drugs that lower blood pressure.
- you have a history of congestive heart failure, heart attack, or stroke.
- you are subject to disturbances of heart rhythm (such as atrial fibrillation).
- you have a narrowing (stenosis) of the aorta.
- your stomach is blocked or works very quickly (extended-release forms— GI hypermotility or obstruction).
- you develop a skin reaction while taking this medicine.
- you have circulatory impairment to the fingers.
- you have muscular dystrophy or myasthenia gravis.
- you have a history of impaired liver or kidney function.

Possible Side Effects (natural, expected and unavoidable drug actions)
Swelling of feet and ankles, flushing and sensation of warmth.

▷ **Possible Adverse Effects** (unusual, unexpected and infrequent reactions)
If any of the following develop, consult your physician promptly for guidance.

Mild Adverse Effects
Allergic reactions: skin rash—rare.
Headache—frequent.
Dizziness, fatigue or sleep disorders—infrequent.
Indigestion, nausea, stomach pain, constipation or diarrhea—all rare.
Increased liver enzymes—possible.
Palpitations or fast heart rate (tachycardia)—infrequent to frequent.
Dose-related flushing—possible.
Impaired sense of smell—possible.
Cough or pharyngitis—infrequent.
Increased urination—possible.
Abnormal growth of the gums (gingival hyperplasia)—rare.

Serious Adverse Effects
Allergic reactions: serious skin reactions.
Idiosyncratic reactions: none reported.
Aggravation of angina—possible.
Decreased hemoglobin, hematocrit and red blood cell count (reported with other drugs in the same family)—case reports.
Stroke—case reports.

▷ **Possible Effects on Sexual Function:** Impotence (0.5-1.5%)—rare. Swelling of male breast tissue (gynecomastia) reported for some other calcium channel blockers.

▷ **Adverse Effects That May Mimic Natural Diseases or Disorders**
An allergic rash and swelling of the legs may resemble erysipelas.

Possible Effects on Laboratory Tests
Liver function tests: minor and short-term increases.

CAUTION
1. Tell your health care providers that you take this drug. Carry a note in your purse or wallet saying you take it.
2. You may use nitroglycerin and other nitrate drugs to ease acute episodes of angina pain. Call your doctor if angina attacks become more frequent or intense.

Precautions for Use
By Those Over 60 Years of Age: You may be more susceptible to the development of weakness, dizziness, fainting and falling. Take necessary precautions to prevent injury.

▷ **Advisability of Use During Pregnancy**
Pregnancy Category: C. See Pregnancy Risk Categories at the back of this book.
Animal studies: No information available.
Human studies: Adequate studies of pregnant women are not available.
Avoid this drug during the first 3 months. Use during the final 6 months only if clearly needed. Ask your physician for guidance.

Advisability of Use If Breast-Feeding
Presence of this drug in breast milk: Unknown.
Avoid drug or refrain from nursing.

Habit-Forming Potential: None. An increased severity and/or frequency of angina may occur if the drug is stopped quickly, but it is not a result of addiction.

Effects of Overdose: Weakness, fainting, fast pulse, low blood pressure, shortness of breath, flushed and warm skin, tremors.

Possible Effects of Long-Term Use: None reported.

Suggested Periodic Examinations While Taking This Drug (at physician's discretion)
Heart function tests (electrocardiograms) and blood pressure checks in supine, sitting and standing positions.

▷ **While Taking This Drug, Observe the Following**
Foods: Avoid eating grapefruit for 1 hour after taking this medicine. Avoid excessive salt intake.
Herbal Medicines or Minerals: Ginseng may increase blood pressure, blunting the benefits of these medicines. Hawthorn, saw palmetto, ma huang, goldenseal, yohimbe and licorice may also increase blood pressure. Calcium and garlic may help lower blood pressure. Indian snakeroot has a German Commission E monograph indication for hypertension—talk to your doctor. Eleuthero root and ephedra should be avoided by people living with hypertension.
Beverages: Grapefruit juice can cause **a serious increase** in the absorption of this drug—levels may be increased by over 400%. Do NOT take this drug with grapefruit juice. May be taken with milk or water.

▷ *Alcohol:* Use with caution—alcohol may exaggerate the drop in blood pressure experienced by some people.

   Tobacco Smoking: Nicotine may reduce effectiveness. I advise everyone to quit smoking.

▷ *Other Drugs*

   Felodipine *taken concurrently* with
   - adenosine may result in an extended slowing of the heart.
   - amiodarone (Cordarone) may lead to slowing of heart rate or worsening atrioventricular (AV) block if both drugs are used in people with partial AV block or "sick sinus" syndrome.
   - beta-blocker drugs or digitalis preparations (see Drug Classes) may affect heart rate and rhythm adversely. Careful monitoring by your physician is necessary if these drugs are taken concurrently.
   - carbamazepine (Tegretol) may decrease felodipine benefits.
   - cyclosporine (Sandimmune) may change levels of either drug.
   - delavirdine (Rescriptor) may lead to felodipine toxicity.
   - digoxin (Lanoxin) may increase digoxin levels and result in toxicity.
   - itraconazole, fluconazole or ketoconazole (see Antifungal Drugs in Drug Classes) may lead to felodipine toxicity.
   - magnesium (particularly in high doses) may cause low blood pressure (not specifically reported for felodipine, but another drug in the calcium-channel-blocker class does this).
   - nonsteroidal anti-inflammatory drugs (NSAIDs) or oral anticoagulants (Coumadin) may increase risk of stomach or intestinal (GI) bleeding.
   - phenobarbital can cause decreased felodipine benefits.
   - phenytoin (Dilantin) or fosphenytoin (Cerebyx) may cause decreased phenytoin or fosphenytoin levels.
   - quinupristin/dalfopristin (Synercid) may lead to felodipine toxicity.
   - rifampin (Rifadin) may cause decreased felodipine benefits (reported with other calcium channel blockers).
   - ritonavir (Norvir) and perhaps other protease inhibitors (see Drug Classes) may lead to toxicity.
   - saquinavir (Invirase) may lead to felodipine toxicity. Lower felodipine doses are prudent if these medicines are combined.
   - theophylline (Theo-Dur, others) may lower theophylline levels, requiring theophylline dose changes.

   The following drugs may **increase** the effects of felodipine:
   - cimetidine (Tagamet).
   - erythromycin—may also occur with other macrolide antibiotics (see Drug Classes), since they are structurally similar.

▷ *Driving, Hazardous Activities:* Usually no restrictions. This drug may cause dizziness. Restrict activities as necessary.

   Aviation Note: Hypertension *is a disqualification* for piloting. Consult a designated Aviation Medical Examiner.

   Exposure to Sun: No restrictions.

   Exposure to Heat: Caution is advised. Hot environments can exaggerate the blood-pressure-lowering effects of this drug. Observe for light-headedness or weakness.

   Discontinuation: Do not stop this drug abruptly. Ask your physician about gradual withdrawal. Watch for development of rebound hypertension.

FENAMATE (NONSTEROIDAL ANTI-INFLAMMATORY DRUG) FAMILY

Meclofenamate (MEK low fen a mate)   **Mefenamic Acid** (MEF en amik a sid)
Introduced: 1977, 1966   **Class:** Analgesic, mild; NSAIDs   **Prescription:** USA: Yes   **Controlled Drug:** USA: No; Canada: No   **Available as Generic:** Yes

Brand Names: *Meclofenamate:* Meclodium, Meclofenaf, Meclomen; *Mefenamic Acid:*✳Apo-Mefanamic, ✳Novo-Mefanamic Ponstel, ✳Ponstan

BENEFITS versus RISKS	
Possible Benefits	*Possible Risks*
EFFECTIVE RELIEF OF MILD TO MODERATE PAIN AND INFLAMMATION	Diarrhea (frequent for meclofenamate) Gastrointestinal pain, ulceration, bleeding Kidney damage Fluid retention Bone marrow depression (mefenamic acid) Hemolytic anemia (mefenamic acid) Systemic lupus erythematosus (mefenamic acid) Pancreatitis (mefenamic acid)

Author's Note: Risks more serious than diarrhea are rare.

▷ **Principal Uses**

As a Single Drug Product: Uses currently included in FDA-approved labeling: (1) Meclofenamate is used to relieve pain of osteoarthritis and rheumatoid arthritis; (2) mefenamic acid is used to relieve chronic pain, painful menstruation (dysmenorrhea) (meclofenamate as well) and general and post-operative pain; (3) meclofenamate also treats menorrhagia.

Other (unlabeled) generally accepted uses: (1) Meclofenamate is used to treat temporal arteritis and the nephrotic syndrome; (2) mefenamic acid is used to treat PMS and osteoarthritis (maximum 1 week).

How These Drugs Work: These drugs reduce prostaglandins (and related substances), chemicals involved in producing inflammation and pain.

Available Dosage Forms and Strengths

Meclofenamate (Meclomen):
    Capsules — 50 mg, 100 mg
    Gel capsules — 50 mg, 100 mg
Mefenamic acid (Ponstel):
    Capsule — 250 mg

▷ **Usual Adult Dosage Ranges:**

Meclofenamate: Osteoarthritis or rheumatoid arthritis—200 to 400 mg daily, in three or four equally divided doses. Total daily dose should not be more than 400 mg. Dysmenorrhea or menorrhagia—100 mg three times a day for up to 6 days.

Mefenamic acid: 500 mg initially and then 250 mg every 6 hours, taken with food for up to a week.

Note: Actual dose and schedule must be determined for each patient individually.

Conditions Requiring Dosing Adjustments

Liver Function: Dosing changes not presently recommended.

Kidney Function: Meclofenamate is removed by the kidneys, and a low starting dose and close patient monitoring are prudent. Mefenamic acid not to be used by patients with compromised kidneys.

▷ **Dosing Instructions:** Take with food or milk to prevent stomach irritation. Take with a full glass of water or milk and remain upright (do not lie down) for 30 minutes. Meclofenamate can be taken with an antacid such as Mylanta to help avoid stomach upset. DO NOT take mefenamic acid with antacids. The capsules may be opened to take them.

Usual Duration of Use: Meclofenamate: Use on a regular schedule for 2 to 3 weeks usually determines its effectiveness in arthritis therapy. The smallest effective dose should be used. Long-term use (months to years) requires physician supervision and periodic evaluation.

Mefenamic acid: Peak levels occur in up to 4 hours. Use beyond 7 days is not recommended.

▷ **These Drugs Should Not Be Taken If**
- you have had an allergic reaction to them previously.
- you get asthma or nasal polyps caused by aspirin.
- you have active peptic ulcer disease, regional enteritis, ulcerative colitis or gastrointestinal bleeding.
- you have a bleeding disorder or a blood cell disorder.
- you have severe impairment of kidney function (mefenamic acid).
- you have systemic lupus erythematosus (mefenamic acid).
- you have recently had pancreatitis (mefenamic acid).

▷ **Inform Your Physician Before Taking These Drugs If**
- you are allergic to aspirin or to other aspirin substitutes.
- you have a history of peptic ulcer disease, regional enteritis or ulcerative colitis.
- you have a history of any type of bleeding disorder.
- you have impaired liver or kidney function.
- you have high blood pressure or a history of heart failure.
- you take acetaminophen, aspirin or other aspirin substitutes; anticoagulants; oral antidiabetic drugs; or cortisonelike drugs.

Possible Side Effects (natural, expected and unavoidable drug actions)

Ringing in ears, fluid retention or drowsiness.

▷ **Possible Adverse Effects** (unusual, unexpected and infrequent reactions)

If any of the following develop, consult your physician promptly for guidance.

Mild Adverse Effects

Allergic reactions: skin rash, hives, itching.

Headache, dizziness, altered or blurred vision, depression—possible.

Mouth sores, indigestion, nausea, vomiting, diarrhea (10–33%, sometimes severe for meclofenamate).

Serious Adverse Effects

Allergic reactions: severe skin reactions, drug fever (see Glossary)—case reports.

Active peptic ulcer, with or without bleeding—possible.

Kidney damage with painful urination, bloody urine, reduced urine formation—case reports.

Liver damage—case reports.

Bone marrow depression (see Glossary): fatigue, weakness, fever, sore throat, abnormal bleeding or bruising—case reports (mefenamic acid, blood dyscrasias rare for meclofenamate).

Mefenamic acid is the NSAID most often associated with immune hemolytic anemia, and also can cause seizures, porphyria, liver damage, pancreatitis and systemic lupus erythematosus.

▷ **Possible Effects on Sexual Function:** None reported.

Possible Delayed Adverse Effects: Mild anemia due to "silent" blood loss from the stomach (less than that caused by aspirin).

Natural Diseases or Disorders That May Be Activated by These Drugs
Peptic ulcer disease, ulcerative colitis.

Possible Effects on Laboratory Tests
Complete blood cell counts: decreased red cells, hemoglobin, white cells and platelets—all rare.
For mefenamic acid, also add SLE test.

CAUTION
1. The smallest dose that offers improvement should be used.
2. May hide early signs of infection. Call your doctor if you think you are developing an infection.
3. Mefenamic acid should be used for a maximum of 7 days.

Precautions for Use
By Infants and Children: Safety and effectiveness for those under 14 years of age have not been established for meclofenamate and under 18 years of age for mefenamic acid.

By Those Over 60 Years of Age: Small doses are advisable. Watch for indications of liver or kidney toxicity, fluid retention, dizziness, confusion, stomach bleeding or diarrhea.

▷ **Advisability of Use During Pregnancy**
Pregnancy Category: Meclofenamate: D. Mefenamic acid: C. See Pregnancy Risk Categories at the back of this book.

Animal studies: Some minor birth defects reported in rodents for meclofenamate. Increased fetal resorption in rabbits with 2.5 times the human mefenamic acid dose.

Human studies: Adequate studies of pregnant women are not available.

The manufacturer does not recommend the use of meclofenamate during pregnancy.

Use of mefenamic acid in late pregnancy should be avoided. Ask your doctor for help regarding mefenamic acid use in pregnancy.

Advisability of Use If Breast-Feeding
Presence of these drugs in breast milk: Yes.
Avoid drug or refrain from nursing.

Habit-Forming Potential: None.

Effects of Overdose: Drowsiness, nausea, vomiting, diarrhea, marked agitation, irrational behavior, metabolic acidosis and seizures.

Possible Effects of Long-Term Use: Possible gastrointestinal damage and/or bleeding. Bone marrow depression for mefenamic acid.

Suggested Periodic Examinations While Taking These Drugs (at physician's discretion)
Complete blood cell counts.
Kidney function tests.
Complete eye examinations if vision is altered in any way.

▷ **While Taking These Drugs, Observe the Following**
Foods: No restrictions.
Herbal Medicines or Minerals: Ginseng, ginkgo, alfalfa, clove oil, feverfew, cinchona bark and garlic may also change clotting, so combining those herbals with these medicines is not recommended. NSAIDs may decrease feverfew effects. Hay flower, mistletoe herb and white mustard seed carry German Commission E monograph indications for arthritis. Talk to your doctor BEFORE combining any medicines.
Beverages: No restrictions. May be taken with milk.
▷ *Alcohol:* Use with caution. Alcohol and these drugs both irritate the stomach. May increase risk of stomach ulcers or bleeding.
Tobacco Smoking: No interactions expected. I advise everyone to quit smoking.
▷ *Other Drugs*
Meclofenamate *taken concurrently* with the following drugs may increase the risk of bleeding. Avoid these combinations:
- aspirin (various).
- dipyridamole (Persantine).
- ketorolac (Toradol).
- sulfinpyrazone (Anturane).
- valproic acid (Depakene).
- warfarin (Coumadin).
Mefenamic acid *taken concurrently* with
- aspirin, dipyridamole or sulfinpyrazone may result in increased bleeding risk.
- cyclosporine (Sandimmune) may result in increased cyclosporine levels and toxicity.
- magnesium-type antacids may cause rapid mefenamic acid toxicity.
Meclofenamate or mefenamic acid *taken concurrently* with
- alendronate (Fosamax) may increase risk of stomach irritation.
- angiotensin converting enzyme (ACE) inhibitors (see Drug Classes) may lead to decreased therapeutic benefits of the ACE.
- anticoagulants (Coumadin, etc.) increases the risk of bleeding; monitor INR (prothrombin time) and adjust dose accordingly.
- any high blood pressure medicine (beta or calcium channel blockers, thiazides, etc.; see Drug Classes) blunts BP benefits.
- diuretics (see Drug Classes) or other medicines for high blood pressure may result in decreased blood pressure control.
- enoxaparin (lovenox) or other low molecular weight heparins may result in increased surgical blood loss if patients receiving this combination undergo surgery.
- lithium (Lithobid, others) will increase blood lithium levels over time and may result in toxicity.

- methotrexate (Mexate) can result in serious methotrexate toxicity.
- ofloxacin (Floxin) may increase seizure risk.
- sulfonylureas (see Drug Classes) may increase hypoglycemia risk.
- tacrolimus (Prograf) may lead to sudden (acute) kidney (renal) failure.

▷ *Driving, Hazardous Activities:* This drug may cause dizziness or altered vision. Restrict activities as necessary.

Aviation Note: The use of these drugs *may be a disqualification* for piloting. Consult a designated Aviation Medical Examiner.

Exposure to Sun: No restrictions.

FENOPROFEN (fen oh PROH fen)

Please see the propionic acid (nonsteroidal anti-inflammatory drug) family profile.

FENTANYL (FEN ta nil)

Introduced: 1991   **Class:** Analgesic, strong   **Prescription:** USA: Yes
Controlled Drug: USA: C-II*; Canada: Yes   **Available as Generic:** USA: No; Canada: No

Brand Names: Actiq, Duragesic, ✦Innovar, Oralet, Sublimaze

BENEFITS versus RISKS	
Possible Benefits	*Possible Risks*
EFFECTIVE PAIN RELIEF	Habit-forming potential with
SKIN PATCH APPLICATION	prolonged use
NEEDED ONLY ONCE EVERY	Impairment of mental function
3 DAYS	Methemoglobinemia
EFFECTIVE RELIEF OF	Respiratory depression
BREAKTHROUGH CANCER PAIN	
WITH A MEDICINE TAKEN BY	
MOUTH (Actiq)	

▷ **Principal Uses**

As a Single Drug Product: Uses currently included in FDA-approved labeling: (1) Treatment of chronic pain; (2) Actiq approved for treatment of breakthrough cancer pain (contains the same medicine as Oralet) for people ALREADY taking or who are tolerant to opioid therapy for cancer pain. Other (unlabeled) generally accepted uses: None at present.

How This Drug Works: Acts at specific pain receptors (Mu agonist) to block pain.

Available Dosage Forms and Strengths

Buccal lozenge (Actiq) — 400 mcg, 600 mcg, 800 mcg, 1,200 mcg, 1,600 mcg
Transdermal patch — 2.5 mg, 5 mg, 7.5 mg, 10 mg
Lozenge on a handle — 200 mcg, 300 mcg, 400 mcg

Author's Note: Injectable forms are not presented in this profile.

*See Schedules of Controlled Drugs at the back of this book.

▷ **Recommended Dosage Ranges** (Actual dose and schedule must be determined for each patient individually.)

Infants and Children: Sucker form: Based on weight for those over 10 kg, 5–15 mcg/kg range. Those 40 kg or greater are given 400 mcg.

18 to 60 Years of Age:

Patch: Not indicated for patients 18 years old who weigh less than 50 kg (110 lb). In patients who have not been using opioids such as morphine, the 25 mcg per hour (2.5 mg) patch should be used. In people who used opioids previously, the amount needed to control pain on a 24-hour basis is calculated, converted to an equal amount of morphine (morphine equianalgesic dose) and then converted to fentanyl.

Oralet form: Used to treat pain/anxiety before surgery; 400 mcg for those with a body mass of 50 kg or more.

Buccal lozenge (Actiq)—used for patients with breakthrough cancer pain: 200 mcg (in cancer patients already receiving and who are tolerant to opioid treatment). They can subsequently be given another of the same dose (IF NEEDED) in 30 minutes. No more than 2 units should be taken for each breakthrough cancer pain episode. When the medicine is being added to the baseline opioid and a dose that works is found, patients should take no more than 4 units in a single day. Current pain treatment dictates that if more than 4 units are needed, the dose of the ongoing long-acting opioid should be increased.

Over 60 Years of Age: Should receive 25 mcg per hour (2.5 mg) patch, unless already receiving equivalent of 135 mg of oral morphine daily. Intravenous fentanyl clears more slowly in those over 60 than in younger patients. Watch carefully for overdose. If a decision is made to use the Actiq form, 200 mcg is used as a starting dose, and those over 75 generally require lower total doses than younger patients.

Conditions Requiring Dosing Adjustments

Liver Function: The dose must be decreased in liver compromise.

Kidney Function: In moderate to severe kidney failure, 75% of the usual dose. Dose reduced by 50% in severe kidney failure. People in end-stage kidney disease may be more sensitive to this medicine.

Dosing Instructions:

Patch: Take the patch from pouch. Remove stiff protective liner from sticky side of patch. Do not cut the system. Place sticky side on a hair-free, dry area (back, chest, side or upper arm). Avoid burned, irritated or oily areas. Wash hands after patch is applied. Apply a new patch to a different area after 3 days. Fold the old patch onto itself and flush it down the toilet. Avoid heat such as electric blankets or heating pads.

Lozenge or sucker: Slowly dissolve in the mouth. Do not bite or chew it. For Actiq, place medicine between cheek and lower gum, and rotate occasionally using the handle.

If the patient feels sleepy or otherwise has signs of excessive fentanyl effects, the medicine should be removed. Subsequent doses MUST be decreased if the above effects occur.

Usual Duration of Use: Regular use for 1 to 3 days determines benefits in pain control. Immediate-release morphine or similar drug should be available while this drug reaches peak effect (patch form). Long-term use (months) requires evaluation by your doctor. If you forget a dose: apply the missed patch as soon as you remember it, and then continue on the same three-day schedule or on the schedule that your doctor has prescribed. DO NOT double doses or apply two patches at the same time unless your doctor has told you to do so.

Typical Treatment Goals and Measurements (Outcomes and Markers)

Pain: Most clinicians treating pain use a device called an algometer to check your pain. This looks like a small ruler, but lets the clinician better understand your pain. The goals of treatment then relate to where the level of pain started (for example, a rating of 7 on a zero to ten scale) and what the cause of the pain was. Pain medicines may also be used together (in combination) in order to get the best result or outcome. If your pain control is not acceptable to YOU (remember, in hospitals and outpatient settings, etc., pain control is a patient right and the fifth vital sign) or if after applying the patch or using the sucker form, and if there is no other pain contingency, ask your doctor about a different rescue medicine. If pain treatment results are not what you expect, be sure to call your doctor as you may need a different medicine or combination. Cancer pain can vary, and it is not unusual to need different doses.

Possible Advantages of This Drug Effective pain relief with patch placement once every 3 days and no injections. Effective pain relief with a medicine used by mouth. Effective rescue pain relief.

▷ **This Drug Should Not Be Taken If**
- you had an allergic reaction to any form of it previously.
- you have had an allergic reaction to the adhesive in the patch.
- you are less than 12 years old. Oralet should NOT be used in children weighing less than 22 pounds (10 kg).
- you are at home and a Fentanyl Oralet is prescribed—these are only to be used in hospital settings.
- you weigh less than 50 kg and are less than 18 years old.
- you have mild pain.
- you have acute or postoperative pain without opportunity for proper dose adjustment.

▷ **Inform Your Physician Before Taking This Drug If**
- you have liver or kidney compromise.
- you have chronic lung disease (such as COPD).
- you have an abnormally slow heartbeat or other heart disease.
- you develop a high fever.
- you have not taken narcotic pain medicines before and you are given a dose more than 25 mcg per hour.
- you take, or took in the last two weeks, an MAO inhibitor (see Drug Classes).
- you have a brain tumor or seizure disorder.
- you are elderly or debilitated.
- a benzodiazepine (such as diazepam or Valium—see Drug Classes) has been prescribed for you.
- you are anemic or have heart disease.
- you have a history of alcoholism or drug abuse.
- you take prescription or nonprescription drugs not discussed with your doctor when fentanyl was prescribed.

Possible Side Effects (natural, expected and unavoidable drug actions)
Constipation, dry mouth.
Sleepiness (somnolence) or euphoria—infrequent to frequent.

▷ **Possible Adverse Effects** (unusual, unexpected and infrequent reactions)
If any of the following develop, consult your physician promptly for guidance.

Mild Adverse Effects
Allergic reactions: skin rash and itching.
Blurred vision or amblyopia—rare to infrequent.
Nausea or vomiting—infrequent.
Urinary retention—infrequent.
Tremor or muscular rigidity—possible.
Sweating or itching (transdermal)—infrequent to frequent.

Serious Adverse Effects
Allergic reactions: exfoliative dermatitis and/or anaphylactic reactions—case reports.
Arrhythmias—rare.
Paranoid reaction, depersonalization, speech problems (aphasia)—rare, dose-related.
Increased or decreased blood pressure—possible.
Seizures or hallucinations—case reports.
Methemoglobinemia or porphyrias—rare.
Paresthesias—rare.
Respiratory depression (this effect may last longer than the pain-relieving effect)—dose-related and possible.

▷ **Possible Effects on Sexual Function:** Impotence and blunted orgasm sensation in men. Irregular menstrual periods and blunted orgasm sensation in women.

Possible Delayed Adverse Effects: Dependence and tolerance.

Possible Effects on Laboratory Tests
Screening tests for opioids: positive.

CAUTION
1. Extreme caution should be used if this drug is combined with other opioids, narcotic drugs, benzodiazepines or alcohol.
2. May cause serious constipation in older patients. Many clinicians use an appropriate drug to PREVENT constipation in older patients.
3. Do not expose the patch site to external sources of heat such as heating pads or electric blankets, as an increased rate of drug release may occur.
4. If there are children living in the same house as someone using Actiq, great care must be taken to avoid accidentally having a child take one of the lozenges, as the dose would be fatal. A child-resistant container is provided in case a lozenge is not fully taken.
5. If this medicine is to be stopped, gradual withdrawal is required.

Precautions for Use
By Infants and Children: Safety and effectiveness for those under 12 years of age are not established.
By Those Over 60 Years of Age: The 2.5-mg patch should NOT be used as a starting dose unless you are already taking more than 135 mg of morphine

daily. Those with cardiac, respiratory, kidney or liver compromise or dehydration should be given low doses and carefully monitored.

▷ **Advisability of Use During Pregnancy**

Pregnancy Category: C, D if used in high doses when the baby is born or for prolonged periods. See Pregnancy Risk Categories at the back of this book.

Animal studies: Some fetal death data with intravenous use in rats.

Human studies: Adequate studies of pregnant women are not available.
Ask your doctor for guidance.

Advisability of Use If Breast-Feeding

Presence of this drug in breast milk: Yes.
Avoid drug or refrain from nursing.

Habit-Forming Potential: Fentanyl is a Schedule II narcotic and can cause
dependence resembling morphine dependence. Physical and psychological
dependence and tolerance can occur with repeated use.

Effects of Overdose: Dizziness, amnesia and stupor. Respiratory depression and
apnea may occur.

Possible Effects of Long-Term Use: Tolerance and physical or psychological
dependence.

Suggested Periodic Examinations While Taking This Drug (at physician's discretion)

Liver function tests.
Check for constipation.

▷ **While Taking This Drug, Observe the Following**

Foods: No restrictions.

Herbal Medicines or Minerals: Valerian and kava kava may interact additively
(drowsiness). Avoid these combinations. St. John's wort can change
(inducing or increasing) P450 3A4 or 2D6 enzymes, blunting the effects of
fentanyl. Talk to your doctor BEFORE you combine any herbal medicines
with fentanyl.

Beverages: No restrictions.

▷ *Alcohol:* **DO NOT DRINK ALCOHOL** while you are taking this drug—leads to
additive loss of mental status, respiratory depression and confusion.

Tobacco Smoking: No interactions expected. I advise everyone to quit smoking.

Marijuana Smoking: Additive adverse effects; however, marijuana may block
the vomiting effect of fentanyl.

▷ *Other Drugs*

Fentanyl may *increase* the effects of
• benzodiazepines such as diazepam (Valium) and alprazolam (Xanax).
• central nervous system depressants such as opiates, barbiturates, tranquilizers and tricyclic antidepressants.

Fentanyl *taken concurrently* with
• amiodarone (Cordarone) may result in heart (cardiac) toxicity.
• clonidine (Catapres, others) may result in greater than expected fentanyl
effects. The fentanyl dose may need to be decreased if these medicines are
to be combined.
• MAO inhibitors (see Drug Classes) may worsen the lowering of blood pressure and depression of breathing seen with fentanyl.
• rifabutin (Mycobutin) may decrease pain control by fentanyl.

- ritonavir (Norvir) and perhaps other protease inhibitors (see Drug Classes) can lead to major fentanyl toxicity.
- sibutramine (Meridia) may increase risk of serotonin syndrome. DO NOT COMBINE.
- sildenafil (Viagra) may lead to changes in sildenafil or in fentanyl levels. Caution is advised (both drugs are removed by CYP450 3A4).

▷ *Driving, Hazardous Activities:* This drug may cause drowsiness, sedation and respiratory depression. Restrict activities as necessary.

Aviation Note: The use of this drug *is a disqualification* for piloting. Consult a designated Aviation Medical Examiner.

Exposure to Sun: No restrictions.

Discontinuation: Once the patch is removed, fentanyl will still be released from the site for 17 hours or more. If pain medicine is still needed, the alternative should be substituted once the fentanyl level is low enough. The level from the lozenge declines more rapidly, and replacement medicine is required sooner if the fentanyl lozenge is stopped. If the lozenge has been used routinely, the drug should be slowly tapered, NOT stopped abruptly.

FILGRASTIM (fil GRA stim)

Other Name: Recombinant G-CSF

Introduced: 1991　**Class:** Hematopoietic agent　**Prescription:** USA: Yes　**Controlled Drug:** USA: No; Canada: No　**Available as Generic:** USA: No; Canada: No

Brand Name: Neupogen

BENEFITS versus RISKS	
Possible Benefits	*Possible Risks*
PREVENTION OF INFECTIONS DUE TO LOWERED WHITE BLOOD CELL COUNTS: FOLLOWING CHEMOTHERAPY FOLLOWING BONE MARROW TRANSPLANT IN PATIENTS WITH CHRONIC OR CYCLIC NEUTROPENIA INCREASED BLOOD CELLS IN AIDS PATIENTS CORRECTION OF DRUG-INDUCED LOWERING OF WHITE BLOOD CELLS	Bone pain Changes in heart waves

▷ **Principal Uses**

As a Single Drug Product: Uses currently included in FDA-approved labeling: (1) Used to help white blood cell counts recover after chemotherapy and bone marrow transplants; (2) used subcutaneously or intravenously to reduce or prevent low white blood cell counts that occur after cancer chemotherapy; (3) treats patients who have an absence of white blood cells at birth; (4) used to help patients with Kostmann syndrome have improved white blood cell counts; (5) used to help patients who have low white blood cell counts (neutropenia) of unknown cause (idiopathic); (6) used to treat low white blood cells (neutropenia) in HIV-positive people or in those with AIDS; (7) used in adults to decrease the time it takes for their white blood cells (neutrophils) to recover from chemotherapy treatment for sudden (acute) myelogenous leukemia; (8) used in adults to move blood-forming cells (hematopoietic progenitors) into the blood stream (peripheral blood) so that they can be collected by leukopharesis.

Other (unlabeled) generally accepted uses: (1) Helps patients recover from a particular kind of lack of white blood cells (agranulocytosis) that has been caused by medicines (drug-induced); (2) used in AIDS (orphan drug status) patients (taking ganciclovir) to help restore white blood cell counts; (3) used to treat patients with severe long-term (chronic) low white blood cell counts; (4) used to treat patients with abnormally low white blood cell and neutrophil counts (myelodysplastic syndrome).

How This Drug Works: Regulates proliferation and release of early (progenitor) forms of white blood cells. Can tell bone marrow to increase rate in which it makes white blood cells. Filgrastim may also work with other factors to increase the production of blood platelets.

Available Dosage Forms and Strengths

Solution for injection — 300 mcg/ml (supplied as a 300- or 480-mcg vial)

How to Store

The prepared solution should be stored at 36 to 46 degrees F (2 to 8 degrees C). This medicine should not be frozen. Some centers draw up a 7-day supply of syringes that are then stored in a refrigerator.

▷ **Recommended Dosage Ranges** (Actual dose and schedule must be determined for each patient individually.)

Infants and Children: Studied doses of 0.6 to 120 mcg per kg of body mass per day for up to 3 years have been well tolerated in children 3 months to 18 years of age. In chronic low white blood cell counts (chronic neutropenia), doses of 5 to 10 mcg per kg of body mass per day have been used. Safety and efficacy in pediatric patients with neutropenia that is a result of one's own immune system working against you (autoimmune) have not been established.

18 to 60 Years of Age: Patients having bone marrow destroyed (myeloablative treatment) and getting a bone marrow transplant: Wait 24 hours after chemo was given and 24 hours after bone marrow transplant. Then 10 mcg per kg of body mass per day to start. Ongoing daily dosing is adjusted to increase of white blood cells (absolute neutrophil count).

Patients receiving bone marrow suppression should wait until 24 hours after or before the chemotherapy is given. Filgrastim is started with 5 mcg per kg of body mass per day, increased by 5 mcg per kg per day for each cycle of chemotherapy. Dosing is based on severity of white blood cell count decrease (nadir) and how long lowered white cell (absolute neutrophil) count lasts. Drug can be given daily for up to 14 days.

Guidelines released by the Infectious Disease Society of America talk about using this medicine (on a non-routine basis) to reverse low white blood cell counts (neutropenia) associated with HIV infection. The dose noted there was 5–10 mcg/square meter per day. The use period listed was two to four weeks.

Over 60 Years of Age: Same as 18 to 60 years of age.

Conditions Requiring Dosing Adjustments

Liver Function: Not significantly involved in the elimination of this drug.

Kidney Function: Roughly 90% of a given filgrastim dose is eliminated by the kidneys. Changes in dosing are not defined.

▷ **Dosing Instructions:** The solution in the reconstituted vial should be colorless and clear. Once your doctor or nurse has taught you how to inject the medicine:

- Make certain the solution has not expired (check the expiration date).
- Make certain that albumin (human) has been added to the 2 mg per ml Neupogen to protect it from attaching (adsorbing) to the plastic material of the container.
- Make certain you have the correct kind of syringe (talk this over with your doctor, nurse or nurse practitioner).
- Follow the provided patient instructions carefully.
- If you are using a syringe, make certain you inject the medicine under the skin (subcutaneously or Sub Q), not into a vein.
- This medicine can also be given intravenously over a period of 15 to 30 minutes.
- If you forget a dose: call your doctor and ask what he or she would like you to do.

Usual Duration of Use: Ten to 14 days of regular use may be needed to see benefits in correcting low white blood cell (absolute neutrophil) counts after chemotherapy. Bone marrow transplant patients may take still longer to respond. Long-term problems with white blood cells (such as chronic neutropenia) may require years of therapy. Long-term use requires periodic evaluation of response and dose adjustment. Consult your physician on a regular basis.

Typical Treatment Goals and Measurements (Outcomes and Markers)

Neutropenia: Most clinicians will check white blood cell counts with differentials two to three times per week and adjust dosing to results. Additionally, bone marrow tests (aspiration) will be done periodically to check granulocyte-macrophage counts, morphology, myeloid/erythroid ratios and even colony forming unit counts.

Possible Advantages of This Drug

Effective recombinant product with few side effects.

▷ **This Drug Should Not Be Taken If**

- you had an allergic reaction to it previously.
- you have a known allergy to products derived from E. coli (a bacteria).

▷ **Inform Your Physician Before Taking This Drug If**

- you have a history of gout or psoriasis.
- you have received chemotherapy within the last 24 hours.
- you have a history of heart problems (heart rhythm should be closely monitored).
- you have a history of leukemia (myeloid type). The safety and efficacy of this medicine are not established in that condition.
- you have a history of cancer (with myeloid characteristics). There is a possibility that this drug may act as a growth factor for these tumors. Use,

however, in a small number of leukemia patients has not resulted in worsening of their leukemia.

- you have an excessive increase in white blood cells (leukocytosis).

Possible Side Effects (natural, expected and unavoidable drug actions)
Pain on injection.
Bone pain (up to 33%).

▷ **Possible Adverse Effects** (unusual, unexpected and infrequent reactions)
If any of the following develop, consult your physician promptly for guidance.

Mild Adverse Effects
Allergic reactions: skin rash or itching—infrequent.
Mild decreases in blood pressure or increases in uric acid—case reports.
Drug-induced fever—infrequent to frequent.
Nausea and anorexia—rare.
Irritation of the eye (iridocyclitis, conjunctival erythema)—case reports.
Enlargement of the spleen: reported in patients with chronic lowering of the white blood cells (chronic neutropenia)—frequent, though asymptomatic in these patients.

Serious Adverse Effects
Allergic reactions: anaphylaxis—case report.
Sweet syndrome (acute neutrophilic dermatosis)—possible.
Worsening of psoriasis—case report.
Low oxygen in the blood (hypoxemia)—very rare.
Depression of part of the heart action (ST depression)—rare to infrequent.
Myocardial infarction (heart attack) happened in 11 of 375 cancer patients in one study, but the relationship to filgrastim is unclear.
Potential for this medicine to act as a growth factor for certain cancers (malignancies of the myeloid type)—possible.
Capillary leak syndrome—possible, case reports.
Respiratory distress syndrome in patients with serious (septic) infections, because white blood cells may travel to the infected area—possible.
Hypothyroidism—case report.

▷ **Possible Effects on Sexual Function:** None reported.

Possible Delayed Adverse Effects: Increased uric acid. Formation of neutralizing antibodies.

▷ **Adverse Effects That May Mimic Natural Diseases or Disorders**
None reported.

Natural Diseases or Disorders That May Be Activated by This Drug
Gout.

Possible Effects on Laboratory Tests
Absolute neutrophil count: increased.
Alkaline phosphatase: increased markedly.
Uric acid: increased mildly.
Lactate dehydrogenase (LDH): increased.
Formation of neutralizing antibodies—possible.

CAUTION
1. Bone pain may be prevented by taking acetaminophen (Tylenol, others) BEFORE this medicine is injected.

2. Call your doctor if you have chills, fever or any other sign of infection.
3. Be certain to follow up with your laboratory testing as scheduled.
4. The solution in the vial should be clear. Do not inject any discolored or cloudy solution.
5. Make sure you have the correct kind of syringe before you inject this medicine.
6. This medicine can be given intravenously when it is appropriately prepared. If your doctor has instructed you on how to give yourself an injection using a syringe, the medicine should be given under the skin. Be certain you understand the technique.
7. Always change the site in which you inject this medicine, as your doctor instructed.

Precautions for Use
By Infants and Children: This medicine has been used in children with long-term lowering of white blood cell counts (chronic neutropenia) in doses of 5 to 10 mcg per kg of body mass per day.
By Those Over 60 Years of Age: No specific precautions.

▷ ### Advisability of Use During Pregnancy
Pregnancy Category: C. See Pregnancy Risk Categories at the back of this book.
Animal studies: In rabbits given 80 mcg per kg of body mass per day (very high doses), increased abortion and death of embryos were observed.
Human studies: Information from adequate studies of pregnant women is not available.
Ask your doctor for help with this benefit-to-risk decision.

Advisability of Use If Breast-Feeding
Presence of this drug in breast milk: Unknown.
Ask your doctor for guidance.

Habit-Forming Potential: None.

Effects of Overdose: No maximum tolerated dose has been identified.

Possible Effects of Long-Term Use: Enlarged spleens may occur in up to 25% of patients (splenomegaly) with severe chronic neutropenia. Skin rashes may occur in up to 6% of patients.

Suggested Periodic Examinations While Taking This Drug (at physician's discretion)
Complete blood cell counts and platelet counts should be obtained prior to chemotherapy and twice weekly during filgrastim therapy.

▷ ### While Taking This Drug, Observe the Following
Foods: No restrictions.
Herbal Medicines or Minerals: Echinacea: Some patients use echinacea to attempt to boost their immune systems. Unfortunately, use of echinacea is not recommended in people with damaged immune systems. This herb may also actually weaken any immune system if it is used too often or for too long a time. Caution: St. John's wort may also cause extreme reactions to the sun. Additive photosensitivity may be possible.
Beverages: No restrictions.
▷ *Alcohol:* No restrictions.
Tobacco Smoking: No interactions expected. I advise everyone to quit smoking.

▷ *Other Drugs*
   Filgrastim *taken concurrently* with
   - lithium (Lithobid, others) may (in theory) result in additive release of white blood cells.
   - topotecan (Hycamtin) may cause extended low white blood cells.
   - vincristine (Oncovin) has led to nerve problems (peripheral neuropathy).
▷ *Driving, Hazardous Activities:* No restrictions presently attributed to this medicine.
   Aviation Note: The use of this drug is ***probably not a disqualification*** for piloting. Consult a designated Aviation Medical Examiner.
   Exposure to Sun: SEVERE intolerance of sunlight (photophobia) has been a treatment-limiting factor. **Caution:** See the "Herbal Medicines" note on St. John's wort above.
   Occurrence of Unrelated Illness: Report development of chills, fever or other signs or symptoms of infection immediately to your doctor.
   Discontinuation: In people taking bone marrow suppressing drugs: Filgrastim is usually stopped when white blood cell (absolute neutrophil count) reaches 10,000 per cubic mm (once the lowest white blood cell count was reached for the chemotherapy given).
   In people taking bone marrow destroying medicine who then have a bone marrow transplant: The drug is started as described. If white blood cell count reaches 1,000 per cubic mm, dose is decreased to 5 mcg per kg of body mass per day. Once white cell count reaches 1,000 per cubic mm for 6 consecutive days, filgrastim can be stopped.
   Special Storage Instructions: This drug should be stored at 36 to 46 degrees F (2 to 8 degrees C) once it has been reconstituted. Care should be taken **not to shake** the prepared drug, as it may lose activity. Care should also be taken **not to freeze** the prepared medicine, as it will clump and lose therapeutic activity.
   Observe the Following Expiration Times: Once the medicine is prepared, it is stable for 1 day (24 hours) if it is refrigerated. If the drug is stored at room temperature, it is stable for 6 hours. Medicine left at room temperature for more than 6 hours should be returned.

FINASTERIDE (fin ASS tur ide)

Introduced: 1992   **Class:** 5-alpha reductase inhibitor   **Prescription:** USA: Yes   **Controlled Drug:** USA: No; Canada: No   **Available as Generic:** USA: No; Canada: No
Brand Names: Propecia, Proscar

BENEFITS versus RISKS	
Possible Benefits	*Possible Risks*
NONSURGICAL TREATMENT OF SYMPTOMATIC BENIGN PROSTATIC HYPERPLASIA	Impotence (small percentage) Decreased libido (small percentage) Gynecomastia (rare)
Shrinkage of prostatic tissue and increase in urine flow	
RETENTION OF HAIR OR INCREASED HAIR GROWTH IN MEN	

▷ **Principal Uses**

As a Single Drug Product: Uses currently included in FDA-approved labeling: (1) Treats symptomatic benign prostatic hyperplasia (BPH)—peak decrease in prostate size has occurred after 6 months of therapy; (2) approved to decrease risk of urine retention and need for prostate surgery in BPH; (3) used as Propecia brand (1 mg) to retain or regrow hair.

Other (unlabeled) generally accepted uses: Reduces excessive hair in women (hirsutism).

How This Drug Works: Blocks an enzyme (5-alpha reductase) that decreases change of testosterone to dihydrotestosterone (in liver); this causes the prostate to shrink. Symptoms such as urgency and trouble urinating improve. Inhibiting 5-alpha reductase also leads to hair growth.

Available Dosage Forms and Strengths

Proscar tablets — 5 mg

Propecia tablets — 1 mg

▷ **Recommended Dosage Ranges** (Actual dose and schedule must be determined for each patient individually.)

Infants and Children: Not indicated.

12 to 60 Years of Age: Symptomatic benign prostatic hyperplasia often does not occur in the younger end of this adult dosing range; however, the dose for this age range is 5 mg each day, taken by mouth.

Hair-restoring agent: 1 mg daily dose.

Over 60 Years of Age: Same as 12 to 60 years of age, unless liver function has decreased.

Conditions Requiring Dosing Adjustments

Liver Function: People with abnormal liver tests should be closely followed by their doctors.

Kidney Function: No changes needed.

▷ **Dosing Instructions:** May be taken without regard to food. Food changes time to peak blood concentration only. If you forget a dose: Take the missed dose as soon as you remember it, unless it is nearly time for your next dose—if that is the case, omit the missed dose and take the next scheduled dose right on schedule. DO NOT double doses.

Usual Duration of Use: Use on a regular schedule for at least 6 months is needed to see this drug's peak benefit in shrinking the prostate and decreasing symptoms. Use for 1 year may be required to demonstrate hair regrowth.

Typical Treatment Goals and Measurements (Outcomes and Markers)

Hair loss: Most clinicians use hair counts, or lack of further hair loss, to define results. Use for that indication will be ongoing.

BPH: Urologists use improvement in urinary flow as well as subjective measures such as relief of difficulty urinating and lowered feeling of urgency. Digital rectal examination for prostate cancer should be done periodically.

Possible Advantages of This Drug: May give you symptomatic relief of benign prostatic hyperplasia (BPH) without surgery. May be more effective than other available agents in helping hair regrowth. No clinically significant drug interactions.

▷ **This Drug Should Not Be Taken If**
* you had an allergic reaction to it previously and you are a woman or child.
* you are pregnant.

▷ **Inform Your Physician Before Taking This Drug If**
* you have impaired liver function or liver disease.
* you are a woman or a child.
* you have kidney problems of any nature.
* your sexual partner is pregnant.

Possible Side Effects (natural, expected and unavoidable drug actions)

May or may not increase testosterone levels; however, the significance of this effect is not known.

▷ **Possible Adverse Effects** (unusual, unexpected and infrequent reactions)

If any of the following develop, consult your physician promptly for guidance.

Mild Adverse Effects

Allergic reactions: skin rash, hives—rare.

Plasma testosterone—decreased.

Serious Adverse Effects

Allergic reactions: hypersensitivity reactions—case reports.

Handling Propecia or Proscar tablets by pregnant females may harm male fetuses.

▷ **Possible Effects on Sexual Function:** Gynecomastia (most frequent adverse effect)—rare.

Impotence, decreased libido or decreased volume of ejaculate—infrequent.

Adverse sexual effects may resolve in more than 60% of patients who continue this medication.

Possible Delayed Adverse Effects: Possible enlargement of male breast tissue (gynecomastia).

Possible Effects on Laboratory Tests

Decreased PSA (prostate specific antigen).

CAUTION

1. A digital rectal exam and other prostate cancer exams are prudent before this medicine is started. PSA will be falsely decreased by this medicine.
2. If you have a change in liver function, inform your doctor.
3. If your sexual partner is pregnant, avoid exposing your partner to your semen. Exposure to finasteride-containing semen may cause genital abnormalities in male offspring.

Precautions for Use

By Infants and Children: Safety and effectiveness for infants and children are not established.

By Those Over 60 Years of Age: No specific precautions other than changes related to decreased liver function.

▷ **Advisability of Use During Pregnancy**

Pregnancy Category: X. See Pregnancy Risk Categories at the back of this book.

Animal studies: When administered to pregnant rats, the male offspring developed hypospadias. The offspring experienced decreased prostatic and seminal vesicular weight, slow preputial separation and transient nipple problems.

Human studies: Contraindicated in women who are pregnant or who plan to become pregnant. Women who are pregnant must avoid exposure to crushed tablets and semen of a sexual partner who is on finasteride.

Ask your physician for guidance.

Advisability of Use If Breast-Feeding

Refrain from nursing if you have been exposed to finasteride or finasteride-containing semen.

Habit-Forming Potential: None.

Effects of Overdose: Multiple doses of up to 80 mg per day have been taken without adverse effect.

Possible Effects of Long-Term Use: Adverse effects of long-term use are similar to short-term use effects.

Suggested Periodic Examinations While Taking This Drug (at physician's discretion)

Patients should be monitored for signs and symptoms of hypersensitivity.

Patients should be monitored for improvement in symptoms of BPH.

▷ **While Taking This Drug, Observe the Following**

Foods: This medicine is best taken on an empty stomach.

Herbal Medicines or Minerals: Saw palmetto works by anti-androgenic and anti-inflammatory actions. The combination of this herb and finasteride has not been studied, but both drugs appear to work by different mechanisms. Talk to your doctor before combining. Autumn crocus should be avoided in alopecia.

Beverages: No restrictions.

▷ *Alcohol:* No restrictions.

Tobacco Smoking: No interactions expected. I advise everyone to quit smoking.

Marijuana Smoking: No interactions expected.

▷ *Other Drugs*

Finasteride *taken concurrently* with

- tirilazad (Freedox) will be increased by up to 29% if combined with finasteride. Caution is advised.

▷ *Driving, Hazardous Activities:* No restrictions.

Aviation Note: No restrictions.

Exposure to Sun: No restrictions.

Special Storage Instructions Keep at room temperature. Avoid exposure to extreme humidity.

FLUCONAZOLE (flu KOHN a zohl)

Introduced: 1985   **Class:** Antifungal (triazole)   **Prescription:** USA: Yes
Controlled Drug: USA: No; Canada: No   **Available as Generic:** USA: No; Canada: No
Brand Names: Apo-Fluconazole, Diflucan, Nu-Flucon

BENEFITS versus RISKS

Possible Benefits	*Possible Risks*
EFFECTIVE PREVENTION OF YEAST (CANDIDIASIS) INFECTIONS	Severe skin reactions
	Possible liver damage

EFFECTIVE PREVENTION OF
  YEAST (CANDIDIASIS)
  INFECTIONS
EFFECTIVE TREATMENT AND
SUPPRESSION OF CRYPTOCOCCAL
  MENINGITIS
EFFECTIVE TREATMENT OF
  CANDIDA INFECTIONS OF THE
  MOUTH, THROAT AND
  ESOPHAGUS
EFFECTIVE TREATMENT OF
  SYSTEMIC *CANDIDA* INFECTIONS
EFFECTIVE SINGLE-DOSE
  TREATMENT OF VAGINAL
  YEAST INFECTIONS

▷ **Principal Uses**

As a Single Drug Product: Uses currently included in FDA-approved labeling: (1) Candida (yeast) infections of the mouth, throat and esophagus (may be AIDS related); (2) systemic Candida infections: lungs, peritonitis, urinary tract infections (may be AIDS related); (3) treats vaginal yeast infections.

Other (unlabeled) generally accepted uses: (1) Prevention of yeast infections in patients with low white blood cell counts or cancer or those taking steroids; (2) treatment and suppression of cryptococcal meningitis; (3) treatment of some fungal eye infections (endophthalmitis); (4) single-dose treatment of vaginal yeast infections; (5) treatment of Aspergillus pneumonia; (6) treatment of candidal urinary tract infections; (7) used to treat some fungal infections that may occur in people who have received transplanted organs; (8) may be a drug of choice for Sporothrix schenckii infections or for prevention of relapse of some Histoplasma infections.

How This Drug Works: By damaging cell walls and blocking essential cell enzymes, this drug inhibits cell growth and reproduction (with low drug concentrations) and destroys fungal cells (with high drug concentrations).

Available Dosage Forms and Strengths
      Injection — 2 mg in 1 ml
      Tablets — 50 mg, 100 mg, 150 mg, 200 mg
  Oral suspension — 10 mg in 5 ml,
         — 40 mg in 5 ml

▷ **Recommended Dosage Ranges** (Actual dose and schedule must be determined for each patient individually.)

Infants and Children: From 3 to 13 years of age: 3–6 mg per kg of body mass daily, depending on the kind and site of infection.

Cryptococcal meningitis: 12 mg per kg on the first day and then 6 mg per kg daily for 10 to 12 weeks after cerebrospinal fluid culture becomes negative.

13 to 60 Years of Age: Cryptococcal meningitis: 400 mg once daily until improvement occurs; then 200 to 400 mg once daily for 10 to 12 weeks after cerebrospinal fluid culture becomes negative.

Suppression of cryptococcal meningitis: 200 mg once daily.

Candida infections of mouth and throat: 200 mg first day and then 100 mg once daily for 2 weeks.

Candida infection of the esophagus: 200 mg first day and then 100 mg once daily for at least 3 weeks; treat for 2 weeks after all signs of infection are gone. Doses up to 400 mg daily may be used. Some patients with chronic mucocutaneous *Candida* infections have benefited from 50 mg/day of this medicine.

Systemic *Candida* infections: 400 mg daily for at least 4 weeks; treating for 2 weeks after all symptoms of infection are gone.

Vaginal yeast infections (*Candida*): One 150-mg tablet by mouth.

Over 60 Years of Age: Same as 13 to 60, adjusted if kidneys are impaired.

Conditions Requiring Dosing Adjustments

Liver Function: Caution: Rare cause of hepatitis.

Kidney Function: Mild to moderate failure—usual dose every 48 hours. In severe kidney failure—half (50%) of usual dose every 48 hours.

▷ **Dosing Instructions:** The tablet may be crushed; may be taken with or after food to reduce stomach upset. Use a measuring spoon for suspension forms. If you forget a dose: take the missed dose as soon as you remember it—unless it is nearly time for your next dose. If that is the case, skip the missed dose and take the next pill right on schedule. DO NOT double doses. Fungal infections will return if you do not take this medicine as long as you are supposed to.

Usual Duration of Use: Use on a regular schedule for 2 to 4 weeks is usually needed to see this drug's benefit in controlling candidal or cryptococcal infections. Actual cures or long-term suppression often requires continual treatment for many months. May be continuous therapy in AIDS patients.

Typical Treatment Goals and Measurements (Outcomes and Markers)

Candida infections: Goals for treatment of infections include resolution of signs and symptoms (such as sore throat and white coloration in candidal throat infections), return of white blood cell count and differential to normal (for systemic infections), and failure of the infection to return in prophylactic use.

Currently a Drug of Choice

For maintenance therapy to prevent relapse following control of AIDS-related candidal esophagitis. Because oral absorption is so complete, oral and intravenous dosing are the same.

▷ **This Drug Should Not Be Taken If**
- you have had an allergic reaction to it previously.
- you have active liver disease.

▷ **Inform Your Physician Before Taking This Drug If**
- you are allergic to clotrimazole, itraconazole, ketoconazole or miconazole.
- you have impaired liver or kidney function.
- you are currently taking any other drugs.
- you tend to have low blood potassium.
- you get a skin rash while taking this medicine.

Mild Adverse Effects
  Allergic reactions: skin rash—rare.
  Hair loss—very rare with usual doses. Reversible hair loss (alopecia) may be
    more common with high doses of fluconazole given for 2 months or longer.
  Headache—rare.
  Nausea, vomiting, stomach pain, diarrhea—frequent.
Serious Adverse Effects
  Allergic reactions: severe dermatitis (Stevens-Johnson syndrome)—very rare.
  Anaphylactic reactions—case reports.
  Liver toxicity—rare.
  Abnormally low platelet counts: abnormal bruising/bleeding or low white
    blood cell counts—rare.
  Seizures or adrenal suppression—case reports, rare.
  Low blood potassium (hypokalemia)—case reports in 3 acute myeloid
    leukemia patients.
  Abnormal heart rhythm (torsade de pointes)—case report.

▷ **Possible Effects on Sexual Function:** Amenorrhea—one case report.

Possible Delayed Adverse Effects: Liver toxicity.

▷ **Adverse Effects That May Mimic Natural Diseases or Disorders**
  Possible liver reaction may suggest viral hepatitis.

Possible Effects on Laboratory Tests
  Blood platelet counts: decreased.
  Liver function tests: increased liver enzymes (ALT/GPT, AST/GOT and alka-
    line phosphatase), increased bilirubin.
  Blood potassium: lowered—case reports.

Precautions for Use
  By Infants and Children: Safety and effectiveness for those under 13 years of
    age are not established.
  By Those Over 60 Years of Age: Age-related decrease in kidney function may
    require adjustment of dose.

▷ **Advisability of Use During Pregnancy**
  Pregnancy Category: C. See Pregnancy Risk Categories at the back of this book.
  Animal studies: Rat studies revealed significant abnormalities in bone growth
    and development.
  Human studies: Adequate studies of pregnant women are not available.
    Use this drug only if clearly needed. Ask your doctor for help.

Advisability of Use If Breast-Feeding
  Presence of this drug in breast milk: Yes.
  Avoid drug or refrain from nursing.

Habit-Forming Potential: None.

Effects of Overdose: Possible nausea, vomiting, diarrhea.

Possible Effects of Long-Term Use: None reported.

Suggested Periodic Examinations While Taking This Drug (at physician's dis-
    cretion)
  Liver and kidney function tests.

▷ **While Taking This Drug, Observe the Following**
  Foods: Caution is advised regarding grapefruit or grapefruit juice. Avoid eating
    grapefruit for an hour after taking this medicine.

Herbal Medicines or Minerals: Echinacea: Some patients use echinacea to attempt to boost their immune systems. Unfortunately, use of echinacea is not recommended in people with damaged immune systems. This herb may also actually weaken any immune system if it is used too often or for too long a time.

Beverages: Grapefruit juice should be avoided. May be taken with milk.

▷ *Alcohol:* No interactions expected.

Tobacco Smoking: No interactions expected. I advise everyone to quit smoking.

▷ *Other Drugs*

Fluconazole may ***increase*** the effects of

- benzodiazepines (see Drug Classes).
- celecoxib (Celebrex).
- cyclosporine (Sandimmune).
- dofetilide (Tikosyn).
- felodipine (Plendil).
- oral antidiabetic drugs (chlorpropamide, glipizide, glyburide, tolbutamide, others) and cause hypoglycemia; check sugar levels carefully.
- phenytoin (Dilantin, etc.) or fosphenytoin (Cerebyx) and cause
- phenytoin or fosphenytoin toxicity; monitor blood levels.
- serolimus (Rapamune), and tacrolimus (Prograf). Serolimus and tacrolimus levels should be used to guide dosing.
- triazolam (Halcion), leading to toxicity.
- tricyclic antidepressants (see Drug Classes).
- trimetrexate (Neutrexin).
- warfarin (Coumadin) and cause unwanted bleeding. Dosing changes and more frequent INRs are prudent.
- zidovudine (AZT) and result in toxicity. The zidovudine dose may need to be decreased if this combination is to be continued.
- zolpidem (Ambien) and result in toxicity. The zolpidem dose may need to be decreased if this combination is to be continued.

The following drugs may ***decrease*** the effects of fluconazole:

- cimetidine (Tagamet).
- rifampin (Rifadin, Rimactane, etc.).

Fluconazole ***taken concurrently*** with

- amphotericin B (Amphotec, others) may decrease amphotericin benefits.
- astemizole (Hismanal—now removed from the US market) may result in fatal toxicity to the heart.
- atorvastatin (Lipitor), and other HMG-CoA inhibitors, may increase risk of muscle toxicity.
- cisapride (Propulsid) may lead to adverse effects on the heart. DO NOT COMBINE.
- hydrochlorothiazide (Esidrix, others) may increase potassium loss.
- loratadine (Claritin) may result in increased blood levels of loratadine, but to date, toxicity to the heart has not been reported. Since blood levels may be increased if combined use is undertaken, it is prudent to decrease the dose of loratadine.
- losartan (Cozaar) may blunt blood pressure control.
- oral contraceptives (birth control pills) may blunt contraception and result in pregnancy.
- quetiapine (Seroquel) may lead to quetiapine toxicity.

- ritonavir (Norvir) may increase ritonavir blood levels.
- terfenadine (Seldane—now removed from the US market) may result in toxicity to the heart.

▷ *Driving, Hazardous Activities:* No restrictions.

Aviation Note: The use of this drug *is probably not a disqualification* for piloting. Consult a designated Aviation Medical Examiner.

Exposure to Sun: No restrictions.

Discontinuation: Take all of the medicine. Ongoing therapy for months may be needed. Ask your doctor when it is okay to stop this medicine.

FLUCYTOSINE (flu SI toh seen)

Other Names: 5-fluorocytosine, 5-FC   **Introduced:** 1977   **Class:** Antifungal   **Prescription:** USA: Yes   **Controlled Drug:** USA: No; Canada: No   **Available as Generic:** USA: No; Canada: No

Brand Names: Ancobon, ✤Ancotil, ✤Novo-triphyl

BENEFITS versus RISKS	
Possible Benefits	*Possible Risks*
EFFECTIVE ADJUNCTIVE TREATMENT OF CERTAIN INFECTIONS CAUSED BY *CANDIDA, CRYPTOCOCCUS* FUNGI AND *ASPERGILLUS*	BONE MARROW DEPRESSION DRUG-INDUCED LIVER DAMAGE Peripheral neuritis
Effective adjunctive treatment of chromomycosis infection	

▷ **Principal Uses**

As a Single Drug Product: Uses currently included in FDA-approved labeling: (1) Treats endocarditis, osteomyelitis, arthritis, meningitis, pneumonia, septicemia and urinary tract infections caused by *Candida*; (2) treats meningitis, pneumonia, septicemia, endocarditis and urinary tract infections caused by *Cryptococcus*.

Other (unlabeled) generally accepted uses: (1) Treatment of disseminated candidiasis, chromomycosis and cryptococcosis (these infections may be AIDS related); (2) treatment of general fungal infections.

Author's Note: Flucytosine is usually used together with amphotericin B to treat disseminated fungal infections.

How This Drug Works: This drug goes into fungal cells and blocks production of RNA and DNA, inhibiting fungal development and reproduction.

Available Dosage Forms and Strengths

Capsules — 250 mg, 500 mg

▷ **Recommended Dosage Ranges** (Actual dose and schedule must be determined for each patient individually.)

Infants and Children: 50 to 150 mg per kg of body mass, divided into four equal doses and given every 6 hours.

12 to 60 Years of Age: 50 to 150 mg per kg of body mass, divided into equal doses and given every 6 hours. Some severe infections have required 250

mg per kg of body mass per day. Capsules are often taken a few at a time and the total dose taken over 15 minutes.

Over 60 Years of Age: Same as 12 to 60 years of age. If kidney function is impaired, dose reduction is mandatory.

Conditions Requiring Dosing Adjustments

Liver Function: No changes needed in mild to moderate liver compromise. This drug may cause liver toxicity (with blood levels greater than 100 mcg/ml). Used with caution in liver compromise.

Kidney Function: In mild to moderate kidney failure, the usual dose can be given every 12–24 hours. In severe kidney failure, the usual dose can be given every 24–48 hours.

▷ **Dosing Instructions:** If a single dose requires more than one capsule, space doses over a period of 15 minutes to reduce stomach upset and nausea. The capsule may be opened and taken with or after food. If you forget a dose: Take the omitted dose as soon as you remember it, unless it is nearly time for your next dose—if that is the case, skip the missed dose and take the next scheduled dose right on time. DO NOT double doses.

Usual Duration of Use: Use on a regular schedule for 4 to 6 weeks is needed to see effectiveness in controlling Candida or cryptococcal infection. Long-term use (months to years) requires periodic physician evaluation.

Typical Treatment Goals and Measurements (Outcomes and Markers)

Fungal infections: Goals for treatment of infections include resolution of signs and symptoms, return of white blood cell count and differential to normal (for systemic infections), and checks of blood levels of flucytosine.

▷ **This Drug Should Not Be Taken If**
- you have had an allergic reaction to it previously.
- you have an active blood cell or bone marrow disorder.
- you have active liver disease.

▷ **Inform Your Physician Before Taking This Drug If**
- you have a history of drug-induced bone marrow depression.
- you have a history of peripheral neuritis.
- you have impaired liver or kidney function.

Possible Side Effects (natural, expected and unavoidable drug actions)
Dose-related nausea and vomiting.

▷ **Possible Adverse Effects** (unusual, unexpected and infrequent reactions)
If any of the following develop, consult your physician promptly for guidance.

Mild Adverse Effects
Allergic reactions: skin rash, itching.
Headache, dizziness, drowsiness, confusion, hallucinations—infrequent.
Loss of appetite, nausea, vomiting, stomach pain, diarrhea—possible and dose-related.

Serious Adverse Effects
Allergic reactions: anaphylactic reactions.
Bone marrow depression (see Glossary): fatigue, weakness, fever, sore throat, abnormal bleeding or bruising—rare.
Liver damage, with or without jaundice (see Glossary)—case reports.
Peripheral neuritis (see Glossary)—possible.
Bowel perforation or kidney damage—rare.

▷ **Possible Effects on Sexual Function:** None reported.

▷ **Adverse Effects That May Mimic Natural Diseases or Disorders**
    Drug-induced hepatitis may suggest viral hepatitis.

Natural Diseases or Disorders That May Be Activated by This Drug
    Crohn's disease, ulcerative colitis.

Possible Effects on Laboratory Tests
    Complete blood counts: decreased red cells, hemoglobin, white cells and
      platelets.
    Liver function tests: increased liver enzymes (ALT/GPT, AST/GOT and alka-
      line phosphatase), increased bilirubin.
    Kidney function tests: increased blood urea nitrogen (BUN) and creatinine.
    Serum creatinine: may be falsely increased if tested by some methods.

CAUTION
    1. When this drug is used alone, resistance can occur rapidly. It is usually
       used concurrently with amphotericin B (Abelcet) (given intravenously).
    2. This drug may cause false increases in creatinine laboratory values
       tested by the Ektachem method. DuPont ACA does not appear to have
       this problem.

Precautions for Use
    By Infants and Children: No information available.
    By Those Over 60 Years of Age: If necessary, adjust dose for age-related
    decrease in kidney function.

▷ **Advisability of Use During Pregnancy**
    Pregnancy Category: C. See Pregnancy Risk Categories at the back of this book.
    Animal studies: Rat studies reveal drug-induced birth defects.
    Human studies: Adequate studies of pregnant women are not available.
    Use this drug only if clearly needed. Ask your physician for guidance.

Advisability of Use If Breast-Feeding
    Presence of this drug in breast milk: Yes.
    Avoid drug or refrain from nursing.

Habit-Forming Potential: None.

Effects of Overdose: Nausea, vomiting, stomach pain, diarrhea, confusion.

Possible Effects of Long-Term Use: Bone marrow depression, liver or kidney
    damage.

Suggested Periodic Examinations While Taking This Drug (at physician's dis-
    cretion)
    Measurement of blood levels of flucytosine.
    Complete blood cell counts.
    Liver and kidney function tests.

▷ **While Taking This Drug, Observe the Following**
    Foods: No restrictions.
    Herbal Medicines or Minerals: Echinacea: Some patients use echinacea to
      attempt to boost their immune systems. Unfortunately, use of echinacea is
      not recommended in people with damaged immune systems. This herb
      may also actually weaken any immune system if it is used too often or for
      too long a time. Caution: St. John's wort may also cause extreme reactions
      to the sun. Additive photosensitivity may be possible.
    Beverages: No restrictions. May be taken with milk.

▷   *Alcohol:* No interactions expected.
     Tobacco Smoking: No interactions expected. I advise everyone to quit smoking.
▷   *Other Drugs*
        The following drugs may *decrease* the effects of flucytosine:
        • antacids.
        • cytarabine (Cytosar).
        Flucytosine *taken concurrently* with
        • amphotericin B may result in increased risk of kidney toxicity; lipid-associated form (Abelcet) may help avoid this.
        • zidovudine (AZT) may result in additive and serious blood (hematological) toxicity.
▷   *Driving, Hazardous Activities:* This drug may cause dizziness, drowsiness or confusion. Limit activities as necessary.
     Aviation Note: The use of this drug *may be a disqualification* for piloting. Consult a designated Aviation Medical Examiner.
     Exposure to Sun: Use caution—may cause photosensitivity (see Glossary). See "Herbal Medicines" note above.
     Discontinuation: This drug may be needed for an extended period. Your doctor must decide when to stop it.

FLUNISOLIDE (flu NIS oh lide)

Introduced: 1980   **Class:** Antiasthmatic, cortisonelike drugs   **Prescription:** USA: Yes   **Controlled Drug:** USA: No; Canada: No   **Available as Generic:** No

Brand Names: AeroBid, AeroBid-M, ✤Bronalide, Nasalide, Nasarel, ✤Nu-Flunisolide, ✤Rhinalar

BENEFITS versus RISKS	
Possible Benefits	*Possible Risks*
EFFECTIVE CONTROL OF SEVERE, CHRONIC BRONCHIAL ASTHMA	Yeast infections of mouth and throat (inhaler form)
	Increased susceptibility to respiratory tract infections (inhaler form)
	Localized areas of "allergic" pneumonia (inhaler form)

Principal Uses

As a Single Drug Product: Uses currently included in FDA-approved labeling: (1) Treats chronic bronchial asthma in people requiring cortisonelike drugs for asthma control; (2) treats various kinds of hay fever (seasonal or perennial allergic rhinitis).

Other (unlabeled) generally accepted uses: (1) Treatment of nasal polyps; (2) treats bronchopulmonary dysplasia; (3) may have a role in acute or chronic sinusitis in combination with an antibiotic (amoxicillin/clavulanate in one study).

How This Drug Works: Increases cyclic AMP, which may increase epinephrine, an effective bronchodilator and antiasthmatic. Also reduces local allergic reaction and inflammation.

Available Dosage Forms and Strengths

Inhalation aerosol — 0.25 mg (250 mcg) per metered spray

Nasal solution — 25 mcg per actuation

▷ **Recommended Dosage Ranges** (Actual dose and schedule must be determined for each patient individually.)

Infants and Children:

Oral inhalation: Up to 6 years old—not recommended. Six to 15 years old—two inhalations or 500 mcg twice a day. Maximum daily dose is 1 mg.

Nasal inhalation: Up to 6 years old—not recommended. Six to 15 years old—0.25 mcg (one spray in each nostril) three times a day. Once the peak effect is seen, the dose should be reduced to the smallest dose and frequency that works. Maximum is four sprays in each nostril (200 mcg/day).

Aqueous nasal form: Up to 6 years old—not recommended. Six to 14 years old—two sprays in each nostril twice daily or one spray in each nostril three times a day. Once the peak effect is seen, the dose should be reduced to the smallest dose and frequency that works.

15 to 60 Years of Age:

Oral inhalation: 0.5 to 1 mg (two to four metered sprays) twice a day, morning and evening. Limit total daily dose to 2 mg (four inhalations twice daily). Once the peak effect is seen, the dose should be reduced to the smallest dose and frequency that works.

Nasal inhalation: Two sprays (50 mcg) per nostril twice daily. The dose may be increased to two sprays in each nostril three times a day (300 mcg/day). Maximum dose with this route is eight sprays (400 mcg) in each nostril daily. Once the peak effect is seen, the dose should be reduced to the smallest dose and frequency that works.

Aqueous nasal form: Two sprays in each nostril twice daily to start. Maintenance dosing is continued with the lowest dose that is effective. This may be as low as one spray in each nostril daily.

Over 60 Years of Age: Same as 15 to 60 years of age.

Conditions Requiring Dosing Adjustments

Liver Function: Specific guidelines are not available.

Kidney Function: No specific changes needed—dual kidney and fecal elimination (Nasalide).

▷ **Dosing Instructions:** May be used as needed without regard to eating. Shake the container well before using. Carefully follow the printed patient instructions provided with the inhaler; rinse the mouth and throat (gargle) with water thoroughly after each inhalation. A decongestant is prudent BEFORE flunisolide is used in people with blocked nose (nasal) passages. If you forget a dose: take the next dose as soon as you remember it, unless it is nearly time for your next dose—if that is the case, skip the dose you forgot, and take the next dose right on schedule. DO NOT double doses.

Usual Duration of Use: Use on a regular schedule for 1 to 3 weeks is necessary to see effectiveness in controlling allergic rhinitis. It may take 4 weeks to see the greatest benefit in severe, chronic asthma. Long-term use requires physician supervision and guidance.

Typical Treatment Goals and Measurements (Outcomes and Markers)

Asthma: Frequency and severity of asthma attacks should ease. Some clinicians also use decreased frequency of rescue inhaler use as a further clinical indicator. It is critical that this medicine is used regularly to get the best results. An additional goal of therapy is to use the lowest effective dose. Some people keep their improvements when doses are lowered, while others relapse. Specific testing goals include improvement in PEFR and other lung (pulmonary) function tests. Wheezing and difficulty breathing (Dyspnea) should ease as well as asthma caused (induced) by exercise. If the usual benefit is not realized, call your doctor.

Allergic rhinitis: Signs and symptoms of allergic rhinitis such as runny or stuffy nose, postnasal drip and sneezing should ease. Scratch testing for a specific immune substance (IgE) can also be done to check progress at a cellular level.

▷ **This Drug Should Not Be Taken If**
- you have had an allergic reaction to it previously.
- you are having severe acute asthma or status asthmaticus that requires more intense treatment for prompt relief.
- you have a form of nonallergic bronchitis with asthmatic features.

▷ **Inform Your Physician Before Taking This Drug If**
- you are now taking or have recently taken any cortisone-related drug (including ACTH by injection; see Drug Classes) for any reason.
- you have a history of tuberculosis (inhalation form).
- you have herpes simplex infection of the eye.
- you have chicken pox or measles or have been exposed to them.
- you have had recent surgery of the nose or have ulcers of the nose or nosebleeds—this medicine should be used cautiously until the site has healed.
- you are a child and your growth has slowed.
- you have chronic bronchitis or bronchiectasis.
- you think you may have an active infection of any kind, especially a respiratory infection (such as tuberculosis).

Possible Side Effects (natural, expected and unavoidable drug actions)
Yeast infections (thrush) of the mouth and throat.
Unpleasant taste. Orally inhaled flunisolide can cause flu-like symptoms occasionally in people taking the drug by oral inhalation. Nasal form most frequent adverse effect is irritation of the nose (nasal mucosa).

▷ **Possible Adverse Effects** (unusual, unexpected and infrequent reactions)
If any of the following develop, consult your physician promptly for guidance.
Mild Adverse Effects
Allergic reactions: skin rash, hives, itching.
Headache, dizziness, nervousness, moodiness, insomnia, loss of smell or taste—rare to infrequent.
Aftertaste (nasal form)—frequent.
Upper respiratory infections, cough—possible.
Heart palpitation, increased blood pressure, swelling of feet and ankles (inhalation form)—possible to infrequent.
Loss of appetite, indigestion, nausea, vomiting, stomach pain, diarrhea—infrequent.
Sore throat, stinging of the nose—infrequent to frequent.
Nasal irritation—infrequent to frequent (less common with the aqueous form).

Slowing of growth rate in children—possible.

Impaired sense of smell—possible.

Serious Adverse Effects

Allergic reaction: localized areas of "allergic" pneumonitis (lung inflammation).

Bronchospasm, asthmatic wheezing—rare with the inhalation form.

Tachycardia or hypertension—rare with the inhalation form.

Osteoporosis—possible with long-term use (alendronate may prevent this).

Increased risk of cataracts (posterior subcapsular)—possible.

▷ **Possible Effects on Sexual Function:** None reported.

Natural Diseases or Disorders That May Be Activated by This Drug

Cortisone-related drugs (used by inhalation) that produce systemic effects can impair immunity and lead to reactivation of "healed" or quiescent tuberculosis. People with a history of tuberculosis should be watched closely during use of cortisonelike drugs by inhalation.

Possible Effects on Laboratory Tests

None reported.

CAUTION

1. Does NOT act primarily as a bronchodilator. **Should not be used for immediate relief of acute asthma**.
2. If you were using any cortisone-related drugs for treatment of your asthma before changing to this inhaler, the cortisone-related drug may be required if you are injured, have an infection or require surgery. Tell your doctor about prior use of cortisone-related drugs.
3. If severe asthma returns while using this drug, call your doctor immediately.
4. If you have used cortisone-related drugs in the past year, carry a card that says so.
5. Five to ten minutes should separate the inhalation of bronchodilators, such as albuterol, epinephrine, pirbuterol, etc. (which should be used first), and the inhalation of this drug. This lets more flunisolide reach the bronchial tubes and reduces risk of adverse effects from the propellants used in the two inhalers.
6. A decongestant may be a good idea in people with blocked nasal passages. Talk with your doctor or pharmacist.
7. Osteoporosis risk is increased with long-term use of this medicine. Bone mineral density tests are prudent as well as the use of alendronate (Fosamax) as a preventive (prophylactic) medicine in some high-risk patients
8. Up to 50% of an intranasal dose may reach the rest of the body (systemic circulation).

Precautions for Use

By Infants and Children: Safety and effectiveness for those under 4 years of age are not established. To obtain maximal benefit, the use of a spacer device is recommended for inhalation therapy in children.

By Those Over 60 Years of Age: People with chronic bronchitis or bronchiectasis should be watched closely for the development of lung infections.

▷ **Advisability of Use During Pregnancy**

Pregnancy Category: C. See Pregnancy Risk Categories at the back of this book.

Animal studies: Rat and rabbit studies reveal significant birth defects due to this drug.

Human studies: Adequate studies of pregnant women are not available.

Avoid drug during the first 3 months. Use infrequently and only as clearly needed during the final 6 months.

Advisability of Use If Breast-Feeding

Presence of this drug in breast milk: Unknown.

Avoid drug or refrain from nursing.

Habit-Forming Potential: With recommended dose, a state of functional dependence (see Glossary) is not likely to develop.

Effects of Overdose: Indications of cortisone excess (due to systemic absorption)—fluid retention, flushing of the face, stomach irritation, nervousness.

Possible Effects of Long-Term Use: Development of acne, cataracts, altered menstrual pattern. Osteoporosis (periodic bone mineral density tests are prudent).

Suggested Periodic Examinations While Taking This Drug (at physician's discretion)

Inspection of mouth and throat for evidence of yeast infection.

Check of adrenal function in people who have used cortisone-related drugs for an extended period of time before using this drug.

X-ray of the lungs of people with a prior history of tuberculosis.

Bone mineral density testing (osteoporosis test DEXA or PDEXA) with long-term use.

▷ **While Taking This Drug, Observe the Following**

Foods: No specific restrictions beyond those advised by your physician.

Herbal Medicines or Minerals: Fir or pine needle oil should NOT be used by asthmatics. Ephedra alone does carry a German Commission E monograph indication for asthma treatment. If you are allergic to plants in the Asteraceae family (aster, chrysanthemum, daisy or ragweed), you may also be allergic to echinacea, chamomile, feverfew and St. John's wort. Increased calcium and vitamin D are prudent while taking this medicine. Talk to your doctor BEFORE adding any herbals to this medicine.

Beverages: No specific restrictions.

▷ *Alcohol:* No direct interactions expected, but excessive alcohol use may be a risk factor for osteoporosis. Since long-term use of this medicine may lead to osteoporosis, excessive use of alcohol must be avoided.

Tobacco Smoking: No direct drug interactions expected; however, smoking can worsen asthma and reduce benefits of flunisolide. I advise everyone to quit smoking.

▷ *Other Drugs*

The following drugs may *increase* the effects of flunisolide:

• inhalant bronchodilators—albuterol, bitolterol, epinephrine, etc.

• oral bronchodilators—aminophylline, ephedrine, terbutaline, theophylline, etc.

Flunisolide *taken concurrently* with

• stanozolol (Winstrol) may result in increased risk of acne or edema.

• some antiepileptic medicines such as phenytoin (Dilantin) may increase risk of osteoporosis.

- inhalant bronchodilators—epinephrine, isoetharine, isoproterenol—may offer improved results in asthma treatment.
- methylphenidate (Ritalin) may cause increased risk of growth suppression.

▷ *Driving, Hazardous Activities:* No restrictions.

Aviation Note: The use of this drug and the disorder for which this drug is prescribed **may be disqualifications** for piloting. Consult a designated Aviation Medical Examiner.

Exposure to Sun: No restrictions.

Occurrence of Unrelated Illness: Acute infections, serious injuries or surgical procedures can create an urgent need for cortisone-related drugs given by mouth and/or injection. Call your doctor immediately in the event of new illness or injury.

Special Storage Instructions: Store at room temperature. Avoid exposure to temperatures above 120 degrees F (49 degrees C). Do not store or use this inhaler near heat or open flame.

Discontinuation: If this drug has made it possible to reduce or discontinue cortisonelike drugs by mouth, do not stop this drug abruptly. If you must stop this drug, call your doctor promptly. Cortisone preparations and other measures may be necessary.

FLUOROQUINOLONE ANTIBIOTIC FAMILY

Ciprofloxacin (sip roh FLOX a sin) **Gatifloxacin** (GAT ih flox a sin) **Grepafloxacin** (GREP ah flox a sin) **Levofloxacin** (leev oh FLOX a sin) **Lomefloxacin** (loh me FLOX a sin) **Norfloxacin** (nor FLOX a sin) **Ofloxacin** (oh FLOX a sin) **Sparfloxacin** (SPAR flox a sin) **Trovafloxacin** (TROV ah flox a sin)

Introduced: 1984, 2000, 1997, 1996, 1992, 1986, 1984, 1996, 1997, respectively **Class:** Anti-infective, fluoroquinolone **Prescription:** USA: Yes **Controlled Drug:** USA: No **Available as Generic:** USA: No; Canada: Yes (IV)

Brand Names: Ciprofloxacin: Ciloxan, Cipro, Cipro Cystitis pack, Cipro HC [CD]; Gatifloxacin: Tequin; Grepafloxacin: (removed from the market); Levofloxacin: Levaquin, Maxaquin, Quixin; Moxifloxacin: Avelox; Norfloxacin: Chibroxin, Noroxin, Noroxin Ophthalmic; Ofloxacin: Floxin, Floxin Otic, Floxin Uropak, Ocuflox; Sparfloxacin: Zagam; Trovafloxacin: Trovan

Author's Note: Information in this profile will be broadened to include data on gatifloxacin and moxifloxacin once more data are available. It does carry a precautionary note regarding QTc interval prolongation and avoidance in people with QTc prolongation and in those taking other medicines that can cause QTc prolongation.

Warning: Some prescribers use "Norflox" to identify norfloxacin. This is not an accepted name in any setting for any reason. Using this name has resulted in serious medication errors—that is, the dispensing of Norflex, the generic drug orphenadrine, a skeletal muscle relaxant. Check to be sure you get the right drug.

Warning: There have been reports for some drugs in this class that find tendon rupture as a rare adverse effect. Ask your doctor about limits on strenuous exercise while you are taking this medicine. A rare idiosyncratic

reaction has also been reported that presents as mental confusion and disorientation. Use of these medicines after head trauma may be a risk factor. If you have suffered a fall, ask your doctor if a medicine in a different antibiotic class should be substituted. If you are taking this drug and notice a change in your thinking, call your doctor. **THE FDA HAS RESTRICTED TROVAFLOXACIN USE TO EMERGENCIES AND THE DRUG WILL NO LONGER BE SOLD IN DRUGSTORES.**

BENEFITS versus RISKS	
Possible Benefits	*Possible Risks*
HIGHLY EFFECTIVE TREATMENT FOR INFECTIONS OF THE LOWER RESPIRATORY TRACT (ciprofloxacin and ofloxacin), URINARY TRACT, BONES, JOINTS AND SKIN TISSUES due to susceptible organisms	TROVAFLOXACIN PATIENTS WERE WARNED (IN EUROPE) TO STOP TROVAFLOXACIN IF THEY DEVELOP SKIN RASH OR HIVES, YELLOWING OF THE SKIN OR EYES, DARK URINE OR NAUSEA AND VOMITING WITH STOMACH PAIN AND THE DRUG IS NO
EFFECTIVE TREATMENT OF BACTERIAL (EYE) INFECTIONS	LONGER SOLD IN DRUG STORES
Effective treatment for some forms of bacterial gastroenteritis (diarrhea)	SOME OF THESE MEDICINES CAN CAUSE SEVERE SUN SENSITIVITY
Effective treatment for some infections of the prostate gland	Nausea, indigestion
	Drug-induced colitis
	Hallucination or seizure
	Tendon rupture

▷ **Principal Uses**

As a Single Drug Product: Uses currently included in FDA-approved labeling: Treats responsive infections (in adults) of (1) the lower respiratory tract (lungs and bronchial tubes); (2) the urinary tract (kidneys, bladder, urethra [including uncomplicated gonorrhea] and prostate gland); (3) the digestive tract (small intestine and colon); (4) bones and joints (ciprofloxacin; ofloxacin—unlabeled); (5) skin and related tissues; (6) used in an ophthalmic preparation to treat bacterial conjunctivitis caused by susceptible organisms; (7) ciprofloxacin has been approved to treat mild to moderate acute sinusitis caused by Streptococcus pneumoniae, Haemophilus influenzae or Moraxella catarrhalis; (8) sparfloxacin is very active against Streptococcus; (9) ciprofloxacin/hydrocortisone is used for sudden infections of the outside of the ear (acute otitis externa); (10) ciprofloxacin is used in post-exposure anthrax cases.

Other (unlabeled) generally accepted uses: (1) Can have a role in treating cholera where the organisms are resistant to doxycycline (ciprofloxacin); (2) lessens symptoms or prevents traveler's diarrhea; (3) ciprofloxacin can be of use in treating some unusual organisms such as Aeromonas, catscratch fever or chancroid; (4) ofloxacin and sparfloxacin may help in combination therapy of leprosy.

Author's Note: A study in Britain of 3,315 first-time heart attack victims found that people who had been given fluoroquinolones had a 55% lower risk for a first heart attack. More research is needed.

How These Drugs Work: These medicines block the bacterial enzyme DNA gyrase (required for DNA synthesis and cell reproduction), arrest bacterial growth (in low concentrations) and kill bacteria (in high concentrations).

Available Dosage Forms and Strengths

Ciprofloxacin:

Ophthalmic solution — 0.3%

Suspension — 250 mg and 500 mg per 5 ml

Tablets — 250 mg, 500 mg, 750 mg

Tablets Ciprocystitis pack — 100 mg

Levofloxacin:

Ophthalmic solution — 0.5%

Solution for injection — 5 mg per ml, 25 mg per ml

Tablets — 250 mg, 500 mg

Lomefloxacin:

Tablets — 400 mg

Norfloxacin:

Ophthalmic solution — 3 mg/ml

Tablets — 400 mg

Ofloxacin:

Ophthalmic solution — 3 mg/ml

Tablets — 200 mg, 300 mg, 400 mg

Sparfloxacin:

Tablet — 200 mg

Trovafloxacin:

Tablet — 100 mg, 200 mg

▷ **Recommended Dosage Ranges** (Actual dose and schedule for all these medicines must be determined for each patient individually.)

Infants and Children: None of these medicines are recommended.

18 to 60 Years of Age:

Ciprofloxacin: 250 mg to 750 mg every 12 hours (depends on nature and severity of infection). Daily maximum is 1,500 mg. Mild to moderate sinusitis (caused by organisms outlined above) treated with 500 mg every 12 hours for 10 days in adults. Ophthalmic—one or two drops instilled in the eye every 2 hours while awake for 2 days and then one or two drops for 5 more days (given every 4 hours while awake).

Levofloxacin: 500 mg orally every 24 hours for 7–14 days for community acquired pneumonia.

Ophthalmic: On the first and second day—one to two drops in the affected eye every 2 hours (up to 8 times a day) while you are awake. On the 3rd through 7th day—1–2 drops every 4 hours (up to 4 times a day) while you are awake.

Lomefloxacin: For bronchitis—400 mg daily for 10 days. For bladder infections (cystitis)—400 mg daily for 10 days. For complicated urinary tract infections—400 mg daily for 14 days. For preoperative prevention of urinary tract infection—400 mg (single dose) taken 2 to 6 hours before surgery.

Norfloxacin: Uncomplicated urinary tract infections—400 mg every 12 hours for 3 days. Complicated urinary tract infections—400 mg every 12 hours for 10 to 21 days. Total daily dose should not exceed 800 mg. Ophthalmic dosing—one to two drops to the affected eye four times daily.

Ofloxacin: 200 mg to 400 mg every 12 hours (for 10 days for lower respiratory infections), depending on nature and severity of infection. Daily maximum is 800 mg. Ophthalmic dosing (conjunctivitis)—one to two drops every 2 to 4 hours for 2 days and then four times a day for 7 to 10 days.

Sparfloxacin: 400 mg now; then 200 mg a day for 10 days for pneumonia.

Trovafloxacin: Varies with the infection. Bronchitis—100 mg once daily for 7–10 days. Community acquired pneumonia—200 mg once daily for 7–14 days. Prostatitis—200 mg once a day for 28 days.

Over 60 Years of Age: Same as 18 to 60 years of age unless kidney function is an issue.

Conditions Requiring Dosing Adjustments

Liver Function: Use ciprofloxacin, norfloxacin and trovafloxacin with caution in severe liver failure. Trovafloxacin may pose increased risk in liver compromise. No changes for ofloxacin or sparfloxacin.

Kidney Function: Ciprofloxacin, levofloxacin, lomefloxacin, norfloxacin, ofloxacin and sparfloxacin **must** be decreased (or time between doses increased) in kidney compromise. For moderate to severe kidney compromise, ofloxacin dose is decreased to 400 mg daily. For patients with moderate kidney failure, the usual ofloxacin dose can be taken every 24 hours. For patients with severe failure, one-half the usual dose should be taken every 24 hours. Since some of these medicines can form crystals in urine, drink adequate quantities of water. Trovafloxacin is removed in the feces and by the liver.

Cystic Fibrosis: A loading dose for ciprofloxacin, as well as ongoing doses of 750 mg every 8 hours, is taken by cystic fibrosis patients. This dosing gives blood levels that are more aggressive versus the bacteria that usually cause infections in these patients. No changes for the other drugs are presented.

▷ **Dosing Instructions:** Ciprofloxacin, levofloxacin, lomefloxacin, norfloxacin, sparfloxacin or trovafloxacin may be taken with or without food (NOT dairy products), and all may be crushed. Ofloxacin is best taken 2 hours after eating. Drink large amounts of fluids while taking any of these drugs. Avoid aluminum or magnesium antacids, iron, zinc or calcium for 2 hours before and after drug doses. If you forget a dose: take the missed dose as soon as you remember it, unless it is nearly time for your next dose—then skip the missed dose and take the next dose right on schedule. Then return to your usual schedule. If you are taking one of the every-12-hour quinolones, take any remaining doses for the day at an evenly spaced time period. If you miss more than one dose, please call your doctor.

Usual Duration of Use: Regular use for 7 to 14 days is needed to see benefits in eradicating infection. Dosing should be continued for at least 2 days after all indications of infection have disappeared. Bone and joint infections (ciprofloxacin or ofloxacin) or prostate gland infections may be treated for 6 weeks or longer. Long-term use requires periodic evaluation of response.

Typical Treatment Goals and Measurements (Outcomes and Markers)

Infections: The most commonly used measures of serious infections are white blood cell counts and differentials (the kind of blood cells that occur most often in your blood), and temperature. Many clinicians look for positive changes in 24–48 hours. NEVER stop an antibiotic because you start to feel better. For many infections, a full 14 days is REQUIRED to kill the bacteria. The goals and time frame (see peak benefits above) should be discussed with you when the prescription is written.

Possible Advantages of These Drugs: Ciprofloxacin and ofloxacin have very broad spectrums of antibacterial activity of all currently available oral antimicrobial drugs. Highly effective in treating numerous types of infection caused by a wide spectrum of bacteria. Provide effective drug levels in the prostate gland (a difficult place to penetrate). Lomefloxacin has not had significant effects on kidney function. Sparfloxacin has better gram positive (Strep and Staph) activity than other medicines in this family.

▷ **These Drugs Should Not Be Taken If**
- you take an antiarrhythmic drug (see Drug Classes) or have a prolonged QTc (heartbeat interval) or take medicines known to cause torsades de pointes. Talk with your doctor (gatifloxacin, moxifloxacin, sparfloxacin—perhaps others).
- you had an allergic reaction to any quinolone antibiotic.
- you have swelling (inflammation), pain or bursting (rupture) of a tendon.
- you are pregnant or breast-feeding.
- you have a poorly controlled seizure disorder.
- you are less than 18 years of age.

▷ **Inform Your Physician Before Taking These Drugs If**
- you are allergic to cinoxacin (Cinobac), nalidixic acid (NegGram) or other quinolone drugs.
- you have a seizure disorder or a brain circulatory disorder.
- you have increased lipids (dyslipidemia) as this may increase risk of tendonitis.
- you have impaired liver or kidney function.
- you have a history of mental disorders (psychosis).
- you are taking any form of probenecid, theophylline or steroids.
- your work requires you to be in the sun. Sparfloxacin can cause severe phototoxicity.
- your work requires heavy manual labor. (Several cases of tendon rupture have been reported with fluoroquinolone use. Heavy exercise or work may be contraindicated. Call your doctor immediately if you develop inflammation or pain in a tendon.)

Possible Side Effects (natural, expected and unavoidable drug actions)
Superinfections (see Glossary). Permanent greenish tooth discoloration if used in infants (ciprofloxacin).

▷ **Possible Adverse Effects** (unusual, unexpected and infrequent reactions)
If any of the following develop, consult your physician promptly for guidance.
Mild Adverse Effects
Allergic reactions: rash, itching, localized swelling—rare.
Dizziness, headache (frequent with lomefloxacin), weakness, migraine, anxiety, abnormal vision—rare.
Nausea, diarrhea, vomiting, indigestion—rare to frequent.
Muscle aches—case reports.
Burning feeling in the eye when the ophthalmic solutions are used—possible.
Decreased vision (with ophthalmic use)—case reports.

Serious Adverse Effects

Allergic reactions: anaphylaxis—case reports.

Serious skin rashes—case reports for some (for example, ciprofloxacin has a case report of bullous pemphigoid). Call your doctor immediately if you develop a rash.

Idiosyncratic reactions—central nervous system stimulation (restlessness, tremor, confusion, hallucinations, seizures). One medication of this class has had reports of severe neurological compromise. Stop the drug immediately and call your doctor if you become confused or have trouble speaking while taking this drug—case reports. An idiosyncratic reaction between levofloxacin and warfarin leading to increased INR has been reported. Careful consideration of alternative antibiotics is advisable, more frequent INR checks and patient instruction on self-monitoring of possible bleeding is prudent if those medicines must be combined.

Kidney disease (interstitial nephritis)—case reports.

Tendon rupture—case reports for some family members.

Abnormal heartbeats (even torsades de pointes) or palpitations—rare, but may be additive or worse with other medicines that change QT interval.

Liver toxicity—rare (trovafloxacin availability changed because of this).

Blood sugar disturbances—possible (more likely in diabetics taking insulin or an oral hypoglycemic medicine).

Bone marrow depression—case reports with ciprofloxacin, norfloxacin and levofloxacin.

Intracranial hypertension (ciprofloxacin or ofloxacin)—case reports.

Worsening of myasthenia gravis—case reports.

▷ **Possible Effects on Sexual Function:** Vaginitis with discharge has been reported. Painful menstruation, excessive menstrual bleeding (ofloxacin only)—case reports. Intermenstrual bleeding—case reports (lomefloxacin).

Natural Diseases or Disorders That May Be Activated by These Drugs

Latent epilepsy, latent gout.

Possible Effects on Laboratory Tests

Kidney function: increased blood creatinine and urea nitrogen (BUN)—rare.

Liver function tests: increased as a sign of liver toxicity—rare.

Red and white blood cell counts: rarely decreased (norfloxacin and ciprofloxacin)—case reports.

Blood glucose levels: rare fluctuations.

CAUTION

1. If you develop skin rash, hives, fatigue or skin yellowing with nausea and vomiting while taking these medicines (especially trovafloxacin), call your doctor immediately.

2. With high doses or prolonged use, crystal formation in the kidneys may occur. This can be prevented by drinking large amounts of water, up to 2 quarts daily.

3. These drugs may decrease saliva formation, making dental cavities or gum disease more likely. Consult your dentist if dry mouth persists.

4. Changes in heart rhythm have been reported (QT interval). Sparfloxacin, gatifloxacin and moxifloxacin appear to cause this problem more often than ciprofloxacin.

5. Strenuous exercise is NOT recommended while these medicines are being taken.
6. If a sudden change in mental status is noticed, call your doctor immediately.
7. The ciprofloxacin suspension must be reconstituted with the special diluent that comes with the powder. DO NOT reconstitute with water.
8. Two case reports of bone marrow depression have been made in patients taking ciprofloxacin. This drug should be suspect if white blood cell counts and platelets fall while taking this medicine.
9. Sun sensitivity which may be severe (phototoxicity) is possible with sparfloxacin (Zagam), lomefloxacin (Maxaquin) and ciprofloxacin. Sun should be avoided while sparfloxacin is being taken and for 5 days after the medicine is stopped. Sun sensitivity may be minimized by taking lomefloxacin in the evening. Excessive sunlight exposure should be avoided with levofloxacin.

Precautions for Use

By Infants and Children: Avoid the use of these drugs completely. Impairs normal bone growth and development.

By Those Over 60 Years of Age: Impaired kidney function may require dose reduction.

▷ **Advisability of Use During Pregnancy**

Pregnancy Category: C. See Pregnancy Risk Categories at the back of this book.

Animal studies: Rabbit studies showed maternal weight loss and increased abortions (ciprofloxacin). Mild skeletal defects due to ofloxacin were found in rat studies; toxic effects on the fetus were shown in rat and rabbit studies. These drugs can impair normal bone development in immature dogs.

Human studies: Adequate studies of pregnant women are not available.

The potential for adverse effects on fetal bone development contraindicates the use of these drugs during entire pregnancy.

Advisability of Use If Breast-Feeding

Presence of these drugs in breast milk: Ofloxacin, trovafloxacin—yes. Probably for the rest.

Avoid drug or refrain from nursing.

Habit-Forming Potential: None.

Effects of Overdose: Confusion, headache, abdominal pain, diarrhea, liver toxicity, seizures, kidney toxicity, hallucinations.

Possible Effects of Long-Term Use: Superinfections (see Glossary); crystal formation in kidneys.

Suggested Periodic Examinations While Taking These Drugs (at physician's discretion)

Liver function tests. (Baseline and regular liver function tests may be prudent for trovafloxacin as it appears to pose more risk of liver damage than the other medicines in this class.)

Urine analysis.

While Taking These Drugs, Observe the Following

Foods: Caffeine may remain in your system longer than usual. Use care in the amount of caffeine consumed. Dairy foods will decrease the effectiveness of these drugs by decreasing the amount absorbed.

Herbal Medicines or Minerals: Calcium supplements, iron pills or zinc will decrease the amount of these medicines that go to work fighting infection. Separate doses by one hour before or two hours after the antibiotic. Use of St. John's wort may lead to additive sensitivity to the sun. Some patients use echinacea to attempt to boost their immune systems. Unfortunately, use of echinacea is not recommended in people with damaged immune systems. This herb may also actually weaken any immune system if it is used too often or for too long a time. Do NOT take mistletoe herb, oak bark or F.C. of marshmallow root and licorice.

Beverages: No restrictions (see "Foods" note on caffeine above).

▷ *Alcohol:* No interactions expected, but since heavy alcohol intake can blunt the immune system, limit alcohol if you are ill enough to require an antibiotic.

Tobacco Smoking: No interactions expected. I advise everyone to quit smoking.

▷ *Other Drugs*

The following drug may ***increase*** the effects of fluoroquinolones:
- probenecid (Benemid).

Fluoroquinolones ***taken concurrently*** with
- azlocillin may result in toxicity.
- caffeine will result in increased caffeine levels.
- cyclosporine (Sandimmune) may result in increased risk of kidney toxicity.
- dofetilide (Tikosyn) may lead to prolonged QT intervals and even possible torsade de pointes.
- foscarnet (Foscavir) may result in an increased risk of seizures.
- ibutilide (Corvert) may lead to prolonged QT intervals and even possible torsade de pointes.
- live typhoid vaccine (Vivotif Bernia) may lead to blunted immunological response.
- olanzapine (Zyprexa) may lead to increased olanzapine levels (reported for ciprofloxacin, but caution advised for all quinolones acting on CYP1A2).
- phenytoin (Dilantin) or fosphenytoin (Cerebyx) may result in increased or decreased phenytoin levels.
- theophylline (Theo-Dur, others) may lead to theophylline toxicity over time (norfloxacin or ciprofloxacin).
- warfarin (Coumadin) can result in increased risk of bleeding or blunted warfarin response (not yet reported for levofloxacin). More frequent INR testing is needed.

The following drugs may ***decrease*** the effects of fluoroquinolones:
- antacids containing aluminum or magnesium, reducing absorption and lessening effectiveness.
- calcium supplements.
- didanosine (ciprofloxacin only).
- iron salts.
- magnesium, decreasing therapeutic benefits.
- morphine (only reported for trovafloxacin).
- nitrofurantoin (Macrodantin, etc.), which may antagonize the antibacterial action in the urinary tract. Avoid this combination.
- sucralfate (Carafate).
- zinc salts.

Sparfloxacin *taken concurrently* with the following drugs may cause abnormal heartbeats (also to be used with extreme caution with any new medicines that can prolong the QTc interval):

- amiodarone (Cordarone).
- astemizole (Hismanal).
- bepridil (Vascor).
- beta blockers (see Drug Classes).
- chlorpromazine (Thorazine).
- cisapride (Propulsid).
- disopyramide (Norpace).
- macrolide antibiotics (erythromycin, dirithromycin, others).
- phenothiazines (see Drug Classes).
- procainamide (Pronestyl) (see Drug Classes).
- quinidine (Quinaglute, various).
- tricyclic antidepressants (see Drug Classes).

Moxifloxacin *taken concurrently* with

- class 1A or class III antiarrhythmic agents (see Drug Classes) may lead to abnormal heart changes (QT prolongation or even torsades de pointes). DO NOT combine.

Norfloxacin *taken concurrently* with

- dofetilide (Tikosyn) may lead to dofetilide toxicity via inhibition of CYP 3A4.

▷ *Driving, Hazardous Activities:* May cause dizziness or impair vision. Restrict activities as necessary.

Aviation Note: The use of these drugs *may be a disqualification* for piloting. Consult a designated Aviation Medical Examiner.

Exposure to Sun: Some members of this class have caused photosensitivity (see Glossary) and have limiting sun warnings. Sunglasses are advised if eyes are overly sensitive to bright light. A strong sun block is advised for your skin. Sparfloxacin users should avoid the sun while taking that medicine and for five days after the medicine is stopped. Lomefloxacin sun sensitivity may be reduced by taking the medicine at night. Excessive sun exposure should be avoided by levofloxacin users.

Heavy Exercise or Exertion: Several reports have surfaced regarding tendon rupture in patients with some of the medicines in this class. It is prudent to avoid heavy exercise or exertion while you are taking a fluoroquinolone.

Discontinuation: If you experience no adverse effects from these drugs, take the full course prescribed for best results. Ask your doctor when to stop treatment.

FLUOXETINE (flu OX e teen)

Introduced: 1978   **Class:** Antidepressant   **Prescription:** USA: Yes
Controlled Drug: USA: No   **Available as Generic:** USA: Yes
Brand Name: ❦Apo-Fluoxetine, ❦Gen-Fluoxetine, ❦Med-Fluoxetine, Prozac, Prozac Weekly, Sarafem

---

BENEFITS versus RISKS

Possible Benefits	*Possible Risks*
EFFECTIVE TREATMENT OF MAJOR DEPRESSIVE DISORDERS	Serious allergic reactions
	Conversion of depression to mania in manic-depressive (bipolar) disorders
EFFECTIVE PREVENTION OF RECURRENCE OF DEPRESSION	
EFFECTIVE IN SEVERE PMS (premenstrual dysphoric syndrome or PMDS)	
TREATS BULIMIA NERVOSA	
TREATS OBSESSIVE-COMPULSIVE DISORDER	
ONCE-WEEKLY FORMULATION WILL HELP ADHERENCE	
May reduce hot flashes in some cancer survivors	

▷ **Principal Uses**

As a Single Drug Product: Uses currently included in FDA-approved labeling: Treats (1) major forms of depression (including depression in HIV-positive patients and in geriatric depression); (2) obsessive-compulsive disorder; (3) bulimia; (4) approved for use in severe PMS (PMDS).

Other (unlabeled) generally accepted uses: (1) Refractory diabetic neuropathy; (2) may help control kleptomania; (3) can be of help in treating obesity, especially when obesity is accompanied by depression; (4) eases symptoms of panic attacks; (5) used to treat seasonal affective disorder (such as depression limited to winter months); (6) treats some forms of sexual problems; (7) some data for use of childhood anxiety disorder; (8) may ease ringing in the ears (tinnitus) that has not responded to other medicines; (9) may reduce the severity and frequency of hot flashes (by about half) in cancer survivors.

How This Drug Works: It slowly restores normal levels of a nerve transmitter (serotonin).

Available Dosage Forms and Strengths

> Capsules — 10 mg, 20 mg, 40 mg
> Capsules — 90 mg (Prozac Weekly form)
> Capsules — 10 mg and 20 mg (28-pill blister packs Sarafem form)
> Oral solution — 20 mg/5 ml
> Tablet — 10 mg

▷ **Usual Adult Dosage Ranges:**

Depression: Starts with 20 mg in the morning; if no improvement after several weeks, dose may be increased by 20 mg/day. Doses over 20 mg/day should be divided into two equal doses and taken twice daily. Maximum daily dose is 80 mg. Prozac Weekly form is intended for people who are already stabilized on the daily 20 mg form.

Bulimia: 60 mg once daily in the morning.

PMDS (severe PMS): A 28-pill blister pack is available (Sarafem form). In clinical studies, some patients used 20–60 mg during the entire month to check sign and symptom decreases. One part of the study group obtained an 86% symp-

tom reduction using 20 mg a day on days 14–28 of each menstrual cycle. Your doctor may adjust dosing strategies to the severity of your symptoms.
Hot flashes in cancer survivors: 20 mg per day.
Obsessive-compulsive disorder: 20 to 80 mg daily.
Note: Actual dose and schedule must be determined for each patient individually.

Conditions Requiring Dosing Adjustments
Liver Function: The dose should be decreased or the dosing interval lengthened for patients with liver compromise. Some clinicians decrease the dose by 50% in compensated cirrhosis. This drug is also a rare cause of liver toxicity and should be used with caution by this patient population.
Kidney Function: Dosing changes do not appear to be needed. Patients should be closely watched for adverse effects.

▷ **Dosing Instructions:** The capsule may be opened and the contents mixed with any convenient food. To make smaller doses, the contents may be mixed with orange juice or apple juice (NOT GRAPEFRUIT JUICE) and refrigerated; doses of 5–10 mg may prove effective and better tolerated. If you forget a dose: take the dose you missed as soon as you remember it, unless it is nearly time for your next dose—if that is the case, skip the missed dose and take the next dose right on schedule. DO NOT DOUBLE DOSES. If you find yourself missing doses—talk to your doctor.

Usual Duration of Use: Use on a regular schedule for 1 to 2 weeks may reveal start of benefits in depression. Up to 5 weeks may be needed for peak effects in (1) relieving depression and (2) the pattern of both favorable and unfavorable effects. Since there is an active metabolite and a long half-life, it may take several weeks before the benefits of a change in dose are seen. Long-term use (months to years) requires periodic physician evaluation. Some clinical guidelines suggest that 4 to 9 months of treatment should continue after the symptoms of depression go away. Some clinicians use lower doses to prevent or prophylax depression. People who take their medicine regularly are least likely to have a recurrence. Will often take several weeks to work in reducing hot flashes in cancer survivors. PMDS use is expected to be cyclic (in relation to menstrual cycles) and may not involve use during the entire month.

Typical Treatment Goals and Measurements (Outcomes and Markers)
Depression: The general goal is to lessen the degree and severity of depression, letting patients return to their daily lives. Specific measures of depression involve testing or inventories and can be valuable in helping check benefits from this medicine. The Hamilton depression scale is widely used to assess depression. In the case of PMDS, control of irritability and decreased number and/or severity of symptoms and the ability of the patient to return to normal activities or not have them interrupted is a hallmark of successful treatment.
PMDS: The goal is to lessen the degree and severity of menstrual difficulties (such as pain, irritability, etc.) or to prevent menstruation-associated problems altogether.

Possible Advantages of This Drug
Does not cause weight gain, a common side effect of tricyclic antidepressants. May actually cause weight loss. Less likely to cause dry mouth, con-

stipation, urinary retention or orthostatic hypotension (see Glossary) than tricyclic antidepressants. Since a large National Cancer Institute study found that those who suffer depression for 6 years or more have a generally increased risk of cancer, one benefit of effective treatment of depression with this drug may be a generally reduced risk of cancer.

▷ **This Drug Should Not Be Taken If**
- you had an allergic reaction to it previously.
- you take, or took in the last 14 days, a monoamine oxidase (MAO) type A inhibitor (see Drug Classes).

▷ **Inform Your Physician Before Taking This Drug If**
- you have had any adverse effects from antidepressant drugs.
- you have impaired liver or kidney function.
- you have Parkinson's disease.
- you have a seizure disorder.
- you have a history of psychosis.
- you have a history of SIADH (talk with your doctor).
- you are pregnant or plan pregnancy while taking this drug.

Possible Side Effects (natural, expected and unavoidable drug actions)
Decreased appetite, weight loss.
Case reports of orthostatic hypotension (see Glossary).

▷ **Possible Adverse Effects** (unusual, unexpected and infrequent reactions)
If any of the following develop, consult your physician promptly for guidance.
Mild Adverse Effects
Allergic reactions: skin rash, hives, itching—rare.
Headache, nervousness, insomnia, drowsiness, tremor, dizziness, tingling of extremities—rare.
Vivid nightmares—case reports.
Altered taste, nausea—frequent.
Vomiting, diarrhea—possible to rare.
Bruising—rare.
Hair loss—case reports.
Fast heart rate (tachycardia) or palpitations—rare.
Blurred vision—infrequent.
Excessive sweating—frequent.
Serious Adverse Effects
Allergic reactions: serum-sickness-like syndrome (fever, weakness, joint pain and swelling, swollen lymph glands, fluid retention, skin rash and/or hives).
Drug-induced seizures—rare.
Worsening of Parkinson's disease—possible.
Parkinson-like reactions (extrapyramidal effects)—rare.
Neuroleptic malignant syndrome—case reports.
Intense suicidal preoccupation in severe depression that does not respond to this drug—possible.
Mania or hypomania and psychosis or hallucinations—rare.
Abnormal and excessive urination (SIADH)—case reports.
Abnormal heartbeats (even torsades de pointes) or palpitations—rare, but may be additive or worse with other medicines that change QT interval.
Liver toxicity—rare.

▷ **Possible Effects on Sexual Function:** Impaired erection (1.9%), inhibition of ejaculation or inhibited orgasm in men and women—case reports. Worsening of fibrocystic breast disease in a female—case report.

Natural Diseases or Disorders That May Be Activated by This Drug

Latent epilepsy.

Possible Effects on Laboratory Tests

Blood glucose level: decreased.

Blood sodium level: decreased.

CAUTION

1. If any skin reaction develops (rash, hives, etc.), stop this drug and inform your physician promptly.
2. If dry mouth develops and persists for more than 2 weeks, consult your dentist for help.
3. Ask your doctor or pharmacist before taking any other prescription or over-the-counter drug while taking fluoxetine.
4. If you must start any monoamine oxidase (MAO) type A inhibitor (see Drug Classes), allow an interval of 5–6 weeks after stopping this drug before starting the MAO inhibitor.
5. This drug should be withheld if electroconvulsive therapy (ECT, "shock" treatment) is to be used.
6. Be honest with your doctor about how well this medicine is helping you. There are many antidepressants available, and the first one that is tried may or may not work.

Precautions for Use

By Infants and Children: Safety and effectiveness for those under 5 years of age are not established.

For those 5 to 18 years old, some clinicians have used 5–10 mg per day or 10 mg three times a week. The dose is subsequently increased as needed and tolerated to a maximum of 20 mg per day.

By Those Over 60 Years of Age: Lower or less frequent doses are recommended by the manufacturer.

▷ **Advisability of Use During Pregnancy**

Pregnancy Category: C. See Pregnancy Risk Categories at the back of this book.

Animal studies: No birth defects due to this drug found in rat or rabbit studies.

Human studies: Adequate studies of pregnant women are not available. Of the SSRIs, this medicine probably has the largest amount of data on women who have taken fluoxetine during pregnancy without adverse effects. One study of 228 women appeared to show that it was safer to take fluoxetine in the first two trimesters of pregnancy and discontinue it during the last trimester.

Use of this drug during pregnancy is a benefit-to-risk decision that must be discussed with your doctor.

Advisability of Use If Breast-Feeding

Presence of this drug in breast milk: Yes.

Avoid drug or refrain from nursing.

Habit-Forming Potential: Reports of patients using excess doses of fluoxetine or combining the drug with alcohol have surfaced. It appears possible that a euphoric effect and abuse potential exists.

Effects of Overdose: Agitation, restlessness, excitement, nausea, vomiting, seizures.

Possible Effects of Long-Term Use: None reported.

Suggested Periodic Examinations While Taking This Drug (at physician's discretion)

None.

▷ **While Taking This Drug, Observe the Following**

Foods: No restrictions (see Beverages below).

Beverages: Grapefruit juice may lead to increased blood levels. AVOID IT. May be taken with milk.

Herbal Medicines or Minerals: Since fluoxetine and St. John's wort may act to increase serotonin, the combination is not advised. Since part of the way ginseng works may be as a MAO inhibitor, do not combine with fluoxetine. Ma huang, yohimbe, Indian snakeroot and kava kava are also best avoided while taking this medicine. Calcium now has excellent data (1200–1,600 mg per day unless contraindicated) in helping prevent premenstrual dysphoric syndrome (PMS). This may be an intelligent first-line therapy or valuable adjunctive use. Talk to your doctor to see if this makes sense for you.

▷ *Alcohol:* Does not appear to increase the central nervous system effects of fluoxetine or change the metabolism of alcohol.

Tobacco Smoking: No interactions expected, but I advise everyone to quit smoking.

▷ *Other Drugs*

Fluoxetine may *increase* the effects of
- beta blockers (see Drug Classes).
- diazepam (Valium) and other benzodiazepines (see Drug Classes).
- digitalis preparations (digitoxin, digoxin).
- diltiazem (Cardizem).
- dofetilide (Tikosyn), requiring dosing decreases.
- flecainide (Tambocor).
- phenytoin (Dilantin), or fosphenytoin (Cerebyx) by increasing the phenytoin or fosphenytoin levels.
- propafenone (Rythmol).
- propranolol (Inderal).
- quinidine (Quinaglute).
- sildenafil (Viagra), by inhibiting CYP3A4.
- valproic acid (Depakote, others).
- warfarin (Coumadin) and related oral anticoagulants. Test INR more often.

Fluoxetine *taken concurrently* with
- antidiabetic drugs (insulin, oral hypoglycemics) may increase the risk of hypoglycemic reactions; monitor blood sugar levels carefully.
- aspirin (various) caused hives to reappear in a patient allergic to fluoxetine.
- astemizole (Hismanal), terfenadine (Seldane) or similar drugs may result in increased antihistamine levels and risk of heart arrhythmias. **Avoid** combining (these medicines are now removed from the US market).
- azole antifungals (such as fluconazole, itraconazole and ketoconazole) may lead to higher than expected fluoxetine blood levels and increased risk of adverse effects.
- buspirone (Buspar) may increase underlying anxiety. Combination is best avoided, but if deemed clinically necessary, patients should be closely watched for worsening of symptoms.
- carbamazepine (Tegretol) will increase the carbamazepine level. Drug levels are critical if the drugs are combined.

- cimetidine (Tagamet) may theoretically lead to increased fluoxetine levels.
- clarithromycin (Biaxin) may lead to fluoxetine toxicity—avoid the combination.
- clozapine (Clozaril) may result in increased levels of clozapine. The clozapine dose may need to be decreased if both medicines are to be used at the same time.
- delavirdine (Rescriptor) may lead to delavirdine toxicity.
- dextromethorphan (a cough suppressant in many "DM"-labeled nonprescription cough medicines) may result in visual hallucinations if these drugs are combined. DO NOT COMBINE.
- fenfluramine (Pondimin) may lead to serotonin syndrome—DO NOT COMBINE.
- haloperidol (Haldol) will increase haloperidol levels. Dose decrease and blood levels are needed.
- ketorolac (Toradol) may result in hallucinations. DO NOT COMBINE.
- lithium (Lithobid, etc.) will result in increased lithium levels and increased risk of neurotoxicity. AVOID COMBINING.
- loratadine (Claritin) may result in increased loratadine levels. It may be prudent to decrease the loratadine dose if these medicines are to be combined. Unlike some of the other nonsedating antihistamines (see Drug Classes), loratadine has not (to date) resulted in abnormal heart rhythms.
- medicines that inhibit liver metabolism (removal) of this medicine may lead to higher than expected fluoxetine blood levels and increased toxicity risk.
- monoamine oxidase (MAO) type A inhibitor drugs (see Drug Classes) may cause confusion, agitation, high fever, seizures and dangerous elevations of blood pressure. AVOID COMBINING.
- morphine (various) blunted pain management benefits of morphine in one case report.
- naratriptan (Amerge), rizatriptan (Maxalt), sumatriptan (Imitrex) or zolmitriptan may lead to incoordination and abnormal reflexes. Caution is advised.
- selegiline (Eldepryl) can result in serotonin toxicity syndrome. AVOID COMBINING.
- sibutramine (Meridia) may lead to serotonin syndrome. AVOID COMBINING.
- tramadol (Ultram) may increase seizure risk. DO NOT COMBINE.
- any tricyclic antidepressant (amitriptyline, nortriptyline, etc.) will result in increased antidepressant drug levels that will persist for weeks. Avoid the combination.
- tryptophan will result in central nervous system toxicity. AVOID COMBINING.
- zolpidem (Ambien) may increase risk of hallucinations.

▷ *Driving, Hazardous Activities:* This drug may cause drowsiness, dizziness, impaired judgment and delayed reaction time. Restrict activities as necessary.

Aviation Note: The use of this drug *is a disqualification* for piloting. Consult a designated Aviation Medical Examiner.

Exposure to Sun: No restrictions.

Discontinuation: Slow drug elimination makes withdrawal effects unlikely, but call your doctor if you plan to stop this drug for any reason.

Current Controversies in Drug Management: In 1990, six patients being treated with fluoxetine experienced intense and violent suicidal preoccupation. All six had severe depression that had not responded to the use of fluoxetine for 2 to 7 weeks. For most of them, suicidal mentality persisted for 2 to 3 months after stopping the drug. Adverse publicity suggested that this may be characteristic of fluoxetine in contrast to other antidepressant drugs. A review of relevant literature on this subject reveals that the development or intensification of suicidal thoughts during treatment (regardless of the severity of depression) has been documented repeatedly for many antidepressant drugs in wide use. Suicidal thinking may emerge during treatment with any antidepressant. Recent reports establish that some patients who become suicidal while taking one antidepressant can be switched to fluoxetine and experience cessation of suicidal thinking and satisfactory relief of depression.

The most recent study of fluoxetine in the *American Journal of Psychiatry* in February of 1999 found that in 643 Caucasians studied, treatment of affective disorders resulted in suicidal behavior that was marginally lower than in those patients who were not treated.

FLUPHENAZINE (flu FEN a zeen)

Introduced: 1959   **Class:** Strong tranquilizer, phenothiazines   **Prescription:** USA: Yes   **Controlled Drug:** USA: No; Canada: No   **Available as Generic:** USA: Yes; Canada: Yes

Brand Names: ✤Apo-Fluphenazine, ✤Modecate, ✤Moditan, Permitil, PMS-Fluphenazine, Prolixin

BENEFITS versus RISKS	
Possible Benefits	*Possible Risks*
EFFECTIVE CONTROL OF ACUTE MENTAL DISORDERS	SERIOUS TOXIC EFFECTS ON BRAIN with long-term use
Beneficial effects on thinking, mood and behavior	Liver damage with jaundice
Decanoate injection gives long-lasting benefit with one shot	Blood cell disorders: abnormally low white blood cell counts

Author's Note: The information in this profile has been shortened to make room for more widely used medicines.

FLURAZEPAM (flur AZ e pam)

Introduced: 1970   **Class:** Hypnotic, benzodiazepines   **Prescription:** USA: Yes   **Controlled Drug:** USA: C-IV*; Canada: No   **Available as Generic:** USA: Yes; Canada: Yes

*See Schedules of Controlled Drugs at the back of this book.

Brand Names: ❋Apo-Flurazepam, Dalmane, Durapam, ❋Novo-Flupam, ❋ Somnol

BENEFITS versus RISKS	
Possible Benefits	*Possible Risks*
EFFECTIVE HYPNOTIC	Habit-forming potential with
NO SUPPRESSION OF REM (RAPID	long-term use
EYE MOVEMENT) SLEEP	Minor impairment of mental
NO REM SLEEP REBOUND after	functions ("hangover" effect)
discontinuation	Jaundice
Wide margin of safety with	Blood cell disorder
therapeutic doses	Suppression of stage 4 sleep with
	reduced "quality" of sleep

▷ **Principal Uses**

As a Single Drug Product: Uses currently included in FDA-approved labeling: Short-term treatment of insomnia consisting of difficulty in falling asleep, frequent nighttime awakenings and/or early morning awakenings.

Other (unlabeled) generally accepted uses: None at present.

Author's Note: Information in this profile has been shortened to make room for more widely used medicines.

Author's Note: The National Institute of Mental Health has an information Web page on anxiety. It can be found at www.nimh.nih.gov/anxiety.

FLURBIPROFEN (flur BI proh fen)

Please see the propionic acids (nonsteroidal anti-inflammatory drug) family profile.

FLUTAMIDE (FLUTE a myde)

Introduced: 1983   **Class:** Anticancer (antineoplastic)   **Prescription:** USA: Yes   **Controlled Drug:** USA: No; Canada: No   **Available as Generic:** USA: Yes; Canada: Yes

Brand Names: ❋Apo-flutamide, ❋Euflex, Eulexin, Flutamex (Germany)

BENEFITS versus RISKS	
Possible Benefits	*Possible Risks*
EFFECTIVE ADJUNCTIVE	Rare drug-induced hepatitis
TREATMENT OF PROSTATE	Breast enlargement and tenderness
CANCER	Hot flashes

▷ **Principal Uses**

As a Single Drug Product: Uses currently included in FDA-approved labeling: Treatment of metastatic prostate cancer, used concurrently with leuprolide (given by injection) or with removal of the testicles (orchiectomy).

Other (unlabeled) generally accepted uses: (1) Some early data on use in bulimia; (2) can help excessive hair growth in women (hirsutism).

How This Drug Works: Flutamide suppresses effects of testosterone (a male sex hormone) by blocking uptake and binding target tissues (such as the prostate gland). Used in conjunction with leuprolide (a drug that suppresses testosterone from testicles by damping the pituitary gland's testicular stimulation). The combination of these two drug actions—chemical castration by leuprolide and testosterone blockage by flutamide—significantly reduces hormonal stimulation of cancerous prostate tissue.

Available Dosage Forms and Strengths
　　Capsules — 125 mg (US)
　　Tablets — 250 mg (Canada, Germany)

▷ **Recommended Dosage Ranges** (Actual dose and schedule must be determined for each patient individually.)

Infants and Children: Not used in this age group.

12 to 60 Years of Age: In stage B2-C prostate cancer: 250 mg by mouth every 8 hours. Flutamide is to be taken concurrently with an LHRH agonist such as leuprolide; the usual dose of leuprolide is 7.5 mg given by injection once a month—starting 8 weeks before radiation treatment. The medicine is also continued during radiation treatment.

Stage D2 prostate cancer: 250 mg by mouth every 8 hours in conjunction with an LHRH agonist. It is continued until there is evidence of progression.

Over 60 Years of Age: Same as 12 to 60 years of age.

Conditions Requiring Dosing Adjustments

Liver Function: Use with caution by patients with liver compromise. It is also a rare cause of cholestatic jaundice.

Kidney Function: Primarily eliminated by the kidneys. Use with caution in kidney compromise.

▷ **Dosing Instructions:** May be taken without regard to food. The capsule may be opened, and the tablet may be crushed. If you forget a dose: take the missed dose as soon as you remember it, unless it is nearly time for your next dose—if that is the case, skip the missed dose and take the next dose right on schedule. DO NOT double doses. Use a condom to keep your semen from contacting your sexual partner.

Warning: Since this medicine is an antineoplastic agent, proper disposal of urine or vomit MUST be undertaken (ask your doctor).

Usual Duration of Use: Regular use for 2 to 3 months usually needed to see drug's benefits in controlling prostate cancer. Long-term use (months to years) requires periodic physician evaluation.

Typical Treatment Goals and Measurements (Outcomes and Markers)

Prostate cancer: The goal is to decrease bone pain, increase urine outflow and increase survival time in D2 prostate cancer. Remissions have been gained from this medicine. PSA tests may serve as a marker of success.

Possible Advantages of This Drug
　　Ease of use. Less toxicity than other chemotherapeutic drugs.

Currently a "Drug of Choice"
　　For the management of prostate cancer (in combination with leuprolide) and coupled with castration.

▷ **This Drug Should Not Be Taken If**
　　• you have had an allergic reaction to it previously.
　　• your liver is severely impaired.

▷ **Inform Your Physician Before Taking This Drug If**
   • you have a history of liver disease or impaired liver function.
   • you have high blood pressure (hypertension).
   • you have a history of anemia, low white blood cells or low blood platelets.
   • you have a history of lupus erythematosus.

Possible Side Effects (natural, expected and unavoidable drug actions)
   Hot flashes (61%), loss of libido (with combination LHRH therapy), impotence, breast enlargement and tenderness. Bright yellow urine color.

▷ **Possible Adverse Effects** (unusual, unexpected and infrequent reactions)
   If any of the following develop, consult your physician promptly for guidance.
   Mild Adverse Effects
   Allergic reactions: skin rash.
   Drowsiness, confusion, nervousness, depression—rare.
   Indigestion, nausea/vomiting, diarrhea—infrequent.
   Blurred vision—rare.
   Fluid retention (edema) of legs—possible.
   Serious Adverse Effects
   Drug-induced hepatitis with jaundice (see Glossary)—rare to infrequent.
   Low blood platelets, white blood cells or anemia—rare.
   Lupus erythematosus-like skin rash—case reports.
   Heart attack—rare.
   Methemoglobinemia—case report.

▷ **Possible Effects on Sexual Function:** See "Possible Side Effects" above. Flutamide itself does not presently appear to change libido, sexual performance or the ability to have an erection. Combination therapy does appear to carry the risks of these adverse effects. Swelling and tenderness of male breast tissue (gynecomastia) may be frequent.

▷ **Adverse Effects That May Mimic Natural Diseases or Disorders**
   Drug-induced hepatitis may suggest viral hepatitis.

Possible Effects on Laboratory Tests
   Complete blood counts: decreased red and white cells, hemoglobin and platelets.
   Liver function tests: increased liver enzymes (ALT/GPT, AST/GOT and alkaline phosphatase), increased bilirubin.
   PSA: reduced (a marker for cancer treatment results).
   Sperm counts and testosterone levels: decreased.

CAUTION
   1. For best results, flutamide and leuprolide should be started together and continued for the duration of therapy.
   2. During combination therapy with flutamide and leuprolide, symptoms of prostate cancer (difficult urination, bone pain, etc.) may worsen temporarily; these are transient and not significant.

Precautions for Use
   By Those Over 60 Years of Age: Drug is more slowly excreted. If digestive symptoms or edema are troublesome, ask your doctor about adjusting dose.

▷ **Advisability of Use During Pregnancy**
   Pregnancy Category: D. See Pregnancy Risk Categories at the back of this book.

Animal studies: Rat studies reveal malformation of bone structures and feminization of male fetuses.

Human studies: Adequate studies of pregnant women are not available.
Discuss this benefit-to-risk decision with your doctor.

Advisability of Use If Breast-Feeding
Presence of this drug in breast milk: Unknown.
Stop nursing.

Habit-Forming Potential: None.

Effects of Overdose: Possible drowsiness, unsteadiness, nausea, vomiting.

Possible Effects of Long-Term Use: None reported.

Suggested Periodic Examinations While Taking This Drug (at physician's discretion)
Prostate-specific antigen (PSA) assays.
Complete blood cell counts.
Liver function tests.

▷ **While Taking This Drug, Observe the Following**
Foods: No restrictions.

Herbal Medicines: Since St. John's wort may also lead to increased sensitivity to the sun, DO NOT COMBINE. There are no data about use of echinacea with this medicine and the combination cannot be recommended.

Beverages: No restrictions. May be taken with milk.

▷ *Alcohol:* No interactions expected.

Tobacco Smoking: No interactions expected, but I advise everyone to quit smoking.

Marijuana Smoking: Animal studies have shown this combination to result in additive suppression of the immune system. The combination therefore is not advisable.

▷ *Other Drugs*
Flutamide *taken concurrently* with
- influenza, pneumococcal or yellow fever vaccine may result in blunting of immune response to the vaccine.
- warfarin (Coumadin, others) may cause an increased bleeding risk. More frequent INRs are prudent.

▷ *Driving, Hazardous Activities:* This drug may cause drowsiness. Restrict activities as necessary.

Aviation Note: The use of this drug *may be a disqualification* for piloting. Consult a designated Aviation Medical Examiner.

Exposure to Sun: This drug may cause photosensitivity (see Glossary).

Discontinuation: To be determined by your physician.

FLUTICASONE (flu TIC a zone)

Introduced: 1994   **Class:** Adrenocortical steroids   **Prescription:**
USA: Yes   **Controlled Drug:** USA: No; Canada: No   **Available as**
Generic: USA: No; Canada: No

Brand Names: ✤ Advair [CD], Advair Diskus [CD], Cutivate, Flonase, Flovent, Flovent Diskus, Flovent Rotadisc

Author's Note: Some of the side effects are specific to or more likely with a particular dosing form (product).

BENEFITS versus RISKS	
Possible Benefits	*Possible Risks*
EFFECTIVE, ONCE-DAILY RELIEF OF SEASONAL ALLERGIC RHINITIS	Reversible adrenal gland suppression
	Irritation of the nose (nasal form)
EFFECTIVE ONCE-DAILY ECZEMA TREATMENT	
EFFECTIVE ASTHMA TREATMENT	

▷ **Principal Uses**

As a Single Drug Product: Uses currently included in FDA-approved labeling: (1) Helps perennial and seasonal (hay fever) allergic or nonallergic rhinitis in adults or children who are 12 years of age or older; (2) the topical form is used for a variety of skin conditions from sunburn to lupus erythematosus; (3) asthma (inhaler form); (4) cream approved for once-daily treatment of eczema.

Other (unlabeled) generally accepted uses: Oral form may have a role in Crohn's disease.

As a Combination Drug Product [CD]: Combined with salmeterol in (see drug profile later in this book). These drugs complement each other, making the combination a more effective antiasthmatic.

How This Drug Works: Corticosteroid-type medicines work to ease inflammation, suppress reaction of certain cells and slow the inflammatory process. Halomethyl carbothionates have very potent anti-inflammatory and blood-vessel-contracting (vasoconstrictive) activity.

Available Dosage Forms and Strengths

Amber glass bottle — 16 g (120 actuations) and 9 g (60 actuations)

Cream — 0.05 mg/g

Inhalation — 44 mcg, 110 mcg, 220 mcg

Inhalation powder (US, Canada)— 50 mcg of salmeterol and 100, 250 or 500 mcg fluticasone per actuation

Nasal spray — 0.05%

▷ **Recommended Dosage Ranges** (Actual dose and schedule must be determined for each patient individually.)

Infants and Children: Safety and efficacy for those less than 4 have not yet been defined. Nasal dosing for those 4 to 12—start with one spray (50 mcg in each spray) in each nostril once a day. If symptoms are severe, the dose can be increased to two sprays in each nostril (50 mcg each spray) or 200 micrograms a day. After a few days, the dose should be reduced to 50 micrograms in each nostril once daily.

12 to 60 Years of Age:

Nasal dosing: Started with two sprays (50 mcg in each spray) in each nostril once daily. The same dose can also be given as 100 mcg twice daily (8 a.m. and 8 p.m.). After a few days, the dose can often be decreased to 100 mcg (one spray in each nostril) daily.

Inhalation for asthma: Starting dose is 88 mcg twice a day for patients who were previously treated with bronchodilators alone. Maximum daily dose is 440 mcg. Patients who required an inhaled corticosteroid previously are given 88 to 220 mcg twice daily. This dose is increased up to 440 mcg twice a day as needed and tolerated. Those taking a corticosteroid by mouth are given 880 mcg twice daily. Once the asthma is under control, the dose is reduced to the lowest effective dose.

Fluticasone/salmeterol combination: The starting dose is 100 mcg fluticasone and 50 mcg of salmeterol in people who are not presently taking an inhaled steroid (corticosteroid). If they are taking an inhaled corticosteroid such as budesonide and the steroid dose is less than or equal to 400 mcg a day, then the combination inhaler containing 100 mcg of fluticasone and 50 mcg of salmeterol is substituted and is taken twice a day. Other doses of budesonide or other corticosteroids require different combinations of fluticasone/salmeterol to get the best results.

Over 60 Years of Age: Same as 12 to 60 years of age.

Conditions Requiring Dosing Adjustments

Liver Function: This drug is extensively changed in the liver; however, no specific dosing changes are defined for patients with compromised livers.

Kidney Function: No changes in dosing are needed.

▷ **Dosing Instructions:** A patient instruction sheet will always accompany this medicine. The instructions should be followed closely. Your doctor should be called if the condition worsens or does not improve. Once an inhalation treatment is completed, rinse your mouth with water. If you forget a dose: use the spray or inhaler as soon as you remember it, unless it's nearly time for your next dose—if this is the case, skip the missed dose and just take the next scheduled dose right on time. DO NOT double doses. This medicine is not used for sudden asthma episodes or status asthmaticus.

Usual Duration of Use: Continual use on a regular schedule for several days is usually necessary to determine this drug's effectiveness in treating seasonal and perennial allergic rhinitis. For the inhaled form, a beneficial response may happen in a day, but it may take two weeks to realize the maximum benefits. Long-term use (months to years) requires periodic evaluation of response and dose adjustment. Keep appointments with your doctor.

Typical Treatment Goals and Measurements (Outcomes and Markers)

Asthma: Frequency and severity of asthma attacks should ease. Some clinicians also use decreased frequency of rescue inhaler use as a further clinical indicator. It is critical that this medicine is used regularly to get the best results. An additional goal of therapy is to use the lowest effective dose. Some people keep their improvements when doses are lowered, while others relapse. Specific testing goals include improvement in PEFR and other lung (pulmonary) function tests. Wheezing and difficulty breathing (dyspnea) should ease as well as asthma caused (induced) by exercise. If the usual benefit is not realized, call your doctor.

Allergic rhinitis: Signs and symptoms of allergic rhinitis such as runny or stuffy nose, postnasal drip and sneezing should ease. Scratch testing for a specific immune substance (IgE) can also be done to check progress at a cellular level.

Possible Advantages of This Drug
Once-a-day dosing for the nasal form.

▷ **This Drug Should Not Be Taken If**
- you have had an allergic reaction to any dose form of it previously.
- you have sudden onset asthma or status asthmaticus. (Fluticasone or fluticasone/salmeterol WON'T WORK.)

▷ **Inform Your Physician Before Taking This Drug If**
- you are already taking systemic prednisone.
- you are exposed to measles or chicken pox.
- you are unsure how much to take or how often to take it.
- you take prescription or nonprescription medicines not discussed when fluticasone was prescribed.
- you have diabetes.
- you have signs or symptoms of an infection in your nose.
- your skin is shrunken (atrophied) or you have acne, warts or other skin problems (topical form).
- you've had fungal infections, herpes simplex of the eye, tuberculosis or other infections.
- you have damage from an accident or surgery to your nose while you are taking this medicine.
- your allergic rhinitis does not improve or worsens.

Possible Side Effects (natural, expected and unavoidable drug actions)
Irritation of the nose, nosebleeds. Systemic steroid effects—possible.

▷ **Possible Adverse Effects** (unusual, unexpected and infrequent reactions)
If any of the following develop, consult your physician promptly for guidance.
Mild Adverse Effects
Allergic reactions: contact dermatitis.
Nosebleeds or nasal burning—case reports to infrequent.
Dizziness or headache—rare to infrequent.
Unpleasant taste, nausea or vomiting—rare.
Increased heart rate—case reports.
Serious Adverse Effects
Allergic reactions: anaphylaxis—case report.
Suppression of the hypothalamic pituitary adrenal (HPA) axis—rare.
Increased risk from viral infections—possible.
Increased pressure in the head (more likely in children)—possible.
Yeast infections of the nose—rare.
Loss of control of blood sugar—possible in diabetics and others.
Glaucoma or cataracts—case reports (inhaled form).
Cushing's syndrome (with excessive doses or very sensitive patients)—possible.
Growth suppression in children—possible.
Osteoporosis—increased risk with long-term use.

▷ **Possible Effects on Sexual Function:** None defined.

Possible Delayed Adverse Effects: Yeast infections of the nose—rare. Osteoporosis—increased risk.

▷ **Adverse Effects That May Mimic Natural Diseases or Disorders**
None defined.

Natural Diseases or Disorders That May Be Activated by This Drug

If systemic effects occur, the patient may be more susceptible to infections, or dormant infections may become active. This drug increases osteoporosis risk even in those not predisposed to developing osteoporosis.

Possible Effects on Laboratory Tests

Cortisol levels: decreased.

CAUTION

1. Call your doctor if you are exposed to measles or chicken pox.
2. Long-term use requires periodic evaluation for yeast infection of the nose.
3. Call your doctor if your condition does not improve or worsens.

Precautions for Use

By Infants and Children: Safety and effectiveness for use by those under 12 years of age have not been established for the intranasal form. Many adolescents can be started successfully with one spray in each nostril per day (100 mcg). Maximum total daily dose should not exceed 200 mcg. Children in general are at greater risk for suppression of the HPA axis and glucocorticosteroid insufficiency than adults.

By Those Over 60 Years of Age: No specific precautions.

▷ **Advisability of Use During Pregnancy**

Pregnancy Category: C. See Pregnancy Risk Categories at the back of this book.

Animal studies: High-dose studies in rats revealed fetal toxicity consistent with changes caused by other steroids.

Human studies: Information from adequate studies of pregnant women is not available.

Ask your doctor for guidance.

Advisability of Use If Breast-Feeding

Presence of this drug in breast milk: Unknown.

Monitor nursing infant closely and discontinue drug or nursing if adverse effects develop.

Habit-Forming Potential: Not defined.

Effects of Overdose: Not defined.

Possible Effects of Long-Term Use: Rare nasal yeast infections.

Suggested Periodic Examinations While Taking This Drug (at physician's discretion)

Nasal exams, check for osteoporosis (DEXA, PDEXA) with long term use.

▷ **While Taking This Drug, Observe the Following**

Foods: No restrictions.

Herbal Medicines or Minerals: Fir or pine needle oil should NOT be used by asthmatics. Ephedra alone does carry a German Commission E monograph indication for asthma treatment. If you are allergic to plants in the Asteraceae family (aster, chrysanthemum, daisy or ragweed), you may also be allergic to echinacea, chamomile, feverfew and St. John's wort. Increased calcium and vitamin D are prudent while taking this medicine. Talk to your doctor BEFORE adding any herbals to this medicine.

Beverages: No restrictions.

▷ *Alcohol:* No interactions expected.

Tobacco Smoking: No interactions expected. I advise everyone to quit smoking.

▷   *Other Drugs*
Fluticasone ***taken concurrently*** with
* ketoconazole (Nizoral) and perhaps other azole antifungals may increase fluticasone blood levels.
* medicines that inhibit CYP 3A4 will lead to increased fluticasone effects and those that induce 3A4 will decrease fluticasone benefits.
* ritonavir (Norvir) may increase fluticasone blood levels and lead to Cushing's syndrome. A check of cortisol levels may help make the diagnosis.
* systemic steroids (such as prednisone) may increase the likelihood of suppression of the hypothalamic pituitary adrenal (HPA) axis.

▷   *Driving, Hazardous Activities:* This drug may cause dizziness. Restrict activities as necessary.
Aviation Note: The use of this drug ***may be a disqualification*** for piloting. Consult a designated Aviation Medical Examiner.
Exposure to Sun: No restrictions.
Discontinuation: This medicine should not be stopped abruptly. Talk with your doctor before stopping this drug.

FLUVASTATIN (flu va STAT in)

Introduced: 1994   **Class:** Cholesterol-reducing drug, HMG-CoA reductase inhibitor   **Prescription:** USA: Yes   **Controlled Drug:** USA: No; Canada: No   **Available as Generic:** USA: No; Canada: No
Brand Name: Lescol, Lescol XL

BENEFITS versus RISKS	
Possible Benefits	*Possible Risks*
EFFECTIVE REDUCTION OF TOTAL BLOOD CHOLESTEROL	Increased liver enzymes
REDUCES TRIGLYCERIDES AND APOLIPOPROTEIN B	Muscle pain or weakness
SLOWS PROGRESSION OF CORONARY ATHEROSCLEROSIS	Decreased coenzyme Q10

▷ **Principal Uses**
As a Single Drug Product: Uses currently included in FDA-approved labeling: (1) Manages abnormally high cholesterol and triglycerides and apolipoprotein B in people with type 2 hypercholesterolemia; (2) slows progression of atherosclerosis in patients with coronary heart disease.
Other (unlabeled) generally accepted uses: (1) One case of blue toe syndrome was successfully reversed; (2) worked to lower LDL cholesterol in one study of Type II hyperlipoproteinemia; (3) may have a role in stroke prevention, but further studies are needed; (4) helps prevent clogging (restenosis) of coronary stents; (4) like other HMG-CoA reductase inhibitors—may have a role in reducing risk of bone fractures.

How This Drug Works: This medicine is changed (hydrolyzed) to a beta-hydroxy-acid form. The beta-hydroxy-acid inhibits HMG-CoA reductase. This enzyme is critical for cholesterol formation. Once inhibited, cholesterol formation slows.

Available Dosage Forms and Strengths
Tablets — 10 mg, 20 mg, 40 mg

▷ **Recommended Dosage Ranges** (Actual dose and schedule must be determined for each patient individually.)

Infants and Children: Safety and efficacy for those less than 18 years of age have not been established.

18 to 60 Years of Age: Dosing is started with 20 mg a day, taken with the evening meal. This dose is increased as needed and tolerated to 80 mg with each evening (24 hours apart) meal. Any needed increases are made at intervals of 4 weeks. Patients who take immunosuppressant medicines are started on 10 mg of lovastatin daily and should not receive more than 20 mg daily with the evening meal. If 80 mg is required to achieve cholesterol and HDL goals—a single evening dose of 80 mg of the Lescol XL form can be taken.

Over 60 Years of Age: Same as 18 to 60 years of age.

Conditions Requiring Dosing Adjustments
Liver Function: This drug is extensively changed in the liver. Lower doses appear prudent in liver disease.

Kidney Function: Patients with severe failure (creatinine clearance less than 30 ml/min) should be closely followed if given over 20 mg daily.

▷ **Dosing Instructions:** This medicine is best taken with the EVENING MEAL, as it produces the best cholesterol-lowering results or outcomes. If you forget a dose: Take the next dose as soon as you remember it, unless it is nearly time for your next dose—then skip the dose you missed and just take the next scheduled dose. DO NOT double doses. If you find yourself omitting doses, call your doctor for some added ways to help remember your medicine.

Usual Duration of Use: Continual use on a regular schedule for 4 to 6 weeks may be needed to determine this drug's effectiveness in helping lower low-density lipoprotein (LDL) level. Long-term use (months to years) requires evaluation of response by your doctor. Know your cholesterol numbers and try to achieve NCEP goals.

Typical Treatment Goals and Measurements (Outcomes and Markers)
Cholesterol: The National Institutes of Health has released ATP III as part of the update to the National Cholesterol Education Program or NCEP. Key points in these new guidelines include acknowledging diabetes as one of the conditions that increases risk of heart disease, modifying risk factors and recommending routine testing for all of the cholesterol fractions (lipoprotein profile) versus total cholesterol alone. These new guidelines also recommend a desirable total cholesterol of 200 mg/dl as before, but change optimal LDL to 100 mg/dl, 130–159 mg/dl as borderline high, 160 mg/dl as high and cite 190 mg/dl as very high. One other noteworthy change is that "good cholesterol" or HDL has been made more important. The "too low" measure for HDL has been increased to 40 mg/dl. Take your medicine and reach these new targets! Electron beam computed tomography (EBCT) is an important tool to use in conjunction with these laboratory studies because even patients who meet cholesterol goals (particularly females over 55) can still be at risk.

Possible Advantages of This Drug
Recent studies indicate that drugs of this class (HMG-CoA reductase inhibitors) are more effective and better tolerated than other drugs currently available for reducing total and LDL-C cholesterol.

▷ **This Drug Should Not Be Taken If**
  • you had an allergic reaction to it previously.
  • you have active liver disease or your liver enzymes become elevated (talk to your doctor).
  • you are pregnant or breast-feeding your infant.

▷ **Inform Your Physician Before Taking This Drug If**
  • you have previously taken any other drugs in this class: lovastatin (Mevacor), pravastatin (Pravachol).
  • another doctor prescribes niacin, cyclosporine, erythromycin or fibrate-type medicines.
  • you have a history of liver disease or impaired liver function.
  • you are not using birth control or you are planning pregnancy.
  • you regularly consume substantial amounts of alcohol.
  • you have cataracts or impaired vision.
  • you have any type of chronic muscular disorder.
  • you develop muscle pain, weakness or soreness that is unexplained while taking this medicine.
  • you plan to have major surgery in the near future.

Possible Side Effects (natural, expected and unavoidable drug actions)
  Development of abnormal liver function tests without associated symptoms.

▷ **Possible Adverse Effects** (unusual, unexpected and infrequent reactions)
  If any of the following develop, consult your physician promptly for guidance.
  Mild Adverse Effects
  Allergic reactions: rash.
  Headache, insomnia or dizziness—infrequent.
  Indigestion, nausea, excessive gas, constipation, diarrhea—infrequent.
  Lowering of the blood pressure—possible.
  Serious Adverse Effects
  Marked and persistent abnormal liver function tests with focal hepatitis (without jaundice)—case reports.
  Acute myositis (muscle pain and tenderness)—occurred rarely during long-term use.
  Rhabdomyolysis and sudden kidney failure—rare.
  Vision changes—possible, case report.
  Lichen planus skin rash—rare.
  Neuropathy—case reports.
  Systemic lupus erythematosus–like syndrome—case reports.

▷ **Possible Effects on Sexual Function:** None reported.

Possible Delayed Adverse Effects: Vision change. Doses of 15 to 33 times the human dose of another drug in this class given to rats caused an increase in liver cancers.

Natural Diseases or Disorders That May Be Activated by This Drug
  Latent liver disease.

Possible Effects on Laboratory Tests
  Blood alanine aminotransferase (ALT) enzyme level: increased (with higher doses of drug).
  Blood total cholesterol, LDL cholesterol and triglyceride levels: decreased.
  Blood HDL cholesterol level: increased.

CAUTION

1. If pregnancy occurs while taking this drug, stop taking the drug immediately and call your doctor.
2. Report promptly any development of muscle pain or tenderness, especially if accompanied by fever or weakness (malaise).
3. Report promptly altered or impaired vision so that appropriate evaluation can be made.

Precautions for Use

By Infants and Children: Safety and effectiveness for those under 20 years of age are not established.

By Those Over 60 Years of Age: Tell your doctor about any personal or family history of vision problems. If periodic eye examinations are recommended, get them. Promptly report any vision changes.

▷ **Advisability of Use During Pregnancy**

Pregnancy Category: X. See Pregnancy Risk Categories at the back of this book.

Animal studies: Mouse and rat studies reveal skeletal birth defects due to a closely related drug of this class.

Human studies: Adequate studies of pregnant women are not available.

This drug should be avoided during entire pregnancy.

Advisability of Use If Breast-Feeding

Presence of this drug in breast milk: Unknown, but not thought to be safe.

Avoid drug or refrain from nursing.

Habit-Forming Potential: None.

Effects of Overdose: Increased indigestion, stomach distress, nausea, diarrhea.

Possible Effects of Long-Term Use: Abnormal liver function with focal hepatitis. Abnormal liver function tests. Decreased coenzyme Q10 (co-Q10 or ubiquinone).

Suggested Periodic Examinations While Taking This Drug (at physician's discretion)

Blood cholesterol studies: total cholesterol, HDL and LDL fractions (usually every 4 weeks with dose changes).

Liver function tests before treatment, every 6 weeks during the first 3 months of use, every 8 weeks for the rest of the first year, and at 6-month intervals thereafter.

Author's Note: A related medicine called cerivastatin (Baycol) was removed from the market because of liver changes. It is unknown at the time of this writing if the FDA will review similar medicines and ask for more frequent checks of liver function.

Complete eye examination at beginning of treatment and at any time that significant change in vision occurs. Ask your physician for guidance.

Electron beam computed tomography (EBCT) can help predict silent ischemia and other problems with blood vessels that supply the heart itself. This also may help define the results (outcomes) you are getting from this medicine.

▷ **While Taking This Drug, Observe the Following**

Foods: Follow a standard low-cholesterol diet.

Herbal Medicines or Minerals: No data exist from well-designed clinical studies about garlic and fluvastatin combinations and can not presently be recommended. Additionally, garlic may inhibit blood clotting (platelet) aggregation—something to consider if you are already taking a platelet inhibitor. The FDA will allow one dietary supplement called Cholestin to be sold. Because this product actually contains lovastatin, and the use of two HMG-Co-A inhibitors may increase risk of rhabdomyolysis or myopathy, the combination is NOT advised. Some products containing plant sterols (Benecol) may be useful as complimentary care to lower total and LDL cholesterol. Substituting soy for some of the meat in your diet can help avoid cardiovascular problems. Lastly, because this medicine can deplete co-Q10, supplementation may be needed.

Beverages: No restrictions. May be taken with milk.

▷ *Alcohol:* No interactions expected. Use sparingly.

Tobacco Smoking: No interactions expected. I advise everyone to quit smoking.

▷ *Other Drugs*

Fluvastatin may ***increase*** the effects of
- digoxin (Lanoxin).
- warfarin (Coumadin); more frequent testing of INR (prothrombin time) will be needed.

Fluvastatin ***taken concurrently*** with
- amprenavir (Agenerase) and ritonavir (Norvir) and perhaps other protease inhibitors may increase fluvastatin levels and the risk of muscle damage (myopathy).
- clofibrate (Atromid-S) or other fibrate compounds may result in increased risk of serious muscle toxicity.
- clopidogrel (Plavix) may result in increased fluvastatin levels (because of possible CYP 450 2C9 inhibition. Careful patient follow up is prudent.
- cyclosporine (Sandimmune) can result in kidney failure and myopathy.
- erythromycin and perhaps other macrolide antibiotics (see Drug Classes) may increase risk of muscle damage (myopathy or rhabdomyolysis).
- fluconazole (Diflucan), itraconazole (Sporanox) or ketoconazole (Nizoral) increases myopathy or rhabdomyolysis risk.
- gemfibrozil (Lopid) may alter the absorption and excretion of fluvastatin; these drugs should not be taken concurrently.
- levothyroxine (various) may blunt the effects of levothyroxine.
- medicines that change cytochrome P450 3A4 (inhibitors will increase fluvastatin levels and inducers will blunt atorvastatin therapeutic effects).
- niacin may cause an increased frequency of muscle problems (myopathy) when combined with a related medicine (lovastatin). Caution is advised. Niacin may also increase homocysteine levels—a risk factor for heart disease.
- omeprazole (Prilosec) and possible esomeprazole (Nexium) may increase fluvastatin levels and lead to toxicity.
- quinupristin/dalfopristin (Synercid) may increase the risk for myopathy by increasing cerivastatin blood levels.
- ranitidine (Zantac) may increase peak blood levels of fluvastatin.
- ritonavir (Norvir) may lead to fluvastatin toxicity.
- sildenafil (Viagra) may change levels of either drug as they both use CYP3A4 to be removed from the body.

The following drug may ***decrease*** the effects of fluvastatin:
- cholestyramine (Questran), by possibly reducing absorption of fluvastatin; take fluvastatin 1 hour before or 4 hours after cholestyramine.

▷ *Driving, Hazardous Activities:* No restrictions.
Aviation Note: No restrictions.
Exposure to Sun: No restrictions.
Discontinuation: Do not stop this drug without your physician's knowledge and guidance. There may be significant increase in blood cholesterol levels following discontinuation of this drug.

FLUVOXAMINE (FLU vox a meen)

Introduced: 1995   **Class:** Antidepressant, selective serotonin reuptake inhibitor   **Prescription:** USA: Yes   **Controlled Drug:** USA: No; Canada: No   **Available as Generic:** USA: Yes; Canada: Yes
Brand Names: ✦ Apo-Fluvoxamine, Luvox, ✦Novo-Fluvoxamine, ✦PMS-Fluvoxamine, ✦Riva-Fluvoxamine
Warning: Do not combine this medicine with terfenadine (Seldane) or astemizole (Hismanal). No longer on the US market, but may still be in some foreign countries.

BENEFITS versus RISKS

Possible Benefits	*Possible Risks*
TREATMENT OF OBSESSIVE-COMPULSIVE DISORDER IN ADULTS	Nausea and vomiting (often resolve with time)
TREATMENT OF OBSESSIVE-COMPULSIVE DISORDER IN CHILDREN	
Treatment of depression	
Treatment of panic disorder	
May have a role in helping to control binge eating	
May have a role in helping to treat social anxiety disorder	

▷ **Principal Uses**
As a Single Drug Product: Uses currently included in FDA-approved labeling: Treatment of obsessive-compulsive disorder in adults and children.
Other (unlabeled) generally accepted uses: (1) May have a role in helping compulsive exhibitionism; (2) treats depression; (3) may be useful in eating problems where binge behaviors are a key factor; (4) can help panic attacks; (5) helps prevent long-standing (chronic) tension headaches; (6) eases social anxiety disorder; (7) may help pathological gambling.
How This Drug Works: Inhibits reuptake of the neurotransmitter 5-HT, easing symptoms of treated behaviors or conditions.
Available Dosage Forms and Strengths
Tablets — 25 mg, 50 mg, 100 mg
▷ **Recommended Dosage Ranges** (Actual dose and schedule must be determined for each patient individually.)
Infants and Children: Safety and efficacy have been established in pediatrics (children and adolescents). Dosing is started with 25 mg at bedtime for 3

days. The dose is then increased by 25-mg steps every 3 to 4 days until a maximum of 200 mg is reached. If the required dose is larger than 75 mg, the total daily dose is divided into two equal doses and given twice daily.

18 to 60 Years of Age: Therapy is started with 50 mg taken at bedtime. The dose may then be increased as needed and tolerated by 50-mg intervals every 4 to 7 days to a maximum dose of 300 mg daily. The prescriber should remember that the drug may take from 4 to 14 days to begin to work. If patient needs a daily dose greater than 100 mg, dose is divided in half and taken twice daily.

Over 60 Years of Age: This medicine is removed half as slowly as in younger patients. Plasma concentrations are also roughly 40% higher than in younger patients. Slower time frames for any increases beyond the starting dose and lower maintenance doses are indicated.

Conditions Requiring Dosing Adjustments

Liver Function: This drug is extensively changed by the liver. If it is used by patients with liver disease, lower starting doses, slow dose increases, and careful patient monitoring are indicated.

Kidney Function: A lower starting dose and careful patient monitoring are needed.

▷ **Dosing Instructions:** Take this medicine exactly as prescribed and at the same time. This medicine may be taken with or without food. Call your doctor if vomiting (a possible side effect) continues for more than 2 days after you start treatment. If you forget a dose: take the missed dose as soon as you remember it, unless it's nearly time for your next dose—if that is the case, skip the missed dose and take the next dose right on time. DO NOT double doses.

Usual Duration of Use: Continual use on a regular schedule for 4 to 14 days is usually necessary to determine effectiveness in helping obsessive-compulsive disorder. Long-term use (months to years) requires evaluation by your doctor.

Typical Treatment Goals and Measurements (Outcomes and Markers)

Depression: The general goal: to lessen the degree and severity of depression, letting patients return to their daily lives. Specific measures of depression involve testing or inventories and can be valuable in helping check benefits from this medicine.

Possible Advantages of This Drug

Requires once-daily dosing and has a good side-effect profile.

▷ **This Drug Should Not Be Taken If**

- you had an allergic reaction to it previously.
- you have taken or are taking astemizole or cisapride.

▷ **Inform Your Physician Before Taking This Drug If**

- you continue to have a problem with vomiting 2 days after starting this medicine.
- you feel light-headed when you get up from a sitting position.
- you have a history of seizures.
- you are unsure how much to take or how often to take it.
- you have taken a MAO inhibitor (see Drug Classes) within the last 14 days.
- you have a history of heart problems.
- you take prescription or nonprescription medicines not discussed when fluvoxamine was prescribed.

Possible Side Effects (natural, expected and unavoidable drug actions)
> Nausea and vomiting (usually stops after a few days of treatment). Dose-related orthostatic hypotension.

▷ **Possible Adverse Effects** (unusual, unexpected and infrequent reactions)
> **If any of the following develop, consult your physician promptly for guidance.**

Mild Adverse Effects
> Allergic reactions: skin rash.
> Somnolence, headache, agitation, sleep disorders—infrequent to frequent.
> Change in heart waves (R-R, QT and QTc intervals).
> Bruising—possible.
> Liver toxicity—rare.
> Patchy baldness (alopecia)—case report.
> Dry mouth, anorexia or constipation—possible to frequent.

Serious Adverse Effects
> Allergic reactions: anaphylactic reaction—case reports.
> Serious skin rash—case reports.
> Liver toxicity—rare.
> Seizures or mania—rare.
> Parkinson-like reactions—case reports with SSRI-type medicines.
> Tourette's syndrome—case reports.
> Serotonin syndrome—case report.
> Excessive urination (SIADH)—case reports.

▷ **Possible Effects on Sexual Function:** Delayed or absent orgasm, failure to ejaculate—case reports.
> Galactorrhea—case reports with SSRIs.

Possible Delayed Adverse Effects: Not reported.

▷ **Adverse Effects That May Mimic Natural Diseases or Disorders**
> Increased liver enzymes may mimic hepatitis.

Natural Diseases or Disorders That May Be Activated by This Drug
> None defined.

Possible Effects on Laboratory Tests
> Liver function tests: increased.
> Melatonin level: increased.

CAUTION
> 1. This medicine has several important drug-drug interactions. Be certain to tell all health care professionals that you take this medicine.
> 2. If nausea and vomiting continue for more than 2 days after you start this medicine, call your doctor.

Precautions for Use
> *By Infants and Children:* Safety and effectiveness for use by those under 18 years of age have not been established.
> *By Those Over 60 Years of Age:* Lowering starting and maintenance doses is indicated.

▷ **Advisability of Use During Pregnancy**
> *Pregnancy Category:* C. See Pregnancy Risk Categories at the back of this book.
> *Animal studies:* Consistent with category C.

Human studies: Information from adequate studies of pregnant women is not available.

Ask your doctor for help.

Advisability of Use If Breast-Feeding

Presence of this drug in breast milk: Yes, in small amounts.

Monitor nursing infant closely and discontinue drug or nursing if adverse effects develop.

Habit-Forming Potential: None, but a withdrawal syndrome has been reported if the medicine is stopped abruptly (moderate to high occurrence rate).

Effects of Overdose: Nausea, vomiting, seizures.

Possible Effects of Long-Term Use: Not defined.

Suggested Periodic Examinations While Taking This Drug (at physician's discretion)

Liver function tests.

▷ **While Taking This Drug, Observe the Following**

Foods: No restrictions. Vitamin C (500 mg daily) may stop bruising that is possible with this medicine.

Herbal Medicines or Minerals: Since fluvoxamine and St. John's wort may both act to increase serotonin, the combination is not advised. Since part of the way ginseng works may be as a MAO inhibitor, do not combine ginseng with fluvoxamine. Ma huang and yohimbe are also best avoided while taking this medicine. Valerian and kava kava may interact additively (drowsiness). Avoid these combinations. Indian snakeroot is also best avoided while taking this medicine. Talk to your doctor BEFORE adding any herbal medicine to this medicine.

Beverages: No restrictions.

▷ *Alcohol:* No significant interaction. Ask your doctor for guidance.

Tobacco Smoking: Fluvoxamine stays in the body of smokers up to one-quarter less time than in nonsmokers, and fluvoxamine benefits may be blunted. I advise everyone to quit smoking.

Marijuana Smoking: Additive somnolence.

▷ *Other Drugs*

Fluvoxamine *taken concurrently* with

- amitriptyline (Elavil, others) can result in amitriptyline toxicity.
- astemizole (Hismanal) may cause *serious heart arrhythmias.* DO NOT COMBINE.
- benzodiazepines (see Drug Classes) may result in benzodiazepine toxicity.
- beta blockers (see Drug Classes) may result in decreased drug clearance and toxicity.
- buspirone (Buspar) may lead to very slow heart rates in some patients. One later study found doubling of buspirone levels but no clinical effects. The combination is best avoided, but if deemed clinically necessary, clinical effects on the patient should be closely followed.
- carbamazepine (Tegretol) may cause toxicity.
- cimetidine (Tagamet) may lead to toxicity.
- cisapride (Propulsid) may cause heart toxicity. DO NOT COMBINE.
- clomipramine (Anafranil) may cause toxicity.
- clozapine (Clozaril) can result in higher clozapine levels and toxicity.

- cyclosporine (Sandimmune, others) may increase cyclosporine levels.
- dextromethorphan may cause hallucinations (reported with similar medicines).
- diltiazem (Cardizem) may cause diltiazem toxicity.
- dofetilide (Tikosyn) may lead to dofetilide toxicity via inhibition of CYP 3A4 inhibition.
- imipramine (Tofranil, others) may result in imipramine toxicity.
- lithium (Lithobid) can cause serotonin syndrome.
- MAO inhibitors (see Drug Classes) can cause toxicity. DO NOT COMBINE.
- maprotiline can cause maprotiline toxicity.
- methadone may result in increased opioid effects.
- monoamine oxidase inhibitors (see Drug Classes) may lead to central nervous system toxicity or frank serotonin syndrome.
- olanzapine (Zyprexa) may lead to olanzapine toxicity via inhibition of CYP 1A2.
- oral antidiabetic drugs (see Drug Classes) may remain in the body longer than expected, requiring a dose decrease. This has not been reported with fluvoxamine, but has been reported with sertraline, a medicine in the same pharmacological family.
- phenytoin (Dilantin) or fosphenytoin (Cerebyx) may lead to toxicity. Patients should be watched closely for problems walking (ataxia) or drowsiness (early toxicity signs), and their doctor notified at once if these occur.
- ritonavir (Norvir) and perhaps other protease inhibitors may lead to toxicity.
- sibutramine (Meridia) may lead to serotonin syndrome.
- sumatriptan (Imitrex) may lead to weakness and confusion.
- tacrine (Cognex) may lead to tacrine toxicity.
- terfenadine (Seldane) may cause **serious heart arrhythmias.** DO NOT COMBINE.
- theophylline may result in theophylline toxicity.
- tramadol (Ultram) may increase seizure risk. DO NOT COMBINE.
- tricyclic antidepressants (imipramine, others) may lead to tricyclic toxicity.
- triptans, such as naratriptan (Amerge), rizatriptan (Maxalt), sumatriptan (Imitrex) or zolmitriptan (Zomig), may lead to weakness and incoordination.
- tryptophan may increase serotonin effects of fluvoxamine and cause severe vomiting.
- warfarin (Coumadin) can result in increased warfarin concentrations and may lead to bleeding; more frequent INR testing is needed.

▷ *Driving, Hazardous Activities:* This drug may cause drowsiness. Restrict activities as necessary.

Aviation Note: The use of this drug *is probably a disqualification* for piloting. Consult a designated Aviation Medical Examiner.

Exposure to Sun: No restrictions.

Discontinuation: A withdrawal syndrome has been reported if this medicine is abruptly stopped. The doses should be slowly tapered.

FORMOTEROL (for MOT er all)

Introduced: 2001　**Class:** Bronchodilator　**Prescription:** USA: Yes
Controlled Drug: USA: No; Canada: Not available in Canada　**Available as Generic:** USA: No
Brand Names: Foradil Aerolizer
Author's Note: Information in this profile will be broadened in subsequent editions if evolving patient benefit and research data warrant.

FOSINOPRIL (FOH sin oh pril)

Introduced: 1986　**Class:** Antihypertensive, ACE inhibitor
Please see the angiotensin converting enzyme (ACE) inhibitor family profile.

FUROSEMIDE (fur OH se mide)

Introduced: 1964　**Class:** Antihypertensive, diuretic　**Prescription:** USA: Yes　**Controlled Drug:** USA: No; Canada: No　**Available as Generic:** USA: Yes; Canada: Yes
Brand Names: ♥Albert Furosemide, ♥Apo-Furosemide, Fumide MD, Furomide MD, Furocot, Furosemide-10, ♥Furoside, Lasaject, Lasimide, Lasix, ♥Lasix Special, Lo-Aqua, Luramide, Myrosemide, Novo-Semide, Ro-Semide, SK-Furosemide, ♥Uritol

BENEFITS versus RISKS	
Possible Benefits	*Possible Risks*
PROMPT, EFFECTIVE, RELIABLE DIURETIC	WATER AND ELECTROLYTE DEPLETION with excessive use
MODEST ANTIHYPERTENSIVE IN MILD TO MODERATE HYPERTENSION	Excessive potassium and magnesium loss
ENHANCES EFFECTIVENESS OF OTHER ANTIHYPERTENSIVES	Increased blood sugar level
	Decreased blood calcium level
	Liver damage
	Blood cell disorder

▷ **Principal Uses**
　As a Single Drug Product: Uses currently included in FDA-approved labeling: (1) Increases urine and removes excessive water (edema), as in congestive heart failure or some forms of liver, lung and kidney disease; (2) lowers high blood pressure, usually with other drugs.
　Other (unlabeled) generally accepted uses: (1) Inhaled furosemide may help protect the lungs in people with asthma; (2) can have a role in helping infants with lung problems (chronic bronchopulmonary dysplasia); (3) one study found furosemide beneficial in helping lung mechanics of infants after heart surgery.
　How This Drug Works: By increasing the elimination of salt and water through increased urine production, this drug reduces fluid in the blood and body tissues. These changes also contribute to lowering blood pressure.

Available Dosage Forms and Strengths
Injection — 10 mg/ml
Solution — 10 mg/ml
Tablets — 20 mg, 40 mg, 80 mg

▷ **Usual Adult Dosage Ranges:** *As antihypertensive:* 40 mg every 12 hours initially; increase dose as needed and tolerated. *As diuretic:* 20 to 80 mg in a single dose initially; if necessary, increase the dose by 20 to 40 mg every 6 to 8 hours. The smallest effective dose should be used. Daily maximum is 640 mg. In general, other medicines for high blood pressure should be added before daily dose is increased beyond 80 mg per day. **Note: Actual dose and schedule must be determined for each patient individually.**

Conditions Requiring Dosing Adjustments
Liver Function: Larger doses may be needed for patients with liver compromise, and extreme care must be used to maintain critical electrolytes.
Kidney Function: Larger initial doses may be needed before any benefit is seen. Drug may cause kidney stones and protein in urine.
Cystic Fibrosis: Patients with this disease may be more sensitive to the drug, and smaller starting doses are indicated.

▷ **Dosing Instructions:** The tablet may be crushed and taken with or following meals to reduce stomach irritation. Best taken in the morning to avoid nighttime urination. If you forget a dose: take the missed dose as soon as you remember it, unless it's nearly time for your next dose—if that is the case, skip the missed dose and take the next dose right on time. DO NOT double doses. Call your doctor if you find yourself having problems remembering to use this medicine.

Usual Duration of Use: Use on a regular schedule for 2 to 3 weeks is best to see effectiveness in lowering high blood pressure. Long-term use (months to years) requires periodic physician evaluation of response. Some cases of mild hypertension may remain normal after therapy with furosemide, lowering blood pressure to goals and gradual furosemide withdrawal.

Typical Treatment Goals and Measurements (Outcomes and Markers)
Blood pressure: The most recent treatment guidelines (JNC VI) actually define optimal blood pressure (BP) as less than 120/80 and high normal as 139/89. The American Diabetes Association has chosen a target of 130/80 as the blood pressure goal for people living with diabetes. Most clinicians try to achieve a BP that achieves the best balance of lower cardiovascular risk while avoiding the problem of too low a blood pressure. Because this medicine works to remove excess fluid, additional markers of response include increased urination (intake and output may be checked) as well as decreased swelling (edema) of the ankles. The goals and time frame should be discussed with you when the prescription is written. In high blood pressure patients, this medicine is usually reserved as additional (adjunctive) treatment in patients with kidney problems.
Congestive heart failure: Used to remove excessive fluid which builds up in the body. Typical treatment markers include resolution of ankle swelling and increased output of fluid (diuresis).

▷ **This Drug Should Not Be Taken If**
- you had an allergic reaction to it previously.
- you have extremely low potassium or sodium.

- your kidneys are not making urine.
- you are in a coma caused by liver failure.

▷ **Inform Your Physician Before Taking This Drug If**
- you are allergic to any form of "sulfa" drug.
- you are pregnant or planning pregnancy.
- you have a history of kidney or liver disease.
- you have diabetes, gout or lupus erythematosus.
- you have impaired hearing.
- you have low blood potassium or other electrolytes (talk with your doctor).
- you take cortisone, digitalis, oral antidiabetic drugs or insulin.
- you will have surgery with general anesthesia.

Possible Side Effects (natural, expected and unavoidable drug actions)

Light-headedness on arising from sitting or lying position (see orthostatic hypotension in Glossary).

Increase in blood sugar level, affecting control of diabetes.

Increase in blood uric acid level, affecting control of gout.

Decrease in blood potassium level, causing muscle weakness and cramping.

Decreased magnesium level.

▷ **Possible Adverse Effects** (unusual, unexpected and infrequent reactions)

If any of the following develop, consult your physician promptly for guidance.

Mild Adverse Effects

Allergic reactions: skin rashes, hives, drug fever—case reports.

Headache, dizziness, blurred or yellow vision, ringing in ears, numbness and tingling—rare to infrequent.

Reduced appetite, indigestion, nausea, vomiting, diarrhea—possible.

Metabolic alkalosis—possible.

Serious Adverse Effects

Allergic reactions: hepatitis with jaundice (see Glossary), anaphylactic reaction (see Glossary), severe skin reactions—case reports.

Idiosyncratic reaction: fluid in lungs—case reports.

Temporary hearing loss—case reports.

Inflammation of the pancreas (severe abdominal pain)—rare.

Bone marrow depression (see Glossary): fatigue, weakness, fever, sore throat, abnormal bleeding or bruising—case reports.

Low blood pressure on standing or abnormal heartbeat (arrhythmias)—rare.

Drug-induced porphyria or excessive parathyroid gland action (hyperparathyroidism)—case reports.

Low blood potassium or magnesium—possible.

Vitamin deficiency (thiamine)—possible.

Kidney stones (calcium-containing)—case reports.

Liver toxicity (cholestatic jaundice)—rare.

Fever in infants—case reports.

Skin lesions (erythema multiforme or Stevens-Johnson syndrome)—case reports.

Hip fractures (may increase risk).

▷ **Possible Effects on Sexual Function:** Impotence using recommended dose of 20 to 80 mg per day—infrequent.

▷ **Adverse Effects That May Mimic Natural Diseases or Disorders**
Liver reaction may suggest viral hepatitis.

Natural Diseases or Disorders That May Be Activated by This Drug
Diabetes, gout, systemic lupus erythematosus.

Possible Effects on Laboratory Tests
Complete blood counts: reduced red cells, hemoglobin, white cells and platelets.
Blood amylase and lipase levels: increased (possible pancreatitis).
Blood sodium and chloride levels: decreased.
Blood levels of total cholesterol, LDL and VLDL cholesterol and triglycerides: increased.
Blood glucose level: increased.
Glucose tolerance test (GTT): decreased tolerance.
Blood potassium or magnesium level: decreased.
Blood thyroid hormone (T3 and T4) levels: decreased.
Blood uric acid level or blood urea nitrogen (BUN): increased.
Urine sugar tests: no drug effect (Tes-Tape); false low (Clinistix, Diastix).

CAUTION
1. Take exactly the dose that was prescribed. Increased doses can cause serious loss of sodium and potassium, with resultant loss of appetite, nausea, fatigue, weakness, confusion and tingling in the extremities.
2. If you take a digitalis preparation (digitoxin, digoxin), ensure an adequate intake of high potassium foods to prevent potassium deficiency. (See Table 13, "High Potassium Foods," Section Six.) Magnesium is also important.

Precautions for Use
By Infants and Children: Significant potassium loss can occur within the first 2 weeks of drug use.
By Those Over 60 Years of Age: Small starting doses are critical. Increased risk of impaired thinking, orthostatic hypotension, potassium loss and blood sugar increase. Overdose and extended use of this drug can cause excessive loss of body water, thickening (increased viscosity) of the blood and an increased tendency for the blood to clot—predisposing to stroke, heart attack or thrombophlebitis (vein inflammation with blood clot).

▷ **Advisability of Use During Pregnancy**
Pregnancy Category: C. See Pregnancy Risk Categories at the back of this book.
Animal studies: Significant birth defects have been reported.
Human studies: Adequate studies of pregnant women are not available.
It should not be used during pregnancy unless a very serious complication occurs for which this drug is significantly beneficial. Avoid completely during the first 3 months. Ask your physician for guidance.

Advisability of Use in Breast-Feeding
Presence of this drug in breast milk: Yes.
Avoid drug or refrain from nursing.

Habit-Forming Potential: None.

Effects of Overdose: Dry mouth, thirst, lethargy, weakness, muscle cramping, nausea, vomiting, drowsiness progressing to stupor or coma.

Possible Effects of Long-Term Use: Impaired water, salt, magnesium and potassium balance; dehydration and increased blood coagulability, with risk of blood clots.

Development of glucose intolerance or hyperglycemia in predisposed individuals.

Suggested Periodic Examinations While Taking This Drug (at physician's discretion)

Complete blood counts.

Measurements of blood levels of sodium, potassium, chloride, sugar and uric acid.

Kidney and liver function tests.

▷ **While Taking This Drug, Observe the Following**

Foods: Ask your doctor if it would benefit you to eat foods rich in potassium. If so advised, see Table 13, "High Potassium Foods," Section Six. Follow your physician's advice regarding the use of salt. Food decreases absorption of furosemide by up to 30%. Take this medicine 1 hour before or 2 hours after a meal.

Herbal Medicines or Minerals: Ginseng may increase blood pressure, blunting the benefits of this medicine. Eleuthero root, hawthorn, saw palmetto, ma huang, goldenseal and licorice may also cause increased blood pressure. Couch grass may worsen edema due to heart or kidney problems. Indian snakeroot, calcium and garlic may help lower blood pressure. CAUTION: St. John's wort may also lead to photosensitivity. Magnesium levels should be checked and magnesium replaced if needed. Talk to your doctor BEFORE adding any herbal medicines or minerals.

Beverages: No restrictions. This drug may be taken with milk.

▷ *Alcohol:* Use with caution—alcohol may exaggerate the blood-pressure-lowering effects of this drug and cause orthostatic hypotension.

Tobacco Smoking: No interactions expected. I advise everyone to quit smoking.

▷ *Other Drugs*

Furosemide may increase the effects of

• other antihypertensive drugs; dose adjustments may be necessary to prevent excessive lowering of blood pressure.
• digoxin (Lanoxin) and result in digoxin toxicity.
• lithium (Lithobid, others) and cause lithium toxicity.

Furosemide may *decrease* the effects of

• oral antidiabetic drugs (sulfonylureas); dose adjustments may be necessary for proper control of blood sugar.

Furosemide *taken concurrently with*

• activated charcoal (various) will blunt absorption of oral furosemide.
• adrenocortical steroids (see Drug Classes) may cause additive loss of potassium.
• amikacin, gentamicin, tobramycin or other aminoglycosides may cause hearing toxicity (ototoxicity).
• bepridil (Vascor) may lead to abnormal heart effects if potassium is low.
• cephalosporin antibiotics (see Drug Classes) may increase risk of kidney problems (nephrotoxicity).
• cholestyramine (Questran) may cause loss of furosemide effectiveness.
• clofibrate (Atromid-S) may lead to muscle stiffness and increased diuretic effects.
• colestipol (Colestid) may cause loss of furosemide effectiveness.
• cortisone (various) may lead to excessive potassium loss.

- cyclosporine (Sandimmune) may cause elevated uric acid levels (hyperuricemia) and gout.
- digitalis preparations (digitoxin, digoxin) requires blood tests or dose changes to maintain potassium levels and avoid heart rhythm problems.
- lomefloxacin (Maxaquin) may increase lomefloxacin levels and lead to toxicity.
- metformin (Glucophage) may increase metformin and decrease furosemide effects.
- NSAIDs (see Drug Classes) may cause loss of diuretic effectiveness.
- phenytoin (Dilantin) or fosphenytoin (Cerebyx) may decrease furosemide diuretic effects.

▷ *Driving, Hazardous Activities:* Use caution until the possible occurrence of orthostatic hypotension, dizziness or impaired vision has been determined.

Aviation Note: The use of this drug *may be a disqualification* for piloting. Consult a designated Aviation Medical Examiner.

Exposure to Sun: Use caution—this drug may cause photosensitivity (see Glossary). See "Herbal Medicines" warning on St. John's wort above.

Exposure to Heat: Avoid excessive perspiring, which could cause additional loss of salt and water from the body.

Heavy Exercise or Exertion: Avoid exertion that produces light-headedness, excessive fatigue or muscle cramping. Ask your doctor for help about participation in exercise.

Occurrence of Unrelated Illness: Vomiting or diarrhea can produce a serious imbalance of important body chemistry. Ask your doctor for guidance.

Discontinuation: It may be best to discontinue this drug 5 to 7 days before major surgery. Ask your physician, surgeon and/or anesthesiologist for guidance regarding dose adjustment or drug withdrawal.

GABAPENTIN (GAB ah pen tin)

Introduced: 1981   **Class:** Anticonvulsant, pain syndrome modifier   **Prescription:** USA: Yes   **Controlled Drug:** USA: No; Canada: No   **Available as Generic:** USA: No; Canada: No

Brand Name: Neurontin

BENEFITS versus RISKS	
Possible Benefits	*Possible Risks*
ADJUNCTIVE THERAPY OF PARTIAL SEIZURES	Sleepiness
EFFECTIVE TREATMENT OF A VARIETY OF PAIN SYNDROMES	Movement problems
PREVENTION OF MIGRAINES	
May have a role in reducing symptoms of social phobia	

▷ **Principal Uses**

As a Single Drug Product: Uses currently included in FDA-approved labeling: As an antiepileptic drug adjunctive to other medicines to control partial seizures.

Other (unlabeled) generally accepted uses: (1) widely used in chronic pain syndromes, such as diabetic nerve damage (diabetic neuropathy); (2) may have a role in spasticity; (3) possible role in combination treatment of resistant bipolar disorder; (4) low-dose gabapentin eased spasms seen in multiple sclerosis in one study; (5) a small study found that gabapentin reduced symptoms of social phobia; (6) may be of help in essential tremor; (7) helps prevent migraines.

How This Drug Works: Similar in chemistry to an inhibitory substance called gamma-aminobutyric acid (GABA). Gabapentin appears to increase GABA levels in the brain. Works in preventing migraines by stabilizing actions of the nerves.

Available Dosage Forms and Strengths
Capsules — 100 mg, 300 mg, 400 mg
Tablets — 100 mg, 300 mg, 400 mg, 600 mg and 800 mg

▷ **Usual Adult Dosage Ranges**
Seizures: Initially 100 mg three times a day. Dose may be increased to 900 mg a day by the third day. Doses up to 2,400 mg have been well-tolerated and 3,600 mg used in some patients.
Pain syndromes: 100 mg a day, increased as needed and tolerated. Maximum doses are as those seen in seizure patients.
Note: Actual dose and schedule must be determined for each patient individually.

Conditions Requiring Dosing Adjustments
Liver Function: Not changed by the liver. No dosing changes needed.
Kidney Function: 300 mg twice daily is given to those with a creatinine clearance of 30–60 ml/min. For creatinine clearance 15–30 ml/min, 300 mg is given daily.

▷ **Dosing Instructions:** May be taken with or after food to reduce stomach irritation. The capsule may be opened, and the tablet may be crushed. If you forget a dose: take the missed dose as soon as you remember it, unless it's nearly time for your next dose—if that is the case, skip the missed dose and take the next dose right on time. DO NOT double doses. Call your doctor if you find yourself having problems remembering this medicine or if you miss two doses.

Usual Duration of Use: Use on a regular schedule for 2 to 3 weeks usually determines benefit in reducing frequency and severity of seizures. Optimal control will require careful dose adjustments. Use in pain syndromes may take a similar time. Long-term use requires ongoing physician supervision.

Typical Treatment Goals and Measurements (Outcomes and Markers)
Pain: Most clinicians treating pain use a device called an algometer to check your pain. This looks like a small ruler, but lets the clinician better understand your pain. The goals of treatment then relate to where the level of pain started (for example, a rating of 7 on a zero to ten scale) and what the cause of the pain was. Pain medicines may also be used together (in combination) in order to get the best result or outcome. If your pain control is not acceptable to YOU (remember, in hospitals and outpatient settings, etc. pain control is a patient right) and if after a week of pain treatment results are not acceptable, be sure to call your doctor as you may need a different medicine or combination.

▷ **This Drug Should Not Be Taken If**
  • you have pancreatitis.
  • you have had an allergic reaction to this drug.

▷ **Inform Your Physician Before Taking This Drug If**
  • you are taking any other drugs at this time.
  • you have a history of kidney disease or impaired kidney function.
  • you are less than 12 years old (not studied).
  • you have low blood pressure.

Possible Side Effects (natural, expected and unavoidable drug actions)
  Mild fatigue, sluggishness, drowsiness—may be frequent.

▷ **Possible Adverse Effects** (unusual, unexpected and infrequent reactions)
  If any of the following develop, consult your physician promptly for guidance.

Mild Adverse Effects
  Allergic reactions: skin rashes, hives—possible.
  Weight gain—infrequent.
  Accumulation of fluid in the ankles (edema)—infrequent.
  Nausea, vomiting, constipation—infrequent.
  Vision changes—infrequent.
  Purpura—may be frequent.
  Lowering or increasing of blood pressure—infrequent.
  Bedwetting—case reports, mild and resolved with ongoing therapy.

Serious Adverse Effects
  Allergic reactions: none reported.
  Idiosyncratic reactions: none reported.
  Seizures—case reports.
  Movement disorders—possible, case reports.
  Lowered white blood cell counts—rare.

▷ **Possible Effects on Sexual Function:** Impotence—rare.

▷ **Adverse Effects That May Mimic Natural Diseases or Disorders**
  Drug-induced hepatitis may suggest viral hepatitis.
  Skin reactions may resemble lupus erythematosus.

Natural Diseases or Disorders That May Be Activated by This Drug
  Partial seizures.

Possible Effects on Laboratory Tests
  Complete blood cell counts: decreased white cells—rare.

CAUTION
  1. When used for the treatment of epilepsy, **this drug must not be stopped abruptly**.
  2. Regularity of drug use is essential. Take this drug at the same time each day.
  3. Carry a personal identification card noting that you are taking this drug.

Precautions for Use
  By Infants and Children: Not indicated unless 12 or older.
  By Those Over 60 Years of Age: You may be more sensitive to all of the actions of this drug and require smaller doses. Some clinicians start with 100 mg at bedtime and slowly increase the dose as needed and tolerated. Observe closely for any adverse effects: drowsiness, fatigue, confusion, "cogging" of arms, vision changes.

▷ **Advisability of Use During Pregnancy**

Pregnancy Category: C. See Pregnancy Risk Categories at the back of this book.

Human studies: Information from adequate studies of pregnant women is not available. Discuss use of this drug during pregnancy with your doctor.

Advisability of Use If Breast-Feeding

Presence of this drug in breast milk: Unknown.

Monitor nursing infant closely and discontinue drug or nursing if adverse effects develop.

Habit-Forming Potential: None.

Effects of Overdose: Drowsiness, slurred speech, double vision and diarrhea.

Possible Effects of Long-Term Use: None defined.

Suggested Periodic Examinations While Taking This Drug (at physician's discretion)

Checks of seizure control. Check for "cogging" of arms.

▷ **While Taking This Drug, Observe the Following**

Foods: No restrictions.

Herbal Medicines or Minerals: Ma huang may cause increased blood pressure and excessive sympathetic stimulation. Ginseng, eleuthero root, hawthorn, saw palmetto, goldenseal and licorice may also cause increased blood pressure.

Nutritional Support: None required.

Beverages: No restrictions. May be taken with milk.

▷ *Alcohol:* Use extreme caution. Alcohol (in large quantities or with continual use) may reduce effectiveness in preventing seizures.

Tobacco Smoking: No interactions expected. I advise everyone to quit smoking.

▷ *Other Drugs*

Gabapentin *taken concurrently* with

- antacids (various) may lower beneficial effects.
- cimetidine (Tagamet) may increase blood levels of gabapentin.
- phenytoin (Dilantin) or fosphenytoin (Cerebyx) may lead to phenytoin or fosphenytoin toxicity.

▷ *Driving, Hazardous Activities:* This drug may impair mental alertness, vision and coordination. Restrict activities as necessary.

Aviation Note: The use of this drug *is a disqualification* for piloting. Consult a designated Aviation Medical Examiner.

Exposure to Sun: No restrictions at present.

Discontinuation: **This drug must not be discontinued abruptly**. Sudden withdrawal can precipitate severe and repeated seizures. If this drug is to be discontinued, gradual reduction in dose should be made. Discuss this with your doctor.

GALANTAMINE (ga LAN tah meen)

Introduced: 1981   **Class:** Anticholinesterase inhibitor, allosteric nicotinic receptor agonist, anti-Alzheimer's   **Prescription:** USA: Yes   **Controlled Drug:** USA: No; Canada: No   **Available as Generic:** USA: No; Canada: No   **Brand Name:** Reminyl

BENEFITS versus RISKS	
Possible Benefits	*Possible Risks*
TREATMENT OF MILD TO MODERATE ALZHEIMER'S INHIBITS EFFECTIVE CHOLINESTERASE AS WELL AS ACTING AS AN ALLOSTERIC NICOTINIC RECEPTOR AGONIST	CHOLINERGIC ADVERSE EFFECTS SUCH AS NAUSEA AND VOMITING Benefits may decrease as disease progresses Metabolized by cytochrome P-450 system in the liver

▷ **Principal Uses**

   As a Single Drug Product: Uses currently included in FDA-approved labeling: Treatment of mild to moderate Alzheimer's.

Author's Note: Information in this profile will be broadened as clinical studies define the role in therapy.

GANCICLOVIR (gan SIGH klo veer)

Introduced: 1995 (tablet)   **Class:** Antiviral   **Prescription:** USA: Yes
Controlled Drug: USA: No; Canada: No   **Available as Generic:** USA: No; Canada: No

Brand Names: Cytovene, Vitrasert

Warning: The oral form of this medicine should be used only by patients not candidates for intravenous dosing and for whom the risk of more rapid cytomegalovirus (CMV) retinitis progression is outweighed by the benefit of avoiding the intravenous route.

BENEFITS versus RISKS	
Possible Benefits	*Possible Risks*
Oral, intravenous or implanted treatment of cytomegalovirus (CMV) retinitis	More rapid progression of CMV disease (capsules)
Decreased side effects with the oral form	Bone marrow suppression
Transition to an oral form following intravenous induction	Reproductive toxicity (see "Infants and Children" section)
	Possible increased cancer risk (see "Infants and Children" section)

▷ **Principal Uses**

   As a Single Drug Product: Uses currently included in FDA-approved labeling: (1) Treatment of cytomegalovirus (CMV) retinitis; (2) prevention of CMV retinitis in a variety of patients such as liver, kidney, lung, bone marrow and heart transplant patients; (3) implantation of the ocular implant into the diseased area—this form may work for 5 months or more; (4) prevention of CMV disease in patients with advanced HIV infection.

   Other (unlabeled) generally accepted uses: (1) Treatment of pediatric CMV; (2) may have a role in treating Epstein-Barr virus infection; (3) can have a role in treating leukoplakia; (4) may help outer retinal necrosis.

How This Drug Works: Changed to an active (triphosphate) in infected cells. The active form interferes with DNA and the survival of the virus.

Available Dosage Forms and Strengths
Capsules — 250 mg
Intravenous — 500 mg/10 ml
Intravitreal insert — 4.5 mg

▷ **Recommended Dosage Ranges** (Actual dose and schedule must be determined for each patient individually.)
Infants and Children: **Author's Note: This drug has potential for reproductive toxicity and the risk of causing cancer. It is used in children only after careful evaluation and with extreme caution.**
Induction: 2.5 mg per kg of body mass given intravenously three times daily.
Maintenance dose: 6.5 mg per kg of body mass given intravenously once daily five to seven times a week.
12 to 60 Years of Age:
Induction: 5 mg per kg of body mass intravenously (infused over 1 hour) every 12 hours for 14 to 21 days.
Maintenance dose: 2.1 to 6 mg per kg of body mass infused into a vein over 1 hour each day. Some centers have used 6 mg per kg of body mass given once daily 5 days per week. If retinitis progresses, the patient can be restarted on the twice-daily-dosing approach. Maximum dose is 6 mg per kg of body mass infused over 1 hour.
Oral: Once the intravenous induction dosing has been accomplished, oral ganciclovir is given at 1,000 mg three times daily. Some centers have opted for 500 mg six times per day, given every 3 hours while the patient is awake. If retinitis progresses, intravenous induction therapy should be given.
Intravitreous: This device is surgically implanted and has been effective for 5 or more months.
Over 60 Years of Age: Kidney function must be checked, and the dose appropriately adjusted.

Conditions Requiring Dosing Adjustments
Liver Function: The liver is only minimally involved in the elimination of this drug, and dosing changes in liver compromise are not needed.
Kidney Function: The dose must be decreased in kidney compromise. This adjustment is accomplished based on creatinine clearance (see Glossary).
Induction: 5 mg per kg of body mass every 12 hours (70 ml/min or higher); 2.5 mg per kg of body mass every 12 hours (50–69); 2.5 mg per kg of body mass every 24 hours (25–49); 1.25 mg per kg of body mass every 24 hours (10–24); 1.25 mg per kg of body mass three times per week (less than 10).
Maintenance: 5 mg per kg of body mass every 24 hours (70 ml/min or higher); 2.5 mg per kg of body mass every 24 hours (50–69); 1.25 mg per kg of body mass every 24 hours (25–49); 0.625 mg per kg of body mass every 24 hours (10–24); 0.625 mg per kg of body mass three times per week (less than 10).

▷ **Dosing Instructions:** This medicine should be taken with food if taken by mouth (orally). It is best to take the medicine at the same time each day. Capsule form should not be opened or crushed, because you may have adverse reactions from the toxic powder. If you are taking the capsule form and your vision declines, call your doctor immediately. If you miss a dose: take it as soon as you remember it, unless it's nearly time for your next dose—if that is the case, skip the missed dose and return to taking the medicine on your usual schedule. DO NOT double doses. Call your doctor if you miss more than one dose.

Usual Duration of Use: Continual use on a regular schedule for up to 16 days is usually needed to determine this drug's effectiveness in treating retinitis. Because of a very high frequency of relapse, most centers recommend ongoing maintenance therapy. Long-term use (months to years) requires periodic evaluation of response and dose adjustment. The ocular implant form may work for 5 months or more. Keep your follow-up appointments with your doctor.

Typical Treatment Goals and Measurements (Outcomes and Markers)

CMV infections: Goals for treatment of CMV include response to the treatment and avoidance of bone marrow depression and kidney problems. Markers for the infection itself include eye sight improvement, eye exam for retinopathy, slit lamp tests and eye pressure. Additionally, many patients have been found to gain weight and improve albumin levels.

Possible Advantages of This Drug

Transition from the intravenous form to the oral form (if successful in treatment) offers a clear quality-of-life advantage.

Currently a "Drug of Choice"

For patients with liver failure and CMV.

▷ **This Drug Should Not Be Taken If**
- you had an allergic reaction to it previously.
- your absolute neutrophil count (a specific kind of white blood cell) is less than 500 per cubic mm.
- your platelet count is less than 25,000 per cubic mm.

▷ **Inform Your Physician Before Taking This Drug If**
- you think you are dehydrated (this drug is primarily removed by the kidneys).
- you have a sore throat or fever.
- you have a history of blood cell disorders.
- you are planning pregnancy.
- you are male and are planning pregnancy (attempted conception should be avoided for at least 3 months after ganciclovir therapy).
- you are uncertain of how much ganciclovir to take, how often to take it or how to handle the intravenous solution.
- you take other prescription or nonprescription medicines that were not discussed with your doctor when ganciclovir was prescribed. This includes natural extracts or herbal remedies and "underground" therapies for AIDS.

Possible Side Effects (natural, expected and unavoidable drug actions)

Pain at the injection site with the IV form. Possible phlebitis.

▷ **Possible Adverse Effects** (unusual, unexpected and infrequent reactions)

If any of the following develop, consult your physician promptly for guidance.

Mild Adverse Effects

Allergic reactions: skin rash and itching.

Confusion, headache, nervousness, tremor, somnolence, abnormal dreams, ataxia, "pins-and-needles" sensations of the hands (paresthesias)—infrequent.

Muscle aches—rare.
Fever—may be frequent with oral therapy.
Decreased blood glucose or potassium—rare.
Nausea, vomiting or diarrhea—infrequent to frequent.
Serious Adverse Effects
Allergic reactions: anaphylactic reaction—case reports.
Bone marrow suppression—rare.
Lowered white blood cell (neutropenia) counts—frequent.
Lowered blood platelets—infrequent.
Arrhythmias—rare.
Coma, psychosis or seizures—case reports.
Neuropathy—infrequent to frequent.
Liver toxicity—rare to infrequent.
Retinal detachment—infrequent.
Visual decline—infrequent to frequent with intravitreal implant.
This drug is a potential cancer-causing (carcinogenic) agent—no percentage defined.

▷ **Possible Effects on Sexual Function:** Reversible infertility in men.

Possible Delayed Adverse Effects: Lowered white blood cell counts or platelets.

▷ **Adverse Effects That May Mimic Natural Diseases or Disorders**
Increased liver enzymes may mimic hepatitis.

Natural Diseases or Disorders That May Be Activated by This Drug
None defined.

Possible Effects on Laboratory Tests
Liver enzymes: increased.
Serum bilirubin or creatinine: increased.
Blood glucose, platelets or white blood cells: decreased.

CAUTION
1. The oral form may be less effective than the intravenous form. Call your doctor immediately if your vision declines.
2. May cause bone marrow suppression. Call your doctor if you get a sore throat, start to bruise easily or develop fever.

Precautions for Use
By Infants and Children: Safety and effectiveness for use by those under 18 years of age have not been established. The drug has been used selectively in patients as young as 36 weeks.
By Those Over 60 Years of Age: Because of the age-related decline in kidney function, a creatinine clearance should be obtained and dosing adjusted appropriately.

▷ **Advisability of Use During Pregnancy**
Pregnancy Category: C. See Pregnancy Risk Categories at the back of this book.
Animal studies: Rabbits have developed cleft palate, exhibited poorly developed organs and have experienced fetal death.
Human studies: Information from adequate studies of pregnant women is not available.
Use of this drug during pregnancy is not recommended.

Advisability of Use If Breast-Feeding

Presence of this drug in breast milk: Unknown.

Avoid drug or refrain from nursing.

Habit-Forming Potential: None.

Effects of Overdose: Nausea and vomiting, excessive salivation, increased liver function tests, bone marrow suppression, kidney failure.

Possible Effects of Long-Term Use: Not defined.

Suggested Periodic Examinations While Taking This Drug (at physician's discretion)

Platelet counts and complete blood counts: every 2 days during induction and weekly thereafter.

Liver function tests: monthly.

Kidney function tests: every 2 weeks.

Eye (ophthalmologic) exams: weekly during induction and every 2 weeks thereafter. These exams may be needed more frequently if the optic nerve or macula of the eye is involved.

▷ **While Taking This Drug, Observe the Following**

Foods: No restrictions—the oral form should be taken with food.

Herbal Medicines or Minerals: Some patients use echinacea to attempt to boost their immune systems. Unfortunately, use of echinacea is not recommended in people with damaged immune systems. This herb may also actually weaken any immune system if it is used too often or for too long a time. Caution: St. John's wort may also cause extreme reactions to the sun. Additive photosensitivity may be possible.

Beverages: No restrictions.

▷ *Alcohol:* No restrictions; however, alcohol may blunt the immune system.

Tobacco Smoking: No interactions expected. I advise everyone to quit smoking.

Marijuana Smoking: May increase somnolence.

▷ *Other Drugs*

Ganciclovir *taken concurrently* with

- amphotericin B (Fungizone, Abelcet) may result in increased bone marrow suppression.
- cancer chemotherapy may result in additive bone marrow suppression.
- cotrimoxazole (Septra) may result in added bone marrow suppression problems.
- cyclosporine (Sandimmune) can result in increased kidney toxicity.
- dapsone is a benefit-to-risk decision, as additive bone marrow suppression may occur.
- flucytosine (Ancobon) can cause additive bone marrow toxicity.
- imipenem/cilastatin (Primaxin) can cause seizures.
- pentamidine may result in additive bone marrow suppression.
- tacrolimus (Prograf) can result in increased risk of kidney toxicity.
- zidovudine (AZT) will often cause a serious increase in bone marrow suppression.

The following drug may *increase* the effects of ganciclovir:

- probenecid (Benemid)—by interfering with elimination by the kidney.

▷ *Driving, Hazardous Activities:* This drug may cause somnolence. Restrict activities as necessary.

Aviation Note: The use of this drug *may be a disqualification* for piloting. Consult a designated Aviation Medical Examiner.

Exposure to Sun: Caution is advised. Photosensitivity has been reported (with IV or oral use). See "Herbal Medicines" caution on St. John's wort above.

Discontinuation: Talk with your doctor before stopping this medicine.

Special Storage Instructions: Store the intravenous form at 39 degrees F (4 degrees C) and use within 12 hours after it has been reconstituted.

Observe the Following Expiration Times: The intravenous form will be stamped or labeled with a specific expiration time if this has been provided by a home infusion company; it should be used within 12 hours after it has been reconstituted.

GEMFIBROZIL (jem FI broh zil)

Introduced: 1976   **Class:** Anticholesterol   **Prescription:** USA: Yes
Controlled Drug: USA: No; Canada: No   **Available as Generic:** USA: Yes; Canada: No
Brand Names: ✦Apo-Gemfibrozil, Gemcor, ✦Gem-Gemfibrozil, Lopid, ✦Med-Gemfibrozil, ✦Novo-Gemfibrozil, ✦PMS-Gemfibrozil

BENEFITS versus RISKS	
Possible Benefits	*Possible Risks*
EFFECTIVE REDUCTION OF TRIGLYCERIDE BLOOD LEVELS	Possible myopathy or rhabdomyolysis
INCREASE IN HIGH-DENSITY LIPOPROTEIN (HDL) BLOOD LEVELS	
REDUCES RISK OF CORONARY HEART DISEASE	

▷ **Principal Uses**

As a Single Drug Product: Uses currently included in FDA-approved labeling: (1) Reduces abnormally high blood levels of triglycerides in Types IV and V blood lipid (fat) disorders or Type IIb patients who do not have symptoms or history of existing heart disease (coronary); (2) decreases risk for developing coronary artery heart disease.

Other (unlabeled) generally accepted uses: Used by diabetics as combination therapy with oral hypoglycemic agents to further increase desirable HDLs.

How This Drug Works: Reduces triglycerides by inhibiting the liver from making them. Decreases VLDL and LDL. Increases HDL more than clofibrate.

Available Dosage Forms and Strengths
Capsules — 300 mg
Tablets — 600 mg

▷ **Usual Adult Dosage Ranges:** 1,200 to 1,600 mg daily in two divided doses (30 minutes before the morning and evening meal). The average dose is 1,200 mg daily. Dose increases should be made gradually over a period of 2 to 3 months. **Note: Actual dose and schedule must be determined for each patient individually.**

Conditions Requiring Dosing Adjustments

Liver Function: This drug is contraindicated in primary biliary cirrhosis and severe liver failure.

Kidney Function: For patients with moderate kidney failure, 50% of the usual dose should be taken at the usual interval. Patients with severe kidney failure should take 25% of the usual dose at the usual dosing interval.

▷ **Dosing Instructions:** The capsule may be opened and taken 30 minutes before the morning and evening meals. If you forget a dose: take it as soon as you remember it, unless its nearly time for your next dose—if that is the case, skip the missed dose and return to taking the medicine on your usual schedule. DO NOT double doses. Call your doctor if you find yourself missing doses.

Usual Duration of Use: Regular use for 4 to 8 weeks determines effectiveness in reducing triglycerides. Results in reducing coronary heart disease showed up during the second year of treatment in one study. Long-term use (months to years) requires periodic evaluation by your doctor. **Author's Note: One study found that niacin increased good cholesterol (HDL) more than gemfibrozil. These medicines can be used together and may offer valuable benefits.**

Typical Treatment Goals and Measurements (Outcomes and Markers)

Cholesterol: The National Cholesterol Education Program (NCEP) recommends low-density lipoprotein cholesterol levels (LDL-C) according to this schedule: (a) patients with coronary artery disease: LDL-C less than 100 mg/dL; (b) those with 2 or more risk factors: LDL-C less than 130 mg/dL; (c) people with none or one risk factor: LDL-C less than 160 mg/dL. Using EBCT to get your calcium score relates well to potential cardiovascular problems.

▷ **This Drug Should Not Be Taken If**
- you have had an allergic reaction to it previously.
- you have biliary cirrhosis of the liver or liver disease.
- you have gallbladder disease.
- you have severe kidney compromise.

▷ **Inform Your Physician Before Taking This Drug If**
- you have impaired liver or kidney function.
- you have gallbladder disease or gallstones.
- you are a diabetic (conflicting reports).
- you are obese and increased exercise and diet have not been attempted.
- you are taking an anticoagulant medicine.
- you have an underactive thyroid (hypothyroidism).

Possible Side Effects (natural, expected and unavoidable drug actions)
Moderate increase in blood sugar levels.

▷ **Possible Adverse Effects** (unusual, unexpected and infrequent reactions)
If any of the following develop, consult your physician promptly for guidance.

Mild Adverse Effects
Allergic reactions: skin rash, hives, itching.

Headache, dizziness, blurred vision, fatigue, muscle aches and cramps—infrequent.

Indigestion, excessive gas, stomach discomfort, nausea, vomiting, diarrhea—rare to infrequent.

Paresthesias—very rare.

Serious Adverse Effects

Abnormally low white blood cell count: fever, chills, sore throat—rare.

Formation of gallstones with long-term use—possible.

Low blood potassium—possible.

Raynaud's phenomenon—case report.

Liver toxicity—possible.

Myopathy (muscle weakness) or rhabdomyolysis (inability to walk)—case reports to rare.

Kidney failure with muscle damage (rhabdomyolysis with renal failure)—case reports.

▷ **Possible Effects on Sexual Function:** Decreased libido or impotence—rare to infrequent.

Natural Diseases or Disorders That May Be Activated by This Drug

Latent diabetes, latent urinary tract infections.

Possible Effects on Laboratory Tests

Complete blood counts: decreased red cells, hemoglobin, white cells and platelets.

Blood HDL cholesterol levels: increased.

Blood triglyceride levels: decreased.

Liver function tests: increased liver enzymes (ALT/GPT, AST/GOT and alkaline phosphatase), increased bilirubin.

CAUTION

1. Gemfibrozil is used only after diet has NOT worked to lower triglyceride levels.
2. If you used the drug clofibrate (Atromid-S) in the past, tell your physician fully regarding your experience.
3. Periodic triglyceride and cholesterol levels are critical.

Precautions for Use

By Infants and Children: Safety and effectiveness for those under 12 years of age are not established.

By Those Over 60 Years of Age: Watch for increased tendency to infection; treat all infections promptly.

▷ **Advisability of Use During Pregnancy**

Pregnancy Category: C. See Pregnancy Risk Categories at the back of this book.

Animal studies: Produces adverse effects in rabbits and rats.

Human studies: Adequate studies of pregnant women are not available.

Ask your physician for guidance.

Advisability of Use If Breast-Feeding

Presence of this drug in breast milk: Yes.

Avoid drug or refrain from nursing.

Habit-Forming Potential: None.

Effects of Overdose: Abdominal pain, nausea, vomiting, diarrhea.

Possible Effects of Long-Term Use: Formation of gallstones.

Suggested Periodic Examinations While Taking This Drug (at physician's discretion)

Complete blood cell counts and liver function tests.

Measurements of blood levels of total cholesterol, HDL and LDL cholesterol fractions, triglycerides and sugar.

▷ **While Taking This Drug, Observe the Following**

Foods: Follow the diet prescribed by your physician.

Herbal Medicines or Minerals: No data exist from well-designed clinical studies about garlic and gemfibrozil combinations and can not presently be recommended. The FDA allowed one dietary supplement called Cholestin to continue to be sold. This preparation actually contains lovastatin. Since use of an HMG-CoA inhibitor with gemfibrozil may increase risk of rhabdomyolysis or myopathy, the combination is NOT advised. One study found that niacin (Niaspan form) worked to increase HDL levels more than gemfibrozil. This may represent a complementary combination. Talk to your doctor to see if this makes sense for you.

Beverages: No restrictions. May be taken with milk.

▷ *Alcohol:* No interactions expected.

Tobacco Smoking: No interactions expected. I advise everyone to quit smoking.

▷ *Other Drugs*

Gemfibrozil *taken concurrently* with

• ritonavir (Norvir) may risk gemfibrozil toxicity.

Gemfibrozil may *increase* the effects of

• glyburide (Micronase) and other oral antidiabetic drugs (see Drug Classes).

• lovastatin and HMG-CoA type drugs (see Drug Classes), which may increase muscle damage risk (myopathy) if taken at the same time.

• warfarin (Coumadin) and increase the risk of bleeding; increased frequency of INR (prothrombin time or protime) measurements and dose changes based on results are critical.

Gemfibrozil may *decrease* the effects of

• chenodiol (Chenix), reducing its benefit in gallstone therapy.

• colestipol (Colestid); separate doses by two hours.

▷ *Driving, Hazardous Activities:* This drug may cause dizziness and blurred vision. Restrict activities as necessary.

Aviation Note: The use of this drug *is usually not a disqualification* for piloting. Consult a designated Aviation Medical Examiner.

Exposure to Sun: No restrictions.

Discontinuation: If triglyceride lowering does not occur after 3 months, this drug should be stopped.

GLIMEPIRIDE (glim EP er ide)

Introduced: 1996   **Class:** Antidiabetic,   sulfonylureas   **Prescription:** USA: Yes   **Controlled Drug:**   USA: No   **Available as Generic:**   No   **Brand Name:**   Amaryl

```
┌─────────────────────────────────────────────────────────────┐
│                   BENEFITS versus RISKS                       │
│        Possible Benefits              Possible Risks          │
│   TIGHTER CONTROL OF BLOOD      Allergic skin reactions       │
│     SUGAR (adjunctive to appropriate  Possible increased risk of heart │
│     diet and weight control)      (cardiovascular) mortality  │
│   DECREASED RISK OF HEART                                      │
│     DISEASE, KIDNEY DISEASE,                                   │
│     ETC., BY ATTAINING TIGHTER                                 │
│     CONTROL OF BLOOD SUGAR                                     │
│   ONCE-A-DAY DOSING                                            │
│   DECREASED RISK OF INCREASED                                  │
│     INSULIN LEVELS                                             │
│   DECREASED RISK OF                                            │
│     HYPOGLYCEMIA                                               │
│   MAY BE COMBINED WITH                                         │
│     METFORMIN IF BLOOD SUGAR                                   │
│     GOALS ARE NOT ACHIEVED                                     │
│     WITH SINGLE MEDICINE                                       │
│     TREATMENT                                                  │
│   MAY BE USED IN COMBINATION                                   │
│     WITH INSULIN IN SECONDARY                                  │
│     FAILURE                                                    │
└─────────────────────────────────────────────────────────────┘
```

▷ **Principal Uses**

As a Single Drug Product: Uses currently included in FDA-approved labeling: (1) Used in type 2 diabetes (adult, maturity-onset) not requiring insulin, but not adequately controlled by diet alone; (2) approved for combination use with insulin or metformin if diet and exercise and this drug are not adequate and in secondary failures (USED WITH INSULIN).

Other (unlabeled) generally accepted uses: None at present.

How This Drug Works: This drug (1) stimulates insulin secretion; (2) enhances use of insulin by tissues (increased sensitivity); and (3) binds to a receptor on the pancreas (beta cell sulfonylurea-inhibiting K-ATP) and activating the L-type calcium channel.

Available Dosage Forms and Strengths

Tablets — 1 mg, 2 mg, 4 mg, 6 mg

▷ **Usual Adult Dosage Ranges:** Started with 1 or 2 mg once daily, with breakfast or the first meal. Once a dose of 2 mg is reached, further dose increases should be made at 1- to 2-week intervals in increments of no more than 2 mg; the maximum daily dose is 8 mg. Typical ongoing doses have ranged from 1 to 4 mg a day. Some doctors say that patients who fail treatment with an oral blood-sugar lowering agent should be considered for combined glimepiride and insulin therapy. If fasting blood sugar (glucose) is greater than 150 mg/dl and insulin/glimepiride is used, 8 mg is taken with the first main meal. Low-dose insulin is started and increased as needed/tolerated weekly based on blood sugar. **Note: Actual dose and schedule must be determined for each patient individually.**

Conditions Requiring Dosing Adjustments

Liver Function: Starting dose is 1 mg daily in mild liver failure. Further dose changes are based on results of blood sugar testing. No data on use in more severe liver compromise.

Kidney Function: Starting dose is 1 mg daily. Further dose changes are based on results of blood sugar testing.

▷ **Dosing Instructions:** The tablet may be crushed. Follow doctor's instructions about dosing and diet closely. If meals are skipped, hypoglycemia may result. Know the signs and symptoms of hypoglycemia.

Usual Duration of Use: Use on a regular schedule for 1 to 2 weeks determines effectiveness in controlling diabetes. Failure to respond to maximal doses within 1 month constitutes a primary failure. Insulin or metformin may then be combined with glimepiride to reach blood sugar goals. Blood sugars must be measured, and your doctor will decide if the drug should be continued. If you forget a dose: take it as soon as you remember it, unless its nearly time for your next dose—if that is the case, skip the missed dose and return to taking the medicine on your usual schedule. DO NOT double doses. Call your doctor if you find yourself missing doses. There are reminder services (beeper-based) that can help.

Typical Treatment Goals and Measurements (Outcomes and Markers)

Blood sugar: The general goal for blood sugar is to return it to the usual "normal" range (generally 80–120 mg/dl), while avoiding risks of excessively low blood sugar. One study (UKPDS) used a fasting plasma sugar (glucose) of less than 108 mg/dl.

Fructosamine and glycosylated hemoglobin: Fructosamine levels (a measure of the past two to three weeks of blood sugar control) should be less than or equal to 310 micromoles per liter. Glycosylated hemoglobin or hemoglobin A1C (a measure of the past 2–3 months of blood sugar control) should be less than or equal to 7.0%.

Possible Advantages of This Drug

Effective with once-daily dosing.

May be less likely to cause excessive lowering of the blood sugar (hypoglycemia).

May cause less excessive insulin in the bloodstream (hyperinsulinemia).

May be combined with insulin in secondary failure.

▷ **This Drug Should Not Be Taken If**
- you have had an allergic reaction to it previously.
- you have diabetic ketoacidosis (insulin is the drug of choice).

▷ **Inform Your Physician Before Taking This Drug If**
- you are allergic to other sulfonylurea drugs or to "sulfa" drugs.
- you have been experiencing prolonged vomiting.
- you are pregnant or are breast-feeding your infant.
- you do not know how to recognize or treat hypoglycemia (see Glossary).
- you have a history of congestive heart failure, peptic ulcer disease, cirrhosis of the liver, kidney disease or hypothyroidism.
- you are malnourished or have a high fever, infection or pituitary or adrenal insufficiency.

Possible Side Effects (natural, expected and unavoidable drug actions)
> Hypoglycemia will occur if drug dose is excessive or if meals are missed or inadequate. The risk of hypoglycemia may be increased if this medicine is combined with insulin.

▷ **Possible Adverse Effects** (unusual, unexpected and infrequent reactions)
> **If any of the following develop, consult your physician promptly for guidance.**

Mild Adverse Effects
> Allergic reactions: skin rash, hives, itching (may subside over time).
> Headache, dizziness or blurred vision—rare.
> Nausea—rare.
> Increased liver enzymes—infrequent.

Serious Adverse Effects
> Allergic reactions: not reported to date.
> Lowering of sodium—case reports.
> Low blood sugar (hypoglycemia)—possible.

▷ **Possible Effects on Sexual Function:** None reported.

▷ **Adverse Effects That May Mimic Natural Diseases or Disorders**
> Increased liver enzymes may suggest viral hepatitis.

Possible Effects on Laboratory Tests
> Hemoglobin A1C (glycosylated hemoglobin): trending toward normal if tight control of blood sugar has been achieved.
> Glycated hemoglobin (fructosamine) checks will trend toward normal.
> Blood glucose levels: decreased.
> Liver function tests: increased liver enzymes (ALT/GPT, AST/GOT and alkaline phosphatase), increased bilirubin.

CAUTION
> 1. This drug is only one part of a diabetes program. It is not a substitute for a proper diet and regular exercise.
> 2. Over time (usually several months) this drug may not work. Periodic follow-up examinations are mandatory.

Precautions for Use
> *By Infants and Children:* Safety and effectiveness in pediatrics have not been established.
> *By Those Over 60 Years of Age:* Use with caution, and start with 1 mg/day. Dose should be increased slowly as needed and tolerated and glucose checked often. Repeated hypoglycemia in the elderly can cause brain damage.

▷ **Advisability of Use During Pregnancy**
> *Pregnancy Category:* C. See Pregnancy Risk Categories at the back of this book.
> *Human studies:* Adequate studies of pregnant women are not available.
> Because uncontrolled blood sugar levels during pregnancy are dangerous for the fetus, many experts recommend insulin instead of an oral agent.

Advisability of Use If Breast-Feeding
> Presence of this drug in breast milk: Yes, in animal data; unknown, in humans.
> Avoid drug or refrain from nursing.

Habit-Forming Potential: None.

Effects of Overdose: Symptoms of mild to severe hypoglycemia: headache, light-headedness, faintness, nervousness, confusion, tremor, sweating, heart palpitation, weakness, hunger, nausea, vomiting, stupor progressing to coma.

Possible Effects of Long-Term Use: Reports of increased frequency and severity of heart and blood vessel diseases with long-term use of this class of drugs are highly controversial and inconclusive. A direct cause-and-effect relationship (see Glossary) is tenuous. Ask your doctor for help.

Suggested Periodic Examinations While Taking This Drug (at physician's discretion)

Hemoglobin A1C and/or fructosamine.

Liver function tests.

Evaluation of heart and circulatory system.

Blood sugar levels.

▷ **While Taking This Drug, Observe the Following**

Foods: Follow the diabetic diet and portion control.

Herbal Medicines or Minerals: Using chromium may change the way your body is able to use sugar. Some health food stores advocate vanadium as mimicking the actions of insulin, but possible toxicity and need for rigorous studies presently preclude recommending it. Caution: St. John's wort may cause photosensitivity, and this drug may too.

DHEA may change sensitivity to insulin or insulin resistance. Hawthorn, ginger, garlic, ginseng and licorice, nettle and yohimbe may change blood sugar. Since this may require adjustment of hypoglycemic medicine dosing, talk to your doctor BEFORE combining any of these herbal medicines with this medicine. Echinacea pupurea (injectable) and blonde psyllium seed or husk should NOT be taken by people living with diabetes.

Beverages: As directed in the diabetic diet. May be taken with milk.

▷ *Alcohol:* Use with extreme caution—alcohol can prolong this drug's hypoglycemic effect. Other drugs in this class can also cause a disulfiramlike reaction (see Glossary).

Tobacco Smoking: No interactions expected. I advise everyone to quit smoking.

▷ *Other Drugs*

The following drugs may *increase* the effects of glimepiride:

- aspirin and other salicylates.
- chloramphenicol.
- cimetidine (Tagamet).
- clofibrate (Atromid-S).
- cotrimoxazole (Septra).
- fenfluramine (Pondimin).
- miconazole (Lotrimin).
- monoamine oxidase (MAO) type A inhibitors (see Drug Classes).
- NSAIDs (see Drug Classes).
- probenecid (SK-Probenecid).
- ranitidine (Zantac).
- sulfa drugs such as Septra.

The following drugs may *decrease* the effects of glimepiride:

- beta-blocker drugs (see Drug Classes).
- birth control pills.
- bumetanide (Bumex).

- conjugated estrogens (Premarin).
- diazoxide (Proglycem).
- ethacrynic acid (Edecrin).
- furosemide (Lasix).
- phenothiazines (see Drug Classes).
- phenytoin (Dilantin) or fosphenytoin (Cerebyx).
- rifampin (Rifadin, others).
- steroids (betamethasone, prednisone, others).
- thiazide diuretics (see Drug Classes).

Glimepiride *taken concurrently* with

- antacids (magnesium hydroxide-containing) may result in increased risk of excessively lowered blood sugar.
- antifungal agents (such as itraconazole or other azoles) may result in severe lowering of blood sugar.
- calcium channel blockers (see Drug Classes) may cause excessive lowering of blood glucose.
- cyclosporine (Sandimmune) may result in cyclosporine toxicity.

▷ *Driving, Hazardous Activities:* Dosing schedule, eating schedule and physical activities must be coordinated to prevent hypoglycemia. Know the early symptoms of hypoglycemia so that you can avoid hazardous activities and take corrective measures.

Aviation Note: Diabetes *is a disqualification* for piloting. Consult a designated Aviation Medical Examiner.

Exposure to Sun: Some drugs of this class can cause photosensitivity (see Glossary).

Occurrence of Unrelated Illness: Acute infections, vomiting or diarrhea, serious injuries and surgical procedures can worsen diabetic control and may require insulin. If any of these conditions occur, call your doctor.

Discontinuation: Because of secondary failures, the continued benefit of this drug should be evaluated every 6 months.

GLIPIZIDE (GLIP i zide)

Introduced: 1972   **Class:** Antidiabetic, sulfonylureas   **Prescription:** USA: Yes   **Controlled Drug:** USA: No   **Available as Generic:** Yes
Brand Names: Glucotrol, Glucotrol XL

BENEFITS versus RISKS	
Possible Benefits	*Possible Risks*
TIGHTER CONTROL OF BLOOD SUGAR (adjunctive to appropriate diet and weight control)	HYPOGLYCEMIA, severe and prolonged
	Allergic skin reactions (some severe)
DECREASED RISK OF HEART DISEASE, KIDNEY DISEASE, ETC., BY ATTAINING TIGHTER CONTROL OF BLOOD SUGAR	Blood cell and bone marrow disorders
	Possible increased risk of heart (cardiovascular) mortality
ONCE-A-DAY DOSING	

▷ **Principal Uses**

As a Single Drug Product: Uses currently included in FDA-approved labeling: Type 2 diabetes (adult, maturity-onset) not requiring insulin but not adequately controlled by diet alone.

Other (unlabeled) generally accepted uses: Delay of abnormal metabolism and blood vessel disease if given early in diabetes.

How This Drug Works: This drug (1) stimulates the secretion of insulin and (2) enhances the use of insulin by appropriate tissues.

Available Dosage Forms and Strengths

Tablets — 5 mg, 10 mg

Tablets, extended release — 2.5 mg, 5 mg, 10 mg

▷ **Usual Adult Dosage Ranges:** Starts with 5 mg daily before a meal. At 3- to 7-day intervals, dose may be increased (by 2.5 to 5 mg daily) as needed and tolerated. Daily maximum is 40 mg. If the daily dose is more than 15 mg, it should be divided into two equal doses given twice a day (immediate-release form). Extended-release form starts at 5 mg, taken with breakfast. Dose increases are made at 7-day intervals. Most patients have a favorable response to 10 mg daily. Maximum daily extended-release-form dose is 20 mg.

Note: Actual dose and schedule must be determined for each patient individually.

Conditions Requiring Dosing Adjustments

Liver Function: Patients with liver failure should take a starting dose of 2.5 mg and be closely followed.

Kidney Function: Some clinicians DO NOT recommend use of glipizide in severe renal compromise. Patients should be monitored closely if the drug is used in mild to moderate renal (kidney) compromise. It is a rare cause of kidney stones.

▷ **Dosing Instructions:** If the daily maintenance dose is found to be 15 mg or more (immediate-release form), the total dose should be divided into two equal doses—the first taken with the morning meal, the second with the evening meal. The tablet may be crushed. If you forget a dose: take it as soon as you remember it, unless it's nearly time for your next dose—if that is the case, skip the missed dose and return to taking the medicine on your usual schedule. DO NOT double doses. Call your doctor if you find yourself missing doses because the best results are achieved by taking exactly the right dose and keeping your blood sugar in "tight" control.

Usual Duration of Use: Use on a regular schedule for 1 to 2 weeks determines effectiveness in controlling diabetes. Failure to respond to maximal doses within 1 month constitutes a primary failure. Up to 10% who respond initially may fail later (secondary failure). Blood sugars must be checked. Tight sugar control is best!

Typical Treatment Goals and Measurements (Outcomes and Markers)

Blood sugar: The general goal for blood sugar is to return it to the usual "normal" range (generally 80–120 mg/dl), while avoiding risks of excessively low blood sugar. One study (UKPDS) used a fasting plasma sugar (glucose) of less than 108 mg/dl.

Fructosamine and glycosylated hemoglobin: Fructosamine levels (a measure of the past two to three weeks of blood sugar control) should be less than or equal to 310 micromoles per liter. Glycosylated hemoglobin or hemoglobin A1C (a measure of the past 2–3 months of blood sugar control) should be less than or equal to 7.0%.

Possible Advantages of This Drug

Effective with once-daily dosing.

Onset of action within 30 minutes. Near-normal insulin response to eating.

Well tolerated by the elderly diabetic.

Currently a Drug of Choice

For starting therapy in non-insulin-dependent diabetes if diet and weight control fail.

▷ **This Drug Should Not Be Taken If**

- you have had an allergic reaction to it previously.
- you have diabetic ketoacidosis.

▷ **Inform Your Physician Before Taking This Drug If**

- you are allergic to other sulfonylurea drugs or to "sulfa" drugs.
- your diabetes has been unstable or "brittle" in the past.
- you do not know how to recognize or treat hypoglycemia (see Glossary).
- you have severe impairment of liver or kidney function.
- you have an infection or fever.
- you are pregnant.
- you have a history of congestive heart failure, peptic ulcer disease, cirrhosis of the liver, bone marrow depression, hypothyroidism or porphyria.

Possible Side Effects (natural, expected and unavoidable drug actions)

If drug dose is excessive or if meals are missed or inadequate, abnormally low blood sugar (hypoglycemia) will occur as a drug effect.

▷ **Possible Adverse Effects** (unusual, unexpected and infrequent reactions)

If any of the following develop, consult your physician promptly for guidance.

Mild Adverse Effects

Allergic reactions: skin rash, hives, itching.

Headache, drowsiness, dizziness, fatigue, sweating—rare to infrequent.

Indigestion, nausea, vomiting, diarrhea—rare to infrequent.

Increased liver enzymes—case reports.

Serious Adverse Effects

Allergic reactions: severe skin reactions—case reports.

Idiosyncratic reaction: hemolytic anemia (see Glossary).

Disulfiramlike reaction (see Glossary) with alcohol use.

Low blood sodium or drug-induced urinary stones—possible.

Bone marrow depression (see Glossary): fatigue, weakness, fever, sore throat, abnormal bleeding or bruising—case reports.

Risk of cardiovascular mortality (based on an old study with a different drug)—possible.

▷ **Possible Effects on Sexual Function:** None reported.

▷ **Adverse Effects That May Mimic Natural Diseases or Disorders**

Liver reaction may suggest viral hepatitis.

Possible Effects on Laboratory Tests

Complete blood counts: decreased red cells, hemoglobin, white cells and platelets.

Glycated hemoglobin or protein: trending toward normal.

Blood glucose levels: decreased.

Liver function tests: increased liver enzymes (ALT/GPT, AST/GOT and alkaline phosphatase), increased bilirubin.

CAUTION

1. This drug is only part of a diabetes program. It is not a substitute for a proper diet and regular exercise.
2. Over time (usually months), this drug may not work. Periodic follow-up examinations are needed.
3. If you develop an infection, insulin may be required to control your blood sugar.

Precautions for Use

By Infants and Children: This drug does not work in type 1 (juvenile, growth-onset) insulin-dependent diabetes.

By Those Over 60 Years of Age: Use with caution, and start with 2.5 mg/day. Dose should be increased slowly and glucose checked often. Repeated hypoglycemia in the elderly can cause brain damage.

▷ **Advisability of Use During Pregnancy**

Pregnancy Category: C. See Pregnancy Risk Categories at the back of this book.

Animal studies: No birth defects reported in rats and rabbits.

Human studies: Adequate studies of pregnant women are not available.

Because uncontrolled blood sugar levels during pregnancy are associated with a higher incidence of birth defects, many experts recommend that insulin (instead of an oral agent) be used as necessary to control diabetes during the entire pregnancy.

Advisability of Use If Breast-Feeding

Presence of this drug in breast milk: Unknown.

Avoid drug or refrain from nursing.

Habit-Forming Potential: None.

Effects of Overdose: Symptoms of mild to severe hypoglycemia: headache, light-headedness, faintness, nervousness, confusion, tremor, sweating, heart palpitation, weakness, hunger, nausea, vomiting, stupor progressing to coma.

Possible Effects of Long-Term Use: Reduced thyroid function (hypothyroidism). Reports of increased frequency and severity of heart and blood vessel diseases with long-term use of this class of drugs are highly controversial and inconclusive. A direct cause-and-effect relationship (see Glossary) is tenuous. Ask your doctor for help.

Suggested Periodic Examinations While Taking This Drug (at physician's discretion)

Complete blood cell counts.

Liver function tests.

Thyroid function tests.

Periodic evaluation of heart and circulatory system.

▷ **While Taking This Drug, Observe the Following**

Foods: Follow the diabetic diet prescribed by your physician.

Herbal Medicines or Minerals: Using chromium may change the way your body is able to use sugar. Some health food stores advocate vanadium as mimicking the actions of insulin, but possible toxicity and need for rigorous studies presently preclude recommending it. Caution: St. John's wort may cause photosensitivity, and this drug may too.

DHEA may change sensitivity to insulin or insulin resistance. Hawthorn, ginger, garlic, ginseng and licorice, nettle and yohimbe may change blood sugar. Since this may require adjustment of hypoglycemic medicine dosing, talk to your doctor BEFORE combining any of these herbal medicines with this medicine. Echinacea pupurea (injectable) and blonde psyllium seed or husk should NOT be taken by people living with diabetes.

Beverages: As directed in the diabetic diet. May be taken with milk.

▷ *Alcohol:* Use with extreme caution—alcohol can prolong this drug's hypoglycemic effect. This drug can also cause a disulfiramlike reaction (see Glossary): facial flushing, sweating, palpitation.

Tobacco Smoking: No interactions expected. I advise everyone to quit smoking.

▷ *Other Drugs*

The following drugs may ***increase*** the effects of glipizide:
- acarbose (Precose) may increase risk of excessive lowering of blood sugar.
- aspirin and other salicylates.
- chloramphenicol (Chloromycetin).
- cimetidine (Tagamet).
- clofibrate (Atromid-S).
- cotrimoxazole (Septra).
- fenfluramine (Pondimin).
- itraconazole (Sporanox) and other azole antifungal medicines.
- levothyroxine (and other thyroid products).
- magnesium (increased absorption into the body).
- monoamine oxidase (MAO) type A inhibitors (see Drug Classes).
- NSAIDs (see Drug Classes).
- probenecid (Benemid).
- ranitidine (Zantac).
- sulfa drugs such as trimethoprim/sulfamethoxazole (Septra) or erythromycin/sulfisoxazole (Pediazole).

The following drugs may ***decrease*** the effects of glipizide:
- beta-blocker drugs (see Drug Classes).
- birth control pills (oral contraceptives).
- bumetanide (Bumex).
- cholestyramine (Questran).
- conjugated estrogens (Premarin).
- diazoxide (Proglycem).
- ethacrynic acid (Edecrin).
- furosemide (Lasix).
- phenothiazines (see Drug Classes).
- phenytoin (Dilantin).
- rifampin (Rifadin, others).
- ritonavir (Norvir).
- steroids (betamethasone, prednisone, others).
- thiazide diuretics (see Drug Classes).

Glipizide ***taken concurrently*** with
- antacids (containing magnesium hydroxide) may result in increased risk of excessively lowered blood sugar.

- antifungal agents (such as itraconazole or other azoles) may result in severe lowering of blood sugar.
- calcium channel blockers (see Drug Classes) may cause excessive lowering of blood glucose.
- cyclosporine (Sandimmune) may result in cyclosporine toxicity.
- sildenafil (Viagra) one case report of an interaction. Talk to your doctor about current data regarding combined use.
- warfarin (Coumadin) can cause an increased hypoglycemic effect.

▷ *Driving, Hazardous Activities:* Dosing schedule, eating schedule and physical activities must be coordinated to prevent hypoglycemia. Know the early symptoms of hypoglycemia so that you can avoid hazardous activities and take corrective measures.

Aviation Note: Diabetes **is a disqualification** for piloting. Consult a designated Aviation Medical Examiner.

Exposure to Sun: Some drugs of this class can cause photosensitivity (see Glossary).

Occurrence of Unrelated Illness: Acute infections, vomiting or diarrhea, serious injuries and surgical procedures can worsen diabetic control and may require insulin. If any of these conditions occur, call your doctor.

Discontinuation: Because of secondary failures, the continued benefit of this drug should be evaluated every 6 months.

GLYBURIDE (GLI byoor ide)

Other Name: Glibenclamide   **Introduced:** 1970   **Class:** Antidiabetic, sulfonylureas   **Prescription:** USA: Yes   **Controlled Drug:** USA: No; Canada: No   **Available as Generic:** Yes

Brand Names: ✤Albert-Glyburide, ✤Apo-Glyburide, Diabeta, ✤Euglucon, ✤ Gen-Glybe, Glubate, Glucovance [CD], Glynase Prestab, Micronase, ✤ Novo-Glyburide

BENEFITS versus RISKS	
Possible Benefits	*Possible Risks*
HELPS REGULATE BLOOD SUGAR IN TYPE 2 DIABETES (NON-INSULIN DEPENDENT DIABETES) ADJUNCTIVE TO APPROPRIATE DIET AND WEIGHT CONTROL COMBINED WITH METFORMIN IN THE GLUCOVANCE FORM TO GIVE ADDED AND TIGHTER BLOOD SUGAR (GLUCOSE) CONTROL	HYPOGLYCEMIA, SEVERE AND PROLONGED LACTIC ACIDOSIS (A RARE RISK WITH GLUCOVANCE FORM) Possible anemia with long-term use (added as a rare risk with Glucovance form) Liver damage Blood cell and bone marrow disorders Allergic skin reactions (some severe) Possible increased risk of heart (cardiovascular) mortality

▷ **Principal Uses**

As a Single Drug Product: Uses currently included in FDA-approved labeling: Type 2 diabetes mellitus (adult, maturity-onset) that does not require insulin but can't be adequately controlled by diet alone.

Other (unlabeled) generally accepted uses: None.

How This Drug Works: This drug (1) stimulates the secretion of insulin, (2) decreases glucose production in the liver and (3) enhances insulin use.

Available Dosage Forms and Strengths

Tablets — 1.25 mg, 1.5 mg, 2.5 mg, 3 mg, 5 mg, 6 mg

Tablets, combination — 250 mg metformin and 1.25 mg glyburide, 500 mg metformin and 2.5 or 5.0 mg glyburide

▷ **Usual Adult Dosage Ranges:** *Regular-release products:* 2.5 to 5 mg daily with breakfast. At 7-day intervals the dose may be increased by increments of 2.5 mg daily as needed and tolerated. Total daily dose should not exceed 20 mg. Prudent to start sensitive patients on 1.25 mg daily.

Micronized products: 1.5 to 3 mg daily taken with breakfast. (Patients more sensitive to oral agents should be started at 0.75 mg daily.) If the daily dose required is more than 6 mg daily, twice daily dosing may be needed. Maximum dose is 12 mg daily.

Note: Actual dose and schedule must be determined for each patient individually.

Conditions Requiring Dosing Adjustments

Liver Function: Glyburide may cause catastrophic hypoglycemia (low blood sugar) if it is used by patients with liver disease. Very low starting doses should be taken and the patient closely followed. It is also a rare cause of hepatitis and cholestatic jaundice.

Kidney Function: Glyburide should be used with caution in mild renal compromise, with low initial doses and careful patient monitoring. The drug SHOULD NOT be used by patients with moderate kidney failure (creatinine clearances less than 50 ml/min) or in severe kidney failure.

▷ **Dosing Instructions:** If the daily maintenance dose is 10 mg or more, the total dose should be divided into two equal doses: the first taken with the morning meal, the second with the evening meal. The tablet may be crushed. If you forget a dose: take it as soon as you remember it, unless it's nearly time for your next dose—if that is the case, skip the missed dose and return to taking the medicine on your usual schedule. DO NOT double doses. Call your doctor if you find yourself missing doses—the best results are achieved by taking exactly the right dose and keeping your blood sugar in "tight" control.

Usual Duration of Use: Use on a regular schedule for 1 to 2 weeks determines effectiveness in controlling diabetes. No response to peak doses in 1 month constitutes a primary failure. Up to 10% of those who respond initially may develop secondary failure. The duration of effective use can only be determined by periodic measurement of the blood sugar.

Typical Treatment Goals and Measurements (Outcomes and Markers)

Blood sugar: The general goal for blood sugar is to return it to the usual "normal" range (generally 80–120 mg/dl), while avoiding risks of excessively low blood sugar. One study (UKPDS) used a fasting plasma sugar (glucose) of less than 108 mg/dl.

Fructosamine and glycosylated hemoglobin: Fructosamine levels (a measure of the past two to three weeks of blood sugar control) should be less than or equal to 310 micromoles per liter. Glycosylated hemoglobin or hemoglobin A1C (a measure of the past 2–3 months of blood sugar control) should be less than or equal to 7.0%.

▷ **This Drug Should Not Be Taken If**
- you have had an allergic reaction to it previously.
- you have severe impairment of liver and kidney function.
- you have diabetic ketoacidosis.
- you are pregnant.

▷ **Inform Your Physician Before Taking This Drug If**
- you are allergic to other sulfonylurea drugs or to "sulfa" drugs.
- your diabetes has been unstable or "brittle" in the past.
- you do not know how to recognize or treat hypoglycemia (see Glossary).
- you have a history of problems with blood clotting or have a glucose-6-phosphate dehydrogenase (G6PD) deficiency.
- you have a history of congestive heart failure, peptic ulcer disease, cirrhosis of the liver, hypothyroidism or porphyria.
- you have an infection or a fever.

Possible Side Effects (natural, expected and unavoidable drug actions)

If drug dose is excessive or food intake is delayed or inadequate, abnormally low blood sugar (hypoglycemia) will occur as a predictable drug effect.

▷ **Possible Adverse Effects** (unusual, unexpected and infrequent reactions)

If any of the following develop, consult your physician promptly for guidance.

Mild Adverse Effects

Allergic reactions: skin rash, hives, itching.

Headache, drowsiness, dizziness, fatigue—possible.

Indigestion, heartburn, nausea—rare.

Bedwetting at night (nocturnal enuresis), especially in young adults—case reports.

Serious Adverse Effects

Allergic reactions: hepatitis with jaundice (see Glossary), severe skin reactions (exfoliative dermatitis)—case reports.

Idiosyncratic reaction: hemolytic anemia (see Glossary).

Disulfiramlike reaction with concurrent use of alcohol (see Glossary)—possible.

Bone marrow depression (see Glossary): fatigue, fever, sore throat, abnormal bleeding—case reports.

Thrombocytopenic purpura—case report

Liver toxicity (granulomatous or intrahepatic cholestasis)—case reports.

Blood clotting defects (coagulation)—rare.

Cardiovascular mortality (based on an old study of a different medicine)—increased risk.

▷ **Possible Effects on Sexual Function:** None reported.

▷ **Adverse Effects That May Mimic Natural Diseases or Disorders**

Liver reactions may suggest viral hepatitis.

Possible Effects on Laboratory Tests
Blood platelet counts: decreased.
Blood cholesterol and triglyceride levels: decreased.
Glycated hemoglobin or protein: trending toward normal.
Blood glucose levels: decreased.
Liver function tests: increased liver enzymes (ALT/GPT, AST/GOT and alkaline phosphatase).

CAUTION
1. This drug is only part of diabetes management. Much of the damage from diabetes can be delayed or avoided if you keep your blood sugar in the normal range. Ask your doctor about a proper diet and regular exercise.
2. Over time (usually several months), this drug may not work. Periodic follow-up examinations are necessary.

Precautions for Use
By Infants and Children: This drug does not work in type 1 (juvenile, growth-onset) insulin-dependent diabetes.
By Those Over 60 Years of Age: Use with caution, and start with 1.25 mg/day of the regular form. Dose should be slowly increased and glucose closely followed. Repeated hypoglycemia in the elderly can cause brain damage.

▷ **Advisability of Use During Pregnancy**
Pregnancy Category: C. See Pregnancy Risk Categories at the back of this book.
Animal studies: No birth defects reported in rats and rabbits.
Human studies: Adequate studies of pregnant women are not available.
Uncontrolled blood sugar levels during pregnancy are associated with a higher incidence of birth defects, so many experts recommend insulin (instead of an oral agent) to control diabetes during the entire pregnancy.

Advisability of Use If Breast-Feeding
Presence of this drug in breast milk: Unknown.
Avoid drug or refrain from nursing.

Habit-Forming Potential: None.

Effects of Overdose: Symptoms of mild to severe hypoglycemia: headache, light-headedness, faintness, nervousness, confusion, tremor, sweating, heart palpitation, weakness, hunger, nausea, vomiting, stupor progressing to coma.

Possible Effects of Long-Term Use: Reduced thyroid gland function (hypothyroidism). Reports of increased frequency and severity of heart and blood vessel diseases associated with long-term use of this class of drugs are highly controversial and inconclusive. A direct cause-and-effect relationship (see Glossary) is tenuous. Ask your physician for guidance.

Suggested Periodic Examinations While Taking This Drug (at physician's discretion)
Complete blood cell counts.
Liver function tests.
Thyroid function tests.
Periodic evaluation of heart and circulatory system.
Self assessment of blood sugar is prudent as well as periodic glycosylated hemoglobin and/or fructosamine tests.

▷ **While Taking This Drug, Observe the Following**

Foods: Follow the diabetic diet prescribed by your physician.

Herbal Medicines or Minerals: Using chromium may change the way your body is able to use sugar. Some health food stores advocate vanadium as mimicking the actions of insulin, but possible toxicity and need for rigorous studies presently preclude recommending it. Caution: St. John's wort may cause photosensitivity, and this drug may too.

DHEA may change sensitivity to insulin or insulin resistance. Hawthorn, ginger, garlic, ginseng and licorice, nettle and yohimbe may change blood sugar. Since this may require adjustment of hypoglycemic medicine dosing, talk to your doctor BEFORE combining any of these herbal medicines with this medicine. Echinacea pupurea (injectable) and blonde psyllium seed or husk should NOT be taken by people living with diabetes.

Beverages: As directed in the diabetic diet. May be taken with milk.

▷ *Alcohol:* Use with extreme caution—alcohol can exaggerate this drug's hypoglycemic effect. This drug can cause a disulfiramlike reaction (see Glossary): facial flushing, sweating, palpitation.

Tobacco Smoking: No interactions expected. I advise everyone to quit smoking.

▷ *Other Drugs*

The following drugs may *increase* the effects of glyburide:
• acarbose (Precose).
• aspirin and other salicylates (aspirin may also block disulfiram effect).
• chloramphenicol (Chloromycetin).
• cimetidine (Tagamet).
• ciprofloxacin (Cipro).
• clofibrate (Atromid-S).
• cotrimoxazole (various).
• fenfluramine (Pondimin).
• gemfibrozil (Lopid).
• monoamine oxidase (MAO) type A inhibitors (see Drug Classes).
• phenylbutazone (Butazolidin).
• ranitidine (Zantac).
• ritonavir (Norvir).
• sulfa drugs such as trimethoprim/sulfamethoxazole (Septra) or erythromycin/sulfisoxazole (Pediazole).

The following drugs may *decrease* the effects of glyburide:
• beta-blocker drugs (see Drug Classes).
• bumetanide (Bumex).
• diazoxide (Proglycem).
• ethacrynic acid (Edecrin).
• furosemide (Lasix).
• phenytoin (Dilantin).
• rifampin (Rifadin, others).
• thiazide diuretics (see Drug Classes).
• thyroid hormones (see Drug Classes).

Glyburide *taken concurrently* with
• antacids (containing magnesium hydroxide) or magnesium supplements may result in increased risk of excessively lowered blood sugar.
• antifungal agents (such as itraconazole or other azoles) may result in severe lowering of blood sugar.

- cyclosporine (Sandimmune) may increase cyclosporine levels by up to 57%.
- enalapril (Vasotec) may enhance blood sugar lowering effect.
- MAO inhibitors (see Drug Classes) may increase risk of hyperglycemia.
- steroids (betamethasone, prednisone, others) blunts glyburide benefits.
- warfarin (Coumadin) may result in bleeding; more frequent INR (pro-thrombin time) testing is needed.

▷ *Driving, Hazardous Activities:* Regulate dosing, eating and physical activities carefully to prevent hypoglycemia. Know the early symptoms of hypo-glycemia so that you can avoid hazardous activities and take corrective measures.

Aviation Note: Diabetes *is a disqualification* for piloting. Consult a designated Aviation Medical Examiner.

Exposure to Sun: Use caution until sensitivity has been determined. Some drugs of this class can cause photosensitivity (see Glossary).

Occurrence of Unrelated Illness: Acute infections, vomiting or diarrhea, serious injuries and surgical procedures can worsen diabetic control and may require insulin. If any of these conditions occur, consult your physician promptly.

Discontinuation: Because of the possibility of secondary failure, it is advisable to evaluate the continued benefit of this drug every 6 months.

GUANFACINE (GWAHN fa seen)

Introduced: 1980   **Class:** Antihypertensive   **Prescription:** USA: Yes
Controlled Drug: USA: No   **Available as Generic:** USA: Yes
Brand Name: Tenex

BENEFITS versus RISKS	
Possible Benefits	*Possible Risks*
EFFECTIVE ANTIHYPERTENSIVE IN MILD TO MODERATE HIGH BLOOD PRESSURE	Amnesia
EFFECTIVE IN HIGH BLOOD PRESSURE IN PREGNANCY	

▷ **Principal Uses**

As a Single Drug Product: Uses currently included in FDA-approved labeling: (1) Used to treat mild to moderate high blood pressure; (2) used alone or in combination to treat high blood pressure caused by kidney problems.

Other (unlabeled) generally accepted uses: (1) Heroin withdrawal; (2) may be useful in problem pregnancies; (3) could have a role in treating atten-tion deficit hyperactivity disorder (ADHD); (4) may help some sleep disor-ders; (5) one report of benefit in Tourette's syndrome in a child.

How This Drug Works: By reducing sympathetic nervous system output (alpha-2-receptors), this drug causes blood vessels to relax and blood pressure to lower.

Available Dosage Forms and Strengths

Tablets — 1 mg, 2 mg

▷ **Usual Adult Dosage Ranges:** Starts with 1 mg taken at bedtime. Dose may be increased after 3 to 4 weeks to 2 mg daily, as needed and tolerated. Dose may then be further increased after another 3 to 4 weeks to 3 mg daily. Total daily dose may be taken in two divided doses if needed. Usual maximum is 6 mg daily. **Note: Actual dose and schedule must be determined for each patient individually.**

Conditions Requiring Dosing Adjustments
Liver Function: Should be used with caution by patients with liver compromise.
Kidney Function: Used with caution.

▷ **Dosing Instructions:** Tablets may be crushed and taken without regard to eating. Taking daily dose at bedtime reduces daytime drowsiness. If you forget a dose: take it as soon as you remember it, unless it's nearly time for your next dose—if that is the case, skip the missed dose and return to taking the medicine on your usual schedule. DO NOT double doses. Call your doctor if you forget two doses in a row.

Usual Duration of Use: Regular use for 4 to 6 weeks is usually needed to see drug's effect in controlling high blood pressure. Peak benefit may not be seen for 12 weeks. Even though high blood pressure often does not have any symptoms, it is CRITICAL to keep it under control. Long-term use (months to years) requires follow-up by your doctor.

Typical Treatment Goals and Measurements (Outcomes and Markers)
Blood pressure: The most recent treatment guidelines (JNC VI) actually define optimal blood pressure (BP) as less than 120/80 and high normal as 139/89. The American Diabetes Association has chosen a target of 130/80 as the blood pressure goal for people living with diabetes. Most clinicians try to achieve a BP that achieves the best balance of lower cardiovascular risk while avoiding the problem of too low a blood pressure. The goal and time frame (see peak benefits above) should be discussed with you when the prescription is written.

▷ **This Drug Should Not Be Taken If**
  • you have had an allergic reaction to it previously.

▷ **Inform Your Physician Before Taking This Drug If**
  • you have a circulatory disorder of the brain.
  • you have angina, coronary artery disease or a recent heart attack.
  • you have or have had serious emotional depression.
  • you have impaired liver or kidney function.
  • you are a diabetic.
  • you have a history of orthostatic hypotension.
  • you are taking any sedative or hypnotic drugs or an antidepressant.
  • you will have surgery with general anesthesia.

Possible Side Effects (natural, expected and unavoidable drug actions)
Drowsiness—frequent.
Dry nose and mouth—frequent.
Constipation—infrequent to frequent.
Mild lowering of blood pressure on standing (orthostatic hypotension; see Glossary).

▷ **Possible Adverse Effects** (unusual, unexpected and infrequent reactions)
If any of the following develop, consult your physician promptly for guidance.
Mild Adverse Effects
Allergic reactions: skin rash, itching.
Dermatitis or hair loss—case reports.
Headache, dizziness, fatigue, sedation or insomnia—rare to infrequent.
Urination at night or incontinence—case reports.
Reduced insulin release in response to sugar—possible.
Indigestion, nausea, diarrhea—infrequent.
Edema or leg cramps—rare.
Serious Adverse Effects
Depression—infrequent.
Slow heartbeat (bradycardia)—infrequent.
Liver toxicity—rare.
Amnesia—infrequent.
Rebound hypertension (if abruptly stopped).

▷ **Possible Effects on Sexual Function:** Dose-related decreased libido, impotence—case reports.

Possible Effects on Laboratory Tests
Liver function tests: increased.
Blood sugar (glucose): increased.

CAUTION
1. **Do not stop this drug suddenly.** Sudden withdrawal can produce anxiety, nervousness, tremors, fast or irregular heart action, nausea, stomach cramps, vomiting and rebound hypertension.
2. Hot weather and fever can reduce blood pressure significantly. Dose adjustments may be necessary.
3. Report the development of any tendency to emotional depression.

Precautions for Use
By Infants and Children: Safety and effectiveness for use by those under 12 years of age have not been established.
By Those Over 60 Years of Age: **Proceed cautiously.** Pressure should be reduced without creating the risks associated with excessively low blood pressure. Watch for light-headedness, dizziness, unsteadiness, fainting and falling. Sedation and dry mouth occur commonly in elderly users. Report promptly any changes in mood or behavior: depression, delusions, hallucinations.

▷ **Advisability of Use During Pregnancy**
Pregnancy Category: B. See Pregnancy Risk Categories at the back of this book.
Animal studies: No birth defects due to this drug reported in rat and rabbit studies.
Human studies: Adequate studies of pregnant women are not available.
Use this drug only if clearly needed. Ask your physician for guidance.

Advisability of Use If Breast-Feeding
Presence of this drug in breast milk: Probably.
Avoid drug or refrain from nursing.

Habit-Forming Potential: None.

Effects of Overdose: Marked drowsiness, dry mouth, slow pulse, low blood pressure, vomiting, stupor progressing to coma.

Possible Effects of Long-Term Use: Development of tolerance (see Glossary) with loss of drug effectiveness.

Suggested Periodic Examinations While Taking This Drug (at physician's discretion)

Blood pressure measurements.

▷ **While Taking This Drug, Observe the Following**

Foods: Avoid excessive salt, and ask your doctor about degree of salt restriction.

Herbal Medicines or Minerals: Ginseng may increase blood pressure, blunting the benefits of this medicine. Hawthorn, saw palmetto, ma huang, goldenseal, yohimbe and licorice may also increase blood pressure. Valerian and kava kava may cause additive drowsiness. Calcium and garlic may help lower blood pressure. Indian snakeroot has a German Commission E monograph indication for hypertension—talk to your doctor. Eleuthero root and ephedra should be avoided by people living with hypertension.

Beverages: No restrictions. May be taken with milk.

▷ *Alcohol:* Use with extreme caution—can cause marked drowsiness or exaggerated reduction of blood pressure.

Tobacco Smoking: No interactions expected. I advise everyone to quit smoking.

▷ *Other Drugs*

Guanfacine *taken concurrently* with

• amitriptyline (Elavil) and other tricyclic antidepressants (see Drug Classes) can cause decreased effectiveness as an antihypertensive.
• bupropion (Wellbutrin) led to seizures in one case report.
• phenobarbital can lead to loss of therapeutic effect of guanfacine.

▷ *Driving, Hazardous Activities:* Use caution. This drug can cause drowsiness and can impair mental alertness, judgment and coordination.

Aviation Note: Hypertension (high blood pressure) *is a disqualification* for piloting. Consult a designated Aviation Medical Examiner.

Exposure to Sun: No restrictions.

Exposure to Heat: Use caution. Hot environments may reduce the blood pressure significantly; be alert to the possibility of orthostatic hypotension (see Glossary).

Heavy Exercise or Exertion: Use caution. Isometric exercises can raise blood pressure significantly. This drug may intensify the hypertensive response to isometric exercise. Ask your physician for guidance.

Occurrence of Unrelated Illness: Fever may lower blood pressure significantly. Vomiting may prevent regular use of this drug and result in acute withdrawal reactions. Call your doctor.

*Discontinuation: **Do not stop this drug suddenly.*** Withdrawal reactions occur within 2 to 7 days after the last dose. It is best to reduce dose gradually (over 3 to 4 days), with periodic monitoring of the blood pressure.

HALOPERIDOL (hal oh PER i dohl)

Introduced: 1958   **Class:** Antipsychotic; tranquilizer, strong   **Prescription:** USA: Yes   **Controlled Drug:** USA: No; Canada: No   **Available as Generic:** USA: Yes; Canada: Yes

Brand Names: ❧Alti-Haloperidol, ❧Apo-Haloperidol, Haldol, ❧Haldol LA, Halperon, ❧Novo-Peridol, ❧Peridol, ❧PMS Haloperidol

BENEFITS versus RISKS	
Possible Benefits	*Possible Risks*
EFFECTIVE CONTROL OF PSYCHOSES	FREQUENT PARKINSON-LIKE side effects
BENEFICIAL EFFECTS ON THINKING, MOOD AND BEHAVIOR	SERIOUS TOXIC EFFECTS ON BRAIN with long-term use
EFFECTIVE CONTROL OF SOME CASES OF TOURETTE'S SYNDROME	Rare blood cell disorders Abnormally low white blood cell count
Beneficial in management of some hyperactive children	
Decanoate form treats schizophrenia for a month with a single injection	

▷ **Principal Uses**

As a Single Drug Product: Uses currently included in FDA approved labeling: (1) Helps control psychotic thinking and abnormal behavior in acute psychosis of unknown nature, acute schizophrenia, paranoid states and the manic phase of manic-depressive disorders; (2) helps control outbursts of aggression and agitation; (3) used to treat Tourette's syndrome.

Other (unlabeled) generally accepted uses: (1) Helps control refractory hiccups; (2) used to lessen delirium in LSD flashbacks and phencyclidine intoxication; (3) used as combination (adjuvant) therapy in chronic pain syndromes; (4) may be helpful in autistic patients; (5) may have a role in refractory vomiting caused by cancer chemotherapy; (6) can ease symptoms in refractory sneezing; (7) may be helpful as adjunctive therapy in stuttering.

How This Drug Works: By interfering with a nerve impulse transmitter (dopamine), this drug reduces anxiety and agitation, improves coherence and thinking and abolishes delusions and hallucinations.

Available Dosage Forms and Strengths

Concentrate — 2 mg/ml

Injection — 5 mg/ml, 50 mg/ml, and 100 mg/ml

Tablets — 0.5 mg, 1 mg, 2 mg, 5 mg, 10 mg, 20 mg

▷ **Usual Adult Dosage Ranges:** Initially 0.5 to 2 mg two or three times daily. Dose may be increased by 0.5 mg/day at 3- to 4-day intervals as needed and tolerated. The usual dose range is 0.5 to 30 mg daily. The total daily dose should not exceed 100 mg. Decanoate form may relieve schizophrenia for a month with a single injection. **Note: Actual dose and schedule must be determined for each patient individually.**

Conditions Requiring Dosing Adjustments

Liver Function: The dose, dosing interval and titration interval (time to adjust the drug to desired effect) should be adjusted for liver compromise.

Kidney Function: High doses used with caution in kidney compromise.

▷ **Dosing Instructions:** The tablet may be crushed and taken with or following food to reduce stomach irritation. The concentrate may be diluted in 2 ounces of water or fruit juice; do not add it to coffee or tea. If you forget a dose: take it as soon as you remember it, unless it's nearly time for your next dose—if that is the case, skip the missed dose and return to taking the medicine on your usual schedule. DO NOT double doses. Call your doctor if you find yourself forgetting doses.

Usual Duration of Use: Use on a regular schedule for several weeks determines this drug's effectiveness in controlling psychotic behavior. If it doesn't provide significant benefit in 6 weeks, it should be stopped. Long-term use requires supervision and periodic physician evaluation.

Typical Treatment Goals and Measurements (Outcomes and Markers)

Psychosis: The general goal: to lessen the degree and severity of abnormal thinking, letting patients return to their daily lives. Specific measures of psychosis may involve testing or inventories and can be valuable in helping check benefits from this medicine.

This Drug Should Not Be Taken If
- you had an allergic reaction to it previously.
- you are experiencing severe mental depression.
- you have any form of Parkinson's disease.
- you have severe active liver disease.
- you are presently experiencing central nervous system (CNS) depression due to alcohol or narcotics.
- you currently have a bone marrow or blood cell disorder.

▷ **Inform Your Physician Before Taking This Drug If**
- you are allergic or abnormally sensitive to phenothiazine drugs.
- you have a history of mental depression.
- you have any type of heart disease.
- you have impaired liver or kidney function.
- you have cancer of the breast.
- you have thyroid disease.
- you are allergic to the dye tartrazine.
- you are pregnant or are planning pregnancy.
- you have a history of neuroleptic malignant syndrome.
- you have low blood pressure, epilepsy or glaucoma.
- you are taking any drugs with a sedative effect.
- you plan to have surgery and general or spinal anesthesia soon.

Possible Side Effects (natural, expected and unavoidable drug actions)
Mild drowsiness, low blood pressure, blurred vision, dry mouth, constipation, marked and frequent Parkinson-like reactions (see Glossary).

▷ **Possible Adverse Effects** (unusual, unexpected and infrequent reactions)
If any of the following develop, consult your physician promptly for guidance.

Mild Adverse Effects
Allergic reactions: skin rash, hives.
Dizziness, weakness, agitation, insomnia—case reports to infrequent.
Loss of appetite, indigestion, nausea, vomiting, diarrhea—case reports.
Decreased white blood cell count—possible.

Serious Adverse Effects
Allergic reactions: rare liver reaction with jaundice, asthma, spasm of vocal cords.

Idiosyncratic reactions: Neuroleptic malignant syndrome (see Glossary).
Nervous system reactions: rigidity of extremities, tremors, seizures, constant movement, facial grimacing, eye-rolling, spasm of neck muscles, tardive dyskinesia (see Glossary)—case reports to infrequent.
Rhabdomyolysis—case report.
Abnormal heartbeat (premature ventricular contractions)—possible with aggressive dosing.
Torsades de pointes—possible.
Worsening of psychosis—possible.
Low blood sugar or abnormal and frequent urination (SIADH)—case reports.
Liver toxicity—possible.
Bronchospasm or myasthenia gravis—case reports.

▷ **Possible Effects on Sexual Function:** Decreased libido; impotence—infrequent to frequent; painful ejaculation; priapism (see Glossary). Tender and enlarged breast tissue in men (gynecomastia); breast enlargement with milk production in women.
Altered timing and pattern of menstruation—case reports.

▷ **Adverse Effects That May Mimic Natural Diseases or Disorders**
Liver reaction may suggest viral hepatitis. Nervous system reactions may suggest Parkinson's disease or Reye's syndrome.

Natural Diseases or Disorders That May Be Activated by This Drug
Latent epilepsy, glaucoma, diabetes.

Possible Effects on Laboratory Tests
Complete blood counts: decreased red cells, hemoglobin and white cells; increased eosinophils.
INR (prothrombin time): decreased.
Blood cholesterol level: decreased.
Blood glucose level: increased.
Liver function tests: increased liver enzymes (ALT/GPT, AST/GOT and alkaline phosphatase), increased bilirubin.

CAUTION
1. The smallest effective dose should be used for long-term therapy.
2. Use with extreme caution in epilepsy; can alter seizure patterns.
3. Those with lupus erythematosus or who are taking prednisone have more nervous system reactions.
4. Levodopa should not be used to treat Parkinson-like reactions; it can cause agitation and worsening of the psychotic disorder.
5. Obtain prompt evaluation of any change or disturbance in vision.

Precautions for Use
By Infants and Children: This drug should not be used in children under 3 years of age or 15 kg in weight. Avoid this drug in the presence of symptoms suggestive of Reye's syndrome. Children are quite susceptible to nervous system reactions caused by this drug.
By Those Over 60 Years of Age: Small doses are indicated when therapy is started. This drug can cause significant changes in mood and behavior; watch for confusion, disorientation, agitation, restlessness, aggression, and paranoia. You may be more susceptible to the development of drowsiness, lethargy, orthostatic hypotension (see Glossary), hypothermia (see Glossary), Parkinson-like reactions and prostatism (see Glossary).

▷ **Advisability of Use During Pregnancy**
Pregnancy Category: C. See Pregnancy Risk Categories at the back of this book.
Animal studies: Cleft palate reported in mouse studies.
Human studies: No increase in birth defects reported in 100 exposures. Adequate studies of pregnant women are not available.
Avoid during the first 3 months (trimester). Use only if clearly needed. Ask your physician for guidance.

Advisability of Use If Breast-Feeding
Presence of this drug in breast milk: Yes.
Monitor nursing infant closely and discontinue drug or nursing if adverse effects develop.

Habit-Forming Potential: Reports of recreational use have been filed. If the drug is stopped suddenly, patient may experience a withdrawal syndrome.

Effects of Overdose: Marked drowsiness, weakness, tremor, unsteadiness, agitation, stupor, coma, convulsions.

Possible Effects of Long-Term Use: Eye damage-deposits in cornea, lens or retina; tardive dyskinesia (see Glossary).

Suggested Periodic Examinations While Taking This Drug (at physician's discretion)
Complete blood counts.
Liver function tests.
Eye examinations.
Electrocardiograms.
The tongue should be watched for fine, involuntary, wavelike movements that could be the beginning of tardive dyskinesia.

▷ **While Taking This Drug, Observe the Following**
Foods: No restrictions.
Herbal Medicines or Minerals: St. John's wort may also lead to increased sensitivity to the sun—DO NOT COMBINE. Since part of the way ginseng works may be as an MAO inhibitor, do not combine.
Beverages: No restrictions. May be taken with milk.
▷ *Alcohol:* Avoid completely. Alcohol can increase the sedative action of haloperidol and accentuate its depressant effects on brain function. Haloperidol can increase the intoxicating effects of alcohol.
Tobacco Smoking: Combination with nicotine actually increased suppression of tics in Tourette's syndrome in one study. I advise everyone to quit smoking.
Marijuana Smoking: Moderate increase in drowsiness; accentuation of orthostatic hypotension; increased risk of precipitating latent psychosis, confusing interpretation of mental status and of drug response.
▷ *Other Drugs*
Haloperidol may ***increase*** the effects of
• all drugs with sedative actions and cause excessive sedation.
• some antihypertensive drugs and cause excessive lowering of blood pressure; monitor the combined effects carefully.
• fluvoxamine (Luvox) and result in toxicity (altered mental status, GI side effects).

Haloperidol may *decrease* the effects of
- guanethidine (Esimil, Ismelin) and reduce its antihypertensive effect.

Haloperidol *taken concurrently* with
- anticholinergic drugs (see Drug Classes) can cause additive anticholinergic effects (dry mouth, constipation or sedation).
- beta-blocker drugs may cause excessive lowering of blood pressure.
- dextromethorphan (common cough suppressant in cough medicines) may lead to dextromethorphan toxicity.
- fluoxetine (Prozac) can result in an increased risk of haloperidol toxicity.
- fluvoxamine (Luvox) can result in an increased risk of haloperidol toxicity.
- lithium (Lithobid, others) may cause toxic effects on the brain and nervous system.
- MAO inhibitors (see Drug Classes) may exaggerate low blood pressure and brain (CNS) effects.
- methyldopa (Aldomet) may cause serious dementia.
- olanzapine (Zyprexa) may lead to Parkinson-like symptoms.
- paroxetine (Paxil) may lead to haloperidol toxicity.
- quinidine (Quinaglute, others) may lead to haloperidol toxicity.
- ritonavir (Norvir) and perhaps other protease inhibitors (see Drug Classes) may lead to toxicity.
- sertraline (Zoloft) may lead to haloperidol toxicity.
- sparfloxacin (Zagam) may lead to abnormal heartbeats.
- tacrine (Cognex) may lead to Parkinson-like symptoms.
- tramadol (Ultram) may lead to seizures.
- venlafaxine (Effexor) may lead to haloperidol toxicity.

The following drugs may *decrease* the effects of haloperidol:
- antacids containing aluminum and/or magnesium, which may reduce its absorption.
- barbiturates.
- benztropine (Cogentin).
- buspirone (Buspar)
- carbamazepine (Tegretol).
- phenytoin (Dilantin) or fosphenytoin (Cerebyx).
- rifampin (Rifater, others).
- trihexyphenidyl (Artane).

▷ *Driving, Hazardous Activities:* This drug may impair mental alertness, judgment and physical coordination. Restrict activities as necessary.

Aviation Note: The use of this drug *is a disqualification* for piloting. Consult a designated Aviation Medical Examiner.

Exposure to Sun: Use caution—this drug can cause photosensitivity. See "Herbal Medicines" note on St. John's wort above.

Exposure to Heat: Use caution in hot environments. This drug may impair the regulation of body temperature and increase the risk of heatstroke.

Exposure to Cold: This drug can increase the risk of hypothermia (see Glossary) in the elderly.

Discontinuation: This drug should not be stopped abruptly following long-term use. Gradual withdrawal over a period of 2 to 3 weeks is advised. Ask your doctor for help.

HISTAMINE (H2) BLOCKING DRUG FAMILY

Cimetidine (si MET i deen)   **Famotidine** (fa MOH te deen)   **Nizatidine** (ni ZA te deen)   **Ranitidine** (ra NI te deen)

Introduced: 1977, 1986, 1988, 1983, respectively   **Class:** Histamine (H2) blocking drugs   **Prescription:** USA: Yes   **Controlled Drug:** USA: No; Canada: No   **Available as Generic:** USA: Yes (prescription forms cimetidine and ranitidine) and Tagamet HB; Canada: Yes

Brand Names: *Cimetidine:* ✳Apo-Cimetidine, ✳Enlon, ✳Novo-Cimetine, ✳Nu-Cimet, ✳Peptol, Tagamet, Tagamet HB 200 (nonprescription); *Famotidine:* Pepcid, Pepcid AC (nonprescription), Pepcid Complete [CD] (nonprescription); *Nizatidine:* Axid, Axid AR (nonprescription); *Ranitidine:* ✳Apo-Ranitidine, Novo-Ranidine, Nu-Ranit, Zantac, Zantac 75 (nonprescription), ✳Zantac-C, Zantac 75 EFFERdose (nonprescription)

Warning: The brand names Zantac and Xanax are similar and can be mistaken. These are very different drugs, and a mix-up can lead to serious problems. Check the color chart insert of drugs and verify that you are taking the correct drug.

```
                        BENEFITS versus RISKS
         Possible Benefits                    Possible Risks
EFFECTIVE TREATMENT OF GERD      Drug-induced hepatitis
   AND PEPTIC ULCERS IN          Bone marrow depression (lowered
   CHILDREN (FAMOTIDINE ONLY)       white blood cells or hemoglobin)
EFFECTIVE TREATMENT OF           Confusion (particularly in
   PEPTIC ULCER DISEASE: relief of   compromised elderly with some of
   symptoms, acceleration of healing,  these drugs)
   prevention of recurrence      Low blood platelet counts
CONTROL OF HYPERSECRETORY        (All of the above are case report to
   STOMACH DISORDERS                 rare effects.)
TREATMENT OF REFLUX
   ESOPHAGITIS
TREATMENT OF HEARTBURN
PREVENTION OF HEARTBURN
   (cimetidine, famotidine and
   nizatidine)
```

Author's Note: The nonprescription heartburn-preventing or treating forms of these medicines have, in general, side effects or adverse effects that occur less frequently or not at all when compared to the already well-tolerated prescription forms. Some doctors are using proton pump inhibitors (see Drug Classes) during the day combined with a dose of a histamine H2 blocker at night.

▷ **Principal Uses**

As a Single Drug Product: Uses currently included in FDA-approved labeling: (1) Treatment and prevention of recurrence of peptic ulcer in adults; (2) all are used for both duodenal and gastric ulcers; (3) cimetidine, ranitidine and famotidine are used in conditions where extreme production of stomach acid occurs (Zollinger-Ellison syndrome); (4) all four medicines are used to control excess acid moving from the stomach into the lower throat (gastroesophageal reflux disease—GERD); (5) cimetidine is approved for use in preventing upper stomach/intestinal bleeding; (6) all have been used with antibiotics and bismuth compounds (Pepto-Bismol and others) in refractory ulcers where Helicobacter pylori has been found; (7) cimetidine is approved to prevent ulcers caused by stress (stress ulcer prophylaxis); (8) all are approved in nonprescription forms for treatment of heartburn—cimetidine (Tagamet HB 200), famotidine (Pepcid AC) and nizatidine (Axid AR) are also approved for prevention of heartburn; (9) famotidine is approved for treatment of peptic ulcers and GERD in children.

Other (unlabeled) generally accepted uses: (1) Ranitidine, famotidine and nizatidine have been used in the prevention of upper stomach/intestinal bleeding; (2) cimetidine has been used prior to surgery to prevent aspiration pneumonitis caused by anesthesia, and ranitidine has shown some benefit here as well; (3) ranitidine and famotidine have been used to help prevent ulcers that may occur in acutely and seriously ill patients; (4) cimetidine appears to have a role in helping patients with colorectal cancer live longer, but further research is needed; (5) famotidine may have a role in treating anaphylactic reactions; (6) cimetidine also may have a role in helping recurrent and resistant warts in some children; (7) cimetidine intravenously has been helpful in cases of resistant drug-induced anaphylactic shock.

How These Drugs Work: They block the action of histamine and, by doing this, inhibit the ability of the stomach to make acid. Once acid is decreased, the body is able to heal itself. Ulcers resistant to healing have now been shown to have an infectious component (Helicobacter pylori), and antibiotics combined with a histamine (H2) blocking drug can work.

Available Dosage Forms and Strengths

Cimetidine:

Injection — 300 mg/2 ml, 300 mg/50 ml (single dose in 0.9% sodium chloride)

Liquid — 300 mg/5 ml (2.8% alcohol)

Oral solution — 300 mg/5 ml

Tablets — 100 mg, 200 mg, 300 mg, 400 mg, 600 mg, 800 mg

Tablets (nonprescription) — 200 mg

Famotidine:

Injection — 10 mg/ml (in 2-and 4-ml vials)

Oral suspension — 40 mg/5 ml

Tablets — 20 mg, 40 mg

Tablets (nonprescription) — 10 mg

Nizatidine:

Pulvules (capsules) — 75 mg, 150 mg, 300 mg

Tablets (nonprescription) — 75 mg

Ranitidine:

Gelcap — 168 mg, 336 mg (Canada only)

GELdose capsules — 150 mg, 300 mg

Injection — 0.5 mg/ml (single dose in 100 ml)

— 25 mg/ml (in 2-, 10- and 40-ml vials and 2-ml syringes)

Oral solution (Canada) — 84 mg/5 ml
Syrup — 15 mg/ml (7.5% alcohol)
Tablets — 150 mg, 300 mg (effervescent)
— 150 mg
Tablets (nonprescription) — 5 mg

▷ **Recommended Dosage Ranges** (Actual dose and schedule must be determined for each patient individually.)

Infants and Children:

Cimetidine: Routine use is not recommended in those less than 16 years old. Doses of 20 to 40 mg per kg of body mass per day have been used.

Famotidine: GERD—1 mg per kg per day separated into two equal daily doses. Peptic ulcer—0.5 mg per kg of body mass at bedtime or divided into two equal doses up to a total of 40 mg per day (children).

Nizatidine: No data.

Ranitidine: For those 2 to 18 years old—1.25 to 2 mg per kg of body mass per dose given every 12 hours, or 37.5 mg per dose.

16 to 60 Years of Age:

Peptic ulcer and hypersecretory states:

Cimetidine: 300 mg by mouth four times daily, taken with meals and at bedtime, or 800 mg at bedtime. A maintenance dose of 400 mg at bedtime is useful for some patients.

Famotidine: 40 mg by mouth at bedtime for 4 or up to 8 weeks. Maintenance doses of 20 mg at bedtime have been used. Up to 640 mg daily for hypersecretory states.

Nizatidine: 300 mg by mouth at bedtime, or 150 mg twice a day for up to 8 weeks. A maintenance dose of 150 mg at bedtime is useful for some patients. Not used for hypersecretory states.

Ranitidine: 150 mg by mouth twice daily, or 300 mg at bedtime. Maintenance doses of 150 mg at bedtime may be of benefit for some patients. Up to 6 g in hypersecretory states.

Heartburn (nonprescription forms):

Cimetidine: 200 mg by mouth 30 minutes or less before eating foods or drinking liquids that cause you problems. May also be taken once heartburn has started.

Famotidine: 10 mg by mouth before eating foods or drinking liquids that cause you problems or once heartburn has started.

Nizatidine: 75 mg up to twice daily before eating foods or drinking liquids that cause you problems or once heartburn has started.

Ranitidine: 75 mg by mouth.

Over 60 Years of Age:

Cimetidine: Half the usual adult dose to start. Cimetidine may be more likely to cause confusion in the elderly than the other medicines in this family.

Ranitidine, famotidine and nizatidine: Same dose as 16 to 60 years of age. All pose a risk for formation of masses (phytobezoars) of undigested vegetable fibers. Watch for nervousness, confusion, loss of appetite, stomach fullness, nausea and vomiting.

Conditions Requiring Dosing Adjustments:

Liver Function: Cimetidine and famotidine are most dependent on the liver for elimination. Dose must be decreased in liver failure.

    Kidney Function: All of these H2 blockers are primarily eliminated by the kidneys. Doses must be decreased in moderate kidney failure.

▷ **Dosing Instructions:** Cimetidine and ranitidine should be taken immediately after meals to obtain the longest decrease in stomach acid when treating peptic ulcers. Cimetidine, ranitidine and famotidine should be taken after meals when used in hypersecretory states. If you forget a dose: take it as soon as you remember it, unless it's nearly time for your next dose—if that is the case, skip the missed dose and return to taking the medicine on your usual schedule. DO NOT double doses. Call your doctor if you find yourself forgetting doses.

Usual Duration of Use: Use on a regular schedule for 4 to 6 weeks usually determines effectiveness in healing active peptic ulcer disease. Long-term use (months to years) for prevention requires periodic individualized consideration by your physician. Continual use for 6 to 12 weeks is needed to heal the esophagus when cimetidine, ranitidine, famotidine or nizatidine is used in gastroesophageal reflux disease (GERD). Since nonprescription forms are available for heartburn, if heartburn relief has not occurred in 2 hours, call your doctor, as there may be another reason for your symptoms.

Typical Treatment Goals and Measurements (Outcomes and Markers)

    Ulcers: The role of *Helicobacter pylori* in ulcers is no longer questioned and omeprazole (a proton pump inhibitor) is widely recognized as the standard for short-term treatment of stomach ulcers. When *H. pylori* is present, single medicine therapy is not recommended. Additionally, an antibiotic is often used with other agents. The goal is to heal the ulcer area and prevent re-occurrence of the ulceration. Sign and symptom relief as well as endoscopic examination help define success of treatment.

    Heartburn: The general goal: to lessen the degree or severity of or to prevent heartburn. Some patients take the nonprescription forms BEFORE they eat foods that historically have given them heartburn.

Possible Advantages of These Drugs: Nonprescription forms offer relief of heartburn discomfort. Famotidine is approved for nonprescription prevention of heartburn.

These Drugs Should Not Be Taken If
* you had an allergic reaction to it previously.

▷ **Inform Your Physician Before Taking These Drugs If**
* you have impaired liver or kidney function.
* you have a low sperm count (cimetidine).
* you are taking any anticoagulant drug.
* you do not tolerate or should not take phenylalanine (ranitidine EFFERdose tablets or granules).
* you have had low white blood cell counts.
* you have a history of acute porphyria (ranitidine).

Possible Side Effects (natural, expected and unavoidable drug actions)
    None reported.

▷ **Possible Adverse Effects** (unusual, unexpected and infrequent reactions)
    If any of the following develop, consult your physician promptly for guidance.

Mild Adverse Effects

   Allergic reactions: skin rash, hives.

   Headache: ranitidine—rare; cimetidine—rare; famotidine—infrequent; nizatidine—frequent.

   Abnormal dreams: nizatidine—rare.

   Diarrhea: ranitidine, nizatidine, cimetidine, famotidine—all rare.

   Joint pain (arthralgia): cimetidine, ranitidine, famotidine—all rare.

   Depression: cimetidine—case reports.

   Muscle pain: cimetidine, nizatidine, famotidine—rare.

Serious Adverse Effects

   Allergic reactions: cimetidine and ranitidine can be rare causes of pancreatitis and anemia. Cimetidine and nizatidine can cause exfoliative dermatitis. There have been some case reports of serious skin rashes with all of these medicines. Most recently, ranitidine received a second case report of toxic epidermal necrolysis (TEN).

   Anaphylactic reactions: cimetidine, nizatidine—rare.

   Idiosyncratic reactions: nervousness, confusion, hallucinations.

   Worsening of Alzheimer's: cimetidine—case reports.

   Liver damage—case reports.

   Abnormal heart rhythm changes (slow heartbeat or atrioventricular block): cimetidine, ranitidine, famotidine, nizatidine—case reports.

   Bone marrow depression: cimetidine, ranitidine, famotidine—rare.

   Decreased platelets: cimetidine, ranitidine, nizatidine—rare; famotidine—case reports and questionable.

   Bronchospasm: cimetidine and ranitidine—rare; famotidine—rare and questionable.

▷ **Possible Effects on Sexual Function:** Impotence: ranitidine, famotidine, cimetidine, nizatidine—case reports.

   Decreased libido: cimetidine—rare.

   Male breast enlargement (gynecomastia): nizatidine, cimetidine—case reports.

Possible Delayed Adverse Effects: Male breast enlargement (nizatidine and cimetidine).

▷ **Adverse Effects That May Mimic Natural Diseases or Disorders**

   Liver changes may mimic viral hepatitis. Mental status changes from cimetidine in older patients may mimic organic causes.

Possible Effects on Laboratory Tests

   Blood platelet counts: may be decreased by all histamine (H2) blockers.

   Complete blood counts: rare white blood cell (granulocytes) decrease by cimetidine, ranitidine and famotidine.

   Urine protein tests (Multistix): false positive with ranitidine use.

   Urine urobilinogen: false positive with nizatidine.

   Thyroid hormones: T4, free T4 may be low with ranitidine use.

   Liver enzymes (SGPT, OT, etc.): can be increased with liver damage.

   Sperm count: decreased with cimetidine.

CAUTION

1. Ulcer rebound/perforation may occur if you stop these drugs abruptly when they are being used to treat ulcers.
2. Once medicines are stopped, call your doctor promptly if symptoms recur.

3. Use of these medicines and symptom relief does not absolutely remove possibility of cancer of the stomach (gastric malignancy).
4. The nonprescription forms of these medicines should NOT be used to treat ulcers.
5. Some of cimetidine is removed by hemodialysis. Additional doses are needed.
6. Cimetidine may worsen thinking ability (mental status) in those older patients with pre-existing mental status problems.

Precautions for Use
By Infants and Children:
  Cimetidine: Routine use is not recommended in those less than 16 years old. Doses of 20 to 40 mg per kg of body mass per day have been used.
  Famotidine: 0.5 mg per kg of body mass twice a day for 8 weeks in those 6 to 15 years old.
  Nizatidine: No data.
  Ranitidine: For those 2 to 18 years old—1.25 to 2 mg per kg of body mass per dose given every 12 hours, or 37.5 mg per dose.
By Those Over 60 Years of Age: Increased risk of masses of partially digested vegetable fibers (phytobezoars), especially in people who can't chew well. Watch closely for decreased appetite, stomach fullness, nausea and vomiting. Watch those in this age range who are taking cimetidine for changes in thinking (mental status changes).

▷ **Advisability of Use During Pregnancy**
  Pregnancy Category: B for all. See Pregnancy Risk Categories at the back of this book.
  Animal studies: No birth defects for cimetidine, ranitidine and famotidine. Rabbit studies of nizatidine showed abortions, while rat studies showed no effects.
  Human studies: Adequate studies of pregnant women are not available.
  Use only if clearly needed. Ask your doctor for advice.

Advisability of Use If Breast-Feeding
  Presence of these drugs in breast milk: Yes.
  Avoid drugs or refrain from nursing.

Habit-Forming Potential: None.

Effects of Overdose:
  Cimetidine (rarely documented): confusion, tachycardia, sweating, drowsiness, muscle twitching, seizures, respiratory failure, severe CNS symptoms such as coma (after 20–40 g).
  Nizatidine (rarely documented): increased tearing of the eyes, salivation, vomiting and diarrhea.
  Ranitidine and famotidine: no documentation of overdose changes. Adverse effects of the usual dose. Symptomatic and supportive care would be indicated (nonprescription forms do not have documentation of overdoses).

Possible Effects of Long-Term Use: Rare liver damage with cimetidine, ranitidine and nizatidine. Swelling and tenderness of breast tissue with cimetidine, ranitidine and nizatidine.

Suggested Periodic Examinations While Taking These Drugs (at physician's discretion)
  Complete blood counts.

Liver and kidney function tests.

More frequent tests of INR (prothrombin time) if an anticoagulant is also taken.

Sperm counts (cimetidine).

Mental status check.

▷ **While Taking These Drugs, Observe the Following**

Foods: Protein-rich foods increase stomach acid secretion. Garlic, onions, citrus fruits and tomatoes may also increase acid secretion. Many people know the kinds of foods that are likely to result in significant heartburn. Ask your doctor or pharmacist for help in timing the dose of a nonprescription agent for heartburn.

Herbal Medicines or Minerals: Kola and ma huang may increase stomach acid, blunting the benefits of these medicines. Black cohosh root, ginkgo and squill are contraindicated in gastrointestinal disturbances. Licorice root has a German Commission E monograph indication for gastrointestinal ulcers, but use with H2 blockers has not been studied. Some members of this family have increased sun sensitivity. Caution is advised if St. John's wort is being considered. Talk to your doctor BEFORE adding any herbals to these medicines.

Nutritional Support: Diet as prescribed by your doctor.

Beverages: The caffeine in caffeine-containing beverages such as coffee, tea and some sodas may stay in the body up to 50% longer than usual with cimetidine (Tagamet) use. Milk may increase acid secretion.

▷ *Alcohol:* Stomach acidity is increased by alcohol—avoid use. Cimetidine may produce a drug interaction with higher than expected levels.

Tobacco Smoking: Smoking is a clear risk factor for peptic ulcer disease. I advise everyone to quit smoking.

Marijuana Smoking: Possible additive reduction in sperm counts with cimetidine use.

▷ *Other Drugs*

Cimetidine may *increase* the effects of

- amiodarone (Cordarone).
- amitriptyline (Elavil) and perhaps other tricyclic antidepressants (see Drug Classes). Decreased doses may be needed if the medicines are to be combined.
- benzodiazepines (Librium, etc.; see Drug Classes).
- carbamazepine (Tegretol), with increased toxicity risk. Blood levels are recommended and ongoing carbamazepine doses adjusted to blood levels.
- cyclosporine (Sandimmune, others) may result in increased blood levels and cyclosporine toxicity.
- dofetilide (Tikosyn) may result in increased blood levels and dofetilide toxicity.
- flecainide (Tambocor) and require dosing changes and more frequent blood level checks.
- loratadine (Claritin), by causing a large increase in blood levels. A study did NOT report any adverse effects on the heart from these levels, but since excessive blood levels of any medicine may be more likely to cause undesirable effects, it appears prudent to lower loratadine doses if these medicines are to be combined.

- meperidine (Demerol, others) and result in toxicity with potential respiratory depression and low blood pressure.
- metformin (Glucophage).
- metoprolol (Lopressor, others), and perhaps other beta blockers (see Drug Classes), and result in very slow heartbeat and excessively low blood pressure.
- morphine (MS Contin, MSIR, others) and result in central nervous system depression and respiratory depression.
- oral anticoagulants, with increased risk of bleeding; increased frequency of INR testing is recommended.
- phenytoin (Dilantin).
- procainamide (Procan, Pronestyl).
- propranolol (Inderal).
- quinidine (Quinaglute).
- sertraline (Zoloft).
- sildenafil (Viagra) may increase blood levels of sildenafil by up to 56% (800 mg cimetidine dose). Talk to your doctor about this BEFORE using these medicines together.
- sirolimus (Rapamune) may result in increased blood levels and sirolimus toxicity.
- tacrolimus (Prograf) may result in increased blood levels and tacrolimus toxicity.
- tamsulosin (Flomax) may result in increased blood levels and tamsulosin.
- terbinafine (Lamisil).
- theophylline (Theo-Dur, etc.).
- venlafaxine (Effexor).
- warfarin (Coumadin).
- zaleplon (Sonata) may result in increased blood levels and zaleplon toxicity.
- zolmitriptan (Zomig) may result in increased blood levels and zolmitriptan toxicity.

Ranitidine may *increase* the effects of
- diazepam (Valium).
- fluvastatin (Lescol).
- glipizide (Glucotrol) and perhaps other oral antidiabetic drugs (see Drug Classes).
- metformin (Glucophage).
- midazolam (Versed).
- procainamide (Procan, Pronestyl).
- theophylline (Theo-Dur, etc.).
- warfarin (Coumadin)—rarely; increased INR testing is recommended.

Nizatidine, ranitidine and famotidine (prescription forms) may *increase* the effects of
- amoxicillin.
- high-dose aspirin (may increase level and toxicity risk).
- pentoxifylline (Trental); however, this interaction has only been documented with cimetidine.
- theophylline (Theo-Dur, others); ongoing theophylline dosing should be based on more frequent blood levels if these medicines are to be taken together.

Cimetidine *taken concurrently* with
- most calcium channel blockers (see Drug Classes) may result in increased blood levels of the calcium channel blockers and potential toxicity; decreased calcium-channel-blocker doses may be needed. This may also occur with other H2 blockers, and caution is advised.
- carmustine (BiCNU) may cause severe bone marrow depression.
- carvedilol (Coreg) may result in increased blood levels and carvedilol toxicity.
- chloroquine may result in toxicity and may cause cardiac arrest.
- cisapride (Propulsid) may result in increased cisapride levels and a potential serious increase in heart rate.
- clozapine (Clozaril) may result in increased blood levels and clozapine toxicity.
- digoxin (Lanoxin) may result in changes in digoxin levels.
- oral hypoglycemic agents such as glipizide (Glucotrol), glyburide (DiaBeta, Micronase) and tolbutamide (Tolinase, others) may result in severe low blood sugars and seizures.
- paroxetine (Paxil) and perhaps other SSRI antidepressants (see Drug Classes) may result in increased blood levels of the SSRI and require dosing changes.
- pentoxifylline (Trental) may result in increases in blood levels of pentoxifylline; pentoxifylline dose changes may be needed.
- ritonavir (Norvir), amprenavir (Agenerase) and perhaps other protease inhibitors may result in increased cimetidine levels.
- zalcitabine (Hivid) may result in increased blood levels of zalcitabine and result in toxicity; decreased doses of zalcitabine may be needed.

Cimetidine, ranitidine, famotidine and nizatidine *taken concurrently* with
- antacids will result in a decreased histamine blocker level; it may be prudent to separate the dosing of these medicines (prescription forms).

Cimetidine may *decrease* the effects of
- indomethacin (Indocin) and perhaps other NSAIDs, by decreasing absorption.
- iron salts, by decreasing absorption.
- ketoconazole, itraconazole and fluconazole.
- tetracyclines, by decreasing absorption.

Ranitidine, nizatidine and famotidine may *decrease* the effects of
- indomethacin, by decreasing absorption.
- ketoconazole, itraconazole and fluconazole.
- sucralfate (Carafate).

▷ *Driving, Hazardous Activities:* Use caution until the degree of confusion, dizziness or other effect is seen.

Aviation Note: The use of these drugs (prescription forms) *may be a disqualification* for piloting. Consult a designated Aviation Medical Examiner.

Exposure to Sun: Rare and questionable association with ranitidine; use caution with sun exposure when first starting this medicine.

Occurrence of Unrelated Illness: Idiopathic thrombocytopenic purpura (ITP), a rare lowering of blood platelets, is a contraindication for use of any of these medicines. Aplastic anemia, whatever the cause, may be worsened by cimetidine. If symptoms of heartburn get worse, you experience unexplained weight loss and are over 45 years old, talk with your doctor—this may be an indication of stomach cancer.

Discontinuation: **Do not stop these medicines suddenly if they are being taken for peptic ulcer disease.** Ask your doctor for withdrawal instructions. Be alert to the recurrence of ulcers any time after these drugs are stopped. Recurrent or refractory ulcers may also represent an infectious disease caused by Helicobacter pylori. If this is the case, combination therapy with an antibiotic may be indicated.

HYDRALAZINE (hi DRAL a zeen)

Introduced: 1950   **Class:** Antihypertensive   **Prescription:** USA: Yes
Controlled Drug: USA: No; Canada: No   **Available as Generic:** USA: Yes; Canada: No

Brand Names: Alazine, Alphapress, Apo-Hydralazine, Apresazide [CD], Apresoline, Apresoline-Esidrix [CD], Cam-Ap-Es, Dralserp, Dralzine, H-H-R, Hydroserpine [CD], Hyserp [CD], Lo-Ten, Marpres, Novo-Hylazin, Nu-Hydral, Ser-A-Gen [CD], Ser-Ap-Es [CD], Serpasil-Apresoline [CD], Serprex [CD], Supres [CD], Tri-Hydroserpine, Unipres [CD], Uniserp [CD]

BENEFITS versus RISKS	
Possible Benefits	*Possible Risks*
EFFECTIVE ADJUNCT IN MODERATE TO SEVERE HYPERTENSION	DRUG-INDUCED LUPUS ERYTHEMATOSUS-LIKE SYNDROME
Possibly beneficial in severe congestive heart failure	Intensification of angina pectoris
	Rare blood cell disorders
	Rare liver damage

▷ **Principal Uses**
As a Single Drug Product: Uses currently included in FDA-approved labeling: (1) Used with other drugs in moderate to severe high blood pressure or hypertensive crisis; (2) therapy of hypertension caused by abnormal changes in kidney blood vessels.
    Other (unlabeled) generally accepted uses: (1) Therapy for aortic or mitral heart valve insufficiency, providing support until surgery can be performed; (2) treatment of acute congestive heart failure in combination with dobutamine; (3) help in anorexia or cachexia; (4) therapy of high blood pressure in pregnancy; (5) painful erections that may occur in sickle cell disease (sickle cell priapism).
As a Combination Drug Product [CD]: Available combined with hydrochlorothiazide (a diuretic) and with reserpine (another type of antihypertensive). When used in combination, several different types of drug action occur at the same time and result in a more beneficial decrease in blood pressure.
How This Drug Works: Causing direct relaxation of arterial walls, lowering blood pressure. Dilation can also help in some cases of heart failure by reducing workload and increasing the output of the heart. Combination with a diuretic reduces sodium and water in the body and combination

with reserpine reduces the rate and force of contraction of the heart and increases blood vessel expansion.

Available Dosage Forms and Strengths
Tablets — 10 mg, 25 mg, 50 mg, 100 mg

Author's Note: The information in this profile has been shortened to make room for more widely used medicines.

HYDROCHLOROTHIAZIDE (hi droh klor oh THI a zide)

Please see the thiazide diuretics family profile.

HYDROCODONE (hi droh KOH dohn)

Other Name: Dihydrocodeinone

Introduced: 1951   **Class:** Analgesic, strong; cough suppressant; opioid
Prescription: USA: Yes   **Controlled Drug:** USA: C-III*; Canada: Yes
Available as Generic: USA: Yes, hydrocodone/APAP; Canada: No

Brand Names: Allay [CD], Allure 5/500 [CD], Anaplex, Anexsia [CD], Anexsia 7.5 [CD], Anolor DH5, Atuss [CD], Azdone [CD], Ban-Tuss-HC [CD], ✤Biohisdex DHC [CD], ✤Biohisdine DHC [CD], Chemdal-HD [CD], Codone, Detussin [CD], DHC Plus, Dicoril, Dimetane Expectorant-DC [CD], Dolacet [CD], Duocet [CD], Duratuss HD [CD], Endagen HD [CD], Endal-HD, Entuss-D, Histinex-HC [CD], Histussin HC [CD], ✤Hycodan, Hycodan [CD], ✤Hycomine [CD], Hycomine Compound [CD], Hycomine Pediatric Syrup [CD], ✤Hycomine-S [CD], Hycomine Syrup [CD], Hyco-tuss Expectorant [CD], Lorcet-HD [CD], Lorcet Plus [CD], Lortab [CD], Lortab ASA [CD], Medipain 5, Norcet 7 [CD], ✤Novahistex DH [CD], ✤Novahistine DH [CD], Polygesic, Protuss, ✤Robidone, Ru-Tuss [CD], T-Gesic [CD], Triaminic Expectorant DH [CD], ✤Tussaminic Expectorant DH [CD], Tussend [CD], Tussend Expectorant [CD], Tussionex [CD], Tycolet [CD], Vanex [CD], Vicodin [CD], Vicodin ES [CD], Vicoprofen [CD], Zydone [CD]

BENEFITS versus RISKS	
Possible Benefits	*Possible Risks*
EFFECTIVE RELIEF OF MILD TO MODERATE PAIN	Mild allergic reactions—infrequent
	Nausea, constipation
EFFECTIVE CONTROL OF COUGH	Small potential for addiction

▷ **Principal Uses**
As a Single Drug Product: Uses currently included in FDA-approved labeling: (1) Controls cough; (2) relieves mild to moderate pain.
   Other (unlabeled) generally accepted uses: May be a benefit for some patients with chronic obstructive lung disease (COPD).
As a Combination Drug Product [CD]: Often added to cough mixtures containing antihistamines, decongestants and expectorants to increase effectiveness in reducing cough. Also combined with analgesics, such as

*See Schedules of Controlled Drugs at the back of this book.

acetaminophen and aspirin and other nonsteroidal anti-inflammatory (NSAID) compounds, to enhance pain relief.

How This Drug Works: Decreases pain perception, calming emotional responses to pain and reducing cough reflex sensitivity. Vicoprofen form combines an NSAID with hydrocodone.

Available Dosage Forms and Strengths

Syrup — 5 mg/5 ml

Tablets — 5 mg

Tablets (combination) — 10 mg hydrocodone, 650 mg acetaminophen

▷ **Usual Adult Dosage Ranges:** *As analgesic:* 5 to 10 mg every 6 hours to start and may later be reduced as needed. Maximum for pain is 40 mg. *For cough:* 5 mg every 6 to 8 hours as needed.

Lorcet: One tablet every four to six hours as directed by your doctor. Total daily dose of hydrocodone should not exceed 40 mg.

Vicoprofen: Short-term (less than 10 days) management of sudden pain—one tablet every 4–6 hours. Dose should NOT exceed 5 tablets in any 24-hour period. The lowest effective dose should be used.

Note: Actual dose and schedule must be determined for each patient individually.

Conditions Requiring Dosing Adjustments

Liver Function: Use with caution by patients with severe liver compromise, with decreases in dose or longer time between doses.

Kidney Function: This drug may cause urinary retention, and a benefit-to-risk decision should be made for patients with renal (kidney) outflow problems. Up to 20% of this drug is eliminated by the kidneys. Consideration for reduced doses should be given, especially for longer-term therapy. Combination products containing NSAIDs are a benefit-to-risk decision in kidney compromise.

▷ **Dosing Instructions:** Tablet may be crushed and taken with or following food to reduce stomach irritation or nausea. If you forget a dose: take it as soon as you remember it, unless it's nearly time for your next dose—if that is the case, skip the missed dose and return to taking the medicine on your usual schedule. DO NOT double doses. Call your doctor if you find yourself forgetting doses.

Usual Duration of Use: As long as needed, to control pain or cough. Continual use should not exceed 5 to 7 days without interruption and reassessment of need.

Typical Treatment Goals and Measurements (Outcomes and Markers)

Pain: Most clinicians treating pain use a device called an algometer to check your pain. This looks like a small ruler, but lets the clinician better understand your pain. The goals of treatment then relate to where the level of pain started (for example, a rating of 7 on a zero to ten scale) and what the cause of the pain was. Pain medicines may also be used together (in combination) in order to get the best result or outcome. If your pain control is not acceptable to YOU (remember, in hospitals and outpatient settings, etc. pain control is a patient right) and if results are not acceptable, be sure to call your doctor as you may need a different medicine or combination.

▷ **This Drug Should Not Be Taken If**
- you had an allergic reaction to it previously.
- you have a lesion in your head (intracranial) that causes increased pressure.
- you are among those who should not take NSAIDs (may be in combination products).
- you are having an acute attack of asthma.

▷ **Inform Your Physician Before Taking This Drug If**
- you had an unfavorable reaction to any narcotic drug.
- you have a history of drug abuse or alcoholism.
- you have chronic lung disease with impaired breathing.
- you have impaired liver or kidney function.
- you have gallbladder disease, a seizure disorder or an underactive thyroid gland.
- you have difficulty emptying the urinary bladder.
- you are prone to constipation.
- you are allergic to sulfites (some preparations contain sulfites).
- this drug is being considered for a child with whooping cough (pertussis).
- you are taking any other drugs that have a sedative effect.
- you will have surgery with general anesthesia.

Possible Side Effects (natural, expected and unavoidable drug actions)
Drowsiness, light-headedness, dry mouth, urinary retention, constipation—infrequent to frequent.

▷ **Possible Adverse Effects** (unusual, unexpected and infrequent reactions)
If any of the following develop, consult your physician promptly for guidance.

Mild Adverse Effects
Allergic reactions: skin rash, hives, itching.
Dizziness, impaired concentration, sensation of drunkenness, confusion, depression, blurred or double vision, facial flushing, sweating—infrequent to frequent.
Nausea, vomiting—infrequent to frequent (may also be dose related).
Abnormal constriction of the pupils of the eye (miosis)—possible.

Serious Adverse Effects
Allergic reactions: anaphylaxis, severe skin reactions—case reports.
Idiosyncratic reactions: delirium, hallucinations, excitement, increased sensitivity to pain after the analgesic effect has worn off.
Seizures—possible.
Impaired breathing (respiratory depression)—dose-related.
Liver or kidney toxicity—case reports (some noted with acetaminophen-containing combination products).
Psychological and physical dependence—possible.

▷ **Possible Effects on Sexual Function:** Blunting of sexual response or drive—possible.

▷ **Adverse Effects That May Mimic Natural Diseases or Disorders**
Paradoxical behavioral disturbances may suggest psychotic disorder.

Possible Effects on Laboratory Tests
Blood amylase and lipase levels: increased (natural side effect).
Urine screening tests for drug abuse: initial test result may be falsely posi-

tive; confirmatory test result will be negative. (Test results depend upon amount of drug taken and testing method used.)

CAUTION

1. People with asthma, chronic bronchitis or emphysema may have breathing problems with extended use of this drug. The secretions of the bronchi may thicken, and cough will be suppressed.
2. Combination of this drug with atropinelike drugs can increase the risk of urinary retention and reduced intestinal function.
3. Do not take this drug following acute head injury.

Precautions for Use

By Infants and Children: Do not use this drug in children under 2 years of age because of their vulnerability to life-threatening respiratory depression.

By Those Over 60 Years of Age: Small doses and short-term treatment are indicated. Patients in this group may have increased susceptibility to drowsiness, dizziness, unsteadiness, falling, urinary retention and constipation (often leading to fecal impaction).

▷ ### Advisability of Use During Pregnancy

Pregnancy Category: B. D if in high doses or near the time of birth. Listed as C by the manufacturer. See Pregnancy Risk Categories at the back of this book.

Animal studies: Birth defects reported in hamster studies.

Human studies: Adequate studies of pregnant women are not available. Hydrocodone taken repeatedly during the final few weeks before delivery may cause withdrawal symptoms in the newborn infant.

Use this drug only if clearly needed and in small, infrequent doses.

Advisability of Use If Breast-Feeding

Presence of this drug in breast milk: Unknown.

Monitor nursing infant closely and discontinue drug or nursing if adverse effects develop. Ask your doctor for guidance.

Habit-Forming Potential: Psychological and/or physical dependence can develop with use of large doses for an extended period of time. True dependence is infrequent and unlikely with prudent use.

Effects of Overdose: Drowsiness, restlessness, agitation, nausea, vomiting, dry mouth, vertigo, weakness, lethargy, stupor, coma, seizures.

Possible Effects of Long-Term Use: Psychological and physical dependence, chronic constipation.

Suggested Periodic Examinations While Taking This Drug (at physician's discretion)

Liver function tests.

Check for constipation.

▷ ### While Taking This Drug, Observe the Following

Foods: No restrictions.

Herbal Medicines or Minerals: Valerian and kava kava may interact additively (drowsiness). Avoid these combinations. Ginseng, ginkgo, alfalfa, clove oil, feverfew, cinchona bark and garlic may also change clotting, so combining those herbals with the NSAID combination form of this medicine is not recommended. Talk to your doctor BEFORE combining any medicines. NSAIDs may decrease feverfew effects.

Beverages: No restrictions. May be taken with milk.

▷ *Alcohol:* Use extreme caution. Hydrocodone can intensify the intoxicating effects of alcohol, and alcohol can intensify the depressant effects of hydrocodone on brain function, breathing and circulation.

Tobacco Smoking: No interactions expected. I advise everyone to quit smoking.

Marijuana Smoking: Increased drowsiness and pain relief; impaired mental and physical status.

▷ *Other Drugs*

Hydrocodone may *increase* the effects of
- atropinelike drugs and increase the risk of constipation and urinary retention.
- other drugs with sedative effects.

Hydrocodone *taken concurrently* with
- cimetidine (Tagamet) may result in increased risk of breathing problems and central nervous system suppression.
- MAO inhibitors (see Drug Classes) may result in an increased effect and the need to decrease the dose of hydrocodone.
- naltrexone (ReVia) may cause (precipitate) withdrawal symptoms. DO NOT COMBINE.
- ritonavir (Norvir) and perhaps other protease inhibitors (see Drug Classes) can lead to toxicity.
- tramadol (Ultram) may result in increased risk of breathing problems and central nervous system suppression.

▷ *Driving, Hazardous Activities:* This drug can impair mental alertness, judgment, reaction time and physical coordination. Avoid hazardous activities accordingly.

Aviation Note: The use of this drug *is a disqualification* for piloting. Consult a designated Aviation Medical Examiner.

Exposure to Sun: No restrictions.

Discontinuation: This drug is best limited to short-term use. If used for extended periods, discontinuation should be gradual to minimize withdrawal (usually mild with this drug).

HYDROXYCHLOROQUINE (hi drox ee KLOR oh kwin)

Introduced: 1967   **Class:** Antimalaria, immunosuppressant   **Prescription:** USA: Yes   **Controlled Drug:** USA: No; Canada: No   **Available as Generic:** USA: Yes; Canada: No

Brand Names: ♣Dermoplast, Plaquenil

BENEFITS versus RISKS	
Possible Benefits	*Possible Risks*
EFFECTIVE PREVENTION AND TREATMENT OF CERTAIN FORMS OF MALARIA	INFREQUENT DAMAGE OF CORNEAL AND RETINAL EYE TISSUES
Possibly effective in the management of acute and chronic rheumatoid arthritis and juvenile arthritis	BONE MARROW DEPRESSION
	Heart muscle damage
Possibly effective in the management of chronic discoid and systemic lupus erythematosus	Ear damage: hearing loss, ringing in ears

▷ **Principal Uses**
  As a Single Drug Product: Uses currently included in FDA-approved labeling:
  (1) Prevention and therapy of acute attacks of certain types of malaria; (2)
  reduces disease activity in rheumatoid arthritis; (3) suppresses disease
  activity in chronic discoid and systemic lupus erythematosus.

  Other (unlabeled) generally accepted uses: (1) Treatment of Sjögren's syndrome; (2) treats refractory Lyme arthritis; (3) therapy of sarcoidosis, poly-
  morphous light eruption, porphyria, solar urticaria and chronic vasculitis;
  (4) may help decrease steroid requirements in asthma; (5) can help
  decrease insulin needs when an oral hypoglycemic agent is taken with
  insulin; (6) combination therapy of Weber-Christian disease.

How This Drug Works: In malaria, this drug impairs DNA in the organisms. As
  an antiarthritic and antilupus drug, acts as a mild immunosuppressant.
  Accumulates in white blood cells and inhibits many enzymes involved in
  tissue destruction.

Available Dosage Forms and Strengths
  Tablets — 200 mg

▷ **Usual Adult Dosage Ranges**
  For malaria suppression: 400 mg once every 7 days.
  For malaria treatment: (1) 800 mg as a single dose or (2) initially 800 mg, followed by 400 mg in 6 to 8 hours; then 400 mg once a day on the second
  and third days.
  For pediatric malaria treatment: 10 mg per kg of body mass followed in 6 hours
  by 5 mg per kg of body mass, with 5 mg per kg of body mass given 18 hours
  after the second dose; then 5 mg per kg of body mass taken 24 hours after
  the first dose.
  For lupus erythematosus: 400 mg once or twice daily. This is used for several
  weeks or cautiously until remission. Ongoing dose is 200–400 mg daily.
  For rheumatoid arthritis: Starting dose of 400 to 600 mg and an ongoing dose of
  200–400 mg a day.
  **Note: Actual dose and schedule must be determined for each patient
  individually.**

Conditions Requiring Dosing Adjustments
  Liver Function: Benefit-to-risk decision by patients with liver compromise or
  who take liver-toxic drugs.
  Kidney Function: Use with caution in kidney compromise.

▷ **Dosing Instructions:** Take with food or milk to reduce stomach irritation. The
  tablet may be crushed and mixed with jam, jelly or gelatin. Take it exactly
  as prescribed.
  **Author's Note: For malaria prevention, begin medication 2 weeks before
  entering malarious area; continue medication while in the area and
  for 4 weeks after leaving the area.**
  For treating arthritis and lupus, take medication on a regular schedule
  daily; continual use for 6 months may be necessary to determine maximal benefit. If you forget a dose: take it as soon as you remember it,
  unless it's nearly time for your next dose—if that is the case, skip the
  missed dose and return to taking the medicine on your usual schedule.
  DO NOT double doses. If you only take one dose a week, call your doctor
  for instructions.

Usual Duration of Use: Use on a regular schedule for 2 weeks before exposure, during period of exposure and 4 weeks after exposure determines this drug's effectiveness in preventing attacks of malaria. Use on a regular schedule for up to 6 months may be required to evaluate benefits in reducing rheumatoid arthritis and lupus erythematosus. If significant improvement is not achieved, this drug should be stopped. Long-term use (months to years) requires periodic physician evaluation.

Possible Advantages of This Drug

Considered to have less potential for retinal toxicity than chloroquine.

Typical Treatment Goals and Measurements (Outcomes and Markers)

Rheumatoid arthritis: Most rheumatologists use sign and symptom control, joint mobility and pain as indicators of success of therapy. For clinicians treating pain, a device called an algometer is used to check your pain. This looks like a small ruler, but lets the clinician better understand your pain. The goals of treatment then relate to where the level of pain started (for example, a rating of 7 on a zero to ten scale) and what the cause of the pain was. Pain medicines may also be used together (in combination) in order to get the best result or outcome. If your pain control is not acceptable to YOU (remember, in hospitals and outpatient settings, etc. pain control is a patient right) and if results are not acceptable, be sure to call your doctor as you may need a different medicine or combination.

Currently a Drug of Choice

For the treatment of chronic discoid and systemic lupus erythematosus.

▷ **This Drug Should Not Be Taken If**
- you had past allergies to chloroquine or hydroxychloroquine.
- you have an active bone marrow or blood cell disorder.
- it was prescribed for long-term treatment in children (should not be used in that way).

▷ **Inform Your Physician Before Taking This Drug If**
- you are pregnant or planning pregnancy.
- you have had bone marrow depression or a blood cell disorder.
- you have a deficiency of glucose-6-phosphate dehydrogenase (G6PD)—talk with your doctor.
- you have any disorder of the eyes, especially disease of the cornea or retina or visual field changes.
- you have impaired hearing or ringing in the ears.
- you have a seizure disorder of any kind.
- you have a history of peripheral neuritis.
- you have low blood pressure or a heart rhythm disorder.
- you have peptic ulcer disease, Crohn's disease or ulcerative colitis.
- you have impaired liver or kidney function.
- you have a history of porphyria.
- you have any form of psoriasis.
- you are taking antacids, cimetidine, digoxin or penicillamine.

Possible Side Effects (natural, expected and unavoidable drug actions)

Light-headedness (low blood pressure); blue-black discoloration of skin, fingernails or mouth lining with long-term use.

▷ **Possible Adverse Effects** (unusual, unexpected and infrequent reactions)
   If any of the following develop, consult your physician promptly for guidance.

Mild Adverse Effects

   Allergic reactions: skin rash, itching (more common in African Americans).
   Loss of hair color, loss of hair.
   Headache, blurring of near vision (reading), ringing in ears—possible to infrequent.
   Loss of appetite, nausea, vomiting, stomach cramps, diarrhea—infrequent.
   Dizziness—case reports.

Serious Adverse Effects

   Allergic reactions: severe skin rash, exfoliative dermatitis.
   Idiosyncratic reactions: hemolytic anemia in those with glucose-6-phosphate dehydrogenase (G6PD) deficiency in red blood cells.
   Emotional or psychotic mental changes; seizures—case reports.
   Loss of hearing, porphyria—case reports.
   Eye tissue damage, specifically cornea and retina, with significant impairment of vision—case reports.
   Aplastic anemia (see Glossary): abnormally low red blood cell counts (fatigue and weakness); abnormally low white blood cell counts (fever, sore throat, infections); abnormally low platelet counts (abnormal bruising or bleeding)—case reports.
   Muscle damage (myopathy)—case report.

▷ **Possible Effects on Sexual Function:** None reported.

Possible Delayed Adverse Effects: Irreversible eye (retinal) damage has developed 7 years after discontinuation of chloroquine, a closely related drug. Retinal damage is more likely to occur following high-dose and/or long-term use.

▷ **Adverse Effects That May Mimic Natural Diseases or Disorders**
   Central nervous system toxicity may suggest unrelated neuropsychiatric disorder. Seizures may suggest the onset of epilepsy.

Natural Diseases or Disorders That May Be Activated by This Drug
   Porphyria, psoriasis.

Possible Effects on Laboratory Tests
   Complete blood cell counts: decreased red cells, hemoglobin, white cells and platelets.
   Liver function tests: increased liver enzymes (ALT/GPT, AST/GOT and alkaline phosphatase), increased bilirubin.
   Electrocardiogram: conduction abnormalities, prolonged QRS interval, T-wave changes and heart block have all been reported for chloroquine, a closely related drug.

CAUTION
   1. Does not prevent relapses in certain types of malaria.
   2. High-dose and/or long-term use of this drug may cause irreversible retinal damage, significant visual impairment or hearing loss due to nerve damage. Report promptly any changes in vision or hearing so appropriate evaluation can be made.

Precautions for Use

By Infants and Children: This age group is very sensitive to the effects of this drug. Doses should be determined and therapy should be monitored by a qualified pediatrician.

By Those Over 60 Years of Age: Tolerance for this drug may be reduced. Watch for behavioral changes, low blood pressure, heart rhythm disturbances, muscle weakness and changes in vision or hearing.

▷ **Advisability of Use During Pregnancy**

Pregnancy Category: C. See Pregnancy Risk Categories at the back of this book.

Animal studies: No information available.

Human studies: Adequate studies of pregnant women are not available. However, closely related drugs of this class are known to cause abnormal retinal pigmentation and hemorrhage and congenital deafness in the fetus.

Avoid use during pregnancy except for the suppression or treatment of malaria. Other use is a benefit-to-risk decision.

Advisability of Use If Breast-Feeding

Presence of this drug in breast milk: Yes.

Avoid drug or refrain from nursing (controversial).

Habit-Forming Potential: None.

Effects of Overdose: Drowsiness, headache, blurred vision, excitability, low blood pressure, seizures, coma.

Possible Effects of Long-Term Use: Irreversible eye damage (cornea and retina), hearing loss, muscle weakness, aplastic anemia.

Suggested Periodic Examinations While Taking This Drug (at physician's discretion)

Complete blood cell counts.

Liver and kidney function tests.

Serial blood pressure readings and electrocardiograms.

Neurological examinations for significant muscle weakness.

Complete eye examinations before starting high-dose and/or long-term treatment and every 3 to 6 months during drug use.

Hearing tests as indicated.

▷ **While Taking This Drug, Observe the Following**

Foods: No restrictions.

Herbal Medicines or Minerals: Caution: St. John's wort may also cause extreme reactions to the sun. Additive photosensitivity may be possible. Hay flower, mistletoe herb and white mustard seed carry German Commission E monograph indications for arthritis, but have not been studied with this medicine. Talk to your doctor BEFORE combining any herbal with hydroxychloroquine.

Beverages: No restrictions. May be taken with milk.

▷ *Alcohol:* Use sparingly to minimize stomach irritation.

Tobacco Smoking: No interactions expected, but I advise everyone to quit smoking.

▷ *Other Drugs*

Hydroxychloroquine may ***increase*** the effects of

- aurothioglucose (Solganol), which increases risk of blood problems.
- digoxin (Lanoxin) and increase its toxic potential.
- penicillamine (Cuprimine, Depen) and increase its toxic potential.

The following drug may *increase* the effects of hydroxychloroquine:
- cimetidine (Tagamet).

The following drugs may **decrease** the effects of hydroxychloroquine:
- magnesium salts and antacids.

▷ *Driving, Hazardous Activities:* This drug may cause light-headedness, blurred vision or impaired hearing. Restrict activities as necessary.

Aviation Note: The use of this drug *may be a disqualification* for piloting. Consult a designated Aviation Medical Examiner.

Exposure to Sun: Use caution until sensitivity has been determined. Closely related drugs of this class may cause photosensitivity (see Glossary and previous St. John's wort entry).

Discontinuation: This drug should be stopped and prompt evaluation should be made if any of the following develop—changes in vision or hearing, seizures, unusual muscle weakness, indications of infection (fever, sore throat, etc.), abnormal bruising or bleeding.

HYDROXYUREA (hi DROX EE yur ia)

Introduced: 1995 (AIDS or sickle cell)   **Class:** Anti-AIDS, anticancer, anti-sickle-cell anemia   **Prescription:** USA: Yes   **Controlled Drug:** USA: No; Canada: No   **Available as Generic:** USA: Yes; Canada: No

Brand Names: Droxia, Hydrea

Warning: **This drug is a cytotoxic agent. Appropriate precautions must be taken, as with other chemotherapy.**

BENEFITS versus RISKS	
Possible Benefits	*Possible Risks*
COMBINATION TREATMENT OF AIDS	BONE MARROW SUPPRESSION
DECREASED SEVERITY AND FREQUENCY OF SICKLE CELL CRISES	Hepatitis
Treatment of chronic myelocytic leukemia, melanoma and other cancers	Possible secondary leukemia-causing agent (long-term—7–10 years of therapy)

▷ **Principal Uses**

As a Single Drug Product: Uses currently included in FDA-approved labeling: (1) Blast crisis; (2) chronic myelogenous leukemia; (3) head, neck and ovarian cancers; (4) chronic leukemias; (5) cancers of certain cell types (squamous cell); (6) decreases frequency and severity of sickle cell crises; (7) malignant melanoma.

Other (unlabeled) generally accepted uses: (1) Used to treat certain diseases of the red blood cells (polycythemia vera); (2) used in combination with other medicines to treat HIV-positive patients (possible first-line or salvage therapy); (3) brain cancer.

How This Drug Works: When used in cancer, this medicine is a cell-cycle-specific drug. It works in the S phase of mitosis. When used in HIV-positive patients, the exact mechanism of action is not fully understood. When used in sickle cell patients, the specific mechanism has not been identified.

Available Dosage Forms and Strengths
Capsules (Droxia) — 200 mg, 300 mg, 400 mg
Capsule (Hydrea) — 500 mg

▷ **Recommended Dosage Ranges** (Actual dose and schedule must be determined for each patient individually.)

Infants and Children: Safety and effectiveness have not been defined in this age group.

18 to 60 Years of Age: All doses are decided based on ideal or actual body mass, whichever is less.

Oral dosing: Usual oral doses range from 20 to 30 mg per kg of body mass per day, which is given as a single daily dose. Some centers give 80 mg per kg of body mass every third day. If a patient is in blast crisis, up to 12 g per day has been given to rapidly decrease white blood cell counts.

In the sickle cell studies: Patients were started on 15 mg per kg of body mass and had their dose increased by 5 mg per kg of body mass every 12 weeks unless toxicity occurred or the maximum dose of 35 mg per kg of body mass per day was reached.

In AIDS: The protocols are still changing.

Over 60 Years of Age: Same as 18 to 60 years of age.

Conditions Requiring Dosing Adjustments

Liver Function: No changes in dosing are anticipated.

Kidney Function: The dose must be decreased for patients with kidney compromise. Decreases of up to 80% are needed in severe compromise.

▷ **Dosing Instructions:** This medicine is best taken on an empty stomach. Call your doctor if you vomit after taking this medicine. If you forget a dose: take it as soon as you remember it, unless it's nearly time for your next dose—if that is the case, skip the missed dose and return to taking the medicine on your usual schedule. DO NOT double doses. Adherence with this medicine is very important. Call your doctor if you find yourself forgetting doses.

Usual Duration of Use: Continual use on a regular schedule for up to 16 weeks may be needed to treat cancers of the head and neck. Treatment in sickle cell disease is ongoing, using the lowest effective dose.

Treatment in HIV-positive patients is yet to be defined.

Long-term use (months to years) requires periodic evaluation of response and dose adjustment. Consult your physician on a regular basis.

Typical Treatment Goals and Measurements (Outcomes and Markers)

Sickle cell anemia: The severity and number of sickle cell attacks is used as a marker for success when treating sickle cell anemia. This medicine can also help decrease the number of sudden (acute) visits to the emergency room and subsequent hospitalizations for sickle cell crisis.

Currently a Drug of Choice

For reducing the frequency and severity of sickle cell crises in patients with sickle cell disease.

▷ **This Drug Should Not Be Taken If**
- you had an allergic reaction to it previously.
- you have severely depressed bone marrow. This is seen in very low white

blood cell, platelet or hemoglobin levels (neutrophils less than 2,000, platelets less than 100,000 or severe anemia).

▷ **Inform Your Physician Before Taking This Drug If**
- you have signs or symptoms of cancer.
- you are considering pregnancy (males or females).
- you have had chemotherapy or radiation therapy previously.
- you have compromised kidneys.
- you have herpes zoster (shingles).
- you have recently been exposed to chicken pox.
- you are having unusual bruising or bleeding.
- you are unsure how to dispose of urine or vomit.
- you are unsure how much to take or how often to take it.
- you plan to breast-feed your baby.
- you take prescription or nonprescription medicines not discussed when hydroxyurea was prescribed.

Possible Side Effects (natural, expected and unavoidable drug actions)
Hair loss, painful mouth sores, sensitivity to the sun, hair loss—rare.

▷ **Possible Adverse Effects** (unusual, unexpected and infrequent reactions)
If any of the following develop, consult your physician promptly for guidance.
Mild Adverse Effects
Allergic reactions: skin rash and itching or fever.
Dizziness, disorientation, headaches or fever—rare.
Nausea, vomiting or diarrhea—frequent (vomiting usually mild).
Difficulty urinating—rare.
Ulceration of the skin—rare.
Serious Adverse Effects
Allergic reactions: skin ulceration—case reports.
Idiosyncratic reactions: not reported.
Bone marrow depression—possible.
Convulsions or hallucinations—rare.
Hepatitis or kidney problems—rare.
Drug-induced lupus erythematosus—case report.
Lung problems (acute interstitial lung disease)—rare.
Squamous cancer (carcinoma) or leukemia—possible increased risk.

▷ **Possible Effects on Sexual Function:** None reported.

Possible Delayed Adverse Effects: Bone marrow suppression, temporary decrease in kidney function.

▷ **Adverse Effects That May Mimic Natural Diseases or Disorders**
Liver toxicity may be similar to acute hepatitis.

Natural Diseases or Disorders That May Be Activated by This Drug
Not defined.

Possible Effects on Laboratory Tests
Liver function tests: increased.
Complete blood counts: decreases in several components.

CAUTION
1. This medicine is toxic to cells. Be certain your doctor has carefully explained how to dispose of urine or vomit.

2. Call your doctor at once if you have a seizure.
3. Both women and men should avoid conception for several months after taking this medicine.
4. Wash your hands after taking this medicine before you touch your eyes or your nose.

Precautions for Use

By Infants and Children: Safety and effectiveness for use by those under 18 years of age have not been established.

By Those Over 60 Years of Age: Lower doses are prudent, as increased sensitivity to any dose may occur. Natural declines in kidney function may require dose decrease.

▷ **Advisability of Use During Pregnancy**

Pregnancy Category: D. See Pregnancy Risk Categories at the back of this book.

Animal studies: Causes birth defects in animals.

Human studies: Adequate studies of pregnant women are not available.

Talk with your doctor about this benefit-to-risk decision.

Advisability of Use If Breast-Feeding

Presence of this drug in breast milk: Yes.

Avoid drug or refrain from nursing.

Habit-Forming Potential: None.

Effects of Overdose: Bone marrow depression, increased heart rate, liver cell and testicular damage.

Possible Effects of Long-Term Use: Bone marrow depression.

Suggested Periodic Examinations While Taking This Drug (at physician's discretion)

Complete blood cell counts.

Dental exams.

▷ **While Taking This Drug, Observe the Following**

Foods: No restrictions.

Herbal Medicines or Minerals: Some patients use echinacea to attempt to boost their immune systems. Unfortunately, use of echinacea is not recommended in people with damaged immune systems. This herb may also actually weaken any immune system if it is used too often or for too long a time. Caution: St. John's wort may also cause extreme reactions to the sun. Additive photosensitivity may be possible.

Beverages: No restrictions. May be taken with milk.

▷ *Alcohol:* Do not drink alcohol.

Tobacco Smoking: No interactions expected. I advise everyone to quit smoking.

▷ *Other Drugs*

Hydroxyurea *taken concurrently* with

• amphotericin (Abelcet) may increase risk of kidney toxicity and spasm of bronchi.
• fluorouracil (Efudil) may increase toxicity to nerves.
• other medicines that cause bone marrow depression (see Table 5, Section Six) may lead to additive toxicity to bone marrow.
• vaccines (live virus, such as rotavirus vaccine) may result in undesirable or life-threatening effects if immune system is depressed.

▷ *Driving, Hazardous Activities:* This drug may cause light-headedness, blurred vision or impaired hearing. Restrict activities as necessary.

Aviation Note: The use of this drug *may be a disqualification* for piloting. Consult a designated Aviation Medical Examiner.

Exposure to Sun: Use caution until sensitivity has been determined. Closely related drugs of this class may cause photosensitivity (see Glossary). See "Herbal Medicines" caution on St. John's wort above.

Discontinuation: This drug should be stopped and prompt evaluation should be made if any of the following develop—changes in vision or hearing, seizures, unusual muscle weakness, indications of infection (fever, sore throat, etc.), abnormal bruising or bleeding.

IBUPROFEN (i byu PROH fen)

Please see the propionic acid (nonsteroidal anti-inflammatory drug) family profile.

IMATINIB (im ah TIN ib)

Introduced: 2001   **Class:** Protein-tyrosine kinase inhibitor, signal transduction inhibitor, pharmacogenomic, anti-cancer   **Prescription:** USA: Yes
Controlled Drug: USA: No; Canada: No   **Available as Generic:** No
Brand Names: Gleevec

BENEFITS versus RISKS	
Possible Benefits	*Possible Risks*
EFFECTIVE TREATMENT OF CHRONIC MYELOID LEUKEMIA (IN BLAST CRISIS, ACCELERATED PHASE OR IN CHRONIC PHASE AFTER FAILURE OF INTERFERON-ALPHA THERAPY) May have a role in treating gastrointestinal stromal tumors (GIST)	HEMATOLOGICAL TOXICITY EDEMA (MAY BE SEVERE) Liver toxicity Opportunistic infections (with long-term use in animals)

▷ **Principal Uses**

As a Single Drug Product: Uses currently included in FDA-approved labeling: (1) Treats patients with chronic myeloid leukemia (CML) who are in blast crisis, accelerated phase or who are in chronic phase after failure of interferon-alpha therapy.

Other (unlabeled) generally accepted uses: (1) Shows promise against gastrointestinal stromal tumors (GIST).

How This Drug Works: By inhibiting protein kinase, this medicine inhibits the Bcr-Abl abnormal kinase required by Philadelphia chromosome–positive chronic myelogenous leukemia cells. This works to stop the abnormal and excessive number of white blood cells seen in that kind of leukemia. In GIST tumors, this signal transduction inhibitor (STI) interferes with a gene named c-kit which makes cells divide and multiply when the gene is stuck in the "on" position.

Available Dosage Forms and Strengths

Capsules — 100 mg

▷ Usual Adult Dosage Ranges

Chronic phase chronic myelogenous leukemia (CML): 400 mg is given daily. This dose should be taken at the same time each day with a meal and a large glass of water.

Blast crisis or accelerated phase CML: 600 mg daily. The dose should be taken at the same time each day with a meal and a large glass of water. **Note: Actual dose and schedule must be determined for each patient individually.**

Conditions Requiring Dosing Adjustments

Liver Function: Not studied in patients with compromised liver function. If liver bilirubin increases by three times the upper limit of normal (ULN), or if other liver function tests (liver transaminases) increase by five times the ULN, imatinib should be held until bilirubin levels have lowered to 1.5 ULN or transaminases levels to less than 2.5 ULN. Once those conditions are met, therapy can continue at a reduced daily dose.

Kidney Function: Not studied in patients with decreased kidney (renal function). Clinical trials specifically excluded those with serum creatinine levels more than 2 times the upper limit of normal. Metabolites and imatinib itself are not significantly removed by the kidney.

▷ Dosing Instructions:

Doses should be taken at the same time each day with a meal and a large glass of water (lessens gastrointestinal tract irritation). If increases in bilirubin or liver enzymes develops, dosing instructions above should be followed. If severe lowering of white blood cells (neutropenia) or severe lowering of platelets happens, specific steps MUST be taken (see cautions). If you forget a dose: take it as soon as you remember it, unless it's nearly time for your next dose—if that is the case, skip the missed dose and return to taking the medicine on your usual schedule. DO NOT double doses. Call your doctor for instructions if you miss more than one dose.

Usual Duration of Use:

Duration of use will be decided by your doctor based on response of the condition being treated. For example, in CML, resolution of blast crisis and lowering of abnormally elevated white blood cell counts as well as development of any adverse effects will determine the course of therapy. In GIST, tumor response and adverse effect development will determine therapy steps to be taken. Follow up of many patients treated with this medicine has been short (less than 6 months). Long-term safety information of treatment with this medicine is lacking. Talk to your doctor on a regular basis.

Typical Treatment Goals and Measurements (Outcomes and Markers)

CML: The number and type of white blood cells are used to describe the kind of leukemia. For example, in blast crisis, a certain amount and a certain kind of white blood cell predominates the cells seen in the blood/bone marrow. Resolution of the kind and number of cells toward normal levels indicate response of the condition to the medicine. Usual terms used are: no evidence of leukemia (NEL) or return to chronic phase of CML.

GIST: Shrinkage of the tumor and lack of tumor progression are indicators that the situation is resolving.

Possible Advantages of This Drug

Response of GIST where responses to other chemotherapy was poor. Response of CML where other treatment has failed and blast crisis resulted and return to chronic phase is an excellent result.

Currently a "Drug of Choice"

For use in CML in blast crisis, accelerated phase or chronic phase after interferon-alpha failure.

▷ **This Drug Should Not Be Taken If**

- you have had an allergic reaction to it previously.
- your absolute neutrophil count and/or platelets have dropped or bilirubin or liver transaminases have increased to unacceptable levels.

▷ **Inform Your Physician Before Taking This Drug If**

- you have an increase in bilirubin or liver transaminases that your doctor is not aware of.
- your white blood cells (neutrophils) have lowered to less than 1.0×10^9 per liter or your platelets have dropped to less than 50×10^9 per liter.
- you are taking medicines that change or are removed by cytochrome P450 3A4 or 2C9.
- you have any type of heart disease, especially congestive heart failure that may be worsened by fluid accumulation.
- you have impaired liver or kidney function.
- you have a history of alcoholism.

Possible Side Effects (natural, expected and unavoidable drug actions)

Weakness and headache—possible (may be more pronounced in women).

▷ **Possible Adverse Effects** (unusual, unexpected and infrequent reactions)

If any of the following develop, consult your physician promptly for guidance.

Mild Adverse Effects

Allergic reactions: possible.

Nausea, vomiting, diarrhea—possible to infrequent.

Fluid retention/edema—may be frequent.

Fever—infrequent.

Serious Adverse Effects

Allergic reactions: possible.

Idiosyncratic reactions: not reported as yet.

Liver or kidney toxicity—infrequent.

Carcinogenicity studies not yet performed, but positive genotoxic effects were seen in an in vitro mammalian cell assay (Chinese hamster ovary).

Fluid retention/edema (including rapid weight gain and/or pulmonary edema—possible (some cases have been life threatening).

Abnormally low white blood cell and platelet counts: fever, sore throat, infections, abnormal bleeding or bruising—possible and dose related.

▷ **Possible Effects on Sexual Function:** Not reported.

▷ **Adverse Effects That May Mimic Natural Diseases or Disorders**
Liver toxicity may suggest viral hepatitis.

Natural Diseases or Disorders That May Be Activated by This Drug
Not defined.

Possible Effects on Laboratory Tests
Complete blood cell counts: decreased white cells (neutropenia) and platelets (depends on the stage of the disease).
Kidney function tests: increased BUN or creatinine.
Liver function tests: increased liver enzymes (ALT/GPT, AST/GOT and alkaline phosphatase), increased bilirubin.

CAUTION
1. Look for early signs of liver, kidney or hematologic toxicity.
2. If a different doctor than the one prescribing imatinib wants to start a new prescription medicine—make certain you tell him or her that you are taking this medicine.
3. Talk to your doctor if you have an unexplained weight gain or swelling of the ankles.
4. Be certain to keep appointments for any follow-up laboratory testing that your doctor orders.
5. Specific interruptions of therapy steps should be taken if platelet counts or the absolute neutrophil count (ANC) is in the range of: white blood cells (neutrophils) have lowered to less than 1.0×10^9 per liter or your platelets have dropped to less than 50×10^9 per liter.

Precautions for Use
By Infants and Children: Safety and effectiveness for pediatric use not established.
By Those Over 60 Years of Age: Efficacy was similar to younger patients. Edema happened more often in older patients than younger ones.

▷ **Advisability of Use During Pregnancy**
Pregnancy Category: D. See Pregnancy Risk Categories at the back of this book.
Human studies: Information from adequate studies of pregnant women is not available.
Talk to your doctor if you become pregnant while taking this medicine and ask your doctor for guidance about the risk of fetal damage versus the benefits this medicine brings to you.

Advisability of Use If Breast-Feeding
Presence of this drug in breast milk: Unknown in humans, yes in rats.
Breast-feeding is NOT recommended.

Habit-Forming Potential: Not defined, not expected.

Effects of Overdose: Limited experience. An oral dose of 2.5 times the human dose given to rats was not lethal after 14 days. A dose equal to 7.5 times the human dose was lethal to rats after 7–10 days.

Possible Effects of Long-Term Use: Hematologic toxicity—possible, immunosuppression, liver or kidney toxicity.

Suggested Periodic Examinations While Taking This Drug (at physician's discretion)
Complete blood cell counts.
Liver and kidney function tests.
Weight.

Pedal edema checks.

Check of GIST tumor progression or regression.

▷ **While Taking This Drug, Observe the Following**

Foods: No specific restrictions, and food may help lessen GI irritation.

Herbal Medicines or Minerals: Some people take echinacea or mistletoe to try to boost their immune systems, Since neither herb was studied with imatinib, this is NOT recommended. Because St. John's wort acts on the cytochrome P450 system—DO NOT COMBINE. Talk to your doctor BEFORE combining any herbal medicine with imatinib.

Beverages: No restrictions. Should be taken with a full glass of water.

▷ *Alcohol:* May increase stomach and intestinal irritation that can be caused by this drug. Talk to your doctor about this.

Tobacco Smoking: No specific interactions, but I advise everyone to quit.

Marijuana Smoking: Increased chance of opportunistic fungal infections and possible drug level changes.

▷ *Other Drugs*

Imatinib may *increase* the effects of
- all drugs requiring cytochrome P450 3A4 for removal from the body.
- carbamazepine (Tegretol).
- dihydropyridine calcium channel blockers.
- dofetilide (Tikosyn).
- medicines removed by cytochrome P450 2C9.
- triazolo benzodiazepines.
- warfarin (Coumadin). Patients who require a blood thinner (anticoagulant) would more prudently be given a low molecular weight heparin (see Drug Classes).

Imatinib *taken concurrently* with
- anticonvulsants requires careful monitoring for changes in seizure patterns and need to adjust anticonvulsant dose.
- cyclosporine (Sandimmune) should have more frequent cyclosporine blood levels and dosing adjusted to blood levels.
- fosphenytoin (Cerebyx) or phenytoin (Dilantin) may excessively lower the blood level of imatinib.
- medicines with hematologic toxicity may lead to additive toxicity if combined with imatinib.
- ritonavir (Norvir) and perhaps other protease inhibitors (see Drug Classes) may lead to toxicity.

The following drugs may *increase* the effects of imatinib:
- azole antifungals (such as fluconazole, itraconazole and ketoconazole) may lead to higher than expected imatinib blood levels and increased risk of adverse effects.
- macrolide antibiotics (Erythromycin [various] or clarithromycin [Biaxin].

The following drugs may *decrease* the effects of imatinib:
- barbiturates (see Drug Classes).
- carbamazepine (Tegretol).
- dexamethasone (various).
- fosphenytoin (Cerebyx) or phenytoin (Dilantin) may excessively lower the blood level of imatinib.
- rifampin (various).

▷ *Driving, Hazardous Activities:* Fatigue from this medicine or from the underlying condition may make operating hazardous equipment dangerous. Restrict activities as necessary.

Aviation Note: The use of this drug *is probably a disqualification* for piloting. Consult a designated Aviation Medical Examiner.

Exposure to Heat: Use caution. This drug can cause temperature increases.

Discontinuation: Talk to your doctor before stopping this medicine for any reason.

IMIPRAMINE (im IP ra meen)

Introduced: 1955   **Class:** Antidepressant   **Prescription:**   USA: Yes
Controlled Drug: USA: No; Canada: No   **Available as Generic:**   USA: Yes; Canada: Yes

Brand Names: Antipress, ✤Apo-Imipramine, ✤Impril, Imprin, Janimine, ✤Novo-Pramine, ✤PMS Imipramine, Presamoine, SK-Pramine, Tipramine, Tofranil, Tofranil-PM, W.D.D.

BENEFITS versus RISKS

Possible Benefits	*Possible Risks*
EFFECTIVE RELIEF OF NEUROSES AND PSYCHOTIC DEPRESSION	ADVERSE BEHAVIORAL EFFECTS
EFFECTIVE TREATMENT FOR CHILDHOOD BEDWETTING (enuresis)	CONVERSION OF DEPRESSION TO MANIA in manic-depressive (bipolar) disorders
Helps manage chronic, severe pain	Aggravation of schizophrenia and paranoia
Aids cocaine withdrawal	Induction of serious heart rhythm abnormalities
Relieves symptoms of attention deficit disorder	Abnormally low white blood cell and platelet counts
Helps prevent panic attacks	
Helps control binge eating and purging in bulimia	

▷ **Principal Uses**

As a Single Drug Product: Uses currently included in FDA-approved labeling: (1) Relieves severe emotional depression and initiates gradual restoration of normal mood; (2) helps prevent childhood bedwetting in children over 6 years of age; (3) used to treat delusions.

Other (unlabeled) generally accepted uses: (1) Helps treat agoraphobia; (2) some case evidence of help in treating aspermia; (3) can be of help in chronic pain syndromes; (4) eases diabetic neuropathy; (5) inappropriate emotionalism (such as pathological crying) can be controlled by this drug; (6) of use in globus hystericus; (7) may have a role in treating panic disorder; (8) can help posttraumatic stress disorder; (9) may help control retrograde ejaculation; (10) can be of adjunctive benefit in helping control schizophrenia; (11) shows some benefit in patients who fail ear, nose, or throat surgery or weight reduction as treatment of sleep apnea; (12) may be of help as a second-line agent in attention deficit disorder (ADD).

How This Drug Works: By increasing nerve impulse transmitters (norepinephrine and serotonin), this drug relieves the depression. Beneficial effects in treating bedwetting are thought to be due partially to this drug's atropine-like action.

Available Dosage Forms and Strengths

    Capsules — 75 mg, 100 mg, 125 mg, 150 mg

    Injection — 25 mg/2 ml

    Tablets — 10 mg, 25 mg, 50 mg, 75 mg

▷ **Usual Adult Dosage Ranges**

Depression: Initially 75 mg daily, divided into three doses. Dose may be increased cautiously as needed and tolerated by 10 mg to 25 mg daily at intervals of 1 week. The usual maintenance dose is 50 mg to 150 mg every 24 hours. The total daily dose should not exceed 200 mg for outpatient therapy. (When determined, the optimal daily requirement may be given at bedtime as a single dose.)

Diabetic neuropathy: Same starting doses, with titration as needed and tolerated to 125–350 mg per day. Some clinicians adjust (titrate) doses to a dose that results in a plasma level (checked from a blood test) of 100–200 nmol/L.

Enuresis: Children over 6 are started at 25 mg given an hour before bedtime. If progress does not happen in 7 days, the dose can be increased by 25 mg to total 50 mg at bedtime. Children over 12 may be given 75 mg at bedtime if needed and tolerated.

Note: Actual dose and schedule must be determined for each patient individually.

Conditions Requiring Dosing Adjustments

Liver Function: Used with caution and in decreased dose by patients with liver compromise. It is also a rare cause of hepatic necrosis.

Kidney Function: No changes in dosing are anticipated in kidney compromise.

▷ **Dosing Instructions:** May be taken without regard to meals. If necessary, may be taken with food to reduce stomach irritation. The capsule may be opened, and the tablet may be crushed. Note: Tofranil-PM capsules should not be used to treat childhood bedwetting. If you forget a dose: take it as soon as you remember it, unless it's nearly time for your next dose—if that is the case, skip the missed dose and return to taking the medicine on your usual schedule. If you only take this medicine at bedtime, and you've forgotten your dose, skip the missed dose and take the next dose on schedule at bedtime. DO NOT double doses. Call your doctor for instructions if you miss more than one dose.

Usual Duration of Use: Continual use on a regular schedule for 3 to 4 weeks is usually necessary to determine this drug's effectiveness in relieving depression; optimal response may require 3 or more months of use. Long-term use (months to years) requires periodic evaluation of response and dose adjustment. Benefits in diabetic neuropathy may be seen in one week. Talk to your doctor on a regular basis.

Typical Treatment Goals and Measurements (Outcomes and Markers)

Enuresis: The number of bedwetting episodes as well as the ability to recognize bladder fullness and urinate in the toilet are used as indicators of acceptable results. Continuation of enuresis after 7 days at the same dose will prompt a dose increase.

Possible Advantages of This Drug

Less likely to increase the heart rate than other tricyclic antidepressants.

Currently a "Drug of Choice"

For adjunctive use in treating childhood bedwetting when organic causes for this disorder have been eliminated.

▷ **This Drug Should Not Be Taken If**

- you have had an allergic reaction to it previously.
- you are taking, or have taken within the past 14 days, any monoamine oxidase (MAO) type A inhibitor drug (see Drug Classes).
- you have had a recent heart attack (myocardial infarction).
- you have angina, abnormal heartbeats or congestive heart failure.
- you are pregnant.

▷ **Inform Your Physician Before Taking This Drug If**

- you have had an adverse reaction to any other antidepressant drug.
- you have any type of seizure disorder.
- you have increased internal eye pressure.
- you have narrow-angle glaucoma.
- you have any type of heart disease, especially coronary artery disease or a heart rhythm disorder.
- you are subject to bronchial asthma.
- you have impaired liver or kidney function.
- you have any type of thyroid disorder or are taking thyroid medication.
- you have diabetes or sugar intolerance.
- you have prostatism (see Glossary).
- you have a history of alcoholism.
- you plan to have surgery under general anesthesia in the near future.

Possible Side Effects (natural, expected and unavoidable drug actions)

Moderate drowsiness; abnormally low blood pressure on standing (orthostatic hypotension); light-headedness (low blood pressure); blurred vision; dry mouth (xerostomia)—frequent; constipation; impaired urination; increased appetite; weight gain.

▷ **Possible Adverse Effects** (unusual, unexpected and infrequent reactions)

If any of the following develop, consult your physician promptly for guidance.

Mild Adverse Effects

Allergic reactions: skin rash, hives, swelling of face or tongue, drug fever (see Glossary).

Headache, dizziness, nervousness, weakness, unsteadiness, tremors, fainting—possible to rare.

Sleep disturbances, ringing in the ears—case reports.

Irritation of tongue or mouth, dental cavities, altered taste, indigestion, nausea—possible.

Fluctuations of blood sugar—case reports.

Serious Adverse Effects

Allergic reactions: drug-induced hepatitis, with or without jaundice; anaphylactic reaction (see these terms in Glossary).

Idiosyncratic reactions: neuroleptic malignant syndrome (see Glossary).

Adverse behavioral effects: delirium, delusions, hallucinations, precipitation of Tourette's syndrome—case reports.

Porphyria or abnormal urine excretion (SIADH)—rare.

Liver or kidney toxicity—rare.

Drug-induced myasthenia gravis—case reports.

Seizures, reduced control of epilepsy—possible.

Eye changes (glaucoma, ophthalmoplegia)—case reports.

Heart rhythm disturbances or spasm of blood vessels—case reports.

Abnormally low white blood cell and platelet counts: fever, sore throat, infections, abnormal bleeding or bruising—case reports.

▷ **Possible Effects on Sexual Function:** Decreased libido, increased libido (antidepressant effect)—possible.

Impaired erection or ejaculation—frequent; impotence, inhibited male orgasm—case reports to infrequent; inhibited female orgasm—may be frequent.

Male breast enlargement and tenderness (gynecomastia), female breast enlargement with milk production, swelling of testicles—case reports.

▷ **Adverse Effects That May Mimic Natural Diseases or Disorders**

Liver toxicity may suggest viral hepatitis.

Natural Diseases or Disorders That May Be Activated by This Drug

Latent diabetes, epilepsy, glaucoma, prostatism.

Possible Effects on Laboratory Tests

Complete blood cell counts: decreased white cells and platelets; increased eosinophils (allergic reaction).

Blood glucose levels: increased and decreased (fluctuations).

Liver function tests: increased liver enzymes (ALT/GPT, AST/GOT and alkaline phosphatase), increased bilirubin.

CAUTION

1. Look for early signs of toxicity or overdose: confusion, agitation, rapid heart rate, heart irregularity. Measurement of the drug blood level will clarify the situation.
2. Use with caution in treating depression associated with schizophrenia. Watch for deterioration of thinking or behavior.
3. It is advisable to withhold this drug if electroconvulsive therapy (ECT) is to be used to treat depression.
4. Tolerance to beneficial effects of this medicine may happen after a few weeks or months. Follow-up of continued response and dose adjustments are prudent.

Precautions for Use

By Infants and Children: Safety and effectiveness for use by those under 6 years of age have not been established. Children (6 to 12 years of age) may be more susceptible than adults to heart toxicity from this or related drugs.

Bedwetting (enuresis): Children 6 or older have been given 25 mg by mouth an hour before bedtime. Dose and management should be supervised by a properly trained pediatrician.

By Those Over 60 Years of Age: Treatment is started with 25 mg at bedtime. Dose may be increased gradually as needed and tolerated to 100 mg daily in divided doses. During the first 2 weeks of treatment, observe for behavioral reactions: restlessness, agitation, forgetfulness, disorientation, delusions or hallucinations. Also observe for unsteadiness and instability that may predispose to falling. This drug may aggravate prostatism.

▷ **Advisability of Use During Pregnancy**
Pregnancy Category: D. See Pregnancy Risk Categories at the back of this book.
Animal studies: Skeletal defects reported in rabbit studies. No defects reported in mouse, rat and monkey studies.
Human studies: Information from adequate studies of pregnant women is not available. Case reports of fetal respiratory distress, convulsions.
Ask your doctor for guidance.

Advisability of Use If Breast-Feeding
Presence of this drug in breast milk: Yes, in small amounts.
Monitor nursing infant closely and discontinue drug or nursing if adverse effects develop.

Habit-Forming Potential: Psychological or physical dependence is possible. A withdrawal syndrome has been described.

Effects of Overdose: Confusion, hallucinations, drowsiness, tremors, heart irregularity, seizures, stupor, hypothermia (see Glossary) early, fever later.

Possible Effects of Long-Term Use: Neuroleptic malignant syndrome (see Glossary): fever, fast or irregular heartbeat, fast breathing, sweating, weakness, muscle stiffness, seizures, loss of bladder control—possible.

Suggested Periodic Examinations While Taking This Drug (at physician's discretion)
Monitoring of blood drug levels as appropriate.
Complete blood cell counts.
Liver and kidney function tests.
Serial blood pressure readings and electrocardiograms.
Measurement of internal eye pressure.

▷ **While Taking This Drug, Observe the Following**
Foods: No specific restrictions. May need to limit food intake to avoid excessive weight gain. Vitamin C in large doses (more than 2 g per day) may require higher imipramine doses.
Herbal Medicines or Minerals: Since imipramine and St. John's wort may both act to increase serotonin, the combination is not advised. St. John's wort may also lead to increased sensitivity to the sun—DO NOT COMBINE. Since part of the way ginseng works may be as a MAO inhibitor, do not combine ginseng with imipramine.
Beverages: No restrictions. May be taken with milk.
▷ *Alcohol:* Avoid completely. This drug can markedly increase the intoxicating effects of alcohol; the combination can depress brain function significantly.
Tobacco Smoking: May accelerate the elimination of this drug and require increased dose. I advise everyone to quit.
Marijuana Smoking: Increased drowsiness and mouth dryness; possible reduced effectiveness of this drug. Excessive increases in heart rate.
▷ *Other Drugs*
Imipramine may ***increase*** the effects of
• all drugs with atropinelike effects (see Drug Classes).
• all drugs with sedative effects; observe for excessive sedation.

- amphetaminelike drugs.
- norepinephrine.
- phenytoin (Dilantin) or fosphenytoin (Cerebyx).
- warfarin (Coumadin) and require more frequent INR testing.

Imipramine may *decrease* the effects of
- clonidine (Catapres).
- guanadrel (Hylorel).
- guanethidine (Ismelin, Esimil).
- guanfacine (Tenex).

Imipramine *taken concurrently* with
- anticonvulsants requires careful monitoring for changes in seizure patterns and need to adjust anticonvulsant dose.
- antihistamines (see Drug Classes) may result in urinary retention, acute glaucoma or excessive anticholinergic actions.
- baclofen (Lioresal) may lead to short-term memory loss.
- bepridil (Vascor) may increase risk of abnormal heartbeats.
- cisapride (Propulsid) may increase risk of abnormal heartbeats.
- citalopram (Celexa) may increase risk of abnormal heartbeats.
- dofetilide (Tikosyn) may increase risk of abnormal heartbeats and possibly cardiac arrest.
- ethchlorvynol (Placidyl) may cause delirium; avoid concurrent use.
- gatifloxacin (Tequin) may increase risk of abnormal heartbeats. DO NOT combine.
- meperidine (Demerol) may result in increased meperidine-caused depression of breathing.
- monoamine oxidase (MAO) type A inhibitor drugs (see Drug Classes) may cause high fever, seizures and excessive rise in blood pressure; avoid concurrent use of these drugs and provide periods of 14 days between dosing of either.
- ritonavir (Norvir) and perhaps other protease inhibitors (see Drug Classes) may lead to toxicity.
- sparfloxacin (Zagam) increases risk of abnormal heartbeats.
- stimulant drugs (amphetamine, cocaine, epinephrine, phenylpropanolamine, etc.) may cause severe high blood pressure and/or high fever.
- thyroid preparations may increase the risk of heart rhythm disorders.
- tramadol (Ultram) can increase seizure risk.

The following drugs may *increase* the effects of imipramine:
- cimetidine (Tagamet).
- diltiazem (Cardizem).
- estrogens (various) (birth control pills).
- fluoxetine (Prozac).
- fluvoxamine (Luvox).
- labetalol (Normodyne).
- methylphenidate (Ritalin).
- oral contraceptives.
- phenothiazines (see Drug Classes).
- quinidine (Quinaglute, others).
- ranitidine (Zantac).
- venlafaxine (Effexor) and increases imipramine metabolite.

The following drugs may *decrease* the effects of imipramine:
- barbiturates (see Drug Classes).
- carbamazepine (Tegretol).
- chloral hydrate (Noctec, Somnos, etc.).
- lithium (Lithobid, Lithotab, etc.).
- reserpine (Serpasil, Ser-Ap-Es, etc.).
- vitamin C (if more than 2 g per day are taken).

▷ *Driving, Hazardous Activities:* This drug may impair mental alertness, judgment, physical coordination and reaction time. Restrict activities as necessary.

Aviation Note: The use of this drug *is a disqualification* for piloting. Consult a designated Aviation Medical Examiner.

Exposure to Sun: Use caution until sensitivity has been determined. This drug may cause photosensitivity (see Glossary). See "Herbal Medicines" warning on St. John's wort above.

Exposure to Heat: Use caution. This drug can inhibit sweating and impair the body's adaptation to hot environments, increasing the risk of heatstroke. Avoid saunas.

Exposure to Cold: The elderly should use caution and avoid conditions conducive to hypothermia (see Glossary).

Exposure to Environmental Chemicals: This drug may mask the symptoms of poisoning due to handling certain insecticides (organophosphorus types). Read their labels carefully.

Discontinuation: It is advisable to discontinue this drug gradually over a period of 3 to 4 weeks. Abrupt withdrawal after prolonged use may cause nausea, vomiting, diarrhea, headache, malaise, disturbed sleep and vivid dreaming. When this drug is stopped, it may be necessary to adjust the doses of other drugs taken concurrently.

INDAPAMIDE (in DAP a mide)

Introduced: 1974   **Class:** Antihypertensive, diuretic   **Prescription:** USA: Yes   **Controlled Drug:** USA: No; Canada: No   **Available as Generic:** Yes
Brand Names: ✤Lozide, Lozol

BENEFITS versus RISKS	
Possible Benefits	*Possible Risks*
EFFECTIVE ONCE-A-DAY TREATMENT OF MILD TO MODERATE HYPERTENSION EFFECTIVE, MILD DIURETIC COMBINATION USE WITH AN ACE INHIBITOR (PERINDOPRIL OR ACEON) REDUCED RISK OF RECURRENT STROKE BY NEARLY HALF IN ONE STUDY	Excessive loss of blood potassium or magnesium Increased blood sugar level Increased blood uric acid level

▷ **Principal Uses**
As a Single Drug Product: Uses currently included in FDA-approved labeling:
(1) Increases urine output (diuresis) to correct fluid retention seen in con-

gestive heart failure (edema); (2) used as starting therapy in high blood pressure (hypertension).

Other (unlabeled) generally accepted uses: (1) Helps ease the excessive elimination of calcium in the urine (hypercalciuria); (2) may help protect the heart after blood-flow problems (preserves ischemic heart from reperfusion injury); combination use with perindopril (Aceon) reduced risk of repeat stroke by nearly 50% in one study.

How This Drug Works: Increases elimination of salt and water (through increased urine production). Relaxes the walls of smaller arteries and decreases pressure reactions (calcium channel action). The combined effects lower blood pressure.

Available Dosage Forms and Strengths
Tablets — 1.25 mg, 2.5 mg

▷ **Usual Adult Dosage Ranges:** *Hypertension:* 1.25 mg per day, as a single dose in the morning. If needed, the dose may be increased to 2.5 mg/day after 4 weeks. Use in treating edema may require a starting dose of 2.5 mg. Maximum total daily dose is 5 mg. (In Canada, the total daily dose limit is given as 2.5 mg.) **Note: Actual dose and dosing schedule must be determined for each individual patient.**

Conditions Requiring Dosing Adjustments
Liver Function: Should be used with caution and in decreased doses by patients with liver problems. Blood chemistry (electrolytes) should be closely followed.
Kidney Function: Must be stopped if kidney failure progresses after indapamide is started.

▷ **Dosing Instructions:** The tablet may be crushed and taken with or following food to reduce stomach upset. Take in the morning to avoid nighttime urination. If you forget a dose: take it as soon as you remember it, unless it's nearly time for your next dose—if that is the case, skip the missed dose and return to taking the medicine on your usual schedule. DO NOT double doses. Call your doctor for instructions if you miss more than one dose.

Usual Duration of Use: Use on a regular schedule for 2 to 4 weeks determines peak effect in lowering blood pressure. Long-term use (months to years) requires periodic physician evaluation.

Typical Treatment Goals and Measurements (Outcomes and Markers)
Blood pressure: The most recent treatment guidelines (JNC VI) actually define optimal blood pressure (BP) as less than 120/80 and high normal as 139/89. The American Diabetes Association has chosen a target of 130/80 as the blood pressure goal for people living with diabetes. Most clinicians try to achieve a BP that achieves the best balance of lower cardiovascular risk while avoiding the problem of too low a blood pressure. The goal and time frame (see peak effect above) should be discussed with you when the prescription is written.

Possible Advantages of This Drug
Causes no significant increase in blood cholesterol levels. Less likely to cause significant loss of potassium. Increased good cholesterol (HDL). ONCE-DAILY DOSING will encourage people to take this medicine regularly.

▷ **This Drug Should Not Be Taken If**
  • you have had an allergic reaction to it previously.
  • your kidneys are not making any urine.

▷ **Inform Your Physician Before Taking This Drug If**
  • you are allergic to any form of "sulfa" drug.
  • you are pregnant or planning pregnancy.
  • you presently have an excessively low blood potassium.
  • you have a history of kidney or liver disease.
  • you have diabetes, gout or systemic lupus erythematosus.
  • you take any form of cortisone, digoxin, oral antidiabetic drug or insulin.
  • you have had a sympathectomy.
  • you plan to have surgery under general anesthesia in the near future.

Possible Side Effects (natural, expected and unavoidable drug actions)
  Light-headedness on arising from sitting or lying position (see orthostatic hypotension in Glossary). Increase in blood sugar level, affecting control of diabetes. Increase in blood uric acid level, affecting control of gout. Decrease in blood potassium level, causing muscle weakness and cramping. Low blood sodium and magnesium.

▷ **Possible Adverse Effects** (unusual, unexpected and infrequent reactions)
  If any of the following develop, consult your physician promptly for guidance.
  Mild Adverse Effects
  Allergic reactions: skin rashes, hives, itching—infrequent.
  Headache, dizziness, drowsiness, weakness, lethargy, visual disturbance—case reports.
  Reduced appetite, indigestion, nausea, vomiting, diarrhea—rare.
  Paresthesias—rare.
  Urination at night—possible, especially with evening dosing.
  Serious Adverse Effects
  Abnormal heartbeat (premature ventricular contractions)—rare.
  Liver or kidney toxicity—rare.
  Serious skin rashes (Stevens-Johnson syndrome, toxic epidermal necrolysis)—case reports.
  Inhibition of platelet aggregation—possible.

▷ **Possible Effects on Sexual Function:** Decreased libido—infrequent; impotence—rare.

Natural Diseases or Disorders That May Be Activated by This Drug
  Diabetes, gout, systemic lupus erythematosus.

Possible Effects on Laboratory Tests
  Total cholesterol and LDL cholesterol levels: no effect or slightly decreased.
  Blood HDL cholesterol level: increased.
  Blood potassium, magnesium or sodium level: decreased.
  Blood uric acid level or blood sugar (glucose): increased.

CAUTION
  1. Take exactly as prescribed—excessive doses can cause excessive sodium and potassium loss (decreased appetite, nausea, fatigue, confusion or tingling extremities).
  2. If you take a digitalis preparation (digitoxin, digoxin), ensure intake of

high-potassium foods to help avoid digitalis toxicity (see Table 13, "High-Potassium Foods").

Precautions for Use

By Infants and Children: Safety and effectiveness for those under 12 years of age are not established.

By Those Over 60 Years of Age: It is best to start with small doses. You may be more susceptible to impaired thinking, orthostatic hypotension, potassium loss and blood sugar increase. Overdose or extended use causes excessive loss of body water, thickening (increased viscosity) of blood and an increased tendency for the blood to clot—predisposing to stroke, heart attack or thrombophlebitis (vein inflammation with blood clot).

▷ Advisability of Use During Pregnancy

Pregnancy Category: B. D by one researcher. See Pregnancy Risk Categories at the back of this book.

Animal studies: No birth defects reported.

Human studies: Data from studies of pregnant women are not available.

This drug should not be used during pregnancy unless a very serious complication occurs for which this drug is significantly beneficial. Ask your physician for guidance.

Advisability of Use If Breast-Feeding

Presence of this drug in breast milk: Unknown.

Avoid drug or refrain from nursing.

Habit-Forming Potential: None.

Effects of Overdose:
Dry mouth, thirst, lethargy, weakness, muscle cramping, nausea, vomiting, drowsiness progressing to stupor or coma.

Possible Effects of Long-Term Use:
Impaired balance of water, salt and potassium in blood and body tissues. Development of diabetes in predisposed individuals.

Suggested Periodic Examinations While Taking This Drug (at physician's discretion)

Measurements of blood levels of sodium, potassium, chloride, sugar and uric acid.

▷ While Taking This Drug, Observe the Following

Foods: Ask your doctor about a high-potassium diet. If so advised, see Table 13, "High-Potassium Foods," in Section Six. Follow your doctor's advice about salt use.

Herbal Medicines or Minerals: Ginseng may increase blood pressure, blunting the benefits of these medicines. Hawthorn, saw palmetto, ma huang, goldenseal, yohimbe and licorice may also increase blood pressure. Calcium and garlic may help lower blood pressure. Indian snakeroot has a German Commission E monograph indication for hypertension—talk to your doctor. Eleuthero root and ephedra should be avoided by people living with hypertension.

Beverages: No restrictions. This drug may be taken with milk.

▷ *Alcohol:* Alcohol may exaggerate the blood-pressure-lowering effects of this drug and cause orthostatic hypotension.

Tobacco Smoking: No interactions expected. I advise everyone to quit smoking.

▷ *Other Drugs*

Indapamide may *increase* the effects of
- ACE inhibitors (see Drug Classes) and cause SEVERE lowering of blood pressure on standing (postural hypotension).
- other antihypertensive drugs; dose adjustments may be necessary to prevent excessive lowering of blood pressure.
- lithium (Lithobid, others) and cause lithium toxicity.

Indapamide may *decrease* the effects of
- oral antidiabetic drugs (sulfonylureas); dose adjustments may be needed for proper control of blood sugar.

Indapamide *taken concurrently* with
- digitalis preparations (digitoxin, digoxin) must be followed closely and adjustments made to prevent fluctuations of blood potassium levels and serious disturbances of heart rhythm.
- NSAIDs (see Drug Classes) may blunt the therapeutic benefit of indapamide.

The following drugs may *decrease* the effects of indapamide:
- cholestyramine (Cuemid, Questran)—may interfere with its absorption.
- colestipol (Colestid)—may interfere with its absorption.

Take cholestyramine and colestipol 1 hour before any oral diuretic.

▷ *Driving, Hazardous Activities:* Use caution until the possible occurrence of orthostatic hypotension, drowsiness, dizziness or impaired vision has been determined.

Aviation Note: The use of this drug *may be a disqualification* for piloting. Consult a designated Aviation Medical Examiner.

Exposure to Sun: No restrictions.

Exposure to Heat: Excessive perspiring could cause additional loss of salt and water.

Heavy Exercise or Exertion: Isometric exercises can raise blood pressure significantly. Ask your physician for help.

Occurrence of Unrelated Illness: Vomiting or diarrhea can produce a serious imbalance of important body chemistry. Consult your physician for guidance.

Discontinuation: It may be advisable to discontinue this drug 5 to 7 days before major surgery. Ask your physician, surgeon and/or anesthesiologist for guidance.

INDOMETHACIN (in doh METH a sin)

Please see the acetic acid (nonsteroidal anti-inflammatory drug) family profile.

INFLIXIMAB (IN FLIX ih mab)

Other Names: Anti-TNF monoclonal antibody, chimeric monoclonal antibody to TNF alpha, cA2

Introduced: 1998 (Crohn's, 1999 rheumatoid arthritis combination approval)

Class: Disease-modifying antirheumatic drug (DMARD), biologic response

modifier   **Prescription:** USA: Yes   **Controlled Drug:** USA: No; Canada:
No   **Available as Generic:** No
Brand Name: Remicade

BENEFITS versus RISKS	
Possible Benefits	*Possible Risks*
GIVEN ORPHAN PRODUCT DESIGNATION FOR USE IN CROHN'S DISEASE	POSSIBLE LOWERED RESISTANCE TO INFECTIONS AND OPPORTUNISTIC INFECTIONS
EASES RHEUMATOID ARTHRITIS (RA) IN COMBINATION WITH METHOTREXATE	Injection site reactions
MAY GIVE A RESPONSE IN RA WHERE OTHER AGENTS HAVE FAILED	Possible development of antibodies
COULD HAVE A ROLE IN CONGESTIVE HEART FAILURE AND IN DECREASING RISK OF REPEAT HEART ATTACKS	

▷ **Principal Uses**

> *As a Single Drug Product:* Uses currently included in FDA-approved labeling: (1) Treatment of moderately to severely active Crohn's disease or fistulizing Crohn's disease; (2) Use in combination with methotrexate in rheumatoid arthritis (RA) patients to lower signs and symptoms when patients have not responded to methotrexate alone.

> Other (unlabeled) generally accepted uses: (1) May have a role in some kinds of wasting (cachexia) where tumor necrosis factor (TNF) is involved; (2) data from the cholesterol and recurrent events (CARE) trial found that decreasing tumor necrosis factor (TNF) (see "How This Drug Works," below) reduces risk of repeat heart attacks; (3) may ease congestive heart failure.

How This Drug Works: Binds with both soluble and transmembrane tumor necrosis factor alpha (TNF-alpha) in the body. Inhibits binding of existing TNF alpha to p55 and p75 receptors. Both effects act to stop the biologic actions of TNF alpha. Works to change the body's responses that are caused or regulated by TNF, such as increased levels of matrix metalloproteinase-3, serum levels of cytokines and release of substances that control white blood cell migration.

Author's Note: The company that makes this product has added a more stringent (black box) warning about opportunistic infections to the product label. The FDA will review this medicine and etanercept (Enbrel) in late August 2001. Information in this profile may be broadened in subsequent editions if warranted.

INFLUENZA VACCINE (IN flu en za VAX ceen)

Other Name: Flu vaccine
Introduced: Specific formulation for each year   **Class:** Antiviral   **Prescription:** USA: Yes   **Controlled Drug:** USA: No; Canada: No   **Available as Generic:** USA: No; Canada: No

Brand Names: Flu-Immune, FluMist (investigational), Fluoge, Flu-Shield, Fluzone

Author's Note: For the 2001–2002 flu season the shot (vaccine) will have three strains: A/Moscow/10/99-like (H3N2), A/New Caledonia/20/99-like (H1N1) and B/Sichuan/379/99-like. US makers of flu vaccines will use the antigenically equivalent A/Panama/2007/99 (H3N2) virus for the Moscow strain and B/Johannesburg/05/99, B/Victoria/504/2000 or Bguangdong/120/2000. Like last year, the Advisory Committee suggests that people ages 50–64 get a flu shot. From 20,000 to 40,000 people die from the flu each year. Don't become a statistic. Unfortunately, for this influenza season, vaccines could still be in somewhat shorter supply—though not as limited or delayed as last year when some high-risk people had to be prioritized by the CDC. If you would like a copy of the ACIP recommendations, call 1-888-232-3228.

Warning: Since the vaccine is formulated to contain the viral strains expected to cause the most serious problems in a given year, the side effects or adverse effects may differ each year.

BENEFITS versus RISKS	
Possible Benefits	*Possible Risks*
PREVENTION OF INFLUENZA CAUSED BY THE MOST SERIOUS OR PREVALENT VIRAL STRAINS IDENTIFIED FOR A GIVEN YEAR	GUILLAIN-BARRÉ SYNDROME (questionable causation) Hypersensitivity
FLUMIST FORM AVOIDS INJECTION AND IS A NASAL SPRAY	
Possible cross-protection from other similar virus strains	

▷ **Principal Uses**

As a Single Drug Product: Uses currently included in FDA-approved labeling: Prevention of influenza.

Other (unlabeled) generally accepted uses: (1) Used in patients with compromised immune systems (such as HIV-positive, cancer and bone marrow transplant patients); (2) can be of use in isolated outbreaks such as in nursing homes or military camps; (3) may decrease the number of middle ear infections in children who attend day-care centers.

How This Drug Works: Vaccine made of purified parts of the virus surface, split virus or whole virus, which has been inactivated. When injected, it stimulates the immune system to make antibodies. The antibodies (2 weeks after vaccination) act to reduce disease severity or decrease probability of infection by the expected flu viruses.

Available Dosage Forms and Strengths

Typical split virus: 15 mcg/0.5 ml of each of the three selected strains.

▷ **Recommended Dosage Ranges** (Actual dose and schedule must be determined for each patient and each flu season individually.)

Infants and Children: Those 6 to 35 months old should be given 0.25 ml of a split-dose vaccine. If this is the first vaccination, two doses should be given

1 month apart. Split dose is suggested for children because it tends to cause fewer undesirable effects. For infants and young children, the vaccine is usually given in the thigh muscle.

Children 3 to 8 years old should be given 0.5 ml of the selected split-virus vaccine. Children in this age range who have not been previously vaccinated should be given two vaccinations, 1 month apart.

Children 9 years old or older should be given a single vaccination of 0.5 ml of split-virus vaccine in the deltoid muscle.

13 to 60 Years of Age: Should be given 0.5 ml of whole or split-virus vaccine in the deltoid muscle.

Over 60 Years of Age: Same as 13 to 60 years of age.

Conditions Requiring Dosing Adjustments

Liver Function: Not involved.

Kidney Function: Not involved.

▷ **Dosing Instructions:** Prior vaccination **does not** mean you are immune to the current year's virus strains. Some tenderness at the injection site is possible. Fever and muscular aches or pains are also possible and may be treated with acetaminophen (Tylenol, others). If you forget to get the shot: timing of vaccination (enough time to let your body build up immunity) before the flu season is important. If you get the flu because you did NOT get vaccinated, a neuramidase inhibitor (see drug profile) may be an option for you. Talk to your doctor.

Usual Duration of Use: Single vaccination confers relative immunity to the expected viral strains in 2 weeks. This does not confer immunity to all strains of virus capable of causing an influenzalike (flu-like) syndrome. Annual vaccination is strongly suggested.

Typical Treatment Goals and Measurements (Outcomes and Markers)

Influenza: Prevention of a serious viral illness. In a typical season some 20,000 Americans die from influenza. Years with virulent strains can see 40,000 people lose their lives. This vaccination can avoid illness, hospitalization and death.

Possible Advantages of This Drug

Allows the prevention of a viral syndrome that can cause loss of several weeks of work in younger, otherwise healthy patients or serious illness in older or compromised patients. Once FluMist form is available, a nasal spray will replace an injection.

Currently a Drug of Choice

For prevention of type A and B influenza due to the viral strains that are of the greatest concern in the current flu season.

▷ **This Drug Should Not Be Taken If**
- you have had an allergic reaction to any dose form of it previously.
- you are allergic to eggs (the virus is grown on eggs).
- you have an acute illness and a fever.

▷ **Inform Your Physician Before Taking This Drug If**
- you are HIV positive.
- you have a history of blood disorders.
- you have had Guillain-Barré syndrome.
- you have a history of seizures.
- you have been receiving cancer therapy (chemotherapy).

Possible Side Effects (natural, expected and unavoidable drug actions)

Pain at the vaccination site. Muscle aches, fever or bothersome tiredness (malaise). This is **not** the flu. The vaccine contains viral fragments or non-infectious virus. These symptoms are a reaction to the components of the vaccine.

▷ **Possible Adverse Effects** (unusual, unexpected and infrequent reactions)

If any of the following develop, consult your physician promptly for guidance.

Mild Adverse Effects

Allergic reactions: swelling and redness—possible.

Muscle aches or fever—infrequent.

Fatigue, nausea and headache—infrequent.

Vasculitis (joint pain, weakness, fever and rash)—rare.

Serious Adverse Effects

Allergic reactions: anaphylactic reactions.

Low blood platelets or pericarditis—case reports.

Guillain-Barré syndrome (only reported during the 1976–1977 flu season and of questionable causation).

Kidney toxicity—case report.

Vision changes—case report.

▷ **Possible Effects on Sexual Function:** None reported.

Possible Delayed Adverse Effects: None reported.

▷ **Adverse Effects That May Mimic Natural Diseases or Disorders**

Reaction to vaccine contents may mimic the flu.

Natural Diseases or Disorders That May Be Activated by This Drug

None reported.

Possible Effects on Laboratory Tests

Hepatitis B test: false positive.

Hepatitis C test: false positive.

HTLV-1 test: false positive.

CAUTION

1. A vaccine in the previous year **does not** confer immunity to the flu in following years.
2. The flu vaccine confers immunity to viruses predicted to cause influenza in a particular flu season. Vaccine does not confer immunity to all strains of virus capable of causing a flu-like syndrome.
3. If muscle aches or fever occur after vaccination, acetaminophen (Tylenol, others) is recommended. **Do not** take aspirin, and especially do not give aspirin to children. It may be prudent to take acetaminophen BEFORE vaccination to prevent such reactions.
4. Call your doctor immediately if you develop hives, facial swelling or difficulty breathing after the vaccination.
5. It is ALWAYS better to prevent a disease or condition than to have to treat it. Additionally, **when the Type-A flu is prevalent, some 20,000 people usually die** from the flu or its complications in that particular flu season. Talk with your doctor or pharmacist. If you do not have a medical reason for avoiding flu vaccination—get the shot! In many states, your pharmacist can actually give you a flu shot.

Precautions for Use

By Infants and Children: Safety and effectiveness for use by those under 6 months of age have not been established.

By Those Over 60 Years of Age: The vaccine is especially **valuable** in this age group, as the effects of the flu may be devastating.

▷ **Advisability of Use During Pregnancy**

Pregnancy Category: C. See Pregnancy Risk Categories at the back of this book.

Animal studies: Animal studies have not been conducted.

Human studies: Information from adequate studies of pregnant women is not available.

Ask your doctor for guidance.

Advisability of Use If Breast-Feeding

Presence of this drug in breast milk: Not defined.

Monitor nursing infant closely and contact your doctor if adverse effects develop. The CDC has not listed breast-feeding as a precaution against receiving this vaccine.

Habit-Forming Potential: None.

Effects of Overdose: No specific cases reported. Treatment would be consistent with any symptoms of the patient.

Possible Effects of Long-Term Use: Not indicated for long-term use.

Suggested Periodic Examinations While Taking This Drug (at physician's discretion)

None indicated.

▷ **While Taking This Drug, Observe the Following**

Foods: No restrictions.

Herbal Medicines or Minerals: Some patients use echinacea to attempt to boost their immune systems. Unfortunately, use of echinacea is not recommended in people with damaged immune systems. This herb may also actually weaken any immune system if it is used too often or for too long a time.

Beverages: No restrictions.

▷ *Alcohol:* No restrictions.

Tobacco Smoking: No interactions expected. I advise everyone to quit smoking.

▷ *Other Drugs*

Influenza vaccine may *increase* the effects of

- carbamazepine (Tegretol), by decreasing the elimination of the drug.
- phenobarbital, by increasing the half-life of the drug.
- theophylline (Theo-Dur, others), by increasing the blood level of the drug.
- warfarin (Coumadin) and pose an increased risk of bleeding; more frequent INR (prothrombin time or protime) testing is suggested.

Influenza vaccine *taken concurrently* with

- cyclosporine (Sandimmune) can cause blunting of the immune response to the vaccine.
- immunosuppressive agents (chemotherapy, corticosteroids) may impair or blunt immune response to the vaccine.
- methotrexate (Rheumatrex) can result in blunting of the immune response to this vaccine.

- neuramidase inhibitors (see Drug Classes) has not been found to cause differences in hemagglutination inhibition antibody levels (titers).
- phenytoin (Dilantin) and fosphenytoin (Cerebyx) has had variable effects on the blood levels of this drug.

▷ *Driving, Hazardous Activities:* This drug may cause excessive tiredness and muscle aches. Restrict activities as necessary.

Aviation Note: The use of this drug *may be a short-term disqualification* for piloting. Consult a designated Aviation Medical Examiner.

Exposure to Sun: No restrictions.

Exposure to Heat: Since this vaccine may cause short-duration fevers, it is wise to avoid hot environments for a day after vaccination.

Heavy Exercise or Exertion: A fever may result, and it is wise to avoid strenuous exercise for a day after vaccination.

Special Storage Instructions: This vaccine is ideally stored in the refrigerator. If this is how storage is accomplished, the outdate specified by the manufacturer is valid. If the vaccine is stored at room temperature, it is stable for up to 7 days.

Observe the Following Expiration Times: If the vaccine is stored at room temperature, it is stable for up to 7 days.

Author's Note: There is a Vaccine Adverse Event Reporting System (VAERS). The toll-free number is 1-800-822-7967.

INSULIN (IN suh lin)

Introduced: 1922, insulin lispro 1996, insulin glargine 2000   **Class:** Antidiabetic   **Prescription:** USA: No   **Controlled Drug:** USA: No; Canada: No   **Available as Generic:** Yes

Brand Names: Humalog, Humalog Mix 75/25, Humulin BR, Humulin L, Humulin N, Humulin R, Humulin 70/30, Humulin 30/70, Humulin U, Humulin U Ultralente, Iletin I NPH, Iletin II Pork, Iletin U—40, Iletin U—500, ✦Initard, Insulatard NPH, ✦Insulin Human, ✦Insulin-Toronto, Lantus (insulin glargine), Lente Iletin I, Lente Iletin II Beef, Lente Iletin II Pork, Lente Insulin, Lente Purified Pork, Mixtard, Mixtard Human 70/30, NovoLog, Novolin L, ✦Novolin-Lente, Novolin N, ✦Novolin-NPH, NovolinPen, Novolin R, ✦Novolinset, ✦Novolinset NPH, ✦Novolinset 30/70, ✦Novolinset Toronto, Novolin—70/30, Novolin 70/30, Novolin 70/30 Penfill, Novolin 30/70, ✦Novolin-Toronto, ✦Novolin-Ultralente, NPH Iletin I, NPH Iletin II Beef, NPH Iletin II Pork, NPH Insulin, NPH Purified Pork, Protamine, Zinc & Iletin I, Protamine, Zinc & Iletin II Beef, Protamine, Zinc & Iletin II Pork, Regular Concentrated Iletin II, Regular Iletin I, Regular Iletin II Beef, Regular Iletin II Pork, Regular Iletin II U—500, Regular Insulin, Regular Purified Pork Insulin, Semilente Iletin I, Semilente Insulin, Semilente Purified Pork, Ultralente Iletin I, Ultralente Insulin, Ultralente Purified Beef, Velosulin, ✦Velosulin Cartridge, Velosulin Human

```
┌────────────────────────────────────────────────────────────────┐
│                     BENEFITS versus RISKS                        │
│        Possible Benefits              Possible Risks             │
│  EFFECTIVE CONTROL OF TYPE 1    HYPOGLYCEMIA WITH EXCESSIVE       │
│     (INSULIN-DEPENDENT)            DOSE                           │
│     DIABETES MELLITUS           Infrequent allergic reactions    │
│  EFFECTIVE COMBINATION OF       Lipodystrophy                    │
│     TYPE 2 DIABETES THAT DOES                                    │
│     NOT RESPOND (MEET BLOOD                                      │
│     SUGAR GOALS) TO DIET AND                                     │
│     ORAL HYPOGLYCEMIC AGENT                                      │
│     ALONE                                                        │
│  EFFECTIVE CONTROL OF A TYPE                                     │
│     OF BLOOD SUGAR PROBLEM                                       │
│     (GESTATIONAL DIABETES) THAT                                  │
│     HAPPENS IN PREGNANCY                                         │
│  TIGHT CONTROL OF BLOOD                                          │
│     SUGAR MAY AVOID OR DELAY                                     │
│     DEVELOPMENT OF HIGH                                          │
│     BLOOD PRESSURE AND KIDNEY,                                   │
│     HEART, NERVE, EYE OR OTHER                                   │
│     DAMAGE THAT HAPPENS WHEN                                     │
│     BLOOD SUGAR IS OUT OF                                        │
│     CONTROL                                                      │
│  ONCE-DAILY DOSING (Lantus                                      │
│     form—insulin glargine only)                                 │
└────────────────────────────────────────────────────────────────┘
```

▷ **Principal Uses**

    As a Single Drug Product: Uses currently included in FDA-approved labeling: (1) Used in diabetes mellitus that is insulin-dependent and by people who have non-insulin-dependent diabetes who are experiencing stress such as illness or who do not meet blood sugar goals; (2) used to control blood sugar in critically ill patients who are being fed by intravenous nutrient mixtures; (3) used to control blood sugar in pregnancy (gestational diabetes).

    Other (unlabeled) generally accepted uses: (1) Insulin in combination with glucagon has been used in alcoholic hepatitis; (2) may have a role in combination therapy with an oral hypoglycemic agent in some diabetics; (3) helps diabetic ketoacidosis; (4) can help diabetic neuropathy and retinopathy; (5) can be of help in critically ill patients with maple syrup urine disease; (6) used in implantable pumps to control blood sugar; (7) intensive therapy (more than 3 injections daily) may decrease risk of small blood vessel disease, retinopathy and kidney problems (nephropathy); (8) one study used a combination of insulin and sugar (glucose) intravenously after a heart attack and found that death decreased by 30% in the following year.

How This Drug Works: Insulin helps sugar get through the cell wall to the inside of the cell (action on cell membranes), where it is used for energy.

Available Dosage Forms and Strengths

        Injections — 40, 100 and 500 units per ml

    Penfill cartridges — 100 units per ml

▷ **Usual Adult Dosage Ranges:** According to individual requirements for the best regulation of blood sugar on a 24-hour basis. **Note: Actual dose and schedule must be determined for each patient individually.**

Conditions Requiring Dosing Adjustments

Liver Function: Specific adjustment guidelines are not available.

Kidney Function: Caution should be used by patients with compromised kidneys. Requirements become extremely variable.

Thyrotoxicosis: Glucose utilization is typically increased, and insulin requirements may actually decrease.

▷ **Dosing Instructions:** Inject insulin subcutaneously according to the schedule prescribed by your physician. The timing and frequency of injections will vary with the type of insulin prescribed. The following table of insulin actions (according to type) will help you understand the treatment schedule prescribed for you. If you forget a dose: Please call your doctor. It is critical that this medicine be taken exactly as prescribed.

Insulin Type	Action Onset	Peak	Duration
Insulin glargine	1.0 hr	none	24 hrs
Insulin lispro	0.25 hr	0.5–1.5 hrs	3–4 hrs
Regular	0.5–1 hr	2–4 hrs	5–7 hrs
Isophane (NPH)	3–4 hrs	6–12 hrs	18–28 hrs
Regular 30%/NPH 70%	0.5 hr	4–8 hrs	24 hrs
Semilente	1–3 hrs	2–8 hrs	12–16 hrs
Lente	1–3 hrs	8–12 hrs	18–28 hrs
Ultralente	4–6 hrs	18–24 hrs	36 hrs
Protamine Zinc	4–6 hrs	14–24 hrs	36 hrs

Usual Duration of Use: In Type 1 insulin-dependent (juvenile-onset) diabetes mellitus, insulin therapy is usually required for life. Type 2 non-insulin-dependent (maturity-onset) diabetes may be controlled by oral antidiabetic drugs and/or diet, but can require insulin when you have a serious infection, injuries, burns, surgical procedures and other physical stress. See your doctor on a regular basis.

Typical Treatment Goals and Measurements (Outcomes and Markers)

Blood sugar: The general goal for blood sugar is to return it to the usual "normal" range (generally 80–120 mg/dl), while avoiding risks of excessively low blood sugar. One study (UKPDS) used a fasting plasma sugar (glucose) of less than 108 mg/dl.

Fructosamine and glycosylated hemoglobin: Fructosamine levels (a measure of the past two to three weeks of blood sugar control) should be less than or equal to 310 micromoles per liter. Glycosylated hemoglobin or hemoglobin A1C (a measure of the past 2–3 months of blood sugar control) should be less than or equal to 7.0%.

Possible Advantages of This Drug: Allows tight control of blood sugar that can help avoid microvascular, visual, kidney and cardiovascular effects of diabetes. The insulin lispro provides extremely rapid onset, which may be more forgiving in the sense of timing of the shot itself (goes to work faster) as well as offering a more physiologic response to blood sugar. The new insulin glargine actually does NOT have a peak effect. The kinetics of that formulation offer a great advantage in providing a relatively constant (baseline) insulin level. Some prescribers use Lantus as a baseline insulin and Humalog with meals—avoiding use of a pump in some patients. An experimental form of insulin sprayed into the mouth (Oralin) is now in phase three studies.

▷ **This Drug Should Not Be Taken If**
- the need for insulin and its dose schedule have not been established by a qualified clinician.
- you are hypoglycemic.

▷ **Inform Your Physician Before Taking This Drug If**
- you have an insulin allergy.
- you do not know how to recognize and treat abnormally low blood sugar (see Hypoglycemia in Glossary).
- you are pregnant.
- you take aspirin, beta-blockers, fenfluramine (Pondimin) or monoamine oxidase (MAO) type A inhibitors (see Drug Classes).

Possible Side Effects (natural, expected and unavoidable drug actions)
In stable diabetes, no side effects occur when insulin dose, diet and physical activity are correctly balanced and maintained. In unstable ("brittle") diabetes, unexpected drops in blood sugar levels can occur, resulting in hypoglycemia (see Glossary). Weight gain.

▷ **Possible Adverse Effects** (unusual, unexpected and infrequent reactions)
If any of the following develop, consult your physician promptly for guidance.
Mild Adverse Effects
Allergic reactions: local redness, swelling and itching at site of injection or hives—infrequent.
Taste disorders—possible.
Thinning of subcutaneous tissue at sites of injection (lipodystrophy)—infrequent.
Serious Adverse Effects
Allergic reaction: anaphylactic reactions (see Glossary).
Severe, prolonged hypoglycemia—possible to infrequent.
Inflammation of the parotid (parotitis)—case reports.
Hemolytic anemia or porphyria—case reports.
Arrhythmias (associated with hypoglycemia) or very fast heart rate (with intravenous use)—case reports.
Insulin resistance—possible to rare.

▷ **Possible Effects on Sexual Function:** May resolve sexual problems (dysfunction) in patients who have this prior to starting insulin therapy. May also cause decrease in libido and erectile dysfunction—case reports (may also be a result of nerve/blood vessel damage as part of diabetes progressive effect).

▷ **Adverse Effects That May Mimic Natural Diseases or Disorders**
The early signs of hypoglycemia may be mistaken for alcoholic intoxication.

Possible Effects on Laboratory Tests
Blood cholesterol level: decreased.
Blood glucose level: decreased.
Blood potassium level: decreased.
Glycosylated hemoglobin (hemoglobin A1-C) or fructosamine: decreased.

CAUTION
1. Carry a card in your purse or wallet saying that you have diabetes and are taking insulin.
2. Know how to recognize hypoglycemia and how to treat it. Always carry a readily available form of sugar, such as hard candy or sugar cubes. Report all episodes of hypoglycemia to your doctor.
3. Your vision may improve during the first few weeks of insulin therapy. Postpone eye exams for eyeglasses for 6 weeks after starting insulin.
4. Insulin is absorbed more quickly or slowly depending on where it is injected. Absorption is 80% greater from the abdominal wall than from the leg and 30% greater than from the arm. It is advisable to rotate the injection site within the same body region than from one site to another.
5. Insulin glargine is CLEAR, not cloudy. This may be confusing to some patients because in the past, diabetics have been taught that short-acting insulins are clear and long acting insulins are cloudy. Lantus form should NOT be mixed with other insulins.
6. The American Diabetic Association (ADA) now says that a person is considered diabetic if two fasting blood sugars in a row are more than 125 mg/dl. This more conservative approach reflects new information saying that complications start at lower blood sugar levels than previously thought.

Precautions for Use
By Infants and Children: Insulin doses and schedules are modified according to patient's size. Adhere strictly to the physician's prescribed routine.
By Those Over 60 Years of Age: Insulin needs may change with age. Periodic individual evaluation is needed to identify the best dose and schedule. The aging brain adapts well to higher blood sugar levels. Rigid attempts at "tight" sugar control may result in hypoglycemia that shows as confusion and abnormal behavior. Repeated hypoglycemia (especially if severe) may cause brain damage.

▷ **Advisability of Use During Pregnancy**
Pregnancy Category: B. See Pregnancy Risk Categories at the back of this book.
Animal studies: Inconclusive.
Human studies: Adequate studies of pregnant women are not available. Birth defects occur two to four times more frequently in infants of diabetic mothers than in infants of mothers who do not have diabetes. The exact causes of this are not known.
Insulin is the drug of choice for managing diabetes during pregnancy. To preserve the health of the mother and fetus, every effort must be made to establish the best dose of insulin necessary for "good control" and to prevent episodes of hypoglycemia.

Advisability of Use If Breast-Feeding
Presence of this drug in breast milk: No.
Insulin treatment of the mother has no adverse effect on the nursing infant. Breast-feeding may decrease insulin requirements; dose adjustment may be necessary.

Habit-Forming Potential: None, but cases of surreptitious insulin injection have been reported.

Effects of Overdose: Hypoglycemia: fatigue, weakness, headache, nervousness, irritability, sweating, tremors, hunger, confusion, delirium, abnormal behavior (resembling alcoholic intoxication), loss of consciousness, seizures.

Possible Effects of Long-Term Use: Thinning of subcutaneous fat tissue at sites of insulin injection. Insulin resistance.

Suggested Periodic Examinations While Taking This Drug (at physician's discretion)

Routine testing of blood sugar levels at intervals recommended by your physician is prudent. Historically, estimates of blood sugar were obtained by checking urine sugar. This method has been replaced by finger stick testing of blood glucose. Finger stick testing accurately reflects the blood sugar and helps ensure better control (tighter control) of blood glucose. One new blood sugar machine can also test glycated protein (fructosamine). If you are ill, increased frequency of finger stick blood glucose testing may be indicated. A new handheld machine called A1cNow enables pharmacists and physicians to check hemoglobin A1C in the office or pharmacy in 8 minutes!

▷ **While Taking This Drug, Observe the Following**

Foods: Follow your diabetic diet conscientiously. Blood sugar control can help avoid or delay diabetes problems! Vitamin C in high dose may worsen blood sugar control. Do not omit snack foods in mid-afternoon or at bedtime if they help prevent hypoglycemia.

Herbal Medicines or Minerals: Using chromium may change the way your body is able to use sugar. Some health food stores advocate vanadium as mimicking the actions of insulin, but possible toxicity and need for rigorous studies presently preclude recommending it. DHEA may change sensitivity to insulin or insulin resistance. Hawthorn, ginger, garlic, ginseng and licorice, nettle and yohimbe may change blood sugar. Since this may require adjustment of hypoglycemic medicine dosing, talk to your doctor BEFORE combining any of these herbal medicines with this medicine. Echinacea pupurea (injectable) and blonde psyllium seed or husk should NOT be taken by people living with diabetes.

Beverages: Use according to prescribed diabetic diet.

▷ *Alcohol:* Used excessively, alcohol can cause severe hypoglycemia, resulting in brain damage.

Tobacco Smoking: Regular smoking can decrease insulin absorption and increase insulin requirements by 30%. It is advisable to stop smoking altogether.

Marijuana Smoking: Possible increase in blood sugar levels.

▷ *Other Drugs*

The following drugs may *increase* the effects of insulin:
- acarbose (Precose)—by decreasing the amount of sugar that insulin has to work on.
- aspirin and other salicylates.
- some beta-blocker drugs (especially the nonselective ones; see Drug Classes)—may prolong insulin-induced hypoglycemia.
- clofibrate (Atromid-S).
- disopyramide (Norpace).

- fenfluramine (Pondimin).
- monoamine oxidase (MAO) type A inhibitors (see Drug Classes).
- oral antidiabetic drugs (see Drug Classes)—results in additive hypoglycemia.

The following drugs may *decrease* the effects of insulin (by raising blood sugar levels):

- birth control pills (oral contraceptives).
- chlorthalidone (Hygroton).
- cortisonelike drugs (see Drug Classes).
- furosemide (Lasix).
- phenytoin (Dilantin, etc.) or fosphenytoin (Cerebyx).
- thiazide diuretics (see Drug Classes).
- thyroid preparations (various).

▷ *Driving, Hazardous Activities:* Be prepared to stop and take corrective action if hypoglycemia develops.

Aviation Note: Diabetes and the use of this drug *are disqualifications* for piloting. Consult a designated Aviation Medical Examiner.

Exposure to Sun: No restrictions.

Exposure to Heat: Use caution. Sauna baths can significantly increase the rate of insulin absorption and cause hypoglycemia.

Heavy Exercise or Exertion: Use caution. Periods of unusual or unplanned heavy physical activity will use up sugar more quickly and predispose to hypoglycemia.

Occurrence of Unrelated Illness: Omission of meals as a result of nausea, vomiting or injury may lead to hypoglycemia. Infections can increase insulin needs. Ask your doctor for help.

Discontinuation: Do not stop this drug without asking your doctor. Omission of insulin may result in life-threatening coma.

Special Storage Instructions: Keep in a cool place, preferably in the refrigerator. Protect from freezing. Protect from strong light and high temperatures when not refrigerated.

Observe the Following Expiration Times: Do not use this drug if it is older than the expiration date on the vial. Always use fresh, "within date" insulin.

IPRATROPIUM (i pra TROH pee um)

Introduced: 1975   **Class:** Bronchodilator   **Prescription:** USA: Yes
Controlled Drug: USA: No; Canada: No   **Available as Generic:** USA: No;
Canada: No

Brand Names: Atrovent, ❧Apo-Atrovent, Atrovent Nasal Spray, Combivent, Dom-Ipratropium, PMS-Ipratropium

BENEFITS versus RISKS	
Possible Benefits	*Possible Risks*
EFFECTIVE BRONCHODILATOR FOR TREATMENT OF CHRONIC BRONCHITIS AND EMPHYSEMA	Mild and infrequent adverse effects (see "Possible Adverse Effects")
EFFECTIVE TREATMENT OF RUNNY NOSE (RHINORRHEA)	
Effective adjunctive treatment in some bronchial asthma	

▷ **Principal Uses**

As a Single Drug Product: Uses currently included in FDA-approved labeling: (1) Helps prevent or relieve episodes of difficult breathing in chronic bronchitis, chronic obstructive pulmonary disease (COPD) and emphysema (should not be used to treat acute attacks of asthma because it takes a while to work); (2) used in nasal spray to relieve symptoms of runny nose (rhinorrhea) from allergic or nonallergic perennial rhinitis (including runny nose from colds) in adults and children more than 12 years old.

Other (unlabeled) generally accepted uses: (1) Relief of asthma symptoms; (2) lung symptoms of congestive heart failure.

How This Drug Works: Through its atropinelike (anticholinergic) action, it blocks bronchial constriction and opens bronchi. Nasal form keeps acetylcholine from working (antagonizes it) and decreases production and secretion of mucus.

Available Dosage Forms and Strengths

Inhalation aerosol — 14-g metered dose inhaler; 18 mcg per inhalation
Nasal inhaler — 20 mcg per actuation
Nasal spray — 0.03 and 0.06%
Nebulizer — 250 mcg/ml solution

▷ **Usual Adult Dosage Ranges:** *Inhalation form:* Initially two inhalations (36 mcg) four times a day, 4 hours apart. If needed, the dose may be increased to four inhalations (72 mcg) at one time to get optimal relief. Maintain 4-hour intervals between doses. Maximum daily dose is 12 inhalations (216 mcg). *Nasal spray:* 0.03%-two sprays (21 mcg each) in each nostril two to three times a day for up to 4 days ; 0.06%-two sprays (42 mcg each) in each nostril three to four times a day for up to 4 days. **Note: Actual dose and dosing schedule must be determined for each patient individually.**

Conditions Requiring Dosing Adjustments

Liver Function: Specific guidelines not developed.

Kidney Function: Used with caution by patients with bladder neck obstructions.

▷ **Dosing Instructions:** Carefully follow the patient instructions provided with the inhaler. Shake well before using. Many people do NOT take the time to learn the best inhaler technique for them; take the time to do this. The pump of the nasal form must be primed before the unit is used. Read the package insert carefully, and ask your pharmacist for help if you don't understand the directions. If you forget a dose: use the inhaler or nasal spray as soon as you remember it, unless it's nearly time for your next dose—then skip the missed dose, space the remaining doses for the day at regularly separated times and continue the next day right on schedule. DO NOT double doses. Call your doctor if you find yourself missing doses or if you do not get the usual benefits from this medicine.

Usual Duration of Use:

Inhalation form: Continual use on a regular schedule for 48 to 72 hours is usually necessary to determine this drug's effectiveness. Long-term use (months to years) requires check of response and dose adjustment. See your doctor.

Nasal spray: The nasal form helps some people feel better right away and may take a week for others. The nasal spray may only be used for up to 4 days.

Typical Treatment Goals and Measurements (Outcomes and Markers)

Asthma: Frequency and severity of asthma attacks should ease. Some clinicians also use decreased frequency of rescue inhaler use as a further clinical indicator. It is critical that this medicine is used regularly to get the best results. If the usual benefit is not realized, call your doctor.

Possible Advantages of This Drug

Inhalation form produces a greater degree of bronchodilation than theophylline in patients with chronic bronchitis and emphysema. Causes minimal adverse effects. Repeated use does not lead to tolerance and loss of effectiveness. Suitable for long-term maintenance therapy.

Nasal spray eases a very annoying symptom (rhinorrhea or runny nose) seen with common cold.

Currently a "Drug of Choice"

For difficult breathing associated with chronic bronchitis and emphysema. Nasal form makes the common cold much easier to deal with.

▷ **This Drug Should Not Be Taken If**

- you have had an allergic reaction to it previously.
- you are allergic to soybeans or peanuts (inhalation form).
- you are allergic to atropine or to aerosol propellants (fluorocarbons) (inhalation form).
- you are allergic to benzalkonium chloride or edetate disodium (nasal spray).

▷ **Inform Your Physician Before Taking This Drug If**

- you have had an adverse effect from any belladonna derivative previously.
- you have a history of glaucoma.
- you have any form of urinary retention or prostatism (see Glossary).

Possible Side Effects (natural, expected and unavoidable drug actions)

Throat dryness, cough, irritation from aerosol—rare.

Blurred vision, dry mouth.

Bad or bitter taste—frequent.

▷ **Possible Adverse Effects** (unusual, unexpected and infrequent reactions)

If any of the following develop, consult your physician promptly for guidance.

Mild Adverse Effects

Allergic reactions: skin rash, hives—rare.

Headache, dizziness, nervousness—rare.

Palpitations—rare.

Nosebleeds (with nasal spray)—infrequent to frequent.

Serious Adverse Effects

Allergic reactions: rare first-dose angioedema or bronchospasm.

Author's Note: Other than the rare allergic reactions, the nasal spray does not have any serious adverse effects.

Abnormal heartbeat (supraventricular tachycardia)—case report.

Intraocular pressure changes—rare.

▷ **Possible Effects on Sexual Function:** None reported.

Natural Diseases or Disorders That May Be Activated by This Drug

Angle-closure glaucoma, prostatism (see Glossary).

Possible Effects on Laboratory Tests: None reported.

CAUTION

1. This drug won't start to work for 5 to 15 minutes. It should not be used alone to treat acute attacks of asthma needing a fast result.
2. When used as combination therapy with beta-adrenergic antiasthmatic drugs (albuterol, terbutaline, metaproterenol, etc.), the beta-adrenergic aerosol should be used about 5 minutes before using ipratropium to prevent fluorocarbon toxicity.
3. When used as an adjunct to steroid or cromolyn aerosols (beclomethasone, Intal), ipratropium should be used about 5 minutes before using the steroid or cromolyn aerosol to prevent fluorocarbon toxicity.
4. Contact with the eyes can cause temporary blurring of vision.
5. Call your doctor if you are using the nasal spray and your runny nose (rhinorrhea) continues or gets worse and you develop a fever.

Precautions for Use

By Infants and Children: Nasal spray is now approved for use for those 6 to 11 years old. Dosing is the same as for adults for the 0.03% form. Safety and effectiveness for those under 6 are not established.

By Those Over 60 Years of Age: Watch for possible development of prostatism and adjust dose as necessary.

▷ **Advisability of Use During Pregnancy**

Pregnancy Category: B. See Pregnancy Risk Categories at the back of this book.

Animal studies: No drug-induced birth defects in mouse, rat or rabbit studies.

Human studies: Adequate studies of pregnant women are not available.

Use this drug during pregnancy only if clearly needed.

Advisability of Use If Breast-Feeding

Presence of this drug in breast milk: Possibly yes, but in very small amounts. Watch nursing infant closely and stop drug or nursing if adverse effects start.

Habit-Forming Potential: None.

Effects of Overdose: This drug is not well absorbed into the circulation when it is taken by aerosol inhalation. No systemic effects of overdose are expected.

Possible Effects of Long-Term Use: Drying of the nose with nasal form.

Suggested Periodic Examinations While Taking This Drug (at physician's discretion)

Internal eye pressure measurements if appropriate.

▷ **While Taking This Drug, Observe the Following**

Foods: No restrictions.

Herbal Medicines or Minerals: Fir or pine needle oil should NOT be used by asthmatics. Ephedra alone does carry a German Commission E monograph indication for asthma treatment. If you are allergic to plants in the Asteraceae family (aster, chrysanthemum, daisy or ragweed), you may also be allergic to echinacea, chamomile, feverfew and St. John's wort. Talk to your doctor BEFORE adding any herbals to this medicine.

Beverages: No restrictions.

▷ *Alcohol:* No interactions expected.

Tobacco Smoking: No interactions expected, but smoking should be avoided completely if you have chronic bronchitis or emphysema. I advise everyone to quit smoking.

Marijuana Smoking: Possible excessive increase in heart rate (tachycardia).

▷ *Other Drugs*

Ipratropium may *increase* the effects of
- albuterol (Proventil, others).
- other atropinelike drugs (see Drug Classes).

Ipratropium *taken concurrently* with
- cisapride (Propulsid) may lessen benefits of cisapride.
- procainamide (Procan, others) may lead to additive effects on the vagal nerve and heart conduction (atrioventricular).
- tricyclic antidepressants (see Drug Classes) may result in additive anticholinergic effects.

▷ *Driving, Hazardous Activities:* May cause dizziness or blurred vision. Restrict activities as necessary.

Aviation Note: The use of this drug *may be a disqualification* for piloting. Consult a designated Aviation Medical Examiner.

Exposure to Sun: No restrictions.

Exposure to Cold: Inhaling cold air may cause bronchospasm and induce asthmatic breathing and cough; dose adjustment of this drug may be necessary.

Heavy Exercise or Exertion: This drug is not considered to be consistently effective in preventing or treating exercise-induced asthma.

Discontinuation: Ask your doctor for help. Substitute medication may be advisable.

ISONIAZID (i soh NI a zid)

Other Names: Isonicotinic acid hydrazide, INH

Introduced: 1956   **Class:** Antituberculosis   **Prescription:** USA: Yes
Controlled Drug: USA: No; Canada: No   **Available as Generic:**   USA: Yes; Canada: Yes

Brand Names: INH, ✚Isotamine, Laniazid, Nydrazid, P-I-N Forte [CD], ✚PMS-Isoniazid, Rifamate [CD], Rifater [CD], Rimactane/INH Dual Pack [CD], Seromycin w/Isoniazid [CD], Teebaconin, Teebaconin and Vitamin B6 [CD]

BENEFITS versus RISKS	
Possible Benefits	*Possible Risks*
EFFECTIVE PREVENTION AND TREATMENT OF ACTIVE TUBERCULOSIS	ALLERGIC LIVER REACTION—RARE Peripheral neuropathy (see Glossary) Bone marrow depression (see Glossary) Mental and behavioral disturbances

Principal Uses

As a Single Drug Product: Uses currently included in FDA-approved labeling: (1) Used alone to prevent the development of tuberculous infection (prophylaxis) in people who are at high risk because of exposure to infection or recent conversion of a negative tuberculin skin test to positive; (2) used in combination with other drugs to treat tuberculosis in a variety of body sites.

Other (unlabeled) generally accepted uses: May have a role in treating atypical mycobacteria that can be associated with Crohn's disease.

As a Combination Drug Product [CD]: Available in combination with rifampin, another antitubercular drug that works in a different way. This combination is more effective than either drug used alone and also encourages patients to take their medicine (adherence). Isoniazid can cause low pyridoxine (vitamin B6); for this reason, a combination of the two drugs is available in tablet form.

How This Drug Works: By interfering with metabolism or cell walls, this drug kills (bactericidal) or inhibits (bacteriostatic) susceptible tuberculosis organisms.

Available Dosage Forms and Strengths

    Injection — 100 mg/ml

     Syrup — 50 mg/5 ml

    Tablets — 50 mg, 100 mg, 300 mg

▷ **Usual Adult Dosage Ranges:** *For prevention:* 300 mg once daily (usually for 6 to 12 months). *For treatment:* 5 mg per kg of body mass daily. The total daily dose should not exceed 300 mg. Some clinicians use 5 mg/kg daily (up to 300 mg) for two weeks and then give 15 mg per kg (up to 900 mg) twice weekly. **Note: Actual dose and dosing schedule must be determined on an individual basis.**

Conditions Requiring Dosing Adjustments

Liver Function: This drug should not be used in sudden (acute) liver disease. It should be discontinued if liver function tests become increased to three times the normal value.

Kidney Function: This drug is a rare cause of nephrosis. For severe kidney failure (creatinine clearance less than 10 ml/min), daily dose is lowered by 50%.

▷ **Dosing Instructions:** The tablet may be crushed and taken with food to prevent stomach irritation. If you forget a dose: take the missed dose as soon as you remember it, unless it's nearly time for your next dose, then skip the missed dose and take the next dose right on schedule. DO NOT double doses. Call your doctor if you find yourself missing doses.

Usual Duration of Use: Use on a regular schedule for one year or more is often necessary, depending upon the nature of the infection. Shorter courses of intermittent high doses may work. See your doctor regularly.

Typical Treatment Goals and Measurements (Outcomes and Markers)

Infections: The most commonly used measures of serious infections are white blood cell counts and differentials (the kind of blood cells that occur most often in your blood), and temperature or night sweats. Because of the nature of this infection, therapy will be long-term. NEVER stop a medicine for tuberculosis because you start to feel better. The goals and time frame should be discussed with you when the prescription is written.

▷ **This Drug Should Not Be Taken If**

- you have had an allergic reaction (especially a liver reaction) to any dose form of it previously.
- you have active liver disease.

▷ **Inform Your Physician Before Taking This Drug If**

- you have serious impairment of liver or kidney function.
- you drink an alcoholic beverage daily.

- you are an alcoholic.
- you are pregnant or breast-feeding your baby.
- you have a seizure disorder.
- you take other drugs on a long-term basis, especially phenytoin (Dilantin).
- you plan to have surgery under general anesthesia in the near future.

Possible Side Effects (natural, expected and unavoidable drug actions)

Toxic fever—rare.

▷ **Possible Adverse Effects** (unusual, unexpected and infrequent reactions)

If any of the following develop, consult your physician promptly for guidance.

Mild Adverse Effects

Allergic reactions: skin rash, fever, swollen glands, painful muscles and joints.

Dizziness, indigestion, nausea, vomiting.

Peripheral neuritis (see Glossary): numbness, tingling, pain, weakness in hands and/or feet—frequent in adults, rare in children (may be prevented with pyridoxine).

Serious Adverse Effects

Allergic reactions: drug-induced hepatitis (see Glossary) (loss of appetite, nausea, fatigue, itching, dark-colored urine, yellowing of eyes and skin, hypersensitivity, meningitis)—case reports.

Severe skin reactions (Stevens-Johnson syndrome, pellagra)—case reports.

Acute mental/behavioral disturbances, psychosis, impaired vision, increase in epileptic seizures—rare.

High or low blood sugars (hyperglycemia or hypoglycemia)—possible.

Porphyria, pancreatitis or kidney toxicity—case reports.

Lupus erythematosus-like syndrome or abnormal muscle changes (rhabdomyolysis)—case reports.

Pellagra—rare.

Disseminated intravascular coagulation (DIC)—case report.

Bone marrow depression (see Glossary): fatigue, weakness, fever, sore throat, abnormal bleeding or bruising—case reports.

▷ **Possible Effects on Sexual Function:** Male breast enlargement and tenderness (gynecomastia)—rare.

Possible Delayed Adverse Effects: Increased frequency of liver cirrhosis has been reported.

▷ **Adverse Effects That May Mimic Natural Diseases or Disorders**

Drug-induced hepatitis may suggest viral hepatitis. Collagen vascular changes may mimic rheumatoid arthritis or systemic lupus erythematosus. Pseudolymphoma may occur.

Natural Diseases or Disorders That May Be Activated by This Drug

Latent epilepsy, systemic lupus erythematosus (questionable).

Possible Effects on Laboratory Tests

Complete blood cell counts: decreased red cells, hemoglobin, white cells and platelets; increased eosinophils (allergic reaction).

Blood amylase level: increased (possible pancreatitis).

Blood antinuclear antibodies (ANA): positive.

Blood lupus erythematosus (LE) cells: positive.

Blood glucose level: increased (with large doses).

Liver function tests: increased liver enzymes (ALT/GPT, AST/GOT and alkaline phosphatase), increased bilirubin.

Urine sugar tests: increased; false positive results with Benedict's solution and Clinitest.

CAUTION

1. **The FDA has required a new warning for Laniazid: "A recent report suggests an increased risk of fatal hepatitis associated with isoniazid among women, particularly African American and Hispanic women. The risk may also be increased during the postpartum period."** Increased laboratory testing is also suggested.

2. Ask your doctor about determining if you are a "slow" or "rapid" inactivator (acetylator) of isoniazid. This has a bearing on your predisposition to developing adverse effects.

3. Copper sulfate tests for urine sugar may give a false-positive test result. (Diabetics, please note.)

4. Because multidrug-resistant (MDR) tuberculosis is now more common in many areas, four-drug combination therapy (isoniazid, pyrazinamide, ethambutol and rifampin) is often used.

Precautions for Use

By Infants and Children: Use with caution in children with seizure disorders. "Slow acetylators" are more prone to adverse drug effects. It is advisable to give supplemental pyridoxine (vitamin B$_6$).

Prevention: Infants and children are given 10 mg per kg per day up to 300 mg for 6–12 months.

By Those Over 60 Years of Age: There is a greater incidence of liver damage in this age group, and liver status should be closely watched. Observe for any indications of an "acute brain syndrome" consisting of confusion, delirium and seizures.

▷ **Advisability of Use During Pregnancy**

Pregnancy Category: C. See Pregnancy Risk Categories at the back of this book.

Animal studies: No birth defects reported in mice, rats or rabbits.

Human studies: Data from adequate studies of pregnant women are not available.

If clearly needed, this drug is now used at any time during pregnancy. Ask your physician for guidance.

Advisability of Use If Breast-Feeding

Presence of this drug in breast milk: Yes.

Talk to your doctor about benefits and risks.

Habit-Forming Potential: None.

Effects of Overdose: Nausea, vomiting, dizziness, blurred vision, hallucinations, slurred speech, stupor, coma, seizures.

Possible Effects of Long-Term Use: Peripheral neuritis due to a deficiency of pyridoxine (vitamin B6).

Suggested Periodic Examinations While Taking This Drug (at physician's discretion)

Complete blood cell counts.

Liver function tests.

Complete eye examinations.

▷ **While Taking This Drug, Observe the Following**

Foods: Eat the following foods cautiously until your tolerance is determined: Swiss and Cheshire cheeses, tuna fish, skipjack fish and Sardinella species. These may interact with the drug to produce skin rash, itching, sweating, chills, headache, light-headedness or rapid heart rate. Taking this drug with food also acts to decrease absorption and lessen therapeutic benefits. Some red wines and aged cheeses also contain high levels of tyramine. This may result in an undesirable increase in blood pressure if consumed. Avoid this combination.

Nutritional Support: It is advisable to take a supplement of pyridoxine (vitamin B6) to prevent peripheral neuritis. Ask your physician for help.

Herbal Medicines or Minerals: Echinacea: Some patients use echinacea to attempt to boost their immune systems. Unfortunately, use of echinacea is not recommended in people with damaged immune systems. This herb may also actually weaken any immune system if it is used too often or for too long a time. DO NOT take mistletoe herb, oak bark or F.C. of marshmallow root and licorice.

Beverages: No restrictions. May be taken with milk.

▷ *Alcohol:* Alcohol may reduce the effectiveness of this drug and increase the risk of liver toxicity.

Tobacco Smoking: No interactions expected. I advise everyone to quit smoking.

▷ *Other Drugs*

Isoniazid may ***increase*** the effects of
- carbamazepine (Tegretol) and cause toxicity.
- disulfiram (Antabuse) and change behavior.
- phenytoin (Dilantin) or fosphenytoin (Cerebyx) and cause toxicity.

The following drugs may ***decrease*** the effects of isoniazid:
- cortisonelike drugs (see Drug Classes).

Isoniazid ***taken concurrently*** with
- acetaminophen (Tylenol) may increase the risk of liver damage (hepatoxicity).
- antacids may decrease the absorption of this medicine. Separate antacid dosing by 2 hours from dosing of this medicine.
- BCG vaccine will result in decreased vaccine effectiveness.
- cyclosporine (Sandimmune) may blunt cyclosporine benefits.
- diazepam and perhaps other benzodiazepines (see Drug Classes) may result in increased blood levels and toxicity.
- ketoconazole, itraconazole or related compounds may result in decreased therapeutic benefits of the antifungal.
- meperidine (Demerol) may result in excessive lowering of blood pressure.
- niacin (various) may lead to a need for increased niacin.
- oral antidiabetic drugs (see Drug Classes) may result in loss of control of blood glucose.
- propranolol (Inderal, others) may lead to isoniazid toxicity.
- rifampin (Rifadin, others) can result in a serious increased risk of liver toxicity.
- theophylline (Theodur, others) may result in theophylline toxicity.
- valproic acid (Depakene) can result in isoniazid or valproic acid toxicity.
- warfarin (Coumadin) may result in increased bleeding risk; more frequent INR (prothrombin time or protime) testing is needed.

▷ *Driving, Hazardous Activities:* This drug may cause dizziness. Restrict activities
    as necessary.
    Aviation Note: The use of this drug *may be a disqualification* for piloting.
    Consult a designated Aviation Medical Examiner.
    Exposure to Sun: No restrictions.
    Discontinuation: Long-term treatment is required. Do not stop this drug with-
    out asking your physician.

ISOSORBIDE DINITRATE (i soh SOHR bide di NI trayt)

Other Name: Sorbide nitrate   **Introduced:** 1959   **Class:** Anti-anginal,
nitrates   **Prescription:** USA: Yes   **Controlled Drug:** USA: No; Canada:
No   **Available as Generic:** USA: Yes; Canada: No

Brand Names: ❧Apo-ISDN, ❧Cedocard-SR, ❧Coradur, ❧Coronex, Dilatrate-
    SR, Iso-BID, Isonate, Isordil, Isordil Tembids, Isordil Titradose, Isotrate
    Timecelles, ❧Novo-Sorbide, Sorbitrate, Sorbitrate-SA

**Warning: The brand names Isordil and Isuprel sound similar; this can lead
to serious errors. Isordil is isosorbide dinitrate, used to treat angina.
Isuprel is isoproterenol, used for asthma. Make sure you are taking the correct drug.**

BENEFITS versus RISKS	
Possible Benefits	*Possible Risks*
EFFECTIVE RELIEF AND	Orthostatic hypotension (see Glossary)
PREVENTION OF ANGINA	Rare skin reactions (severe peeling)
EFFECTIVE ADJUNCTIVE	
TREATMENT IN SOME CASES	
OF CONGESTIVE HEART FAILURE	

▷ **Principal Uses**
    As a Single Drug Product: Uses currently included in FDA-approved labeling:
        (1) The sublingual (under-the-tongue) tablets and the chewable tablets are
        used to prevent and relieve acute attacks of anginal pain; (2) the longer-act-
        ing tablets and capsules are used to prevent the development of angina,
        but are not effective in relieving acute episodes of anginal pain (nitroglyc-
        erin is the drug of choice in those cases).
      Other (unlabeled) generally accepted uses: (1) This drug is also used to
        improve heart function in selected cases of congestive heart failure; (2) can
        help ease the pressure in esophageal varices in alcoholics; (3) can help
        painful leg cramping (intermittent claudication); (4) may be of use topi-
        cally as an ointment to avoid surgery (sphincterotomy) or to ease symp-
        toms of anal fissures; (5) may help diagnose syndrome X (angina resulting
        from exercise in people with normal epicardial coronary arteries); (6) used
        after a heart attack intravenously to help address congestive heart failure.
    How This Drug Works: This drug relaxes and dilates arteries and veins. Benefits
        in treating angina and heart failure are due to dilation of coronary arteries
        and dilation of systemic veins. Net effects are improved heart blood flow
        and reduced workload.

Available Dosage Forms and Strengths

Capsules — 40 mg

Capsules, prolonged action — 40 mg

Tablets — 5 mg, 10 mg, 20 mg, 30 mg, 40 mg

Tablets, chewable — 5 mg, 10 mg

Tablets, prolonged action — 20 mg, 40 mg

Tablets, sublingual — 2.5 mg, 5 mg, 10 mg

▷ **Recommended Dosage Ranges** (Actual dose and schedule must be determined for each patient individually.)

Infants and Children: Dose not established.

12 to 60 Years of Age:

Sublingual tablets: 5 to 10 mg dissolved under tongue every 2 to 3 hours; use for relief of acute attack and for prevention of anticipated attack.

Chewable tablets: initially 5 mg chewed to evaluate tolerance; increase dose to 5 or 10 mg every 2 to 3 hours as needed and tolerated. Use for relief of acute attack and for prevention of anticipated attack.

Tablets: 5 to 20 mg four times daily to prevent acute attack, with at least a 12-hour nitrate-free period.

Prolonged-action capsules and tablets: 40 mg to start and then 40–80 mg every 8 to 12 hours as needed to prevent acute attacks.

Author's Note: Dosing for all forms is set up to give a 12-hour nitrate-free period in order to avoid tolerance to the therapeutic benefits of this medicine.

Over 60 Years of Age: Same as 12 to 60 years of age, although excessive lowering of blood pressure on standing (postural hypotension) may be more likely in this population.

Conditions Requiring Dosing Adjustments

Liver Function: Used with caution and in decreased doses by patients with liver compromise, as increased blood levels will occur.

Kidney Function: No specific dosing changes are needed for compromised kidneys. This drug can discolor urine (brown to black).

▷ **Dosing Instructions:** Capsules and tablets to be swallowed are best taken on an empty stomach to achieve maximal blood levels. Regular tablets may be crushed; prolonged-action capsules and tablets should be taken whole, NOT chewed. If you forget a dose: take the missed dose as soon as you remember it, unless it's nearly time for your next dose skip the missed dose, take the next dose right on schedule. DO NOT double doses. Call your doctor if you find yourself missing doses.

Usual Duration of Use: Use on a regular schedule for 3 to 7 days is needed to (1) identify this drug's peak effect in preventing or relieving acute anginal pain and (2) to find the optimal dose schedule. Long-term use (months to years) requires physician supervision.

Typical Treatment Goals and Measurements (Outcomes and Markers)

Angina: The most commonly used markers are prevention or relief of chest pain (angina). Many cardiologists look for easing of frequency and severity of angina attacks as well as pulmonary capillary wedge pressure as measures of successful therapy. If your chest pain does not go away after using the maximum dose at the recommended time interval, have someone drive you to the hospital or call 911. Ask your doctor on the next office visit if it would make sense for you to chew a regular release full-dose aspirin prior to going to the hospital if that situation occurs.

▷ **This Drug Should Not Be Taken If**
- you had an allergic reaction to any form of it previously.
- you have severe anemia.
- you have increased intraocular pressure.
- you have suffered trauma to the head.
- you have an overactive thyroid gland.
- you have abnormal growth of the heart muscle (hypertrophic cardiomyopathy).
- you have already taken or take sildenafil (Viagra).
- you have had a very recent heart attack (myocardial infarction) and have elevated blood pressure or very rapid heart rate (tachycardia).

▷ **Inform Your Physician Before Taking This Drug If**
- you have had an unfavorable response to other nitrate drugs or vasodilators in the past.
- you have a history of low blood pressure.
- you are anemic and are being prescribed the under-the-tongue (sublingual) form.
- you have any form of glaucoma.
- you have had a cerebral hemorrhage recently.
- you are pregnant or are planning pregnancy.
- you are allergic to the dye tartrazine.
- you have a glucose-6-phosphate dehydrogenase (G6PD) deficiency (ask your doctor).
- you have excessive thyroid function (hyperthyroidism), cardiomyopathy or have suffered head trauma.

Possible Side Effects (natural, expected and unavoidable drug actions)
Flushing of face, throbbing in head, palpitation, rapid heart rate, orthostatic hypotension (see Glossary).

▷ **Possible Adverse Effects** (unusual, unexpected and infrequent reactions)
If any of the following develop, consult your physician promptly for guidance.
Mild Adverse Effects
Allergic reaction: skin rash.
Headache (may be severe and persistent)—infrequent to frequent.
Dizziness, fainting—possible.
Nausea, vomiting—possible.
Bad breath (halitosis)—case reports.
Urine discoloration—possible and not clinically significant.
Serious Adverse Effects
Allergic reaction: severe dermatitis with peeling of skin—case reports.
Transient ischemic attacks (TIAs) in presence of impaired circulation within the brain: dizziness, fainting, impaired vision or speech, localized numbness or weakness—possible.
Anemia (in those with G6PD deficiency)—possible.
Abnormal heart rates or conduction—case reports.
Abnormally low blood pressure on standing (postural hypotension)—possible.
Myocardial ischemia or infarction—possible.

Methemoglobinemia—case report.

Tolerance-possible with 24-hour use (daily 12-hour drug-free period is used to prevent this).

▷ **Possible Effects on Sexual Function:** None reported.

▷ **Adverse Effects That May Mimic Natural Diseases or Disorders**

Spells of low blood pressure (due to this drug) may mimic late-onset epilepsy.

Possible Effects on Laboratory Tests

Methemoglobin: increased.

CAUTION

1. Tolerance (see Glossary) to long-acting forms of nitrates may cause sublingual tablets of nitroglycerin to be less effective in relieving acute anginal attacks. Anti-anginal effectiveness is restored after 1 week of abstinence from long-acting nitrates. Daily 12-hour periods without use of the drug are needed.

2. Many over-the-counter (OTC) medicines for allergies, colds and coughs contain drugs that may counteract the desired drug effects. Ask your physician or pharmacist for help before using such medicines.

Precautions for Use

By Those Over 60 Years of Age: Small starting doses are advisable. You may be more susceptible to the development of low blood pressure and associated "blackout" spells, fainting and falling. Throbbing headaches and flushing may be more apparent.

▷ **Advisability of Use During Pregnancy**

Pregnancy Category: C. See Pregnancy Risk Categories at the back of this book.

Animal studies: No information available.

Human studies: Adequate studies of pregnant women are not available.

Use this drug only if clearly needed.

Advisability of Use If Breast-Feeding

Presence of this drug in breast milk: Unknown.

If this drug is thought to be necessary, monitor the nursing infant for low blood pressure and poor feeding.

Habit-Forming Potential: None.

Effects of Overdose: Headache, dizziness, marked flushing of face and skin, vomiting, weakness, fainting, difficult breathing, coma.

Possible Effects of Long-Term Use: Development of tolerance with temporary loss of effectiveness at recommended doses. Development of abnormal hemoglobin (red blood cell pigment).

Suggested Periodic Examinations While Taking This Drug (at physician's discretion)

Measurement of internal eye pressure.

Red cell counts and hemoglobin and methemoglobin tests.

▷ **While Taking This Drug, Observe the Following**

Foods: Oral doses are best taken on an empty stomach to insure quick absorption. Vitamin C may help ease nitrate tolerance. More study is needed.

Herbal Medicines or Minerals: Hawthorn and co-enzyme Q10 (co-Q10) can affect the way the heart works. Co-Q10 may also interact badly with aspirin. Soy (milk, tofu, etc.) contains phytoestrogens that have led to an FDA-approved health claim for reducing risk of heart disease (if they have at least 6.25 grams of soy protein per serving). Couch grass or nettle should NOT be taken by patients who have increased fluid (edema) caused by heart weakness. Hawthorn (Crataegus variety) has been used to help heart failure, but should not be combined with heart medicines as combination use has not been studied. BE CERTAIN to tell your doctor that you are taking or are considering taking these herbs if you are taking a nitrate.

Beverages: No restrictions. May be taken with milk.

▷ *Alcohol:* Use extreme caution and avoid alcohol completely in the presence of any side effects or adverse effects of this drug. Alcohol may exaggerate the blood-pressure-lowering effect of this drug.

Tobacco Smoking: Nicotine can reduce benefits. Avoid all forms of tobacco.

Marijuana Smoking: Possible reduced effectiveness of this drug; mild to moderate increase in angina; possible changes in electrocardiogram, confusing interpretation.

▷ *Other Drugs*

Isosorbide dinitrate **taken concurrently** with

- antihypertensive drugs may cause excessive lowering of blood pressure; dose adjustments may be necessary.
- hydralazine (Apresoline) may work well to help control angina.
- propranolol (Inderal) can help improve exercise time without angina.
- sildenafil (Viagra) may result in LIFE-THREATENING lowering of blood pressure. NEVER COMBINE.

▷ *Driving, Hazardous Activities:* Usually no restrictions. This drug may cause dizziness or spells of low blood pressure. Restrict activities as necessary.

Aviation Note: Coronary artery disease **is a disqualification** for piloting. Consult a designated Aviation Medical Examiner.

Exposure to Sun: No restrictions.

Exposure to Heat: Use caution. Hot environments can cause a significant drop in blood pressure.

Exposure to Cold: Cold environments can increase the need for this drug and limit its benefits.

Heavy Exercise or Exertion: This drug may improve your ability to be more active without anginal pain. Use caution and avoid excessive exertion.

Discontinuation: It is advisable to gradually withdraw this drug after long-term use. Dose and frequency of prolonged-action dose forms should be reduced gradually over a period of 4 to 6 weeks.

ISOSORBIDE MONONITRATE (i soh SOHR bide mon oh NI trayt)

Introduced: 1983   **Class:** Anti-anginal, nitrates   **Prescription:** USA: Yes   **Controlled Drug:** USA: No   **Available as Generic:** USA: Yes

Brand Names: Elan (Italy), Elantan, Imdur, Ismo, Monoket

BENEFITS versus RISKS	
Possible Benefits	*Possible Risks*
EFFECTIVE PREVENTION OF ANGINA	Orthostatic hypotension (see Glossary) Headache

▷ **Principal Uses**

As a Single Drug Product: Uses currently included in FDA-approved labeling:
(1) To reduce the frequency and severity of recurrent angina; not effective
in acute anginal pain.

Other (unlabeled) generally accepted uses: (1) May have a role in treating
congestive heart failure (intravenous); (2) can help in decreasing the number of attacks and time spent in silent myocardial ischemia; (3) may be of
help in heart attacks (myocardial infarction); (4) may help stomach bleeding in people with cirrhosis of the liver.

How This Drug Works: Relaxes and dilates arteries and veins. Benefits in angina
are due to dilation of coronary arteries and dilation of systemic veins. Net
effects are improved blood flow to the heart and reduced workload of the
heart.

Available Dosage Forms and Strengths

Capsules, sustained release — 60 mg

Capsules, sustained release (Italy) — 50 mg

Tablets — 10 mg, 20 mg

Tablets, sustained release — 30 mg, 60 mg, 120 mg

▷ **Recommended Dosage Ranges** (Actual dose and schedule must be determined
for each patient individually.)

Infants and Children: Dose not established.

12 to 60 Years of Age:

Regular release: 20 mg (one tablet), taken twice daily. Take the first tablet on
arising; take the second tablet 7 hours later. Do not take additional doses
during the balance of the day. Total daily dose should not exceed 40 mg.

**Author's Note: Dosing is set up to give a 12-hour nitrate-free period to
avoid tolerance to the therapeutic benefits of this medicine.**

Sustained release: 30 mg (one half-tablet) or 60 mg (a whole tablet) once
daily, taken in the morning when you get up. Total daily dose should not
exceed 240 mg.

Over 60 Years of Age: Same as 12 to 60 years of age.

Conditions Requiring Dosing Adjustments

Liver Function: This drug should be used with caution by patients with liver
compromise. No specific guidelines for dose reduction are available.

Kidney Function: No dosing changes in kidney compromise. Drug turns urine
brown to black in color.

▷ **Dosing Instructions:** The tablet may be crushed and is preferably taken on an
empty stomach to achieve the best blood levels. Sustained-release forms
should not be chewed or crushed. If you forget a dose: take the missed
dose as soon as you remember it, unless it's nearly time for your next dose,
then skip the missed dose and take the next dose right on schedule. DO
NOT double doses. Call your doctor if you find yourself missing doses.

Usual Duration of Use: Use on a regular schedule for 3 to 7 days is needed to (1)
identify this drug's peak effect in preventing or relieving acute anginal pain
and (2) to find the optimal dose schedule. Long-term use (months to years)
requires physician supervision.

Typical Treatment Goals and Measurements (Outcomes and Markers)

Angina: The most commonly used markers are prevention or relief of chest
pain (angina). Many cardiologists look for easing of frequency and severity

of angina attacks as well as pulmonary capillary wedge pressure as measures of successful therapy. If your chest pain does not go away after using the maximum dose at the recommended time interval, have someone drive you to the hospital or call 911. Plan for this possibility and ask your doctor on the next office visit if it would make sense for you to chew a regular release full-dose aspirin prior to going to the hospital if you do not get relief from maximum nitrate doses and have to go to the hospital.

Possible Advantages of This Drug

Designed to provide the best possible prevention of acute angina with minimal development of tolerance (loss of effectiveness—see Glossary). The nitrate-free interval during the evening and night prevents the development of tolerance.

▷ This Drug Should Not Be Taken If

- you have had an allergic reaction to it previously.
- you currently have congestive heart failure or a severe anemia.
- you have taken or are currently taking sildenafil (Viagra).
- your thyroid is overactive.
- you have a hypertrophic cardiomyopathy.

▷ Inform Your Physician Before Taking This Drug If

- you have had an unfavorable response to other nitrate drugs or vasodilators in the past.
- you have a history of low blood pressure.
- you have had a very recent heart attack (myocardial infarction) and your heart is beating quickly (tachycardia) or your blood pressure is excessively high.
- you have had a cerebral hemorrhage recently.
- you are pregnant or planning pregnancy or breast-feeding your baby.
- you have any form of glaucoma.
- you have excessive thyroid function (hyperthyroidism) or cardiomyopathy or have suffered head trauma.

Possible Side Effects (natural, expected and unavoidable drug actions)

Flushing of face, throbbing in head, palpitation, rapid heart rate, orthostatic hypotension (see Glossary).

▷ Possible Adverse Effects (unusual, unexpected and infrequent reactions)

If any of the following develop, consult your physician promptly for guidance.

Mild Adverse Effects

Allergic reactions: skin rash, itching—infrequent.

Headache—frequent, but decreases over time.

Dizziness, fainting or blurred vision—possible.

Nausea, vomiting or bad breath (halitosis seen with isosorbide dinitrate)—possible.

Urine discoloration—possible and not clinically significant.

Increased liver enzymes—possible.

Serious Adverse Effects

Transient ischemic attacks (TIAs) in presence of impaired circulation within the brain: dizziness, fainting, impaired vision or speech, localized numbness or weakness—possible.

Bone marrow depression—infrequent and of uncertain relationship.

Anemia (in patients with glucose-6-phosphate dehydrogenase (G6PD) deficiency)—possible.

Abnormally low blood pressure—possible.

Abnormal heartbeat—case reports.

Tolerance—possible with 24-hour use (daily 12-hour drug-free period is used to prevent this).

Worsening of angina or abnormal heartbeats—case reports.

▷ **Possible Effects on Sexual Function:** Decreased libido and impotence—infrequent.

▷ **Adverse Effects That May Mimic Natural Diseases or Disorders**

Spells of low blood pressure with fainting (due to this drug) may be mistaken for late-onset epilepsy.

Possible Effects on Laboratory Tests

Liver function tests: increased.

CAUTION

1. Take this drug exactly as prescribed. If headaches are frequent or troublesome, call your doctor. Aspirin or acetaminophen may be taken to relieve headaches.

2. Many over-the-counter (OTC) medicines for allergies, colds and coughs contain drugs that may counteract the desired effects of this drug. Ask your doctor or pharmacist for help before using such medicines.

Precautions for Use

By Those Over 60 Years of Age: Small starting doses are advisable. Increased risk of low blood pressure and associated "blackout" spells, fainting and falling. Throbbing headaches and flushing may be more apparent.

▷ **Advisability of Use During Pregnancy**

Pregnancy Category: Ismo: C. Imdur: B. Monoket: B. See Pregnancy Risk Categories at the back of this book.

Animal studies: Rat and rabbit studies reveal embryo deaths due to large doses of Ismo. Rat and rabbit studies did not reveal embryo deaths from Imdur.

Human studies: Adequate studies of pregnant women are not available.

Use this drug only if clearly needed. Ask your physician for guidance.

Advisability of Use If Breast-Feeding

Presence of this drug in breast milk: Unknown.

If this drug is thought to be necessary, watch the nursing infant for low blood pressure and poor feeding.

Habit-Forming Potential: None.

Effects of Overdose: Headache, dizziness, marked flushing of face and skin, vomiting, weakness, fainting, difficult breathing, coma.

Possible Effects of Long-Term Use: Development of abnormal hemoglobin (red blood cell pigment).

Suggested Periodic Examinations While Taking This Drug (at physician's discretion)

Measurement of internal eye pressure.

▷ **While Taking This Drug, Observe the Following**

Foods: No restrictions. Vitamin C may help ease nitrate tolerance. More study is needed.

Herbal Medicines or Minerals: Hawthorn and co-enzyme Q10 (co-Q10) can affect the way the heart works. Co-Q10 may also interact badly with aspirin. Soy (milk, tofu, etc.) contains phytoestrogens that have led to an FDA-approved health claim for reducing risk of heart disease (if they have at least 6.25 grams of soy protein per serving). Couch grass or nettle should NOT be taken by patients who have increased fluid (edema) caused by heart weakness. Hawthorn (*Crataegus* variety) has been used to help heart failure, but should not be combined with heart medicines as combination use has not been studied. BE CERTAIN to tell your doctor that you are taking or are considering taking these herbs if you are taking a nitrate.

Beverages: No restrictions. May be taken with milk.

▷ *Alcohol:* Use extreme caution. Avoid alcohol completely in the presence of any side effects or adverse effects of this drug. Alcohol may exaggerate the blood-pressure-lowering effect of this drug.

Tobacco Smoking: Nicotine can reduce effectiveness. Avoid all forms of tobacco.

Marijuana Smoking: Possible reduced effectiveness of this drug; mild to moderate increase in angina and possible changes in electrocardiogram confusing interpretation.

▷ *Other Drugs*

Isosorbide mononitrate *taken concurrently* with

- antihypertensive drugs may cause excessive lowering of blood pressure; dose adjustments may be necessary.
- calcium-channel-blocking drugs (see Drug Classes) may cause marked orthostatic hypotension (see Glossary).
- hydralazine (Apresoline) may work well to help control angina.
- propranolol (Inderal) can help improve exercise time without angina.
- sildenafil (Viagra) may result in LIFE-THREATENING lowering of blood pressure. NEVER COMBINE.

▷ *Driving, Hazardous Activities:* Usually no restrictions. This drug may cause dizziness or spells of low blood pressure. Restrict activities as necessary.

Aviation Note: Coronary artery disease *is a disqualification* for piloting. Consult a designated Aviation Medical Examiner.

Exposure to Sun: No restrictions.

Exposure to Heat: Use caution. Hot environments can cause a significant drop in blood pressure.

Exposure to Cold: Cold environments can increase the need for this drug and limit its effectiveness.

Heavy Exercise or Exertion: This drug may improve your ability to be more active without anginal pain. Use caution and avoid excessive exertion.

Discontinuation: It is best to withdraw this drug gradually (over a period of 2 to 4 weeks) after long-term use.

ISOTRETINOIN (i soh TRET i noy in)

Introduced: 1979　**Class:** Antiacne　**Prescription:** USA: Yes　**Controlled Drug:** USA: No; Canada: No　**Available as Generic:** Yes
Brand Name: Accutane

BENEFITS versus RISKS

Possible Benefits	*Possible Risks*
EFFECTIVE TREATMENT OF SEVERE CYSTIC ACNE	DEPRESSION
Treatment of other skin conditions	MAJOR BIRTH DEFECTS
	Initial worsening of acne (transient)
	Inflammation of lips
	Dry skin, nose and mouth
	Musculoskeletal discomfort
	Corneal opacities

▷ **Principal Uses**

As a Single Drug Product: Uses currently included in FDA-approved labeling: (1) Reserved to treat severe, disfiguring nodular and cystic acne that has failed to respond to all other forms of therapy—*it should not be used to treat mild forms of acne;* (2) it is also used to treat some less common conditions of the skin that are due to disorders of keratin production.

Other (unlabeled) generally accepted uses: (1) May be helpful in refractory hypertrophic lupus erythematosus; (2) can help control resistant oral leukoplakia; (3) used in Apert's syndrome facial treatment; (4) used adjunctively to surgery in some cervical cancers; (5) treats mycosis fungoides; (6) eases symptoms in Darier's disease; (7) may have a role in treating dysplastic nevi; (8) eases symptoms of Grover's disease; (9) can help treat the abnormal gum growth (gingival hyperplasia) that can occur with phenytoin therapy; (10) treats severe and refractory rosacea; (11) has been combined with interferon alpha treatment in squamous cell skin cancer.

How This Drug Works: Reduces the size of sebaceous glands and inhibits sebum (skin oil) production. This helps to correct acne and complications.

Available Dosage Forms and Strengths

Capsules — 10 mg, 20 mg, 40 mg

▷ **Usual Adult Dosage Ranges:** Starting dose is based on the patient's weight and severity of acne; the usual dose is 0.5 to 2 mg per kg of body mass daily, taken in two divided doses for 15 to 20 weeks. After weeks of treatment, the dose should be adjusted according to response of the acne and the development of adverse effects. **Note: Actual dose and schedule must be determined for each patient individually.**

Conditions Requiring Dosing Adjustments

Liver Function: The dose should be decreased when isotretinoin is used by patients with compromised livers.

Kidney Function: Isotretinoin should be used with caution in kidney compromise.

Dosing Instructions: Begin treatment only on the second or third day of your next normal menstrual period. Serum pregnancy test should be checked BEFORE treatment is started. Take this medicine with meals (morning and evening) to achieve optimal blood levels. The capsule should not be opened for administration. If you forget a dose: take the missed dose as soon as you remember it, unless it's nearly time for your next dose, then skip the missed dose and take the next dose right on schedule. DO NOT double doses. Call your doctor if you find yourself missing doses.

Author's Note: A new patient consent form must be filled out before starting this medicine. The new form will ask you to tell your doctor if they or family members have had symptoms of depression and/or other psychological symptoms. Female patients will also be reminded about pregnancy risks (severe birth defects) possible if they become pregnant while taking this medicine. Stronger warnings will also be present in labeling about depression and suicide in patients taking Accutane.

Usual Duration of Use: Use on a regular schedule for 15 to 20 weeks best determines effectiveness in clearing or improving severe cystic acne. The drug may be stopped earlier if the total cyst count is reduced by more than 70%. If a repeat course of treatment is necessary, it should not be started for 2 months. Long-term use (months to years) requires physician supervision.

Typical Treatment Goals and Measurements (Outcomes and Markers)

Acne: Many dermatologists look for improvement or decrease in the lesions being treated as the measure of response. Blood fat (lipid) levels are tested before isotretinoin is given and then are rechecked periodically until reaction to the medicine is seen (often in a month).

▷ **This Drug Should Not Be Taken If**
- you have had an allergic reaction to it previously.
- you are allergic to parabens (preservatives used in this drug product).
- you have mild acne.
- you are not able or willing to follow contraception.
- you have not gotten verbal and written warnings about this medicine and fetal damage.
- you have not had a negative urine or serum pregnancy test (at least 50 mIU/ml sensitivity) 1 week before starting this medicine.
- you are pregnant or planning pregnancy.
- you are not starting treatment on the second or third day of a subsequent normal menstrual period.

▷ **Inform Your Physician Before Taking This Drug If**
- you have a history of depression or become depressed while taking this medicine.
- you had an allergic reaction to vitamin A in the past.
- you routinely take a nonprescription form of vitamin A.
- you have diabetes mellitus.
- you are considering giving blood (you will NOT be eligible for 1 month after the last isotretinoin dose).
- you have a cholesterol or triglyceride disorder.
- you are considering having a child or are breast-feeding your infant.
- you wear contact lenses (your tolerance for these may decrease while you take this medicine).
- you have a history of liver or kidney disease.

Possible Side Effects (natural, expected and unavoidable drug actions)

Frequent dryness of the nose and mouth, inflammation of the lips (cheilitis), dryness of the skin with itching, peeling of the palms and soles. Dose-related increase in triglycerides—frequent.

▷ **Possible Adverse Effects** (unusual, unexpected and infrequent reactions)
If any of the following develop, consult your physician promptly for guidance.
Mild Adverse Effects
Allergic reaction: skin rash—may resemble pityriasis rosea.
Thinning of hair, conjunctivitis, intolerance of contact lenses, decreased night vision, muscular and joint aches, headache, fatigue, indigestion—infrequent.
Chest pain (usually reversible if medicine is stopped)—rare.
Serious Adverse Effects
Depression—case reports to infrequent.
Skin infections, arthritis flare, inflammatory bowel disorders—case reports.
Abnormal acceleration of bone development in children—possible.
Development of opacities in the cornea of the eye—possible.
Reduced red blood cell and white blood cell counts; increased blood platelet count—infrequent.
Seizures—case reports.
Myopathy—case reports.
Tendonitis—case reports.
Kidney toxicity, liver toxicity or pancreatitis—rare.
Abnormal blood glucose control—infrequent.
Increased pressure within the head (headache, visual disturbances, nausea/vomiting)—case reports.
Pancreatitis (secondary to increased triglycerides)—case report.
▷ **Possible Effects on Sexual Function:** Decreased male or female libido—possible.
Ejaculatory failure—case report.
Decreased vaginal secretions—possible.
Altered timing and pattern of menstruation—case reports.
Possible Effects on Laboratory Tests
Complete blood cell counts: infrequently decreased red cells and white cells.
Sedimentation rate: increased.
Blood total cholesterol, LDL cholesterol, VLDL cholesterol and triglyceride levels: increased.
Blood HDL cholesterol levels: decreased.
Blood thyroid hormones (T3, T4 and free T4 index): decreased.
Liver function tests: infrequently increased liver enzymes (ALT/GPT, AST/GOT and alkaline phosphatase), increased bilirubin.
Blood calcium level: increased.
Protein in the urine: positive, though infrequent.
CAUTION
1. This medicine has caused a number of verified cases of depression. Your prescriber should ask you about mood changes at each office visit, and you should call if depression starts.
2. This drug should not be used to treat mild forms of acne.
3. Worsening of your acne may occur during the first few weeks of treatment; this will subside with continued use of the drug.
4. Do not take any other form of vitamin A while taking this drug. (Check contents of multiple vitamin preparations.)
5. Women who may become pregnant should have a blood pregnancy test 2 weeks before taking this drug and need two effective forms of contra-

ception simultaneously during its use. Contraception should be continued until normal menstruation resumes after stopping this drug.

6. May increase blood levels of cholesterol and triglycerides.
7. If repeated courses of this drug are prescribed, wait a minimum of 2 months between courses before resuming medication.

Precautions for Use

By Infants and Children: Long-term use (6 to 12 months) may cause abnormal acceleration of bone growth and development. Your physician can monitor this possibility by periodic X-ray examination of long bones.

▷ **Advisability of Use During Pregnancy**

Pregnancy Category: X. See Pregnancy Risk Categories at the back of this book.

Animal studies: Birth defects of skull, brain and vertebral column found in rats; skeletal birth defects found in rabbits.

Human studies: Adequate studies of pregnant women are not available. However, many serious birth defects (thought to be due to this drug) have been reported. These include major abnormalities of the head, brain, heart, blood vessels and hormone-producing glands.

Avoid this drug completely during entire pregnancy.

Advisability of Use If Breast-Feeding

Presence of this drug in breast milk: Unknown.

Avoid drug or refrain from nursing.

Habit-Forming Potential: None.

Effects of Overdose: Increased blood pressure, lethargy, nausea, vomiting, mild gastrointestinal bleeding, elevated blood calcium, hallucinations and psychosis.

Suggested Periodic Examinations While Taking This Drug (at physician's discretion)

Complete blood cell counts, including platelet counts.

Measurements of blood cholesterol and triglyceride levels.

Complete eye examinations.

Liver and kidney function tests.

▷ **While Taking This Drug, Observe the Following**

Foods: Increases absorption and may be a good mechanism to maintain blood levels.

Herbal Medicines or Minerals: **Caution:** St. John's wort may also cause extreme reactions to the sun. Additive photosensitivity may be possible. Medicinal yeast has a German Commission E monograph indication for acne, but has not been studied with isotretinoin. Talk to your doctor BEFORE combining any herbals with prescription medicines.

Beverages: No restrictions.

▷ *Alcohol:* A disulfiramlike reaction was described in one case report.

Tobacco Smoking: No interactions expected. I advise everyone to quit smoking.

▷ *Other Drugs*

Isotretinoin *taken concurrently* with

- carbamazepine (Tegretol) may cause subtherapeutic carbamazepine levels.
- medicines known to increase sensitivity to the sun (see Table 2) as these may additively increase sun sensitivity if taken with isotretinoin.

- minocycline may increase risk of severe headache, papilledema and visual changes.
- tetracyclines may cause increased risk of pseudotumor cerebri.

▷ *Driving, Hazardous Activities:* No restrictions.

Exposure to Sun: Caution: This drug can cause photosensitivity (see Glossary). See "Herbal Medicines" caution above.

ISRADIPINE (is RA di peen)

Introduced: 1984   **Class:** Antihypertensive, calcium channel blocker
Prescription: USA: Yes   **Controlled Drug:** USA: No   **Available as Generic:** USA: No

Brand Names: DynaCirc, DynaCirc CR

Controversies in Medicine: Medicines in this class have had many conflicting reports. The FDA has held hearings on the calcium channel blocker (CCB) class. **Amlodipine got the first FDA approval to treat high blood pressure or angina in people with congestive heart failure.** Early research at New York University found that nifedipine is a cause of reversible male infertility. CCBs are currently second-line agents for high blood pressure according to the JNC VI (see Glossary).

BENEFITS versus RISKS	
Possible Benefits	*Possible Risks*
EFFECTIVE TREATMENT OF MILD TO MODERATE HYPERTENSION	Headache, dizziness, fluid retention, palpitations
May prevent progression of early atherosclerotic damage in blood vessels	
Might slow how quickly new atherosclerotic lesions are developed	

▷ **Principal Uses**

As a Single Drug Product: Uses currently included in FDA-approved labeling: (1) Treats mild to moderate hypertension, alone or in combination; (2) treats hypertension in pregnancy.

Other (unlabeled) generally accepted uses: (1) Treatment of chronic, stable angina; (2) may help prevent progression of early lesions and rate of development of new lesions in atherosclerosis.

How This Drug Works: Blocks passage of calcium through cell walls, inhibiting contraction of coronary arteries and peripheral arterioles. As a result:
- promotes dilation of the coronary arteries (anti-anginal effect);
- reduces the degree of contraction of peripheral arterial walls, resulting in lowering of blood pressure. This further reduces heart workload and helps prevent angina.

Available Dosage Forms and Strengths

Capsules — 2.5 mg, 5 mg

Tablets (timed release) — 5 mg and 10 mg

▷ **Usual Adult Dosage Ranges:** *Hypertension:* Initially 2.5 mg twice daily, 12 hours apart, for a trial period of 2 to 4 weeks. If needed, the dose may be increased by 5 mg per day at intervals of 2 to 4 weeks. The usual maintenance dose is 5 to 10 mg daily. The total daily dose should not exceed 20 mg. Sustained release form is started at 5 mg once a day and increased slowly if needed. **Note: Actual dose and dosing schedule must be determined for each patient individually.**

Conditions Requiring Dosing Adjustments

Liver Function: Empiric decreases in dosing are prudent in liver damage.

Kidney Function: Use with caution in kidney compromise. Initial dose should be 2.5 mg twice a day or 5 mg once daily (sustained release).

▷ **Dosing Instructions:** May be taken with or following food to reduce stomach irritation. The capsule may be opened, mixed with food and swallowed promptly. The sustained release tablets MUST NOT be altered. If you forget a dose: take the missed dose as soon as you remember it, unless it's nearly time for your next dose—if that is the case, skip the missed dose and take the next dose right on schedule. DO NOT double doses. Call your doctor if you find yourself missing doses.

Usual Duration of Use: Use on a regular schedule for 2 to 4 weeks determines this drug's effectiveness in controlling hypertension or in reducing the frequency and severity of angina. The smallest effective dose should be used for long-term (months to years) therapy. Periodic physician evaluation is essential.

Typical Treatment Goals and Measurements (Outcomes and Markers)

Blood pressure: The most recent treatment guidelines (JNC VI) actually define optimal blood pressure (BP) as less than 120/80 and high normal as 139/89. The American Diabetes Association has chosen a target of 130/80 as the blood pressure goal for people living with diabetes. Most clinicians try to achieve a BP that achieves the best balance of lower cardiovascular risk while avoiding the problem of too low a blood pressure. The goal and time frame (see peak benefits above) should be discussed with you when the prescription is written.

Possible Advantages of This Drug

Does not cause orthostatic hypotension (see Glossary). No adverse effects on heart or kidney function. No adverse effects on blood cholesterol levels.

▷ **This Drug Should Not Be Taken If**
- you have had an allergic reaction to it previously.
- you have symptomatic low blood pressure (hypotension).
- you have severe problems in the left side of your heart (left ventricular dysfunction).

▷ **Inform Your Physician Before Taking This Drug If**
- you have had an unfavorable response to any calcium-channel-blocker drug in the past (see Drug Classes).
- you take any beta-blocker drug (see Drug Classes).
- you are taking any drugs that lower blood pressure.
- you have a history of congestive heart failure, heart attack or stroke.
- you have narrowing of the aorta.
- you are subject to disturbances of heart rhythm.
- you have muscular dystrophy or myasthenia gravis.
- you develop a skin reaction while taking this drug.
- you have impaired liver or kidney function.
- you will have surgery with general anesthesia in the near future.

Possible Side Effects (natural, expected and unavoidable drug actions)

Rapid heart rate—rare.

Swelling of the feet and ankles, cough, flushing and sensation of warmth—infrequent.

Small weight loss—possible.

▷ **Possible Adverse Effects** (unusual, unexpected and infrequent reactions)

If any of the following develop, consult your physician promptly for guidance.

Mild Adverse Effects

Allergic reactions: skin rash, hives, itching—rare.

Headache—frequent.

Dizziness, weakness—infrequent.

Nervousness, blurred vision—rare.

Decreased skin sensation—rare.

Palpitation, shortness of breath—infrequent.

Indigestion, nausea, vomiting, constipation—infrequent.

Cramps in legs and feet—rare.

Increased urination—rare.

Abnormal growth of the gums (gingival hyperplasia)—frequent with some drugs in the same class.

Serious Adverse Effects

Allergic reactions: erythema multiforme, exfoliative dermatitis—case reports.

Heart rhythm disturbances—infrequent.

Increased frequency or severity of angina (when therapy is started or dose increased)—possible.

Marked drop in blood pressure with fainting—rare.

Low white blood cell counts—rare.

▷ **Possible Effects on Sexual Function:** Decreased libido, impotence (less than 1%).

▷ **Adverse Effects That May Mimic Natural Diseases or Disorders**

Flushing and warmth may resemble menopausal "hot flashes."

Possible Effects on Laboratory Tests

White blood cell counts: decreased (less than 1% of users).

Liver function tests: increased enzyme levels—infrequent.

Electrocardiogram: slight increase in QT interval.

CAUTION

1. If you check your blood pressure, check it just before each dose and 2 to 3 hours after each dose. Even though high blood pressure usually has no symptoms, high blood pressure MUST be treated to avoid serious complications.

2. Tell health care professionals who treat you that you take this drug. List this drug on a card in your purse or wallet.

3. Nitroglycerin and other nitrate drugs may be used as needed to relieve acute episodes of angina pain. However, if your angina attacks are becoming more frequent or intense, notify your physician promptly.

Precautions for Use

By Infants and Children: Safety and effectiveness under 18 years of age not established.

By Those Over 60 Years of Age: Usually well tolerated by this age group. However, watch for weakness, dizziness, fainting and falling. Take necessary precautions to prevent injury.

▷ **Advisability of Use During Pregnancy**

Pregnancy Category: C. See Pregnancy Risk Categories at the back of this book.

Animal studies: Embryo and fetal toxicity reported in small animals, but no birth defects due to this drug.

Human studies: Adequate studies of pregnant women are not available.

Avoid this drug during the first 3 months. Use during the final 6 months only if clearly needed. Ask your physician for guidance.

Advisability of Use If Breast-Feeding

Presence of this drug in breast milk: Unknown.

Avoid drug or refrain from nursing.

Habit-Forming Potential: None.

Effects of Overdose: Weakness, light-headedness, fainting, fast pulse, low blood pressure, shortness of breath, flushed and warm skin, tremors, abnormal heartbeats.

Possible Effects of Long-Term Use: None reported.

Suggested Periodic Examinations While Taking This Drug (at physician's discretion)

Evaluations of heart function, including electrocardiograms.

Measurements of blood pressure in supine, sitting and standing positions.

▷ **While Taking This Drug, Observe the Following**

Foods: DO NOT take this medicine with grapefruit or grapefruit juice. Avoid excessive salt intake.

Herbal Medicines or Minerals: Ginseng may increase blood pressure, blunting the benefits of these medicines. Hawthorn, saw palmetto, ma huang, goldenseal, yohimbe and licorice may also increase blood pressure. Calcium and garlic may help lower blood pressure. Indian snakeroot has a German Commission E monograph indication for hypertension—talk to your doctor. Eleuthero root and ephedra should be avoided by people living with hypertension. Talk to your doctor before combining any herbal medicine or mineral with isradipine.

Beverages: DO NOT take this medicine with grapefruit or grapefruit juice. May be taken with milk.

▷ *Alcohol:* Use caution. Alcohol may exaggerate the drop in blood pressure in some people.

Tobacco Smoking: Nicotine may reduce the effectiveness of this drug. I advise everyone to quit smoking.

Marijuana Smoking: Possible reduced effectiveness; mild to moderate increase in angina; possible changes in electrocardiogram, confusing interpretation.

▷ *Other Drugs*

Isradipine *taken concurrently* with

- amiodarone (Cordarone) should be avoided in people with certain kinds of heart conduction problems (partial atrioventricular block or "sick sinus" syndrome).
- antifungals (triazoles) such as fluconazole (Diflucan), itraconazole (Sporanox) or ketoconazole (Nizoral) may lead to toxicity.

- beta-blocker drugs or digitalis preparations (see Drug Classes) may affect heart rate and rhythm adversely. Careful monitoring by your physician is needed if these drugs are taken concurrently.
- carbamazepine (Tegretol) has resulted in decreased blood levels of carbamazepine with calcium channel blockers from the same pharmacological family. Caution is advised.
- delavirdine (Rescriptor) may lead to isradipine toxicity.
- digoxin (Lanoxin) may increase blood levels. Laboratory testing of blood levels should be performed more often if these drugs are combined.
- erythromycin (various) may increase the free (active) form of isradipine, resulting in a larger than expected effect.
- magnesium (various)—especially in doses used in premature labor, can cause very low and abnormal blood pressure.
- nonsteroidal anti-inflammatory drugs (NSAIDs; see Drug Classes) may blunt benefits of isradipine.
- oral anticoagulant medicines (such as Coumadin or warfarin) may lead to increased risk of bleeding from the stomach or intestines.
- phenytoin (Dilantin) may result in loss of isradipine's effectiveness. Caution is advised.
- rifampin (Rifadin, others) may result in a decreased therapeutic benefit from isradipine.
- ritonavir (Norvir) and perhaps other protease inhibitors (see Drug Classes) can lead to toxicity.

▷ *Driving, Hazardous Activities:* Usually no restrictions. This drug may cause drowsiness or dizziness. Restrict activities as necessary.

Aviation Note: Coronary artery disease and hypertension ***are disqualifications*** for piloting. Consult a designated Aviation Medical Examiner.

Exposure to Sun: No restrictions.

Exposure to Heat: Caution is advised. Hot environments can exaggerate the blood-pressure-lowering effects of this drug. Observe for light-headedness or weakness.

Heavy Exercise or Exertion: This drug may improve your ability to be more active without resulting in angina pain. Use caution and avoid excessive exercise that could impair heart function in the absence of warning pain.

Discontinuation: Do not stop this drug abruptly. Ask your doctor about gradual withdrawal. Watch for the development of rebound angina.

KETOCONAZOLE (kee toh KOHN a zohl)

Introduced: 1981   **Class:** Antifungal   **Prescription:** USA:Yes
Controlled Drug: USA: No; Canada: No   **Available as Generic:** USA: Yes; Canada: No
Brand Name: ✣Apo-Ketoconazole, Nizoral, ✣Nu-Ketocon

```
                    BENEFITS versus RISKS
        Possible Benefits                Possible Risks
EFFECTIVE TREATMENT OF THE      SERIOUS DRUG-INDUCED LIVER
  FOLLOWING FUNGUS                 DAMAGE
  INFECTIONS: blastomycosis,     Allergic reactions
  candidiasis, chromomycosis,    Low blood platelets and anemia
  coccidioidomycosis, histoplasmosis,  Some serious drug interactions
  paracoccidioidomycosis, tinea
  (ringworm)
Beneficial short-term treatment of
  advanced prostate cancer
Beneficial auxiliary treatment of
  Cushing's syndrome
```

▷ **Principal Uses**

As a Single Drug Product: Uses currently included in FDA-approved labeling: Treatment of (1) lung and systemic blastomycosis; (2) Candida (yeast) infections of the skin, mouth, throat and esophagus (may be AIDS-related); (3) systemic Candida infections—pneumonia, peritonitis, urinary tract infections (may be AIDS-related); (4) chromomycosis (auxiliary); (5) lung and systemic coccidioidomycosis; (6) lung and systemic histoplasmosis; (7) paracoccidioidomycosis; (8) tinea infections—groin (jock itch) and feet (athlete's foot); (9) tinea versicolor (pityriasis); (10) fungal dandruff (topical).

Other (unlabeled) generally accepted uses: Treatment of (1) Candida infections of the vulva and vagina; (2) prostate cancer (short-term); (3) Cushing's syndrome (excessive adrenal hormones); (4) systemic sporotrichosis; (5) fungal toenail infections; (6) visceral leishmaniasis.

How This Drug Works: As an antifungal: By damaging cell walls and impairing critical cell enzymes, this drug inhibits cell growth and reproduction (with low drug levels) and destroys fungal cells (with high drug concentrations).

In treating prostate cancer: Decreases testosterone (male hormone) levels—and prostate cancer needs testosterone to grow.

In treating Cushing's syndrome: This drug suppresses the excessive production of adrenal corticosteroid hormones.

Available Dosage Forms and Strengths

Cream — 2% (for local application to Candida or tinea skin infections)

Oral suspension — 100 mg/5 ml (Canada)

Shampoo — 2%

Tablets — 200 mg (U.S. and Canada)

▷ **Recommended Dosage Ranges** (Actual dose and schedule must be determined for each patient individually.)

Infants and Children: Up to 2 years of age—Dose not established.

Over 2 years of age—3.3 to 6.6 mg per kg of body mass, once daily; the dose depends upon the nature of the infection.

12 to 60 Years of Age: For fungus infections—200 to 400 mg once daily; 800 mg maximum daily dose.

For prostate cancer—400 mg three times daily; 1,200 mg maximum daily dose. For Cushing's syndrome—600 to 1,200 mg once daily; total daily dose should not exceed 1,200 mg.

Over 60 Years of Age: Same as 12 to 60 years of age.

Conditions Requiring Dosing Adjustments

Liver Function: Dose empirically decreased for patients with liver compromise.

Kidney Function: Decreased doses are not needed in kidney compromise.

Achlorhydria (lack of acid in the stomach): This medicine requires an acid environment in the stomach to be absorbed. Talk with your doctor about making a dilute acid solution to drink prior to taking the tablet form.

▷ **Dosing Instructions:** The tablet may be crushed and is best taken with or after food to enhance absorption and reduce stomach irritation. Do not take with antacids. Take the full course prescribed. If you forget a dose: Take the missed dose as soon as you remember it, unless it's nearly time for your next dose—if that is the case, skip the missed dose and take the next dose right on schedule. Talk with your doctor if you find yourself missing doses.

Usual Duration of Use: Use on a regular schedule for 2 to 4 weeks determines effectiveness in controlling fungal infections. Actual cures or long-term suppression often requires continual treatment for many months. Periodic physician evaluation of response and dose adjustment are essential.

Typical Treatment Goals and Measurements (Outcomes and Markers)

Fungal infections: Resolution of signs and symptoms of infection (such as sore throat and white coloration in candidal throat infections), return of white blood cell count and differential to normal (for systemic infections), and failure of the infection to return in prophylactic use. Blood levels can be used to guide dosing in serious infections or in the case of relapses.

▷ **This Drug Should Not Be Taken If**
- you have had an allergic reaction to it previously.
- you have active liver disease.
- you take astemizole, cisapride, triazolam or sildenafil.

▷ **Inform Your Physician Before Taking This Drug If**
- you are allergic to related antifungal drugs: clotrimazole, fluconazole, itraconazole or miconazole.
- you have a liver disease or impaired liver function.
- you take loratadine. Heart problems have not been reported as with other nonsedating antihistamines, but the blood level does increase if the drugs are combined; the dose of loratadine may need to be decreased.
- you have a history of adrenal gland problems (adrenal insufficiency).
- you have a history of low blood platelets or anemia.
- you have a history of alcoholism.
- you have a deficiency of stomach hydrochloric acid.
- you are taking any other drugs currently.

Possible Side Effects (natural, expected and unavoidable drug actions)

Suppression of testosterone and adrenal corticosteroid hormone production (more pronounced with high drug doses).

▷ **Possible Adverse Effects** (unusual, unexpected and infrequent reactions)

If any of the following develop, consult your physician promptly for guidance.

Mild Adverse Effects

Allergic reactions: skin rash, hives, itching—rare.

Headache, dizziness, drowsiness, photophobia—infrequent.

Nausea (helped by taking with meals) and vomiting, stomach pain, diarrhea—rare.

Increased blood pressure—possible.

Hair loss (alopecia) or ringing in the ears—case reports.

Muscle and joint aches—infrequent.

Serious Adverse Effects

Allergic reactions: anaphylactic reaction (see Glossary).

Severe liver toxicity: loss of appetite, nausea, yellow skin or eyes, dark urine, light-colored stools (see Jaundice in Glossary)—rare.

Suppression of the adrenal gland or low thyroid function—case reports.

Mental depression—rare.

Hemolytic anemia or abnormally low platelet counts (abnormal bruising or bleeding)—rare.

▷ **Possible Effects on Sexual Function:** Decreased testosterone blood levels: reduced sperm counts, decreased libido, impotence, male breast enlargement and tenderness (gynecomastia)—case reports.

Altered menstrual patterns—case reports.

Possible Delayed Adverse Effects: Deficiency of adrenal corticosteroid hormones (cortisone related); this could be serious during stress resulting from illness or injury.

▷ **Adverse Effects That May Mimic Natural Diseases or Disorders**

Drug-induced liver reaction may suggest viral hepatitis.

Possible Effects on Laboratory Tests

Complete blood cell counts: decreased red cells, white cells and platelets.

Liver function tests: increased liver enzymes (ALT/GPT, AST/GOT and alkaline phosphatase), increased bilirubin.

Thyroid function tests: decreased—rare.

Adrenal corticosteroid blood levels: decreased.

Testosterone blood levels: decreased.

CAUTION

1. This drug inhibits several liver enzymes (CYP 3A4, 1A2, 2C9 and 2C19). If you combine medicines with ketoconazole that are removed by these liver enzymes, there may be serious increases in effect or blood levels (toxicity) of those drugs.

Precautions for Use

By Infants and Children: Safety and effectiveness for under 2 years old not established.

By Those Over 60 Years of Age: This drug requires an acid stomach to enter the body. Talk with your doctor if achlorhydria (gastric) has been diagnosed.

▷ **Advisability of Use During Pregnancy**

Pregnancy Category: C. See Pregnancy Risk Categories at the back of this book.

Animal studies: Rat studies revealed significant embryo toxicity and birth defects due to this drug.

Human studies: Adequate studies of pregnant women are not available.

Use this drug only if clearly needed. Ask your physician for guidance.

Advisability of Use If Breast-Feeding
Presence of this drug in breast milk: Yes.
Avoid drug or refrain from nursing.

Habit-Forming Potential: None.

Effects of Overdose: Possible nausea, vomiting, diarrhea.

Possible Effects of Long-Term Use: Suppression of adrenal corticosteroid hormone production, requiring replacement therapy during periods of stress.

Suggested Periodic Examinations While Taking This Drug (at physician's discretion)
Liver function tests should be obtained BEFORE long-term therapy is started and checked monthly during treatment.
Sperm counts.

▷ **While Taking This Drug, Observe the Following**
Foods: No restrictions.
Herbal Medicines or Minerals: Some patients use echinacea to attempt to boost their immune systems. Unfortunately, use of echinacea is not recommended in people with damaged immune systems. This herb may also actually weaken any immune system if it is used too often or for too long a time. If you are considering St. John's wort, caution is advised as it can alter the liver enzymes involved in ketoconazole removal and can also cause sun sensitivity.
Beverages: No restrictions. May be taken with milk.
▷ *Alcohol:* Avoid completely. Alcohol can cause a disulfiramlike reaction (see Glossary). In addition, alcohol may cause liver toxicity.
Tobacco Smoking: No interactions expected. I advise everyone to quit smoking.

▷ **Other Drugs**
Ketoconazole may *increase* the effects of
- alprazolam (Xanax) and other benzodiazepines (see Drug Classes).
- carbamazepine (Tegretol).
- cortisonelike drugs (prednisone, etc.).
- cyclosporine (Sandimmune).
- delavirdine (Rescriptor).
- dihydropyridine calcium channel blockers (nifedipine, nicardipine, amlodipine, isradipine and felodipine). Caution is advised.
- HMG-CoA reductase inhibitors (atorvastatin, cerivastatin, etc.; see Drug Classes), increasing risk of myopathy.
- loratadine (Claritin) and fexofenadine (Allegra), which are also minimally sedating antihistamines, but HAVE NOT been associated with heart rhythm problems when combined with ketoconazole. The blood level does appear to increase, and lower doses of both medicines may be prudent if these medicines are to be combined.
- oral antidiabetic drugs (see Drug Classes) and result in very low blood sugars.
- medicines removed by liver cytochrome P450 3A4 because ketoconazole inhibits this medicine removing enzyme system. Extreme caution is advised.
- nonsedating antihistamines, such as astemizole (Hismanal) and terfenadine (Seldane) (now removed from the US market) and may cause large

increases in blood levels and result in serious heart rhythm problems. DO NOT COMBINE.

- protease inhibitors (see Drug Classes).
- quetiapine (Seroquel).
- quinidine (Quinaglute) and cause toxicity; blood levels are needed.
- ritonavir (Norvir) and other liver-removed (such as amprenavir [Agenerase]) protease inhibitors.
- sibutramine (Meridia) can lead to sibutramine toxicity. Caution is advised.
- sildenafil (Viagra)—talk to your doctor BEFORE using these medicines together.
- serolimus (Rapamune) or tacrolimus (Prograf) can lead to serolimus or tacrolimus toxicity. More frequent blood levels and dosing adjustments are prudent.
- sucralfate (Carafate), which may decrease the blood levels of ketoconazole.
- tolterodine (Detrol) can lead to tolterodine toxicity. Caution is advised.
- tretinoin (Vesanoid), which may increase risk of tretinoin toxicity.
- trimexate (Neutrexin).
- warfarin (Coumadin) and cause bleeding; increased testing of INR (prothrombin time or protime) are needed.

Ketoconazole may *decrease* the effects of
- amphotericin B (Abelcet).
- didanosine (Videx).
- theophyllines (aminophylline, Theo-Dur, etc.).

The following drugs may *decrease* the effects of ketoconazole:
- antacids; if needed, take antacids 2 hours after ketoconazole.
- histamine (H2) blocking drugs: cimetidine, famotidine, nizatidine, ranitidine; if needed, take 2 hours after ketoconazole.
- isoniazid (Laniazid, Nydrazid, etc.).
- lansoprazole (Prevacid).
- omeprazole (Prilosec), or other proton pump inhibitors.
- rifampin (Rifadin, Rifater, Rimactane, etc.).

Ketoconazole *taken concurrently* with
- cisapride (Propulsid) can lead to serious heart toxicity. DO NOT COMBINE.
- dofetilide (Tikosyn) can lead to serious heart toxicity. DO NOT COMBINE.
- miconazole (Monistat) may increase the blood levels of ketoconazole or miconazole.
- phenytoin (Dilantin) or fosphenytoin (Cerebyx) may change the levels of both drugs.

▷ *Driving, Hazardous Activities:* This drug may cause dizziness or drowsiness. Restrict activities as necessary.

Aviation Note: The use of this drug *may be a disqualification* for piloting. Consult a designated Aviation Medical Examiner.

Exposure to Sun: This drug may cause photophobia; wear sunglasses if appropriate.

Discontinuation: Take the full course prescribed. Continual treatment for several months may be needed. Ask your doctor when the drug should be stopped.

KETOPROFEN (kee toh PROH fen)

Please see the propionic acid (nonsteroidal anti-inflammatory drug) family profile.

LABETALOL (la BET a lohl)

Introduced: 1978   **Class:** Antihypertensive, alpha- and beta-adrenergic blocker   **Prescription:** USA: Yes   **Controlled Drug:** USA: No; Canada: No   **Available as Generic:** Yes

Brand Names: Normodyne, Normozide [CD], Trandate, Trandate HCT [CD]

<table>
<tr><td colspan="2" align="center">BENEFITS versus RISKS</td></tr>
<tr><td align="center">Possible Benefits</td><td align="center">Possible Risks</td></tr>
<tr><td>EFFECTIVE, WELL-TOLERATED ANTIHYPERTENSIVE in mild to moderate high blood pressure
PROLONGS LIFE AFTER A HEART ATTACK</td><td>CONGESTIVE HEART FAILURE in advanced heart disease
Worsening of angina in coronary heart disease (if drug is abruptly withdrawn)
Masking of low blood sugar (hypoglycemia) in drug-treated diabetes
Liver toxicity</td></tr>
</table>

▷ **Principal Uses**

As a Single Drug Product: Uses currently included in FDA-approved labeling: (1) Treats mild to moderate high blood pressure; (2) treats hypertension in pregnancy.

Other (unlabeled) generally accepted uses: (1) Combination therapy of hypertension in heart attacks (acute MI)—beta blockers have also been shown to decrease the risk of repeat heart attacks, limit the size of the original heart attack damage and help control arrhythmias; (2) treatment of cocaine overdose; (3) therapy of phobic anxiety reactions; (4) treatment of angina; (5) therapy of pheochromocytoma, a tumor that releases compounds that increase blood pressure (controversial).

As a Combination Drug Product [CD]: This drug has been combined with hydrochlorothiazide (a thiazide diuretic) to attack high blood pressure in two different ways.

How This Drug Works: By blocking part of the sympathetic nervous system, this drug:

- reduces the rate and contraction force of the heart, thus lowering the ejection pressure of blood leaving the heart.
- reduces the degree of contraction of blood vessel walls, resulting in their expansion and lowering of blood pressure.

Available Dosage Forms and Strengths

Injection — 5 mg/ml

Tablets — 100 mg, 200 mg, 300 mg

▷ **Usual Adult Dosage Ranges:** *High blood pressure*: Initially 100 mg twice daily, 12 hours apart; the dose may be increased by 100 mg twice daily every 2 to 3 days as needed to reduce blood pressure. The usual ongoing dose is 200 to 400 mg twice daily. Maximum daily dose is 2,400 mg daily, given as 800 mg three times daily.

Stable angina: 100 to 400 mg by mouth two to three times daily. Low doses (100 mg) are usually used in people who have normal blood pressure to help avoid excessively low blood pressure on standing up. **Note: Actual dose and dosing schedule must be determined individually.**

Conditions Requiring Dosing Adjustments

Liver Function: The dose must be decreased in liver disease. Average dose for people with long-standing liver disease is 50% of the usual dose. This drug is a rare cause of liver injury.

Kidney Function: No changes presently needed.

▷ **Dosing Instructions:** The tablet may be crushed and is best taken at the same times daily, ideally following morning and evening meals. Do not stop this drug abruptly. If you forget a dose: take the missed dose as soon as you remember it, unless it's within 8 hours of the next scheduled dose—if that is the case, skip the missed dose and take the next dose right on schedule. Talk with your doctor if you find yourself missing doses.

Usual Duration of Use: Use on a regular schedule for 10 to 14 days determines effectiveness in lowering blood pressure. Long-term use (months to years) is determined by individual response to this drug and a program (weight reduction, salt restriction, smoking cessation, etc.).

Typical Treatment Goals and Measurements (Outcomes and Markers)

Blood pressure: The most recent treatment guidelines (JNC VI) actually define optimal blood pressure (BP) as less than 120/80 and high normal as 139/89. The American Diabetes Association has chosen a target of 130/80 as the blood pressure goal for people living with diabetes. Most clinicians try to achieve a BP that achieves the best balance of lower cardiovascular risk while avoiding the problem of too low a blood pressure. The goal and time frame (see peak benefits above) should be discussed with you when the prescription is written.

Possible Advantages of This Drug

Decreases blood pressure more rapidly than other beta-blocker drugs. Can be used to treat hypertensive emergencies.

▷ **This Drug Should Not Be Taken If**
- you have had an allergic reaction to it previously.
- you have active bronchial asthma.
- you have congestive heart failure.
- you are in cardiogenic shock.
- your blood pressure is very low or you have a condition that causes severe lowering of blood pressure for a long time.
- you have an abnormally slow heart rate or a serious form of heart block.

▷ **Inform Your Physician Before Taking This Drug If**
- you have had an adverse reaction to any beta-blocker drug (see Drug Classes).
- you have a history of serious heart disease.

- you have a history of hay fever (allergic rhinitis), asthma, chronic bronchitis or emphysema.
- you have a history of overactive thyroid function (hyperthyroidism).
- you have a history of low blood sugar (hypoglycemia).
- you have sporadic cramping of the leg muscles (intermittent claudication).
- you have a history of spasms of the bronchi of the lungs.
- you have impaired liver or kidney function.
- you have diabetes or myasthenia gravis.
- you take any form of digitalis, quinidine or reserpine or any calcium-channel-blocker drug (see Drug Classes).
- you will have surgery with general anesthesia.

Possible Side Effects (natural, expected and unavoidable drug actions)
Lethargy and fatigability—frequent.
Light-headedness in upright position (see orthostatic hypotension in Glossary).

▷ **Possible Adverse Effects** (unusual, unexpected and infrequent reactions)
If any of the following develop, consult your physician promptly for guidance.
Mild Adverse Effects
Allergic reactions: skin rash, itching.
Headache, drowsiness, dizziness—frequent.
Scalp tingling (during early treatment)—possible.
Vivid dreams, nightmares, depression—infrequent.
Urine retention, difficulty urinating—case reports.
Indigestion, nausea, diarrhea—infrequent.
Joint and muscle discomfort, fluid retention (edema)—rare.
Serious Adverse Effects
Allergic reactions: anaphylaxis—case reports.
Chest pain, shortness of breath, precipitation of congestive heart failure—possible.
Induction of bronchial asthma (in asthmatic individuals)—possible.
Hypertensive crisis in people with pheochromocytoma—case reports.
Lichen planus—case reports.
Muscle toxicity (toxic myopathy, worsening of intermittent claudication)—possible.
Drug-induced systemic lupus erythematosus—rare.
Aggravation of myasthenia gravis—case reports.
Liver damage with jaundice—rare and often reversible.

▷ **Possible Effects on Sexual Function:** Impotence, inhibited ejaculation, prolonged erection following orgasm (related to higher doses), Peyronie's disease (see Glossary)—rare to infrequent.
Decreased vaginal secretions (with low doses), inhibited female orgasm (higher doses)—possible.

Possible Effects on Laboratory Tests
Blood potassium or glucose: slight increase.
Liver function tests: rare increases.

CAUTION
1. ***Do not stop this drug suddenly*** without the knowledge and help of your doctor. Carry a note or wear a labetalol drug-identification bracelet.

2. Ask your physician or pharmacist before using nasal decongestants, which are usually present in over-the-counter cold preparations and nose drops. These can cause sudden increases in blood pressure if combined with labetalol.
3. Report the development of any tendency to emotional depression.

Precautions for Use

By Infants and Children: Safety and effectiveness for those under 12 years of age are not established. If this drug is used, however, watch for low blood sugar (hypoglycemia) during periods of reduced food intake.

By Those Over 60 Years of Age: Proceed *cautiously* with all antihypertensive drugs. Therapy should be started with small doses, with frequent checks of blood pressure. Sudden, rapid or excessive lowering of blood pressure can increase stroke or heart attack risk. Watch for dizziness, unsteadiness, tendency to fall, confusion, hallucinations, depression or urinary frequency.

▷ **Advisability of Use During Pregnancy**

Pregnancy Category: C. See Pregnancy Risk Categories at the back of this book.

Animal studies: No significant increase in birth defects found in rats or rabbits; some increase in fetal deaths reported.

Human studies: Adequate studies of pregnant women are not available.

Use this drug only if clearly needed. Ask your physician for guidance.

Advisability of Use If Breast-Feeding

Presence of this drug in breast milk: Yes, in very small amounts.

Avoid drug or refrain from nursing.

Habit-Forming Potential: None.

Effects of Overdose: Weakness, slow pulse, low blood pressure, fainting, cold and sweaty skin, congestive heart failure, possible coma and convulsions.

Possible Effects of Long-Term Use: Reduced heart reserve and eventual heart failure in susceptible individuals with advanced heart disease.

Suggested Periodic Examinations While Taking This Drug (at physician's discretion)

Measurements of blood pressure.

Evaluation of heart function.

▷ **While Taking This Drug, Observe the Following**

Foods: May increase the absorption of labetalol and result in a larger than expected blood level. Patients taking this medicine should also avoid excessive salt intake.

Herbal Medicines or Minerals: Ginseng may increase blood pressure, blunting the benefits of these medicines. Hawthorn, saw palmetto, ma huang, goldenseal, yohimbe and licorice may also increase blood pressure. Calcium and garlic may help lower blood pressure. Indian snakeroot has a German Commission E monograph indication for hypertension—talk to your doctor. Eleuthero root and ephedra should be avoided by people living with hypertension.

Beverages: No restrictions. May be taken with milk.

▷ *Alcohol:* Use with caution. Alcohol may exaggerate this drug's ability to lower blood pressure and may increase its mild sedative effect.

Tobacco Smoking: Nicotine may reduce this drug's effectiveness. I advise everyone to quit smoking.

▷   *Other Drugs*

Labetalol may ***increase*** the effects of

- oral antidiabetic drugs (see Drug Classes) and prolong recovery from any hypoglycemia (low blood sugar) that may occur.
- other antihypertensive drugs and cause excessive lowering of blood pressure. Dose adjustments may be necessary.

Labetalol ***taken concurrently*** with

- amiodarone (Cordarone) may result in extremely slow heart rates and cardiac arrest.
- cimetidine (Tagamet) can cause elevated labetalol levels and low blood pressure or heart rate.
- clonidine (Catapres) must be closely watched for rebound high blood pressure if clonidine is withdrawn while labetalol is still being taken.
- digoxin's (Lanoxin) atrioventricular node conduction time extension may cause heart block and digoxin toxicity.
- dihydropyridine calcium channel blockers (nifedipine, others) may lead to impaired heart performance or excessively lowered blood pressure.
- epinephrine may result in severe increases in blood pressure.
- fluoxetine (Prozac) may increase labetalol effects.
- fluvoxamine (Luvox) may result in excessive lowering of blood pressure or excessive slowing of the heart.
- imipramine and other tricyclic antidepressants may result in increases in antidepressant blood levels and toxicity.
- insulin must be watched for development of hypoglycemia (see Glossary).
- NSAIDs (see Drug Classes) may result in blunting of the therapeutic effects of labetalol.
- paroxetine (Paxil) may increase labetalol effects.
- phenothiazines (see Drug Classes) may cause additive lowering of the blood pressure.
- ritodrine (Yutopar) may blunt the beneficial effects of ritodrine.
- venlafaxine (Effexor) may increase labetalol effects.
- zileuton (Zyflo) may increase labetalol effects.

▷   *Driving, Hazardous Activities:* Use caution until the full extent of fatigue, dizziness and blood pressure change has been determined.

Aviation Note: The use of this drug ***is a disqualification*** for piloting. Consult a designated Aviation Medical Examiner.

Exposure to Sun: No restrictions.

Exposure to Heat: Caution is advised. Hot environments can lower the blood pressure and exaggerate the effects of this drug.

Exposure to Cold: Caution is advised. Cold environments can increase blood flow problems in the extremities that may occur with beta-blocker drugs. The elderly should take precautions to prevent hypothermia (see Glossary).

Heavy Exercise or Exertion: It is prudent to avoid exertion that produces light-headedness, excessive fatigue or muscle cramping. Use of this drug may intensify hypertensive response to isometric exercise.

Occurrence of Unrelated Illness: Fever can lower blood pressure and require decreased doses. Nausea or vomiting may interrupt scheduled doses. Ask your doctor for help.

Discontinuation: If possible, gradual reduction of dose over a period of 2 to 3 weeks is recommended—otherwise rebound increases in blood pressure may occur. Ask your doctor for help.

LAMIVUDINE (LAM iv u deen)

Introduced: 1995   **Class:** Antiviral, antiretroviral, reverse transcriptase inhibitor, nucleoside analog   **Prescription:** USA: Yes   **Controlled Drug:** USA: No   **Available as Generic:** No
Brand Names: Combivir, Epivir, Epivir HBV, Trizivir (Investigational)

BENEFITS versus RISKS	
Possible Benefits	*Possible Risks*
IMPRESSIVE SUPPRESSION OF VIRAL LOAD WHEN USED IN COMBINATION THERAPY TREATING HIV	DECREASED WHITE BLOOD CELL COUNTS
	Peripheral neuropathy
DOES NOT LEAD TO SUPPRESSION OF THE BONE MARROW	Pancreatitis
	Lactic acidosis
EFFECTIVE TREATMENT OF HEPATITIS B INFECTION	

▷ **Principal Uses**

As a Single Drug Product: Uses currently included in FDA-approved labeling: (1) Used to treat HIV infection. Used in combination because of possible resistance; this medicine was one of the three drugs used together—indinavir (a protease inhibitor) and AZT (a nucleoside analog)—that resulted in decrease of HIV virus levels to undetectable amounts. (2) Used with zidovudine (AZT) and other antiretrovirals to reduce the risk of disease progression and death in HIV. **Author's Note:** *The Panel on Clinical Practices for Treatment of HIV Infection Report* **rejected single-agent therapy.** (3) FDA-approved (in a lower dose than that used for treating HIV) to treat hepatitis B.

Other (unlabeled) generally accepted uses: None at present.

As a Combination Drug Product [CD]: Available in combination with zidovudine, a nucleoside analog. This combination along with a protease inhibitor (indinavir) was one of the first regimens to decrease HIV viral burden to undetectable levels.

How This Drug Works: Potent reverse transcriptase inhibitor—interferes with ability of HIV and the hepatitis B virus to create genetic material.

Available Dosage Forms and Strengths

Solution (Epivir) — 10 mg/ml
Solution (Epivir HBV) — 5 mg/ml
Tablets (Combivir) — 150 mg lamivudine and 300 mg zidovudine
Tablets (Trizivir) — 150 mg lamivudine, 300 mg zidovudine and abacavir (investigational)
Tablets (Epivir) — 150 mg
Tablets (Epivir HBV) — 100 mg

▷ **Recommended Dosage Ranges** (Actual dose and schedule must be determined for each patient individually.)

Infants and Children: 3 months to 12 years old: 4 mg per kg of body mass twice daily (300 mg maximum a day).

Combivir (for those over 12 years old): One tablet twice a day.

12 to 65 Years of Age:

HIV: Usual dose is 150 mg twice daily. 2 mg per kg of body mass twice daily for adults weighing less than 110 lb or 50 kg.

Combivir: One tablet twice a day.

Hepatitis B (Epivir HBV): 100 mg daily.

Over 65 Years of Age: If decision is made to use it in this population, blood levels may be prudent, as up to 70% is removed by the kidneys.

Conditions Requiring Dosing Adjustments

Liver Function: No changes expected.

Kidney Function: Up to 70% of a given dose is removed by the kidneys. Those with creatinine clearances (see Glossary) of 5 to 14 ml/min should take a first dose of 150 mg and then 50 mg once daily.

▷ **Dosing Instructions:** Lamivudine tablets and solution can be taken without regard to meals. A solution is available for patients who can't swallow the tablets. If you forget a dose: take the missed dose as soon as you remember it, unless it's nearly time for your next dose—if that is the case, skip the missed dose and take the next dose right on schedule. Talk with your doctor if you find yourself missing doses.

Author's Note: Adherence or taking medicines for HIV exactly on time and in the right amount is ABSOLUTELY critical to getting the best possible results or outcomes. The new antiretroviral therapy guidelines from NIAID take into account how easily the medicine treating HIV can fit into a patient's life.

Usual Duration of Use: *HIV*: Measurement of viral load (burden) and/or CD4 counts are used to decide the effectiveness of treatment and help in the decision to continue or change medications.

Hepatitis B: Clinical studies saw use of lamivudine for one year. The optimal duration of use is yet decided. The question of combination treatment (such as with interferon) of hepatitis B also has yet to be decided.

Typical Treatment Goals and Measurements (Outcomes and Markers)

HIV: Goals for HIV treatment presently are maximum suppression of viral replication, maximum lowering of the amount of virus in your body (viral load or burden), and maximum patient survival. Markers of successful therapy include undetectable viral load, increased CD4 cells, absence of indicator or opportunistic infections (OIs) and in the case of the HIV-positive patient, failure of the infection to progress to AIDS.

Possible Side Effects (natural, expected and unavoidable drug actions)

Paresthesias and/or peripheral neuropathy (12% in a study in children taking lamivudine monotherapy).

▷ **Possible Adverse Effects** (unusual, unexpected and infrequent reactions)

If any of the following develop, consult your physician promptly for guidance.

Mild Adverse Effects

Skin rash—infrequent.

Headache—frequent.

Dizziness—infrequent.

Sleep disorders—infrequent to frequent.

Nausea, vomiting or diarrhea—infrequent to frequent.

Cough—frequent.

Muscle aches—infrequent.

Serious Adverse Effects

Lowered white blood cell counts—infrequent in adults, frequent in pediatrics.

Lactic acid buildup—possible.

Pancreatitis (more common in children receiving lamivudine monotherapy)—infrequent.

Liver toxicity—infrequent.

Seizures—case reports.

▷ **Possible Effects on Sexual Function:** None reported.

Possible Delayed Adverse Effects: Anemia or lowering of white blood cell counts. Pancreatitis. Peripheral neuropathy.

▷ **Adverse Effects That May Mimic Natural Diseases or Disorders**: Seizures may suggest the possibility of epilepsy.

Possible Effects on Laboratory Tests

Complete blood cell counts: decreased red cells.

Increased amylase and lipase (if pancreatitis occurs).

Lactic acidosis—possible.

CAUTION

1. This drug is not a cure for HIV or AIDS; nor does it protect completely against other infections or complications. Follow your doctor's instructions. Take exactly as prescribed.
2. AIDS can still be spread through sexual contact or blood. Use of an effective condom is mandatory. Don't share needles.

Precautions for Use

By Infants and Children: Patients from 3 months to 12 years old are dosed on a mg-per-kg-of-body-mass basis.

By Those Over 60 Years of Age: Probable age-related decline in kidney function requires blood levels to check need for dose reduction.

▷ **Advisability of Use During Pregnancy**

Pregnancy Category: C. See Pregnancy Risk Categories at the back of this book.

Animal studies: Rat and rabbit studies reveal no birth defects.

Human studies: Adequate studies of pregnant women are not available.

Your physician should call 1-800-722-9292, ext. 38465, if the decision is made to use this medicine while you are pregnant.

Advisability of Use If Breast-Feeding

Presence of this drug in breast milk: Unknown.

Refrain from nursing (HIV may be transferred via breast milk).

Habit-Forming Potential: None.

Effects of Overdose: Nausea, vomiting, diarrhea, bone marrow depression.

Possible Effects of Long-Term Use: Anemia and loss of white blood cells.

Pancreatitis or peripheral neuropathy.

Suggested Periodic Examinations While Taking This Drug (at physician's discretion)

Complete blood counts.

Periodic CD4 counts or viral load tests are needed. Increasing viral load or decreasing CD4 are indicators that therapy is failing and demand change of antiretroviral therapy.

Amylase and lipase. Check for peripheral neuropathy.

Tests for lactic acidosis.

Liver biopsy may need to be taken periodically to assess the success of this medicine in treating hepatitis. Slightly more than half of patients responded in clinical trials.

▷ **While Taking This Drug, Observe the Following**

Foods: No restrictions.

Herbal Medicines or Minerals: Milk thistle has some data to support its role as an antioxidant and may help promote liver cell regeneration. Talk to your doctor if lamivudine is being used to treat the infection of hepatitis B and you are considering milk thistle. Echinacea: Some patients use echinacea to attempt to boost their immune systems. Unfortunately, use of echinacea is not recommended in people with damaged immune systems. This herb may also actually weaken any immune system if it is used too often or for too long a time.

Beverages: No restrictions. May be taken with milk.

▷ *Alcohol:* No interactions expected.

Tobacco Smoking: No interactions expected. I advise everyone to quit smoking.

▷ *Other Drugs*

Lamivudine *taken concurrently* with

- cotrimoxazole (Septra, Bactrim) may increase lamivudine blood levels.
- indinavir (Crixivan) and zidovudine (AZT) resulted in undetectable HIV levels in some HIV-positive patients.
- nelfinavir (Viracept) may increase lamivudine levels.
- other medicines capable of causing pancreatitis may result in increased pancreatitis risk.
- other medicines capable of lowering white or red cell counts may cause additive risks.
- sulfamethoxazole (various) may increase lamivudine levels.
- trimethoprim (various) may increase lamivudine levels.
- trimexate (Mexate) may cause additive blood (hematological) toxicity.

▷ *Driving, Hazardous Activities:* This drug may cause dizziness or fainting. Restrict activities as necessary.

Aviation Note: The use of this drug *is a disqualification* for piloting. Consult a designated Aviation Medical Examiner.

Exposure to Sun: No restrictions.

Discontinuation: Do not stop this drug without your physician's knowledge and guidance.

LAMOTRIGINE (la MOH tri jean)

Introduced: 1995   **Class:** Anticonvulsant,   phenyltriazine   **Prescription:** USA: Yes   **Controlled Drug:** USA: No; Canada: No   **Available as Generic:** USA: No

Brand Name: Lamictal

BENEFITS versus RISKS

Possible Benefits	*Possible Risks*
EFFECTIVE MANAGEMENT OF SEIZURES THAT RESIST THERAPY	RASHES THAT CAN BE LIFE-THREATENING
INCREASE IN SEIZURE-FREE DAYS	Changes in vision
MANAGEMENT OF PARTIAL SEIZURES	Dizziness
MANAGEMENT OF SEIZURES ASSOCIATED WITH LENNOX-GASTAUT SYNDROME	

▷ **Principal Uses**

As a Single Drug Product: Uses currently included in FDA-approved labeling: Adjunctive combination therapy of partial seizures in adults who have not responded to treatment with other medicines.

Other (unlabeled) generally accepted uses: (1) May have a role in treating epilepsy in children who have not responded to more established treatment; (2) could have a role in treating status epilepticus; (3) of use in treating Lennox-Gastaut syndrome; (4) could have a role in some pain syndromes (trigeminal neuralgia).

How This Drug Works: The exact mechanism of action is not known, but animal models appear to show that this medicine blocks voltage-dependent sodium channels. This causes a decreased amount of glutamate and aspartate transmitters and a decreased likelihood of seizures.

Available Dosage Forms and Strengths

Chewable tablets — 5 mg, 25 mg

Tablets — 25 mg, 100 mg, 150 mg, 200 mg

▷ **Recommended Dosage Ranges** (Actual dose and schedule must be determined for each patient individually.)

Infants and Children: Safety and efficacy in those less than 16 years old have not been established. Some researchers used lamotrigine in treating intractable epilepsy: 2 to 15 mg per kg of body mass divided into two equal doses and given every 12 hours.

16 to 65 Years of Age: In patients receiving medicines known to interact (phenytoin, primidone, carbamazepine or phenobarbital but not valproic acid), starting dose is 50 mg a day for 2 weeks and then 50 mg twice a day as needed or tolerated (increases made at 100 mg a day each week). Most patients end up taking 300–500 mg a day in two equal doses. Some centers have used doses as high as 700 mg a day.

Patients only taking valproic acid and/or the above drugs: 25 mg every other day for 2 weeks and then 25 mg once daily for 2 weeks, with increases of 25 to 50 mg per day at 1- to 2-week intervals to a maximum of 150 mg daily as needed and tolerated.

Over 65 Years of Age: Same dosing as 16 to 65 (single-dose pharmacokinetics were similar to younger adults). Few patients over 65 were included during premarketing studies.

Conditions Requiring Dosing Adjustments

Liver Function: This drug is mostly changed in the liver, but guidelines are not available for adjusting the dose.

Kidney Function: Most of this medicine (once changed or glucuronidated) is removed by the kidneys. Used with caution and with blood levels (in severe kidney failure).

▷ **Dosing Instructions:** Take this medicine exactly as prescribed. Food does not affect how much medicine gets into your body. Talk with your doctor IMMEDIATELY if you get a rash, swollen lymph glands and fever. If you forget a dose: take the missed dose as soon as you remember it, unless it's nearly time for your next dose—if that is the case, skip the missed dose and take the next dose right on schedule. Talk with your doctor if you find yourself missing doses.

Usual Duration of Use: Regular use for 3 months in children with resistant seizures may be needed to see peak benefits. Long-term use (months to years) will be determined by individual response.

Typical Treatment Goals and Measurements (Outcomes and Markers)

Seizures: The general goal for this medicine is effective seizure control. Neurologists tend to define effective on a case by case basis depending on the seizure type and patient factors.

Possible Advantages of This Drug

May work where single medicines have failed.

▷ **This Drug Should Not Be Taken If**

- you have developed a rash with swollen lymph glands while taking this medicine.
- you are allergic to this medicine or ones similar to it.

▷ **Inform Your Physician Before Taking This Drug If**

- you develop a rash.
- your heart function is compromised.
- you do not understand how much or how often to take it.
- you have liver or kidney damage.

Possible Side Effects (natural, expected and unavoidable drug actions)

Somnolence.

Weight gain.

▷ **Possible Adverse Effects** (unusual, unexpected and infrequent reactions)

If any of the following develop, consult your physician promptly for guidance.

Mild Adverse Effects

Allergic reactions: skin rash (should be reported to your doctor), itching—infrequent.

Dizziness and headache—most common adverse effects.

Problems coordinating movements (ataxia)—infrequent.

Muscle tremor, chills or nerve tingling (peripheral neuropathy)—infrequent.

Nausea and vomiting—dose-related and may be frequent.

Blurred vision—dose-related.

Increased liver enzymes—case reports.

Serious Adverse Effects

Allergic reactions: anaphylaxis—case reports.

Serious rashes (Stevens-Johnson syndrome, toxic epidermal necrolysis)—case reports.

Hostility—rare.

Lowered blood platelets (thrombocytopenia) or sudden (acute) disseminated intravascular coagulation—case reports.

Anemia (aplastic and hemolytic)—case reports and questioned cause.

Pure red cell aplasia (PRCA)—case report.

Blood in the urine—infrequent.

Peripheral neuropathy—rare and of questionable cause.

Sudden unexplained death (SUDEP). The rate of SUDEP was similar to that of another agent also tested and appears to be a population effect—case reports.

▷ **Possible Effects on Sexual Function:** None reported.

Possible Effects on Laboratory Tests Blood levels of interacting medicines may be changed.

CAUTION

1. **DO NOT** stop this medicine suddenly, as seizures may occur.

Precautions for Use

By Infants and Children: This medicine is approved for add-on therapy in children over 16 years of age.

By Those Over 60 Years of Age: No specific changes.

▷ **Advisability of Use During Pregnancy**

Pregnancy Category: C. See Pregnancy Risk Categories at the back of this book.

Animal studies: No evidence of drug-related changes were found in mice or rabbits that were given up to 1.2 times the human dose.

Human studies: This medicine has been shown to cause toxicity to the mother and, because of this, toxicity to the fetus. Adequate studies of pregnant women are not available.

Discuss benefits and risks with your doctor.

Advisability of Use If Breast-Feeding

Presence of this drug in breast milk: Yes.

Avoid drug or refrain from nursing.

Habit-Forming Potential: None.

Effects of Overdose: Sleepiness, changes in muscular reflexes, coma. Keep a seizure diary to check for decrease in seizure frequency.

Possible Effects of Long-Term Use: Weight gain.

Suggested Periodic Examinations While Taking This Drug (at physician's discretion)

Examinations for nystagmus, muscular coordination.

Blood counts.

Check for rash.

▷ **While Taking This Drug, Observe the Following**

Foods: No restrictions. Can be taken with or without food.

Herbal Medicines or Minerals: Using St. John's wort, ma huang or kola may result in unacceptable central nervous system stimulation and worsen possible nervousness as a side effect of lamotrigine. Since part of the way that ginseng may work is as an MAO inhibitor, combination with this medicine is not recommended. Valerian and kava kava may interact to increase drowsiness.

Beverages: No restrictions. May be taken with milk.

▷ *Alcohol:* Avoid alcohol use, unless you discuss this with your doctor.

Tobacco Smoking: No interactions expected. I advise everyone to quit smoking.

▷ *Other Drugs*

Lamotrigine *taken concurrently* with

- long-standing use of acetaminophen (Tylenol, others) may result in decreases in blood levels of this medicine and a potential decrease in seizure control. Periodic use should not cause problems.
- carbamazepine (Tegretol) may increase the removal of lamotrigine from the body and require dosing adjustments.
- phenobarbital may result in faster removal of lamotrigine from the body and require dosing changes.
- phenytoin (Dilantin) and fosphenytoin (Cerebyx) may result in faster removal of lamotrigine from the body and require dosing changes.
- primidone (Mysoline) may result in faster removal of lamotrigine from the body and require dosing changes.
- ritonavir (Norvir) may lead to decreased lamotrigine levels and increased risk of seizure.
- sertraline (Zoloft) may lead to lamotrigine toxicity.
- valproic acid (Depakene) may slow removal of lamotrigine from the body, requiring lamotrigine dose decreases to avoid toxicity.

▷ *Driving, Hazardous Activities:* Use caution until the full extent of fatigue, dizziness or coordination or vision changes have been determined.

Aviation Note: The use of this drug *is a disqualification* for piloting. Consult a designated Aviation Medical Examiner.

Exposure to Sun: No restrictions.

Exposure to Heat: Use caution. Muscular coordination problems may be worsened by excessive heat.

Discontinuation: DO NOT stop this medicine abruptly without talking with your doctor first. Abrupt discontinuation without first starting another antiseizure medicine may result in seizures.

LANSOPRAZOLE (lan SO pra sole)

Introduced: 1995   **Class:** Anti-ulcer, proton pump inhibitor   **Prescription:** USA: Yes   **Controlled Drug:** USA: No; Canada: No   **Available as Generic:** USA: No; Canada: No

Brand Name: Prevacid, Prevpac [CD]

BENEFITS versus RISKS	
Possible Benefits	*Possible Risks*
VERY EFFECTIVE TREATMENT OF	Liver enzyme increases
CONDITIONS ASSOCIATED WITH	Protein in the urine
EXCESSIVE PRODUCTION OF	
STOMACH (GASTRIC) ACID:	
ZOLLINGER-ELLISON	
SYNDROME, MASTOCYTOSIS,	
ENDOCRINE ADENOMA	
VERY EFFECTIVE TREATMENT OF	
REFLUX ESOPHAGITIS	
VERY EFFECTIVE TREATMENT OF	
DUODENAL ULCER	
EFFECTIVE MAINTENANCE	
THERAPY OF HEALED	
DUODENAL ULCERS	

▷ **Principal Uses**

As a Single Drug Product: Uses currently included in FDA-approved labeling: (1) Used to treat duodenal and stomach (gastric) ulcers; (2) treats erosive esophagitis; (3) used in syndromes (such as Zollinger-Ellison) where excessive amounts of stomach acid are produced; (4) maintains healed duodenal ulcers; (5) treats gastroesophageal reflux disease; (6) part of dual (with amoxicillin) or triple (with amoxicillin and clarithromycin) treatment of Helicobacter pylori.

Other (unlabeled) generally accepted uses: None.

As a Combination Drug Product [CD]: This drug is available in combination with two antibiotics—clarithromycin and amoxicillin. Since refractory ulcers are often actually Helicobacter pylori infections, the combination works to kill the bacteria and lower acid production.

How This Drug Works: Inhibits an enzyme system (H/K adenosine triphosphate) in the stomach (parietal cells) lining and stops production of stomach acid. By doing this, it eliminates the principal cause of ulcers or esophagitis and creates an environment conducive to healing. Taking this medicine 15–30 minutes before the morning meal makes best use of the fact that this will allow the medicine to be at its peak just when the largest number of proton pumps are working. Use of this drug with one or two antibiotics attacks Helicobacter pylori and also decreases acid.

Available Dosage Forms and Strengths

Capsules — 15 mg, 30 mg

Capsules (Prevpac) — 30 mg lansoprazole, 500 mg amoxicillin and clarithromycin

▷ **Recommended Dosage Ranges** (Actual dose and schedule must be determined for each patient individually.)

Infants and Children: Not studied in this age group.

18 to 60 Years of Age: For duodenal ulcer: 15 mg daily, taken before a meal. Some patients require 30 mg daily. Four weeks of therapy are needed.

For ongoing therapy of healed duodenal ulcers: 15 mg daily.

For erosive esophagitis: 30 mg daily, taken before a meal. Up to 8 weeks of treatment can be given. If healing does not occur, an additional 8 weeks may be considered.

For excessive acid production syndromes: Dosing is started at 60 mg daily. The dose is increased as needed and tolerated. Doses up to 90 mg twice daily have been used. Once the condition is under control, dose usually slowly reduced to 30 mg a day.

For *Helicobacter pylori*: Seven-day regimen for duodenal ulcers and *H. pylori* of lansoprazole 30 mg twice daily, plus amoxicillin 1,000 mg twice daily, plus clarithromycin 500 mg twice daily.

Eradication: The above regimen is used for 14 days.

Over 60 Years of Age: Same as 18 to 60 years of age.

Conditions Requiring Dosing Adjustments

Liver Function: The manufacturer strongly suggests a dose of 15 mg daily for people with significant liver problems.

Kidney Function: No dosing changes are needed.

▷ **Dosing Instructions:** The capsules contain enteric-coated granules that protect the medicine in the stomach's acid. Take the capsules whole. Some studies have found that lansoprazole **taken in the morning** worked the best in controlling stomach acid. It should be taken 15–30 minutes before the morning meal so that the peak level of lansoprazole happens just when the largest number of proton pumps are working. If swallowing is a problem, the capsule may be opened and the intact granules sprinkled into applesauce. Take this medicine exactly as prescribed. If you forget a dose: take the missed dose as soon as you remember it, unless it's nearly time for your next dose—if that is the case, skip the missed dose and take the next dose right on schedule. Talk with your doctor if you find yourself missing doses.

Usual Duration of Use: Use on a regular schedule for 7 days resulted in a 90–94% decrease in acid release. Patients with stomach (gastric) or duodenal ulcers had a decrease in symptoms in about 1 week—this DOES NOT mean that the ulcer is gone. Especially with maintenance of healing of duodenal ulcers, therapy may be ongoing. Eradication regimen with three drugs (see above) took 14 days. People with reflux esophagitis had decreases in heartburn after 7 to 28 days. Some esophagitis patients needed a second 8-week course to bring symptoms under control. Long-term use requires periodic physician follow-up.

Typical Treatment Goals and Measurements (Outcomes and Markers)

Ulcers: The role of *Helicobacter pylori* in ulcers is no longer questioned and a proton pump inhibitor is widely recognized as the standard for short-term treatment of stomach ulcers. When *H. pylori* is present, single-medicine therapy is not recommended. Additionally, an antibiotic is often used with other agents. The goal is to heal the ulcer area and prevent re-occurrence of the ulceration. Sign and symptom relief as well as endoscopic examination help define success of treatment.

▷ **This Drug Should Not Be Taken If**
- you are allergic to the medicine or any of its components.

▷ **Inform Your Physician Before Taking This Drug If**
- you have a history of liver disease.
- you smoke and expect to continue smoking (worsens acid secretion).

Possible Side Effects (natural, expected and unavoidable drug actions)

Increased serum gastrin levels (clinical significance is unknown). There have been six cases of black tongue and mouth inflammation reported in people who took antibiotics and lansoprazole to treat *Helicobacter pylori*.

▷ **Possible Adverse Effects** (unusual, unexpected and infrequent reactions)

If any of the following develop, consult your physician promptly for guidance.

Mild Adverse Effects

Allergic reactions: skin rash.

Headache, dizziness or tiredness—infrequent.

Diarrhea or nausea—infrequent.

Ringing in the ears—rare.

Serious Adverse Effects

Allergic reaction: not defined.

Protein in the urine—rare.

Liver toxicity or low blood platelets—rare and of questionable cause.

▷ **Possible Effects on Sexual Function:** None reported.

▷ **Adverse Effects That May Mimic Natural Diseases or Disorders**

Drug-induced liver reaction may suggest viral hepatitis.

Possible Effects on Laboratory Tests

Liver function tests: increased.

CAUTION

1. Follow your doctor's advice on how long to take this drug.
2. This drug effectively treats ulcers but does not preclude the chance of cancer of the stomach.

Precautions for Use

By Infants and Children: Not indicated in this age group.

By Those Over 60 Years of Age: This medicine may cause dizziness. Use caution until you've seen the effects it has on you.

▷ **Advisability of Use During Pregnancy**

Pregnancy Category: B. See Pregnancy Risk Categories at the back of this book.

Advisability of Use If Breast-Feeding

Presence of this drug in breast milk: Unknown.

Avoid drug or refrain from nursing.

Habit-Forming Potential: None.

Effects of Overdose: Possible nausea, vomiting, dizziness, lethargy and abdominal pain.

Possible Effects of Long-Term Use: Serum gastrin levels are increased by this medicine, but the clinical significance is not known. Presently it is indicated for a maximum of two 8-week courses in erosive esophagitis. Maintenance of healed ulcers will further define effects of longer-term treatment.

Suggested Periodic Examinations While Taking This Drug (at physician's discretion)

Complete blood counts.

Liver function tests.

▷ **While Taking This Drug, Observe the Following**

Foods: Lansoprazole is best taken on an empty stomach. Follow your doctor's instructions regarding the types of foods you eat.

Herbal Medicines or Minerals: Kola and ma huang may increase stomach acid, blunting the benefits of this medicine. Black cohosh root, ginkgo and squill are contraindicated in gastrointestinal disturbances. Licorice root has a German Commission E monograph indication for gastrointestinal ulcers, but use with proton pump inhibitors has not been studied. Talk to your doctor BEFORE adding any herbals to these medicines.

Beverages: No restrictions.

▷ *Alcohol:* No specific interactions, but alcohol stimulates the secretion of stomach acid and may lessen the therapeutic benefits of this medicine.

Tobacco Smoking: Smoking can stimulate stomach acid and lessen benefits of this drug. I advise everyone to quit smoking.

▷ *Other Drugs*

Lansoprazole *taken concurrently* with

- antacids may blunt how much lansoprazole gets into your body, blunting lansoprazole benefits.
- clarithromycin (Biaxin) may lead to a blackening of the tongue or stomatitis. Lower lansoprazole doses and stopping the clarithromycin may be required.
- ritonavir (Norvir) may change lansoprazole blood levels.
- sucralfate (Carafate) may decrease lansoprazole absorption; separate doses by 2 hours.
- theophylline (Theo-Dur, others) may decrease blood theophylline level, requiring dosing adjustments.

▷ *Driving, Hazardous Activities:* Caution—this medicine may cause drowsiness. Limit activities as necessary.

Aviation Note: The use of this drug *may be a disqualification* for piloting. Consult a designated Aviation Medical Examiner.

Exposure to Sun: No restrictions.

Discontinuation: Talk with your doctor before stopping this medicine for any reason. Taking the medicine for a shorter time than needed may result in incomplete ulcer healing and continuation of the original problem.

LATANOPROST (la TAN oh prost)

Introduced: 1996   **Class:** Prostaglandin F-2 analogue, antiglaucoma
Prescription: USA: Yes   **Controlled Drug:** USA: No; Canada: No
Available as Generic: No
Brand Name: Xalatan

BENEFITS versus RISKS	
Possible Benefits	*Possible Risks*
EFFECTIVE REDUCTION OF INTERNAL EYE PRESSURE FOR CONTROL OF ACUTE AND CHRONIC GLAUCOMA	Mild side effects with systemic absorption
	Joint or back pain
CONTROL OF OCULAR HYPERTENSION	Minor eye discomfort
	Altered vision
Formation of eyelashes	Iris pigmentation

▷ **Principal Uses**

> *As a Single Drug Product:* Uses currently included in FDA-approved labeling: (1) Used to manage glaucoma; (2) lowers increased pressure in the eye (intraocular pressure).
>
> Other (unlabeled) generally accepted uses: (1) Used to attempt to encourage eyelash formation in patients who previously did not have any.

How This Drug Works: This medicine lowers pressure in the eye by increasing outflow from the uveoscleral area without changing aqueous flow.

Available Dosage Forms and Strengths

> Eyedrop solutions — 0.005% or 50 mcg per ml

▷ **Usual Adult Dosage Ranges:** For open-angle glaucoma or ocular hypertension: One drop (0.005%) in the eye each evening.

> **Note: Actual dose and dosing schedule must be determined for each patient individually.**

Conditions Requiring Dosing Adjustments

> *Liver Function:* The drug is changed in the liver and removed by the kidneys. Dose changes in liver disease are not defined.
>
> *Kidney Function:* Changed drug (metabolites) removed by the kidney, but dosing changes in kidney failure are not defined.

▷ **Dosing Instructions:** Remove contact lenses and do not replace them for at least 15 minutes after putting this medicine into your eye. To avoid excessive absorption into the body, press finger against inner corner of the eye (to close off the tear duct) during and for 1 minute after dropping the medicine in. Be careful not to touch the dropper to the eye. If you forget a dose: Take the missed dose as soon as you remember it, unless it's nearly time for your next dose—if that is the case, skip the missed dose and take the next dose right on schedule. DO NOT double doses. Talk with your doctor if you find yourself missing doses.

Usual Duration of Use: Use on a regular schedule for a day usually sees an effect in lowering the pressure in the eye. A week may be required for the full benefits of the medicine to be realized. Long-term use (months to years) requires physician supervision.

Typical Treatment Goals and Measurements (Outcomes and Markers)

> *Glaucoma*: Ophthalmologists measure intraocular pressure (IOP), and then check IOP lowering once this medicine is started. The chamber angle can be checked prior to treatment.

▷ **This Drug Should Not Be Taken If**

- you have had an allergic reaction to it previously.

▷ **Inform Your Physician Before Taking This Drug If**

- you wear contact lenses.
- you have had an eye infection in the last three months.
- you have sudden (acute) angle closure of the eye.

Possible Side Effects (natural, expected and unavoidable drug actions)

> Burning of the eyes or irritation—frequent (usually mild).
>
> Pigmentation of the eye (iridial) has been reported.
>
> Growth of eyelashes in patients who previously did not have any has been reported.

▷ **Possible Adverse Effects** (unusual, unexpected and infrequent reactions)

If any of the following develop, consult your physician promptly for guidance.

Mild Adverse Effects

Allergic reactions: itching of the eyes, eyelid itching and/or swelling or rash.

Headache—infrequent.

Nausea—case reports.

Muscle or back pain—rare to infrequent.

Serious Adverse Effects

Pigmentation of the iris—infrequent, though may be frequent (up to 16%) with therapy ongoing for more than a year.

▷ **Possible Effects on Sexual Function:** None reported.

Possible Effects on Laboratory Tests

None reported.

Precautions for Use

By Those Over 60 Years of Age: No age-specific changes presently needed.

▷ **Advisability of Use During Pregnancy**

Pregnancy Category: C. See Pregnancy Risk Categories at the end of book.

Human studies: Adequate studies of pregnant women are not available.

Discuss use with your doctor BEFORE using this drug.

Advisability of Use If Breast-Feeding

Presence of this drug in breast milk: Unknown.

Watch infant closely and stop drug or nursing if adverse effects develop.

Habit-Forming Potential: None.

Effects of Overdose: Not defined.

Possible Effects of Long-Term Use: Pigmentation of the iris.

Suggested Periodic Examinations While Taking This Drug (at physician's discretion)

Measurement of internal eye pressure on a regular basis.

Check for early signs of pigmentation.

▷ **While Taking This Drug, Observe the Following**

Foods: No restrictions.

Herbal Medicines or Minerals: Scopolia root has glaucoma as a possible side effect. DO NOT COMBINE. Henbane, ephedra and belladonna should also be avoided.

Beverages: No restrictions.

▷ *Alcohol:* No restrictions except prudence in alcohol use.

Tobacco Smoking: No interactions expected. I advise everyone to quit smoking.

Marijuana Smoking: Sustained additional decrease in internal eye pressure.

▷ *Other Drugs*

Latanoprost **taken concurrently** with

- pilocarpine (various) may blunt latanoprost benefits. Dose pilocarpine one hour after latanoprost.
- thimerosal (various) can cause a precipitation. DO NOT combine eyedrops containing thimerosal with latanoprost. Separate doses by 5 minutes or more.

▷ *Driving, Hazardous Activities:* This drug may cause blurry vision for a time. Restrict activities as necessary.

Aviation Note: The use of this drug *may be a disqualification* for piloting. Consult a designated Aviation Medical Examiner.

Exposure to Sun: This medicine may make your eyes sensitive to the sun. Wear sunglasses.

Discontinuation: Do not stop regular use of this drug without consulting your physician.

LEFLUNOMIDE (LEH flew no myde)

Introduced: 1998   **Class:** Disease-modifying antirheumatic drug (DMARD), pyrimidine synthesis inhibitor, immunosuppressant (T-cell)   **Prescription:** USA: Yes   **Controlled Drug:** USA: No; Canada: No   **Available as Generic:** No

Brand Name: Arava

BENEFITS versus RISKS	
Possible Benefits	*Possible Risks*
TREATS RHEUMATOID ARTHRITIS BY A NOVEL MECHANISM	LIVER TOXICITY
	LOW BLOOD CELLS (LEUKOPENIA)
RETARDS DAMAGE TO JOINTS	Increased blood pressure

▷ **Principal Uses**

As a Single Drug Product: Uses currently included in FDA-approved labeling: Treatment of rheumatoid arthritis in adults.

Other (unlabeled) generally accepted uses: May have a role in organ transplants because it can suppress the immune system in a novel way versus current medicines.

How This Drug Works: Works to lower the immune system (via T-cell pyrimidine synthesis inhibition) by blocking an enzyme (dihydroorotate dehydrogenase) required. It acts as an anti-inflammatory medicine and also modifies (immunomodulates) the immune system by inhibiting proliferation of T cells. It probably inhibits responsiveness of the immune system to interleukin-2 and tyrosine kinase.

Available Dosage Forms and Strengths

Tablets — 10 mg, 20 mg, 100 mg

▷ **Usual Adult Dosage Ranges:** *For rheumatoid arthritis*: An initial loading dose of 100 mg is given for three days (this is required because of an extremely long time to reach steady state). Ongoing doses are 20 mg daily. If the 20 mg dose is not tolerated, the dose may be lowered to 10 mg daily. **Note: Actual dose and schedule determined for each patient individually.**

Conditions Requiring Dosing Adjustments

Liver Function: Used with extreme caution. Studies have not been done. Since this medicine must be changed (metabolized) by the liver and activated (to A77 1726-M1) by the liver, use of leflunomide in people with hepatic insufficiency is NOT recommended. In Europe and Canada, use in patients with liver problems is contraindicated.

Kidney Function: Data from limited studies suggest that kidney damage does not significantly interfere with this medicine. More study is needed to confirm this, and caution is advised.

▷ **Dosing Instructions:** The tablet may be crushed and taken with food. IT IS CRITICAL to take the pills EXACTLY as prescribed, especially while the loading dose is being given (otherwise, it will take a long time for the medicine to reach steady state and go to work for you). This medicine stays in the body for a very long time. If pregnancy becomes desirable or if liver enzymes are unacceptably increased, cholestyramine is often used to help remove leflunomide from the body. The cholestyramine procedure is as follows: Eight grams of cholestyramine is taken three times a day for 11 days. Blood is drawn and plasma levels are checked. Levels should be found to be less than 0.02 mg/l (0.02 mcg/ml) by two separate tests from blood samples taken at least 14 days apart. If levels are more than 0.02 mcg/ml, additional cholestyramine treatment should be undertaken. If you forget a dose: take the missed dose as soon as you remember it, unless it's nearly time for your next dose—if that is the case, skip the missed dose and take the next dose right on schedule. Talk with your doctor if you find yourself missing doses.

Usual Duration of Use: Use on a regular schedule for a month determines benefit in rheumatoid arthritis. The effect stabilizes in 3–6 months and then tends to offer the same degree of relief or lack of progression. Long-term use (months to years) requires physician supervision.

Typical Treatment Goals and Measurements (Outcomes and Markers)

Pain: Most clinicians treating pain use a device called an algometer to check your pain. This looks like a small ruler, but lets the clinician better understand your pain. The goals of treatment then relate to where the level of pain started (for example, a rating of 7 on a zero to ten scale) and what the cause of the pain was. Pain medicines may also be used together (in combination) in order to get the best result or outcome. If your pain control is not acceptable to YOU (remember, in hospitals and outpatient settings, etc. pain control is a patient right and the fifth vital sign) and if after a week of arthritis pain treatment, results are not what you expect, be sure to call your doctor as you may need a different medicine or combination.

Arthritis: Control of arthritis symptoms (pain, loss of mobility, decreased ability to accomplish activities of daily living, range of motion, etc.) is paramount in returning patient quality of life and to checking the results (beneficial outcomes) from this medicine. Many arthritis management or pain centers use interdisciplinary teams (physicians from several specialties, nurses, physician's assistants, physical and occupational therapists, pharmacotherapists, psychotherapists, social workers and others) to get the best results.

▷ **This Drug Should Not Be Taken If**
- you have had an allergic reaction to it previously.
- you are pregnant or planning pregnancy in the near future.
- you are breast-feeding your infant.
- you have liver disease, hepatitis C or B, or positive tests for hepatitis.

▷ **Inform Your Physician Before Taking This Drug If**
- you have a chronic infection of any kind.
- you have impaired liver or kidney function.
- you are taking medicines such as methotrexate or nonsteroidal anti-inflammatory drugs (NSAIDS) or other medicines that may have a toxic effect (hepatotoxic) on the liver.

- you have a history of bone marrow impairment of any kind, especially drug-induced bone marrow depression.
- you have an immune deficiency.
- you currently have, or have had a recent exposure to, either chicken pox or shingles (herpes zoster) or have an active infection.

Possible Side Effects (natural, expected and unavoidable drug actions)
Suppression of the immune system.

▷ **Possible Adverse Effects** (unusual, unexpected and infrequent reactions)
If any of the following develop, consult your physician promptly for guidance.
Mild Adverse Effects
Allergic reactions: skin rash—infrequent.
Headache or dizziness—infrequent.
Increased blood pressure—infrequent.
Loss of appetite, nausea, diarrhea—infrequent to frequent.
Weight loss—infrequent.
Loss of hair—infrequent.
Serious Adverse Effects
Allergic reactions: one case report of anaphylaxis.
Liver toxicity—infrequent and dose-related.
Immune suppression (anemia and leukopenia) and subsequent infection—possible.

▷ **Possible Effects on Sexual Function:** None reported, although this medicine SHOULD NOT be taken if you are pregnant.

Possible Delayed Adverse Effects: Increased liver enzymes. Immune system suppression. The risk of malignancy (particularly lymphoproliferative disorders) is increased if people take medicines that suppress the immune system; no such disorders were reported in clinical trials, but larger and longer-term studies are required to show whether there is increased risk of malignancy or lymphoproliferative disorders.

Possible Effects on Laboratory Tests
Complete blood cell counts: decreased red cells, hemoglobin and white cells.
Immune system components: lowered.
Liver function tests: increased liver enzymes (ALT/GPT, AST/GOT and alkaline phosphatase) or bilirubin.

CAUTION
1. This drug must be monitored carefully by a qualified physician. If liver enzymes (ALT) increase to more than 2 times the upper normal limit, the dose should be reduced to 10 mg daily. If the ALT remains between 2 and 3 times the upper normal limit, a liver biopsy is recommended if treatment is to continue. If the ALT still remains elevated after cholestyramine and a decrease in dose, the medicine should be stopped.
2. Appropriate laboratory examinations, performed before and during the use of this drug, are mandatory.
3. Women with potential for pregnancy should have a pregnancy test before taking this drug and should use an effective form of contraception during its use and until after the drug elimination procedure is performed and their doctor says that the blood level has declined to a low enough level.

4. Live-virus vaccines should be avoided during use of this drug. Live-virus vaccines could actually produce infection rather than stimulate an immune response.

Precautions for Use

By Infants and Children: This drug has not been studied in people less than 18 years old. Safety and effectiveness in children are not established.

By Those Over 60 Years of Age: No dose changes are thought to be needed.

▷ **Advisability of Use During Pregnancy**

Pregnancy Category: X. See Pregnancy Risk Categories at the back of this book.

Animal studies: Increased death of embryos in rats.

Human studies: Adequate studies in humans are not available.

Use in pregnancy is contraindicated.

Advisability of Use If Breast-Feeding

Presence of this drug in breast milk: Unknown.

Avoid drug or refrain from nursing.

Habit-Forming Potential: None.

Effects of Overdose: No human experience with overdoses. Cholestyramine or charcoal is advocated via NG tube in the event of significant toxicity or overdose.

Suggested Periodic Examinations While Taking This Drug (at physician's discretion)

Complete blood cell counts.

Liver function tests (LFTs) BEFORE starting leflunomide and then monthly. If clinically stable, LFTs should be checked at intervals appropriate to the individual clinical situation.

▷ **While Taking This Drug, Observe the Following**

Foods: No restrictions.

Herbal Medicines or Minerals: Some patients use echinacea to attempt to boost their immune systems. Unfortunately, use of echinacea is not recommended in people with damaged immune systems (even if a medicine caused the damage). This herb may also actually weaken any immune system if it is used too often or for too long a time. There is no data from scientifically rigorous studies on combination of leflunomide with glucosamine. Hay flower, mistletoe herb and white mustard seed carry German Commission E monograph indications for arthritis and may be complementary. Talk to your doctor BEFORE combining any medicines.

Beverages: No restrictions. This drug may be taken with milk.

▷ *Alcohol:* No restriction defined by the manufacturer.

Tobacco Smoking: Clearance of M1 is lowered, and while the clinical significance of this is not known, I advise everyone to quit smoking.

Marijuana Smoking: May cause additional impairment of immunity.

▷ *Other Drugs*

Leflunomide may *decrease* the effects of

• live-virus vaccines.

Leflunomide *taken concurrently* with

• activated charcoal (various) may result in decreased leflunomide benefits.

• cholestyramine (Questran, others) and other cholesterol-lowering resins may result in decreased leflunomide effectiveness.

• influenza (flu) vaccine may blunt benefits of the vaccine.

- medicines removed by CYP2C9 (such as losartan, phenytoin and S-warfarin) may lead to higher than expected blood levels and effects of those medicines.
- methotrexate (various) may lead to increased liver enzymes, although one study found increased therapeutic benefits of this combination.
- NSAIDs (see Drug Classes) may lead to higher than expected blood levels of the NSAIDs.
- other medicines that blunt the immune system may result in additive effects.
- pneumococcal or smallpox vaccine may result in decreased immune response to the vaccine.
- rifampin (Rifater, others) may increase risk of leflunomide toxicity.
- tolbutamide (Orinase) may increase the active tolbutamide, resulting in a greater response from tolbutamide than expected.
- yellow fever vaccine can result in blunted response and benefit from the vaccine.

▷ *Driving, Hazardous Activities:* This drug may cause dizziness. Restrict activities as necessary.

Aviation Note: The use of this drug *may be a disqualification* for piloting. Consult a designated Aviation Medical Examiner.

Exposure to Sun: No restrictions reported.

LEVODOPA (lee voh DOH pa)

Introduced: 1967   **Class:** Anti-parkinsonism   **Prescription:** USA: Yes
Controlled Drug: USA: No; Canada: No   **Available as Generic:** USA: Yes; Canada: No

Brand Names: ❦Apo-Levocarb, Bendopa, Dopar, Larodopa, ❦Prolopa [CD], Sinemet [CD], Sinemet CR [CD]

BENEFITS versus RISKS	
Possible Benefits	*Possible Risks*
EFFECTIVE SYMPTOM RELIEF IN IDIOPATHIC PARKINSON'S DISEASE	Emotional depression, confusion, abnormal thinking and behavior
Helpful in parkinsonism after encephalitis	Abnormal involuntary movements
	Heart rhythm disturbance
Roughly 6-month benefit in parkinsonism after manganese poisoning	Urinary bladder retention
	Induction of peptic ulcer
	Blood abnormalities: hemolytic anemia, reduced white blood cell count

▷ **Principal Uses**

As a Single Drug Product: Uses currently included in FDA-approved labeling: Treats major types of Parkinson's disease: paralysis agitans ("shaking palsy" of unknown cause), the type that follows encephalitis, parkinsonism that develops with aging (associated with hardening of the brain arteries) and the parkinsonism that follows poisoning by carbon monoxide or manganese.

Other (unlabeled) generally accepted uses: (1) May have a limited role in treating catatonic stupor; (2) can improve conscious level in coma caused by liver failure; (3) can help restless leg or periodic limb movements in sleep; (4) could be helpful in treating severe congestive heart failure.

As a Combination Drug Product [CD]: This drug is available in combination with carbidopa, a chemical that prevents the breakdown of levodopa before it reaches its site of action. The addition of carbidopa reduces levodopa requirements by 75% and also decreases the frequency and severity of adverse effects.

How This Drug Works: Levodopa enters the brain tissue and is converted to dopamine. After sufficient dose, this corrects the dopamine deficiency (thought to be the cause of parkinsonism) and restores a more normal brain chemistry. Carbidopa blocks an enzyme (decarboxylase) that degrades levodopa before it reaches the brain. This allows a lower dose to have a greater benefit. Products containing carbidopa also have fewer adverse effects.

Available Dosage Forms and Strengths

Capsules — 100 mg, 250 mg, 500 mg

Sinemet CR, sustained-release tablets — 25/100 mg, 50/200 mg

Sinemet tablets — 10/100 mg, 25/100 mg, 25/250 mg

Tablets — 100 mg, 250 mg, 500 mg

▷ **Usual Adult Dosage Ranges:** Initially 250 mg two to four times daily. Dose may be increased by increments of 100 to 750 mg at 3- to 7-day intervals as needed and tolerated. Total dose should not exceed 8,000 mg daily. If the combination drug Sinemet is used, the total levodopa requirement will be considerably less. For someone who has not taken levodopa before (levodopa naive and using the sustained-release form): one 50/200 mg tablet twice daily, no more frequently than every 6 hours while awake. The dose is then increased as needed and tolerated by either daily or every-other-day dosing of one tablet, to a maximum of eight tablets daily. **Note: Actual dose and schedule must be determined for each patient individually.**

Conditions Requiring Dosing Adjustments

Liver Function: Dosing changes are not indicated in liver compromise.

Kidney Function: Possible urine retention requires that patients with urine outflow problems should be closely watched. No dose decreases are needed in kidney failure.

Intestinal Parasites: A report of large increases in doses needed by patients with Strongyloides stercoralis has been filed. Cure of this intestinal parasite allowed the levodopa dose to be decreased by 33%.

▷ **Dosing Instructions:** Tablet may be crushed and is best taken with or following carbohydrate foods to reduce stomach upset. When possible, don't take this drug with high-protein foods. Sustained-release tablet (Sinemet CR) may be cut in half, but it should not be crushed or chewed. The last daily dose should be taken before 7 p.m. in order to avoid problems with normal sleeping patterns. "Drug holidays" (periods when no medicine is taken) are controversial, and not all patients benefit from this approach to therapy. If you forget a dose: take the missed dose as soon as you remember it, unless it's nearly time for your next dose—if that is the case, skip the missed dose and take the next dose right on schedule. Talk with your doctor if you find yourself missing doses.

Usual Duration of Use: Use on a regular schedule for 2 to 3 weeks determines effectiveness in relieving the major symptoms of parkinsonism. Peak benefits may require continual use for 6 months. Long-term use (months to years) requires physician supervision.

Typical Treatment Goals and Measurements (Outcomes and Markers)

Parkinson's disease: The general goal is to minimize symptoms (tremor, sluggish movements, analysis of walking or gait, etc.) to the fullest extent possible. Additionally, many neurologists use Hahn-Yahr scores and the time it takes to maximum amount of finger tapping as indicators of the benefits of this drug.

Possible Advantages of This Drug

The slow-release formulation of Sinemet CR allows a 25 to 50% reduction in dosing frequency.

The wearing-off phenomenon and end-of-dose failure seen with standard Sinemet may be reduced or eliminated.

▷ **This Drug Should Not Be Taken If**
- you are allergic to any of the brands listed.
- you have narrow-angle glaucoma (inadequately controlled).
- you have a history of melanoma or skin lesions that have not been diagnosed.
- you are taking, or have taken within the past 14 days, any monoamine oxidase (MAO) type A inhibitor drug (see Drug Classes).

▷ **Inform Your Physician Before Taking This Drug If**
- you have diabetes, epilepsy, heart disease, high blood pressure or chronic lung disease.
- you have impaired liver or kidney function.
- you have problems making blood (hematopoiesis).
- you have had a heart attack and have some abnormal heart rhythms.
- you have a history of ongoing (chronic) wide angle glaucoma.
- you have a history of depression or other mental illness.
- you have a history of peptic ulcer disease or malignant melanoma.
- you will have surgery with general anesthesia.

Possible Side Effects (natural, expected and unavoidable drug actions)

Fatigue, lethargy.

Altered taste, offensive body odor.

Orthostatic hypotension (see Glossary).

Pink- to red-colored urine, which turns black on exposure to air (of no significance).

Gout.

▷ **Possible Adverse Effects** (unusual, unexpected and infrequent reactions)

If any of the following develop, consult your physician promptly for guidance.

Mild Adverse Effects

Allergic reactions: skin rash, itching.

Headache, dizziness, numbness, insomnia, nightmares, blurred or double vision—infrequent.

Nausea and vomiting—frequent.

Dry mouth, difficult swallowing, gas, diarrhea, constipation—infrequent.

Decreased taste sensation—possible.

Loss of hair—case reports.

Serious Adverse Effects

Idiosyncratic reactions: hemolytic anemia (see Glossary).

Neuroleptic malignant syndrome (see Glossary), high blood pressure—case reports.

Confusion, hallucinations, paranoia, depression—infrequent to frequent.

Psychotic episodes, seizures—rare.

Congestive heart failure—rare.

Mania or seizures—rare.

Abnormal involuntary movements of the head, face and extremities—frequent.

Disturbances of heart rhythm—infrequent, low blood pressure—rare.

Development of peptic ulcer, gastrointestinal bleeding—case reports.

Urinary bladder retention—case reports.

Low white blood cell count: increased infection risk, sore throat (transient, but may require you to stop this medicine until the condition clears) or low blood platelets—case reports to rare.

▷ **Possible Effects on Sexual Function:** Increased male or female libido—infrequent.

Inhibited ejaculation, priapism (see Glossary), postmenopausal bleeding—all rare.

▷ **Adverse Effects That May Mimic Natural Diseases or Disorders**

Mental reactions may resemble idiopathic psychosis.

Natural Diseases or Disorders That May Be Activated by This Drug

Latent peptic ulcer, gout.

Possible Effects on Laboratory Tests

Complete blood cell counts: occasionally decreased white cells; occasionally increased eosinophils (without symptoms).

Blood thyroxine (T4) level: increased.

Urine sugar tests: no effect with Tes-Tape; false negative with Clinistix; false positive with Clinitest.

Urine ketone tests: false positive with Ketostix and Phenistix.

Blood uric acid, growth hormone: increased.

Blood potassium or sodium: may be decreased.

CAUTION

1. It is best to begin treatment with small doses, increasing gradually until desired response is achieved.
2. As improvement occurs, avoid excessive and hurried activity (often causes falls and injury).

Precautions for Use

By Infants and Children: This drug can cause precocious puberty in prepubertal boys. Watch for hypersexual behavior and premature growth of genital organs.

By Those Over 60 Years of Age: Therapy should start with half the usual adult dose; dose increases should be made in small increments as needed and tolerated. Watch for significant behavioral changes: depression or inappropriate elation, acute confusion, agitation, paranoia, dementia, nightmares and hallucinations. Abnormal involuntary movements may also occur.

▷ **Advisability of Use During Pregnancy**

Pregnancy Category: C. See Pregnancy Risk Categories at the back of this book.

Animal studies: Significant birth defects reported in rodent studies.

Human studies: Adequate studies of pregnant women are not available.

Avoid use of drug during the first 3 months. Use only if clearly needed during the final 6 months.

Advisability of Use If Breast-Feeding

Presence of this drug in breast milk: Yes.

Avoid drug or refrain from nursing.

Habit-Forming Potential: None.

Effects of Overdose: Muscle twitching, spastic closure of eyelids, nausea, vomiting, diarrhea, weakness, fainting, confusion, agitation, hallucinations.

Possible Effects of Long-Term Use: Development of abnormal involuntary movements involving the head, face, mouth and extremities. May be reversible and gradually subside as the drug is withdrawn.

Suggested Periodic Examinations While Taking This Drug (at physician's discretion)

Complete blood cell counts.

Measurements of internal eye pressure.

Blood pressure measurements in lying, sitting and standing positions.

▷ **While Taking This Drug, Observe the Following**

Foods: Insofar as possible, do not take concurrently with protein foods; proteins compete for absorption.

Herbal Medicines or Minerals: Calabar bean (chop nut, Fabia, ordeal nut, others) is unsafe when taken by mouth (physostigmine is the active ingredient) and should never be taken by people with Parkinson's disease. Octacosanol (a cousin of vitamin E) can worsen movement problems and should also be avoided.

Nutritional Support: If taken alone (without carbidopa), watch for tingling of the extremities (peripheral neuritis). Small (10 mg or less) doses of pyridoxine (vitamin B_6) may help. Larger doses can decrease the effectiveness of levodopa. If taking Sinemet, supplemental pyridoxine is not required. Rare reports of vitamin C (ascorbic acid) decreasing nausea and other side effects have been made.

Beverages: No restrictions. May be taken with milk.

▷   *Alcohol:* No interactions expected.

Tobacco Smoking: No interactions expected. I advise everyone to quit smoking.

Marijuana Smoking: Increased fatigue and lethargy; possible accentuation of orthostatic hypotension (see Glossary).

▷   *Other Drugs*

Levodopa *taken concurrently* with

- benzodiazepines (see Drug Classes) may blunt the therapeutic benefit of levodopa.
- bromocriptine (Parlodel) may result in decreased blood levels of bromocriptine.
- bupropion (Wellbutrin, Zyban) may increase adverse effects.
- cisapride (Propulsid) may increase adverse effects.

- clonidine (Catapres) can result in decreased therapeutic benefit of levodopa; avoid this combination.
- fentanyl/droperidol (Innovar) can cause muscular rigidity.
- indinavir (Crixivan) may lead to severe movement problems (dyskinesias).
- isoniazid (INH) may cause flushing, worsening of symptoms or increased blood pressure. DO NOT COMBINE.
- monoamine oxidase (MAO) type A inhibitor drugs (see Drug Classes) can cause a dangerous rise in blood pressure and body temperature; do not combine these drugs.
- phenothiazines (see Drug Classes) may blunt therapeutic benefits of levodopa. DO NOT COMBINE.
- reserpine (Naquival, others) may blunt the therapeutic benefits of levodopa; avoid this combination.
- risperidone (Risperdal) can blunt the therapeutic benefits of levodopa; avoid this combination.
- tolcapone (Tasmar) may lead to vitiligo (skin lesions).
- tricyclic antidepressants (see Drug Classes) may decrease the therapeutic effect of levodopa.

The following drugs may *decrease* the effects of levodopa:
- amoxapine (Asendin).
- chlordiazepoxide (Librium) or other benzodiazepines (see Drug Classes).
- iron salts.
- papaverine (Cerespan, Pavabid, Vasospan, etc.).
- phenytoin (Dilantin, etc.) or fosphenytoin (Cerebyx).
- pyridoxine (vitamin B$_6$).
- risperidone (Risperdal).

▷ *Driving, Hazardous Activities:* May cause dizziness, impaired vision and orthostatic hypotension. Restrict activities as necessary.

Aviation Note: Parkinson's disease *is a disqualification* for piloting. Consult a designated Aviation Medical Examiner.

Exposure to Sun: No restrictions.

Exposure to Heat: Use caution. This drug can cause flushing and excessive sweating and predispose to heat exhaustion.

Occurrence of Unrelated Illness: Dark-colored skin lesions should be evaluated carefully by your doctor, as they may be malignant melanoma. White blood cell counts should be closely followed if you develop an infection.

LEVOTHYROXINE (lee voh thi ROX een)

Other Names: L-thyroxine, thyroxine, T-4

Introduced: 1953 **Class:** Thyroid hormones **Prescription:** USA: Yes
Controlled Drug: USA: No; Canada: No **Available as Generic:** USA: Yes; Canada: No

Brand Names: Alti-Thyroxine, Armour Thyroid, ✤Eltroxin, Euthroid [CD], Euthyrox, Levo-T, Levotabs, Levothroid, Levoxine, Levoxyl, L-Thyroxine, Proloid, Synthroid, Synthrox, Syroxine, Thyroid USP, Thyrolar [CD]

BENEFITS versus RISKS	
Possible Benefits	*Possible Risks*
EFFECTIVE REPLACEMENT THERAPY IN STATES OF THYROID HORMONE DEFICIENCY (HYPOTHYROIDISM) EFFECTIVE TREATMENT OF SIMPLE GOITER, CHRONIC THYROIDITIS and THYROID GLAND CANCER	Intensification of angina in presence of coronary artery disease Drug-induced hyperthyroidism (with excessive dose) Spasm of the coronary vessels

▷ **Principal Uses**

As a Single Drug Product: Uses currently included in FDA-approved labeling: (1) Replacement therapy to correct thyroid deficiency (drug-induced, hypothyroidism, cretinism, myxedema); (2) treatment of simple (nonendemic) goiter and benign thyroid nodules; (3) treatment of Hashimoto's thyroiditis; (4) adjunctive prevention and treatment of thyroid cancer; (5) treats Grave's disease. **Author's Note: Concern has arisen over levothyroxine medicines that were never approved under current FDA regulations. On July 16, 2001, the FDA issued guidance that said that manufacturers of unapproved hypothyroidism drugs will have to stop distributing their products. See www.fda.gov/bbs/topics/ANSWERS/2001/ANSO1089.html.**

Other (unlabeled) generally accepted uses: (1) Helps amenorrhea caused by (secondary to) low thyroid function; (2) may help fetal lung tissue mature in premature babies; (3) could help long-standing (chronic) hives (urticaria); (4) some clinicians use levothyroxine in combination with triiodothyronine (10–12.5 mcg of triiodothyronine and lowering the levothyroxine dose by 50 mcg).

As a Combination Drug Product [CD]: This thyroid hormone is available in combination with the other principal thyroid hormone, liothyronine, in a preparation (generic name: liotrix) that resembles the natural hormone material produced by the thyroid gland.

How This Drug Works: Alters cellular chemistry, making more energy available and increases metabolism of all tissues. Thyroid hormones are essential to normal growth and development, especially the development of infant brain and nervous systems.

Available Dosage Forms and Strengths

Injections — 100 mcg/ml, 200 mcg/ml, 500 mcg/ml
Tablets — 0.0125 mg, 0.025 mg, 0.037 mg, 0.05 mg, 0.075 mg, 0.088 mg, 0.1 mg, 0.112 mg, 0.125 mg, 0.15 mg, 0.175 mg, 0.2 mg, 0.3 mg

▷ **Recommended Dosage Ranges** (Actual dose and schedule must be determined for each patient individually.)

Infants and Children: Up to 6 months of age—8 to 10 mcg per kg of body mass, in a single daily dose.

6 to 12 months of age—6 to 8 mcg per kg of body mass, in a single daily dose.

1 to 5 years of age—5 to 6 mcg per kg of body mass, in a single daily dose.

6 to 12 years of age—4 to 5 mcg per kg of body mass, in a single daily dose.

Over 12 years of age—2 to 3 mcg per kg of body mass, in a single daily dose, until the usual adult daily dose is reached (150 to 200 mcg).

12 to 60 Years of Age: Start at 0.05 mg as a single daily dose; increase by 0.025 to 0.05 mg at intervals of 2 to 3 weeks as needed and tolerated. Usual maintenance dose is 0.17 mg/day. Total daily dose should not exceed 0.3 mg. If response is not seen at this level, absorption problems or misunderstanding in taking the medicine should be evaluated.

Over 60 Years of Age: Initially 0.0125 to 0.025 mg as a single daily dose; increase gradually at intervals of 3 to 4 weeks, as needed and tolerated. The usual maintenance dose is approximately 0.075 mg daily.

Author's Note: A University of California Medical Center at San Francisco study found the generic to be as effective as the brand name at savings of 50% of the cost of the brand.

Conditions Requiring Dosing Adjustments

Liver Function: Dosing changes are not needed.

Kidney Function: Dosing changes are not indicated in kidney compromise.

▷ **Dosing Instructions:** The tablets may be crushed and are best taken in the morning on an empty stomach. If you forget a dose: take the missed dose as soon as you remember it, unless it's nearly time for your next dose—if that is the case, skip the missed dose and take the next dose right on schedule. Talk with your doctor if you find yourself missing doses.

Usual Duration of Use: Use on a regular schedule for 4 to 6 weeks determines effectiveness in correcting the symptoms of thyroid deficiency. Long-term use (months to years, possibly for life) requires physician supervision.

Typical Treatment Goals and Measurements (Outcomes and Markers)

Hypothyroidism: The goal is to return the thyroid hormone level to normal or euthyroid. Clinicians check easing of low thyroid signs and symptoms (low energy, weight gain, sluggishness, etc.) as well as checking very specific laboratory tests. Tests often used include the thyroid stimulating hormone and T3 and T4 as well as the thyrotropin test. Adjunctive tests include total cholesterol.

Currently a "Drug of Choice"

For treatment of hypothyroidism.

▷ **This Drug Should Not Be Taken If**
- you have had an allergic reaction to it previously.
- you are recovering from a heart attack; ask your doctor for help.
- you have an adrenal insufficiency that has not been corrected.
- you are using it to lose weight and your thyroid function is normal (no deficiency).

▷ **Inform Your Physician Before Taking This Drug If**
- you have high blood pressure, any form of heart disease or diabetes.
- you have a history of Addison's disease or adrenal gland deficiency.
- you are taking any antiasthmatic medications.
- you are taking an anticoagulant.

Possible Side Effects (natural, expected and unavoidable drug actions)

None if dose is adjusted correctly.

▷ **Possible Adverse Effects** (unusual, unexpected and infrequent reactions)

If any of the following develop, consult your physician promptly for guidance.

Mild Adverse Effects
   Allergic reactions: skin rash, hives.
   Headache in sensitive people, even with proper dose adjustment—may be
   frequent.
Serious Adverse Effects
   Increased frequency or intensity of angina in people with coronary artery
   disease—possible.
   Spasm of the arteries that supply blood to the heart and heart attack—rare.
   Seizures, pseudotumor cerebri, drug-induced porphyria or myasthenia
   gravis—case reports to rare.
   Decrease in IgA immune concentration—rare.
   May be a part of the development of osteoporosis. Bone mineral density test-
   ing is recommended.
   Note: Other adverse effects are manifestations of excessive dose. See "Effects
   of Overdose" below.

▷ **Possible Effects on Sexual Function:** Altered menstrual pattern during dose
   adjustments.
   Possibly beneficial in treating impaired sexual function that is associated
   with true hypothyroidism.

Natural Diseases or Disorders That May Be Activated by This Drug
   Latent coronary artery insufficiency (angina), diabetes.

Possible Effects on Laboratory Tests
   Prothrombin time: increased (when taken concurrently with warfarin).
   Blood total cholesterol, HDL and LDL cholesterol levels: decreased.
   Blood triglyceride levels: no effect.
   Blood glucose level: increased.
   Blood thyroid hormone levels: increased T3, T4 and free T4.
   Blood thyroid-stimulating hormone (TSH) level: decreased.

CAUTION
   1. Careful supervision of individual response is needed to identify correct
      dose. Do not change dosing or drug products without asking your
      physician.
   2. This drug should not be used to treat nonspecific fatigue, obesity,
      infertility or slow growth. Such use is inappropriate and could be
      harmful.
   3. If combination levothyroxine and triiodothyronine dosing is used, the
      levothyroxine dose is lowered by 50 mcg.
   4. If a combination levothyroxine and triiodothyronine dosing is used, thy-
      roid extract should be avoided, as it has an elevated amount of T3, which
      can lead to tremors or palpitations.

Precautions for Use
   By Infants and Children: Thyroid-deficient children often require higher doses
      than adults. Transient hair loss may occur during the early months of
      treatment. Follow the child's response to thyroid therapy by periodic
      measurements of bone age, growth and mental and physical develop-
      ment.
   By Those Over 60 Years of Age: Usually requirements for thyroid hormone
      replacement are about 25% lower than in younger adults. Watch closely
      for any indications of toxicity.

▷ **Advisability of Use During Pregnancy**

Pregnancy Category: A. See Pregnancy Risk Categories at the back of this book.

Animal studies: Cataract formation reported in rat studies. Other defects reported in rabbit and guinea pig studies.

Human studies: Thyroid hormones do not reach the fetus (cross the placenta) in significant amounts. Clinical experience has shown that appropriate use of thyroid hormones causes no adverse effects on the fetus.

Use this drug only if clearly needed and with carefully adjusted dose.

Advisability of Use If Breast-Feeding

Presence of this drug in breast milk: Yes, in minimal amounts.

Breast-feeding is considered safe with correctly adjusted dose.

Habit-Forming Potential: None.

Effects of Overdose: Headache, sense of increased body heat, nervousness, increased sweating, hand tremors, insomnia, rapid and irregular heart action, diarrhea, muscle cramping, weight loss, heart attack.

Possible Effects of Long-Term Use: Bone loss (osteoporosis) in the lumbar vertebrae (spine). Worsening of abnormal growth of the left side of the heart.

Suggested Periodic Examinations While Taking This Drug (at physician's discretion)

Measurement of thyroid hormone levels in blood.

Bone mineral density testing.

▷ **While Taking This Drug, Observe the Following**

Foods: Enteral formulas for nutrition support that contain soybeans may increase the fecal elimination of thyroxine.

Herbal Medicines or Minerals: Horseradish root might worsen low thyroid (hypothyroidism) or blunt effectiveness of therapy. Calcium doses (if taken) should be separated from levothyroxine doses by four hours. Cabbage and iodine may worsen goiters and exacerbate hypothyroidism. Gamma oryzanol (extracted from rice bran oil) can lower thyroid stimulating hormone (TSH) and change test results. Tiratricol is a naturally occurring metabolite of thyroxine and triiodothyronine. In theory, tiratricol may enhance the adverse action and effects of bungleweed, wild thyme and balm leaf. Talk to your doctor BEFORE adding any herbal medicines to levothyroxine.

Beverages: No restrictions.

▷ *Alcohol:* No interactions expected.

Tobacco Smoking: No interactions expected. I advise everyone to quit smoking.

▷ *Other Drugs*

Levothyroxine may *increase* the effects of

- warfarin (Coumadin) and increase the risk of bleeding; decreased anticoagulant dose is usually needed. More frequent INR testing (prothrombin time or protime) are needed.

Levothyroxine may *decrease* the effects of

- digoxin (Lanoxin), when correcting hypothyroidism; a larger dose of digoxin may be needed.

Levothyroxine *taken concurrently* with

- antacids may cause decreased levothyroxine absorption and a decreased therapeutic effect.
- all antidiabetic drugs (insulin and oral hypoglycemic agents) may require an increased dose to obtain proper control of blood sugar levels.

- benzodiazepines (Librium and others) can enhance the toxic or therapeutic effects of both drugs.
- conjugated estrogens (Premarin) may require an increased levothyroxine dose.
- tricyclic antidepressants (see Drug Classes) may cause an increase in activity of both drugs.

The following drugs may *decrease* the effects of levothyroxine:
- cholestyramine (Cuemid, Questran)—may reduce its absorption; intake of the two drugs should be separated by 5 hours.
- colestipol (Colestid).
- iron salts—by decreasing absorption.
- lovastatin (Mevacor).
- phenytoin (Dilantin) or fosphenytoin (Cerebyx)—can increase levothyroxine removal (clearance).
- ritonavir (Norvir).
- sodium polystyrene sulfonate (Kayexalate).
- sucralfate (Carafate).

▷ *Driving, Hazardous Activities:* No restrictions.

Aviation Note: The use of this drug is probably not a disqualification for piloting. Consult a designated Aviation Medical Examiner.

Exposure to Sun: No restrictions.

Exposure to Heat: This drug may decrease individual tolerance to warm environments, increasing discomfort due to heat. Consult your physician if you develop symptoms of overdose during the warm months of the year.

Heavy Exercise or Exertion: Use caution if you have angina (coronary artery disease). This drug may increase the frequency or severity of angina during physical activity.

Discontinuation: Must be taken continually on a regular schedule to correct thyroid deficiency. Never stop it without talking to your doctor.

LIDOCAINE (LYE doh kane)

Other Names: None

Introduced: Patch form 1999   **Class:** Analgesic, antiarrhythmic   **Prescription:** USA: Yes   **Controlled Drug:** USA: No; Canada: No   **Available as Generic:**   USA: No; Canada: No

Brand Names: Lidoderm

BENEFITS versus RISKS	
Possible Benefits	*Possible Risks*
EFFECTIVE TREATMENT/ PREVENTION OF THE PAIN WHICH HAPPENS AFTER SHINGLES (POSTHERPETIC NEURALGIA)	Interactions are possible—drug is used with caution in people who are taking other Class I (such as mexiletine or tocainide) antiarrhythmic drugs
WHEN USED AS DIRECTED, ROUGHLY 2 PERCENT OF THE APPLIED DOSE REACHES THE BODY CIRCULATION	Skin irritation where the patch is applied
	Possible allergic reaction (rare)

▷ **Principal Uses**

As a Single Drug Product: Uses currently included in FDA-approved labeling:
(1) Pain relief for pain associated with postherpetic neuralgia.
Other (unlabeled) generally accepted uses: None at present.

Author's Note: This brief profile focused on the only specifically FDA-approved treatment for pain after shingles (postherpetic neuralgia)—not the anti-arhythmic use. This profile will be broadened in future editions.

LIOTHYRONINE (li oh THI roh neen)

Other Names: Triiodothyronine, T-3

Introduced: 1956   **Class:** Thyroid hormone   **Prescription:** USA: Yes
Controlled Drug: USA: No; Canada: No   **Available as Generic:**   USA: Yes;
Canada: No

Brand Names: Armour Thyroid, Cyronine, Cytomel, Euthroid [CD], Thyroid
USP, Thyrolar [CD], Triostat

BENEFITS versus RISKS	
Possible Benefits	*Possible Risks*
EFFECTIVE REPLACEMENT THERAPY IN STATES OF THYROID HORMONE DEFICIENCY (HYPOTHYROIDISM) EFFECTIVE TREATMENT OF SIMPLE GOITER, CHRONIC THYROIDITIS and THYROID GLAND CANCER	Intensification of angina in presence of coronary artery disease Drug-induced hyperthyroidism (with excessive dosing) Rapid heartbeat Heart attack

▷ **Principal Uses**

As a Single Drug Product: Uses currently included in FDA-approved labeling:
(1) Replacement therapy to correct thyroid deficiency (hypothyroidism);
(2) treatment of simple (nonendemic) goiter and benign thyroid nodules;
(3) treatment of Hashimoto's thyroiditis; (4) adjunctive prevention and
treatment of thyroid cancer; (5) therapy of cretinism; (6) used to help diagnose different kinds of thyroid problems; (7) treats low thyroid that comes
from medicines.

Other (unlabeled) generally accepted uses: (1) Can help infertility caused by
low thyroid function; (2) thyroid replacement of choice for thyroid cancer;
(3) may have a role in some kinds of heart problems (cardiomyopathy).

As a Combination Drug Product [CD]: This thyroid hormone is available in
combination with the other principal thyroid hormone, levothyroxine, in a
preparation (generic name: liotrix) that resembles the natural hormone
material produced by the thyroid gland.

How This Drug Works: Alters cellular chemistry, making more energy available.
Increases cellular metabolism in all tissues. Thyroid hormones are essential to normal growth and development, especially the development of the
infant's brain and nervous system.

Available Dosage Forms and Strengths
>   Injection — 10 mcg/ml
>   Tablets — 5 mcg, 25 mcg, 50 mcg

▷ **Recommended Dosage Ranges** (Actual dose and schedule must be determined for each patient individually.)

Infants and Children: Infants several months old may need 20 mcg a day. When they reach 1 year, 50 mcg a day may be needed. Children more than 3 years old may need the full adult dose.

12 to 60 Years of Age: For mild hypothyroidism—initially 25 mcg daily; increase by 12.5 to 25 mcg every 1 to 2 weeks as needed and tolerated. The usual maintenance dose is 20 to 75 mcg daily.

For severe hypothyroidism—initially 2.5 to 5 mcg daily; increase by 5 to 10 mcg at intervals of 1 to 2 weeks. When a dose of 25 mcg is reached, increase by 12.5 to 25 mcg at intervals of 1 to 2 weeks, as needed and tolerated. The usual maintenance dose is 50 to 100 mcg daily.

For simple goiter—initially 5 mcg daily; increase by 5 to 10 mcg at intervals of 1 to 2 weeks. When a dose of 25 mcg is reached, increase by 12.5 to 25 mcg at intervals of 1 week, as needed and tolerated. The usual maintenance dose is 50 to 100 mcg daily.

Over 60 Years of Age: Initially 5 mcg as a single daily dose; increase by 5 mcg at intervals of 1 to 2 weeks, as needed and tolerated. The usual maintenance dose is 12.5 to 37.5 mcg daily.

Conditions Requiring Dosing Adjustments

Liver Function: Dosing changes are not indicated for patients with liver compromise.

Kidney Function: Dosing changes are not indicated in renal compromise. Caution should be used when increasing the dose of this medicine by those with kidney problems.

▷ **Dosing Instructions:** The tablets may be crushed and are preferably taken in the morning on an empty stomach to ensure maximal absorption and uniform results. If you forget a dose: take the missed dose as soon as you remember it, unless it's nearly time for your next dose—if that is the case, skip the missed dose and take the next dose right on schedule. Talk with your doctor if you find yourself missing doses.

Usual Duration of Use: Use on a regular schedule for 2 to 4 days determines effectiveness in correcting the symptoms of thyroid deficiency. Long-term use (months to years, possibly for life) requires physician supervision.

Typical Treatment Goals and Measurements (Outcomes and Markers)

Hypothyroidism: The goal is to return the thyroid hormone level to normal or euthyroid. Clinicians check easing of low thyroid signs and symptoms (low energy, weight gain, sluggishness, etc.) as well as checking very specific laboratory tests. Tests often used include the thyroid stimulating hormone and T3 and T4 as well as the thyrotropin test. Adjunctive tests include total cholesterol.

▷ **This Drug Should Not Be Taken If**
- you have had an allergic reaction to it previously.
- you are recovering from a heart attack; ask your doctor for guidance.
- you have an uncorrected adrenal cortical deficiency.
- you are using it to lose weight and your thyroid function is normal.

▷ **Inform Your Physician Before Taking This Drug If**
- you have high blood pressure, any form of heart disease or diabetes.
- you have a history of Addison's disease or adrenal gland deficiency.
- you are taking any antiasthmatic medications.
- you take digoxin.
- you are taking an anticoagulant.

Possible Side Effects (natural, expected and unavoidable drug actions)
None if dose is adjusted correctly.

▷ **Possible Adverse Effects** (unusual, unexpected and infrequent reactions)
If any of the following develop, consult your physician promptly for guidance.

Mild Adverse Effects
Allergic reactions: skin rash, hives.
Headache in sensitive individuals, even with proper dose adjustment—may be frequent.
Rapid heart rate (tachycardia)—infrequent.
Hair loss—case reports.

Serious Adverse Effects
Allergic reactions: erythema, bullae and papules.
Increased frequency or intensity of angina or abnormal heartbeat—possible to infrequent.
Lowering of blood pressure—rare.
Heart attack—rare.
Osteoporosis—possible increased risk (bone mineral density testing is recommended).
Hyperthyroidism—possible with improper dosing.
Drug fever or drug-induced myasthenia gravis—case reports.
Author's Note: Other adverse effects are manifestations of excessive dose. See "Effects of Overdose" below.

▷ **Possible Effects on Sexual Function:** Altered menstrual pattern during dose adjustments.

Possibly beneficial in treating impaired sexual function that is associated with true hypothyroidism.

Natural Diseases or Disorders That May Be Activated by This Drug
Latent coronary artery insufficiency (angina), diabetes.

Possible Effects on Laboratory Tests
Prothrombin time: increased (when taken concurrently with warfarin).
Blood total cholesterol, HDL and LDL cholesterol levels: decreased.
Blood triglyceride levels: no effect.
Blood glucose level: increased.
Blood thyroid hormone levels: increased T3.
Blood thyroid—stimulating hormone (TSH) level: decreased.

CAUTION
1. Careful supervision of individual response is needed to identify correct dose. Do not change dosing schedule without asking your doctor.
2. This drug should not be used to treat nonspecific fatigue, obesity, infertility or slow growth. Such use is inappropriate and could be harmful.

Precautions for Use

By Infants and Children: Not recommended for treatment of this age group. It must reach the brain and nervous system, and this drug may not do that. Levothyroxine is the drug of choice to treat thyroid deficiency in infants and children.

By Those Over 60 Years of Age: Needs for thyroid hormone are usually about 25% lower than in younger adults. Watch closely for any toxicity.

▷ **Advisability of Use During Pregnancy**

Pregnancy Category: A. See Pregnancy Risk Categories at the back of this book.

Animal studies: No information available.

Human studies: Thyroid hormones do not reach the fetus (cross the placenta) in significant amounts. Clinical experience has shown that appropriate use of thyroid hormones causes no adverse effects on the fetus.

Use this drug only if clearly needed and with carefully adjusted dose.

Advisability of Use If Breast-Feeding

Presence of this drug in breast milk: Yes, in minimal amounts.

Breast-feeding is considered safe with correctly adjusted dose.

Habit-Forming Potential: None.

Effects of Overdose: Headache, sense of increased body heat, nervousness, increased sweating, hand tremors, insomnia, rapid and irregular heart action, diarrhea, muscle cramping, weight loss, heart attack.

Possible Effects of Long-Term Use: Bone loss (osteoporosis) in the lumbar vertebrae (spine). Bone mineral density testing is recommended.

Suggested Periodic Examinations While Taking This Drug (at physician's discretion)

Measurement of thyroid hormone levels in blood.

▷ **While Taking This Drug, Observe the Following**

Foods: No restrictions.

Herbal Medicines or Minerals: Horseradish root might worsen low thyroid (hypothyroidism) or blunt effectiveness of therapy. Calcium doses (if taken) should be separated from levothyroxine doses by four hours. Cabbage and iodine may worsen goiters and exacerbate hypothyroidism. Gamma oryzanol (extracted from rice bran oil) can lower thyroid stimulating hormone (TSH) and change test results. Tiratricol is a naturally occurring metabolite of thyroxine and triiodothyronine. In theory, tiratricol may enhance the adverse action and effects of bungleweed, wild thyme and balm leaf. Talk to your doctor BEFORE adding any herbal medicines to liothyronine.

Beverages: No restrictions.

▷ *Alcohol:* No interactions expected.

Tobacco Smoking: No interactions expected. I advise everyone to quit smoking.

▷ *Other Drugs*

Liothyronine may *increase* the effects of

• warfarin (Coumadin) and increase the risk of bleeding; more frequent INR (prothrombin time or protime) tests are needed.

Liothyronine may *decrease* the effects of

• digoxin (Lanoxin) when correcting hypothyroidism; a larger dose of digoxin may be needed.

Liothyronine *taken concurrently* with

- all antidiabetic drugs (insulin and oral hypoglycemic agents) may require an increased dose to obtain proper control of blood sugar.
- estrogens (including birth control pills and Premarin) may require increased doses of liothyronine.
- monoamine oxidase (MAO) inhibitors (see Drug Classes) may increase the therapeutic benefits of the antidepressant.
- tricyclic antidepressants (see Drug Classes) may cause an increase in the activity of both drugs; watch for signs of toxicity.

The following drugs may *decrease* the effects of liothyronine:

- carbamazepine (Tegretol, others) may decrease free serum T4 and T3.
- cholestyramine (Cuemid, Questran), and perhaps other cholesterol-lowering resins, may reduce its absorption; intake of the two drugs should be separated by 5 hours.

▷ *Driving, Hazardous Activities:* No restrictions.

Aviation Note: The use of this drug is probably not a disqualification for piloting. Consult a designated Aviation Medical Examiner.

Exposure to Sun: No restrictions.

Exposure to Heat: This drug may decrease individual tolerance to warm environments, increasing discomfort due to heat. Consult your physician if you develop symptoms of overdose during the warm months of the year.

Heavy Exercise or Exertion: Use caution if you have angina (coronary artery disease). This drug may increase the frequency or severity of angina during physical activity.

Discontinuation: This drug must be taken continually on a regular schedule to correct thyroid deficiency. Do not stop it without consulting your physician.

LISINOPRIL (Li SIN oh pril)

Introduced: 1988   **Class:** Antihypertensive, ACE inhibitor

Please see the angiotensin converting enzyme (ACE) inhibitor family profile.

LITHIUM (LITH i um)

Introduced: 1949   **Class:** Antidepressant   **Prescription:** USA: Yes
Controlled Drug: USA: No; Canada: No   **Available as Generic:** USA: Yes; Canada: No
Brand Names: ✤Carbolith, Cibalith-S, ✤Duralith, Eskalith, Eskalith CR, Lithane, ✤Lithizine, Lithobid, Lithonate, Lithotabs

---

BENEFITS versus RISKS

Possible Benefits	*Possible Risks*
RAPID REVERSAL OF ACUTE MANIA	VERY NARROW MARGIN OF TREATMENT
STABILIZATION OF MOOD	POTENTIALLY FATAL TOXICITY WITH INADEQUATE MONITORING
Prevention of recurrent depression in "responders"	Infrequent induction of diabetes mellitus, hypothyroidism
	Diabetes insipidus–like syndrome (excessive dilute urine)

▷ **Principal Uses**

As a Single Drug Product: Uses currently included in FDA-approved labeling: (1) Manages bipolar disorder (promptly corrects acute mania and also reduces frequency and severity of recurrent manic-depressive mood swings); (2) used to treat mania; (3) helps control mania.

Other (unlabeled) generally accepted uses: (1) May be helpful in chronic hair-pulling (trichotillomania); (2) can help prevent cluster headaches; (3) may help control aggressive behavior; (4) can have a role in treating Fanconi's aplastic anemia; (5) may be of use in patients who have mood problems that also affect their sex drive.

How This Drug Works: Lithium changes the way nerve signals are transmitted and interpreted, influencing emotional status and behavior.

Available Dosage Forms and Strengths

Capsules — 150 mg, 300 mg, 600 mg
Syrup — 8 mEq/5 ml
Tablets — 300 mg
Tablets, prolonged action — 300 mg, 450 mg

▷ **Usual Adult Dosage Ranges:** *First day*: 900 to 1,200 mg per day, divided into three equal doses, and then increased as needed and tolerated by 300-mg increments to attain a blood level of 1–1.5 mmol/L.

Usual maintenance dose: 1,200 to 1,800 mg daily taken in three divided doses. The total daily dose should not exceed 3,600 mg. Immediate-release forms are often given 3 or 4 times daily, and sustained-release forms are given less often—only TWICE daily. **Note: Actual dose and dosing schedule must be determined for each patient individually.**

Conditions Requiring Dosing Adjustments

Liver Function: The liver is minimally involved in the elimination of lithium.

Kidney Function: Frequent and careful side effect monitoring, decreased doses, and more frequent blood levels are prudent. In moderate to severe kidney failure (creatinine clearance of 10–50 ml/min), 50–75% of the usual dose is taken. In severe kidney failure, 25–50% of the usual dose is taken.

▷ **Dosing Instructions:** The capsules may be opened, and regular tablets crushed, and taken with or after meals to reduce stomach upset. The prolonged-action tablets should be swallowed whole and not altered. If you forget a dose: take the missed dose as soon as you remember it, unless it's nearly time for your next dose—if that is the case, skip the missed dose and take the next dose right on schedule. Talk with your doctor if you find yourself missing doses.

Usual Duration of Use: Use on a regular schedule for 1 to 3 weeks determines effectiveness in correcting acute mania; several months of continual treatment may be required to correct depression. Long-term use (months to years) requires physician supervision and periodic evaluation.

Typical Treatment Goals and Measurements (Outcomes and Markers)

Bipolar disorder: Helps even out the highs and lows often seen in bipolar problems. The general goal is to create a situation where excessive highs or lows no longer feel "normal" and patients are able to return to their appropriate quality of life. Blood levels are kept in a tight range (0.6 to 1.5 mmol/L). Levels are usually checked every two months. Thyroid function tests are checked every three to six months.

Currently a "Drug of Choice"

For the treatment of acute mania in bipolar manic-depressive disorders.

▷ **This Drug Should Not Be Taken If**
- you had an allergic reaction to it previously.
- you have uncontrolled diabetes or uncorrected hypothyroidism.
- you are breast-feeding your infant.
- you will be unable to comply with the need for regular monitoring of lithium blood levels.
- you have severe kidney failure.

▷ **Inform Your Physician Before Taking This Drug If**
- you have a history of a schizophreniclike thought disorder.
- you have any type of organic brain disease or a history of grand mal epilepsy.
- you have diabetes, heart disease, hypothyroidism or impaired kidney function.
- you are on a salt-restricted diet.
- you are pregnant or planning pregnancy.
- you are taking any diuretic drug or a cortisonelike steroid preparation.
- your blood sodium level is low.
- you will have surgery with general anesthesia.

Possible Side Effects (natural, expected and unavoidable drug actions)

Increased thirst and urine volume in 60% of initial users and in 20% of long-term users.

Weight gain in first few months of use.

Drowsiness and lethargy in sensitive individuals.

Metallic taste.

Increased white blood cells—not a sign of infection, but an effect of lithium.

Heart block—frequent but does not usually lead to the medicine being stopped.

Tremor (fine)—frequent (may respond to a beta blocker).

▷ **Possible Adverse Effects** (unusual, unexpected and infrequent reactions)

If any of the following develop, consult your physician promptly for guidance.

Mild Adverse Effects

Allergic reactions: skin rashes, generalized itching.

Skin dryness, loss of hair—case reports.

Headache, joint pain, dizziness, weakness, blurred vision, ringing in ears, unsteadiness—infrequent.

Nausea, vomiting, diarrhea—frequent.

Metallic taste—possible.

Edema—possible.

Serious Adverse Effects

"Blackout" spells, confusion, stupor, slurred speech, spasmodic movements of extremities, epilepticlike seizures—case reports to rare.

Abnormal fixed eye position (oculogyric crisis)—case reports.

Abnormal changes in heart rate, rhythm and wave forms—frequent.

Loss of bladder or rectal control—infrequent.

Diabetes insipidus–like syndrome: excessive dilute urine—infrequent to frequent.

Abnormal movements (may be a sign of toxicity)—rare.

Cerebellar atrophy or neuroleptic malignant syndrome—case reports.

Inflammation of the heart muscle (myocarditis)—case reports.

Pseudotumor cerebri, myasthenia gravis or systemic lupus erythematosus—case reports.

Low thyroid function or abnormally high thyroid function—possible to case reports.

Elevated blood calcium or blood sugar—rare.

Porphyria or inflammation of the parotid gland—case reports.

Seizures—case reports and certainly with toxicity.

Drug-induced low or high potassium—possible.

▷ **Possible Effects on Sexual Function:**

Decreased libido (blood level of 0.7 to 0.9 mEq/L)—case reports.

Inhibited erection (0.6 to 0.8 mEq/L)—frequent.

Male infertility.

Female breast swelling with milk production—case reports.

▷ **Adverse Effects That May Mimic Natural Diseases or Disorders**

Painful discoloration and coldness of the hands and feet may resemble Raynaud's phenomenon.

Natural Diseases or Disorders That May Be Activated by This Drug

Diabetes mellitus may be worsened. Psoriasis may be intensified. Myasthenia gravis may be induced (one case).

Possible Effects on Laboratory Tests

White blood cell and platelet counts: increased.

Blood alkaline phosphatase (bone isoenzyme): markedly increased in up to 66% of users.

Blood cholesterol level: increased.

Blood parathyroid hormone level: increased.

Blood thyroid-stimulating hormone (TSH) level: increased.

Blood thyroid hormone (T3 and T4) levels: decreased.

Blood uric acid level: decreased.

Blood bromide, calcium or glucose levels: increased.

Blood potassium level: increased or decreased.

CAUTION

1. The blood level required for this drug to work is close to the level that can cause toxic effects. Periodic blood lithium levels are mandatory. Follow instructions about drug dose and periodic blood tests.

2. Lithium should be stopped at the first signs of toxicity: drowsiness, sluggishness, unsteadiness, tremor, muscle twitching, vomiting or diarrhea.
3. The major causes of lithium toxicity are:
- accidental overdose (may be due to inadequate blood level checks)
- impaired kidney function
- salt restriction
- inadequate fluid intake, dehydration
- concurrent use of diuretics
- intercurrent illness
- childbirth (rapid decrease in kidney clearance of lithium)
- initiation of treatment with a new drug
- Over-the-counter preparations that contain iodides (some cough products and vitamin-mineral supplements) should be avoided because of the added antithyroid effect when taken with lithium.
- Low blood sodium can lead to toxic lithium effects with a "normal" lithium level.

Precautions for Use
By Infants and Children: Safety and effectiveness for those under 12 years of age are not established. Follow your physician's instructions exactly.

By Those Over 60 Years of Age: Treatment should start with a "test" dose of 75 to 150 mg daily. Observe closely for early indications of toxic effects, especially if on a low-salt diet and using diuretics. Increased risk of parkinsonian reactions (abnormal gait and movements); coma can develop without warning symptoms.

▷ Advisability of Use During Pregnancy
Pregnancy Category: D. See Pregnancy Risk Categories at the back of this book.

Animal studies: Cleft palate reported in mice; eye, ear and palate defects reported in rats.

Human studies: Adequate studies of pregnant women are not available, but cardiovascular defects and goiter in newborn infants (of mothers using lithium) have been reported. If the infant's blood level of lithium approaches the toxic range before delivery, the newborn may suffer the "floppy infant" syndrome: weakness, lethargy, unresponsiveness, low body temperature, weak cry and poor feeding ability.

Avoid use of drug during the first 3 months. Use only if clearly necessary during the final 6 months. Monitor mother's blood lithium levels carefully to avoid possible toxicity.

Advisability of Use If Breast-Feeding
Presence of this drug in breast milk: Yes, in significant amounts.
Avoid drug or refrain from nursing.

Habit-Forming Potential: None.

Effects of Overdose: Drowsiness, weakness, lack of coordination, nausea, vomiting, diarrhea, muscle spasms, blurred vision, dizziness, staggering gait, slurred speech, confusion, stupor, coma, cerebellar atrophy, seizures.

Possible Effects of Long-Term Use: Hypothyroidism (5%), goiter, reduced sugar tolerance, diabetes insipidus-like syndrome, serious kidney damage.

Suggested Periodic Examinations While Taking This Drug (at physician's discretion)

Regular determinations of blood lithium levels are absolutely essential. Time to sample blood for lithium level: 12 hours after evening dose or in the morning, just before next dose. Therapeutic range: 0.8 to 1.5 MEq/L (acute) and 0.6 to 1.2 (maintenance).

Periodic evaluation of thyroid gland size and function.

Complete blood cell counts.

Kidney function tests.

▷ **While Taking This Drug, Observe the Following**

Foods: Maintain a normal diet; do not restrict your use of salt.

Herbal Medicines or Minerals: This drug may cause increased calcium. Talk to your doctor BEFORE taking any calcium supplements. Herbs that have a diuretic or potassium-losing effect may lead to lithium toxicity.

Beverages: No restrictions. Drink at least 8 to 12 glasses of liquids daily. This drug may be taken with milk.

▷ *Alcohol:* Use with caution. May have an increased intoxicating effect. Avoid alcohol completely if any symptoms of lithium toxicity develop.

Tobacco Smoking: Lithium may increase sensitivity to nicotine. I advise everyone to quit smoking.

Marijuana Smoking: Possible increase in apathy, lethargy, drowsiness or sluggishness; accentuation of lithium-induced tremor; possible increased risk of precipitating psychotic behavior.

▷ *Other Drugs*

Lithium may ***increase*** the effects of
- tricyclic antidepressants (see Drug Classes).

Lithium ***taken concurrently*** with
- ACE inhibitors (see Drug Classes) such as captopril (Capoten) may increase lithium levels by as much as three times the level prior to combination therapy.
- calcium channel blockers (see Drug Classes), such as diltiazem, may cause neurotoxicity or mania.
- carbamazepine (Tegretol) may result in neurotoxicity.
- chlorpromazine (Thorazine, etc.) and other phenothiazines (see Drug Classes) may decrease lithium or phenothiazine therapeutic effects.
- cisplatin may cause changes in lithium levels; level checks are prudent.
- citalopram (Celexa) may enhance the effect of citalopram on serotonin.
- clozapine (Clozaril) may result in serious agranulocytosis, delirium and neuroleptic malignant syndrome; do not combine these medicines.
- diazepam (Valium) may cause hypothermia.
- diuretics (see Diuretic Drug Classes) may lead to lithium toxicity.
- filgrastim (Neupogen) may result in a greater than expected increase in white blood cell numbers.
- fludrocortisone (Florinef) may result in loss of the mineralocorticoid benefits of fludrocortisone.
- fluoxetine (Prozac) may result in neurotoxicity.
- fluvoxamine (Luvox) may result in increased lithium levels and toxicity.
- haloperidol (Haldol) or with other neuroleptics may result in decreased beneficial effects from both medicines.

- methyldopa (Aldomet, etc.) is usually well tolerated; however, it may cause a severe neurotoxic reaction in susceptible individuals. These combinations should be used very cautiously.
- metronidazole (Flagyl) may lead to lithium toxicity.
- monoamine oxidase (MAO) inhibitors (see Drug Classes) may result in the serotonin syndrome and potential fatality.
- nicotine (various brands) may cause supersensitivity to nicotine.
- sibutramine (Meridia) may cause an increased risk of serotonin syndrome. DO NOT COMBINE.
- verapamil (Calan, Isoptin) may cause unpredictable effects; both lithium toxicity and decreased lithium blood levels have been reported.

The following drugs may *increase* the effects of lithium:
- aspirin (various).
- bumetanide (Bumex).
- celecoxib (Celebrex) or rofecoxib (Vioxx).
- ethacrynic acid (Edecrin).
- fluoxetine (Prozac).
- furosemide (Lasix, etc.).
- indomethacin (Indocin).
- losartan (Cozaar, Hyzaar) and perhaps other angiotensin II inhibitors.
- piroxicam (Feldene) or any nonsteroidal anti-inflammatory drug (NSAID- see Drug Classes).
- thiazide diuretics (see Drug Classes).

The following drugs may *decrease* the effects of lithium:
- acetazolamide (Diamox, etc.).
- calcitonin (various).
- sodium bicarbonate.
- theophylline (Theo-Dur, etc.) and related drugs.

▷ *Driving, Hazardous Activities:* This drug may impair mental alertness, judgment, physical coordination and reaction time. Restrict activities as necessary.

Aviation Note: The use of this drug *is a disqualification* for piloting. Consult a designated Aviation Medical Examiner.

Exposure to Sun: No restrictions.

Exposure to Heat: Excessive sweating can cause significant depletion of salt and water and resultant lithium toxicity. Avoid sauna baths.

Occurrence of Unrelated Illness: Fever, sweating, vomiting or diarrhea can result in significant alterations of blood and tissue lithium concentrations. Close monitoring of your physical condition and blood lithium levels is needed to prevent serious toxicity.

Discontinuation: Sudden discontinuation does not cause withdrawal symptoms. Avoid premature discontinuation; some individuals may require continual treatment for up to a year to achieve maximal response. Discontinuation by "responders" may result in recurrence of either mania or depression. Lithium should be discontinued if symptoms of brain toxicity appear or if an uncorrectable diabetes insipidus-like syndrome develops.

LOMEFLOXACIN (loh me FLOX a sin)

Please see the fluoroquinolone antibiotic family profile.

LOPERAMIDE (loh PER a mide)

Introduced: 1977   **Class:** Antidiarrheal   **Prescription:** USA: Yes
Controlled Drug: USA: No; Canada: No   **Available as Generic:** Yes
Brand Names: Anti-Diarrheal, Apo-loperamide, Diarrid, Imodium, Imodium AD, Kaopectate 1-D, Maalox A/D, Pepto Diarrhea Control

BENEFITS versus RISKS	
Possible Benefits	*Possible Risks*
EFFECTIVE RELIEF OF INTESTINAL CRAMPING AND DIARRHEA	Drowsiness
	Constipation
	May cause serious colon problems (toxic megacolon)

▷ **Principal Uses**
   As a Single Drug Product: Uses currently included in FDA-approved labeling: (1) Control of cramping and diarrhea associated with acute gastroenteritis and chronic enteritis and colitis; (2) used to reduce the volume of discharge from ileostomies; (3) irritable bowel syndrome that has failed to respond to dietary supplements.
   Other (unlabeled) generally accepted uses: (1) Traveler's diarrhea; (2) decreases unformed stools in Shigella diarrhea.
How This Drug Works: Acts directly on the nerve supply of the gastrointestinal tract, decreases secretions and relieves cramping and diarrhea.
Available Dosage Forms and Strengths
   Capsules — 2 mg
   Liquid (4.07% alcohol) — 0.2 mg/5 ml
   Liquid (5.25% alcohol) — 1 mg/5 ml
   Tablets — 2 mg
▷ **Recommended Dosage Ranges:** *For acute diarrhea*: 4 mg initially (2 capsules) and then 2 mg after each unformed stool until diarrhea is controlled.
   For chronic diarrhea: 4 to 8 mg daily in divided doses, taken 8 to 12 hours apart. Maximum daily dose is 16 mg.
   Pediatric dosing: NOT recommended for children under 2 years old. 2 to 5 year olds can be given 1 mg three times a day on the first day (13–30 kg); 6 to 8 year olds can have 2 mg twice daily on the first day (20–30 kg); 8–12 years old can have 2 mg three times daily (greater than 30 kg). Follow-up doses on the next day are 1 mg per 10 kg of body mass, up to the maximum daily doses on day 1. If diarrhea persists, call your doctor.
   Note: Actual dose and schedule must be determined for each patient individually.
Conditions Requiring Dosing Adjustments
   Liver Function: Dosing adjustments for patients with liver compromise are not needed. Half of a given dose is removed unchanged in the feces.
   Kidney Function: Changes in dosing are not indicated in kidney compromise.
▷ **Dosing Instructions:** The capsule may be opened and taken on an empty stomach or with food if stomach upset occurs. If you forget a dose: Take the missed dose as soon as you remember it, unless it's nearly time for your next dose—if that is the case, skip the missed dose and take the next dose right on schedule. Talk with your doctor if you find yourself missing doses.

Usual Duration of Use: Use on a regular schedule for 48 hours determines effectiveness in controlling acute diarrhea; continual use for 10 days may be needed to evaluate its effectiveness in controlling chronic diarrhea. If diarrhea persists, consult your physician.

Typical Treatment Goals and Measurements (Outcomes and Markers)

Diarrhea: The goal is to at least decrease the frequency of stools and ideally to return "normal" bowel patterns and stool consistency. In patients with ostomies, the amount of drainage should decrease.

▷ **This Drug Should Not Be Taken If**
- you have had an allergic reaction to it previously.
- constipation is never acceptable for you.
- it is prescribed for a child under 2 years of age.

▷ **Inform Your Physician Before Taking This Drug If**
- you have a history of liver disease or impaired liver function.
- you have regional enteritis or ulcerative colitis.
- you develop swelling (distention) of the abdomen while taking this medicine.
- you have acute dysentery.

Possible Side Effects (natural, expected and unavoidable drug actions)
Drowsiness, constipation.

▷ **Possible Adverse Effects** (unusual, unexpected and infrequent reactions)
If any of the following develop, consult your physician promptly for guidance.

Mild Adverse Effects
Allergic reaction: skin rash.
Fatigue, dizziness—rare.
Reduced appetite, cramps, dry mouth, nausea, vomiting, stomach pain, bloating—infrequent.

Serious Adverse Effects
"Toxic megacolon" (distended, immobile colon with fluid retention) may develop while treating acute ulcerative colitis—possible.
Necrotizing enterocolitis or paralytic ileus—rare.

▷ **Possible Effects on Sexual Function:** None reported.

Possible Effects on Laboratory Tests: None reported.

CAUTION
1. Do not exceed recommended doses.
2. If treating chronic diarrhea, promptly report development of bloating, abdominal distention, nausea, vomiting, constipation or abdominal pain.

Precautions for Use

By Infants and Children: Do not use in those under 2 years of age. Follow your physician's instructions exactly regarding dose. Watch for drowsiness, irritability, personality changes and altered behavior.

By Those Over 60 Years of Age: Small starting doses are needed, as you may be more sensitive to the sedative and constipating effects of this drug.

▷ **Advisability of Use During Pregnancy**

Pregnancy Category: B. See Pregnancy Risk Categories at the back of this book.
Animal studies: No birth defects found in rat and rabbit studies.

Human studies: Adequate studies of pregnant women are not available. Use sparingly and only if clearly needed. Ask your physician for guidance.

Advisability of Use If Breast-Feeding
Presence of this drug in breast milk: Small, clinically insignificant amounts. Talk with your doctor about the BENEFITS versus RISKS of using this medicine and nursing.

Habit-Forming Potential: Physical dependence has occurred in monkeys, but there have been no reports in humans.

Effects of Overdose: Drowsiness, lethargy, depression, dry mouth.

Possible Effects of Long-Term Use: None identified.

Suggested Periodic Examinations While Taking This Drug (at physician's discretion)
Decreased frequency of stools within 48 hours.

▷ **While Taking This Drug, Observe the Following**
Foods: No restrictions. Follow prescribed diet.
Herbal Medicines or Minerals: Numerous herbal medicines have German Commission E monograph indications for diarrhea. Examples include: bilberry fruit, oak bark, psyllium seed husk, tormentil root and uzara root. Use of these herbals with loperamide has not been studied. Electrolyte replacement (sodium, potassium, etc.) can be critical in ongoing diarrhea—especially if you are taking digoxin and other electrolyte-sensitive medicines. Talk to your doctor BEFORE adding any herbal medicine to loperamide therapy.
Beverages: No restrictions, other than your doctor's recommendations regarding diet.
▷ *Alcohol:* Use with caution. This drug may increase the depressant action of alcohol on the brain.
Tobacco Smoking: No interactions expected. I advise everyone to quit smoking.
▷ *Other Drugs* No significant drug interactions reported.
▷ *Driving, Hazardous Activities:* This drug may cause drowsiness or dizziness. Restrict activities as necessary.
Aviation Note: The use of this drug *is a disqualification* for piloting. Consult a designated Aviation Medical Examiner.
Exposure to Sun: No restrictions.

LORATADINE (lor AT a deen)

Introduced: 1992   **Class:** Antihistamines, nonsedating
Please see the minimally sedating antihistamines family profile.

LORAZEPAM (lor A za pam)

Introduced: 1977   **Class:** Anxiolytic, mild tranquilizer, hypnotic, benzodiazepine   **Prescription:** USA: Yes   **Controlled Drug:** USA: C-IV*; Canada: No   **Available as Generic:** USA: Yes; Canada: Yes

*See Schedules of Controlled Drugs at the back of this book.

Brand Names: Alzapam, ✤Apo-Lorazepam, Ativan, Loraz, Lorazepam Intensol, ✤Novo-Lorazepam, ✤Nu-Loraz

BENEFITS versus RISKS	
Possible Benefits	*Possible Risks*
RELIEF OF ANXIETY AND NERVOUS TENSION	Habit-forming potential with prolonged use
NOT CHANGED SIGNIFICANTLY INTO ACTIVE DRUG FORMS IN THE LIVER	Minor impairment of mental functions
	Blood cell, movement or liver disorders
	Dose-related respiratory depression
Wide margin of safety with therapeutic doses	Withdrawal symptoms if abruptly stopped

▷ **Principal Uses**

As a Single Drug Product: Uses currently included in FDA-approved labeling: (1) Helps treat anxiety; (2) used in surgical cases to help in delivering effective anesthesia; (3) used intravenously as a sedative.

Other (unlabeled) generally accepted uses: (1) Used to help prevent the severe symptoms of alcohol detoxification (delirium tremens or DTs); (2) used under the tongue to treat serial seizures in children; (3) can be used to promote amnesia in patients who must take chemotherapy and have suffered vomiting; (4) used to relieve insomnia.

How This Drug Works: Attaches to a specific site (GABA-A receptor) in the brain and enables gamma-aminobutyric acid to inhibit activity of nervous tissue. Drugs in this class also reduce the time it takes to fall asleep and the number of awakenings during the night.

Available Dosage Forms and Strengths

Injection — 2 mg/ml, 4 mg/ml

Oral solution — 2 mg/ml

Sublingual tablet — 0.5 mg, 1 mg, 2 mg

Tablet — 0.5 mg, 1 mg, 2 mg

▷ **Recommended Dosage Ranges** (Actual dose and dosing schedule must be determined for each patient individually.)

Infants and Children: Safety and effectiveness in those under 18 years of age are not established for injection. Has been used in 1- to 4-mg doses under the tongue for treatment of serial seizures in children.

18 to 60 Years of Age:

Sedation and anxiety: Therapy is started with 1 to 2 mg per day in two to three divided doses. Doses may be increased as needed and tolerated to the usual maintenance dose of 2 to 6 mg daily in divided doses. The maximum dose is 10 mg daily in two to three divided doses.

Insomnia: 2 to 4 mg at bedtime.

Over 60 Years of Age:

Sedation and anxiety: Therapy is started with 0.5 to 1 mg in divided doses. The initial dose should not exceed 2 mg daily.

Insomnia: 0.5 to 1 mg at bedtime.

Conditions Requiring Dosing Adjustments

Liver Function: The dose must be decreased in liver compromise, and the drug should not be used in liver failure. Use of the lowest effective dose is recommended for those with mild to moderate liver failure.

Kidney Function: The drug should not be used in kidney failure. In mild to moderate kidney compromise, the dose must be decreased and the lowest effective dose is recommended.

▷ **Dosing Instructions:** The tablet may be crushed and taken on an empty stomach or with milk or food. Do not stop this drug abruptly if it has been taken for more than 4 weeks. If you forget a dose: take the missed dose as soon as you remember it, unless it's nearly time for your next dose—if that is the case, skip the missed dose and take the next dose right on schedule. DO NOT double doses. Talk with your doctor if you find yourself missing doses.

Usual Duration of Use: Use on a regular schedule for 3 to 5 days usually determines effectiveness in relieving moderate anxiety or insomnia. Continual use should be limited to 1 to 3 weeks. Consult your physician on a regular basis. **Author's Note: The National Institute of Mental Health has a new information page on anxiety. It can be found on the World Wide Web (www.nimh.nih.gov/anxiety).**

Typical Treatment Goals and Measurements (Outcomes and Markers)
Anxiety: Goals for anxiety tend to be more vague and subjective than hypertension or cholesterol. Frequently, the patient (in conjunction with physician assessment) will largely decide if anxiety has been modified to a successful extent. The ability of the patient to return to normal activities is a hallmark of successful treatment.

Possible Advantages of This Drug
More direct elimination and lack of active forms may be of benefit in the elderly. Increased lipid solubility is of benefit when the drug is used to treat acute alcohol withdrawal.

▷ **This Drug Should Not Be Taken If**
- you have had an allergic reaction to any dose form or any component of the dose previously.
- you have a primary depression or psychosis.
- you have excessively low blood pressure.
- you have narrow-angle glaucoma.

▷ **Inform Your Physician Before Taking This Drug If**
- you are allergic to any benzodiazepine (see Drug Classes).
- you have a history of alcoholism or drug abuse.
- you are prone to respiratory depression.
- you are pregnant or planning pregnancy.
- you have impaired liver or kidney function.
- you have a history of low white blood cell counts.
- you have asthma, emphysema, epilepsy or myasthenia gravis.
- you take other prescription or nonprescription medicines that were not discussed with your doctor when lorazepam was prescribed.

Possible Side Effects (natural, expected and unavoidable drug actions)
Sedation, "hangover" effects on the day following bedtime use.

▷ **Possible Adverse Effects** (unusual, unexpected and infrequent reactions)
If any of the following develop, consult your physician promptly for guidance.

Mild Adverse Effects
> Allergic reactions: rashes, hives—rare.
> Dizziness, amnesia, insomnia (rebound), fainting, confusion, blurred vision, slurred speech, constipation and sweating—infrequent.
> Ringing in the ears (associated with withdrawal), decreased hearing ability—infrequent.

Serious Adverse Effects
> Allergic reactions: liver damage with jaundice (see Glossary)—case reports.
> Low white blood cell counts (leukopenia)—rare.
> Paradoxical excitement and rage—case reports.
> Low blood pressure—rare.
> Hallucinations (transient)—rare.
> Porphyria, seizures or abnormal body movements—case reports.
> Respiratory depression—dose-related.

▷ **Possible Effects on Sexual Function:** Decreased male libido or impotence—case reports.

Possible Effects on Laboratory Tests
> White blood cell counts: decreased.
> Liver function tests: increased SGPT, SGOT and LDH.

CAUTION
1. This drug should **not** be stopped abruptly if it has been taken continually for more than 4 weeks.
2. Over-the-counter medicines with antihistamines can cause excessive sedation if taken with lorazepam.
3. Lorazepam should **not** be combined with alcohol. This combination will worsen adverse mental and coordination decreases and increase lorazepam levels.

Precautions for Use
> *By Infants and Children:* Safety and effectiveness for those under 18 years of age are not established. Lorazepam has been used under the tongue in children with serial seizures.
> *By Those Over 60 Years of Age:* Small doses are indicated. Watch for lethargy, fatigue, weakness and paradoxical agitation, anger, hostility and rage.

▷ **Advisability of Use During Pregnancy**
> *Pregnancy Category:* D. See Pregnancy Risk Categories at the back of this book.
> *Animal studies:* Cleft palate has been reported in mice; skeletal defects in rats with similar drugs in this class.
> *Human studies:* Adequate studies of pregnant women are not available.
> Frequent use in late pregnancy can result in "floppy infant" syndrome in the newborn: weakness, depressed breathing and low body temperature. Avoid use during the entire pregnancy.

Advisability of Use If Breast-Feeding
> Presence of this drug in breast milk: Yes.
> Avoid drug or refrain from nursing.

Habit-Forming Potential: This drug can cause psychological and/or physical dependence (see Glossary).

Effects of Overdose: Marked drowsiness, weakness, feeling of drunkenness, staggering gait, depression of breathing, stupor progressing to coma.

Possible Effects of Long-Term Use: Psychological or physical dependence, rare liver toxicity.

Suggested Periodic Examinations While Taking This Drug (at physician's discretion)

Liver function tests.

Complete blood cell counts.

▷ **While Taking This Drug, Observe the Following**

Foods: No restrictions.

Herbal Medicines or Minerals: Kava and valerian may exacerbate central nervous system depression (avoid this combination). Kola nut, Siberian ginseng, mate, ephedra, hawthorn and ma huang may blunt the benefits of this medicine. While St. John's wort is indicated for anxiety, it is also thought to increase (induce) cytochrome P450 enzymes and will tend to blunt lorazepam effectiveness. St. John's wort may also worsen sun sensitivity.

Beverages: Avoid excessive caffeine-containing beverages: coffee, tea and cola.

▷ *Alcohol:* Avoid this combination. Alcohol increases depression of mental function, further worsens coordination and causes increased lorazepam levels.

Tobacco Smoking: Heavy smoking may reduce the calming action of this drug. I advise everyone to quit smoking.

Marijuana Smoking: Additive drowsiness and impaired physical performance.

▷ *Other Drugs*

Lorazepam *taken concurrently* with

- clozapine (Clozaril) may result in marked sedation and muscular incoordination.
- heparin may result in increased effects of lorazepam (increased free fraction).
- lithium (Lithobid, others) may result in a lowering of body temperature (hypothermic reaction).
- oxycodone (Percocet, others) and other central nervous system depressants may result in additive CNS or respiratory depression.
- phenytoin (Dilantin) or fosphenytoin (Cerebyx) may result in altered phenytoin or lorazepam levels.
- quetiapine (Seroquel) may increase lorazepam levels. Watch for increased drowsiness, dizziness or movement trouble.

The following drugs may *increase* the effects of lorazepam:

- macrolide antibiotics (see Drug Classes).
- probenecid (Benemid)—may result in a 50% increased lorazepam level; decreased lorazepam doses or an increased time between doses are indicated.
- valproic acid (Depakene)—decreased doses or an increased time between doses may be needed.

The following drugs may *decrease* the effects of lorazepam:

- birth control pills (oral contraceptives).
- caffeine, amphetamines or other stimulants.
- theophylline (Theo-Dur, others).

▷ *Driving, Hazardous Activities:* This drug can impair alertness and coordination. Restrict activities as necessary.

Aviation Note: The use of this drug *is a disqualification* for piloting. Consult a designated Aviation Medical Examiner.

Exposure to Sun: No restrictions.
Discontinuation: Do **not** stop this drug suddenly if it has been taken for over 4 weeks. Consult your doctor about a gradual tapering of dose.

LOSARTAN (loh SAR tan)

Please see the angiotensin II receptor antagonist family profile.

LOVASTATIN (loh vah STA tin)

Introduced: 1987   **Class:** Anticholesterol   **Prescription:** USA: Yes
Controlled Drug: USA: No   **Available as Generic:** USA: Yes with new generics approved in June and July of 2001; Canada: Yes
Brand Names: ♣Apo-Lovastatin, Mevacor

BENEFITS versus RISKS	
Possible Benefits	*Possible Risks*
EFFECTIVE REDUCTION OF TOTAL BLOOD CHOLESTEROL	Drug-induced hepatitis (without jaundice)
SLOWS PROGRESSION OF CORONARY ATHEROSCLEROSIS	Drug-induced myositis (muscle inflammation)
PREVENTS CORONARY HEART DISEASE IN PATIENTS WHO DO NOT HAVE SYMPTOMS, BUT DO HAVE INCREASED TOTAL CHOLESTEROL, LDL-C AND LOW HDL-C	Decreased co-enzyme Q10
May reduce risk of stroke, like other medicines in this class	
May lower the risk of some cancers	

▷ **Principal Uses**

As a Single Drug Product: Uses currently included in FDA-approved labeling: (1) Reduces abnormally high total blood cholesterol levels in people with type II hypercholesterolemia—should not be used until nondrug methods have proven to be inadequate; (2) used to **slow progression** of coronary (heart) atherosclerosis in people with coronary heart disease. It was also shown to reduce the number of heart attacks; (3) Prevents coronary heart disease in patients who do not have symptoms, but do have increased total cholesterol, LDL-C and below average HDL-C.

Other (unlabeled) generally accepted uses: (1) May help decrease hypercholesterolemia in cholesterol ester storage disease prior to liver transplant; (2) could have a role in helping blue toe syndrome (peripheral atheroembolism); (3) could help lower cholesterol in secondary hyperlipidemia; (4) may help (low dose) in the nephrotic syndrome; (5) could help hyperlipidemia in transplant recipients; (6) may reduce stroke risk; (7) appears to work in the proteasome pathway to increase cyclin-dependent kinase inhibitors (CDKI) and lower the risk of cancer.

How This Drug Works: It is converted to mevinolinic acid, which inhibits the liver enzyme that starts to make cholesterol. It decreases low-density lipoproteins (LDL), the fraction of total blood cholesterol that increases risk of coronary heart disease. Also increases high-density lipoproteins (HDL), the fraction thought to reduce the risk of heart disease. The original (prodrug) form of this medicine increases CDKI P21 and P27 and may account for the ability of lovastatin to lower the risk of cancer.

Available Dosage Forms and Strengths
> Tablets — 10 mg, 20 mg, 40 mg

▷ **Usual Adult Dosage Ranges:** Initially 20 mg once a day with the evening meal. Dose may be increased up to 40 mg twice a day as needed and tolerated. Dose adjustments should be made at 4-week intervals. Limited data support low-dose therapy, where some patients responded to 20 mg as a single evening dose. Maximum daily dose should not exceed 80 mg. **Note: Actual dose and dosing schedule must be determined for each patient individually.**

Conditions Requiring Dosing Adjustments
> *Liver Function:* This drug should be used with caution by patients with liver compromise. 83% of a dose is removed in the feces.
> *Kidney Function:* Great caution should be used in considering doses above 20 mg per day for patients with severe kidney problems (creatinine clearance less than 30 ml/min).

▷ **Dosing Instructions:** Take with food, preferably with the evening meal for maximal effectiveness. Highest rates of cholesterol production occur between midnight and 5 a.m. Tablet may be crushed. If you forget a dose: Take the missed dose as soon as you remember it, unless it's nearly time for your next dose if that is the case, skip the missed dose and take the next dose right on schedule. Talk with your doctor if you find yourself missing doses. Even though high cholesterol does not have symptoms, taking your medicine lets you take control of the problem.

Usual Duration of Use: Use on a regular schedule for 4 to 6 weeks determines effectiveness in reducing blood levels of total and LDL cholesterol. Long-term use (months to years) requires periodic physician evaluation of response.

Typical Treatment Goals and Measurements (Outcomes and Markers)
> *Cholesterol*: The National Institutes of Health has released ATP III as part of the update to the National Cholesterol Education Program or NCEP. Key points in these new guidelines include acknowledging diabetes as one of the conditions that increases risk of heart disease, modifying risk factors and recommending routine testing for all of the cholesterol fractions (lipoprotein profile) versus total cholesterol alone. These new guidelines also recommend a desirable total cholesterol of 200 mg/dl as before, but change optimal LDL to 100 mg/dl, 130–159 mg/dl as borderline high, 160mg/dl as high and cite 190 mg/dl as very high. One other noteworthy change is that "good cholesterol" or HDL has been made more important. The "too low" measure for HDL has been increased to 40 mg/dl. Take your medicine and reach these new targets! Electron beam computed tomography (EBCT) is an important tool to use in conjunction with these laboratory studies. Findings show that even patients who meet cholesterol goals

(particularly females over 55) can still be at significant cardiovascular risk. EBCT then defines that risk by giving a calcium score and a "virtual tour" of the coronary arteries.

Possible Advantages of This Drug:
   Better tolerated than some of the other drugs in this class. Increases compounds in the body that may reduce the risk of cancer.

▷ **This Drug Should Not Be Taken If**
   • you have had an allergic reaction to it previously.
   • you have active liver disease.
   • you are pregnant or breast-feeding.

▷ **Inform Your Physician Before Taking This Drug If**
   • you have liver disease or impaired liver function.
   • you have had peptic ulcer disease or upper gastrointestinal bleeding.
   • you are not using any method of birth control or you are planning pregnancy.
   • you have a history of kidney compromise.
   • you regularly consume substantial amounts of alcohol.
   • you have cataracts or impaired vision.
   • you have any type of chronic muscular disorder.

Possible Side Effects (natural, expected and unavoidable drug actions)
   Development of abnormal liver function tests without associated symptoms. Increases CDKI P21 and P27 and may decrease cancer risk.

▷ **Possible Adverse Effects** (unusual, unexpected and infrequent reactions)
   If any of the following develop, consult your physician promptly for guidance.
   Mild Adverse Effects
   Allergic reactions: skin rash, itching.
   Headache, insomnia, dizziness, blurred vision, altered taste—rare to infrequent.
   Indigestion, stomach pain, nausea, excessive gas, constipation, diarrhea—infrequent.
   Muscle cramps or pain—infrequent.
   Impaired sense of smell—possible.
   Serious Adverse Effects
   Marked and persistent abnormal liver function tests with focal hepatitis (without jaundice) after 1 year of use—rare.
   Acute myopathy (muscle pain and tenderness) or rhabdomyolysis—case reports.
   Cataracts were a concern based on some early data, but long-term information fails to demonstrate any adverse effect on the lens of the eye.
   Neuropathy or systemic lupus erythematosus-like syndrome—case reports.

▷ **Possible Effects on Sexual Function:** None reported.

Possible Delayed Adverse Effects: Myopathy.

Natural Diseases or Disorders That May Be Activated by This Drug
   Latent liver disease.

Possible Effects on Laboratory Tests
   Blood alanine aminotransferase (ALT) enzyme level: increased (with higher doses of drug).

Blood total cholesterol, LDL cholesterol and triglyceride levels: decreased.
Blood HDL cholesterol level: increased.

CAUTION
1. Stop the drug immediately and call your doctor if you become pregnant.
2. Promptly report development of unexplained muscle pain or tenderness.
3. Call your doctor right away if altered or impaired vision happens.

Precautions for Use
By Infants and Children: Safety and effectiveness for those under 20 years of age are not established.
By Those Over 60 Years of Age: Tell your doctor about any personal or family history of cataracts. Comply with periodic eye examinations. Promptly report any alterations in vision.

▷ **Advisability of Use During Pregnancy**
Pregnancy Category: X. See Pregnancy Risk Categories at the back of this book.
Animal studies: Mouse and rat studies reveal skeletal birth defects due to this drug.
Human studies: Adequate studies of pregnant women are not available.
This drug should be avoided during entire pregnancy.

Advisability of Use If Breast-Feeding
Presence of this drug in breast milk: Probably yes.
Avoid drug or refrain from nursing.

Habit-Forming Potential: None.

Effects of Overdose: Increased indigestion, stomach distress, nausea, diarrhea.

Possible Effects of Long-Term Use: Abnormal liver function with focal hepatitis. Studies in rats with three to four times the human dose have resulted in increases in hepatocellular carcinoma (cancer). Clinical significance in humans is not known. Research published in July in the National Academy of Sciences Proceedings shows that this medicine increases cyclin-dependent kinase inhibitors P21 and P27. This effect may reduce the risk of cancer in humans.

Suggested Periodic Examinations While Taking This Drug (at physician's discretion)
Blood cholesterol studies: total cholesterol, HDL and LDL fractions.
Liver function tests BEFORE starting therapy, every 6 weeks during the first 3 months of use, every 3 months for the remainder of the first year and then every 6 months thereafter.
Author's Note: A related medicine called cerivastatin (Baycol) was removed from the market because of liver changes. It is unknown at the time of this writing if the FDA will review similar medicines and ask for more frequent checks of liver function.
Complete eye examination at beginning of treatment and periodically thereafter. Ask your physician for guidance.

▷ **While Taking This Drug, Observe the Following**
Foods: Follow a standard low-cholesterol diet.
Herbal Medicines or Minerals: No data exist from well-designed clinical studies about garlic and cerivastatin combinations and cannot presently be rec-

ommended. Additionally, garlic may inhibit blood-clotting (platelet) aggregation—something to consider if you are already taking a platelet inhibitor. The FDA has allowed one dietary supplement called Cholestin to continue to be sold. This preparation actually contains lovastatin. Since use of two HMG-CoA inhibitors may increase risk of rhabdomyolysis or myopathy, the combination is NOT advised.

Use of plant stanol ester–containing products (Benecol) can help lower total and LDL cholesterol. Soy (milk, tofu, etc.) contains phytoestrogens that have led to an FDA-approved health claim for reducing risk of heart disease (if there are at least 6.25 g of soy protein per serving). Substituting soy for some of the meat in your diet can also help results in fighting excessive cholesterol. Because lovastatin can deplete coenzyme Q10, supplementation may be needed.

Beverages: Grapefruit juice can increase blood levels. Prudent not to combine. No restrictions. May be taken with milk.

▷ *Alcohol:* No interactions expected. Use sparingly.

Tobacco Smoking: No interactions expected, but I advise everyone to quit smoking.

▷ *Other Drugs*

Lovastatin **taken concurrently** with

- clofibrate (Atromid-S, others) may damage muscles (rhabdomyolysis).
- colesevelam (Welchol) can help further lower cholesterol.
- cyclosporine (Sandimmune) can cause a severe myopathy.
- diltiazem (Cardizem) may increase risk of myopathy.
- erythromycin (E.E.S.) and perhaps other macrolide antibiotics (clarithromycin or dirithromycin) may result in severe rhabdomyolysis.
- fluconazole (Diflucan), itraconazole (Sporanox) or ketoconazole (Nizoral) may increase risk of muscle damage (rhabdomyolysis).
- gemfibrozil (Lopid) and other fibrates may cause myopathy and the combination is not recommended.
- levothyroxine (various) may decrease thyroxine benefits.
- nefazodone (Serzone) may lead to myopathy.
- niacin (various) can increase risk of muscle damage (myopathy). Niacin may also increase homocysteine levels—a risk factor for heart disease.
- quinupristin/dalfopristin (Synercid) may increase risk of muscle damage (rhabdomyolysis).
- ritonavir (Norvir), amprenavir (Agenerase), indinavir (Crixivan) and perhaps other protease inhibitors may lead to lovastatin toxicity.
- warfarin (Coumadin, others) may result in bleeding; increased frequency of INR (prothrombin time or protime) testing is suggested.

▷ *Driving, Hazardous Activities:* This drug may cause dizziness or impaired vision. Restrict activities as necessary.

Aviation Note: The use of this drug **may be a disqualification** for piloting. Consult a designated Aviation Medical Examiner.

Exposure to Sun: No restrictions.

Discontinuation: Do not stop this drug without your physician's knowledge and guidance.

LOW-MOLECULAR-WEIGHT HEPARINS (HEP ar inz)

Introduced: (Europe 1991) 1998, (includes latest PI approval data) **Class:** Anticoagulant **Prescription:** USA: Yes **Controlled Drug:** USA: No; Canada: No **Available as Generic:** USA: No; Canada: No

Brand Names: Ardeparin: Normiflo, Dalteparin: Fragmin; Enoxaparin: Lovenox; Tinzaparin: Innohep

Author's Note: Because potential outpatient use trends are increasing, information in this profile will be broadened in subsequent editions. A new statement has been released from the American Heart Association on heparin use with low-molecular-weight heparins.

MACROLIDE ANTIBIOTIC FAMILY (ma KRO lied)

Azithromycin (a zith roh MY sin) **Clarithromycin** (KLAR ith roh my sin) **Erythromycin** (er ith roh MY sin)

Introduced: 1991, 1991, 1952, respectively **Class:** Anti-infective, antibiotic, macrolide antibiotic **Prescription:** USA: Yes **Controlled Drug:** USA: No; Canada: No **Available as Generic:** Azithromycin: No; clarithromycin: No; erythromycin: Yes

Brand Names: Azithromycin: Zithromax, Clarithromycin: Biaxin, Biaxin XL (Biaxin XL Pac), Prevpac [CD], Erythromycin: AK-Mycin Ophthalmic, Akne-Mycin, ❤Apo-Erythro Base, ❤Apo-Erythro E-C, ❤Apo-Erythro-ES, ❤Apo-Erythro-S, A/T/S, Benzamycin [CD], C-Solve 2, E.E.S., E.E.S. 200, E.E.S. 400, Emgel, E-Mycin, E-Mycin Controlled Release, E-Mycin E, E-Mycin 333, Eramycin, ❤Erybid, ERYC, Erycette, Eryderm, Erygel, Erymax, EryPed, Eryphar, Ery-Tab, Erythrocin, ❤Erythromid, E-Solve 2, Ethril, ETS-2%, Ilosone, Ilotycin, ❤Novo-Rythro, PCE, Pediamycin, ❤Pediazole [CD], ❤PMS-Erythromycin, Robimycin, Sans-Acne, SK-Erythromycin, Staticin, ❤Stievamycin, T-Stat, ❤Wyamycin E, Wyamycin S

BENEFITS versus RISKS	
Possible Benefits	*Possible Risks*
EFFECTIVE TREATMENT OF INFECTIONS due to susceptible microorganisms	Allergic reactions, mild and infrequent Liver reaction (most common with erythromycin estolate)
MAY ACTUALLY HAVE A ROLE IN PREVENTING OR TREATING SOME HEART ATTACKS WHERE *CHLAMYDIA PNEUMONIAE* IS PRESENT	Mild gastrointestinal symptoms Drug-induced colitis Superinfections

▷ **Principal Uses**

As a Single Drug Product: Uses currently included in FDA-approved labeling: Treatment of (1) skin and skin structure infections (such as acne and Streptococcus); (2) upper and lower respiratory tract infections, including "strep" throat, diphtheria and several types of pneumonia; (3) gonorrhea and syphilis; (4) amebic dysentery (erythromycin); (5) Legionnaire's disease (erythromycin); (6) long-term prevention of recurrences of rheumatic fever (erythromycin)—effective use requires the precise identification of the causative organism and determination of its sensitivity to a macrolide antibiotic; (7) treatment of mycoplasma pneumonia; (8) listeriosis; (9) neonatal conjunctivitis (erythromycin); (10) treatment of ear infections (otitis media) (all); (11) treatment of AIDS-related *Mycobacterium avium-intracellulare* (all); (12) treatment of *Chlamydia trachomatis* urethritis (azithromycin); (13) therapy of *Helicobacter pylori* duodenal ulcers in combination with omeprazole (clarithromycin); (14) prevention of bacterial endocarditis in people allergic to penicillin.

Author's Note: An Agency for Health Care Policy and Research (AHCPR) study found that most patients who were 60 or younger obtained the same outcomes and significantly reduced costs when erythromycin was used to treat community-acquired pneumonia versus other antibiotics. The new Biaxin XL is presently only approved for sinusitis and bronchitis in adults.

Other (unlabeled) generally accepted uses: (1) Treatment of early Lyme disease (erythromycin; azithromycin is an alternative drug); (2) erythromycin helps sterilize the bowel before surgical procedures; (3) may help threatened preterm labor if the cause is Ureaplasma organisms (erythromycin); (4) helps impetigo (erythromycin); (5) azithromycin or clarithromycin are second choices for Legionnaire's disease; (6) early azithromycin therapy can reduce severity of gum (gingival) hyperplasia caused by cyclosporine; (7) can help some cases of stomach slowness in diabetics (gastroparesis); (8) may treat or prevent some heart attacks where *Chlamydia pneumoniae* is present.

As a Combination Drug Product [CD]: Clarithromycin is available in combination with amoxicillin and lansoprazole. Since refractory ulcers are often actually *Helicobacter pylori* infections, the combination works to kill the bacteria and lower acid production.

How These Drugs Work: They prevent growth and multiplication of susceptible organisms by interfering with their formation of essential proteins.

Available Dosage Forms and Strengths

Azithromycin:
>Oral suspension — 100 mg/5 ml, 200 mg/5 ml
>Tablet — 600 mg

Clarithromycin:
>Oral suspension granules — 125 mg/5 ml, 185.5 mg/5ml or 250 mg/5 ml
>Tablets — 250 mg, 500 mg
>Tablets, extended release — 500 mg

Erythromycin:
>Capsules — 125 mg, 250 mg
>Capsules, enteric coated — 125 mg, 250 mg
>Drops — 100 mg/ml
>Eye ointment — 5 mg/g
>Gel — 2%
>Oral suspension — 125 mg/5 ml, 250 mg/5 ml
>Skin ointment — 2%
>Tablets — 250 mg, 500 mg

Tablets, chewable — 125 mg, 200 mg, 250 mg
Tablets, delayed release — 250 mg, 333 mg
Tablets, dispersible (Canada) — 500 mg
Tablets, enteric coated — 250 mg, 333 mg, 500 mg
Tablets, film coated — 250 mg, 500 mg
Topical solution — 1.5%, 2%

▷ **Recommended Dosage Ranges** (Actual dose and schedule must be determined for each patient individually.)

Infants and Children:

Azithromycin: For otitis media—10 mg per kg of body mass as a single dose on the first day (up to 500 mg), followed by 5 mg per kg of body mass (up to 250 mg) on days 2–5. For pharyngitis—12 mg per kg of body mass (up to 500 mg) daily for 5 days.

Clarithromycin: When used to treat otitis media (caused by Haemophilus influenzae, M. catarrhalis or Strep. pneumoniae) in children, the dose is 7.5 mg per kg of body mass twice daily, up to a maximum of 500 mg twice a day for 10 days. For Mycobacterium avium-intracellulare complex infections in children, the dose is 7.5 mg per kg of body mass twice daily, to a maximum of 500 mg twice a day. If this dose is successful, therapy is continued for life.

Erythromycin: In pediatrics, oral erythromycin is usually given at a dose of 30 to 50 mg per kg of body mass per day and is divided into three or four doses.

12 to 60 Years of Age:

Azithromycin (16 to 60 years of age): For pharyngitis/tonsillitis, bronchitis, pneumonia and skin infections—500 mg as a single dose on the first day and then 250 mg once daily on days 2–4 for a total dose of 1.5 g. For Helicobacter pylori—500 mg daily for 7 days. For nongonococcal urethritis and cervicitis—a single 1 g (1,000 mg) dose.

Clarithromycin: For pharyngitis/tonsillitis—250 mg every 12 hours for 10 days. For maxillary sinusitis—500 mg every 12 hours for 14 days. For acute bronchitis—250 to 500 mg every 12 hours for 7 to 14 days. For pneumonia—250–500 mg every 12 hours for 7 to 14 days. For skin infections—250 mg every 12 hours for 7 to 14 days. Biaxin XL treats bronchitis (sudden or acute exacerbation of chronic bronchitis) in adults with two 500 mg tablets (1,000 mg), once a day for 7 days. Sudden or acute maxillary sinusitis is treated using two 500 mg tablets for 14 days.

Erythromycin: 250 to 500 mg every 6 hours, according to nature and severity of infection. Total daily dose should not exceed 4 g. For endocarditis prophylaxis (stearate oral form): 1 g 2 hours before procedure and 500 mg 6 hours later.

Over 60 Years of Age:

Azithromycin: Same as 16 to 60 years of age. If liver or kidney function is limited, the dose must be reduced.

Clarithromycin: Same as 12 to 60 years of age. Dose must be reduced in kidney compromise.

Erythromycin: Same as usual adult dosing range. If liver or kidney function is limited, dose must be reduced.

Conditions Requiring Dosing Adjustments

Liver Function: These drugs are metabolized in the liver and will accumulate in patients with liver compromise. Decreased doses may be needed. They should be used with caution by patients with biliary tract disease. Clarithromycin does not need to be adjusted for patients with liver problems if kidney function is normal.

Kidney Function: No dosing changes are needed for azithromycin. The dose of clarithromycin must be decreased or the time between doses (dosing interval) prolonged for patients with compromised kidneys (for example, if the CrCl is less than 30 ml/min, one half of the usual dose could be used in the usual dosing interval). Patients with severe kidney failure can take 50–75% of the usual erythromycin dose at the usual time. Azithromycin and erythromycin are rare causes of interstitial nephritis (inflammation of a specific part of the kidney).

▷ **Dosing Instructions:** Nonenteric-coated preparations should be taken 1 hour before or 2 hours after eating. Enteric-coated preparations may be taken without regard to food. Azithromycin may be better tolerated if taken with food. Do not take azithromycin with antacids containing aluminum or magnesium. Regular uncoated capsules may be opened, and tablets may be crushed; coated and prolonged-action preparations should be swallowed whole. Biaxin XL should be taken WITH food to help increase absorption. Ask your pharmacist for help. If you forget a dose: Take the missed dose as soon as you remember it, unless it's nearly time for your next dose—if that is the case, skip the missed dose and take the next dose right on schedule. Talk with your doctor if you find yourself missing doses.

Usual Duration of Use: Use on a regular schedule for 3 to 5 days is necessary to determine this drug's effectiveness in controlling infections. For streptococcal infections: not less than 10 consecutive (5 consecutive for azithromycin) days (without interruption) to reduce the possibility of developing rheumatic fever or glomerulonephritis. The duration of use should not exceed the time required to eliminate the infection.

Typical Treatment Goals and Measurements (Outcomes and Markers)

Infections: The most commonly used measures of serious infections are white blood cell counts and differentials (the kind of blood cells that occur most often in your blood), and temperature. Many clinicians look for positive changes in 24–48 hours. NEVER stop an antibiotic because you start to feel better. For many infections, a full 14 days is REQUIRED to kill the bacteria. The goals and time frame (see peak benefits above) should be discussed with you when the prescription is written.

Possible Advantages of These Drugs

Azithromycin and clarithromycin: Broader spectrum of infectious microorganism coverage; equivalent to erythromycin, some penicillins and some cephalosporins. Effective with fewer doses (only one dose for azithromycin, two for clarithromycin, and once daily for the Biaxin XL form), which may help pill-taking or adherence. Azithromycin and clarithromycin are very well tolerated; infrequent and minor adverse effects.

▷ **These Drugs Should Not Be Taken If**
- you had an allergic reaction to a macrolide previously.
- you have active liver disease (erythromycin estolate form).
- you are pregnant or planning pregnancy (some forms).
- you are allergic to *para*-aminobenzoic-acid-type anesthetics (intramuscular form of erythromycin).
- you are taking terfenadine (Seldane) or astemizole (Hismanal).

▷ **Inform Your Physician Before Taking These Drugs If**
- you have a history of a previous "reaction" to any macrolide antibiotic.
- you are allergic by nature: hay fever, asthma, hives, eczema.
- you have a blood disorder.
- you have an abnormal heart rhythm.
- you have a history of porphyria.
- you have a history of kidney disorder.
- you have myasthenia gravis.
- you have a hearing disorder.
- you are taking a blood thinner (oral anticoagulant) (clarithromycin).
- you have a history of low blood platelets (some macrolides).
- you have taken the estolate form of erythromycin previously.

Possible Side Effects (natural, expected and unavoidable drug actions)
Superinfections (see Glossary).

▷ **Possible Adverse Effects** (unusual, unexpected and infrequent reactions)
If any of the following develop, consult your physician promptly for guidance.

Mild Adverse Effects
Allergic reactions: skin rash, hives, itching—rare.
Nausea, vomiting, diarrhea, abdominal cramping—infrequent.
Headache—rare.
Visual hallucinations—case report for clarithromycin.
Drug-induced increased liver enzymes (see Jaundice in Glossary)—rare.

Serious Adverse Effects
Allergic reaction: anaphylactic reaction (see Glossary)—rare.
Idiosyncratic reactions: liver reaction—nausea, vomiting, fever, jaundice (usually, but not exclusively, associated with erythromycin estolate).
Prolonging of the QT interval (torsade de pointes or ventricular tachycardia)—possible.
Abnormal heart rhythm—rare.
Decreased white blood cells (erythromycin)—rare.
Lowered blood platelets (clarithromycin)—case report.
Worsening of myasthenia gravis—case reports.
Low body temperature (hypothermia)—rare.
Pseudomembranous colitis—rare.
Pancreatitis (erythromycin)—rare.
Kidney problems (interstitial nephritis) (azithromycin, erythromycin)—case reports.
Abnormal urination (SIADH)—case reports for azithromycin.
Hearing loss (ototoxicity)—case reports.

▷ **Possible Effects on Sexual Function:** None reported.

▷ **Adverse Effects That May Mimic Natural Diseases or Disorders**
Liver toxicity may resemble acute gallbladder disease or viral hepatitis.

Possible Effects on Laboratory Tests
Complete blood cell counts: white cells may increase or decrease; eosinophils increased (allergic reaction); platelets decreased.
INR (prothrombin time): increased (drugs taken concurrently with warfarin).
Liver function tests: liver enzymes increased (ALT/GPT, AST/GOT and alkaline phosphatase), increased bilirubin.

CAUTION
1. Take the **full dose prescribed** to help prevent resistant bacteria.
2. If you have a history of liver disease or impaired liver function, avoid any form of erythromycin estolate.
3. If diarrhea develops and continues for more than 24 hours, consult your physician promptly.

Precautions for Use

By Infants and Children: Watch allergic children closely for indications of developing allergy to this drug. Observe also for evidence of gastrointestinal irritation. Dosing based on body mass is critical.

By Those Over 60 Years of Age: Watch for itching reactions in the genital and anal regions, often due to yeast superinfections. Observe also for evidence of hearing loss. Report such developments promptly. If liver or kidney function is impaired, dose decreases must be considered.

▷ **Advisability of Use During Pregnancy**

Pregnancy Category: C for clarithromycin. B for others. See Pregnancy Risk Categories at the back of this book.

Animal studies: Studies of rats are inconclusive for erythromycin. Monkey, rabbit and rat studies have shown problems in pregnancy outcomes and fetal development.

Human studies: Information from adequate studies of pregnant women is not available.

Generally thought to be safe during entire pregnancy, except for erythromycin estolate; this form of erythromycin can cause toxic liver reactions during pregnancy and should be avoided. Clarithromycin should be avoided unless no other antibiotic option is available.

Advisability of Use If Breast-Feeding

Presence of this drug in breast milk: Yes for others; clarithromycin unknown. Watch nursing infant closely and discontinue drug or nursing if adverse effects develop.

Habit-Forming Potential: None.

Effects of Overdose: Possible nausea, vomiting, hallucinations (clarithromycin), diarrhea and abdominal discomfort.

Possible Effects of Long-Term Use: Superinfections (see Glossary).

Suggested Periodic Examinations While Taking These Drugs (at physician's discretion)

Liver function tests if the erythromycin estolate form is used.

Complete blood counts to measure response of infection.

▷ **While Taking These Drugs, Observe the Following**

Foods: New formulation absorption is decreased by more than 70% (especially with high-fat meals) and effectiveness may be seriously compromised for erythromycin. Azithromycin and clarithromycin are not affected.

Herbal Medicines or Minerals: Echinacea: Some patients use echinacea to attempt to boost their immune systems. Unfortunately, use of echinacea is not recommended in people with damaged immune systems. This herb may also actually weaken any immune system if it is used too often or for too long a time. DO NOT take mistletoe herb, oak bark or F.C. of marshmallow root and licorice. **Caution:** St. John's wort may also cause extreme reactions to the sun. Additive photosensitivity may be possible.

Beverages: Avoid fruit juices and carbonated beverages for 1 hour after taking any nonenteric-coated preparation of erythromycin. May be taken with milk.

▷   *Alcohol:* Avoid if you have impaired liver function or are taking the estolate form of erythromycin.

Tobacco Smoking: No interactions expected. I advise everyone to quit smoking.

▷   *Other Drugs*

Clarithromycin and erythromycin may *increase* the effects of

- benzodiazepines (see Drug Classes).
- buspirone (Buspar) (erythromycin only).
- carbamazepine (Tegretol) and cause toxicity.
- cisapride (Propulsid).
- clozapine (Clozaril).
- digoxin (Lanoxin) and cause toxicity.
- ergotamine (Cafergot, Ergostat, etc.) and cause impaired circulation to extremities.
- methylprednisolone (Medrol) and prednisone and cause excess steroid effects.
- phenytoin (Dilantin or fosphenytoin (Cerebyx).
- quetiapine (Seroquel).
- quinidine (Quinaglute, others).
- sibutramine (Meridia).
- sildenafil (Viagra)—reported up to 182% increased blood level (clarithromycin and erythromycin only).
- tacrolimus (Prograf) or sirolimus (Rapamune).
- theophylline (aminophylline, Theo-Dur, etc.) and cause toxicity.
- tretinoin (Vesanoid).
- valproic acid (Depakote).
- vinblastine (Velban).
- warfarin (Coumadin) and increase the risk of bleeding (azithromycin also).

These medicines may *decrease* the effects of

- clindamycin.
- lincomycin.
- penicillins.

These medicines *taken concurrently* with

- astemizole (Hismanal) may cause serious arrhythmias.
- atorvastatin (Lipitor) and other HMG-CoA reductase inhibitors INCREASES RISK OF MYOPATHY (serious muscle damage) if used with erythromycin or clarithromycin.
- birth control pills (oral contraceptives) can cause loss of effectiveness and result in pregnancy (erythromycin).
- cyclosporine (Sandimmune) may result in cyclosporine toxicity.
- dihydroergotamine and other ergot derivatives can lead to increased levels and ergot toxicity.
- disopyramide may cause heart (cardiac) arrhythmias.
- dofetilide (Tikosyn) may lead to dofetilide toxicity.
- fluoxetine (Prozac) may lead to fluoxetine toxicity.
- grepafloxacin (Raxar) and perhaps gatifloxacin (Tequin) may lead to heartbeat changes (prolonged QTc interval) if combined with erythromycin.
- lansoprazole (Prevacid) may lead to black tongue if combined with clarithromycin.

- loratadine (Claritin) may result in increased loratadine levels (also with fexofenadine [Allegra]), but they do not appear to cause the serious arrhythmia of some of the other nonsedating antihistamines. Since loratadine or fexofenadine levels may be increased, it may be prudent to decrease doses while taking erythromycin.
- midazolam (and probably other benzodiazepines) (see Drug Classes) may lead to excessive central nervous system depression.
- nevirapine (Viramune), delavirdine (Rescriptor) or efavirenz (Sustiva) may lead to nevirapine, efavirenz or delavirdine toxicity.
- omeprazole may increase levels of both medicines.
- prednisone and other corticosteroids may lead to corticosteroid toxicity if combined with clarithromycin or erythromycin.
- rifabutin (Mycobutin) increases risk of low white blood cells (neutropenia) if combined with azithromycin or clarithromycin; clarithromycin also increases risk of rifabutin rash.
- ritonavir (Norvir) and perhaps other protease inhibitors (see Drug Classes) may lead to toxicity.
- sparfloxacin (Zagam) may lead to heartbeat changes (prolonged QTc interval) if combined with erythromycin.
- terfenadine (Seldane) can cause cardiac (heart) arrhythmias.
- triazolam may cause toxicity.
- trimexate (Mexate) decrease trimexate metabolism and can lead to toxicity.
- valproic acid (Depakene, Depakote) can lead to toxic blood levels.
- zidovudine (AZT) may lead to decreased levels and lack of zidovudine effectiveness (clarithromycin and erythromycin).

▷ *Driving, Hazardous Activities:* This drug may cause nausea and/or diarrhea. Restrict activities as necessary.

Aviation Note: The use of these drugs *may be a disqualification* for piloting. Consult a designated Aviation Medical Examiner.

Exposure to Sun: Use caution; some medicines in this class have caused increased sensitivity to the sun (photosensitivity).

Special Storage Instructions: Keep liquid forms refrigerated.

Observe the Following Expiration Times: Freshly mixed oral suspension—14 days for clarithromycin (DO NOT refrigerate). Freshly mixed oral suspensions of erythromycin should be refrigerated to preserve taste. These go bad (outdate) in 14 days. Single-dose azithromycin suspension should be mixed with water and taken right away. Ask your pharmacist for help.

MAPROTILINE (ma PROH ti leen)

Introduced: 1974   **Class:** Antidepressant   **Prescription:** USA: Yes
Controlled Drug: USA: No; Canada: No   **Available as Generic:** Yes
Brand Name: Ludiomil
Author's Note: Because use of this medicine has declined in favor of newer medicines, the information in this profile has been abbreviated.

MECLOFENAMATE (me kloh fen AM ayt)

Please see the fenamate (nonsteroidal anti-inflammatory drug) family profile.

MEDROXYPROGESTERONE (me DROX e proh jess te rohn)

Introduced: 1959   **Class:** Female sex hormones, progestins   **Prescription:** USA: Yes   **Controlled Drug:** USA: No; Canada: No   **Available as Generic:** Yes

Brand Names: ✤Alti-MPA, Amen, Curretab, Cycrin, Depo-Provera, Premphase, Prempro, Provera

---

BENEFITS versus RISKS

Possible Benefits	*Possible Risks*
EFFECTIVE TREATMENT OF ABSENT OR ABNORMAL MENSTRUATION due to hormone imbalance	Thrombophlebitis
	Pulmonary embolism
	Liver reaction with jaundice
	Drug-induced birth defects
EFFECTIVE CONTRACEPTION when given by injection	
Useful adjunctive therapy in selected cases of uterine and kidney cancer	

▷ **Principal Uses**

As a Single Drug Product: Uses currently included in FDA-approved labeling: (1) Used to initiate and regulate menstruation and correct abnormal patterns of menstrual bleeding caused by hormonal imbalance (and not by organic disease); (2) used in combination to treat metastatic, inoperable or recurrent endometrial carcinoma; (3) treatment of renal cell carcinoma; (4) used as a contraceptive injected into the muscle once every 3 months; (5) helps dysfunctional uterine bleeding; (6) used to help infants with alveolar hypoventilation syndrome.

Other (unlabeled) generally accepted uses: (1) Used as a part of combination therapy in breast, refractory prostate, lung and ovarian cancers; (2) therapy of endometriosis; (3) used in osteoporosis to help increase bone mineral density; (4) helps abnormal hair growth in women (hirsutism); (5) can help breast pain (mastodynia); (6) used in combination with estrogen to help symptoms of menopause; (7) can be of use in pelvic congestion and pickwickian syndrome; (8) may help severe PMS; (9) can be of use in male hypersexuality.

How This Drug Works: By inducing and maintaining a lining in the uterus that resembles pregnancy, this drug can prevent uterine bleeding until it is withdrawn. By suppressing the release of the pituitary gland hormone that induces ovulation and by stimulating the secretion of mucus by the uterine cervix (to resist the passage of sperm), this drug can prevent pregnancy.

Available Dosage Forms and Strengths

Injection — 100, 150 and 400 mg/ml

Injection (single-dose vials) — 150 mg

Tablets — 2.5 mg, 5 mg, 10 mg

▷ **Usual Adult Dosage Ranges:** *To initiate menstruation*: 5 to 10 mg daily for 5 to 10 days, started at any time.

To correct abnormal bleeding: 5 to 10 mg daily for 5 to 10 days, started on the 16th or 21st day of the menstrual cycle. Withdrawal bleeding usually begins within 3 to 7 days after stopping the drug.

As a contraceptive: Intramuscular injections of 150 mg every 3 months are needed.

Author's Note: Controversy has erupted based on results from the HERS (Heart and estrogen/progestin Replacement Study) trial regarding benefits of estrogen/progestin combination in preventing a second heart attack (secondary prevention). Controversy results from higher use of statins (HMG-CoA reductase inhibitors—see Drug Classes) in the control group and high use of beta blockers and aspirin in both study and control groups. Additional studies include the Women's Health Initiative (WHI) and the WISDOM research. Newer data from the two-year Women's Health, Osteoporosis, Progestin, Estrogen study (HOPE) points to the use of 1.5 mg of progestin with 0.45 or 0.3 mg of estrogen being equal in benefits to higher doses. Note: Actual dose and schedule must be determined for each patient individually.

Conditions Requiring Dosing Adjustments
Liver Function: This drug should be used with caution and the dose empirically decreased, by patients with liver compromise.
Kidney Function: No dosing changes thought to be needed.

▷ **Dosing Instructions:** The tablet may be crushed and taken on an empty stomach or with food to prevent nausea. If you forget a dose: Take the missed dose as soon as you remember it, unless it's nearly time for your next dose—if that is the case, skip the missed dose and take the next dose right on schedule. If you miss a contraceptive injection, call your doctor about alternative forms of birth control. Talk with your doctor if you find yourself missing doses.

Usual Duration of Use: Use on a regular schedule for two or three menstrual cycles determines effectiveness in correcting abnormal patterns of menstrual bleeding. See your doctor on a regular basis.

Typical Treatment Goals and Measurements (Outcomes and Markers)
Contraception: Used to prevent conception with an injection once every 13 weeks. Ongoing use is required to avoid becoming pregnant.

Possible Advantages of This Drug
Effective contraception with a shot once every 13 weeks.

▷ **This Drug Should Not Be Taken If**
- you have had an allergic reaction to it previously.
- you are pregnant.
- you have experienced a missed abortion.
- you have seriously impaired liver function.
- you have a history of cancer of the breast or reproductive organs.
- you have a history of thrombophlebitis, embolism or stroke.
- you have abnormal and unexplained vaginal bleeding.

▷ **Inform Your Physician Before Taking This Drug If**
- you have impaired kidney function.
- you have any of the following disorders: asthma, diabetes, emotional depression, epilepsy, heart disease, migraine headaches.

Possible Side Effects (natural, expected and unavoidable drug actions)
Fluid retention, weight gain, changes in menstrual timing and flow, spotting between periods.

▷ **Possible Adverse Effects** (unusual, unexpected and infrequent reactions)
   If any of the following develop, consult your physician promptly for guidance.
   Mild Adverse Effects
   Allergic reactions: skin rash, hives, itching.
   Fatigue, weakness, nausea—infrequent.
   Acne, excessive hair growth—case reports.
   Serious Adverse Effects
   Liver toxicity with jaundice (see Glossary): yellow eyes/skin, dark-colored urine, light-colored stools—possible.
   Thrombophlebitis (inflammation of a vein with blood clot formation): pain or tenderness in thigh or leg, with or without swelling of the foot, ankle or leg—case reports.
   Pulmonary embolism (movement of blood clot to lung): sudden shortness of breath, chest pain, cough, bloody sputum—case reports.
   Stroke (blood clot in the brain): sudden headache, weakness or paralysis of any part of the body—possible.
   Retinal thrombosis (blood clot in the eye): sudden impairment or loss of vision—case reports.
   Drug-induced pseudotumor cerebri—possible.
   Pneumonitis, especially in patients who have received radiation therapy—case reports.
   Medroxyprogesterone was NOT found to increase risk of breast cancer in a World Health Organization study of 12,759 women. It was also found NOT to increase risk of ovarian or uterine cancer in a study of 5,000 African American women who received it as a contraceptive for ten years.
   A study in mice found that when progesterone was used in large doses for prolonged periods, it acted as a co-carcinogen.
▷ **Possible Effects on Sexual Function:** Altered timing and pattern of menstruation. Female breast tenderness and secretion. Decreased vaginal secretions. Infertility—case reports.
▷ **Adverse Effects That May Mimic Natural Diseases or Disorders**
   Liver toxicity may suggest viral hepatitis.
   Possible Effects on Laboratory Tests
   Blood total cholesterol, HDL cholesterol, LDL cholesterol and triglyceride levels: decreased.
   Glucose tolerance test (GTT): decreased.
   CAUTION
   1. There is an increased risk of birth defects in children whose mothers take this drug during the first 4 months of pregnancy.
   2. Inform your physician promptly if you think you may be pregnant.
   3. This drug should not be used as a test for pregnancy.
   Precautions for Use
   By Infants and Children: Not used in this age group.
   By Those Over 60 Years of Age: Used as adjunctive therapy in cancer of the breast, uterus, prostate and kidney. Watch for excessive fluid retention.
▷ **Advisability of Use During Pregnancy**
   Pregnancy Category: D. See Pregnancy Risk Categories at the back of this book.
   Animal studies: Genital defects reported in rat and rabbit studies; masculin-

ization of the female rodent fetus; various defects in chick embryos and rabbits.

Human studies: In a study of 1,016 pregnancies, oral doses of 80–120 mg daily used from the 5th to 7th week of pregnancy up to the 18th week were not associated with teratogenic effects. Other data show masculinization of the female genitals: enlargement of the clitoris, fusion of the labia. Increased risk of heart, nervous system and limb defects when used in the second and third trimesters of pregnancy.

The drug is used as a benefit-to-risk decision in the first 3 months of pregnancy. Avoid this drug completely during the final 6 months of pregnancy.

Advisability of Use If Breast-Feeding

Presence of this drug in breast milk: Yes.

Avoid drug or refrain from nursing.

Habit-Forming Potential: None.

Effects of Overdose: Nausea, vomiting, fluid retention, breast enlargement and discomfort, abnormal vaginal bleeding.

Possible Effects of Long-Term Use: There has been considerable controversy regarding use of this drug and cancer. The most recent large patient studies do not show an increased relative risk that is statistically significant.

Suggested Periodic Examinations While Taking This Drug (at physician's discretion)

Regular examinations (every 6 to 12 months) of the breasts and reproductive organs (pelvic examination of the uterus and ovaries, including Pap smear).

▷ **While Taking This Drug, Observe the Following**

Foods: No restrictions.

Herbal Medicines or Minerals: Black cohosh appears to work by (1) suppressing luteinizing hormone; (2) binding to estrogen receptors in the pituitary and inhibiting luteinizing hormone release and (3) binding to estrogen receptors in the pituitary. The net effect is that this herb eases symptoms of menopause, but little is known about long-term use or heart and bone protective effects. Talk to your doctor before starting black cohosh if you are currently taking medroxyprogesterone—particularly if you take it for PMS. Calcium may help ease some PMS symptoms.

Beverages: Do not take this medicine with grapefruit juice. Grapefruit juice inhibits CYP3A4, which helps remove this drug from the body.

▷ *Alcohol:* No interactions expected.

Tobacco Smoking: No direct drug interactions expected. I advise everyone to quit smoking.

▷ *Other Drugs*

The following drugs may *decrease* the effects of medroxyprogesterone:
- nevirapine (Viramune).
- rifampin (Rifadin, Rimactane, etc.) may hasten its elimination.

Medroxyprogesterone *taken concurrently* with
- CYP3A4 inhibitors (such as erythromycin, fluoxetine, fluvoxamine, itraconazole, ketoconazole and ritonavir) may lead to increased medroxyprogesterone levels.
- digitoxin may result in slightly higher than expected digoxin levels.
- ritonavir (Norvir) and perhaps other protease inhibitors (see Drug Classes) may lead to toxicity.

- tamoxifen (Nolvadex) may result in blunting of the therapeutic benefits of tamoxifen.
- warfarin (Coumadin) may increase warfarin effects; increased lab INR (prothrombin time or protime) testing is needed.

▷ *Driving, Hazardous Activities:* Usually no restrictions. Ask your doctor about your individual risk and for guidance regarding specific restrictions.

Aviation Note: The use of this drug *may be a disqualification* for piloting. Consult a designated Aviation Medical Examiner.

Exposure to Sun: No restrictions.

MEFENAMIC ACID (me FEN am ik A sid)

Please see the fenamate (nonsteroidal anti-inflammatory drug) family profile.

MEPERIDINE (me PER i deen)

Other Name: Pethidine   **Introduced:** 1939   **Class:** Strong analgesic, opioids   **Prescription:** USA: Yes   **Controlled Drug:** USA: C-II*; Canada: Yes   **Available as Generic:** Yes

Brand Names: Demerol, Demerol APAP [CD], Mepergan, Pethadol, ❧Pethidine

BENEFITS versus RISKS	
Possible Benefits	*Possible Risks*
EFFECTIVE RELIEF OF MODERATE TO SEVERE PAIN	POTENTIAL FOR HABIT FORMATION (DEPENDENCE) ADVERSE REACTIONS FROM ACCUMULATION OF NORMEPERIDINE METABOLITE Weakness, fainting Disorientation, hallucinations Interference with urination Constipation

Author's Note: This profile has been shortened to make room for more effective medicines.

MERCAPTOPURINE (mer kap toh PYUR een)

Other Names: 6-mercaptopurine, 6-MP

Introduced: 1960   **Class:** Anticancer (antineoplastic), immunosuppressant   **Prescription:** USA: Yes   **Controlled Drug:** USA: No; Canada: No   **Available as Generic:** USA: No; Canada: No

Brand Name: Purinethol

*See Schedules of Controlled Drugs at the back of this book.

BENEFITS versus RISKS

Possible Benefits	*Possible Risks*
EFFECTIVE TREATMENT OF CERTAIN ACUTE AND CHRONIC LEUKEMIAS AND LYMPHOMAS	BONE MARROW DEPRESSION (see Glossary)
Effective treatment of polycythemia vera	DRUG-INDUCED LIVER DAMAGE
Possibly effective treatment of Crohn's disease and ulcerative colitis	Rare gastrointestinal ulceration
Possibly effective treatment of severe psoriatic arthritis	

▷ **Principal Uses**

As a Single Drug Product: Uses currently included in FDA-approved labeling: Combination treatment of acute lymphocytic leukemia.

Other (unlabeled) generally accepted uses: Treatment of (1) inflammatory bowel diseases (Crohn's disease and ulcerative colitis); (2) certain cases of severe psoriatic arthritis; (3) may help in cases of autoimmune hepatitis.

How This Drug Works: This drug interferes with specific stages of cell reproduction (tissue growth) by inhibiting the formation of DNA and RNA.

Available Dosage Forms and Strengths

Tablets — 50 mg

▷ **Recommended Dosage Ranges** (Actual dose and schedule must be determined for each patient individually.)

Infants and Children: For leukemia (induction dose)—2.5 mg per kg of body mass (to the nearest 25 mg) daily (roughly 50 mg for the average 5-year-old), in single or divided doses. If the platelets and white blood cell counts do not fall and clinical improvement is not acceptable after 4 weeks of the induction dosing, the dose may be increased to 5 mg per kg of body mass per day. If there is still no response, some centers give mercaptopurine as 75 mg per square meter on days 29–42. This is combined with vincristine, prednisone and methotrexate. Maintenance therapy then occurs as in adult dosing.

12 to 60 Years of Age: For leukemia (induction)—initially 2.5 mg per kg of body mass (to the nearest 25 mg, usually 100–200 mg) daily, in single or divided doses, for 4 weeks. If the white blood cell or platelet counts do not fall and there is no clinical improvement, the dose may be increased as needed and tolerated to 5 mg per kg of body mass daily. For maintenance, 1.5 to 2.5 mg per kg of body mass daily.

For inflammatory bowel disease—1.5 mg per kg of body mass daily. The dose is subsequently adjusted to keep the platelet count above 100,000 and the white blood cell count above 4,500.

Over 60 Years of Age: Same as 12 to 60 years of age.

Conditions Requiring Dosing Adjustments

Liver Function: Used with caution and in decreased doses by patients with liver compromise. It is also a rare cause of liver toxicity.

Kidney Function: Dose should be decreased in kidney (renal) compromise. It is a rare cause of drug crystals in urine.

TPMT Negatives: Some patients do not have an enzyme called thiopurine methyltransferase (TPMT). The mercaptopurine dose is decreased by 10% for these patients.

▷ **Dosing Instructions:** The tablet may be crushed and taken with or following food to reduce stomach upset. If you forget a dose: Take the missed dose as soon as you remember it, unless it's nearly time for your next dose—if that is the case, skip the missed dose and take the next dose right on schedule. DO NOT double doses. Talk with your doctor if you find yourself missing doses.

Usual Duration of Use: Use on a regular schedule for 4 to 6 weeks determines effectiveness in inducing remission in leukemia; continual use for 2 to 3 months determines benefit in treating inflammatory bowel disease. Long-term use (months to years) requires periodic physician evaluation.

Typical Treatment Goals and Measurements (Outcomes and Markers)

Leukemia: The goal is to improve clinical signs and symptoms, and control leukemia while avoiding myelosuppression and liver toxicity. Checks of blood platelets, hematocrits and white blood cell counts are required. Periodic checks of liver function tests help detect liver problems early. Bone marrow tests help define changes in peripheral blood.

▷ **This Drug Should Not Be Taken If**
- you have had an allergic reaction to it previously.
- you have a solid tumor or lymphoma (this drug is not indicated).
- you have leukemia that has spread to the central nervous system.
- you are pregnant. (Ask your physician for guidance.)

▷ **Inform Your Physician Before Taking This Drug If**
- you have a history of drug-induced bone marrow depression.
- you have impaired liver or kidney function.
- you are not using any contraception.
- you have gout.
- you are taking allopurinol (the mercaptopurine dose must be reduced).
- you have inflammatory bowel disease.
- you do not understand the steps needed to dispose of any vomit or urine.
- you have been exposed recently to chicken pox or herpes zoster (shingles).
- you are taking any of the following drugs: allopurinol, probenecid, sulfinpyrazone, anticoagulants, immunosuppressants.

Possible Side Effects (natural, expected and unavoidable drug actions)

Bone marrow depression (see Glossary). Abnormally increased blood uric acid levels; possible urate kidney stones, hyperpigmentation of the skin. Possible drug fever. Serum sickness.

▷ **Possible Adverse Effects** (unusual, unexpected and infrequent reactions)

If any of the following develop, consult your physician promptly for guidance.

Mild Adverse Effects

Allergic reactions: skin rash, itching, joint pain—case reports.

Headache, weakness—infrequent.

Loss of appetite, mouth and lip sores, nausea, vomiting, diarrhea—infrequent.

Serious Adverse Effects

Liver damage with jaundice (see Glossary)—infrequent.

Kidney damage: fever, cloudy or bloody urine—rare.

Pancreatitis (especially in patients taking this medicine for inflammatory bowel disease)—infrequent.

Gastrointestinal ulceration: stomach pain, bloody or black stools.

Increased cancer risk (carcinogen): one case report of cancer in a patient with bowel disease—possible.

▷ **Possible Effects on Sexual Function:** Suppression of sperm production. Cessation of menstruation—case reports.

Possible Delayed Adverse Effects: Bone marrow depression may not be apparent during early treatment.

▷ **Adverse Effects That May Mimic Natural Diseases or Disorders**
Drug-induced liver damage may suggest viral hepatitis.

Natural Diseases or Disorders That May Be Activated by This Drug
Latent gout, peptic ulcer disease, inflammatory bowel disease.

Possible Effects on Laboratory Tests
Complete blood cell counts: decreased red cells, hemoglobin, white cells and platelets.

Blood glucose levels: falsely increased with SMA testing.

Blood uric acid levels: increased.

Liver function tests: increased enzymes (ALT/GPT, AST/GOT and alkaline phosphatase) or bilirubin.

Kidney function tests: increased blood urea nitrogen (BUN) and creatinine.

Sperm counts: decreased.

CAUTION
1. Make sure you get all laboratory tests ordered.
2. Call your doctor at the first sign of infection or abnormal bleeding or bruising.
3. Inform your physician promptly if you become pregnant.
4. It is best to avoid immunizations while taking this drug and to avoid contact with people who have recently taken oral poliovirus vaccine.

Precautions for Use
By Infants and Children: No specific problems anticipated.
By Those Over 60 Years of Age: Increased risk of bone marrow depression. Periodic blood counts are mandatory.

▷ **Advisability of Use During Pregnancy**
Pregnancy Category: D. See Pregnancy Risk Categories at the back of this book.
Animal studies: Rat studies reveal toxic effects on the embryo.
Human studies: Adequate studies of pregnant women are not available. Known to cause abortions and premature births.
Avoid drug during entire pregnancy if possible. Use a nonhormonal method of contraception.

Advisability of Use If Breast-Feeding
Presence of this drug in breast milk: Unknown.
Avoid drug or refrain from nursing.

Habit-Forming Potential: None.

Effects of Overdose: Headache, dizziness, abdominal pain, nausea.

Possible Effects of Long-Term Use: Development of new malignant diseases.

Suggested Periodic Examinations While Taking This Drug (at physician's discretion)

Complete blood cell counts.

Blood uric acid levels.

Liver and kidney function tests.

▷ **While Taking This Drug, Observe the Following**

Foods: No restrictions.

Herbal Medicines or Minerals: Echinacea: Some patients use echinacea to attempt to boost their immune systems. Unfortunately, use of echinacea is not recommended in people with damaged immune systems. This herb may also actually weaken any immune system if it is used too often or for too long a time.

Beverages: No restrictions. Drink liquids liberally, up to 2 quarts daily.

▷ *Alcohol:* Avoid completely.

Tobacco Smoking: No interactions expected. I advise everyone to quit smoking.

▷ *Other Drugs*

Mercaptopurine may ***decrease*** the effects of

• warfarin (Coumadin); the INR (prothrombin time or protime) should be checked more frequently.

The following drug may ***increase*** the effects of mercaptopurine:

• allopurinol (Zyloprim). Doses must be reduced to 33% or even as low as 25% of the usual dose if these two medicines are to be combined.

Mercaptopurine ***taken concurrently*** with

• amphotericin B (Abelcet) may increase risk of kidney toxicity or spasm of the bronchi.

• live-virus vaccines (such as smallpox) may lead to life-threatening infections.

• methotrexate (Rheumatrex, Mexate) can result in mercaptopurine toxicity.

• olsalazine (Dipentum) may increase risk of bone marrow depression.

▷ *Driving, Hazardous Activities:* No restrictions.

Aviation Note: The use of this drug ***may be a disqualification*** for piloting. Consult a designated Aviation Medical Examiner.

Exposure to Sun: No restrictions.

Discontinuation: To be determined by your physician.

MESALAMINE (me SAL a meen)

Other Names: Mesalazine, 5-aminosalicylic acid, 5-ASA

Introduced: 1982 **Class:** Bowel anti-inflammatory **Prescription:** USA: Yes **Controlled Drug:** USA: No; Canada: No **Available as Generic:** USA: No; Canada: No

Brand Names: Asacol, Pentasa, ✤Quintasa, Rowasa, ✤Salofalk

BENEFITS versus RISKS	
Possible Benefits	*Possible Risks*
EFFECTIVE SUPPRESSION OF INFLAMMATORY BOWEL DISEASE	Allergic reactions: acute intolerance syndrome, drug-induced kidney damage

▷ **Principal Uses**

As a Single Drug Product: Uses currently included in FDA-approved labeling: Treatment of active mild to moderate ulcerative colitis, proctosigmoiditis and proctitis.

Other (unlabeled) generally accepted uses: (1) May help improve semen quality that had been damaged by prior sulfasalazine treatment; (2) can ease canker sores (aphthous ulcers); (3) has a steroid-sparing effect in Crohn's disease; (4) used to maintain remission in ulcerative colitis.

How This Drug Works: Suppresses prostaglandin (and related compounds) formation, chemicals causing inflammation, tissue destruction and diarrhea-the main problems in ulcerative colitis and proctitis.

Available Dosage Forms and Strengths

Capsules, timed-release — 400 mg
    Rectal suspension — 4 g per 60-ml unit
Suppositories (Canada) — 250 mg
    Suppositories — 500 mg
    (U.S. and Canada)
Tablets, enteric-coated — 250 mg, 500 mg
Tablets, sustained-release — 250 mg, 500 mg

▷ **Recommended Dosage Ranges** (Actual dose and schedule must be determined for each patient individually.)

Infants and Children: Dose not established.

12 to 60 Years of Age: Active ulcerative colitis: Immediate-release (Asacol)—800 mg three times a day for 6 weeks. Controlled-release (Pentasa)—1,000 mg four times a day for up to 8 weeks.

Maintenance of ulcerative colitis remission: Immediate-release (Asacol)— 1,600 mg divided into equal doses.

Crohn's disease (Pentasa): 1,000 mg taken three times a day.

Over 60 Years of Age: Same as 12 to 60 years of age.

Conditions Requiring Dosing Adjustments

Liver Function: Guidelines for dose adjustment not available. Drug changed by the liver and colon wall to Ac-5-ASA.

Kidney Function: This drug should be used with caution in kidney compromise.

▷ **Dosing Instructions**

Rectal suspension: Use as a retention enema at bedtime. If possible, empty the rectum before inserting suspension; try to retain the suspension all night.

Tablets: Best taken with 8 ounces of water on an empty stomach, 1 hour before or 2 hours after eating. Also can be taken with or following food to reduce stomach upset. Sustained-release tablet should be swallowed whole without alteration. If you forget a dose: Take the missed dose as soon as you remember it, unless it's nearly time for your next dose—if that is the case, skip the missed dose and take the next dose right on schedule. Talk with your doctor if you find yourself missing doses.

Usual Duration of Use: Regular use for 1 to 3 weeks determines benefits controlling ulcerative colitis. Long-term use (months to years) requires periodic physician evaluation.

Typical Treatment Goals and Measurements (Outcomes and Markers)

Inflammatory bowel disease: The goal is to cause (induce) a remission and maintain it. Symptoms that will resolve include rectal bleeding and diarrhea. More involved exams will reveal an absence of bowel ulceration and easing of friability or granularity of the bowel itself.

Possible Advantages of This Drug
Does not cause bone marrow or blood cell disorders. Does not inhibit sperm production or function. Better side effect profile than sulfasalazine.

▷ **This Drug Should Not Be Taken If**
- you have had an allergic reaction to it previously.
- you have severely impaired kidney function.
- you have a known sulfite allergy. (Rectal suspension should NOT be used.)
- you have active ulcer disease.

▷ **Inform Your Physician Before Taking This Drug If**
- you are allergic to aspirin (or other salicylates), olsalazine or sulfasalazine.
- you are allergic by nature: history of hay fever, asthma, hives, eczema.
- you have impaired liver or kidney function.
- you have a history of a blood-clotting (coagulation) disorder.
- you develop chest pain or trouble while taking this medicine (pericarditis happens rarely).
- you have a history of low white blood cell counts.
- you are taking other medicines that effect the bone marrow. Discuss this with your doctor.
- you are currently taking sulfasalazine (Azulfidine).

Possible Side Effects (natural, expected and unavoidable drug actions)
Anal irritation (with use of rectal suspension or suppositories). Flu-like syndrome with oral mesalamine use.

▷ **Possible Adverse Effects** (unusual, unexpected and infrequent reactions)
If any of the following develop, consult your physician promptly for guidance.

Mild Adverse Effects
Allergic reactions: skin rash.
Headache (may be dose-related), hair loss—rare.
Blurred vision, ringing in the ears—possible.
Paresthesias, neck and joint pain, dizziness, cough—infrequent.
Nausea, stomach pain, excessive gas—infrequent.

Serious Adverse Effects
Allergic reactions: acute intolerance syndrome (fever, skin rash, severe headache, severe stomach pain, bloody diarrhea).
Kidney damage (nephrosis, interstitial nephritis)—rare.
Peripheral neuropathy—rare.
Pancreatitis, peptic ulcers or hepatitis—rare.
Low white blood cell or platelet counts or anemia—rare.
Myocarditis, pericarditis, pericardial effusions—case reports.
Lung toxicity (interstitial infiltrates)—case report.

▷ **Possible Effects on Sexual Function:** Oligospermia and infertility has been reported with sulfasalazine, but NOT with mesalamine.

Possible Effects on Laboratory Tests
Increased liver function tests.

CAUTION
1. Report promptly any signs of acute intolerance syndrome. Stop taking drug.

2. Shake the rectal suspension thoroughly before administering.
3. This medicine is a salicylate and as such is a cousin of aspirin. Avoid taking this medicine in combination with other medicines or during other conditions in which aspirin is contraindicated. Salicylate toxicity is possible.

Precautions for Use

By Infants and Children: Safety and effectiveness by those under 12 years of age are not established.

By Those Over 60 Years of Age: None.

▷ **Advisability of Use During Pregnancy**

Pregnancy Category: B. See Pregnancy Risk Categories at the back of this book.

Animal studies: No drug-induced birth defects found in rat or rabbit studies.

Human studies: Adequate studies of pregnant women are not available.

Use this drug only if clearly needed. Ask your physician for guidance.

Advisability of Use If Breast-Feeding

Presence of this drug in breast milk: Yes.

Avoid drug or refrain from nursing.

Habit-Forming Potential: None.

Effects of Overdose: Headache, dizziness, nausea, vomiting, abdominal cramping.

Possible Effects of Long-Term Use: None reported.

Suggested Periodic Examinations While Taking This Drug (at physician's discretion)

Kidney function tests.

Urinalysis.

▷ **While Taking This Drug, Observe the Following**

Foods: Decreased mesalamine levels. Follow prescribed diet.

Herbal Medicines or Minerals: Flaxseed, peppermint oil and psyllium husk have commission E monograph indications for irritable bowel syndrome. This is NOT the same as ulcerative colitis, and those products have not been studied in ulcerative colitis. Aloe, buckhorn berry or bark, cascara sagrada bark, rhubarb root and senna should not be taken by people living with ulcerative colitis.

Beverages: No restrictions. May be taken with milk.

▷ *Alcohol:* No interactions expected.

Tobacco Smoking: No interactions expected. I advise everyone to quit smoking.

▷ *Other Drugs*

Mesalamine **taken concurrently** with

- alendronate (Fosamax) may increase stomach or intestinal upset risks (because of salicylate).
- ardeparin (Normiflo), dalteparin (Fragmin) or enoxaparin (Lovenox) may increase risk of hemorrhage.
- aspirin or other salicylates may increase risk of salicylate toxicity.
- varicella vaccine (Varivax) may result in Reye's syndrome; avoid taking this medicine for 6 weeks following varicella vaccine.
- warfarin (Coumadin) may blunt warfarin effectiveness. More frequent INRs are prudent.

▷ *Driving, Hazardous Activities:* No restrictions.

Aviation Note: The use of this drug is probably not a disqualification for pilot-ing. Consult a designated Aviation Medical Examiner.
Exposure to Sun: No restrictions.

METAPROTERENOL (met a proh TER e nohl)

Other Name: Orciprenaline

Introduced: 1964   **Class:** Antiasthmatic, bronchodilator   **Prescription:** USA: Yes   **Controlled Drug:**   USA: No; Canada: No   **Available as Generic:** Yes

Brand Names: ♣Alti-Orciprenaline, Alupent, Arm-a-Med, Dey-Dose, Dey-Lute, Metaprel, Metaprel Nasal Inhaler, Prometa

BENEFITS versus RISKS	
Possible Benefits	*Possible Risks*
VERY EFFECTIVE RELIEF OF BRONCHOSPASM	Increased blood pressure
	Fine hand tremor
	Fast heart rate
	Irregular heart rhythm (with excessive use)

▷ **Principal Uses**

As a Single Drug Product: Uses currently included in FDA-approved labeling: (1) Relieves acute bronchial asthma and reduces the frequency and sever-ity of chronic, recurrent asthmatic attacks; (2) used to relieve reversible bronchospasm associated with chronic bronchitis and emphysema; (3) eases symptoms in obstructive bronchial disease.

Other (unlabeled) generally accepted uses: Some threatened abortion use.

How This Drug Works: Dilates those bronchial tubes that are in sustained con-striction, increasing the size of airways and improving breathing.

Available Dosage Forms and Strengths

Nasal inhaler — 0.65 mg per metered dose
Oral suspension — 10 mg/5 ml
Powder for inhalation — 0.65 mg per inhalation
Solution for nebulizer — 0.4%, 0.6%, 5%
Syrup — 10 mg/5 ml
Tablets — 10 mg, 20 mg

▷ **Usual Adult Dosage Ranges:** *Inhaler:* Two or three inhalations as often as every 3 to 4 hours; do not exceed 12 inhalations daily.

Hand nebulizer: 5 to 15 inhalations every 4 hours; do not exceed 40 inhala-tions daily.

Syrup and tablets: 20 mg up to every 6 to 8 hours.

Note: Actual dose and schedule must be determined for each patient individually.

Conditions Requiring Dosing Adjustments

Liver Function: Specific guidelines for dosing adjustment for patients with liver compromise are not usually indicated.

Kidney Function: Dosing changes are not indicated in kidney compromise.

▷ **Dosing Instructions:** May be taken on empty stomach or with food or milk. Tablets should not be crushed. For aerosol and nebulizer, follow the written instructions carefully. Do not overuse. If symptoms are not controlled with most-frequent dosing, call your doctor. If you forget a dose: Take the missed dose as soon as you remember it, then take the remaining daily doses at evenly spaced intervals. If it's nearly time for your next dose, skip the missed dose and take the next dose right on schedule. Talk with your doctor if you find yourself missing doses.

Usual Duration of Use: According to individual requirements. Do not use beyond the time necessary to stop episodes of asthma.

Typical Treatment Goals and Measurements (Outcomes and Markers)
Asthma: Beta-adrenergic medicines like this one are used to prevent or treat reversible spasms of the bronchial tubes. The peak effect happens two to four hours after dosing. Inhaled use often gives improvement in FEV-1 in five to 30 minutes. If the usual benefit is not realized, call your doctor.

▷ **This Drug Should Not Be Taken If**
- you had an allergic reaction to it previously.
- you currently have an irregular heart rhythm.
- you are taking, or have taken within the past 2 weeks, any monoamine oxidase (MAO) type A inhibitor drug (see Drug Classes).

▷ **Inform Your Physician Before Taking This Drug If**
- you are overly sensitive to other sympathetic stimulant drugs.
- you currently use epinephrine (Adrenalin, Primatene Mist, etc.) to relieve asthmatic breathing.
- you have any type of heart or circulatory disorder, especially high blood pressure or coronary heart disease.
- you have diabetes or an overactive thyroid gland (hyperthyroidism).
- you are taking any form of digitalis or any stimulant drug.

Possible Side Effects (natural, expected and unavoidable drug actions)
Aerosol—dryness or irritation of mouth or throat, altered taste.
Tablet—nervousness, palpitation.

▷ **Possible Adverse Effects (unusual, unexpected and infrequent reactions)**
If any of the following develop, consult your physician promptly for guidance.
Mild Adverse Effects
Headache, dizziness, restlessness, insomnia, fine tremor of hands—possible to infrequent.
Increased sweating; muscle cramps in arms and legs—case reports.
Nausea, heartburn, vomiting—possible.
Serious Adverse Effects
Rapid or irregular heart rhythm, intensification of angina, increased blood pressure—possible.
Hallucinations and psychosis—rare.
Paradoxical spasm of the bronchi (bronchospasm)—rare.

▷ **Possible Effects on Sexual Function:** None reported.

Natural Diseases or Disorders That May Be Activated By This Drug
Latent coronary artery disease, diabetes or high blood pressure.

Possible Effects on Laboratory Tests
 Urine sugar tests: positive (unreliable results with Benedict's solution).

CAUTION
 1. Combined use of this drug by aerosol inhalation with beclomethasone aerosol (Beclovent, Vanceril) may increase the risk of toxicity due to fluorocarbon propellants (these propellants are being phased out). Use this aerosol 20 to 30 minutes before beclomethasone aerosol, as this will reduce the risk of toxicity and enhance the penetration of beclomethasone.
 2. ***Avoid excessive use of aerosol inhalation.*** Excessive or prolonged use of this drug by inhalation can reduce its effectiveness and cause serious heart rhythm disturbances, including cardiac arrest.
 3. Do not combine this drug with epinephrine. These two drugs may be used alternately if an interval of 4 hours is allowed between doses.
 4. If you do not respond to your usually effective dose, ask your doctor for help. Do not increase the size or frequency of the dose without your physician's approval.

Precautions for Use
 By Infants and Children: Safety and effectiveness of the aerosol and nebulized solution are not established for children under 12 years of age.
 Oral dosing in children less than 6 years old—1.3 to 2.6 mg per kg of body mass per day, divided into equal doses and given three to four times a day. In children 6 to 9 years old or less than 60 pounds—10 mg per dose three to four times a day. Children more than 9 years old or over 60 pounds—20 mg three or four times a day.
 Safety and effectiveness of the syrup and tablet are not established for children under 6 years of age.
 By Those Over 60 Years of Age: Avoid excessive and continual use. If acute asthma is not relieved promptly, other drugs will have to be tried. Watch for nervousness, palpitations, irregular heart rhythm and muscle tremors. Use with extreme caution if you have hardening of the arteries, heart disease or high blood pressure.

▷ **Advisability of Use During Pregnancy**
 Pregnancy Category: C. See Pregnancy Risk Categories at the back of this book.
 Animal studies: Significant birth defects reported in rabbit studies.
 Human studies: Adequate studies of pregnant women are not available.
 Avoid during first 3 months. Used in final 6 months only if clearly needed.

Advisability of Use If Breast-Feeding
 Presence of this drug in breast milk: Unknown.
 Avoid drug or refrain from nursing.

Habit-Forming Potential: None.

Effects of Overdose: Nervousness, palpitation, rapid heart rate, sweating, headache, tremor, vomiting, chest pain.

Possible Effects of Long-Term Use: Loss of effectiveness (see "CAUTION" above).

Suggested Periodic Examinations While Taking This Drug (at physician's discretion)

Blood pressure measurements.

Evaluation of heart status.

▷ **While Taking This Drug, Observe the Following**

Foods: No restrictions.

Herbal Medicines or Minerals: Using St. John's wort, ma huang, ephedrine-like compounds or kola while taking this medicine may result in unacceptable central nervous system stimulation. Fir or pine needle oil should NOT be used by asthmatics. Ephedra alone does carry a German Commission E monograph indication for asthma treatment. If you are allergic to plants in the Asteraceae family (aster, chrysanthemum, daisy or ragweed), you may also be allergic to echinacea, chamomile, feverfew and St. John's wort.

Beverages: Avoid excessive use of caffeine-containing beverages: coffee, tea, cola, chocolate.

▷ *Alcohol:* No interactions expected.

Tobacco Smoking: No interactions expected. I advise everyone to quit smoking.

▷ *Other Drugs*

Metaproterenol *taken concurrently* with

- albuterol (Proventil, others) may result in increased heart (cardiovascular) side effects.
- monoamine oxidase (MAO) type A inhibitors (see Drug Classes) may cause excessive increase in blood pressure and undesirable heart stimulation.
- phenothiazines (see Drug Classes) may blunt some effects of this drug.

▷ *Driving, Hazardous Activities:* Usually no restrictions. Use caution if excessive nervousness or dizziness occurs.

Aviation Note: The use of this drug *is a disqualification* for piloting. Consult a designated Aviation Medical Examiner.

Exposure to Sun: No restrictions.

Heavy Exercise or Exertion: Use caution. Excessive exercise can induce asthma in sensitive individuals.

METFORMIN (met FOR min)

Introduced: 1995   **Class:** Antidiabetes drug, oral; biguanide   **Prescription:** USA: Yes   **Controlled Drug:** USA: No; Canada: No   **Available as Generic:** USA: No; Canada: No

Brand Names: ❧Apo-Metformin, Glucophage, Glucophage XR, Glucovance [CD]

Warning: Avoid excessive alcohol. Alcohol can cause lactic acidosis, a condition that metformin can also rarely cause. All oral hypoglycemic agents may carry the risk of increased cardiovascular death, based on a 1975 study of tolbutamide and phenformin.

BENEFITS versus RISKS

Possible Benefits	*Possible Risks*
COMBINATION USE WITH ROSIGLITAZONE (AVANDIA) MAY SLOW THE PROGRESSION OF DIABETES	LACTIC ACIDOSIS
	Possible anemia with long-term use

COMBINATION USE WITH
  ROSIGLITAZONE (AVANDIA)
  MAY SLOW THE PROGRESSION
  OF DIABETES
COMBINATION USE WITH
  ROSIGLITAZONE MAY PREVENT
  LONG-TERM COMPLICATIONS
  OF DIABETES
EFFECTIVE GLUCOSE CONTROL
  WITHOUT INSULIN INJECTION
A PRESENTATION AT THE 2001
  AMERICAN DIABETES
  CONFERENCE FOUND
  EXCELLENT RESULTS
  WHEN METFORMIN WAS
  COMBINED WITH AN INSULIN
  SPRAYED INTO THE MOUTH
  (ORALIN)
MAY BE USED CONCURRENTLY
  WITH A SULFONYLUREA
DOES NOT LEAD TO WEIGHT GAIN
TAKEN BY MOUTH, VERSUS
  INJECTION OF INSULIN
Usually avoids excessive lowering of
  blood sugar
Favorable effects on lipids

▷ **Principal Uses**

  As a Single Drug Product: Uses currently included in FDA-approved labeling: (1) Used in combination with diet restrictions to treat non-insulin-dependent diabetes (type 2); (2) can be combined with a sulfonylurea (see Drug Classes) for patients who do not have an adequate response to diet restrictions plus a sulfonylurea; (3) combination use with rosiglitazone may slow progression of diabetes and help avoid long-term complications of diabetes.

  Other (unlabeled) generally accepted uses: (1) May be used as single-agent therapy to overcome insulin resistance; (2) could help nondiabetic, obese women with high blood pressure in helping improve blood pressure and lipid profile; (3) may help insulin-dependent (type 1) diabetics decrease insulin requirements; (4) may have a role in treating polycystic ovary syndrome (PCOS)

  As a Combination Drug Product [CD]: Metformin is available combined with glyburide (Glucovance) as initial treatment of type 2 diabetes or when blood sugar (glucose) control goals are not met by either medicine alone.

How This Drug Works: Decreases sugar (glucose) production in the liver. It also increases sensitivity of the body to insulin.

Available Dosage Forms and Strengths

Tablets — 500 mg, 850 mg

Tablets, combination — 250 mg metformin and 1.25 mg glyburide,
500 mg metformin and 2.5 or 5.0 mg glyburide

Tablets, extended release — 500 mg

▷ **Recommended Dosage Ranges** (Actual dose and schedule must be determined for each patient individually.)

Infants and Children: Not approved for use in this population.

12 to 60 Years of Age: Dosing is started at 500 mg twice daily. It is best to take this medicine with the morning and evening meal. Some clinicians use 850 mg once daily. If the 850 mg dose is used, dosing is increased as needed and tolerated at 14-day intervals. Maximum dose is 2,500 mg if the 500 mg tablets are used, and 2,550 mg if the 850 mg tablets are used. Doses up to 2,000 mg are separated into two doses, but doses higher than this are best divided into three daily doses.

Extended-release form: Dosing is started with 500 mg once daily with the evening meal.

Combination form: Dosing is started with the 1.25 glyburide and 250 mg metformin once a day with meals in people who have a fasting blood sugar more than 200 mg/dl or a glycosylated hemoglobin (hemoglobin A1C) more than 9%.

Over 60 Years of Age: Some patients may have acceptable blood sugar control with as little as 500 mg daily. If this dose is used, take it with the morning meal. Dose may be slowly increased if needed.

Conditions Requiring Dosing Adjustments

Liver Function: This drug should not be used by patients with liver compromise. This is a risk factor for lactic acidosis.

Kidney Function: NOT to be used in kidney disease (renal dysfunction) defined as females with steady-state creatinine levels greater than 1.4 or males with levels greater than 1.5.

▷ **Dosing Instructions:** This drug should be taken with the morning and evening meal if it has been prescribed on a twice-daily basis. One study found that use of metformin with insulin at bedtime not only lowered risk of excessively low blood sugar (hypoglycemia), but also prevented weight gain. If you forget a dose: Take the missed dose as soon as you remember it, unless it's nearly time for your next dose—if that is the case, skip the missed dose and take the next dose right on schedule. Talk with your doctor if you find yourself missing doses.

Usual Duration of Use: Continual use on a regular schedule for a week is usually necessary to determine this drug's effectiveness in establishing tight glucose control. A month of continuous use will be needed before an effect on glycosylated hemoglobin (a measure of past success of glucose control) is seen. Long-term use (months to years) requires periodic evaluation of response and dose adjustment. Consult your physician on a regular basis.

Typical Treatment Goals and Measurements (Outcomes and Markers)

Blood sugar: The general goal for blood sugar is to return it to the usual "normal" range (generally 80–120 mg/dl), while avoiding risks of excessively low blood sugar. One study (UKPDS) used a fasting plasma sugar (glucose) of less than 108 mg/dl.

Possible Advantages of This Drug

Does not lead to weight gain.

Can be used (because of its mechanism of action) in combination with a sulfonylurea.

Can be used to overcome insulin resistance.

Can be used in combination with rosiglitazone to slow diabetes progression and help avoid long-term diabetes complications.

Does not cause excessive lowering of blood sugar (hypoglycemia) when used as monotherapy.

Currently a Drug of Choice

For treatment of hyperglycemia in the elderly.

▷ **This Drug Should Not Be Taken If**

- you had an allergic reaction to it previously.
- you have impaired kidneys (serum creatinine greater than 1.4 for females or 1.5 for males).
- you have liver disease.
- you have a serious infection (increases risk of lactic acidosis).
- you are an alcoholic.
- you have a heart or lung insufficiency (increased lactic acidosis risk).
- you are going to have a radiology test that uses iodinated contrast media (ask your doctor).
- you have chronic metabolic acidosis or ketoacidosis.
- you are breast-feeding your infant.

▷ **Inform Your Physician Before Taking This Drug If**

- you are planning to have surgery soon.
- you have a history of megaloblastic anemia.
- you have seen another doctor and ketoacidosis was diagnosed.
- you are unsure how much to take or how often to take it.

Possible Side Effects (natural, expected and unavoidable drug actions)

Lactic acidosis—rare. Low blood sugar (hypoglycemia) if meals are skipped or if you exercise strenuously without eating.

▷ **Possible Adverse Effects** (unusual, unexpected and infrequent reactions)

If any of the following develop, consult your physician promptly for guidance.

Mild Adverse Effects

Allergic reactions: rash.

Metallic taste—infrequent and usually resolves.

Anorexia, nausea, vomiting or diarrhea—up to 30% when started and then they often subside.

Headache, nervousness, dizziness or tiredness—infrequent.

Serious Adverse Effects

Allergic reactions: not reported.

Idiosyncratic reactions: liver toxicity—rare.

Lactic acidosis—rare.

Lowered vitamin B_{12} levels and resultant anemia (megaloblastic)—rare.

Destruction of red blood cells (hemolysis)—case report.

Drug-induced porphyria—case reports.

All oral hypoglycemic agents carry a label indicating that they may increase risk of cardiovascular death (based on a 1975 study of tolbutamide and phenformin)—possible.

▷ **Possible Effects on Sexual Function:** None reported.

Possible Delayed Adverse Effects: Low vitamin B_{12} levels and anemia (megaloblastic).

▷ **Adverse Effects That May Mimic Natural Diseases or Disorders**

Acidosis may mimic ketoacidosis, which is seen in diabetics.

Natural Diseases or Disorders That May Be Activated by This Drug

None reported.

Possible Effects on Laboratory Tests

Blood glucose: decreased.

Vitamin B_{12}: lowered

CAUTION

1. This drug may cause lactic acidosis. Ask your doctor for signs or symptoms that may occur.
2. Drugs in this class (phenformin) or tolbutamide were reported to increase risk of cardiovascular death. Although there is no data to support that effect for this medicine, patients should be closely followed.

Precautions for Use

By Infants and Children: Safety and effectiveness for use by those under 18 years of age have not been established.

By Those Over 60 Years of Age: Smaller starting doses (500 mg daily) are indicated. People in this age group tend to have an age-related decline in kidney function as well as a more compromised ability to tolerate lower blood sugar levels.

▷ **Advisability of Use During Pregnancy**

Pregnancy Category: B. See Pregnancy Risk Categories at the back of this book.

Animal studies: No birth defects in rats at two times the typical human dose.

Human studies: Information from adequate studies of pregnant women is not available. The manufacturer does not recommend the use of this drug in pregnancy.

Insulin is still considered the drug of choice to control blood sugar in pregnancy.

Advisability of Use If Breast-Feeding

Presence of this drug in breast milk: Yes.

Avoid drug or refrain from nursing.

Habit-Forming Potential: None.

Effects of Overdose: Nausea and vomiting, pulmonary edema, hemorrhage from the stomach, lactic acidosis, seizures, intractable lowering of blood pressure, coma.

Possible Effects of Long-Term Use: Lowering of vitamin B_{12} and resultant anemia (megaloblastic). Possible malabsorption of folic acid and amino acids.

Suggested Periodic Examinations While Taking This Drug (at physician's discretion)

Vitamin B_{12} levels (every 2–3 years in people likely to have low B_{12}).

Tests of kidney function before treatment is started and at least yearly.

Liver function.

▷ **While Taking This Drug, Observe the Following**

Foods: Follow the ADA diet your doctor recommends.

Herbal Medicines or Minerals: Using chromium may change the way your body is able to use sugar. Some health food stores advocate vanadium as mimicking the actions of insulin, but possible toxicity and need for rigorous studies presently preclude recommending it. DHEA may change sensitivity to insulin or insulin resistance. Hawthorn, ginger, garlic, ginseng and licorice, nettle and yohimbe may change blood sugar. Since this may require adjustment of hypoglycemic medicine dosing, talk to your doctor BEFORE combing any of these herbal medicines with acarbose. Echinacea pupurea (injectable) and blonde psyllium seed or husk should NOT be taken by people living with diabetes. Caution: Like this medicine, St. John's wort may increase sensitivity to the sun.

Nutritional Support: Diet as prescribed by your doctor. Check of vitamin B_{12} levels determines need for support.

Beverages: No restrictions.

▷ *Alcohol:* Use with extreme caution. Alcohol worsens the effect of metformin on lactate. Avoid alcohol in excessive amounts.

Tobacco Smoking: No interactions expected, but I advise everyone to quit smoking.

Marijuana Smoking: May worsen dizziness.

▷ *Other Drugs*

Metformin may ***increase*** the effects of

- insulin, in the sense that the lowering of blood sugar will be increased; this may be used to therapeutic advantage in some insulin-dependent diabetics.

Metformin ***taken concurrently*** with

- ACE inhibitors (see Drug Classes) may increase lowering of blood sugar to an undesirable extent.
- azole antifungals (see Drug Classes) may increase lowering of blood sugar to an undesirable extent.
- beta blockers (see Drug Classes) may slow recovery from any hypoglycemia that occurs and can also block symptoms of low blood sugar.
- cationic drugs (cotrimoxazole, procainamide, quinidine, quinine and others) may increase risk of lactic acidosis.
- contrast media for certain X-ray studies may increase risk of lactic acidosis. Metformin should not be combined with these agents. Some clinicians substitute a different agent to control blood sugar, stop the metformin 48 hours before the X-ray and then stop the substituted agent and restart metformin once kidney function is tested and found to be normal.
- cotrimoxazole (Bactrim, others) may increase risk of lactic acidosis.
- digoxin (Lanoxin, others) may pose a problem because it is a cationic drug and may lead to excess metformin levels.
- dofetilide (Tikosyn) may pose a problem because it is a cationic drug and uses the same removal (elimination) pathway that metformin does. This may lead to increased risk of dofetilide toxicity.
- itraconazole (Sporanox) or other azole antifungal agents can result in severe lowering of the blood sugar.
- procainamide (Pronestyl) may lead to toxicity.
- quinidine (Quinaglute) may lead to toxicity.

- thyroid hormones (see Drug Classes) can result in blunting of metformin's therapeutic effect.

The following drugs may *increase* the effects of metformin:
- cimetidine (Tagamet)—may result in toxicity.
- morphine (various)—may lead to toxicity.
- nifedipine (Adalat)—may lead to toxicity.
- oral antidiabetic drugs (see Drug Classes)—this effect may be used to therapeutic advantage.
- ranitidine (Zantac)—may lead to toxicity.
- trimethoprim (Septra)—may lead to toxicity.
- vancomycin (Vancoled)—may lead to toxicity.

▷ *Driving, Hazardous Activities:* This drug may cause drowsiness or dizziness. Restrict activities as necessary.

Aviation Note: Diabetes *is a disqualification for piloting.* Consult a designated Aviation Medical Examiner.

Exposure to Sun: Use caution. Some medicines that are similar in chemical structure can cause increased sensitivity to the sun.

Heavy Exercise or Exertion: Heavy exercise will tend to use up sugar faster than usual. This drug will have an effect on lowering the blood sugar. Be alert to the symptoms of low blood sugar.

Occurrence of Unrelated Illness: Infections or other illness may still require use of insulin to achieve acceptable blood sugar control.

Discontinuation: Periodic physician evaluations of the continued benefit of this medicine are needed.

METHOTREXATE (meth oh TREX ayt)

Other Names: Amethopterin, MTX

Introduced: 1948   **Class:** Anticancer drugs, antipsoriasis   **Prescription:** USA: Yes   **Controlled Drug:** USA: No; Canada: No   **Available as Generic:** Yes

Brand Names: Abitrexate, Folex, Folex PFS, Mexate, Mexate AQ, Rheumatrex Dose Pack

BENEFITS versus RISKS	
Possible Benefits	*Possible Risks*
EFFECTIVE TREATMENT OF SOME CASES OF SEVERE DISABLING PSORIASIS	GASTROINTESTINAL ULCERATION AND BLEEDING MOUTH AND THROAT ULCERATION
EFFECTIVE TREATMENT OF CERTAIN ADULT AND CHILDHOOD CANCERS	SEVERE BONE MARROW DEPRESSION
PREVENTION OF REJECTION OF BONE MARROW TRANSPLANTS	DAMAGE TO LUNGS, LIVER OR KIDNEYS
USEFUL IN RHEUMATOID ARTHRITIS AND RELATED DISORDERS	Loss of hair

▷ **Principal Uses**

As a Single Drug Product: Uses currently included in FDA-approved labeling: (1) Combination therapy of acute lymphocytic leukemia; (2) combination therapy of various types of adult and childhood cancer; (3) severe and widespread forms of disabling psoriasis that have failed to respond to all standard treatment procedures; (4) various types of both adult and childhood cancer; (5) used to prevent rejection of transplanted bone marrow; (6) used in the treatment of connective tissue disorders such as rheumatoid arthritis and related conditions (its use in rheumatoid arthritis is restricted to the treatment of selected adults with severe active disease that has failed to respond to conventional therapy); (7) used in COMBINATION with methotrexate in some cases of refractory rheumatoid arthritis.

Other (unlabeled) generally accepted uses: (1) Used in a variety of neoplastic syndromes in combination therapy; (2) may have a role in helping decrease steroid use in steroid-dependent asthma; (3) helps lessen neutropenia in Felty's syndrome; (4) used in combination with misoprostol to cause abortion; (5) can be of help in chronic granulomatous hepatitis of unknown cause (idiopathic).

How This Drug Works: Blocks normal use of folic acid in cell reproduction and slows abnormally rapid tissue growth (as in psoriasis and cancer).

Available Dosage Forms and Strengths

Injections — 2.5 mg/ml, 10 mg/ml, 25 mg/ml

Injections, preservative free — 25 mg/ml, 50 mg/ml, 100 mg/ml, 250 mg/ml

Powder, intrathecal cryodessicated — 20 mg, 50 mg, 100 mg

Tablets — 2.5 mg

▷ **Usual Adult Dosage Ranges:** *For psoriasis (alternate schedules):* (1) 10 to 50 mg once a week; (2) 2.5 to 5 mg every 12 hours for three doses or every 8 hours for four doses, once a week, up to a maximum of 30 mg/week; (3) 2.5 mg/day for 5 days, followed by 2 days without drug, with gradual increase in dose to a maximum of 6.25 mg/day.

For rheumatoid arthritis (alternate schedules): (1) single oral dose of 7.5 mg once weekly; (2) divided doses of 2.5 mg every 12 hours for three doses per week. Dose may be increased gradually as needed and tolerated. Do not exceed a weekly dose of 20 mg.

For acute lymphocytic leukemia (ALL): Induction—3.3 mg per square meter in combination with corticosteroid treatment is usually taken daily for 4 to 6 weeks. Maintenance—a total weekly dose of 30 mg per square meter is given as two divided oral or intramuscular injections. Some centers also use 2.5 mg per kg of body mass intravenously every 14 days.

Note: Actual dose and schedule must be determined for each patient individually.

Conditions Requiring Dosing Adjustments

Liver Function: Used with caution and in decreased dose in liver disease. Some clinicians use laboratory tests as a guide—for example, when dose is due, if bilirubin is less than 3 mg % and AST (SGOT) is less than 180 IU, 100% of the scheduled dose can be given. If bilirubin is greater than 5.0 mg %, dose SHOULD NOT be given.

Kidney Function: Methotrexate is a benefit-to-risk decision. Increased adverse effects are possible with damaged kidneys. Do not take with severe kidney failure (creatinine clearance less than 10 ml/min). For moderate failure, 50% of the usual dose should be taken in the usual dosing interval.

▷ **Dosing Instructions:** The tablet may be crushed and taken with food to reduce stomach irritation. Drink at least 2 to 3 quarts of liquids daily. Many clinicians using methotrexate in rheumatoid arthritis also give folic acid in order to minimize methotrexate toxicity. If you forget a dose: Take the missed dose as soon as you remember it, unless it's nearly time for your next dose—if that is the case, skip the missed dose and take the next dose right on schedule. Talk with your doctor if you find yourself missing doses.

Usual Duration of Use: Use on a regular schedule for several weeks determines benefit in reducing the severity and extent of psoriasis. Response in rheumatoid arthritis usually begins after 3 to 6 weeks of treatment. Dose should be reduced to smallest amount that will maintain acceptable improvement. Long-term use (months to years) requires physician supervision.

Typical Treatment Goals and Measurements (Outcomes and Markers)

Rheumatoid arthritis: Control of arthritis symptoms (severity of pain, number of swollen joints, loss of mobility, decreased ability to accomplish activities of daily living, range of motion, early morning stiffness [EMS], etc.) is paramount in returning patient quality of life and to checking the results (beneficial outcomes) from this medicine. Many arthritis management or pain centers use interdisciplinary teams (physicians from several specialties, nurses, physician's assistants, physical and occupational therapists, pharmacotherapists, psychotherapists, social workers and others) to get the best results. Blood levels of methotrexate are used to help avoid toxicity. In rheumatoid arthritis, C-reactive protein or sedimentation rate also measures results.

▷ **This Drug Should Not Be Taken If**
- you have had an allergic reaction to it previously.
- you currently have, or have had a recent exposure to, either chicken pox or shingles (herpes zoster).
- you are pregnant or planning pregnancy in the near future and you are taking this drug to treat psoriasis or rheumatoid arthritis.
- you are breast-feeding your infant.
- you have alcoholic liver disease.
- you have an immune deficiency.
- you have fluid in the pleura of the lung (pleural effusions).
- you have active liver disease, peptic ulcer, regional enteritis or ulcerative colitis.
- you are making very small amounts of urine or your creatinine clearance (see Glossary) is less than 40 ml/min.
- you currently have a blood cell or bone marrow disorder.

▷ **Inform Your Physician Before Taking This Drug If**
- you have a chronic infection of any kind.
- you do not understand how to handle vomit or urine while taking chemotherapy.

- you have impaired liver or kidney function.
- you have a history of bone marrow impairment of any kind, especially drug-induced bone marrow depression.
- your white blood cell count is less than 1,500 or your platelet count is less than 75,000.
- you are dehydrated.
- you have a history of gout, peptic ulcer disease, regional enteritis or ulcerative colitis.

Possible Side Effects (natural, expected and unavoidable drug actions)
The following are due to the pharmacological actions of this drug. **Report such developments to your physician promptly.**
Sores on the lips, in the mouth or throat.
Vomiting.
Intestinal cramping.
Diarrhea (may be bloody).
Painful urination.
Bloody urine.
Reduced resistance to infection, fatigue, weakness, fever, abnormal bleeding or bruising (bone marrow depression).

▷ **Possible Adverse Effects** (unusual, unexpected and infrequent reactions)
If any of the following develop, consult your physician promptly for guidance.
Mild Adverse Effects
Allergic reactions: skin rash, hives, itching.
Headache, drowsiness, blurred vision, conjunctivitis—infrequent.
Loss of appetite, nausea, vomiting—infrequent to frequent.
Muscle pain—rare.
Loss of hair, loss of skin pigmentation, acne—infrequent.
Impaired sense of smell or taste—possible.
Serious Adverse Effects
Allergic reactions: drug-induced pneumonia (cough, chest pain, shortness of breath).
Anaphylaxis.
Nervous system toxicity: speech disturbances, paralysis, seizures—infrequent.
Liver toxicity with jaundice (see Glossary)—case reports.
Kidney toxicity: reduced urine volume, kidney failure—more likely with higher doses.
Colitis or toxic megacolon—case report.
Tumor lysis syndrome: uric acid nephropathy; very low potassium, magnesium and calcium—possible.
Fluid buildup in the lung pleura (pleural effusion)—possible.
Immune suppression and subsequent infection with Pneumocystis carinii pneumonia—possible.
Severe skin reactions (toxic epidermal necrolysis)—case reports.
Chromosomal damage (from occupational exposure)—possible.

▷ **Possible Effects on Sexual Function:** Altered timing and pattern of menstruation. Swelling and tenderness of the male breast tissue (gynecomastia)—case reports.

Possible Delayed Adverse Effects: Some reports suggest that methotrexate therapy may contribute to the later development of secondary cancers. Other studies have not confirmed this.

Possible Effects on Laboratory Tests

Complete blood cell counts: decreased red cells, hemoglobin, white cells and platelets.

Blood uric acid level: increased.

Liver function tests: increased liver enzymes (ALT/GPT, AST/GOT and alkaline phosphatase) or bilirubin.

Kidney function tests: increased blood urea nitrogen (BUN) level; increased urine creatinine.

Fecal occult blood test: positive.

Sperm count: decreased.

CAUTION

1. This drug must be monitored carefully by a qualified physician. Request the Patient Package Insert (Rheumatrex Dose Pack) and read it thoroughly.
2. When methotrexate is used to treat rheumatoid arthritis, folic acid can minimize toxicity.
3. Appropriate laboratory examinations, performed before and during the use of this drug, are mandatory.
4. Women with potential for pregnancy should have a pregnancy test before taking this drug and should use an effective form of contraception during its use and for 8 weeks following its discontinuation.
5. Live-virus vaccines should be avoided during use of this drug. Live-virus vaccines could actually produce infection rather than stimulate an immune response.

Precautions for Use

By Those Over 60 Years of Age: Careful evaluation of kidney function should be made before starting treatment and during the entire course of therapy.

▷ **Advisability of Use During Pregnancy**

Pregnancy Category: X. See Pregnancy Risk Categories at the back of this book.

Animal studies: Skull and facial defects reported in mice.

Human studies: This drug is known to cause fetal deaths and birth defects. Its use during pregnancy to treat psoriasis or rheumatoid arthritis cannot be justified.

Advisability of Use If Breast-Feeding

Presence of this drug in breast milk: Yes.

Avoid drug or refrain from nursing.

Habit-Forming Potential: None.

Effects of Overdose: The side effects and adverse effects listed above develop earlier and with greater severity.

Possible Effects of Long-Term Use: Liver compromise (fibrosis and cirrhosis) occurs in 3–5% of long-term users (35 to 49 months).

Suggested Periodic Examinations While Taking This Drug (at physician's discretion)

Complete blood cell counts (CBCs). When methotrexate is used in rheumatoid arthritis, complete blood counts are checked after the first, second and fourth weeks of use. If the CBC is acceptable, after 2 weeks, the dose can be increased to 7.5 mg a week. Usually the CBC is checked each month after this.

Liver and kidney function tests.

Blood uric acid levels.

Chest X-ray examinations.

▷ **While Taking This Drug, Observe the Following**

Foods: Avoid highly seasoned foods that could be irritating. Between courses of treatment, eat liberally of the following foods: beef, chicken, lamb and pork liver, asparagus, navy beans, kale and spinach. Any food will reduce the peak methotrexate level obtained. Folic acid supplementation is suggested for people who will take this medicine on an ongoing basis.

Herbal Medicines or Minerals: Some patients use echinacea to attempt to boost their immune systems. Unfortunately, use of echinacea is not recommended in people with damaged immune systems (even if a medicine caused the damage). This herb may also actually weaken any immune system if it is used too often or for too long a time. Like methotrexate, St. John's wort may cause sensitivity to the sun. Avoid this combination. There are no data regarding combined use of hay flower, mistletoe herb or white mustard seed with methotrexate in rheumatoid arthritis.

Beverages: No restrictions. This drug may be taken with milk.

▷ *Alcohol:* Avoid completely.

Tobacco Smoking: No interactions expected. I advise everyone to quit smoking.

Marijuana Smoking: May cause additional impairment of immunity.

▷ *Other Drugs*

Methotrexate may **decrease** the effects of

- digoxin (Lanoxin).
- folate (various) by blocking the change (conversion) of folate to folic acid.
- phenytoin (Dilantin) or fosphenytoin (Cerebyx).

The following drugs may **increase** the effects of methotrexate and enhance its toxicity:

- aspirin and other salicylates.
- diuretics (see Drug Classes) may result in methotrexate enhanced lowering of granulocyte type white blood cells (myelosuppression).
- NSAIDs (see Drug Classes) (especially with higher NSAID doses).
- omeprazole (Prilosec).
- probenecid (Benemid).
- rofecoxib (Vioxx).

Methotrexate **taken concurrently** with

- amiodarone (Cordarone) may result in methotrexate toxicity.
- asparaginase (Elspar, others) may result in blunted methotrexate activity.
- bismuth subsalicylate (Pepto-Bismol, others) may result in methotrexate toxicity.
- carbenicillin (Geocillin, others) and other penicillins (see Drug Classes) may lead to methotrexate toxicity.
- cholestyramine (Questran, others) and other cholesterol-lowering resins may result in decreased methotrexate effectiveness.

- cotrimoxazole (Bactrim) may result in lowering of all blood cells (pancytopenia).
- cyclosporine (Sandimmune) can result in increased toxicity from both drugs. This combination should be avoided.
- doxycycline (various) may result in methotrexate toxicity.
- etretinate (Tegison) results in increased liver toxicity.
- influenzae vaccine (flu) may blunt benefits of the vaccine.
- leflunomide (Arava) may result in liver toxicity.
- live-virus vaccines (such as RotaShield) may lead to severe infections.
- neomycin (various) may result in decreased methotrexate benefits.
- pneumococcal or smallpox vaccine may result in decreased immune response to the vaccine.
- sulfa drugs, such as sulfamethoxazole, can result in increased hematological toxicity.
- tamoxifen (Nolvadex) may increase risk of blood clots (thromboembolism)—part of a combination regimen that leads to this.
- thiazide diuretics (see Drug Classes) may increase risk of myelosuppression.
- theophylline (Theo-Dur, others) may result in theophylline toxicity; decreased theophylline doses may be needed.
- triamterene (Dyazide, others) may increase risk of bone marrow problems (myelosuppression).
- trimethoprim (Septra, others) may increase risk of toxicity.
- yellow fever vaccine can result in blunted response and benefit from the vaccine.

▷ *Driving, Hazardous Activities:* This drug may cause drowsiness, dizziness or blurred vision. Restrict activities as necessary.

Aviation Note: The use of this drug *is a disqualification* for piloting. Consult a designated Aviation Medical Examiner.

Exposure to Sun: Use caution—this drug can cause photosensitivity. Avoid ultraviolet lamps.

METHYCLOTHIAZIDE (METH i kloh thi a zide)

Please see the thiazide diuretics family profile.

METHYLPHENIDATE (meth il FEN i dayt)

Introduced: 1956   **Class:** Amphetaminelike drug, anti-attention-deficit-disorder drug   **Prescription:** USA: Yes   **Controlled Drug:** USA: C-II*; Canada: Yes   **Available as Generic:** USA: Yes; Canada: Yes

Brand Names: Concerta, Metadate ER, ✿PMS-Methylphenidate, Methylin ER, Ritalin, Ritalin-SR

*See Schedules of Controlled Drugs at the back of this book.

BENEFITS versus RISKS	
Possible Benefits	*Possible Risks*
EFFECTIVE CONTROL OF NARCOLEPSY	POTENTIAL FOR SERIOUS PSYCHOLOGICAL DEPENDENCE (oral dosing reaches brain levels slowly and appears to avoid this effect)
USEFUL AS ADJUNCTIVE TREATMENT IN ATTENTION DEFICIT DISORDERS	
CONCERTA FORM OFFERS ONCE DAILY DOSING	SUPPRESSION OF GROWTH IN CHILDHOOD (recovers when medicine is stopped)
Adjunctive treatment in ADHD	
Useful in treatment of mild to moderate depression	Abnormal behavior
	Rare blood cell disorders
Useful in some cases of emotional withdrawal in the elderly	

▷ **Principal Uses**

As a Single Drug Product: Uses currently included in FDA-approved labeling: Treats (1) narcolepsy—recurrent spells of uncontrollable drowsiness and sleep; (2) attention deficit disorders of childhood, formerly known as the hyperactive child syndrome, with minimal brain damage and minimal brain dysfunction.

Other (unlabeled) generally accepted uses: (1) Treats mild to moderate depression; (2) manages apathetic and withdrawal states in the elderly; (3) combination therapy of chronic pain, particularly cancer pain; (4) could have a role in autism; (5) may help passing out (recurrent neurocardiogenic syncope).

How This Drug Works: Activates the brain stem, improves alertness and concentration, increases learning ability and attention span. A study in Science found that levels of the nerve transmitter serotonin are increased by this medicine, restoring a proper balance between serotonin and other brain chemicals.

Available Dosage Forms and Strengths

Tablets — 5 mg, 10 mg, 20 mg

Tablets, prolonged action — 20 mg

Tablet, osmotic controlled release — 18 mg, 36 mg

▷ **Recommended Dosage Ranges:** *Narcolepsy*: 10 to 60 mg daily, divided into equal doses, given two to three times daily. Ideally, given 30 minutes before meals.

Attention deficit disorder: Pediatric dosing: Children over 6 years old (regular-release form)—5 mg before breakfast and lunch (twice daily). Some clinicians use 0.25 mg per kg per day divided into two doses as a starting dose. Dose is increased as needed and tolerated (weekly intervals) to daily maximum of dose of 60 mg. Sustained-release form lasts 8 hours. Osmotic-release form (Concerta) is given once daily in the morning.

Note: Actual dose and schedule must be determined for each patient individually.

Conditions Requiring Dosing Adjustments

Liver Function: Used with caution and in decreased dose in liver disease.

Kidney Function: No changes currently thought to be needed.

▷ **Dosing Instructions:** The regular tablet may be crushed and taken 30 to 45 minutes before meals. The prolonged-action tablet and the osmotic controlled-release form (Concerta) should be taken whole, not crushed. If you forget a dose: Take the missed dose as soon as you remember it, unless it's nearly time for your next dose—if that is the case, skip the missed dose and take the next dose right on schedule. Talk with your doctor if you find yourself missing doses.

Usual Duration of Use: Regular use for 3 to 4 weeks determines benefits in easing the symptoms of narcolepsy or improving behavior of attention-deficit children. If there is no improvement after this time, the drug should be stopped. Long-term use (months to years) requires supervision by your doctor.

Typical Treatment Goals and Measurements (Outcomes and Markers)
Attention Deficit: The general goal is to achieve the ability to "stay on task." This medicine can also help decrease impulsiveness and socially appropriate behavior. Specific measures of cognitive function, motor performance and educational tasking may help assess response. New treatment guidelines from AHCPR and DSM-IV criteria from the American Psychiatric Association are widely used.

▷ **This Drug Should Not Be Taken If**
- you have had an allergic reaction to it previously.
- you have glaucoma (inadequately treated).
- you have Tourette's syndrome or experience tics while using this medicine.
- you are experiencing a period of severe anxiety, nervous tension or emotional depression.

▷ **Inform Your Physician Before Taking This Drug If**
- you have a history of mental illness.
- you have a seizure disorder.
- you have a history of abnormal heartbeats.
- you have high blood pressure, angina or epilepsy.
- you took a monoamine oxidase (MAO) type A inhibitor (see Drug Classes) within the past 14 days.

Possible Side Effects (natural, expected and unavoidable drug actions)
Nervousness, excitement, insomnia. Reduced appetite. Growth suppression (stopping the medicine in the summer is used to allow a growth spurt). Slight increase in heart rate.

▷ **Possible Adverse Effects** (unusual, unexpected and infrequent reactions)
If any of the following develop, consult your physician promptly for guidance.
Mild Adverse Effects
Allergic reactions: skin rash, hives, drug fever, joint pains—possible.
Headache, dizziness, rapid and forceful heart palpitation—infrequent.
Nausea, abdominal discomfort—infrequent.
Stuttering and hallucinations—case reports.
Serious Adverse Effects
Allergic reactions: severe skin reactions, extensive bruising (allergic destruction of platelets)—case reports.
Idiosyncratic reactions: abnormal patterns of behavior.
Porphyria or muscle damage (rhabdomyolysis)—rare.

Liver toxicity—case reports.

Precipitation of Tourette's syndrome—case reports.

▷ **Possible Effects on Sexual Function:** None reported.

Natural Diseases or Disorders That May Be Activated by This Drug

Latent epilepsy. Increased eye pressure unmasking glaucoma.

Possible Effects on Laboratory Tests

Eosinophils: Increased (IV abuse).

CAUTION

1. This drug should be used ONLY AFTER a careful assessment by a qualified specialist is made. True attention deficit disorder requires careful assessment to differentiate it from behavior problems arising from family tensions or other conditions that do not require methylphenidate therapy.
2. A February 2000 study of 200,000 children coordinated by the University of Maryland found a large increase in Ritalin, Prozac and clonidine prescriptions in patients less than four years old. This retrospective review of Medicaid and HMO records may represent better ability to diagnose, but may also reflect excessive use. The American Academy of Pediatricians issued the first set of guidelines for ADHD to help standardize the diagnosis (see www.aap.org).
3. Careful dose adjustments on an individual basis are mandatory.
4. Paradoxical reactions (see Glossary) can occur, causing aggravation of initial symptoms for which this drug was prescribed.

Precautions for Use

By Infants and Children: Safety and effectiveness for those under 6 years of age are not established. If this drug is not beneficial in managing an attention deficit disorder after a trial of 1 month, it should be stopped. During long-term use, monitor the child for normal growth and development.

By Those Over 60 Years of Age: Start with small doses. Those in this group may be at increased risk for nervousness, agitation, insomnia, high blood pressure, angina or disturbance of heart rhythm.

▷ **Advisability of Use During Pregnancy**

Pregnancy Category: C. See Pregnancy Risk Categories at the back of this book.

Animal studies: No birth defects found in mouse studies.

Human studies: Adequate studies of pregnant women are not available.

Ask your physician for guidance.

Advisability of Use If Breast-Feeding

Presence of this drug in breast milk: Unknown.

Avoid drug or refrain from nursing.

Habit-Forming Potential: This drug can produce tolerance and cause serious psychological dependence (see Glossary), a potentially dangerous characteristic of amphetaminelike drugs (see Drug Classes). The street name for this medicine is R-ball or Vitamin-R. It is one of the top prescription drugs stolen in the United States for recreational use. Caution is needed.

Effects of Overdose: Headache, vomiting, agitation, tremors, dry mouth, sweating, fever, confusion, hallucinations, seizures, coma.

Possible Effects of Long-Term Use: Suppression of growth (in weight and/or height) occurs. Many patients are taken off the drug during summer vacations.

Suggested Periodic Examinations While Taking This Drug (at physician's discretion)

Complete blood cell counts.

Blood pressure measurements.

Height and weight.

Follow up evaluation for beneficial effects of treatment.

▷ **While Taking This Drug, Observe the Following**

Herbal Medicines or Minerals: Using St. John's wort, guarana, ma huang or kola while taking this medicine may result in unacceptable central nervous system stimulation.

Beverages: Avoid beverages prepared from meat or meat extracts. This drug may be taken with milk.

▷ *Alcohol:* Avoid beer, Chianti wines and vermouth (may have high tyramine contents).

Tobacco Smoking: No interactions expected. I advise everyone to quit smoking.

▷ *Other Drugs*

Methylphenidate may ***increase*** the effects of

• tricyclic antidepressants (see Drug Classes) and enhance their toxic effects.

Methylphenidate may ***decrease*** the effects of

• guanethidine (Ismelin) and impair its ability to lower blood pressure.

Methylphenidate **taken concurrently** with

• anticonvulsants (such as carbamazepine or fosphenytoin or phenytoin) may cause a significant change in the pattern of epileptic seizures; dose adjustments may be necessary for proper control.

• monoamine oxidase (MAO) type A inhibitors (see Drug Classes) may cause a significant rise in blood pressure; avoid the concurrent use of these drugs.

• morphine may be used to great therapeutic benefit to increase alertness, especially if high doses of morphine must be used.

• tricyclic antidepressants (see Drug Classes) may result in undesirable increases in blood pressure.

▷ *Driving, Hazardous Activities:* This drug may cause dizziness or drowsiness. Restrict activities as necessary.

Aviation Note: The use of this drug ***is a disqualification*** for piloting. Consult a designated Aviation Medical Examiner.

Exposure to Sun: No restrictions.

Discontinuation: If the drug has been taken for a long time, do not stop it abruptly. Talk to your doctor about how to slowly decrease doses.

METHYLPREDNISOLONE (meth il pred NIS oh lohn)

Introduced: 1957   **Class:** Cortisonelike   drugs   **Prescription:** USA: Yes   **Controlled Drug:** USA: No; Canada: No   **Available as Generic:** USA: Yes; Canada: Yes

Brand Names: A-Methapred, Depmedalone-40, Depmedalone-80, Depo-Medrol, Enpak Refill, Mar-Pred 40, Medrol, ✤Medrol Acne Lotion, Medrol Enpak, ✤Medrol Veriderm Cream, Meprolone, ✤Neo-Medrol Acne Lotion, ✤Neo-Medrol Veriderm, Solu-Medrol

```
┌─────────────────────────────────────────────────────────────┐
│                    BENEFITS versus RISKS                     │
│        Possible Benefits              Possible Risks          │
│   EFFECTIVE RELIEF OF          Use exceeding 2 weeks is associated │
│     SYMPTOMS IN A WIDE VARIETY    with many adverse effects such as: │
│     OF INFLAMMATORY AND        ALTERED MOOD AND               │
│     ALLERGIC DISORDERS           PERSONALITY                  │
│   EFFECTIVE IMMUNO-            CATARACTS, GLAUCOMA            │
│     SUPPRESSION IN SELECTED    HYPERTENSION                   │
│     BENIGN AND MALIGNANT       OSTEOPOROSIS                   │
│     DISORDERS                  ASEPTIC BONE NECROSIS          │
│                                INCREASED SUSCEPTIBILITY TO    │
│                                  INFECTIONS                   │
│                                (See "Possible Adverse Effects" and │
│                                "Possible Effects of Long-Term Use" │
│                                below.)                        │
└─────────────────────────────────────────────────────────────┘
```

▷ **Principal Uses**

As a Single Drug Product: Uses currently included in FDA-approved labeling: (1) Treats a wide variety of allergic and inflammatory conditions (used most commonly in the management of serious skin disorders, asthma, regional enteritis, multiple sclerosis, lupus erythematosus, ulcerative colitis and all types of major rheumatic disorders including bursitis, tendonitis and most forms of arthritis); (2) helps treat low platelet counts of unknown cause (idiopathic thrombocytopenic purpura); (3) treats shock due to adrenal gland insufficiency—Addisonian shock; (4) plays an adjunctive role in anaphylactic shock.

Other (unlabeled) generally accepted uses: (1) Treats refractory anemia; (2) used in therapy of chronic obstructive pulmonary disease; (3) used in combination treatment of acute nonlymphoblastic leukemia; (4) used in combination therapy of severe vomiting caused by chemotherapy; (5) helps prevent rejection of transplanted organs; (6) combination therapy of *Pneumocystis carinii* pneumonia in AIDS patients; (7) helps treat bone cysts in children; (8) has a role in treating croup; (9) can help symptoms in Still's disease; (10) used by intramuscular injection to treat polymyalgia rheumatica; (11) used to help control cancer pain, especially where inflammation is involved.

How This Drug Works: Anti-inflammatory effect is due to its ability to block normal defensive functions of certain white blood cells. Immunosuppressant effect comes from reduced production of lymphocytes (a kind of white blood cell) and antibodies.

Available Dosage Forms and Strengths

Injection, solution (per vial) — 40 mg, 125 mg, 500 mg, 1 g

Injection, suspension — 40 mg/ml, 80 mg/ml

Ointment — 0.25%, 1%

Retention enema (per bottle) — 40 mg

Tablets — 2 mg, 4 mg, 8 mg, 16 mg, 24 mg, 32 mg

▷ **Usual Adult Dosage Ranges:** 4 to 48 mg daily as a single (oral) dose or in divided doses. **Note: Actual dose and schedule must be determined for each patient individually.**

Conditions Requiring Dosing Adjustments

Liver Function: Specific dose adjustments in liver compromise are not defined. This drug is a rare cause of liver changes (hepatomegaly).

Kidney Function: This drug can worsen existing kidney compromise. A benefit-to-risk decision must be made regarding the use of methylprednisolone by these patients.

Obesity: The amount of time this medicine stays in the body is extended in obese patients. Dosing should be calculated based on ideal body weight.

▷ **Dosing Instructions:** The tablet may be crushed and taken with or following food to prevent stomach irritation, preferably in the morning. If you forget a dose: Call your doctor for instructions.

Usual Duration of Use: For sudden (acute) disorders, 4 to 10 days. For long-standing (chronic) disorders, according to individual requirements. Duration of use should not exceed the time necessary to obtain adequate symptomatic relief in acute self-limiting conditions or the time required to stabilize a chronic condition and permit gradual withdrawal. Because of its intermediate duration of action, this drug is appropriate for alternate-day use. See your doctor on a regular basis.

Typical Treatment Goals and Measurements (Outcomes and Markers)

Inflammation: The general goal is to decrease inflammation. Physical signs and symptoms such as hives (urticaria), rash, difficulty breathing and swelling should ease. Tests include sedimentation rate, peak expiratory flow rate, FEV1 for respiratory conditions.

Asthma: Frequency and severity of asthma attacks should ease. Some clinicians also use decreased frequency of rescue inhaler use as a further clinical indicator. It is critical that this medicine is used regularly to get the best results. An additional goal of therapy is to use the lowest effective dose. Some people keep their improvements when doses are lowered, while others relapse. Specific testing goals include improvement in PEFR, FEV1 and other lung (pulmonary) function tests. Wheezing and difficulty breathing (dyspnea) should ease as well as asthma caused (induced) by exercise. If the usual benefit is not realized, call your doctor.

▷ **This Drug Should Not Be Taken If**
- you had an allergic reaction to it previously.
- you have active peptic ulcer disease.
- you have had recent bowel surgery where an anastomosis was performed.
- you have a premature infant and the injection form is ordered (contains benzyl alcohol).
- you have an active eye infection from herpes simplex virus.
- you have active tuberculosis.

▷ **Inform Your Physician Before Taking This Drug If**
- you have had an reaction to any cortisonelike drug.
- you have a history of peptic ulcer disease, thrombophlebitis or tuberculosis.
- you have diabetes, glaucoma, high blood pressure, deficient thyroid function or myasthenia gravis.
- you have been exposed to measles or chicken pox.
- you plan to have surgery of any kind in the near future.
- you have liver compromise.

Possible Side Effects (natural, expected and unavoidable drug actions)

Increased appetite, weight gain, retention of salt and water, excretion of potassium, increased susceptibility to infection. Decreased wound healing. Adrenal gland suppression. Growth retardation with chronic use in children. Increased eye pressure (intraocular). Easy bruising (ecchymosis).

▷ **Possible Adverse Effects** (unusual, unexpected and infrequent reactions)

If any of the following develop, consult your physician promptly for guidance.

Mild Adverse Effects

Allergic reaction: skin rash.

Headache, dizziness, insomnia—infrequent.

Acid indigestion, abdominal distention—infrequent.

Muscle cramping, weakness and joint pain—possible.

Acne, excessive growth of facial hair—case reports.

Serious Adverse Effects

Allergic reactions: anaphylaxis.

Mental and emotional disturbances—infrequent.

Reactivation of latent tuberculosis, Pneumocystis carinii pneumonia—possible, case reports.

Development of peptic ulcer—case reports.

Seizures—possible.

Toxic megacolon—case reports.

Liver or kidney compromise—rare.

Blindness, cataracts—case reports.

Changes in white blood cell counts—possible.

Cushing's syndrome with chronic use (central obesity, buffalo hump and moon-shaped face)—possible.

Osteoporosis, osteonecrosis—possible with long-term use.

Increased blood sugar (hyperglycemia)—possible and dose-related.

Muscle changes (myopathy) or pancreatitis—case reports.

Increased blood pressure—case reports.

Abnormal heartbeat (arrhythmias)—case reports.

Development of inflammation of the pancreas—case reports.

Thrombophlebitis (inflammation of a vein with the formation of blood clot): pain or tenderness in thigh or leg, with or without swelling of the foot, ankle or leg—case reports.

Pulmonary embolism (movement of a blood clot to the lung): sudden shortness of breath, pain in the chest, coughing, bloody sputum—case reports.

▷ **Possible Effects on Sexual Function:** Altered timing and pattern of menstruation—infrequent.

▷ **Adverse Effects That May Mimic Natural Diseases or Disorders**

Pattern of symptoms and signs resembling Cushing's syndrome.

Natural Diseases or Disorders That May Be Activated by This Drug

Latent diabetes, glaucoma, peptic ulcer disease, tuberculosis.

Possible Effects on Laboratory Tests

Blood amylase and lipase levels: increased (possible pancreatitis).

Glucose tolerance test (GTT): decreased.

Blood potassium or testosterone level: decreased.

Cholesterol and LDL: Increased.

HDL: Decreased.

CAUTION

1. Carry a card in your purse or wallet that says you take this drug, if your treatment will exceed 1 week.
2. You have an increased risk of severe infection from viral illnesses, such as measles or chicken pox. Try to avoid being exposed, and call your doctor if exposure occurs.
3. Growth and development of children receiving chronic steroids should be carefully followed.
4. Do not stop this drug abruptly after long-term treatment.
5. If vaccination against measles, rabies, smallpox or yellow fever is required, stop drug 72 hours before vaccination and do not resume it for at least 14 days.
6. Dermatitis around the mouth may occur. Talk with your doctor if this happens.

Precautions for Use

By Infants and Children: Avoid prolonged use if possible. Watch for growth suppression. Long-term use also increases risk of adrenal gland deficiency during stress (up to 18 months after drug is stopped). Pressure in the brain may increase.

By Those Over 60 Years of Age: Cortisonelike drugs should be used very sparingly after 60 and only when the disorder under treatment is unresponsive to adequate trials of unrelated drugs. Avoid prolonged use of this drug. Continual use (even in small doses) can increase the severity of diabetes, enhance fluid retention, raise blood pressure, weaken resistance to infection, induce stomach ulcer and accelerate the development of cataract and osteoporosis.

▷ **Advisability of Use During Pregnancy**

Pregnancy Category: C. See Pregnancy Risk Categories at the back of this book.

Animal studies: Birth defects reported in mice, rats and rabbits.

Human studies: Adequate studies of pregnant women are not available. Avoid completely during the first 3 months. Limit use during the final 6 months as much as possible. If used, the infant should be examined for possible deficiency of adrenal gland function.

Advisability of Use If Breast-Feeding

Presence of this drug in breast milk: Yes.

Avoid drug or refrain from nursing.

Habit-Forming Potential: Use of this drug over an extended period of time may produce a state of functional dependence (see Glossary). Treating asthma and rheumatoid arthritis, the dose should be kept as small as possible, and withdrawal should be attempted after periods of reasonable improvement. Such procedures may reduce "steroid rebound"—return of symptoms as the drug is withdrawn.

Effects of Overdose: Fatigue, muscle weakness, stomach irritation, acid indigestion, excessive sweating, facial flushing, fluid retention, swelling of extremities, increased blood pressure.

Possible Effects of Long-Term Use: Increased blood sugar (possible diabetes), increased fat deposits on the trunk of the body ("buffalo hump"), rounding of the face ("moon face"), thinning and fragility of skin, loss of texture and strength of bones (osteoporosis, aseptic necrosis), cataracts, glaucoma, retarded growth and development in children.

Suggested Periodic Examinations While Taking This Drug (at physician's discretion)

Measurements of blood pressure.

Blood sugar and potassium levels.

Complete eye examinations at regular intervals.

Chest X-ray if history of tuberculosis.

Determination of the rate of development of the growing child to detect retardation of normal growth.

Bone mineral density testing to assess osteoporosis and fracture risk.

▷ **While Taking This Drug, Observe the Following**

Foods: See grapefruit note under beverages. Ask your physician regarding need to restrict salt intake or to eat potassium-rich foods. During long-term use of this drug, it is advisable to eat a high-protein diet.

Herbal Medicines or Minerals: Fir or pine needle oil should NOT be used by asthmatics. Ephedra alone does carry a German Commission E monograph indication for asthma treatment. If you are allergic to plants in the Asteraceae family (aster, chrysanthemum, daisy or ragweed), you may also be allergic to echinacea, chamomile, feverfew and St. John's wort. Added calcium and vitamin D while taking this medicine is prudent. During wound repair, zinc supplementation may be prudent. Talk to your doctor BEFORE adding any herbals to this medicine.

Beverages: Grapefruit juice will increase the plasma levels of methylprednisolone—water is a better liquid to take this medicine with. Drink all forms of milk liberally.

▷ *Alcohol:* No interactions expected. Use caution if you are prone to peptic ulcer disease.

Tobacco Smoking: Nicotine increases the blood levels of naturally produced cortisone and related hormones. I advise everyone to quit smoking.

Marijuana Smoking: May cause additional impairment of immunity.

▷ *Other Drugs*

Methylprednisolone may *decrease* the effects of

• insulin and require higher doses.

• isoniazid (INH, Niconyl, etc.).

• salicylates (aspirin, sodium salicylate, etc.).

Methylprednisolone *taken concurrently* with

• amphotericin B (Fungizone) may increase risk of potassium loss.

• carbamazepine (Tegretol) may blunt methylprednisolone benefits.

• cholestyramine (Questran) may decrease the amount of medicine that is absorbed into your body.

• clarithromycin (Biaxin) can result in increased methylprednisolone levels and toxicity.

• cyclosporine (Sandimmune) can result in increased steroid levels and cyclosporine toxicity.

• ketoconazole (Nizoral) (and other azole antifungals) may increase blood levels of methylprednisolone and result in toxicity (abnormal heartbeats or psychiatric reactions).

- loop diuretics, such as furosemide (Lasix) or bumetanide (Bumex), may result in increased risk of potassium loss.
- neuromuscular blocking agents (such as pancuronium [Pavulon], vecuronium [Norcuron], others) can result in increased risk and or severity of muscle problems (myopathy and flaccid paralysis) and can also antagonize blockade from these medicines. Caution and unparalyzed periods are prudent.
- NSAIDs may cause increased risk of ulceration of the stomach or intestine.
- oral anticoagulants (warfarin [Coumadin]) may either increase or decrease their effectiveness; consult your physician regarding the need for prothrombin time testing and dose adjustment.
- oral antidiabetic drugs (see Drug Classes) or insulin may result in loss of control of blood sugar and require higher doses or more frequent dosing of oral hypoglycemics or insulin in order to control blood sugar.
- primidone (Mysoline) may lead to increased metabolism of methylprednisolone and decreased therapeutic benefits of methylprednisolone.
- quinupristin/dalfopristin (Synercid) can result in increased steroid levels and toxicity.
- rifampin (Rifadin, others) may lead to increased metabolism of methylprednisolone and decreased therapeutic benefits of methylprednisolone.
- ritonavir (Norvir) and perhaps other protease inhibitors (see Drug Classes) may change therapeutic benefits of methylprednisolone.
- tacrolimus (Prograf) can result in increased tacrolimus levels and tacrolimus toxicity.
- theophylline (Theo-Dur) results in variable changes in blood levels; more frequent theophylline blood levels are indicated.
- thiazide diuretics (see Drug Classes) can result in additive potassium loss.
- vaccines (such as flu or pneumococcal) may result in a blunting of the immune response to the vaccine.

The following drugs may *decrease* the effects of methylprednisolone:
- antacids—may reduce its absorption.
- barbiturates (Amytal, Butisol, phenobarbital, etc.).
- phenytoin (Dilantin, etc.) or fosphenytoin (Cerebyx).
- rifampin (Rifadin, Rimactane, etc.).

▷ *Driving, Hazardous Activities:* Usually no restrictions. Be alert to the rare occurrence of dizziness.

Aviation Note: The use of this drug *may be a disqualification* for piloting. Consult a designated Aviation Medical Examiner.

Exposure to Sun: No restrictions.

Occurrence of Unrelated Illness: Decreases resistance to infection. Tell your doctor if you get an infection of any kind. May also reduce ability to respond to stress of acute illness, injury or surgery. Tell your doctor about any significant changes in your state of health.

Discontinuation: After extended use of this drug, do not stop it abruptly. Ask your doctor for help regarding slow withdrawal. For 2 years after stopping this drug, it is essential that you tell medical personnel that you have used this drug if you get sick, are injured or have surgery. Impaired response to stress after taking cortisonelike drugs may last for 1 to 2 years.

METHYSERGIDE (meth i SER jide)

Introduced: 1961   **Class:** Antimigraine drug   **Prescription:** USA: Yes
Controlled Drug: USA: No; Canada: No   **Available as Generic:** USA: No;
Canada: No
Brand Name: Sansert

BENEFITS versus RISKS	
Possible Benefits	*Possible Risks*
EFFECTIVE PREVENTION OF MIGRAINE AND CLUSTER HEADACHES	FIBROSIS (SCARRING) INSIDE CHEST AND ABDOMINAL CAVITIES, OF HEART AND LUNG TISSUES, ADJACENT TO MAJOR BLOOD VESSELS AND INTERNAL ORGANS (see "Effects of Long-Term Use" below)
	Aggravation of hypertension, coronary artery disease and peripheral vascular disease

▷ **Principal Uses**

As a Single Drug Product: Uses currently included in FDA-approved labeling: Prevention of frequent and/or disabling vascular headaches (migraine and cluster neuralgia) that have not responded to other conventional treatment.

Other (unlabeled) generally accepted uses: None at present.

How This Drug Works: Blocks serotonin inflammatory and vasoconstrictor effects, easing blood vessel constriction that causes vascular headaches. (Competitive 5-HT blocker.)

Available Dosage Forms and Strengths

Tablets — 2 mg

▷ **Recommended Dosage Ranges** (Actual dose and schedule must be determined for each patient individually.)

Infants and Children: Use of this drug is not recommended.

12 to 60 Years of Age: 4 to 8 mg daily, in divided doses with meals. A medication-free period of 3 to 4 weeks is REQUIRED after every 6-month course.

Over 60 Years of Age: 2 to 4 mg daily, in divided doses. Use very cautiously, with frequent monitoring for adverse effects.

Conditions Requiring Dosing Adjustments

Liver Function: This drug should not be used by patients with liver compromise.

Kidney Function: This drug should not be used by patients with renal compromise.

▷ **Dosing Instructions:** The tablet may be crushed and taken with food or milk to reduce stomach irritation. Uninterrupted use is limited to 6 months; avoid drug completely for 3 to 4 weeks between courses. If you forget a dose: Call your doctor. It is extremely important that you take this medicine exactly as directed.

▷ **Usual Duration of Use:** Use on a regular schedule for 3 weeks usually determines effectiveness in preventing recurrence of vascular headache. If significant benefit does not occur during this trial, this drug should be stopped. None of this medicine can be given for 3 to 4 weeks after every 6-month course of treatment. Periodic long-term use (months to years) requires periodic physician evaluation.

Typical Treatment Goals and Measurements (Outcomes and Markers)

Pain: Most clinicians treating pain use a device called an algometer to check your pain. This looks like a small ruler, but lets the clinician better understand your pain. The goals of treatment then relate to where the level of pain started (for example, a rating of 7 on a zero to ten scale) and what the cause of the pain was. Specific results in migraine therapy and this medicine relate to decreasing the frequency and/or severity of headaches or avoiding them altogether.

▷ **This Drug Should Not Be Taken If**
- you have had an allergic reaction to it previously.
- you are pregnant.
- you currently have a severe infection.
- you have any of the following conditions:
  - angina pectoris
  - Buerger's disease
  - cellulitis of the lower legs
  - chronic lung disease
  - connective tissue (collagen) disease
  - coronary artery disease
  - hardening of the arteries (arteriosclerosis)
  - heart valve disease
  - high blood pressure (significant hypertension)
  - kidney disease or significantly impaired kidney function
  - liver disease or significantly impaired liver function
  - active peptic ulcer disease
  - peripheral vascular disease
  - phlebitis of any kind
  - Raynaud's disease or phenomenon

▷ **Inform Your Physician Before Taking This Drug If**
- you had an adverse reaction to any ergot.
- you have a history of peptic ulcer disease.

Possible Side Effects (natural, expected and unavoidable drug actions)

Fluid retention, weight gain. Impaired circulation to the extremities (peripheral ischemia).

▷ **Possible Adverse Effects** (unusual, unexpected and infrequent reactions)

If any of the following develop, consult your physician promptly for guidance.

Mild Adverse Effects

Allergic reactions: skin rashes, flushing of the face, transient loss of scalp hair.

Dizziness, drowsiness, agitation, unsteadiness, altered vision—infrequent to frequent.

Heartburn, nausea, vomiting, diarrhea—infrequent.

Transient muscle and joint pains—infrequent.

Serious Adverse Effects

Idiosyncratic reactions: nightmares, hallucinations, acute mental disturbances.

Fibrosis (scar tissue formation) involving the chest and/or abdominal cavities, heart, heart valves, lungs, kidneys, major blood vessels—case reports.

Spasm and narrowing of coronary and peripheral arteries: anginal chest pain, cold and painful extremities, leg cramps on walking—case reports.

Hemolytic anemia (see Glossary) or abnormally low white blood cell counts—case reports.

Heart attack (myocardial infarction)—case reports.

▷ **Possible Effects on Sexual Function:** Fibrosis of penile tissues—case reports.

▷ **Adverse Effects That May Mimic Natural Diseases or Disorders**

Swelling of the hands, lower legs, feet and ankles (peripheral edema) may suggest heart or kidney dysfunction.

Natural Diseases or Disorders That May Be Activated by This Drug

Latent coronary artery insufficiency (angina), Buerger's disease, Raynaud's disease, peptic ulcer disease.

Possible Effects on Laboratory Tests

Complete blood cell counts: decreased white cells (lymphocytes).

Stomach hydrochloric acid: increased.

Kidney function tests: increased blood urea nitrogen (BUN).

CAUTION

1. Continual use limited to 6 months. Gradual dose reduction is prudent during last 2 to 3 weeks of each course to prevent headache rebound. Omit drug for a period of 3 to 4 weeks before resuming. Mandatory "drug-free" period reduces fibrosis risk.

2. Promptly report fatigue, fever, chest pain, difficult breathing, stomach/flank pain or urinary changes.

3. Useful only for prevention of recurring vascular headaches. NOT recommended for acute headaches. Not effective for tension headaches.

Precautions for Use

By Infants and Children: Use of this drug is not recommended.

By Those Over 60 Years of Age: The age-related changes in blood vessels, circulatory functions and kidney function can make you more susceptible to the serious adverse effects of this drug. See the list of diseases and disorders above that are contraindications to the use this drug. Ask your doctor for help.

▷ **Advisability of Use During Pregnancy**

Pregnancy Category: X. See Pregnancy Risk Categories at the back of this book.

Animal studies: No information is available.

Human studies: Adequate studies of pregnant women are not available.

The manufacturer states that this drug is contraindicated during entire pregnancy.

Advisability of Use If Breast-Feeding

Presence of this drug in breast milk: Yes.

Avoid drug or refrain from nursing.

Habit-Forming Potential: None.

Effects of Overdose: Nausea, vomiting, stomach pain, diarrhea, dizziness, excitement, cold hands and feet.

Possible Effects of Long-Term Use: Formation of scar tissue (fibrosis) inside chest cavity and/or abdominal cavity, on heart valves, in lung tissues and surrounding major blood vessels and internal organs. Requires close and continual medical supervision.

Suggested Periodic Examinations While Taking This Drug (at physician's discretion)

Careful examination at regular intervals (6 to 12 months) for scar tissue formation or circulatory complications.

Complete blood cell counts.

Kidney function tests.

▷ **While Taking This Drug, Observe the Following**

Foods: No restrictions except foods you are allergic to. Some vascular headaches are due to food allergy, or have specific food triggers. A headache diary can help you identify triggers and then avoid them.

Herbal Medicines or Minerals: Since methysergide and St. John's wort may act on serotonin, the combination is not advised. Using ma huang or ephedrine-like compounds (ephedra) may result in additive and undesirable vasoconstriction. If you are allergic to plants in the *Asteraceae* family (aster, chrysanthemum, daisy or ragweed), you may also be allergic to echinacea, chamomile, feverfew and St. John's wort. St. John's wort can cause changes in the liver enzymes that help remove this medicine—talk to your doctor before combining any herbal medicine or mineral with methysergide.

Beverages: No restrictions.

▷ *Alcohol:* No interactions expected. Observe closely to determine if alcoholic beverages can initiate a migrainelike headache.

Tobacco Smoking: Avoid completely.

▷ *Other Drugs*

Methysergide *taken concurrently* with

- beta-blocker drugs (see Drug Classes) may cause hazardous constriction of peripheral arteries; watch combined effects on circulation in the extremities. Careful patient monitoring and a selective beta blocker (such as atenolol) is prudent.
- efavirenz (Sustiva) increases risk of methysergide toxicity.
- medicines removed by the cytochrome P450 3A4 enzymes as well as those that inhibit CYP 3A4 may lead to methysergide toxicity. Medicines that increase CYP3A4 will blunt methysergide benefits.
- sibutramine (Meridia) increases serotonin syndrome risk.
- sildenafil (Viagra) may increase risk of methysergide toxicity.
- sumatriptan (Imitrex) and other triptans, such as naratriptan, zolmitriptan or rizatriptan, may cause prolonged spasm of blood vessels—DO NOT COMBINE or use within 24 hours of a "triptan" dose.

▷ *Driving, Hazardous Activities:* This drug may cause dizziness, drowsiness or impaired vision. Restrict activities as necessary.

Aviation Note: The use of this drug *is a disqualification* for piloting. Consult a designated Aviation Medical Examiner.

Exposure to Sun: No restrictions.

Exposure to Cold: Use caution. Cold environments may increase the occurrence of reduced circulation (blood flow) to the extremities.

Discontinuation: Do not stop it abruptly if drug has been taken for a long time. Slowly lowering (tapering) the dose over 2 to 3 weeks can prevent rebound vascular headaches.

METOCLOPRAMIDE (met oh KLOH pra mide)

Introduced: 1973   **Class:** Gastrointestinal drug, antinausea (antiemetic)
Prescription: USA: Yes   **Controlled Drug:** USA: No; Canada: No
Available as Generic: Yes

Brand Names: ✤Apo-Metoclop, ✤Clopra, ✤Emex, ✤Gastrobid, ✤Maxeran, Maxolon, Octamide, Reclomide, Reglan

BENEFITS versus RISKS	
Possible Benefits	*Possible Risks*
EFFECTIVE STOMACH STIMULANT FOR CORRECTING DELAYED EMPTYING	Sedation and fatigue
	Parkinson-like reactions
	Tardive dyskinesia
Symptomatic relief in reflux esophagitis	
Relief of nausea and vomiting associated with migraine headache	

▷ **Principal Uses**

As a Single Drug Product: Uses currently included in FDA-approved labeling: Helps (1) stomach retention (gastroparesis) associated with diabetes; (2) acid reflux from the stomach into the esophagus (esophagitis); (3) nausea and vomiting associated with migraine headaches; (4) nausea and vomiting induced by anticancer drugs (chemotherapy); (5) decrease the time needed to place a tube in the intestine; (6) used prior to cesarean section to decrease postdelivery or postsurgical nausea or vomiting; (7) used in some X-ray (radiologic) tests or tube placements (intubations).

Other (unlabeled) generally accepted uses: (1) Used as a preparatory drug in stomach hemorrhage; (2) may help gastrointestinal symptoms in anorexia nervosa; (3) eases drug-induced slowed functioning of the intestine (adynamic ileus); (4) decreases the frequency of accumulations of food in the stomach (bezoars); (5) can be of benefit in migraine attacks.

How This Drug Works: Inhibits relaxation of stomach muscles and enhances parasympathetic nervous system (responsible for stomach muscle contractions) stimulation, which accelerates emptying of stomach contents into the intestine.

Available Dosage Forms and Strengths

Injection — 5 mg/ml, 10 mg/ml
Intranasal — (investigational)
Solution — 10 mg/ml
  Syrup — 5 mg/5 ml
  Tablets — 5 mg, 10 mg

▷ **Usual Adult Dosage Ranges:** *Diabetic gastroparesis:* Ten mg, taken 30 minutes before breakfast, lunch and dinner and at bedtime (four times a day) for 2 to 8 weeks. Daily maximum is 0.5 mg per kg of body mass. **Note: Actual dose and schedule must be determined for each patient individually.**

Conditions Requiring Dosing Adjustments

Liver Function: No changes appear to be needed.

Kidney Function: For patients with moderate kidney failure, 75% of the usual dose can be taken at the usual dosing interval. In severe kidney failure, 50% of the usual dose can be taken at the usual dosing interval. A benefit-to-risk decision must be made.

▷ **Dosing Instructions:** Take tablet or syrup 30 minutes before each meal and at bedtime. The tablet may be crushed. If you forget a dose: Take the missed dose as soon as you remember it, unless it's nearly time for your next dose—if that is the case, skip the missed dose and take the next dose right on schedule. Talk with your doctor if you find yourself missing doses.

Usual Duration of Use: Use on a regular schedule for 5 to 7 days determines benefit in accelerating stomach emptying and relieving symptoms of heartburn, fullness and belching. Long-term use (months to years) requires physician supervision.

Typical Treatment Goals and Measurements (Outcomes and Markers)

Gastroparesis: The general goal is to decrease feeling of stomach fullness by increasing stomach (gastric) emptying. For other uses, nausea and vomiting is decreased.

▷ **This Drug Should Not Be Taken If**
- you have had an allergic reaction to it previously.
- you have a seizure disorder of any kind.
- you have active gastrointestinal bleeding.
- you are taking, or have taken within the last 14 days, a MAO inhibitor (see Drug Classes).
- you are taking tricyclic antidepressants.
- you have a pheochromocytoma (adrenaline-producing tumor).

▷ **Inform Your Physician Before Taking This Drug If**
- you are allergic or overly sensitive to procaine or procainamide.
- you have impaired liver or kidney function.
- you have Parkinson's disease.
- you have epilepsy.
- you have high blood pressure.
- you have a history of depression.
- you are taking atropinelike drugs, antipsychotics or opioid analgesics (see Drug Classes).

Possible Side Effects (natural, expected and unavoidable drug actions)

Drowsiness and lethargy, breast tenderness and swelling, milk production.

▷ **Possible Adverse Effects** (unusual, unexpected and infrequent reactions)

If any of the following develop, consult your physician promptly for guidance.

Mild Adverse Effects

Allergic reaction: skin rash. Mild decreases in blood pressure.

Headache, dizziness, restlessness, depression, insomnia—infrequent.

Dry mouth, nausea, diarrhea, constipation—infrequent to frequent.

Urinary retention or incontinence—possible.

Serious Adverse Effects
Idiosyncratic reactions: neuroleptic malignant syndrome (see Glossary), bronchospastic reactions in asthmatics.

Parkinson-like reactions (see Glossary) or tardive dyskinesia (see Glossary)—case reports.

Abnormal fixed positioning of the eyes (oculogyric crisis)—case reports.

Depression—case reports.

Severe decrease in white blood cells (agranulocytosis)—case report.

Abnormal heartbeat—possible, case reports with intravenous use.

Severe increases in blood pressure (hypertensive crisis)—case reports.

Drug-induced porphyria—case reports.

Methemoglobinemia—case report in an overdose case.

▷ **Possible Effects on Sexual Function:** Decreased libido, impaired erection, decreased sperm count, sustained painful erection (priapism).

Altered timing and pattern of menstruation, galactorrhea—case reports to infrequent.

Possible Effects on Laboratory Tests
Blood lithium level: increased.

Blood thyroid-stimulating hormone (TSH) level: increased.

Precautions for Use
By Infants and Children: Watch for development of Parkinson-like reactions soon after starting therapy. Use of the smallest effective dose can minimize such reactions. For diabetic gastroparesis, 0.5 mg per kg of body mass per day, divided into three equal doses given every 8 hours has been used. Children less than 6 years old should NOT receive single doses more than 0.1 mg per kg of body mass.

By Those Over 60 Years of Age: Parkinson-like reactions and tardive dyskinesias are more likely to occur with the use of high doses over an extended period of time. The smallest effective dose should be identified and used only when clearly needed.

▷ **Advisability of Use During Pregnancy**
Pregnancy Category: B. See Pregnancy Risk Categories at the back of this book.
Animal studies: No birth defects found due to this drug.
Human studies: Adequate studies of pregnant women are not available.
Use this drug only if clearly needed.

Advisability of Use If Breast-Feeding
Presence of this drug in breast milk: Yes.
But blood levels appear to avoid therapeutic 500 mcg/kg/day in children. Talk to your doctor about BENEFITS versus RISKS and watch your infant closely.

Habit-Forming Potential: None.

Effects of Overdose: Marked drowsiness, confusion, muscle spasms, jerking movements of head and face, tremors, shuffling gait. Methemoglobinemia.

Possible Effects of Long-Term Use: Parkinson-like reactions may appear within several months of use. Tardive dyskinesias usually occur after a year of continual use; they may persist after this drug is discontinued.

Suggested Periodic Examinations While Taking This Drug (at physician's discretion)

> During long-term use, observe for the development of fine, wormlike movements on the surface of the tongue; these may be the first indications of an emerging tardive dyskinesia.

▷ **While Taking This Drug, Observe the Following**

Foods: No restrictions.

Herbal Medicines or Minerals: Valerian and kava kava may intensify drowsiness. Aloe, cascara and senna may increase possibility of diarrhea. Using chromium may change the way your body is able to use sugar. Some health food stores advocate vanadium as mimicking the actions of insulin, but possible toxicity and need for rigorous studies presently preclude recommending it. DHEA may change sensitivity to insulin or insulin resistance. Hawthorn, ginger, garlic, ginseng and licorice, nettle and yohimbe may change blood sugar. Since this may require adjustment of hypoglycemic medicine dosing, talk to your doctor BEFORE combining any of these herbal medicines with metoclopramide. Echinacea pupurea (injectable) and blonde psyllium seed or husk should NOT be taken by people living with diabetes.

Beverages: No restrictions. May be taken with milk.

▷ *Alcohol:* Combined effects can result in excessive sedation and marked intoxication. Alcohol is best avoided.

Tobacco Smoking: No interactions expected. I advise everyone to quit smoking.

▷ *Other Drugs*

Metoclopramide may ***decrease*** the effects of
- cimetidine (Tagamet).
- digoxin (slow-dissolving dose forms) and reduce its effectiveness.

Metoclopramide ***taken concurrently*** with
- acetaminophen may increase the absorption of this drug; decreased doses are prudent if chronic acetaminophen use will continue with metoclopramide therapy.
- major antipsychotic drugs (phenothiazines, thiothixenes, haloperidol, etc.) may increase the risk of developing Parkinson-like reactions.
- cyclosporine (Sandimmune) may result in increased cyclosporine levels and toxicity.
- morphine (slow release) may result in faster onset and increased sedation.
- neuromuscular blocking agents (such as pancuronium-Pavulon, vecuronium-Norcuron, others) can result in extended recovery times from blockade. Caution is prudent.
- penicillin may result in decreased therapeutic benefits of the antibiotic; increased doses may be needed.
- quinidine (Quinaglute, others) may result in decreased therapeutic benefits from quinidine; increased blood level testing and adjustment of dosing to levels is indicated.
- serolimus (Rapamune) or tacrolimus (Prograf) may result in toxicity. Checks of serolimus or tacrolimus levels are prudent.
- sertraline (Zoloft) may increase risk of movement disorders.
- zalcitabine (Hivid) may blunt zalcitabine levels and benefits.

The following drugs may *decrease* the effects of metoclopramide:
- atropinelike drugs.
- opioid analgesics (see Drug Classes).
- ritonavir (Norvir).

▷ *Driving, Hazardous Activities:* This drug may cause drowsiness and dizziness. Restrict activities as necessary.

Aviation Note: The use of this drug *may be a disqualification* for piloting. Consult a designated Aviation Medical Examiner.

Exposure to Sun: No restrictions.

METOLAZONE (me TOHL a zohn)

Please see the thiazide diuretics family profile.

METOPROLOL (me TOH proh lohl)

Introduced: 1974   **Class:** Antihypertensive, beta-adrenergic blocker
Prescription: USA: Yes   **Controlled Drug:** USA: No; Canada: No
Available as Generic: Yes

Brand Names: ✤Apo-Metoprolol, ✤Betaloc, ✤Co-Betaloc [CD], Lopressor, Lopressor Delayed-Release, Lopressor HCT [CD], Lopressor OROS, ✤Novo-Metoprol, ✤Nu-Metop, Toprol, Toprol XL

```
┌─────────────────────────────────────────────────────────────┐
│                   BENEFITS versus RISKS                      │
│      Possible Benefits              Possible Risks           │
│ EFFECTIVE, WELL-TOLERATED     Worsening of angina in coronary heart │
│   ANTIHYPERTENSIVE in mild to    disease (abrupt withdrawal) │
│   moderate high blood pressure Masking of low blood sugar    │
│ MAY HELP REDUCE DEATH FROM       (hypoglycemia) in drug-treated │
│   HEART ATTACKS                  diabetes                    │
│ APPROVED (Toprol XL form) TO   Provocation of asthma (with high │
│   TREAT CONGESTIVE HEART         doses in asthmatics)        │
│   FAILURE                                                    │
└─────────────────────────────────────────────────────────────┘
```

▷ **Principal Uses**

As a Single Drug Product: Uses currently included in FDA-approved labeling: (1) Treats mild to moderate high blood pressure, alone or with other drugs; (2) helps reduce the frequency and severity of angina; (3) used to reduce the risk of a second heart attack; (4) approved (Toprol XL form) to treat congestive heart failure (carvedilol or Coreg is the only other beta blocker approved for this use).

Other (unlabeled) generally accepted uses: (1) Reduces symptoms of heart muscle damage (dilated cardiomyopathy); (2) second-line drug in panic attacks; (3) used to decrease pressure in the eye (intraocular pressure) in open-angle glaucoma; (4) helps prevent migraine headaches.

As a Combination Drug Product [CD]: Metoprolol is available combined with hydrochlorothiazide (Lopressor HCT) which gives the benefits of both a beta blocker and a thiazide diuretic.

How This Drug Works: Blocks some actions of the sympathetic nervous system:
- reducing rate, contraction force and ejection pressure of the heart.
- reducing contraction of blood vessels, resulting in lowering of blood pressure.
- prolonging conduction time of nerve impulses through the heart, managing certain heart rhythm disorders.

Available Dosage Forms and Strengths

Injection — 1 mg/ml

Tablets — 50 mg, 100 mg

Tablets, prolonged action — 25 mg, 50 mg, 100 mg, 200 mg

▷ **Usual Adult Dosage Ranges:** *Hypertension:* Starts with 50 mg once or twice daily (12 hours apart). Dose may be increased gradually at intervals of 7 to 10 days as needed and tolerated, up to 300 mg/day. For ongoing use (maintenance), 100 mg twice a day. The total daily dose should not exceed 450 mg. The sustained-release form is only given once daily.

Migraine prevention: 50 to 200 mg a day.

Heart failure (once symptoms are stable for 2–4 weeks): Clinicians may start patients on a low dose such as 12.5 mg once a day. The dose then can be doubled every two weeks as needed and tolerated up to 200 mg a day.

Note: Actual dose and schedule must be determined for each patient individually.

Conditions Requiring Dosing Adjustments

Liver Function: Used with caution by patients with liver compromise.

Kidney Function: No changes thought to be needed.

▷ **Dosing Instructions:** The regular tablet may be crushed and taken without regard to eating. In general, prolonged-action forms should be swallowed whole (not altered). Toprol XL brand now comes in an updated 25 mg form that is scored so that heart failure patients can take a 12.5 mg dose (talk to your doctor about this). Do not stop this drug abruptly. If you forget a dose: Take the missed dose as soon as you remember it, unless it's within 4 hours (regular release) or 8 hours (extended-release form) of your next dose—if that is the case, skip the missed dose and take the next dose right on schedule. Talk with your doctor if you find yourself missing doses.

Usual Duration of Use: Regular use for 10 to 14 days determines benefits in lowering blood pressure. The long-term use in controlling blood pressure will be determined by your response to a treatment program (weight reduction, restricted salt, smoking cessation, etc.). Secondary cardiovascular disease prevention use (after a heart attack) and use in heart failure will be ongoing. See your doctor regularly.

Typical Treatment Goals and Measurements (Outcomes and Markers)

Blood pressure: The most recent treatment guidelines (JNC VI) actually define optimal blood pressure (BP) as less than 120/80 and high normal as 139/89. The American Diabetes Association has chosen a target of 130/80 as the blood pressure goal for people living with diabetes. Most clinicians try to achieve a BP that achieves the best balance of lower cardiovascular risk while avoiding the problem of too low a blood pressure. The goal and time frame (see peak benefits above) should be discussed with you when the prescription is written.

Migraine prevention: Specific results in migraine therapy and this medicine relate to decreasing the frequency and/or severity of headaches or avoiding them altogether.

Possible Advantages of This Drug: Generic form offers beta blocker advantages at a lower cost than some other medicines in the same class. A small study in the journal *Circulation* found no difference between the generic version of metoprolol and the more expensive carvedilol. The Oros brand of metoprolol works to reduce exercise-induced angina and daily lowering of heart blood flow (ischemia). The Toprol XL form is FDA approved for use in heart failure.

Currently a "Drug of Choice"

For starting hypertension therapy with one drug, especially for those with bronchial asthma or diabetes and to lower cardiovascular morbidity and mortality.

▷ **This Drug Should Not Be Taken If**
- you have had an allergic reaction to it previously.
- you have had a heart attack and your heart rate is less than 45 beats/min.
- you have an abnormally slow heart rate or a serious form of heart block (second or third degree).
- you took any monoamine oxidase (MAO) type A drug (see Drug Classes) in the last 14 days.

▷ **Inform Your Physician Before Taking This Drug If**
- you had an adverse reaction to any beta blocker (see Drug Classes).
- you have a history of serious heart disease.
- you have a history of hay fever (allergic rhinitis), asthma, chronic bronchitis or emphysema. (People with bronchial asthma should generally not take beta blockers. This drug is somewhat heart selective and may be used with caution by asthmatics.)
- you have a history of overactive thyroid function (hyperthyroidism).
- you have a history of low blood sugar (hypoglycemia).
- you have impaired liver or kidney function.
- you have diabetes or myasthenia gravis.
- you currently take digitalis, quinidine or reserpine or any calcium-channel-blocker drug (see Drug Classes).
- you have a history of poor circulation to the extremities (peripheral vascular disease).
- you have a history of periodic cramps of your legs (intermittent claudication).
- you will have surgery with general anesthesia.

Possible Side Effects (natural, expected and unavoidable drug actions)

Lethargy and fatigability, cold extremities, slow heart rate, light-headedness in upright position (see orthostatic hypotension in Glossary). Abnormally slow heartbeat (bradycardia). Mild increase in potassium.

▷ **Possible Adverse Effects** (unusual, unexpected and infrequent reactions)

If any of the following develop, consult your physician promptly for guidance.

Mild Adverse Effects

Allergic reactions: skin rash, itching.

Worsening of psoriasis—case reports.

Headache, fatigue, dizziness, insomnia, abnormal dreams—infrequent.
Indigestion, nausea, vomiting, constipation, diarrhea—infrequent.
Eye and joint pain—case reports.
Joint and muscle discomfort, fluid retention (edema)—possible.

Serious Adverse Effects

Mental depression, hallucinations, anxiety—infrequent.
Chest pain, shortness of breath, precipitation of congestive heart failure—case reports.
Induction of bronchial asthma (in asthmatic patients)—possible.
Rebound hypertension—if the drug is abruptly stopped.
Precipitation of myasthenia gravis—case reports.
Carpal tunnel syndrome—case reports.
Low or high blood sugar (hypoglycemia or hyperglycemia)—possible.
Liver compromise (hepatitis)—case reports.

▷ **Possible Effects on Sexual Function:** Decreased libido (four times more common in men); impaired erection (less common with this drug than with most other beta blockers); Peyronie's disease (see Glossary)—case reports.

Possible Effects on Laboratory Tests

Blood HDL cholesterol level: decreased.
Blood LDL and VLDL cholesterol level: decreased.
Blood glucose level: increased.
Blood triglyceride levels: increased.

CAUTION

1. ***Do not stop this drug suddenly*** without the knowledge and help of your physician. Carry a note with you that says you take this drug.
2. Ask your doctor or pharmacist before using any nasal decongestants. These are often found in nonprescription cold medicines and nose drops. They may increase blood pressure.
3. Report development of emotional depression.
4. When patients are changed from an immediate-release to a sustained-release form, the same total dose is used and is then increased as needed and tolerated.
5. As the dose of this medicine is increased, the heart (beta one) selectivity is lost.

Precautions for Use

By Infants and Children: Safety and effectiveness for use by those under 12 years of age have not been established, but if this drug is used, observe for the development of low blood sugar (hypoglycemia) during periods of reduced food intake.

By Those Over 60 Years of Age: Proceed cautiously with all antihypertensive drugs. Unacceptably high blood pressure should be reduced slowly, to avoid the risks associated with excessively low blood pressure. Therapy should be started with small doses and the blood pressure checked often. Sudden, rapid and excessive reduction of blood pressure can predispose to stroke or heart attack. Watch for dizziness, unsteadiness, tendency to fall, confusion, hallucinations, depression or urinary frequency.

▷ **Advisability of Use During Pregnancy**

Pregnancy Category: C. See Pregnancy Risk Categories at the back of this book.
Animal studies: No significant increase in birth defects due to this drug.

Human studies: Adequate studies of pregnant women are not available. Use this drug only if clearly needed. Ask your physician for guidance.

Advisability of Use If Breast-Feeding
Presence of this drug in breast milk: Yes.
Discuss BENEFITS versus RISKS with your doctor.

Habit-Forming Potential: None.

Effects of Overdose: Weakness, slow pulse, low blood pressure, cold and sweaty skin, congestive heart failure, possible coma and convulsions.

Possible Effects of Long-Term Use: Reduced heart reserve and eventual heart failure in susceptible individuals with advanced heart disease.

Suggested Periodic Examinations While Taking This Drug (at physician's discretion)
Measurements of blood pressure.
Evaluation of heart function.

▷ **While Taking This Drug, Observe the Following**
Foods: Peak drug concentration and peak effect will increase if taken with food. Avoid excessive salt intake. Migraines often have specific food triggers. Keep a headache diary, and then avoid the triggering foods.

Herbal Medicines or Minerals: Valerian and kava kava may intensify drowsiness. Ginseng may increase blood pressure, blunting the benefits of these medicines. Hawthorn, saw palmetto, ma huang, goldenseal, yohimbe and licorice may also increase blood pressure. Calcium and garlic may help lower blood pressure. Indian snakeroot has a German Commission E monograph indication for hypertension—talk to your doctor. Eleuthero root and ephedra should be avoided by people living with hypertension.

Beverages: No restrictions. May be taken with milk.

▷ *Alcohol.* Use with caution. Alcohol may exaggerate this drug's ability to lower the blood pressure and may increase its mild sedative effect.

Tobacco Smoking: Nicotine may reduce this drug's benefit in treating high blood pressure. I advise everyone to quit smoking.

▷ *Other Drugs*
Metoprolol may ***increase*** the effects of
• other antihypertensive drugs, causing excessive lowering of blood pressure; dose adjustments may be necessary.
• reserpine (Ser-Ap-Es, etc.) and cause sedation, depression, slowing of the heart rate and lowering of the blood pressure.
• verapamil (Calan, Isoptin) and cause excessive depression of heart function; monitor this combination closely.

Metoprolol ***taken concurrently*** with
• amiodarone (Cordarone) may result in extremely slow heartbeat and cardiac arrest—NOT ADVISED.
• clonidine (Catapres) requires close monitoring for rebound high blood pressure if clonidine is withdrawn while metoprolol is still being taken.
• digoxin (Lanoxin, others) may increase heart slowing.
• fluoxetine (Prozac) may cause metoprolol toxicity.
• fluvoxamine (Luvox) may lead to metoprolol toxicity.
• insulin requires close monitoring to avoid undetected hypoglycemia (see Glossary).
• lidocaine can lead to lidocaine toxicity (cardiac arrest).

- methyldopa (Aldomet, others) can have a rare paradoxical hypertensive response—caution is advised.
- nifedipine (Adalat, Procardia, others) may result in heart failure.
- oral antidiabetic drugs (see Drug Classes) can result in prolonged hypoglycemia if it occurs.
- phenothiazines (see Drug Classes) can result in low blood pressure or toxicity due to the phenothiazine.
- quinidine (Quinaglute, others) can lead to abnormally slow heartbeat and shortness of breath.
- ritonavir (Norvir) and perhaps other protease inhibitors (see Drug Classes) may cause toxicity.
- tocainide (Tonocard) may lead to depressed contraction ability of the heart (myocardial contractility).
- venlafaxine (Effexor) may lead to metabolic changes and toxic blood levels of both medicines.

The following drugs may *increase* the effects of metoprolol:

- alpha one adrenergic blockers, such as prazosin (Minipres).
- bupropion (Zyban). Metoprolol doses at the lower end of the dosing range are prudent if these drugs must be used together.
- cimetidine (Tagamet).
- ciprofloxacin (Cipro).
- diltiazem (Cardizem) and other dihydroperidine calcium blockers—especially in people with decreased function of the left ventricle.
- MAO inhibitors (see Drug Classes).
- methimazole (Tapazole).
- oral contraceptives (birth control pills); a different (non-first pass) beta blocker is advisable.
- propafenone (Rythmol).
- propoxyphene (Darvocet, others).
- propylthiouracil (Propacil).
- zafirlukast (Accolate) or zileuton (Zyflo); dose decreases of metoprolol may be needed.

The following drugs may *decrease* the effects of metoprolol:

- barbiturates (phenobarbital, etc.).
- indomethacin (Indocin) and possibly other aspirin substitutes or NSAIDs—may impair metoprolol's antihypertensive effect.
- rifampin (Rifadin, Rimactane).

▷ *Driving, Hazardous Activities:* Use caution until the full extent of drowsiness, lethargy and blood pressure change has been determined.

Aviation Note: The use of this drug *is a disqualification* for piloting. Consult a designated Aviation Medical Examiner.

Exposure to Sun: No restrictions.

Exposure to Heat: Caution is advised. Hot environments can lower the blood pressure and exaggerate the effects of this drug.

Exposure to Cold: Caution: Cold environments can increase circulatory deficiency in extremities. The elderly should take care to prevent hypothermia (see Glossary).

Heavy Exercise or Exertion: Best to avoid exertion that produces light-headedness, excessive fatigue or muscle cramping. This drug may intensify the blood pressure response to isometric exercise.

Occurrence of Unrelated Illness: Fever can lower the blood pressure and require adjustment of dose. Nausea or vomiting may interrupt the regular dose schedule. Ask your doctor for help.

Discontinuation: **Do not stop this drug suddenly.** Gradual dose lowering over 1 to 2 weeks is recommended. Ask your doctor for help.

METRONIDAZOLE (me troh NI da zohl)

Introduced: 1960   **Class:** Anti-infective   **Prescription:** USA: Yes   **Controlled Drug:**   USA: No; Canada: No   **Available as Generic:**   Yes

Brand Names: ♣Apo-Metronidazole, Femazole, Flagyl, Flagyl ER (extended-release form), Flagystatin [CD], Helidac [CD], Lagyl, Losec Helicopak [CD], Metizol, MetroGel, Metro IV, Metryl, ♣Neo-Tric, ♣Novo-Nidazole, Protostat, ♣Rho-Metrostatin, SK Metronidazole, ♣Trikacide

BENEFITS versus RISKS	
Possible Benefits	*Possible Risks*
EFFECTIVE TREATMENT FOR TRICHOMONAS INFECTIONS, AMEBIC DYSENTERY AND GIARDIASIS AND SOME ANAEROBIC BACTERIAL INFECTIONS	Superinfection with yeast organisms Peripheral neuropathy Abnormally low white blood cell count (transient) Colitis
TREATMENT OF BACTERIAL VAGINOSIS (ER FORM)	Aggravation of epilepsy
Effective local treatment for rosacea	

▷ **Principal Uses**

As a Single Drug Product: Uses currently included in FDA-approved labeling: (1) Treats *Trichomonas* infections of the vaginal canal and cervix and of the male urethra; (2) also used to treat amebic dysentery and liver abscess, *Giardia* infections of the intestine and serious infections caused by certain strains of anaerobic bacteria; (3) treats *Gardnerella* infections of the vagina; (4) treatment of acne rosacea with local application of a gel dose form; (5) used in therapy of pseudomembranous colitis; (6) has a role in treating bed sores (decubitus ulcers); (7) can help prevent infection (prophylaxis) in gynecological, appendectomy or colorectal surgery; (8) ER form used in bacterial vaginosis.

Other (unlabeled) generally accepted uses: (1) Combination therapy with gentamicin in treating intra-abdominal infections; (2) combination antibiotic treatment of duodenal ulcers caused by *Helicobacter pylori;* (3) can help treat infections caused by *Giardia lamblia;* (4) used to help heal the lesions in Crohn's disease; (5) may help abnormal gum growth (gingival hyperplasia) caused by cyclosporine.

As a Combination Drug Product [CD]: Metronidazole is available combined with 20 mg of omeprazole, 500 mg of amoxicillin and 400 mg of metronidazole for combination treatment of *Helicobacter pylori.*

How This Drug Works: Interacts with DNA, destroying essential component (nucleus) that is needed for life and growth of infecting organisms.

Available Dosage Forms and Strengths
Capsules — 375 mg
Gel — 0.75%
Injection — 500 mg/100 ml
Tablets — 250 mg, 500 mg
Tablets, extended release — 750 mg
Vaginal cream — 10%

▷ **Usual Adult Dosage Ranges:** *For bacterial vaginosis* (ER form): 750 mg once a day for seven days in a row.

For trichomoniasis: 1-day course—2 g as a single dose or 1 g for two doses 12 hours apart. 7-day course—250 mg three times a day for 7 consecutive days. (The 7-day course is preferred.)

For amebiasis: 500 to 750 mg three times a day for 5 to 10 consecutive days.

For giardiasis: 2 g once daily for 3 days, or 250 to 500 mg three times a day for 5 to 7 days.

The total daily dose should not exceed 4 g (4,000 mg).

Note: Actual dose and schedule must be determined for each patient individually.

Conditions Requiring Dosing Adjustments
Liver Function: Dose is decreased by one-third in mild to moderate liver disease. Should not be used in severe liver compromise.

Kidney Function: In severe kidney failure, 50% of the normal dose can be taken at the usual dosing interval. A benefit-to-risk decision must be made for these patients, as there is a risk of systemic lupus erythematosus (SLE) from the metabolites of this drug.

▷ **Dosing Instructions:** The tablet may be crushed and taken with or following food to reduce stomach irritation. If you forget a dose: Take the missed dose as soon as you remember it, unless it's nearly time for your next dose—if that is the case, skip the missed dose and take the next dose right on schedule. Talk with your doctor if you find yourself missing doses.

Usual Duration of Use: Use on a regular schedule as outlined is needed to ensure effectiveness. Do not repeat the course of treatment without your physician's approval.

Typical Treatment Goals and Measurements (Outcomes and Markers)
Infections: The most commonly used measures of serious infections are white blood cell counts and differentials (the kind of blood cells that occur most often in your blood), and temperature. Many clinicians look for positive changes in 24–48 hours. NEVER stop an antibiotic because you start to feel better. For many infections, a full 14 days is REQUIRED to kill the bacteria. The goals and time frame (see peak benefits above) should be discussed with you when the prescription is written.

▷ **This Drug Should Not Be Taken If**
- you have had an allergic reaction to it or any of the parabens contained in the gel form.
- you are pregnant.
- you currently have a bone marrow or blood cell disorder.
- you have any type of central nervous system disorder, including epilepsy.

▷ **Inform Your Physician Before Taking This Drug If**
- you have a history of any type of blood cell disorder, especially one caused by drugs.
- you have a history of seizures or peripheral neuropathy.
- you have impaired liver or kidney function.
- you have a history of alcoholism.
- you are pregnant or breast-feeding.

Possible Side Effects (natural, expected and unavoidable drug actions)
A sharp, metallic, unpleasant taste. Dark discoloration of the urine (of no clinical significance). Superinfection (see Glossary) by yeast organisms in the mouth or vagina. Pseudomembranous colitis.

▷ **Possible Adverse Effects** (unusual, unexpected and infrequent reactions)
If any of the following develop, consult your physician promptly for guidance.
Mild Adverse Effects
Allergic reactions: skin rash, hives, flushing, itching.
Headache, dizziness, incoordination, unsteadiness, incontinence—infrequent.
Loss of appetite, nausea, vomiting, abdominal cramps, diarrhea—infrequent.
Irritation of mouth and tongue, possibly due to yeast infection—possible.
Serious Adverse Effects
Idiosyncratic reactions: abnormal behavior; confusion; depression; Jarisch-Herxheimer's reaction (sweating, diarrhea, vomiting, scalding urination, joint pain and itching)—case reports.
Peripheral neuropathy (see Glossary)—case reports.
Abnormally low white blood cell count (transient): fever, sore throat, infections—case reports.
Disulfiram-type reaction (nausea, vomiting) if alcoholic beverages are consumed—possible.
Seizures—case reports.
Drug-induced pneumonitis, porphyria or pancreatitis—case reports.
Hemolytic-uremic syndrome—case reports.

▷ **Possible Effects on Sexual Function:** Decreased libido; decreased vaginal secretions (difficult or painful intercourse)—case reports.
Abnormal swelling of male breast tissue (gynecomastia)—case report.

Possible Delayed Adverse Effects: Studies have shown that this drug can cause cancer in mice and possibly in rats. Two researchers concluded that the carcinogenic risk is low in doses used to treat episodic vaginitis. High-dose, long-term use may carry increased cancer risk. Follow your doctor's instructions exactly. Avoid unnecessary or prolonged use.

▷ **Adverse Effects That May Mimic Natural Diseases or Disorders**
Behavioral changes may suggest spontaneous psychosis.

Natural Diseases or Disorders That May Be Activated by This Drug
Latent yeast infections.

Possible Effects on Laboratory Tests
White blood cell counts: decreased.
INR (prothrombin time): increased.
Blood theophylline levels: falsely increased by some methods.

CAUTION
1. Troublesome and persistent diarrhea can develop. If diarrhea persists for more than 24 hours, stop this drug and call your physician.
2. Stop this drug immediately if you develop any signs of toxic effects on the brain or nervous system: confusion, irritability, dizziness, incoordination, unsteady stance or gait, muscle jerking or twitching, numbness or weakness in the extremities.

Precautions for Use
By Infants and Children: Avoid use in those with a history of bone marrow or blood cell disorders.
By Those Over 60 Years of Age: Natural changes in the skin may predispose to yeast infections in the genital and anal regions. Report the development of rashes and itching promptly.

▷ **Advisability of Use During Pregnancy**
Pregnancy Category: B. See Pregnancy Risk Categories at the back of this book.
Animal studies: No birth defects reported in rat studies, but this drug is known to cause cancer in mice and possibly in rats.
Human studies: No increase in birth defects reported in 206 exposures to this drug during the first 3 months. However, information from adequate studies of pregnant women is not available.
The manufacturer advises against the use of this drug during the first 3 months. Use during the final 6 months is not advised unless it is absolutely essential to the mother's health.

Advisability of Use If Breast-Feeding
Presence of this drug in breast milk: Yes.
Avoid drug or refrain from nursing.

Habit-Forming Potential: None.

Effects of Overdose: Weakness, stomach irritation, nausea, vomiting, confusion, disorientation.

Possible Effects of Long-Term Use: None reported. Avoid long-term use.

Suggested Periodic Examinations While Taking This Drug (at physician's discretion)
Complete blood cell counts.

▷ **While Taking This Drug, Observe the Following**
Foods: No restrictions.
Herbal Medicines or Minerals: Some patients use echinacea to attempt to boost their immune systems. Unfortunately, use of echinacea is not recommended in people with damaged immune systems (even if a medicine caused the damage). This herb may also actually weaken any immune system if it is used too often or for too long a time. DO NOT take mistletoe herb, oak bark or F.C. of marshmallow root and licorice.
Beverages: No restrictions. May be taken with milk.
▷ *Alcohol:* A disulfiramlike reaction has been reported (see Glossary). It is NOT advisable to drink alcohol while taking metronidazole.
Tobacco Smoking: No interactions expected. I advise everyone to quit smoking.
▷ *Other Drugs*
Metronidazole may ***increase*** the effects of
• carbamazepine (Tegretol) and lead to toxicity.
• warfarin (Coumadin, etc.) and cause abnormal bleeding; the INR (pro-

thrombin time or protime) should be monitored closely, especially during the first 10 days of concurrent use.

Metronidazole *taken concurrently* with

- antacids may decrease absorption of metronidazole.
- birth control pills (oral contraceptives) may block the effectiveness of contraception and result in pregnancy.
- cholestyramine (Questran) or other cholesterol-lowering resins may decrease metronidazole absorption and lower its therapeutic effect.
- cotrimoxazole or other sulfa drugs may result in a disulfiramlike effect.
- cyclosporine (Sandimmune) can lead to cyclosporine toxicity.
- disulfiram (Antabuse) may cause severe emotional and behavioral disturbances.
- lithium (Lithobid, others) can cause lithium toxicity.
- phenytoin (Dilantin) or fosphenytoin (Cerebyx) may result in increased blood levels of phenytoin; more frequent blood level testing is needed, and the phenytoin dose should be adjusted to blood levels.
- ritonavir (Norvir) may increase blood levels of metronidazole.
- sirolimus (Rapamune) may increase risk of sirolimus toxicity.
- sulfamethoxazole (Septra, others) and perhaps other sulfa drugs may lead to a disulfiramlike reaction.
- tacrolimus (Prograf) may increase risk of tacrolimus toxicity.
- trimethoprim (Septra, others) and perhaps other sulfa drugs may lead to a disulfiramlike reaction.

▷ *Driving, Hazardous Activities:* This drug may cause dizziness or incoordination. Restrict activities as necessary.

Aviation Note: The use of this drug *may be a disqualification* for piloting. Consult a designated Aviation Medical Examiner.

Exposure to Sun: No restrictions.

MEXILETINE (mex IL e teen)

Introduced: 1973 **Class:** Antiarrhythmic (Class or Group One) **Prescription:** USA: Yes **Controlled Drug:** USA: No; Canada: No Available as Generic: Yes

Brand Name: Mexitil

BENEFITS versus RISKS	
Possible Benefits	*Possible Risks*
EFFECTIVE TREATMENT IN SELECTED HEART RHYTHM DISORDERS	NARROW TREATMENT RANGE FREQUENT ADVERSE EFFECTS WORSENING OF SOME ARRHYTHMIAS Rare seizures, liver injury and reduced white blood cell count

▷ **Principal Uses**

As a Single Drug Product: Uses currently included in FDA-approved labeling: Helps correct premature beats that arise in the ventricles (lower heart chambers).

Other (unlabeled) generally accepted uses: (1) Eases pain in some pain syndromes (diabetic neuropathy); (2) combination therapy of Wolff-Parkinson-White syndrome.

How This Drug Works: Slows transmission of electrical impulses in the heart, restoring normal heart rate and rhythm in selected types of arrhythmia.

Available Dosage Forms and Strengths

Capsules — 150 mg, 200 mg, 250 mg

Gelcap — 100 mg

Gelcap (Canada) — 200 mg

▷ **Usual Adult Dosage Ranges:** When rapid control of ventricular arrhythmias is required, the manufacturer recommends a loading dose of 400 mg, then 200 mg every 8 hours. Dose can be increased (every 2 to 3 days), as needed and tolerated in 50- or 100-mg steps. Daily maximum is 1,200 mg (doses greater than this can have undesirable central nervous system side effects). Some clinicians try to improve how well patients take this medicine by using an every-12-hours dosing strategy. The strategy is to arrive at an every-8-hours approach (for example, 300 mg every 8 hours). If that dose or less works to control abnormal heartbeats, the same dose is given every 12 hours with careful follow up for rhythm control. Dosing can then be adjusted as needed and tolerated up to 450 mg every 12 hours to get the required suppression of abnormal heartbeats. Testing blood levels is advised (when available). **Note: Actual dose and schedule must be determined for each patient individually.**

Conditions Requiring Dosing Adjustments

Liver Function: Dose should be decreased by one-fourth to one-third in liver disease.

Kidney Function: Dose is decreased and blood levels obtained more often.

▷ **Dosing Instructions:** The capsule may be opened and taken with food or antacid to reduce stomach irritation. Take at same times each day to obtain uniform results (even blood levels). If you forget a dose: and you take this medicine twice a day, take the missed dose as soon as you remember it, unless you are more than 6 hours late—if that is the case, skip the missed dose and take the next dose right on schedule. If you take the mexiletine three times a day, take the missed dose once you remember it, unless you are more than 4 hours late—if that is the case, skip the missed dose and return to your usual schedule. Talk with your doctor if you find yourself missing doses.

Usual Duration of Use: Use on a regular schedule for 1 to 2 weeks determines effectiveness in correcting or preventing responsive rhythm disorders—particularly if a loading dose approach is used. Long-term use requires physician supervision.

Typical Treatment Goals and Measurements (Outcomes and Markers)

Abnormal heartbeats: The general goal is to return the heart to a normal rhythm or at least to markedly reduce the occurrence of abnormal heartbeats. For example, when a loading dose is used to help control ventricular arrhythmias, the effect is usually seen in 30 to 150 minutes. In life-threatening arrhythmias, the goal is to abort the abnormal beats and return the heart rhythm pattern to normal.

▷ **This Drug Should Not Be Taken If**
   • you have had an allergic reaction to it previously.
   • you have shock resulting from the heart (cardiogenic shock).
   • you have second- or third-degree heart block (determined by electrocardiogram), uncorrected by a pacemaker.

▷ **Inform Your Physician Before Taking This Drug If**
   • you had adverse reactions to other antiarrhythmic drugs.
   • you have a history of heart disease of any kind, especially "heart block" or heart failure AND YOU DO NOT HAVE A PACEMAKER.
   • you have impaired liver function.
   • you have Parkinson's disease.
   • you are prone to low blood pressure or have a seizure disorder of any kind.
   • you take digitalis, a potassium supplement or any diuretic drug that can cause potassium loss (ask your doctor).

Possible Side Effects (natural, expected and unavoidable drug actions)
Nervousness, light-headedness. Unpleasant taste.

▷ **Possible Adverse Effects** (unusual, unexpected and infrequent reactions)
If any of the following develop, consult your physician promptly for guidance.

Mild Adverse Effects
Allergic reaction: skin rash.
Headache, dizziness, visual disturbance, fatigue, weakness, tremor—infrequent.
Loss of appetite, indigestion, nausea, vomiting, constipation, diarrhea, abdominal pain—rare.

Serious Adverse Effects
Idiosyncratic reactions: depression, confusion, amnesia, hallucinations, seizures—all rare.
Drug-induced heart rhythm disorders: shortness of breath, palpitations, chest pain, swelling—rare.
Myelofibrosis or systemic lupus erythematosus—case reports.
Seizures—case reports.
Ataxia and confusion—may be frequent.
Congestive heart failure and sinus arrest—rare.
Urinary retention—possible.
Bleeding in the stomach or intestines (gastrointestinal tract)—rare.
Liver damage with jaundice (see Glossary)—case reports.
Low white blood cell or platelet counts: fever, sore throat, abnormal bleeding/bruising—case reports.

▷ **Possible Effects on Sexual Function:** Decreased libido, impotence—rare.

▷ **Adverse Effects That May Mimic Natural Diseases or Disorders**
Liver toxicity may suggest viral hepatitis.

Natural Diseases or Disorders That May Be Activated by This Drug
Latent epilepsy.

Possible Effects on Laboratory Tests
Blood white cell and platelet counts: decreased.
Liver function tests: increased liver enzymes (ALT/GPT, AST/GOT)—increased in less than 1% of users.

CAUTION

1. Thorough evaluation of your heart function (including electrocardiograms) is necessary prior to using this drug.
2. Periodic evaluation of your heart function is needed to determine your response to this drug. Some individuals may experience worsening of their heart rhythm disorder and/or deterioration of heart function. Close monitoring of heart rate, rhythm and overall performance is essential.
3. Dose must be adjusted carefully for each person. Do not change your dose without talking to your doctor.
4. Do not take any other antiarrhythmic drug while taking this drug unless you are directed to do so by your physician.
5. Carry a card in your purse or wallet saying that you take this drug. Tell health care providers that you take it.

Precautions for Use

By Infants and Children: Safety and effectiveness for those under 12 years of age are not established. Initial use of this drug requires hospitalization and supervision by a qualified cardiologist.

By Those Over 60 Years of Age: Reduced liver function may require reduction in dose. Watch carefully for light-headedness, dizziness, unsteadiness and tendency to fall.

▷ **Advisability of Use During Pregnancy**

Pregnancy Category: C. See Pregnancy Risk Categories at the back of this book.

Animal studies: No birth defects reported in mice, rats or rabbits, but an increased rate of fetal resorption was found.

Human studies: Adequate studies of pregnant women are not available. Avoid during first 3 months. Use this drug only if clearly needed. Ask your physician for guidance.

Advisability of Use If Breast-Feeding

Presence of this drug in breast milk: Yes.

Avoid drug or refrain from nursing.

Habit-Forming Potential: None.

Effects of Overdose: Impaired urination, constipation, marked drop in blood pressure, abnormal heart rhythms, congestive heart failure, dizziness, incoordination, seizures.

Possible Effects of Long-Term Use: None reported.

Suggested Periodic Examinations While Taking This Drug (at physician's discretion)

Electrocardiograms.

Complete blood cell counts.

Liver function tests.

Mexiletine blood levels.

▷ **While Taking This Drug, Observe the Following**

Foods: No restrictions. Ask your physician regarding need for salt restriction.

Herbal Medicines or Minerals: Using St. John's wort, ma huang, ephedra or kola while taking this medicine may result in unacceptable heart stimulation. Belladonna, henbane, scopolia, pheasant's eye extract or lily-of-the-valley or squill powdered extracts should NOT be taken if you have abnormal heart rhythms.

Beverages: Caffeine may have an effect on heart rate and may not be desirable. Talk to your doctor about caffeine. Can be taken with milk.

▷ *Alcohol:* Use caution. Alcohol can increase the blood-pressure-lowering effects of this drug.

Tobacco Smoking: Nicotine irritates the heart, reducing drug effectiveness. I advise everyone to quit smoking.

▷ *Other Drugs*

Mexiletine may *increase* the effects of
- antihypertensive drugs and cause excessive lowering of blood pressure.
- beta-blocker drugs (see Drug Classes).
- disopyramide (Norpace).
- lidocaine (various).
- quinidine (Quinaglute, various).
- theophylline (Theo-Dur, others), leading to theophylline toxicity and seizures.

Mexiletine *taken concurrently* with
- amiodarone (Cordarone) may lead to abnormal heartbeat or rhythm (QT changes and torsades de pointes).
- dofetilide (Tikosyn) may lead to prolongation of the QTc interval and undesirable effects. This combination is not recommended.
- drugs that inhibit or are removed by CYP 2D6 (talk to your doctor) may increase mexiletine effects.
- ritonavir (Norvir) and perhaps other protease inhibitors (see Drug Classes) may lead to toxicity.

The following drugs may *decrease* the effects of mexiletine:
- phenytoin (Dilantin, etc.) or fosphenytoin (Cerebyx).
- rifampin (Rifadin, Rimactane).

▷ *Driving, Hazardous Activities:* This drug may cause weakness, dizziness or blurred vision. Restrict activities as necessary.

Aviation Note: The use of this drug *may be a disqualification* for piloting. Consult a designated Aviation Medical Examiner.

Exposure to Sun: No restrictions.

Occurrence of Unrelated Illness: Vomiting, diarrhea or dehydration can affect this drug's action adversely. Report such developments promptly.

Discontinuation: Should not be stopped abruptly after long-term use. Ask your doctor about slowly reducing the dose.

MIBEFRADIL (mi BEF rah dill)

Introduced: 1997 **Class:** Antihypertensive, calcium channel blocker
Author's Note: This medicine has been withdrawn from the market.

MIGLITOL (MIG lit all)

Introduced: 1999 **Class:** Antidiabetic, alpha-glucosidase inhibitor **Prescription:** USA: Yes **Controlled Drug:** USA: No; Canada: No **Available as Generic:** No
Brand Name: Glyset

BENEFITS versus RISKS

Possible Benefits	*Possible Risks*
EFFECTIVE LOWERING OF BLOOD SUGAR	Gas and abdominal pain (often decreases over time)
USE IN TYPE 1 OR TYPE 2 DIABETICS	
DECREASED RISK OF HIGH BLOOD PRESSURE, HEART DISEASE OR OTHER LONG-TERM DAMAGE OF HIGH BLOOD SUGAR (WITH BETTER GLUCOSE CONTROL)	
COMBINED TREATMENT WITH SULFONYLUREA IF NEEDED	

▷ **Principal Uses**

As a Single Drug Product: Uses currently included in FDA-approved labeling: (1) Used with diet in diabetics who don't require insulin, yet don't have good blood sugar control with diet alone; (2) can be combined with a sulfonylurea (see Drug Classes) if diet plus miglitol or diet and sulfonylurea do not control blood sugar as well as needed.

Other (unlabeled) generally accepted uses: Can be used to further lower blood sugar in diabetics who require insulin.

How This Drug Works: By blocking intestinal alpha glucosidase and pancreatic alpha amylase (two enzymes), this medicine impairs sugar digestion and actually keeps sugar low after meals.

Available Dosage Forms and Strengths

Tablets — 25 mg, 50 mg, 100 mg

▷ **Recommended Dosage Ranges** (Actual dose and schedule must be determined individually for each patient.)

Infants and Children: Safety and effectiveness not established in those less than 18 years old.

18 to 65 Years of Age: The most conservative starting dose is 25 mg once a day with the first meal of the day. Subsequently, as needed and tolerated, the dose can be increased to 25 mg three times daily, taken at the start of each meal (after first bite). Dose increases are made at 4-to-8 week intervals to achieve blood sugar control while minimizing intestinal side effects (using 50 mg three times daily at the start of each meal). If response is not acceptable, dose may be increased to 50 mg three times daily. After three months of therapy, a glycosylated hemoglobin should be checked. If this is still abnormal, dose may be increased to 100 mg three times daily. If a dose increase doesn't give better sugar control, consider dose decrease.

Over 65 Years of Age: No specific recommendations unless kidney function is very limited. Smaller doses are prudent.

Conditions Requiring Dosing Adjustments

Liver Function: Specific dosing changes do not appear to be needed.

Kidney Function: Use NOT recommended in kidney disease.

▷ **Dosing Instructions:** Take this pill after starting breakfast, lunch and dinner— after the first bite of a meal has been eaten. Gas (flatulence) and diarrhea are common side effects but often decrease over time. Limiting sucrose can also help. If dose changes are made at 4- to 8-week intervals, the best sugar response and the least potential gas (flatulence) or diarrhea are realized. Often blood sugar is checked one hour after a meal (1 hr postprandial) and the dose adjusted to get the best balance of blood sugar and side effects. If you forget a dose: Take the missed dose as soon as you remember it, if you are still eating your meal. If you've finished eating, the most conservative course is to check your blood sugar and ask the doctor what to do. DO NOT double doses. Return to the next dose right on schedule. Talk with your doctor if you find yourself missing doses.

Usual Duration of Use: Dosing must be individualized. Peak drug response happens in about an hour. Dosing changes are made at 4- to 8-week intervals if needed. Regular use required to give better blood glucose control. Since non-insulin-dependent diabetes is a chronic condition, use of miglitol will be ongoing. Periodic hemoglobin A1C (glycosylated hemoglobin) tests and physician follow-up are needed. Keeping the sugar close to normal can minimize diabetic problems.

Typical Treatment Goals and Measurements (Outcomes and Markers)

Blood sugar: The general goal for blood sugar is to return it to the usual "normal" range (generally 80–120 mg/dl), while avoiding risks of excessively low blood sugar. One study (UKPDS) used a fasting plasma sugar (glucose) of less than 108 mg/dl.

Fructosamine and glycosylated hemoglobin: Fructosamine levels (a measure of the past 2–3 weeks of blood sugar control) should be less than or equal to 310 micromoles per liter. Glycosylated hemoglobin or hemoglobin A1C (a measure of the past 2–3 months of blood sugar control) should be less than or equal to 7.0%.

Possible Advantages of This Drug

May be used in combination with sulfonylurea oral hypoglycemics (see Drug Classes) to get the best control of blood sugar. May be more potent than acarbose (Precose) on a mg-to-mg basis.

▷ **This Drug Should Not Be Taken If**

- you have had an allergic reaction to it previously.
- you are in diabetic ketoacidosis.
- your history includes intestinal obstruction or you have a partial obstruction of the intestine.
- you have inflammatory bowel disease or colon ulceration.
- your serum creatinine is over 2 mg/dl (talk to your doctor).
- you have an intestinal condition that may worsen (such as a megacolon or bowel obstruction) if increased gas (flatus) forms.
- you have a long-standing (chronic) intestinal disease altering digestion or your ability to absorb materials from the intestine.

▷ **Inform Your Physician Before Taking This Drug If**

- you do not know what the symptoms of hypoglycemia are.
- you have an infection (insulin may be required).
- you are pregnant or are breast-feeding your infant (no data exists on use in pregnancy or breast-feeding).
- you have a history of kidney or liver disease.
- you will have surgery with general anesthesia.

- you forgot to tell your doctor about all the drugs you take.
- you are unsure of how much to take or how often to take it.

Possible Side Effects (natural, expected and unavoidable drug actions)

Gas (flatulence) or diarrhea results from bacterial action on sugars and tends to decrease over time.

▷ **Possible Adverse Effects** (unusual, unexpected and infrequent reactions)

If any of the following develop, consult your physician promptly for guidance.

Mild Adverse Effects

Allergic reactions: skin rash, itching.

Sleepiness, headache, dizziness—of questionable causation.

Pain or swelling of the belly (abdomen)—frequent.

Gas (flatulence) or diarrhea—frequent (often eases).

Low serum iron—infrequent.

Serious Adverse Effects

Low blood sugar if combined with sulfonylureas—possible.

Ileus—case reports and in those with prior bowel blockage history.

▷ **Possible Effects on Sexual Function:** None reported.

Possible Effects on Laboratory Tests

Hemoglobin A1C: trending more toward normal (good effect).

Blood sugar one hour after eating (postprandial): decreased.

Liver enzymes: no change in one short-term study.

CAUTION

1. This medicine itself does not cause hypoglycemia. Low sugar may result if combined with insulin or sulfonylureas.
2. Infections may cause loss of sugar control and require temporary insulin use.
3. This medicine is part of the total management of diabetes. A properly prescribed diet and regular exercise are still required for best control of blood sugar.
4. **If** your kidneys fail or worsen, tell your doctor. This drug should not be used if serum creatinine is greater than 2 mg/dl.

Precautions for Use

By Infants and Children: Safety and effectiveness for those under 18 not established.

By Those Over 60 Years of Age: Specific recommendations are not made at this time.

▷ **Advisability of Use During Pregnancy**

Pregnancy Category: B. See Pregnancy Risk Categories at the back of this book.

Human studies: Adequate studies of pregnant women are not available.

Insulin is often the drug of first choice for blood sugar control in pregnancy. Ask your doctor for help.

Advisability of Use If Breast-Feeding

Presence of this drug in breast milk: Yes, in very small amounts.

Avoid drug or refrain from nursing.

Habit-Forming Potential: None.

Effects of Overdose: Temporary gas (flatus), abdominal discomfort and diarrhea.

Possible Effects of Long-Term Use: Beneficial effects on blood sugar.

Suggested Periodic Examinations While Taking This Drug (at physician's discretion)

Periodic blood sugar one hour after eating.

Glycated protein (fructosamine).

Hemoglobin A1C levels.

Liver function tests (transaminases)—do not appear to be required based on one study.

Serum iron or iron-binding capacity prudent if anemia develops.

▷ **While Taking This Drug, Observe the Following**

Foods: Closely follow the diet your doctor has prescribed. Blood sugar control can help avoid or delay diabetes problems!

Herbal Medicines or Minerals: Using chromium may change the way your body is able to use sugar. Some health food stores advocate vanadium as mimicking the actions of insulin, but possible toxicity and need for rigorous studies presently preclude recommending it. DHEA may change sensitivity to insulin or insulin resistance. Hawthorn, ginger, garlic, ginseng and licorice, nettle and yohimbe may change blood sugar. Since this may require adjustment of hypoglycemic medicine dosing, talk to your doctor BEFORE combining any of these herbal medicines with miglitol. Echinacea pupurea (injectable) and blonde psyllium seed or husk should NOT be taken by people living with diabetes.

Beverages: No restrictions. May be taken with milk.

▷ *Alcohol:* No interaction with miglitol. If you also take a sulfonylurea (see Drug Classes), alcohol can exaggerate lowering of blood sugar, blood sugar or cause a disulfiramlike (see Glossary) reaction.

Tobacco Smoking: No interactions expected. I advise everyone to stop smoking.

▷ *Other Drugs*

Miglitol may ***increase*** the effects of

- sulfonylureas (see Drug Classes), causing a lower blood sugar (not a miglitol effect); this may be used for therapeutic benefit.

Miglitol ***taken concurrently*** with

- clofibrate (Atromid-S) may result in hypoglycemia.
- digestive enzyme products that contain amylase or lipase may result in loss of blood sugar control.
- digoxin (Lanoxin) may lead to low digoxin levels and benefits.
- disopyramide (Norpace) may result in hypoglycemia.
- high-dose aspirin or other salicylates and some NSAIDs (see Drug Classes) may result in hypoglycemia.
- insulin (see profile) increases risk of low blood sugar.
- levofloxacin (Levaquin) may increase or decrease blood sugar. Caution and close follow-up on blood sugar are required.
- ranitidine (Zantac) may blunt the benefits of ranitidine.
- sulfonamide antibiotics (see Drug Classes) may pose an increased risk for low blood sugar (hypoglycemia).

The following drugs may **decrease** the effects of miglitol:

- adrenocorticosteroids (see Drug Classes).
- beta blockers (see Drug Classes).
- calcium channel blockers (see Drug Classes).

- furosemide (Lasix) and bumetanide (Bumex).
- isoniazid (INH).
- monoamine oxidase (MAO) inhibitors (see Drug Classes).
- nicotinic acid.
- pancreatin (various).
- phenytoin (Dilantin).
- rifampin (Rifadin, others).
- theophylline (Theo-Dur, others).
- thiazide diuretics (see Drug Classes).
- thyroid hormones (see Drug Classes).

▷ *Driving, Hazardous Activities:* Use caution until degree of drowsiness you may experience is known.

Aviation Note: Diabetes **is a disqualification** for piloting. Consult a designated Aviation Medical Examiner.

Exposure to Sun: No restrictions.

Heavy Exercise or Exertion: Caution advised because this drug lowers peak in blood sugar after meals. Talk over dosing changes with your doctor.

Occurrence of Unrelated Illness: Illness can change blood sugar control. Temporary use of insulin may be required.

Discontinuation: Never stop miglitol before calling your doctor.

MINIMALLY SEDATING ANTIHISTAMINES

Astemizole (a STEM ah zohl)   **Cetirizine** (sa TEER a zeen)   **Fexofenadine** (fex oh FEN a deen)   **Loratadine** (lor AT a deen)   **Terfenadine** (ter FEN a deen)

Introduced: 1982, 1996, 1996, 1992, 1977, respectively   **Class:** Antihistamines, minimally sedating   **Prescription:** USA: Yes   **Controlled Drug:** USA: No; Canada: No   **Available as Generic:** U.S.: astemizole: Yes; cetirizine: No; fexofenadine: No; loratadine: Yes; terfenadine: Yes; Canada: Same as U.S.

Brand Names: Astemizole: Hismanal, Cetirizine: ✤Apo-Cetirizine, ✤Reactine Zyrtec, Zyrtec D [CD], Fexofenadine: Allegra, Allegra-D [CD], Loratadine: ✤Chlor-Tripolon ND [CD], Claritin, Claritin D [CD], ✤Claritin Extra, Claritin Reditabs [CD], Clarinex (investigational), Terfenadine: Seldane, Seldane-D

Author's Note: Astemizole and terfenadine data will be left in this book for another year. Considerable controversy erupted relative to these medicines when an FDA panel voted in overwhelming fashion to make cetirizine (Zyrtec), fexofenadine (Allegra) and loratadine (Claritin) available without a prescription. Historically, manufacturers have requested this switch. In this case, Wellpoint Health Networks—not the manufacturers—petitioned the FDA on the basis of a cost avoidance of $90 million dollars a year if it did not have to pay for the products. The situation has not been resolved at the time of this writing.

```
┌─────────────────────────────────────────────────────────────┐
│                   BENEFITS versus RISKS                      │
│   Possible Benefits              Possible Risks              │
│ EFFECTIVE AND LONG-LASTING     RARE HEART RHYTHM             │
│   RELIEF OF ALLERGIC RHINITIS    DISTURBANCES (HAVE          │
│ EFFECTIVE RELIEF OF SOME         OCCURRED AS A DRUG          │
│   ALLERGIC SKIN DISORDERS        INTERACTION EFFECT OR AS A  │
│ MINIMAL DROWSINESS               DRUG EFFECT) (astemizole,   │
│ MINOR TO NO ANTICHOLINERGIC      fexofenadine [one case report], │
│   SIDE EFFECTS                   loratadine)                 │
│                                Low white blood cell count   │
│                                  (leukopenia) (1.4% of fexofenadine │
│                                  patients)                  │
│                                Slight atropinelike effects (some │
│                                  medicines in this class)   │
│                                Mild sedation or fatigue     │
└─────────────────────────────────────────────────────────────┘
```

▷ **Principal Uses**

As a Single Drug Product: Uses currently included in FDA-approved labeling: (1) Used to treat non-nasal and nasal symptoms of seasonal allergic rhinitis (hay fever); (2) helps ease symptoms of rhinitis; (3) used to treat swellings of unknown origin (idiopathic urticaria) (astemizole, cetirizine, loratadine); (4) helps ease symptoms of pollen-induced asthma (astemizole, cetirizine, loratadine).

Other (unlabeled) generally accepted uses: (1) Lichen nitidus lesions (astemizole); (2) can help control chronic vertigo (astemizole); (3) chronic idiopathic urticaria (astemizole, loratadine); (4) food allergies (cetirizine).

As a Combination Drug Product [CD]: Allegra-D, Claritin-D and Zyrtec-D contain the original minimally sedating antihistamine and add the benefits of pseudoephedrine. Caution should be used when taking the "D" forms if you are also taking a medicine that interacts with pseudoephedrine.

How These Drugs Work: These medicines block histamine, stopping symptoms (caused by histamine), such as swelling and itching of the eyes.

Available Dosage Forms and Strengths

Astemizole:
> Oral suspension (Canada only) — 1 mg/ml, 2 mg/ml
> Tablets — 10 mg

Cetirizine:
> Solution — 5 mg/ml
> Tablets — 5 mg, 10 mg
> Tablets (Canada only) — 20 mg

Fexofenadine:
> Capsules — 60 mg
> Tablet — 30 mg, 60 mg, 180 mg
> Tablets, extended-release — 60 mg fexofenadine,
> — 120 mg pseudoephedrine

Loratadine:
> Syrup — 1 mg/ml
> Tablets — 10 mg

Tablets, extended-release (Claritin-D 24-Hour) — 10 mg loratadine, 240 mg pseudoephedrine
Tablets, rapidly disintegrating (micronized — 10 mg loratadine)
Tablets, repeat-action (Claritin-D [CD]) — 5 mg loratadine, 120 mg pseudoephedrine

▷ **Recommended Dosage Ranges** (Actual dose and schedule must be determined for each patient individually.)

Infants and Children: **Safety and efficacy in children youngeer than 12 years old have been established only for fexofenadine and cetirizine, not for the rest of the medicines in this family.**

Cetirizine (Zyrtec) is approved for children 2 to 5 years old who have seasonal or perennial allergic rhinitis or hives (idiopathic urticaria) of unknown cause.

Fexofenadine (Allegra) is newly approved for children 6 to 11 years old who have seasonal or perennial allergic rhinitis or hives (idiopathic urticaria) of unknown cause using 30 mg twice daily.

12 to 60 Years of Age:

Astemizole: 10 mg per day. This is also the maximum daily dose.

Cetirizine: The starting dose is 5 mg (depending on severity, may be 10 mg) and is increased as needed and tolerated to a maximum of 20 mg daily.

Fexofenadine:

Seasonal allergic rhinitis: 60 mg twice daily or 180 mg once daily.

Chronic idiopathic urticaria: 60 mg twice daily.

Loratadine: A single 10-mg tablet (of the nonrepeat action, noncombination product) is taken once daily.

Loratadine/pseudoephedrine (5 mg/120 mg nonrepeat action): One tablet twice daily.

Loratadine/pseudoephedrine (10 mg/240 mg repeat action): One tablet daily.

Over 60 Years of Age:

Fexofenadine and loratadine (Claritin-D and Claritin-D 24-Hour forms) are NOT recommended for those over 60. Prudent to decrease cetirizine doses, as it is slowly removed at this age.

Conditions Requiring Dosing Adjustments

Liver Function: Astemizole: NOT to be used in severe liver disease. Dosing guidelines are not available.

Cetirizine: A 5-mg dose is recommended.

Fexofenadine: Dosing changes do not appear to be needed.

Loratadine: Patients with liver compromise take a dose of 10 mg (of the non-repeat action, noncombination product) every other day.

Kidney Function: Astemizole: No dosing changes appear to be needed.

Cetirizine: Patients with moderate kidney decline (creatinine clearance 11–31 ml/min) may take 5 mg daily.

Fexofenadine: A daily dose of 60 mg once daily is recommended.

Loratadine: Patients with moderate kidney failure (creatinine clearance less than 30 ml/min) get a starting dose of 10 mg (of nonrepeat action, non-combination product) every other day.

▷ **Dosing Instructions:** Astemizole and loratadine are best taken on an empty stomach. Once the rapidly disintegrating (Reditab) form has dissolved, water may be used to help patients swallow the contents of the pill. The other medicines in this class may be taken with food. Extended-release forms of these medicines should never be crushed. If you forget a dose: Take the missed dose as soon as you remember it, unless it's nearly time for your next dose—if that is the case, skip the missed dose and take the next dose right on schedule. DO NOT double doses. Talk with your doctor if you find yourself missing doses.

Usual Duration of Use: Although all of these medicines may go to work immediately, regular use for up to 1 day (fexofenadine), up to 2 days (astemizole or cetirizine) or up to 3 days (loratadine) may be needed to see substantial symptom improvement. Long-term use requires evaluation of response by your doctor.

Typical Treatment Goals and Measurements (Outcomes and Markers)
Seasonal allergic rhinitis: The general goal is to decrease or eliminate hay fever symptoms such as watery eyes, sneezing and itchy feelings in the throat or eyes and runny nose.

Possible Advantages of These Drugs: Less sedating than previously available antihistamines. Once-daily dosing for some agents in this class. Some medicines in this class do not interact with certain antifungals and macrolide antibiotics (see Drug Classes) or do interact but do not appear to cause side effects on the heart or change the safety profile. Cetirizine has NOT had ANY case reports of QTc prolongation. Tachyphylaxis or tolerance may be less likely to occur to these medicines than with earlier agents. Reditabs do not require water to take them! Fexofenadine did NOT exhibit any driving performance decrease in one study of 24 healthy men when fexofenadine was combined with ethanol. Once a day dosing is a distinct advantage.

Currently "Drugs of Choice"
For patients who must take antihistamine-type medicines and require the best possible balance of symptom relief and minimal sedation.

▷ **These Drugs Should Not Be Taken If**
- you have had an allergic reaction to any dose form of these medicines or any of the ingredients in them previously.
- you are presently being tested (using skin tests) for allergies.
- you are taking medicines that prolong the QT interval, such as quinidine, pentamidine, disopyramide or others (for astemizole, cetirizine, fexofenadine and terfenadine).
- you have urinary retention, liver disease, severe disease of the arteries of the heart (coronary artery disease) or narrow-angle glaucoma (loratadine combination products that contain pseudoephedrine).

▷ **Inform Your Physician Before Taking These Drugs If**
- you have asthma.
- you are at risk for drowsiness or fainting (syncope).
- you have a history of a heart rhythm disorder.
- your electrolytes are not in balance.
- you are taking other medicines metabolized by or that change CYP 3A4 levels (ask your doctor) and one of these medicines is removed by that enzyme.
- you are taking other medicines (especially antifungal or macrolide antibiotics). Blood levels of loratadine or fexofenadine may be increased.

Decreases in loratadine and fexofenadine doses may be prudent. Astemizole should NOT be combined with these medicines.
- you have a history of liver or kidney compromise.
- you are pregnant.
- your work REQUIRES mental alertness.

Possible Side Effects (natural, expected and unavoidable drug actions)

Dry nose, mouth or throat, somnolence (drowsiness): cetirizine—frequent, fexofenadine—rare, loratadine—infrequent.

▷ **Possible Adverse Effects** (unusual, unexpected and infrequent reactions)

If any of the following develop, consult your physician promptly for guidance.

Mild Adverse Effects

Allergic reactions: skin rash, itching.

Headache, fatigue or dizziness—infrequent to frequent, depending on the agent.

Dry mouth—possible to infrequent.

Leg cramps, muscle aches (astemizole or loratadine)—rare.

Weight gain (cetirizine)—uncommon.

Fast heart rate (tachycardia) (loratadine)—rare.

Prolonged QTc interval (fexofenadine, astemizole)—possible if used in people with existing heart disease, case report(s).

Lowering of the blood pressure (loratadine)—rare.

Vision changes (loratadine)—rare.

Serious Adverse Effects

Allergic reactions: anaphylaxis (astemizole or loratadine)—rare.

Idiosyncratic reactions: not reported.

Paresthesia—case report for astemizole.

Serious heart rhythm disorders: astemizole—rare; loratadine and fexofenadine—case report.

Tachycardia—rare.

Lowering of the white blood cell count (fexofenadine)—rare.

Abnormal liver function (loratadine)—case reports.

Depression, confusion, paresthesias—rare.

Passing out (syncope)—rare.

▷ **Possible Effects on Sexual Function:** Vaginitis, painful menses (dysmenorrhea), breast enlargement or breast pain (loratadine)—case reports.

Menstrual disorders (loratadine, fexofenadine)—case reports to rare.

Galactorrhea (loratadine)—case reports.

Impotence (loratadine)—case reports.

Possible Delayed Adverse Effects: None reported.

▷ **Adverse Effects That May Mimic Natural Diseases or Disorders**

Increased liver enzymes may mimic hepatitis of infectious origin.

Natural Diseases or Disorders That May Be Activated by These Drugs

None reported.

Possible Effects on Laboratory Tests

Skin tests for allergies will be blunted and less diagnostic.

Liver function tests: may be increased (loratadine, fexofenadine [mildly] or terfenadine).

White blood cell counts: decreased (leukopenia)—rare in clinical trials (fexofenadine).

CAUTION

1. Loratadine does interact with some antifungals and some macrolide antibiotics—but appears to be free of the heart (cardiac) effects, even though blood levels of loratadine may increase if it is taken with these interacting medicines. Talk to your doctor or pharmacist before taking any medicines that were not discussed when loratadine was prescribed.

2. Some of these medicines HAVE LIFE-THREATENING DRUG INTER-ACTIONS. Talk to your doctor or pharmacist BEFORE combining any prescription, nonprescription or herbal remedies with medicines in this class.

3. Report dizziness, heart palpitation or chest pain promptly when using any of these medicines.

4. Fexofenadine (Allegra) levels may be decreased by roughly 70% if it is taken with orange, apple or grapefruit juice. Current thinking holds that this is due to fruit juice inhibiting a drug "taxi" (transporter) called OATP.

Precautions for Use

By Infants and Children: Safety and effectiveness for use by those under 12 years of age have not been established.

By Those Over 60 Years of Age: Smaller starting and maintenance doses are needed. Longer dosing intervals may be needed as well.

▷ **Advisability of Use During Pregnancy**

Pregnancy Category: B (cetirizine, loratadine); C (astemizole, fexofenadine). See Pregnancy Risk Categories at the back of this book.

Animal studies: No birth defects reported.

Human studies: Information from adequate studies of pregnant women is not available. **These medicines should be used during pregnancy only if clearly needed. Discuss the BENEFITS versus RISKS with your doctor.**

Advisability of Use If Breast-Feeding

Presence of this drug in breast milk: No data (cetirizine, fexofenadine); expected (astemizole); yes (loratadine).

Ask your doctor for guidance regarding stopping the drug or stopping nursing (astemizole, cetirizine, fexofenadine or loratadine).

Habit-Forming Potential: None.

Effects of Overdose: With overdoses greater than 10 mg (40–80 mg): tachycardia, somnolence and headache (loratadine). Usual antihistamine protocols (cetirizine or fexofenadine). Possible life-threatening heart rhythm problems (astemizole).

Possible Effects of Long-Term Use: None defined.

Suggested Periodic Examinations While Taking These Drugs (at physician's discretion)

Examination for relief of the condition(s) being treated.

Electrocardiogram (ECG), especially for those with heart conditions.

▷ **While Taking These Drugs, Observe the Following**

Foods: Astemizole and loratadine are best taken on an empty stomach. DO NOT combine with grapefruit.

Herbal Medicines or Minerals: Valerian and kava kava may intensify drowsiness. St. John's wort may lead to photosensitivity. Combination with medicines in this class that also cause photosensitivity is NOT advised. If you are allergic to plants in the *Asteraceae* family (aster, chrysanthemum, daisy or ragweed), you may also be allergic to echinacea, chamomile, feverfew and St. John's wort.

Beverages: Grapefruit juice may lead to increased blood levels of astemizole and loratadine, leading to toxicity. Fexofenadine (Allegra) levels may be decreased by roughly 70% if it is taken with orange, apple or grapefruit juice. Current thinking holds that this is due to fruit juice inhibiting a drug "taxi" (transporter) called OATP. Water is the best liquid to take with medicines in this class.

▷ *Alcohol:* May cause excessive drowsiness (central nervous system depression).
Tobacco Smoking: No interactions expected. I advise everyone to quit smoking.
Marijuana Smoking: May cause additive drowsiness or lethargy.

▷ *Other Drugs*

These medicines ***taken concurrently*** with

- cimetidine (Tagamet) may produce a significant increase in loratadine blood levels. No serious drug effects have been reported, but since in general the frequency of adverse effects increases with increasing blood levels, it appears prudent to decrease the dose of loratadine if these medicines are to be taken at the same time because of possible loratadine toxicity. The loratadine dose should certainly be decreased if increased frequency of adverse effects occurs if these medicines are combined in usual doses. Astemizole may also react. Cetirizine is mostly removed by the kidneys.
- cisapride (Propulsid) may lead to SERIOUS heart rhythm problems when combined with astemizole.
- efavirenz (Sustiva) may lead to life-threatening heart problems if combined with astemizole.
- fluoxetine (Prozac) produced a serious heart rhythm problem in a patient taking terfenadine—DO NOT COMBINE THESE MEDICINES. Caution is advised for the other drugs in this class.
- fluvoxamine (Luvox) may result in increased blood levels of astemizole, cetirizine or loratadine. Caution is advised.
- grepafloxacin (Raxar) may increase risk of heart rhythm problems (astemizole)—DO NOT COMBINE THESE MEDICINES.
- indinavir (Crixivan) and perhaps ritonavir, saquinavir or nelfinavir may decrease metabolism of astemizole and should NEVER BE COMBINED. Loratadine levels may be increased, and doses may need to be lowered. Other drugs in this family may also be affected.
- itraconazole (and perhaps other similarly structured antifungals, such as ketoconazole) should NEVER be combined with astemizole. These drugs may cause increased blood levels of loratadine or fexofenadine. Although no serious heart rhythm toxicity has been reported to date with this medicine, caution is advised, and it appears prudent to lower the dose of loratadine or fexofenadine.
- macrolide antibiotics such as clarithromycin or erythromycin **MUST NEVER BE COMBINED WITH ASTEMIZOLE.** Although no serious heart rhythm toxicity has been reported to date with loratadine or fexofenadine, caution is advised, as excessive blood levels of any medicine may increase risk of adverse effects; it may be prudent to lower the dose of loratadine.
- medicines that prolong the QT interval should be avoided (such as disopyramide, ibutilide, quinolones [grepafloxacin, sparfloxacin], others); cetirizine is the only medicine in this class without any reports of QTc interval changes.

- nefazodone (Serzone) may lead to life-threatening heart problems if combined with astemizole.
- paroxetine (Paxil) may inhibit the enzymes needed to remove astemizole, cetirizine or loratadine. Caution is advised.
- quinidine (Quinaglute, others) may result in a change in the effect of quinidine and result in undesirable effects on the heart. Caution is advised.
- ritonavir (Norvir) and perhaps other protease inhibitors (see Drug Classes) may increase blood levels and toxicity.
- sertraline (Zoloft) may lead to life-threatening heart problems if combined with astemizole. DO NOT COMBINE.
- sotalol (Betapace) may cause additive adverse effects (QT interval prolongation) on the heart by these medicines—this combination is not recommended.
- theophylline (Theo-Dur, others) may decrease cetirizine clearance. Patients should be closely followed for signs of excessive cetirizine levels.
- zafirlukast (Accolate), and perhaps zileuton (Zyflo) if combined with astemizole, may decrease zafirlukast levels and blunt the therapeutic benefits of zafirlukast.

▷ *Driving, Hazardous Activities:* Although these medicines are much less likely than earlier antihistamines to cause drowsiness, caution should be used until your individual reaction to these medicines is determined. Restrict activities as necessary.

Aviation Note: The use of these drugs is probably not a disqualification for piloting. Consult a designated Aviation Medical Examiner.

Exposure to Sun: Rare cases of photosensitivity have been reported with some medicines (astemizole, loratadine) in this class. Use caution.

MINOXIDIL (min OX i dil)

Introduced: 1972   **Class:** Antihypertensive, hair growth stimulant
Prescription: USA: Yes   **Controlled Drug:** USA: No; Canada: No
Available as Generic: Yes

Brand Names: Alostil, ✤Apo-Gain, Loniten, ✤Med-Minoxidil, Minocalve 5, Minodyl, Minoximen, Rogaine, Rogaine Extra Strength

Author's Note: Rogaine treatment for baldness is available without a prescription.

BENEFITS versus RISKS	
Possible Benefits	*Possible Risks*
POTENT, LONG-ACTING ANTIHYPERTENSIVE	EXCESSIVE BODY HAIR GROWTH SALT AND WATER RETENTION
EFFECTIVE IN CASES OF SEVERE HYPERTENSION, ACCELERATED AND MALIGNANT HYPERTENSION	Excessively rapid heart rate Aggravation of angina Local scalp irritation (topical use)
Moderately effective in treating male pattern baldness and female baldness (alopecia androgenica)	

▷ **Principal Uses**

    As a Single Drug Product: Uses currently included in FDA-approved labeling: (1) Treats severe high blood pressure not controlled by conventional therapy; (2) treats female androgenic baldness or male pattern baldness; (3) effective in patients with high blood pressure and kidney failure.

    Other (unlabeled) generally accepted uses: Supportive therapy in hair transplants.

How This Drug Works: (1) Relaxes constricted muscles in walls of small arteries and permits expansion of the arteries and lower blood pressure. (2) May act directly on the hair follicle and also may increase size of previously closed small scalp blood vessels, restoring small hair follicles to normal size and activity.

Available Dosage Forms and Strengths

        Tablets — 2.5 mg, 10 mg

    Topical solution — 2%,

           — 5% (Extra Strength)

▷ **Usual Adult Dosage Ranges:** *For hypertension:* In severe cases, initially 5 mg once a day. The dose is then gradually increased as needed and tolerated to 10 mg, 20 mg and then 40 mg every 24 hours, taken in one or two divided doses daily. The usual ongoing dose is 10 to 40 mg daily. Daily maximum is 50 mg.

    For male pattern baldness: Apply thinly 1 ml of topical solution to the balding area of the scalp twice daily. The total daily dose should not exceed 2 ml.

    Note: Actual dose and schedule must be determined for each patient individually.

Conditions Requiring Dosing Adjustments

    Liver Function: This drug is metabolized (90%) in the liver. It should be used with caution by patients with liver compromise.

    Kidney Function: In moderate kidney failure, the dose should be decreased empirically.

▷ **Dosing Instructions:** For hypertension: Tablets may be crushed and taken with or following food to prevent nausea. Take at the same time each day. If you forget a dose: Take or apply the missed dose as soon as you remember it, unless it's nearly time for your next dose—if that is the case, skip the missed dose and take or apply the next dose right on schedule. Talk with your doctor if you find yourself missing doses.

    For baldness: The topical solution is for external, local use only; it is not to be swallowed. Begin application at the center of the bald area; apply thinly to cover the entire area. The scalp and hair must be dry at the time of application. Follow instructions carefully.

Usual Duration of Use: Use on a regular schedule for 3 to 7 days usually determines effectiveness in controlling severe hypertension. Continual use of the topical solution for at least 4 months is necessary to determine its ability to promote hair growth. Long-term use (months to years) of both dose forms requires physician supervision.

Typical Treatment Goals and Measurements (Outcomes and Markers)

    Baldness: The goal is to regain hair and maintain existing hair. Some dermatologists use hair counts to assess progress and peak benefits.

    Blood pressure: The most recent treatment guidelines (JNC VI) actually define optimal blood pressure (BP) as less than 120/80 and high normal as

139/89. The American Diabetes Association has chosen a target of 130/80 as the blood pressure goal for people living with diabetes. Most clinicians try to achieve a BP that achieves the best balance of lower cardiovascular risk while avoiding the problem of too low a blood pressure. The goal and time frame (see peak benefits above) should be discussed with you when the prescription is written.

▷ **This Drug Should Not Be Taken If**
- you have had an allergic reaction to it previously.
- you are known to have a pheochromocytoma (an adrenaline-producing tumor).
- you have pulmonary hypertension due to mitral valve stenosis.

▷ **Inform Your Physician Before Taking This Drug If**
- you are pregnant or planning pregnancy.
- you are breast-feeding your infant.
- you have had a heart attack.
- you have angina attacks.
- you have existing blood vessel disease in your head (cerebrovascular disease).
- you have a history of coronary artery disease or impaired heart function.
- you have a history of stroke or impaired brain circulation.
- you have impaired liver or kidney function.

Possible Side Effects (natural, expected and unavoidable drug actions)
Increased heart rate, fluid retention with weight gain, excessive hair growth on face, arms, legs and back (frequent).

▷ **Possible Adverse Effects** (unusual, unexpected and infrequent reactions)
If any of the following develop, consult your physician promptly for guidance.
Mild Adverse Effects
Allergic reactions: skin rash.
Localized dermatitis at site of application of topical solution—rare.
Headache, dizziness, fainting—rare.
Nausea, increased thirst—infrequent.
Hair growth and changes in hair color—case reports.
Weight gain—possible.
Mild increase in liver enzymes—infrequent.
Serious Adverse Effects
Allergic reactions: serious skin rash (Stevens-Johnson syndrome).
Idiosyncratic reaction: fluid formation around the heart (pericardial effusion).
Development of angina pectoris; high blood pressure in the lungs (pulmonary hypertension)—case reports.
Systemic lupus erythematosus—case reports.
Low white blood cells or platelets—rare and transient.
Author's Note: Topical use of this medicine for hair growth avoids most of these adverse effects.

▷ **Possible Effects on Sexual Function:** Male breast tenderness (gynecomastia)—case reports. Some data to support that this drug balances the male ability to ejaculate and have a healthy sex drive that may have been blunted by other drugs that treat high blood pressure.

Natural Diseases or Disorders That May Be Activated by This Drug
Latent coronary artery disease with symptomatic angina.

Possible Effects on Laboratory Tests
Blood HDL cholesterol level: increased.
Blood LDL cholesterol level: decreased.

CAUTION
1. Long-term use for hypertension usually requires use of a diuretic to counteract salt and water retention.
2. The long-term use of this drug for hypertension may require concurrent use of a beta-blocker drug to control excessive acceleration of the heart.
3. It is best to avoid combining this drug and guanethidine; the combination can cause severe orthostatic hypotension (see Glossary).
4. Consult your physician regarding the advisability of using a "no-salt-added" diet.
5. Little of this drug is absorbed into the general circulation when the topical solution is applied to the scalp. However, some systemic effects have been reported. Inform your physician promptly if you experience any unusual symptoms while using the topical solution.
6. The topical form contains alcohol. Avoid getting this baldness medicine into your eyes.

Precautions for Use
By Infants and Children: Dose schedules should be determined by a qualified pediatrician. In children under 12 years old, starting dose is 0.2 mg per kg of body mass in a single dose. Dose is then increased as needed and tolerated by 0.1 to 0.2 mg per kg per day at 3-day intervals. Children over 12 are given the adult dose. Monitor closely for salt and water retention.

By Those Over 60 Years of Age: Treatment with small doses and a limit of total daily dose to 75 mg is indicated. Headache, palpitation and rapid heart rate due to this drug are more common in this age group and can mimic acute anxiety states. Observe for dizziness, unsteadiness, fainting and falling.

▷ **Advisability of Use During Pregnancy**
Pregnancy Category: C. See Pregnancy Risk Categories at the back of this book.
Animal studies: No birth defects reported in rats or rabbits, but studies did reveal decreased fertility and increased fetal deaths.
Human studies: Adequate studies of pregnant women are not available.
Avoid during the first 3 months. Use only if clearly needed during the final 6 months.

Advisability of Use If Breast-Feeding
Presence of this drug in breast milk: Yes.
Avoid drug or refrain from nursing.

Habit-Forming Potential: None.

Effects of Overdose: Headache, dizziness, weakness, nausea, marked low blood pressure, weak and rapid pulse, loss of consciousness.

Possible Effects of Long-Term Use: Excessive growth of body hair occurs in 80% of users after 1 to 2 months of continual treatment for hypertension. Close to 100% of users will experience this effect after 1 year of continual treatment. This may be accompanied by darkening of the skin and coarsening of facial features.

Suggested Periodic Examinations While Taking This Drug (at physician's discretion)

Body weight measurement for insidious gain due to water retention.

Electrocardiographic and echocardiographic heart examinations.

▷ **While Taking This Drug, Observe the Following**

Foods: Avoid excessive salt and heavily salted foods.

Herbal Medicines or Minerals: Ginseng or ma huang may increase blood pressure, blunting the benefits of this medicine if it is being used to lower blood pressure. Hawthorn, saw palmetto and licorice may also cause increased blood pressure. Calcium and garlic may lower blood pressure. Use caution and work with your doctor to make sure blood pressure is not lowered too much. Autumn crocus should be avoided in alopecia.

Beverages: No restrictions. May be taken with milk.

▷ *Alcohol:* Use with extreme caution. Alcohol can exaggerate the blood pressure–lowering effects of this drug.

Tobacco Smoking: Best avoided. Nicotine can contribute significantly to angina. I advise everyone to quit smoking.

▷ *Other Drugs*

Minoxidil may ***increase*** the effects of

• all other antihypertensive drugs; careful dose adjustments are mandatory.

Minoxidil ***taken concurrently*** with

• clonidine (Catapres TTS, others) may help ease fast heart rate and increased sympathetic nervous system activity caused by minoxidil.

• guanethidine (Ismelin, Esimil) may cause severe orthostatic hypotension; avoid this combination.

• NSAIDs may blunt the therapeutic benefit of minoxidil.

• vitamin E (one report of high-dose use) reversing hair growth.

▷ *Driving, Hazardous Activities:* This drug may cause dizziness and fatigue. Restrict activities as necessary.

Aviation Note: The use of this drug ***is a disqualification*** for piloting. Consult a designated Aviation Medical Examiner.

Exposure to Sun: No restrictions.

Discontinuation: This drug should not be stopped abruptly. If it is to be discontinued, consult your physician regarding gradual reduction in dose and appropriate replacement with other drugs for the management of hypertension. Following discontinuation of the topical solution, the pretreatment pattern of baldness may return within 3 to 4 months.

MIRTAZAPINE (mur TAZ a peen)

Introduced: 1996   **Class:** Antidepressant, piperazinoazepine, norepinephrine, serotonin reuptake inhibitor   **Prescription:** USA: Yes   **Controlled Drug:** USA: No; Canada: No   **Available as Generic:** USA: No; Canada: No   **Brand Name:** Remeron

```
┌─────────────────────────────────────────────────────────────────────────┐
│                        BENEFITS versus RISKS                              │
│        Possible Benefits                        Possible Risks            │
│   EFFECTIVE TREATMENT OF            Sleepiness                            │
│     DEPRESSION                      Weight gain                           │
│   BENEFICIAL ACTION ON TWO          Lowering of white blood cells         │
│     NERVE TRANSMITTERS                                                     │
│   HELPS PATIENTS WITH                                                      │
│     DEPRESSION WHO ALSO HAVE                                               │
│     PROBLEMS SLEEPING AND ARE                                             │
│     ANXIOUS                                                                │
└─────────────────────────────────────────────────────────────────────────┘
```

▷ **Principal Uses**

As a Single Drug Product: Uses currently included in FDA-approved labeling: Treatment of depression.

Other (unlabeled) generally accepted uses: (1) Eases presurgical insomnia; (2) may help antidepressant (SSRI)-induced sexual problems (dysfunction); (3) could be useful in tremor or pain syndromes.

How This Drug Works: Enhances the action of two nerve transmitters (norepinephrine and serotonin) that are thought to be low or lowered in cases of depression.

Available Dosage Forms and Strengths

Tablets — 15 mg, 30 mg, 45 mg

▷ **Recommended Dosage Ranges** (Actual dose and schedule must be determined for each patient individually.)

Infants and Children: Dose not established.

Adults to Age 60: For treatment of adult depression, 15 to 45 mg at bedtime. Dosing is started at 15 mg. Increases in dose (as needed and tolerated) are made at one-to-two week intervals.

Over 60 Years of Age: Removed more slowly from the body. Lower doses are prudent.

Conditions Requiring Dosing Adjustments

Liver Function: Lower doses and slow dose increases are needed.

Kidney Function: Lower doses and slow dose increases are needed.

▷ **Dosing Instructions:** The tablet may be crushed and can be taken with or without food. Take it at the same time daily. If you forget a dose: Take the missed dose as soon as you remember it, unless it's morning when you remember it—if that is the case, skip the missed dose and take the next dose right on schedule. Talk with your doctor if you find yourself missing doses.

Usual Duration of Use: Use on a regular schedule for 1 week will usually start to show benefits in relieving depression. Peak effect may take several weeks to be seen. Long-term use (months to years) requires follow-up by your doctor.

Typical Treatment Goals and Measurements (Outcomes and Markers)

Depression: The general goal: to lessen the degree and severity of depression, letting patients return to their daily lives. Specific measures of depression involve testing or inventories and can be valuable in helping check benefits from this medicine.

Pain syndromes: The general goal: to decrease pain to a manageable level. Pain should be appropriately assessed, and progress defined based on lowering of overall pain level.

Possible Advantages of This Drug

Less likely to cause dry mouth, constipation, urinary retention, orthostatic hypotension (see Glossary) and heart rhythm disturbances than tricyclic antidepressants. Does not cause Parkinson-like reactions.

▷ **This Drug Should Not Be Taken If**
- you have had an allergic reaction to it previously.
- you are currently taking, or have taken within the past 14 days, any monoamine oxidase (MAO) type A inhibitor drug (see Drug Classes).

▷ **Inform Your Physician Before Taking This Drug If**
- you have experienced any adverse effects from antidepressant drugs.
- you have impaired liver or kidney function.
- you have Parkinson's disease.
- you have had a recent heart attack or have heart disease.
- you have a seizure disorder.
- you are pregnant or plan pregnancy while taking this drug.

Possible Side Effects (natural, expected and unavoidable drug actions)

Increased appetite, weight gain. Lower blood pressure on standing (see postural hypotension in Glossary).

▷ **Possible Adverse Effects** (unusual, unexpected and infrequent reactions)
If any of the following develop, consult your physician promptly for guidance.

Mild Adverse Effects
Allergic reactions: skin rash, itching—rare.
Headache, nervousness, insomnia—rare to infrequent.
Somnolence—frequent (may be up to 54%).
Fatigue and dry mouth—frequent.
Tremor, dizziness, abnormal dreams—rare.
Abnormal vision, numbness and tingling—rare.
Confusion—rare.
Hallucinations—rare.
Chest pain and increased blood pressure—rare.
Increased heart rate—infrequent.
Altered taste, nausea, vomiting, diarrhea—rare to infrequent.
Constipation—frequent.

Serious Adverse Effects
Allergic reactions: dermatitis (various forms)—rare.
Drug—induced seizures—case reports.
Increased blood cholesterol (hypercholesterolemia)—infrequent.
Cirrhosis or pancreatitis—rare in controlled studies.
Agranulocytosis—case reports.

▷ **Possible Effects on Sexual Function:** Male sexual dysfunction: delayed ejaculation—infrequent.
Female sexual dysfunction: inhibited orgasm—rare.
Swelling and tenderness of male and female breast tissue—case reports.
Dysmenorrhea—rare.

Natural Diseases or Disorders That May Be Activated by This Drug
Latent epilepsy.

Possible Effects on Laboratory Tests
Blood total cholesterol and triglyceride levels: increased—infrequent.
Liver function tests: increased liver enzymes (ALT/GPT, AST/GOT and alkaline phosphatase).
Blood cell counts: decreased (aplastic anemia)—case reports.
Blood sodium: decreased (with rare SIADH).

CAUTION
1. If any type of skin reaction develops (rash, hives, etc.), discontinue this drug and inform your physician promptly.
2. If dryness of the mouth develops and persists for more than 2 weeks, consult your dentist for guidance.
3. Ask your doctor or pharmacist before taking any other prescription or over-the-counter drug while taking mirtazapine.
4. If you are advised to take any monoamine oxidase (MAO) type A inhibitor (see Drug Classes), allow an interval of 5 weeks after discontinuing this drug before starting the MAO inhibitor.
5. It is advisable to withhold this drug if electroconvulsive therapy (ECT, or "shock" treatment) is to be used to treat your depression.

Precautions for Use
By Infants and Children: Safety and effectiveness for those under 12 years of age are not established.
By Those Over 60 Years of Age: The lowest effective dose should be used for maintenance treatment and adjusted as needed for reduced kidney function.

▷ **Advisability of Use During Pregnancy**
Pregnancy Category: C. See Pregnancy Risk Categories at the back of this book.
Animal studies: Delayed bone development due to this drug found in rat and rabbit studies.
Human studies: Adequate studies of pregnant women are not available.
Use this drug only if clearly needed. Ask your physician for guidance.

Advisability of Use If Breast-Feeding
Presence of this drug in breast milk: Unknown.
Avoid drug or refrain from nursing.

Habit-Forming Potential: None.

Effects of Overdose: Agitation, restlessness, excitement, nausea, vomiting, seizures.

Possible Effects of Long-Term Use: None reported.

Suggested Periodic Examinations While Taking This Drug (at physician's discretion)
None.

▷ **While Taking This Drug, Observe the Following**
Foods: No restrictions.
Herbal Medicines or Minerals: Since part of the way ginseng works may be as a MAO inhibitor, do not combine ginseng with mirtazapine. Valerian and kava kava may interact additively (drowsiness). Avoid these combinations. St. John's wort may lead to dangerously increased serotonin activity as

well as additive sensitivity to the sun. Indian snakeroot, ma huang and yohimbe are also best avoided while taking this medicine.

Beverages: No restrictions. May be taken with milk.

▷ *Alcohol:* Avoid completely.

Tobacco Smoking: No interactions expected. I advise everyone to quit smoking.

▷ *Other Drugs*

Mirtazapine *taken concurrently* with

- diazepam (Valium) and perhaps other benzodiazepines (see Drug Classes) may impair movement ability.
- inhibitors of cytochrome CYP 2D6, such as amiodarone, fluoxetine and zileuton, may lead to excessive blood levels and mirtazapine toxicity.
- monoamine oxidase (MAO) type A inhibitor drugs may cause confusion, agitation, high fever, seizures and dangerous elevations of blood pressure; avoid the concurrent use of these drugs.
- ritonavir (Norvir) and perhaps other protease inhibitors (see Drug Classes) may lead to toxicity.

▷ *Driving, Hazardous Activities:* This drug may cause drowsiness, dizziness, impaired judgment and altered vision. Restrict activities as necessary.

Aviation Note: The use of this drug *is a disqualification* for piloting. Consult a designated Aviation Medical Examiner.

Exposure to Sun: Use caution—this drug may (rarely) cause photosensitivity (see Glossary).

Discontinuation: The slow elimination of this drug from the body makes it unlikely that any withdrawal effects will result from abrupt discontinuation. However, call your doctor if you plan to stop this drug for any reason.

MISOPROSTOL (mi soh PROII stohl)

Introduced: 1987   **Class:** Gastrointestinal drug (ulcer preventive), prostaglandin analog   **Prescription:** USA: Yes   **Controlled Drug:** USA: No; Canada: No   **Available as Generic:**   USA: No; Canada: No
Brand Names: Arthotec [CD], Cytotec

BENEFITS versus RISKS	
Possible Benefits	*Possible Risks*
EFFECTIVE PREVENTION OF STOMACH ULCERATION WHILE TAKING ANTI-INFLAMMATORY DRUGS	INCREASED RISK OF ABORTION (IF USED DURING PREGNANCY)
	Diarrhea (transient)
	Neuropathy
Effective treatment of duodenal ulcer	

▷ **Principal Uses**

As a Single Drug Product: Uses currently included in FDA-approved labeling: (1) Prevents development of stomach ulcers during long-term use of anti-inflammatory drugs as therapy for arthritis and related conditions; (2) treatment of duodenal ulcers.

Other (unlabeled) generally accepted uses: (1) Used (in Canada and other countries) for treatment of active duodenal ulcer unrelated to use of anti-inflammatory drugs; (2) has some use in inducing abortions; (3) used in combination with cyclosporine or prednisone to decrease transplanted organ rejection; (4) may have a benefit in helping ripen the cervix in preparation for a vaginal delivery.

As a Combination Drug Product [CD]: Available in combination with diclofenac, an NSAID (see Drug Classes). The misoprostol is used to prevent stomach (gastric) irritation or ulceration from the NSAID.

How This Drug Works: Protects lining of the stomach and duodenum by (1) replacing tissue prostaglandins depleted by anti-inflammatory drugs; (2) inhibiting secretion of stomach acid; (3) increasing local production of bicarbonate (to neutralize acids) and mucus (to protect stomach and duodenal tissues). Combined effects prevent new ulcers and promote healing of existing ulcer(s).

Arthotec form: This combination uses the above mechanism of misoprostol to protect from possible ulcers caused by the NSAID diclofenac.

Available Dosage Forms and Strengths
Tablets — 100 mcg, 200 mcg
Tablets (Arthotec) — misoprostol 0.2 mg (200 mcg) and diclofenac 50 mg

Conditions Requiring Dosing Adjustments
Liver Function: Specific dose adjustments in liver compromise are not defined.
Kidney Function: The dose of misoprostol should be decreased in kidney disease. (See the diclofenac profile for information on diclofenac.)

▷ **Usual Adult Dosage Ranges:** *Prevention of stomach ulcer:* 200 mcg four times daily with food, taken concurrently during the use of any anti-inflammatory drug (see Antiarthritic or NSAIDs Drug Classes).

Treatment of duodenal ulcer: 200 mcg four times daily for 4 to 8 weeks.

Combination abortions: RU-496 600 mg taken once, followed by 400–600 mcg of misoprostol in one dose or two equal doses.

Rheumatoid arthritis (Arthotec form): one tablet 2 to 4 times daily.

Cervical ripening: 100 mcg of extemporaneous gel vaginally.

Note: Actual dose and schedule must be determined for each patient individually.

▷ **Dosing Instructions:** The tablet may be crushed and taken with each of three daily meals; take the last (fourth) dose of the day with food at bedtime. Arthotec form should be taken right after a meal or with food or milk. DO NOT crush or alter. If you forget a dose: Take the missed dose as soon as you remember it, unless it's nearly time for your next dose—if that is the case, skip the missed dose and take the next dose right on schedule. DO NOT double doses. Talk with your doctor if you find yourself missing doses.

Usual Duration of Use: For prevention of stomach ulcer, use is recommended for the entire period of anti-inflammatory drug use. For treatment of duodenal ulcer, continual use on a regular schedule for 4 weeks is recommended; if ulcer healing is not complete, a second course of 4 weeks is advised. Long-term use (months to years) requires periodic physician evaluation of response and dose adjustment.

Typical Treatment Goals and Measurements (Outcomes and Markers)
Prevention of ulcers: The goal is to prevent ulceration from anti-inflammatory drug use, or to heal the ulcer area and prevent re-occurrence of the

ulceration. Sign and symptom prevention or relief as well as endoscopic examination help define success of ulcer treatment or prevention.

Possible Advantages of This Drug: Significantly more effective than histamine (H2) blocking drugs (cimetidine, famotidine, nizatidine, ranitidine) or sucralfate in preventing the development of stomach ulcers. Arthotec form may increase adherence (having people take it as directed).

▷ **This Drug Should Not Be Taken If**
- you have had an allergic reaction to it previously.
- you are allergic to any type of prostaglandin.
- you are pregnant or breast-feeding.
- you are not able or willing to use effective contraception (oral contraceptives or intrauterine device) while taking this drug.

▷ **Inform Your Physician Before Taking This Drug If**
- you have a history of peptic ulcer disease or Crohn's disease.
- you have inflammatory bowel disease.
- you have impaired kidney function.
- you have a seizure disorder.

Possible Side Effects (natural, expected and unavoidable drug actions)
Diarrhea (14–40% of users), usually beginning after 13 days of use and subsiding spontaneously after 8 days.
Abortion (miscarriage) of pregnancy (11% of users); this is often incomplete and accompanied by serious uterine bleeding that may require hospitalization and urgent treatment.

▷ **Possible Adverse Effects** (unusual, unexpected and infrequent reactions)
If any of the following develop, consult your physician promptly for guidance.
Mild Adverse Effects
Allergic reaction: skin rash.
Headache, dizziness—infrequent.
Ringing in the ears—case reports.
Joint pain and muscle aches—rare.
Passing out (syncope)—rare.
Abdominal pain, indigestion, nausea, vomiting, flatulence, constipation—rare to infrequent.
Serious Adverse Effects
Allergic reactions: anaphylaxis—rare.
Anemia and low blood platelets—rare.
Blood in the urine—rare.
Bronchospasm—rare.
Neuropathy—rare.
Autonomic dysreflexia (Arthotec form)—case reports.
Abortion (if taken while pregnant).

▷ **Possible Effects on Sexual Function:** Menstrual irregularity, menstrual cramps, heavy menstrual flow, spotting between periods—all rare.
Postmenopausal vaginal bleeding; this may require further evaluation.
Reduced libido and impotence—rare and causal relationship not established.

▷ **Natural Diseases or Disorders That May Be Activated by This Drug**
Latent epilepsy.

Possible Effects on Laboratory Tests
>   Mild increase in liver function enzymes.

CAUTION
>   1. Do not take this drug if you are pregnant. It can cause abortion.
>   2. Do not make this drug available to others who may be pregnant or who may become pregnant.
>   3. If this drug is prescribed, it is advisable that you have a negative serum pregnancy test within 2 weeks before starting treatment.
>   4. Start taking this drug only on the second or third day of your next normal menstrual period.
>   5. Initiate effective contraceptive measures when you begin to take this drug. Discuss the use of oral contraceptives or intrauterine devices with your physician.
>   6. Should you become pregnant, stop the drug immediately and call your doctor.

Precautions for Use
>   *By Infants and Children:* Safety and effectiveness for those under 18 years of age not established.
>   *By Those Over 60 Years of Age:* This drug is usually well tolerated by this age group, but some forms of prostaglandins can cause drops in blood pressure; watch for light-headedness or faintness that may indicate low blood pressure. Report any such development to your physician.

▷ **Advisability of Use During Pregnancy**
>   *Pregnancy Category:* X. See Pregnancy Risk Categories at the back of this book.
>   *Animal studies:* No birth defects due to this drug found in rat or rabbit studies.
>   *Human studies:* Information from studies of pregnant women confirms that this drug can cause abortion, sometimes incomplete; unpassed products of conception can cause life-threatening complications.
>   Avoid this drug completely.

Advisability of Use If Breast-Feeding
>   Presence of this drug in breast milk: Unknown.
>   Avoid drug or refrain from nursing.

Habit-Forming Potential: None.

Effects of Overdose: Abdominal pain, diarrhea, fever, drowsiness, weakness, tremor, convulsions, difficult breathing.

Possible Effects of Long-Term Use: Unknown at this time.

Suggested Periodic Examinations While Taking This Drug (at physician's discretion)
>   Monitoring for accidental pregnancy.

▷ **While Taking This Drug, Observe the Following**
>   *Foods:* High-fat meals may reduce peak blood concentration.
>   *Herbal Medicines or Minerals:* Kola and ma huang may increase stomach acid, blunting the benefits of these medicines. Black cohosh root, ginkgo and squill are contraindicated in gastrointestinal disturbances. Licorice root has a Commission E monograph indication for gastrointestinal ulcers, but use with misoprostol has not been studied. Talk to your doctor BEFORE adding any herbals to this medicine.
>   *Beverages:* No restrictions. May be taken with milk.

▷ *Alcohol:* No interactions expected, but alcohol can promote the development of stomach ulcer and reduce the effectiveness of this drug.

Tobacco Smoking: No interactions expected. Nicotine is conducive to stomach ulcers. I advise everyone to quit smoking.

▷ *Other Drugs*

Misoprostol *taken concurrently* with

- antacids that contain magnesium may increase the risk of diarrhea; avoid this combination. Antacids in general may decrease misoprostol absorption and lessen its therapeutic benefits.
- phenylbutazone may result in neurosensory problems (movement problems, tingling, etc.).

▷ *Driving, Hazardous Activities:* This drug may cause dizziness, light-headedness, stomach pain or diarrhea. Restrict activities as necessary.

Aviation Note: The use of this drug *may be a disqualification* for piloting. Consult a designated Aviation Medical Examiner.

Exposure to Sun: No restrictions.

Discontinuation: This drug should be taken as combination therapy while you are taking antiarthritic/anti-inflammatory drugs that can cause stomach ulceration. Call your doctor if you have reason to stop it prematurely.

MOLINDONE (moh LIN dohn)

Introduced: 1971   **Class:** Strong tranquilizer, antipsychotic   **Prescription:** USA: Yes   **Controlled Drug:** USA: No; Canada: No   **Available as Generic:** No

Brand Name: Moban

BENEFITS versus RISKS	
Possible Benefits	*Possible Risks*
EFFECTIVE TREATMENT OF SOME CASES OF ACUTE AND CHRONIC SCHIZOPHRENIA	NARROW TREATMENT MARGIN SERIOUS TOXIC EFFECTS ON BRAIN:
May be effective in schizophrenia that has not responded to other drugs	Parkinson-like reactions
	Severe restlessness
	Abnormal involuntary movements
	Tardive dyskinesias
	Liver toxicity, jaundice
	Atropinelike side effects

Author's Note: Information in this profile has been truncated to make room for more widely used medicines.

MORPHINE (MOR feen)

Other Name: MS (morphine sulfate)

Introduced: 1806   **Class:** Strong analgesic, opioids   **Prescription:** USA: Yes   **Controlled Drug:** USA: C-II*; Canada: Yes   **Available as Generic:** Yes

*See Schedules of Controlled Drugs at the back of this book.

Brand Names: Astramorph, Astramorph PF, Duramorph, ✿Epimorph, Infu-
morph, Kadian, ✿Morphine H.P., ✿Morphitec, ✿M.O.S., ✿M.O.S.-S.R.,
MS Contin, MS-IR, OMS Concentrate, Opium Tincture, Oramorph SR,
Paregoric, RMS Uniserts, Roxanol, Roxanol 100, Roxanol SR, ✿Statex

BENEFITS versus RISKS	
Possible Benefits	*Possible Risks*
EFFECTIVE RELIEF OF MODERATE TO SEVERE PAIN WHEN IT IS DOSED CORRECTLY	POTENTIAL FOR HABIT FORMATION (DEPENDENCE) Respiratory depression Disorientation, hallucinations Interference with urination Constipation

▷ **Principal Uses**

As a Single Drug Product: Uses currently included in FDA-approved labeling:
(1) Given by mouth, suppository or injection to relieve moderate to severe
pain of heart attack, cancer, surgical procedures/operations, fluid on the
lungs and other causes; (2) used as an adjunct to anesthesia; (3) used in
treatment-resistant (intractable) cough.

Other (unlabeled) generally accepted uses: (1) Therapy of pain in sickle cell
crisis; (2) used in patient-controlled analgesia pumps to fight pain.

**Author's Note: The FDA and Purdue Pharmaceuticals have worked
together to strengthen warnings for OxyContin because of continuing
reports of abuse and diversion of this medicine. A "Dear Healthcare
Professional" letter has been sent out that explains the strengthening
of the labeling, including proper prescribing information, and also
highlights the problems associated with abuse and diversion of Oxy-
Contin. An important factor that MUST be considered when OxyContin is prescribed is the severity of the pain that is being treated, not
simply the disease that is the root cause of the painful symptoms. The
company has also responsibly undertaken a "Profiles in Pain Management" series in the *Pharmacy Today* journal of the American Pharmaceutical Association to increase awareness of prescription
medication abuse. Because ALL opioids (like morphine) are subject
to abuse, the FDA is also encouraging all makers of opioids sold in
the US to voluntarily review and revise product labeling as needed to
help ensure adequate warnings and precautions regarding risks of
abuse, misuse and diversion are presented and that responsible prescribing practices are promoted.**

How This Drug Works: Acting primarily as a depressant of certain brain functions, this drug suppresses the perception of pain and calms the emotional
response to pain.

Available Dosage Forms and Strengths

Capsules, sustained release (Kadian) — 20 mg, 50 mg, 100 mg

Injection — 0.5 mg/ml, 1 mg/ml, 2 mg/ml, 4 mg/ml,
5 mg/ml, 8 mg/ml, 10 mg/ml, 15 mg/ml,
25 mg/ml, 50 mg/ml

Oral solution — 20 mg/ml; 10 mg/5 ml, 20 mg/5 ml,
100 mg/5 ml

Suppositories — 5 mg, 10 mg, 20 mg, 30 mg

Syrup — 1 mg/ml, 5 mg/ml, 10 mg/ml, 20 mg/ml

Syrup (Canada only) — 50 mg/ml

Tablets — 5 mg, 10 mg, 15 mg, 25 mg, 30 mg, 50 mg

Tablets, soluble — 10 mg, 15 mg, 30 mg

Tablets, sustained release — 15 mg, 30 mg, 60 mg, 100 mg, 200 mg

Tablets, timed release — 15 mg, 30 mg, 60 mg, 100 mg, 200 mg

▷ **Recommended Dosage Ranges** (Actual dose and schedule must be determined for each patient individually.)

Infants and Children: 0.05 to 0.1 mg per kg of body mass have been used every 4 hours. Single dose should not exceed 15 mg, and dosing is adjusted (titrated to pain control goals). Infants and small children should be approached cautiously as they are generally more sensitive to narcotic (opioid) medicines dosed on a body weight basis.

17 to 60 Years of Age: By injection (IV form is used where naloxone [Narcan] and assisted breathing are available): Requirements for analgesia vary with the patient and with the painful condition being treated. For Example: after a heart attack (Acute Myocardial Infarction or MI): When patient symptoms are not helped by 3 appropriately spaced nitroglycerin tablets taken under the tongue or in patients who have symptoms come back (recur) after such treatment: IV morphine 1–5 mg is given every 5 to 30 minutes until the pain is controlled. Limiting factors include patient intolerance or excessive lowering of blood pressure. For general intravenous pain relief (analgesia): 2–10 mg given over 4–5 minutes. Repeat dosing is guided by pain control goals and patient effects. In sickle cell crisis some clinicians have used Patient Controlled Analgesia with or without a constant IV infusion. Constant infusions of 10 to 75 mg per hour were detailed in one case study where the patient had not responded to IV injections. PCA dosing usually combines a loading dose (determined by patient weight, pain being treated and other individual factors) and subsequent patient administered doses (usually a lesser amount than the loading dose with a lock out interval [such as fifteen minutes] to allow for the peak effect of the prior dose to be reached before another dose is given.

By mouth (regular solution, syrup and tablets)—5 to 30 mg every 4 hours.

By mouth (sustained-release forms)—30 mg every 12 hours.

By mouth (Kadian brand extended sustained-release form)—once daily. Dosing here is usually made after pain relief requirements are defined by an immediate-release form of morphine.

By suppository—10 to 30 mg every 4 hours.

Over 60 Years of Age: Same as 12 to 60 years of age, using smaller doses to start. Dose is slowly increased if needed. Many clinicians treat constipation in this age group once the morphine is started.

Author's Note: Current pain treatment theory calls for timed or scheduled dosing. This tends to prevent pain, rather than allowing pain to recur and then having to be treated. Some clinicians will use timed dosing immediately after surgery and then change to regular pain assessment with Patient Controlled Analgesia (PCA), then to regular pain assessment with oral dosing once the most severe period of pain has passed. Pain is now the fifth vital sign.

Conditions Requiring Dosing Adjustments

Liver Function: The dose and frequency **must** be adjusted (decreased) with liver compromise. This medicine is removed (metabolized) by the liver to morphine-6-glucuronide.

Kidney Function: Dose and frequency are prudently reduced in kidney compromise.

▷ **Dosing Instructions:** The regular tablet may be crushed and taken with or following food to reduce stomach irritation or nausea. Sustained-release forms should be swallowed whole; do not break, crush or chew it. Oral liquid may be mixed with fruit juice to improve taste. If you forget a dose: Take the missed dose as soon as you remember it, unless it's nearly time for your next dose—if that is the case, skip the missed dose and take the next dose right on schedule. DO NOT double doses. Talk with your doctor if you find yourself missing doses.

Usual Duration of Use: Used to control pain, hence the duration will be determined by the source of the pain. For short-term, self-limiting conditions, continual use should not exceed 5 to 7 days without interruption and reassessment of need. For the long-term management of severe chronic pain, it is advisable to determine an optimal fixed dose with rescue dose contingency schedule. It is not unusual for additional (adjuvant) medicines such as those usually used for seizures or for depression to be combined with morphine in chronic pain situations.

Typical Treatment Goals and Measurements (Outcomes and Markers)

Pain: Most clinicians treating pain use a device called an algometer to check your pain. This looks like a small ruler, but lets the clinician better understand your pain. The goals of treatment then relate to where the level of pain started (for example, a rating of 7 on a zero to ten scale) and what the cause of the pain was. Pain medicines may also be used together (in combination) in order to get the best result or outcome. If your pain control is not acceptable to YOU (remember, in hospitals and outpatient settings, etc. pain control is a patient right and the fifth vital sign), call your doctor. It is not unusual to have an immediate release rescue dose available and then some percentage of previous day use added back to an extended-release form. Pain can be dynamic and adjustments are often required.

▷ **This Drug Should Not Be Taken If**
  • you had an allergic reaction to it previously.
  • you are having an acute attack of asthma.
  • you have a specific bowel problem (paralytic ileus).
  • you have acute respiratory depression.

▷ **Inform Your Physician Before Taking This Drug If**
  • you took a monoamine oxidase (MAO) type A inhibitor drug (see Drug Classes) in the last 14 days.
  • you are taking atropinelike drugs, antihypertensives, metoclopramide (Reglan) or zidovudine (AZT).
  • you are taking any other drugs that have a sedative effect.
  • you have a history of drug abuse or alcoholism.
  • you have impaired liver or kidney function.
  • you have prostate gland enlargement (see prostatism in Glossary).

- you have a history of asthma, emphysema, epilepsy, gallbladder disease or inflammatory bowel disease.
- you have a tendency toward constipation.
- you have a history of head injury or a seizure disorder.
- you have a history of sickle cell anemia.
- you have a history of low blood pressure.
- you plan to have surgery under general anesthesia in the near future.

Possible Side Effects (natural, expected and unavoidable drug actions)

Drowsiness, light-headedness, weakness, euphoria, dry mouth, urinary retention, dose-related constipation. Temperature changes. Miosis or pin-point pupils. Histamine release if morphine is injected too quickly.

▷ **Possible Adverse Effects** (unusual, unexpected and infrequent reactions)

If any of the following develop, consult your physician promptly for guidance.

Mild Adverse Effects

Allergic reactions: skin rash, hives, itching (especially if the intravenous form is injected too quickly).

Headache, dizziness, impaired concentration, sensation of drunkenness, confusion, depression, blurred or double vision—infrequent to frequent and may be dose-related.

Facial flushing, sweating, heart palpitation—possible.

Nausea, vomiting—possible and may be dose-related.

Spasm of the biliary tract—possible.

Urine retention—possible.

Serious Adverse Effects

Allergic reactions: swelling of throat or vocal cords, spasm of larynx or bronchial tubes—rare.

Hallucinations, psychosis—case reports.

Drop in blood pressure, causing severe weakness and fainting—possible.

Disorientation, hallucinations, unstable gait, tremor, muscle twitching—possible.

Drug-induced myasthenia gravis—case reports.

Respiratory depression—dose-related.

Seizures—possible.

▷ **Possible Effects on Sexual Function:** Reduced libido and/or potency.

Amenorrhea and disruption of ovulation—case reports.

▷ **Adverse Effects That May Mimic Natural Diseases or Disorders**

Paradoxical behavioral disturbances may suggest psychotic disorder.

Possible Effects on Laboratory Tests

Blood amylase and lipase levels: increased (natural side effects).

Liver function tests: increased liver enzymes (ALT/GPT, AST/GOT and alkaline phosphatase), increased bilirubin.

Urine screening tests for drug abuse: may be positive. (Test results depend upon amount of drug taken and testing method used.)

CAUTION

1. If you have asthma, chronic bronchitis or emphysema, excessive use of this drug may cause significant respiratory difficulty, thickening of bronchial secretions and suppression of coughing.

2. Taking this drug with atropinelike drugs can increase the risk of urinary retention and reduced intestinal function.
3. Constipation can be a serious problem, particularly in older patients (as bowel function tends to slow down). Many clinicians prescribe a medicine to promote bowel movements at the same time that morphine is prescribed.
4. Do not take this drug following acute head injury.

Precautions for Use

By Infants and Children: Use very cautiously in infants under 2 years of age because of their vulnerability to life-threatening respiratory depression. Watch for paradoxical excitement in this age group.

By Those Over 60 Years of Age: Small doses and short-term use are indicated. There may be increased risk of drowsiness, dizziness, unsteadiness, falling, urinary retention and constipation (often leading to fecal impaction).

▷ **Advisability of Use During Pregnancy**

Pregnancy Category: B or C. D if used long-term or in high doses at term. See Pregnancy Risk Categories at the back of this book.

Animal studies: Significant skeletal birth defects reported in mouse and hamster studies.

Human studies: Adequate studies of pregnant women are not available, but no significant increase in birth defects was found in 448 exposures to this drug.

Avoid during the first 3 months. Use sparingly and in small doses during the final 6 months only if clearly needed.

Advisability of Use If Breast-Feeding

Presence of this drug in breast milk: Yes.

Avoid drug or refrain from nursing.

Habit-Forming Potential: This drug can cause psychological and physical dependence (see Glossary).

Effects of Overdose: Marked drowsiness, dizziness, confusion, restlessness, depressed breathing, tremors, convulsions, stupor progressing to coma.

Possible Effects of Long-Term Use: Psychological and physical dependence, chronic constipation.

Suggested Periodic Examinations While Taking This Drug (at physician's discretion)

Ask the patient about his or her bowel habits.

▷ **While Taking This Drug, Observe the Following**

Foods: No restrictions.

Herbal Medicines or Minerals: Valerian and kava kava may interact additively (drowsiness). Avoid these combinations. St. John's wort can change (inducing or increasing) P450 3A4 enzymes, blunting the effects of morphine. Talk to your doctor BEFORE you combine any herbal medicines with morphine.

Beverages: No restrictions. May be taken with milk.

▷ *Alcohol:* Alcohol is best avoided. Opioid analgesics can intensify the intoxicating effects of alcohol and alcohol can intensify the depressant effects of opioids on brain function, breathing and circulation.

Tobacco Smoking: No interactions expected. I advise everyone to quit smoking.

Marijuana Smoking: Increase in drowsiness and pain relief; impairment of mental and physical performance.

▷ *Other Drugs*

Morphine may ***increase*** the effects of
* antihypertensives and cause excessive lowering of blood pressure.
* atropinelike drugs and increase the risk of constipation and urinary retention.
* metformin (Glucophage).
* other drugs with sedative effects.

Morphine may *decrease* the effects of
* metoclopramide (Reglan).

Morphine ***taken concurrently*** with
* benzodiazepines (see Drug Classes) may result in increased risk of respiratory depression.
* cimetidine (Tagamet) may result in morphine toxicity.
* fluoxetine (Prozac) may antagonize morphine's pain-relieving effect.
* hydroxyzine (Vistaril) can increase pain relief but carries the risk of increased respiratory depression.
* medicines that increase CYP 3A4 will blunt morphine benefits and those that inhibit or use 3A4 for removal from the body may increase morphine blood levels. Caution and dosing adjustments are prudent.
* metoclopramide (Reglan) may lead to increased morphine effects.
* monoamine oxidase (MAO) type A inhibitors (see Drug Classes) may cause the equivalent of an acute narcotic overdose: unconsciousness and severe depression of breathing, heart rate and circulation. A variation can be excitability, convulsions, high fever and rapid heart action.
* naltrexone (ReVia or Narcan) may lead to sudden withdrawal symptoms.
* phenothiazines (see Drug Classes) may cause excessive and prolonged depression of brain functions, breathing and circulation.
* rifampin (Rifater, others) may lower morphine benefits.
* ritonavir (Norvir) may lead to lower morphine benefits.
* tramadol (Ultram) may increase CNS side effects.
* trovafloxacin (Trovan) may blunt trovafloxacin benefits.
* zidovudine (AZT) may increase the toxicity of both drugs; avoid concurrent use.

▷ *Driving, Hazardous Activities:* This drug can impair mental alertness, judgment, reaction time and physical coordination. Avoid hazardous activities.

Aviation Note: The use of this drug ***is a disqualification*** for piloting. Consult a designated Aviation Medical Examiner.

Exposure to Sun: No restrictions.

Discontinuation: It is advisable to limit this drug to short-term use. Longer-term use requires gradual tapering (decreasing) of doses to minimize possible effects of withdrawal: body aches, fever, sweating, nervousness, trembling, weakness, runny nose, sneezing, rapid heart rate, nausea, vomiting, stomach cramps, diarrhea.

MUPIROCIN (myu PEER oh sin)

Introduced: 1987   **Class:** Antibiotic, topical   **Prescription:** USA: Yes
Controlled Drug: USA: No; Canada: No   **Available as Generic:** USA: No;
Canada: No
Brand Names: Bactroban, Bactroban Nasal

```
┌─────────────────────────────────────────────────────────────────┐
│                      BENEFITS versus RISKS                        │
│        Possible Benefits                    Possible Risks         │
│ EFFECTIVE TOPICAL TREATMENT    Skin irritation                    │
│   OF STAPHYLOCOCCUS AND                                           │
│   STREPTOCOCCUS SKIN                                              │
│   INFECTIONS                                                     │
│ EFFECTIVE ERADICATION OF                                         │
│   STAPHYLOCOCCUS AUREUS                                          │
│   FROM THE NOSE                                                  │
└─────────────────────────────────────────────────────────────────┘
```

▷ **Principal Uses**
   As a Single Drug Product: Uses currently included in FDA-approved labeling:
      (1) Used to treat skin infections caused by staphylococcal and streptococ-
      cal infections such as ecthyma or impetigo; (2) the intranasal form is
      specifically formulated to kill *Staphylococcus aureus* bacteria that have col-
      onized the nasal passages; (3) treats secondary skin infections caused by
      Strep or Staph; (4) treats skin lesions that are traumatic.
   Other (unlabeled) generally accepted uses: (1) Used in burns where resistant
      Staphylococcus aureus is causing infection; (2) helps prevent opportunistic
      infections of venous access devices, such as intravascular cannulas; (3)
      treats cellulitis caused by Gram-positive organisms; (4) has been used in
      some specific situations in skin surgery to prevent infections; (5) used to
      eradicate vaginal *Staphylococcus* infections.

How This Drug Works: Binds to an enzyme (isoleucyl transfer-RNA synthetase)
   and stops susceptible bacteria from being able to make critical proteins.

Available Dosage Forms and Strengths
         Intranasal form (Bactroban Nasal) — 2%
                  Topical cream — 2.15%
         Topical ointment (Bactroban) — 2%
      Topical ointment (Bactroban, Canada) — 20 mg/g

▷ **Recommended Dosage Ranges** (Actual dose and schedule must be determined
      for each patient individually.)
   Infants and Children: Cream (3 months to 16 years)—follow your pediatrician's
      recommendations.
      Nasal (children 12 or over)—one-half of the ointment from the single-use
      tube of mupirocin is applied into one nostril and the other half is applied
      to the second nostril, twice daily, in the morning and evening, for 5 con-
      secutive days.
   16 to 60 Years of Age: 2% ointment—apply three times daily for 5 to 14 days.
      Some more involved or extensive infections have been treated for longer
      periods. If the infection in question has not resolved after the initial course

of the ointment, the site should be evaluated by a physician and systemic antibiotics or other treatment considered.

2% topical cream—for traumatic skin infections caused by Strep pyogenes or Staph aureus, apply (small amount) three times daily for ten days.

Intranasal—one-half of the ointment from the single-use tube of mupirocin is applied into one nostril and the other half is applied to the second nostril, twice daily in the morning and evening for 5 consecutive days.

Over 60 Years of Age: Same as 16 to 60 years of age.

Conditions Requiring Dosing Adjustments

Liver Function: Little of this ointment is usually absorbed into the body. No guidelines exist for liver disease adjustments.

Kidney Function: A substance in this formulation (polyethylene glycol) may be toxic to the kidneys if the ointment is applied over an extensive burn or wound area.

▷ **Dosing Instructions:** This medicine should be applied as a thin film or as described by your doctor. Call your doctor if the condition has not improved or worsens during the course of treatment. Do **not** combine this medicine with other ointments or treatments unless your doctor has prescribed this approach. If you forget a dose: Apply the missed dose as soon as you remember it, unless it's nearly time for your next dose—if that is the case, skip the missed dose and apply the next dose right on schedule. Talk with your doctor if you find yourself missing doses.

Usual Duration of Use: Continual use on a regular schedule for several days is usually necessary to determine this drug's effectiveness in treating skin infections. Wounds not responding in three to five days must be evaluated by your doctor. Longer-term use requires physician evaluation.

Typical Treatment Goals and Measurements (Outcomes and Markers)

Staph colonization or other infection: The goal is to kill the colonizing or infecting organism. Markers for improvement include improvement in signs and symptoms of the infection or in the case of colonization—negative repeat cultures.

Possible Advantages of This Drug

Effective topical treatment of skin infections.

▷ **This Drug Should Not Be Taken If**
- you had an allergic reaction to any form of it previously.
- you have extensive burns or open wounds.

▷ **Inform Your Physician Before Taking This Drug If**
- several days have passed since this medicine was started and there has been no change or worsening of the wound.
- pain at the site of the infection increases.
- you are unsure how much to apply or how often to apply mupirocin.

Possible Side Effects (natural, expected and unavoidable drug actions)

Irritation at the site of infection caused by the polyethylene glycol component.

▷ **Possible Adverse Effects** (unusual, unexpected and infrequent reactions)

If any of the following develop, consult your physician promptly for guidance.

Mild Adverse Effects
   Allergic reactions: skin rash and irritation at the infection site.
   Soreness, stinging or pain at the infection site—possible.
   Headache or taste changes—infrequent (intranasal only).
Serious Adverse Effects
   Allergic reactions: not defined, as the medicine is not appreciably absorbed.
   If this medicine is applied to an extensive skin area, polyethylene glycol may
      be absorbed and cause kidney toxicity—possible.

▷ **Possible Effects on Sexual Function:** Not reported.

Possible Delayed Adverse Effects: This medicine is indicated for short-term use.

▷ **Adverse Effects That May Mimic Natural Diseases or Disorders**
   None reported.

Natural Diseases or Disorders That May Be Activated by This Drug
   None reported.

Possible Effects on Laboratory Tests
   None reported.

CAUTION
   1. Do not apply this medicine to an area of skin larger than what your doc-
      tor prescribed.
   2. Because the Bactroban ointment uses a polyethylene glycol base and
      may cause irritation, the calcium mupirocin (Bactroban Nasal) is rec-
      ommended for intranasal use.

Precautions for Use
   By Infants and Children: Safety and effectiveness for use by some age groups
      varies with the product.
   By Those Over 60 Years of Age: No special changes are needed.

▷ **Advisability of Use During Pregnancy**
   Pregnancy Category: B. See Pregnancy Risk Categories at the back of this book.
   Animal studies: No fetal problems defined.
   Human studies: Information from adequate studies of pregnant women is not
      available.

Advisability of Use If Breast-Feeding
   Presence of this drug in breast milk: Unknown.
   Avoid drug or refrain from nursing.

Habit-Forming Potential: None.

Effects of Overdose: If this medicine is applied to an extensive area of skin,
   excessive amounts of polyethylene glycol may be absorbed and cause kidney toxicity.

Possible Effects of Long-Term Use: None defined.

Suggested Periodic Examinations While Taking This Drug (at physician's discretion)
   None.

▷ **While Taking This Drug, Observe the Following**
   Foods: No restrictions.
   Herbal Medicines or Minerals: Echinacea: Some patients use echinacea to
      attempt to boost their immune systems. Unfortunately, use of echinacea is
      not recommended in people with damaged immune systems. This herb

may also actually weaken any immune system if it is used too often or for too long a time. DO NOT take mistletoe herb, oak bark or F.C. of marshmallow root and licorice.

Beverages: No restrictions.

▷ *Alcohol:* No restrictions.

Tobacco Smoking: No interactions expected. I advise everyone to quit smoking.

▷ *Other Drugs*

Mupirocin *taken concurrently* with

* other medications that are toxic to the kidneys may result in additive kidney toxicity if mupirocin is applied to a large area of skin.

Aviation Note: The use of this drug *does not appear to be a restriction* for piloting. Consult a designated Aviation Medical Examiner.

Exposure to Sun: No restrictions.

NABUMETONE (na BYU me tohn)

Please see the acetic acid (nonsteroidal anti-inflammatory drug) family profile.

NADOLOL (NAY doh lohl)

Introduced: 1976   **Class:** Anti-anginal, antihypertensive, beta blocker
Prescription: USA: Yes   **Controlled Drug:** USA: No; Canada: No   **Available as Generic:** Yes
Brand Names: ❧Alti-Nadol ❧Apo-Nadol, Corgard, Corzide [CD], Syn-Nadol

BENEFITS versus RISKS	
Possible Benefits	*Possible Risks*
EFFECTIVE, WELL-TOLERATED ANTIHYPERTENSIVE for mild to moderate high blood pressure EFFECTIVE ANTI-ANGINAL DRUG IN CLASSICAL CORONARY ARTERY DISEASE with moderate to severe angina	CONGESTIVE HEART FAILURE in advanced heart disease Provocation of asthma (in predisposed patients) Masking of hypoglycemia in drug-dependent diabetes Worsening of angina following abrupt withdrawal

▷ **Principal Uses**

As a Single Drug Product: Uses currently included in FDA-approved labeling: (1) Treats moderate high blood pressure; (2) helps prevent attacks of effort-induced angina (should not be used in Prinzmetal's vasospastic angina).

Other (unlabeled) generally accepted uses: (1) Helps prevent hemorrhage from bulging veins (esophageal varices) in cirrhosis; (2) may have an adjunctive role in helping prevent and reduce migraine severity; (3) may have a role in helping prevent death after a heart attack (myocardial infarction); (4) may help ease tremor in patients taking lithium; (5) helps decrease risk of ruptured blood vessels in the esophagus (esophageal varices) in patients with cirrhosis.

As a Combination Drug Product [CD]: Available in combination with bendroflumethiazide, a diuretic antihypertensive drug. This combination product works better and is more convenient for long-term use.

How This Drug Works: By blocking certain actions of the sympathetic nervous system, this drug:
* reduces the rate and contraction force of the heart, lowering oxygen needs of heart muscle and reducing ejection pressure of blood leaving the heart. This reduces frequency of angina and lowers blood pressure.
* reduces contraction of blood vessel walls, lowering blood pressure.
* prolongs conduction time of nerve impulses through the heart, which is of benefit in the management of certain heart rhythm disorders.

Available Dosage Forms and Strengths
Tablets — 20 mg, 40 mg, 80 mg, 120 mg, 160 mg
Tablets, combination — 40 mg nadolol with 5 mg bendroflumethiazide, 80 mg with 5 mg bendroflumethiazide

▷ **Usual Adult Dosage Ranges:** *For hypertension:* Start with 40 mg daily; this may be increased gradually as needed and tolerated, up to 320 mg daily. The usual ongoing dose is 80 to 320 mg daily. Daily maximum is 320 mg.
For angina: Initially 40 mg daily; increased gradually at intervals of 3 to 7 days up to 240 mg daily. Usual ongoing dose is 80 to 240 mg every 24 hours. Daily maximum is 240 mg of nadolol. **Note: Actual dose and schedule must be determined for each patient individually.**

Conditions Requiring Dosing Adjustments
Liver Function: No dosing changes needed.
Kidney Function: For patients with moderate kidney failure, the usual dose should be taken every 24 to 36 hours. For patients with severe kidney failure, the dose can be taken every 40 to 60 hours.

▷ **Dosing Instructions:** The tablet may be crushed and taken without regard to eating. Do not stop this drug abruptly. If you forget a dose: Take the missed dose as soon as you remember it, unless it's 8 hours or less until your next scheduled dose—if that is the case, skip the missed dose and take the next dose right on schedule. Talk with your doctor if you find yourself missing doses.

Usual Duration of Use: Use on a regular schedule for 10 to 14 days determines this drug's effectiveness in lowering blood pressure and preventing angina. The long-term use of this drug (months to years) will be determined by your response to an overall treatment program (weight reduction, salt restriction, smoking cessation, etc.). Keep follow-up appointments with your doctor.

Typical Treatment Goals and Measurements (Outcomes and Markers)
Blood pressure: The most recent treatment guidelines (JNC VI) actually define optimal blood pressure (BP) as less than 120/80 and high normal as 139/89. The American Diabetes Association has chosen a target of 130/80 as the blood pressure goal for people living with diabetes. Most clinicians try to achieve a BP that achieves the best balance of lower cardiovascular risk while avoiding the problem of too low a blood pressure. The goal and time frame (see peak benefits above) should be discussed with you when the prescription is written.

Possible Advantages of This Drug

Does not reduce blood flow to the kidney. Can be used with other drugs that may reduce blood flow to the kidney (such as most anti-inflammatory aspirin substitutes). May be taken without regard to meals. Once-daily dosing encourages patients to take their medicine (adherence). May have positive effects on lipid peroxidation which then could block processes leading to atherosclerosis.

▷ **This Drug Should Not Be Taken If**
- you have had an allergic reaction to it previously.
- you have congestive heart failure.
- you have an abnormally slow heart rate or a serious form of heart block.
- you have bronchial asthma.
- you are taking, or have taken within the past 14 days, any monoamine oxidase (MAO) type A inhibitor drug (see Drug Classes).

▷ **Inform Your Physician Before Taking This Drug If**
- you have had an adverse reaction to any beta blocker (see Drug Classes).
- you have a history of serious heart disease.
- you have a history of hay fever (allergic rhinitis), asthma, chronic bronchitis or emphysema.
- you have a history of overactive thyroid function (hyperthyroidism).
- you have a history of low blood sugar (hypoglycemia).
- you have impaired liver or kidney function.
- you have diabetes or myasthenia gravis.
- you are pregnant or breast-feeding your infant.
- you have difficulty with blood circulation to the periphery (peripheral vascular disease).
- you are currently taking any form of digitalis, quinidine or reserpine or any calcium-channel-blocker drug (see Drug Classes).
- you will have surgery with general anesthesia.

Possible Side Effects (natural, expected and unavoidable drug actions)

Lethargy and fatigability, cold extremities, slow heart rate, light-headedness in upright position (see orthostatic hypotension in Glossary).

▷ **Possible Adverse Effects** (unusual, unexpected and infrequent reactions)

If any of the following develop, consult your physician promptly for guidance.

Mild Adverse Effects

Allergic reactions: skin rash, itching, drug fever.

Headache, dizziness, vivid dreaming, visual disturbances, ringing in ears, slurred speech, paresthesias—case reports to infrequent.

Hair loss and sweating—case reports to infrequent.

Cough, indigestion, nausea, vomiting, diarrhea, abdominal pain—infrequent.

Increased blood potassium—possible.

Numbness and tingling of extremities—case reports.

Serious Adverse Effects

Allergic reactions: facial swelling, anaphylaxis.

Chest pain, shortness of breath, precipitation of congestive heart failure—possible.

Intensification of heart block or severe slowing of the heart—case reports and may be dose-related.

Bronchospasm—rare.

Carpal tunnel syndrome or pancreatitis—case reports.

Induction of bronchial asthma (in asthmatic individuals)—possible and dose-related.

Masking of warning indications of acute hypoglycemia in drug-treated diabetes—possible.

May precipitate cramping when walking (intermittent claudication)—possible.

Excessively low blood pressure—possible.

▷ **Possible Effects on Sexual Function:** Decreased libido, impotence, impaired erection—case reports to frequent.

▷ **Adverse Effects That May Mimic Natural Diseases or Disorders**

Impaired circulation to the extremities may resemble Raynaud's phenomenon.

Natural Diseases or Disorders That May Be Activated by This Drug

Bronchial asthma, Prinzmetal's variant (vasospastic) angina, latent Raynaud's disease, myasthenia gravis (questionable).

Possible Effects on Laboratory Tests

Blood HDL cholesterol level: decreased.

Blood VLDL cholesterol level: increased.

Blood triglyceride levels: increased.

CAUTION

1. ***Do not stop this drug suddenly*** without the knowledge and help of your doctor. Carry a note stating that you are taking this drug.
2. Ask your physician or pharmacist before using nasal decongestants, which are usually present in over-the-counter cold preparations and nose drops. These can cause rapid blood pressure increases when combined with beta-blocker drugs.
3. Report the development of any tendency to emotional depression.

Precautions for Use

By Infants and Children: Safety and effectiveness for those under 12 years of age are not established. However, if this drug is used, observe for the development of low blood sugar (hypoglycemia) during periods of reduced food intake.

By Those Over 60 Years of Age: Unacceptably high blood pressure should be reduced without creating the risks associated with excessively low blood pressure. Small doses and frequent blood pressure checks are needed. Sudden, rapid and excessive reduction of blood pressure can predispose to stroke or heart attack. Watch for dizziness, unsteadiness, tendency to fall, confusion, hallucinations, depression or urinary frequency.

▷ **Advisability of Use During Pregnancy**

Pregnancy Category: C. See Pregnancy Risk Categories at the back of this book.

Animal studies: No significant increase in birth defects due to this drug, but embryotoxicity reported in rabbits.

Human studies: Adequate studies of pregnant women are not available. Avoid use during the first 3 months if possible. Use this drug only if clearly needed. Ask your physician for guidance.

Advisability of Use If Breast-Feeding

Presence of this drug in breast milk: Yes, in large amounts.

Avoid drug or refrain from nursing.

Habit-Forming Potential: None.

Effects of Overdose: Weakness, slow pulse, low blood pressure, fainting, cold and sweaty skin, congestive heart failure, possible coma and convulsions.

Possible Effects of Long-Term Use: Reduced heart reserve and eventual heart failure in susceptible individuals with advanced heart disease.

Suggested Periodic Examinations While Taking This Drug (at physician's discretion)

Measurements of blood pressure.

Evaluation of heart function.

▷ **While Taking This Drug, Observe the Following**

Foods: Follow the diet your doctor prescribes. Avoid excessive salt intake.

Herbal Medicines or Minerals: Ginseng may increase blood pressure, blunting the benefits of this medicine. Hawthorn, saw palmetto, ma huang, goldenseal, yohimbe and licorice may also increase blood pressure. Calcium and garlic may help lower blood pressure. Indian snakeroot has a German Commission E monograph indication for hypertension—talk to your doctor. Eleuthero root and ephedra should be avoided by people living with hypertension.

Beverages: No restrictions. May be taken with milk.

▷ *Alcohol:* Use with caution. Alcohol may exaggerate this drug's ability to lower blood pressure and may increase its mild sedative effect.

Tobacco Smoking: Nicotine may reduce this drug's effectiveness. I advise everyone to quit smoking.

▷ *Other Drugs*

Nadolol may *increase* the effects of

- other antihypertensive drugs and cause excessive lowering of blood pressure; dose adjustments may be necessary.
- reserpine (Ser-Ap-Es, etc.) and cause sedation, depression, slowing of the heart rate and lowering of blood pressure.
- verapamil (Calan, Isoptin) or other calcium channel blockers (see Drug Classes) and cause excessive depression of heart function; monitor this combination closely.

Nadolol may *decrease* the effects of

- ritodrine (Yutopar), and may result in undesirable heart effects.
- theophyllines (Aminophyllin, Theo-Dur, etc.) and reduce their effectiveness in treating asthma.

Nadolol *taken concurrently* with

- amiodarone (Cordarone) can cause severe slowing of the heart and potentially stop the heart (cardiac arrest).
- antacids containing aluminum can block absorption of this medicine and lessen therapeutic nadolol effects.
- clonidine (Catapres) requires close monitoring for rebound high blood pressure if clonidine is withdrawn while nadolol is still being taken.
- digoxin (Lanoxin) may result in undesirable heart effects.
- dihydropyridine calcium channel blockers may result in undesirable heart effects (bradycardia) or excessively low blood pressure.
- epinephrine can cause serious hypertension and slowing of the heart and, should anaphylaxis occur, epinephrine resistance.
- ergot derivatives (see Drug Classes) can cause decreased blood flow to the extremities (peripheral ischemia).

- insulin requires close monitoring to avoid undetected hypoglycemia (see Glossary).
- lidocaine can lead to lidocaine toxicity (depressed heart function, cardiac arrest).
- oral antidiabetic drugs (see Drug Classes) can cause slowed recovery from any hypoglycemia that may occur.

The following drug may *decrease* the effects of nadolol:

- indomethacin (Indocin), and possibly other "aspirin substitutes" or NSAIDs, and may impair nadolol's antihypertensive effect.

▷ *Driving, Hazardous Activities:* Use caution until the full extent of drowsiness, lethargy and blood pressure change has been determined.

Aviation Note: The use of this drug *is a disqualification* for piloting. Consult a designated Aviation Medical Examiner.

Exposure to Sun: No restrictions.

Exposure to Heat: Caution is advised. Hot environments can lower blood pressure and exaggerate the effects of this drug.

Exposure to Cold: Caution is advised. Cold environments can enhance the circulatory deficiency in the extremities that may occur with this drug. The elderly should take precautions to prevent hypothermia (see Glossary).

Heavy Exercise or Exertion: Prudent to avoid exertion that produces light-headedness, excessive fatigue or muscle cramping.

Occurrence of Unrelated Illness: Fever can lower blood pressure, requiring dose decreases. Nausea or vomiting may interrupt dosing. Ask your doctor for help.

Discontinuation: Best not to stop this drug suddenly. Gradual lowering of doses over 2 to 3 weeks is recommended.

NAFARELIN (NAF a re lin)

Introduced: 1984   **Class:** Hormones, miscellaneous   **Prescription:**
USA: Yes   **Controlled Drug:** USA: No; Canada: No   **Available as**
Generic: USA: No
Brand Name: Synarel

BENEFITS versus RISKS	
Possible Benefits	*Possible Risks*
VERY EFFECTIVE TREATMENT OF ENDOMETRIOSIS (alternative to oophorectomy)	Symptoms of estrogen deficiency (during treatment)
	Masculinizing effects (during treatment)
	Loss of bone density
	White blood cell count lowering

▷ **Principal Uses**

As a Single Drug Product: Uses currently included in FDA-approved labeling: (1) Treats endometriosis: reduction in the size and activity of endometrial implants within the pelvis; relief of pelvic pain associated with menstruation; (2) also used to treat precocious puberty due to excessive production of gonadotropic hormones.

Other (unlabeled) generally accepted uses: (1) Intranasal dosing helps control abnormal hair growth in women; (2) can be injected below the skin (subcutaneously) to help benign prostatic hyperplasia; (3) may be used before surgery to help decrease size of some tumors (myomas); (4) low-dose use for in vitro fertilization.

How This Drug Works: Stimulates the pituitary gland to release two additional hormones that regulate production of estrogen by the ovaries. With continued use, estrogen levels suppress (by a feedback mechanism) ovary-stimulating hormones—thereby lowering estrogen levels. The implants of endometrium (from the lining of the uterus) that are attached to the pelvic wall are stimulated by the rise and fall of estrogen in menstruation. When this drug suppresses estrogen production, the displaced endometrial tissue (endometriosis) becomes dormant and the premenstrual and menstrual pain no longer occurs.

Available Dosage Forms and Strengths
Nasal solution (10-ml bottle) — 2 mg/ml

▷ **Usual Adult Dosage Ranges:** *Endometriosis:* Pregnancy MUST be excluded prior to starting therapy. Dosing starts with 400 mcg daily. Spray one dose of 200 mcg into one nostril in the morning and one dose of 200 mcg into the other nostril in the evening, 12 hours apart. Start dosing between days 2 and 4 of the menstrual cycle. If menstruation persists after 2 months of treatment, the dose may be increased to 800 mcg daily: one spray into each nostril (a total of two sprays, 400 mcg) in the morning and again in the evening.

Note: Actual dose and schedule must be determined for each patient individually.

Conditions Requiring Dosing Adjustments
Liver Function: No dosing changes needed.
Kidney Function: Specific guidelines are not available for dosing. Decreases may be needed in kidney compromise.

▷ **Dosing Instructions:** Carefully read and follow the patient instructions provided with this drug. The solution is to be sprayed directly into the nostrils; it is not to be swallowed. Time the start of therapy and daily dosing exactly as directed. A nasal decongestant (spray or drops) should not be used for at least 30 minutes after dosing with the nafarelin spray; earlier use could impair absorption of nafarelin. If you forget a dose: Take the missed dose as soon as you remember it, unless it's nearly time for your next dose—if that is the case, skip the missed dose and take the next dose right on schedule. DO NOT double doses. Talk with your doctor if you find yourself missing doses.

Usual Duration of Use: Regular use for 2 to 3 months usually determines benefits in easing endometriosis symptoms. The standard course of treatment is limited to 6 months. Safety data does not exist for re-treatment. If re-treatment is considered, a bone mineral density test is prudent.

Typical Treatment Goals and Measurements (Outcomes and Markers)
Endometriosis: The goal most gynecologists use is the resolution of active endometriosis lesions as well as patient relief from pelvic pain, difficulty having intercourse and painful menstruation (dysmenorrhea). A laboratory test (estradiol levels) can be used (when they go below 30 pg/ml) as a guide to expecting patient response.

Possible Advantages of This Drug

Causes fewer masculinizing effects than danazol. Less tendency than dana-zol to increase blood cholesterol levels. Unlike danazol, this drug does not cause abnormally low HDL cholesterol levels or abnormally high LDL cho-lesterol levels. Superb alternative to oophorectomy.

Currently a Drug of Choice

For management of symptoms associated with endometriosis.

▷ **This Drug Should Not Be Taken If**

- you have had an allergic reaction to it previously.
- you are pregnant or breast-feeding.
- you have abnormal vaginal bleeding of unknown cause.

▷ **Inform Your Physician Before Taking This Drug If**

- you have used this drug, danazol or similar drugs previously.
- you are taking any type of estrogen, progesterone or oral contraceptive.
- you are planning pregnancy in the near future.
- you have a family history of osteoporosis.
- you use alcohol or tobacco regularly.
- you have a history of low white blood cells.
- you are using anticonvulsants or cortisonelike drugs.
- you are subject to allergic or infectious rhinitis and use nasal deconges-tants frequently.

Possible Side Effects (natural, expected and unavoidable drug actions)

Effects due to reduced estrogen production: hot flashes (90%), headaches, emotional lability, insomnia. Masculinizing effects: acne, muscle aches, fluid retention, increased skin oil, weight gain, excessive hair growth—rare.

▷ **Possible Adverse Effects** (unusual, unexpected and infrequent reactions)

If any of the following develop, consult your physician promptly for guidance.

Mild Adverse Effects

Allergic reactions: skin rash, hives—rare.

Nasal irritation—frequent.

Vaginal dryness—infrequent to frequent.

Depression—rare.

Hot flashes—when used in men with prostate problems (BPH).

Serious Adverse Effects

Loss of vertebral bone density: at completion of 6 months of treatment, bone density decreases an average of 8.7% and bone mass decreases an average of 4.3%; partial recovery during the post treatment period restores bone density loss to 4.9% and bone mass loss to 3.3%.

Lowering of the white blood cell count—case reports.

Transient prostate enlargement—possible.

Uterine bleeding—case report.

▷ **Possible Effects on Sexual Function:** Decreased libido, vaginal dryness, reduced breast size—infrequent to frequent.

Uterine bleeding—case reports.

Impotence occurred in most men who had used this drug for prostate prob-lems; hot flashes occurred in all of them.

Galactorrhea—case reports.

Natural Diseases or Disorders That May Be Activated by This Drug
Worsening or increased progression of osteoporosis.

Possible Effects on Laboratory Tests
Blood testosterone level: decreased in men with benign enlargement of prostate gland.
Blood estradiol: decreased.
Blood progesterone: decreased to less than 4 ng/ml.
Alkaline phosphatase: increased.
Serum estrone: decreased.

CAUTION
1. With continual use of this drug, menstruation will stop. If regular menstruation persists, call your doctor. Dose changes may be needed.
2. Use this drug consistently on a regular basis. Missed doses can result in breakthrough bleeding and ovulation.
3. It is advisable to avoid pregnancy during the course of treatment. Use a non-hormonal method of birth control; do not use oral contraceptives. Inform your physician promptly if you think you may be pregnant.
4. If you need to use nasal decongestant sprays or drops, delay their use for at least 30 minutes after the intranasal spray of nafarelin.

Precautions for Use
By Infants and Children: Safety and effectiveness for those under 18 years of age are not established.
By Those Over 60 Years of Age: If used for prostatism, impotence is a common side effect. Depression and hot flashes were also often reported.

▷ **Advisability of Use During Pregnancy**
Pregnancy Category: X. See Pregnancy Risk Categories at the back of this book.
Animal studies: Major fetal abnormalities and increased fetal deaths due to this drug have been demonstrated in rat studies.
Human studies: Adequate studies of pregnant women are not available.
Avoid this drug during entire pregnancy.

Advisability of Use If Breast-Feeding
Presence of this drug in breast milk: Unknown.
Avoid drug or refrain from nursing.

Habit-Forming Potential: None.

Effects of Overdose: No significant effects expected.

Possible Effects of Long-Term Use: Continual use should be limited to 6 months. If repeated courses of treatment are considered, bone mineral density testing is prudent.

Suggested Periodic Examinations While Taking This Drug (at physician's discretion)
Blood cholesterol and triglyceride profiles.
Bone density and mass measurements.

▷ **While Taking This Drug, Observe the Following**
Foods: No restrictions.
Herbal Medicines or Minerals: Black cohosh appears to work by: (1) suppressing luteinizing hormone; (2) binding to estrogen receptors in the pituitary and inhibiting luteinizing hormone release; and (3) binding to estrogen receptors in the pituitary. Talk to your doctor before starting black cohosh if you are currently taking nafarelin.

Beverages: No restrictions.

▷ *Alcohol:* No interactions expected.

Tobacco Smoking: No interactions expected. I advise everyone to quit smoking.

▷ *Other Drugs*

The following drugs will **decrease** the effects of nafarelin:
- birth control pills (oral contraceptives).
- estrogens.

▷ *Driving, Hazardous Activities:* No restrictions.

Aviation Note: The use of this drug **is not a disqualification** for piloting. Consult a designated Aviation Medical Examiner for confirmation.

Exposure to Sun: No restrictions.

Special Storage Instructions: Store in an upright position at room temperature. Protect from light.

Discontinuation: Normal ovarian function (ovulation, menstruation, etc.) is usually restored within 4 to 8 weeks after discontinuation of this drug.

NALTREXONE (nahl TREX ohn)

Introduced: 1995   **Class:** Antialcoholism, opioid antagonist   **Prescription:** USA: Yes   **Controlled Drug:** USA: No; Canada: No   **Available as Generic:** USA: Yes; Canada: Yes

Brand Names: Trexan, ReVia

Warning: This medication can cause liver damage if taken in excessive doses. If abdominal pain, white stools or yellowing of the eyes or skin occurs, call your doctor immediately.

BENEFITS versus RISKS

Possible Benefits	*Possible Risks*
CONTROL OF CRAVING FOR ALCOHOL	LIVER DAMAGE IF EXCESSIVE DOSES TAKEN
PART OF AN EFFECTIVE COMBINATION APPROACH TO ALCOHOLISM	
ONCE-DAILY DOSING	

▷ **Principal Uses**

As a Single Drug Product: Uses currently included in FDA-approved labeling: (1) Used as part of a comprehensive program to help alcohol dependence; (2) used to treat narcotic addiction.

Other (unlabeled) generally accepted uses: (1) May help women with a specific type of cessation of menstruation (hypothalamic amenorrhea); (2) helps itching in hemodialysis patients; (3) incidental reports from a detoxification program may yield a use for this drug in smoking cessation.

How This Drug Works: In narcotic addiction, this medicine antagonizes the effects of opioid medicines and blocks the perceived benefit of the drug to the addicted patient. In alcohol addiction, it may interfere with the body's own opioids that are released in response to drinking alcoholic beverages. If the effect of the body's own opioids (endogenous) is blocked, the craving for alcohol is then reduced.

Available Dosage Forms and Strengths
Tablets — 50 mg

▷ **Recommended Dosage Ranges** (Actual dose and schedule must be determined for each patient individually.)

Infants and Children: Not indicated.

18 to 60 Years of Age: 50 mg daily. The best results are gained when this medicine is used as part of a comprehensive approach to curbing alcohol use.

Over 60 Years of Age: Same as 18 to 60 years of age.

Conditions Requiring Dosing Adjustments

Liver Function: This drug is extensively metabolized in the liver and is contraindicated in acute hepatitis or liver failure.

Kidney Function: Metabolites of this drug are removed by the kidneys, but specific guidelines for dosing changes are not available.

▷ **Dosing Instructions:** If there is any question of opioid dependence, a Narcan challenge test must be performed. Naltrexone is almost completely absorbed after oral dosing. This medicine may be taken with or without food. If you forget a dose: Take the missed dose as soon as you remember it, unless it's nearly time for your next dose—if that is the case, skip the missed dose and take the next dose right on schedule. Talk with your doctor if you find yourself missing doses.

Usual Duration of Use: Continual use on a regular schedule for 12 weeks is usually necessary to determine this drug's effectiveness in treating alcoholism. This drug should be a part of a comprehensive alcohol treatment program. Long-term use (months to years) requires periodic evaluation of response and dose adjustment. Consult your physician on a regular basis.

Typical Treatment Goals and Measurements (Outcomes and Markers)

Alcohol or narcotic abuse: The general goal is to gain a patient defined (subjective) decrease in desire for alcohol or narcotics (opioids). Specific markers may include an alcohol abstinence diary or specific urine or blood tests for narcotics.

Possible Advantages of This Drug
Actually decreases the craving for alcohol.

▷ **This Drug Should Not Be Taken If**
- you had an allergic reaction to any form of it previously.
- you have liver failure or acute hepatitis.
- you are in opioid withdrawal.
- you are physically dependent on narcotics.

▷ **Inform Your Physician Before Taking This Drug If**
- you have a history of viral hepatitis.
- you are planning surgery or a diagnostic procedure requiring anesthesia.
- you are unsure how much to take or how often to take it.
- you take prescription or nonprescription medicines not discussed with your doctor when naltrexone was prescribed.

Possible Side Effects (natural, expected and unavoidable drug actions)
None.

▷ **Possible Adverse Effects** (unusual, unexpected and infrequent reactions)
If any of the following develop, consult your physician promptly for guidance.

Mild Adverse Effects
Allergic reactions: rash.
Oily skin, itching, hair loss—case reports.
Nosebleeds—possible.
Joint and muscle pain—infrequent to frequent.
Anorexia, weight loss, fatigue, anxiety, nervousness—case reports to frequent.
Sleep disturbances—infrequent.
Depression—case reports.
Serious Adverse Effects
Allergic reactions: none reported.
Idiosyncratic reactions: none reported.
Liver toxicity (hepatocellular injury)—case reports.
Precipitation of acute withdrawal syndrome in patients dependent on narcotics.
Suicidal ideation—case reports.
Abnormal platelet function (idiopathic thrombocytopenic purpura)—case reports.

▷ **Possible Effects on Sexual Function:** Delayed ejaculation—infrequent.

Possible Delayed Adverse Effects: None reported.

▷ **Adverse Effects That May Mimic Natural Diseases or Disorders**
Liver problems may mimic acute hepatitis.

Natural Diseases or Disorders That May Be Activated by This Drug
None.

Possible Effects on Laboratory Tests
Liver function tests: increased.
Gonadotropins (LH, FSH, ACTH, catecholamines and cortisol): increased.

CAUTION
1. The therapeutic dose and doses that can cause liver damage may be fairly close in some patients. Make certain that you understand how much to take and how often to take it.
2. Self-administration of any narcotic drug may be fatal.
3. If you are taking ongoing narcotic or opioid treatment for pain, this drug could precipitate an acute withdrawal syndrome.

Precautions for Use
By Infants and Children: Safety and effectiveness for use by those under 18 years of age have not been established.
By Those Over 60 Years of Age: None.

▷ **Advisability of Use During Pregnancy**
Pregnancy Category: C. See Pregnancy Risk Categories at the back of this book.
Animal studies: This drug has been shown to be embryocidal in rats and rabbits at roughly 140 times the typical human dose.
Human studies: Information from adequate studies of pregnant women is not available.
Ask your doctor for help with this benefit-to-risk decision.

Advisability of Use If Breast-Feeding
Presence of this drug in breast milk: Unknown.
Avoid drug or refrain from nursing.

Habit-Forming Potential: None.

Effects of Overdose: Human subjects who received over 800 mg daily for a week showed no adverse effects.

Possible Effects of Long-Term Use: None defined.

Suggested Periodic Examinations While Taking This Drug (at physician's discretion)

Liver function tests.

▷ **While Taking This Drug, Observe the Following**

Foods: No restrictions.

Herbal Medicines or Minerals: Ephedra or kola may worsen anxiety associated with abstaining from alcohol. Valerian or kava kava may ease anxiety or difficulty falling asleep, but has not been studied with naltrexone. Talk to your doctor BEFORE you add any herbal medicine.

Beverages: No restrictions.

▷ *Alcohol:* Obviously not recommended, as this medication is part of a combination approach to help problem drinkers.

Tobacco Smoking: No interactions expected. I advise everyone to quit smoking.

Marijuana Smoking: Should not be attempted.

▷ *Other Drugs*

Naltrexone *taken concurrently* with

- narcotic medicines may result in a severe reaction.
- other drugs that are toxic to the liver may result in increased risk of liver toxicity.
- thioridazine (Mellaril) may result in somnolence and lethargy.

▷ *Driving, Hazardous Activities:* This drug may cause fatigue. Restrict activities as necessary.

Aviation Note: Alcoholism *is a disqualification* for piloting. Consult a designated Aviation Medical Examiner.

Exposure to Sun: No restrictions.

Discontinuation: Do not stop this medicine without the knowledge of your doctor.

NAPROXEN (na PROX en)

Please see the propionic acid (nonsteroidal anti-inflammatory drug) family profile.

NATEGLINIDE (na TAG lyn ide)

Introduced: 2000 **Class:** Antidiabetic, D-phenylalanine derivative **Prescription:** USA: Yes **Controlled Drug:** USA: No; Canada: No **Available as Generic:** No
Brand Name: Starlix

```
┌─────────────────────────────────────────────────────────────┐
│                   BENEFITS versus RISKS                       │
│      Possible Benefits              Possible Risks            │
│  HELPS REGULATE BLOOD SUGAR    Hypoglycemia (less common than │
│  IN TYPE 2 DIABETES (adjunctive    sulfonylureas)             │
│  to appropriate diet and weight  Possible increased risk of heart │
│  control)                          (cardiovascular) problems (based │
│  MAY BE COMBINED WITH              on a 1970 UGDP study)      │
│  METFORMIN IF BLOOD SUGAR                                     │
│  CONTROL IS NOT ACCEPTABLE                                    │
│  Absorbed well and cleared quickly                            │
│  from the blood                                               │
└─────────────────────────────────────────────────────────────┘
```

▷ **Principal Uses**

    As a Single Drug Product: Uses currently included in FDA-approved labeling: (1) Type 2 diabetes mellitus (adult, maturity-onset) that does not require insulin but can't be adequately controlled by diet alone; (2) combination treatment with metformin in people who do not have an adequate blood sugar response from nateglinide alone.

    Other (unlabeled) generally accepted uses: None.

    Author's Note: Information in this profile will be broadened if additional data support inclusion in the Essential Guide.

NEDOCROMIL (na DOK ra mil)

Introduced: 1992   **Class:** Antiasthmatic, preventive   **Prescription:** USA: Yes   **Controlled Drug:** USA: No; Canada: No   **Available as Generic:** USA: No; Canada: No

Brand Names: Alocril, Tilade, Tilade Nebulizer Solution

```
┌─────────────────────────────────────────────────────────────┐
│                   BENEFITS versus RISKS                       │
│      Possible Benefits              Possible Risks            │
│  EFFECTIVE PREVENTION OF       Acute bronchospasm—rare        │
│  RECURRENT ASTHMA              Taste disorder                 │
│  Prevention of exercise-induced                               │
│  asthma                                                       │
└─────────────────────────────────────────────────────────────┘
```

▷ **Principal Uses**

    As a Single Drug Product: Uses currently included in FDA-approved labeling: (1) Ongoing therapy of mild to moderate asthma; (2) steroid-sparing effect that may allow reduction or elimination of oral steroids; (3) helps manage asthmatic bronchitis; (4) eases allergic conjunctivitis.

    Other (unlabeled) generally accepted uses: (1) May have a role in helping ease allergic rhinitis; (2) can help vernal conjunctivitis when instilled as an eyedrop; (3) may help exercise-induced asthma.

How This Drug Works: Inhibits release of inflammatory chemical mediators such as histamine, prostaglandins and leukotrienes that constrict the bronchi and cause inflammation seen in acute asthma.

Available Dosage Forms and Strengths

Inhaler — 16.2-g canister

Ophthalmic solution — 2%

Solution for inhalation — 1.75 and 2 mg per actuation

▷ **Recommended Dosage Ranges** (Actual dose and schedule must be determined for each patient individually.)

Infants and Children: See dosing below.

6 to 60 Years of Age:

Asthma Inhaler: Two puffs (inhalations) four times daily, to provide a total of 14 mg per day.

Allergic conjunctivitis: Ophthalmic: one to two drops in each eye twice daily.

Over 60 Years of Age: Same as 6 to 60 years of age.

Conditions Requiring Dosing Adjustments

Liver Function: Adjustments in dose in liver compromise are not defined.

Kidney Function: Adjustments in dose in kidney compromise are not defined.

▷ **Dosing Instructions:** Follow the instructions on the leaflet provided in the medication box carefully. Nedocromil use must be continued, even when you are symptom-free. If you forget a dose: Use the missed dose as soon as you remember it, unless it's nearly time for your next dose—if that is the case, skip the missed dose and use the next dose right on schedule. Take the remaining doses for the day at evenly spaced intervals and then return to your regular schedule. DO NOT double doses. Talk with your doctor if you find yourself missing doses.

Usual Duration of Use: Use on a regular schedule for a week usually determines effectiveness in helping prevent acute asthma. Use during the allergy season determines benefits in controlling patient reaction to prevalent seasonal allergens. Long-term use (months to years) requires periodic physician evaluation of response and dose adjustment.

Typical Treatment Goals and Measurements (Outcomes and Markers)

Asthma: The frequency of asthma attacks as well as the severity of asthma attacks that occur (such as those requiring an emergency department visit) are a benchmark of effectiveness. Some clinicians also use the number of times a rescue inhaler must be used as a clinical fine point. Goals should be communicated and checked.

Possible Advantages of This Drug: Usually well tolerated. Rare serious adverse effects.

▷ **This Drug Should Not Be Taken If**

- you had an allergic reaction to it previously.
- you are having an acute asthma attack.

▷ **Inform Your Physician Before Taking This Drug If**

- you have impaired kidney function.
- you have angina or a heart rhythm disorder.
- you must wear contacts and have been prescribed the ophthalmic form (contacts should not be worn while you have allergic conjunctivitis).
- you are unsure how much to take or how often to take nedocromil.

Possible Side Effects (natural, expected and unavoidable drug actions)

Unpleasant taste. Mild throat irritation or hoarseness. May be lessened by a few swallows of water after each inhalation.

Eye irritation or nasal congestion: infrequent to frequent with Alocril form.

▷ **Possible Adverse Effects** (unusual, unexpected and infrequent reactions)

If any of the following develop, consult your physician promptly for guidance.

Mild Adverse Effects

Allergic reactions: skin rash, hives.

Headache, dizziness—rare to infrequent (headache may be frequent with Alocril).

Unpleasant taste or cough—infrequent to frequent.

Nausea or vomiting—infrequent.

Serious Adverse Effects

Allergic reactions: anaphylactic reaction, allergic pneumonitis (allergic reaction of the lung tissue).

Bronchospasm—case reports.

▷ **Possible Effects on Sexual Function:** None reported.

Possible Delayed Adverse Effects: Pneumonitis—case reports.

Possible Effects on Laboratory Tests: Liver function tests: increased ALT.

CAUTION

1. This drug does **not** act as a bronchodilator and should not be used for immediate relief of acute asthma.
2. If use of this drug has allowed you to stop taking a cortisone-related drug, you may need to resume the cortisone-related drug if you are injured, must stop taking nedocromil, have an infection or need surgery.
3. If severe asthma returns, contact your doctor promptly.
4. If you use a bronchodilator drug by inhalation, it is best to take it about 5 minutes before inhaling nedocromil.

Precautions for Use

By Infants and Children: Safety and effectiveness for those under 12 years of age are not established.

By Those Over 60 Years of Age: This drug does not work in therapy of chronic bronchitis or emphysema.

▷ **Advisability of Use During Pregnancy**

Pregnancy Category: B. See Pregnancy Risk Categories at the back of this book.

Animal studies: Rat, mouse and rabbit studies show no impairment of fertility or harm to the fetus.

Human studies: Adequate studies of pregnant women are not available.

Ask your doctor for guidance.

Advisability of Use If Breast-Feeding

Presence of this drug in breast milk: Unknown.

Avoid drug or refrain from nursing.

Habit-Forming Potential: None.

Effects of Overdose: Head shaking, tremor and salivation were seen in dogs given high doses.

Suggested Periodic Examinations While Taking This Drug (at physician's discretion)

Sputum analysis and X-ray if pneumonitis suspected.

Liver function tests.

▷ **While Taking This Drug, Observe the Following**
Foods: No restrictions.
Herbal Medicines or Minerals: If you are allergic to plants in the Asteraceae family (aster, chrysanthemum, daisy or ragweed), you may also be allergic to echinacea, chamomile, feverfew and St. John's wort. Fir or pine needle oil should NOT be used by asthmatics. Ephedra alone does carry a German Commission E monograph indication for asthma treatment. Talk to your doctor.
Beverages: Avoid all beverages to which you may be allergic.
▷ *Alcohol:* No interaction expected.
Tobacco Smoking: No interaction expected. I advise everyone to quit smoking.
▷ *Other Drugs:* There are no known adverse drug interactions at present. Nedocromil may make it possible to reduce the dose or frequency of use of cortisonelike drugs. Ask your doctor for guidance.
▷ *Driving, Hazardous Activities:* This drug may cause dizziness. Restrict activities as necessary.
Aviation Note: The use of this drug *may be a disqualification* for piloting. Consult a designated Aviation Medical Examiner.
Exposure to Sun: No restrictions.
Heavy Exercise or Exertion: This drug may enable you to partake in exercise. Ask your doctor for guidance.
Discontinuation: If this drug has made it possible to reduce or stop cortisonelike drugs and you must stop nedocromil, you may have to resume the cortisonelike drug as well as other measures to control asthma.

NEFAZODONE (na FAZ oh dohn)

Introduced: 1994　**Class.** Antidepressant　**Prescription:** USA:　Yes
Controlled Drug: USA: No; Canada: No　**Available as Generic:** USA: No; Canada: No
Brand Names: ♣Lin-Nefazodone, Serzone

BENEFITS versus RISKS	
Possible Benefits	*Possible Risks*
EFFECTIVE TREATMENT OF DEPRESSION	Dizziness
Fewer cardiovascular side effects than older agents	Mild blood pressure changes on standing
Minimal anticholinergic side effects	
Decreased sedation versus other medicines used for depression	

▷ **Principal Uses**
As a Single Drug Product: Uses currently included in FDA-approved labeling: Treatment of major depression.
Other (unlabeled) generally accepted uses: (1) May have a role in pain management; (2) successfully treated panic disorder in one case.
How This Drug Works: This antidepressant is unique because it:
- blocks the reuptake of a specific nerve-transmitting chemical (5-HT).
- acts as a 5-HT2 antagonist.

Because of this unique mechanism of action, this drug has fewer cardiovascular and anticholinergic side effects than previously available agents.

Available Dosage Forms and Strengths

Tablets — 100 mg, 150 mg, 200 mg, 250 mg

Tablets (Canada only) — 300 mg

▷ **Recommended Dosage Ranges** (Actual dose and schedule must be determined for each patient individually.)

Infants and Children: Not indicated.

18 to 60 Years of Age: Starting dose is 200 mg daily, taken as 100 mg in the morning and 100 mg in the evening. Dose is increased as needed and tolerated in 100-mg increments (1 week between dose changes). Daily maximum is 600 mg.

Over 60 Years of Age: Dosing in this population starts with 100 mg daily (50 mg twice a day). The medicine is then increased (at a slower rate than in younger patients) as needed and tolerated.

Conditions Requiring Dosing Adjustments

Liver Function: The dose should be decreased for patients with liver compromise.

Kidney Function: No specific dosing changes are presently identified.

▷ **Dosing Instructions:** Food delays the absorption and decreases total absorption, but this effect is not believed to be clinically significant. Water is expected to be the safest liquid to take this medicine with. Grapefruit juice may have an action on some liver enzymes (cytochrome P450) that help remove (metabolize) this medicine. Avoid taking with grapefruit juice. If you forget a dose: Take the missed dose as soon as you remember it, unless it's nearly time for your next dose—if that is the case, skip the missed dose and take the next dose right on schedule. Talk with your doctor if you find yourself missing doses.

Usual Duration of Use: Continual use on a regular schedule for a week will often show some benefits. 4 to 5 weeks usually determines peak effectiveness in treating depression. Long-term use (months to years) requires periodic evaluation of response, dose adjustment and physician follow-up.

Typical Treatment Goals and Measurements (Outcomes and Markers)

Depression: The general goal: to at least help lessen the degree and severity of depression, letting patients return to their daily lives. Specific measures of depression involve testing or inventories (such as the Hamilton Depression) and can be valuable in helping check benefits from this medicine.

Possible Advantages of This Drug

Two different mechanisms of action and decreased side effects versus older TCA type drugs.

▷ **This Drug Should Not Be Taken If**
- you had an allergic reaction to it previously.
- you are taking astemizole, cisapride or terfenadine.
- you are taking an MAO inhibitor (see Drug Classes).

▷ **Inform Your Physician Before Taking This Drug If**
- you take a triazolobenzodiazepine, such as triazolam or alprazolam.
- you have a history of seizure disorder.
- you have a history of heart disease.
- you are unsure how much to take or how often to take it.

- you take other medicines that were not discussed with your doctor when nefazodone was prescribed.

Possible Side Effects (natural, expected and unavoidable drug actions)

Dry mouth, blurred vision or constipation. Lowered blood pressure on standing (postural hypotension).

▷ **Possible Adverse Effects** (unusual, unexpected and infrequent reactions)

If any of the following develop, consult your physician promptly for guidance.

Mild Adverse Effects

Allergic reactions: skin rash.

Nausea—infrequent to frequent.

Ringing in the ears—possible.

Headache, dizziness and tremor—infrequent.

Insomnia, confusion and agitation—rare.

Slowed heart rate—case report.

Serious Adverse Effects

Allergic reactions: not defined.

Idiosyncratic reactions: not identified.

Activation of mania—one case report.

Low blood sugar (hypoglycemia)—case reports.

Seizures—rare.

Subacute liver failure—case reports.

▷ **Possible Effects on Sexual Function:** Impotence, absence of orgasm or abnormal ejaculation have all been rarely reported. Priapism has been reported with a structurally similar drug.

Possible Delayed Adverse Effects: None reported.

▷ **Adverse Effects That May Mimic Natural Diseases or Disorders**

Liver toxicity may mimic hepatitis B.

Natural Diseases or Disorders That May Be Activated by This Drug

None reported.

Possible Effects on Laboratory Tests

None reported.

CAUTION

1. Risk of suicide is present in depressed patients. Small quantities of this medicine should be dispensed at a time when therapy is started. Appropriate suicide precautions should be taken.

2. This medicine **must not** be taken with a MAO inhibitor; there MUST be an interval of 14 days between when a MAO inhibitor is stopped and nefazodone is started.

Precautions for Use

By Infants and Children: Safety and effectiveness for use by those under 18 years of age have not been established.

By Those Over 60 Years of Age: Lower starting doses and more gradual increases in dose are indicated.

▷ **Advisability of Use During Pregnancy**

Pregnancy Category: C. See Pregnancy Risk Categories at the back of this book.

Animal studies: Increased rat pup mortality was seen when doses five times the typical human dose were used.

Human studies: Information from adequate studies of pregnant women is not available.

Ask your doctor for guidance.

Advisability of Use If Breast-Feeding

Presence of this drug in breast milk: Unknown.

Avoid drug or refrain from nursing.

Habit-Forming Potential: None defined at present, but not expected.

Effects of Overdose: Nausea, vomiting and somnolence.

Possible Effects of Long-Term Use: None reported.

Suggested Periodic Examinations While Taking This Drug (at physician's discretion)

Periodic checks of heart rate.

Liver function tests as indicated.

▷ **While Taking This Drug, Observe the Following**

Foods: No restrictions.

Herbal Medicines or Minerals: Since nefazodone and St. John's wort may act to increase serotonin, the combination is not advised. St. John's wort may also worsen sensitivity to the sun. Since part of the way ginseng works may be as a MAO inhibitor, do not combine ginseng with nefazodone. Indian snakeroot, ma huang and yohimbe are also best avoided while taking this medicine. Kava and valerian may worsen drowsiness. The FDA has allowed one dietary supplement called Cholestin to continue to be sold. This preparation actually contains lovastatin. Since use of an HMG-CoA inhibitor with nefazodone may increase risk of rhabdomyolysis or myopathy, the combination is NOT advised.

Beverages: Grapefruit juice may lead to toxicity. DO NOT combine.

▷ *Alcohol:* This combination is not recommended.

Tobacco Smoking: No interactions expected. I advise everyone to quit smoking.

Marijuana Smoking: Increased somnolence.

▷ *Other Drugs*

Nefazodone may ***increase*** the effects of

- alprazolam (Xanax) and potentially other benzodiazepines (see Drug Classes).
- carbamazepine (Tegretol).
- cisapride (Propulsid), leading to possible heart toxicity.
- digoxin (Lanoxin); increased blood level checks are suggested.
- dofetilide (Tikosyn); increased blood level checks are suggested.
- flecainide (Tambocor); blood level checks are prudent.
- haloperidol (Haldol).
- imipramine (Tofranil).
- tacrolimus (Prograf); increased blood level checks are suggested.
- triazolam (Halcion).

Nefazodone ***taken concurrently*** with

- acebutolol (Sectral) and perhaps other beta blockers may result in decreased acebutolol levels and increased nefazodone metabolites.
- astemizole (Hismanal) can cause serious heart toxicity.
- atorvastatin, lovastatin, simvastatin and other HMG-CoA reductase inhibitors (see Drug Classes) may increase risk of muscle damage if combined with nefazodone.

- buspirone (Buspar) resulted in liver enzyme increases with a similar drug (trazodone).
- clozapine (Clozaril) may result in clozapine toxicity since the P450 system in the liver is involved in removing clozapine from the liver.
- cyclosporine (Sandimmune) may result in cyclosporine toxicity. Dosing adjustments may be needed.
- dextromethorphan (in cough medicines with DM on the label) may result in dextromethorphan toxicity since the P450 system in the liver is involved in removing dextromethorphan from the liver.
- MAO inhibitors (see Drug Classes) may cause serious toxicity—DO NOT COMBINE.
- phenytoin (Dilantin) or fosphenytoin (Cerebyx) may result in increased phenytoin or fosphenytoin levels; more frequent blood level checks are needed, and dosing should be adjusted to blood level results.
- ritonavir (Norvir) may lead to toxicity.
- rizatriptan (Maxalt) and other triptans (see Antimigraine Drugs) may lead to loss of coordination, weakness and reflex problems.
- sibutramine (Meridia) increases risk of serotonin syndrome—COMBINATION IS NOT RECOMMENDED.
- terfenadine (Seldane) may cause serious heart rhythm problems.
- tricyclic antidepressants (see Drug Classes) may result in increased tricyclic antidepressant levels and toxicity.
- tryptophan (various) may lead to toxicity.

▷ *Driving, Hazardous Activities:* This drug may cause somnolence. Restrict activities as necessary.

Aviation Note: The use of this drug *is a disqualification* for piloting. Consult a designated Aviation Medical Examiner.

Exposure to Sun: Use caution—photosensitivity is possible.

Discontinuation: Do not stop this medication without discussing this with your doctor.

NEOSTIGMINE (nee oh STIG meen)

Introduced: 1931   **Class:** Antimyasthenic   **Prescription:** USA: Yes
Controlled Drug: USA: No; Canada: No   **Available as Generic:** USA: Yes; Canada: Yes
Brand Names: ❧PMS-Neostigmine, Prostigmin, Viaderm-K.C.

BENEFITS versus RISKS	
Possible Benefits	*Possible Risks*
MODERATELY EFFECTIVE TREATMENT OF OCULAR AND MILD FORMS OF MYASTHENIA GRAVIS (symptomatic relief of muscle weakness) Eases postoperative bowel slowing or block (paralytic ileus)	Cholinergic crisis (overdose): excessive salivation, nausea, vomiting, stomach cramps, diarrhea, shortness of breath (asthmalike wheezing), weakness.

Author's Note: This profile has been shortened to make room for more widely used medicines.

NEURAMIDASE INHIBITOR FAMILY (Nur AM ih dayce)

Oseltamivir   (Oss uhl TAM ih veer)   **Zanamivir**   (Zah NAM ih veer)
Introduced: 1999   **Class:** Antiviral, anti-influenza   **Prescription:** USA:
Yes   **Controlled Drug:**   USA: No; Canada: No   **Available as Generic:**
USA: No; Canada: No
Brand Names: Oseltamivir: Tamiflu, Zanamivir: Relenza

BENEFITS versus RISKS	
Possible Benefits	*Possible Risks*
DECREASED COMPLICATIONS FROM TYPE A OR B FLU (INFLUENZA) DECREASED FLU SEVERITY	Triggering of bronchospasm by zanamivir (may be more likely in those with underlying airway diseases)

▷ **Principal Uses**

As a Single Drug Product: Uses currently included in FDA-approved labeling:
(1) Treatment or prevention of type A or B influenza in people 13 or older
(for oseltamivir) or people 7 or older (for zanamivir).

Other (unlabeled) generally accepted uses: (1) oseltamivir reduced complications (secondary) from the flu in one study.

How These Drugs Work: These medicines preferentially inhibit a critical chemical
called neuramidase in type A or B flu (influenza) viruses. When neuramidase
is blocked, newly formed virus is not released from infected cells (because
sialic acid cleavage is inhibited from cell surface glycoconjugates) and the
flu virus is kept from spreading across the respiratory tract (mucous lining).

Available Dosage Forms and Strengths

Oseltamivir:
Capsule — 75 mg
Suspension — see dosing in mg per ml to get the total dose needed

Zanamivir:
Dry powder inhaler — 5 mg per inhalation

▷ **Usual Adult Dosage Ranges:**

Oseltamivir: Adults: 75 mg is taken twice a day (BID) for 5 days. Best if started
within 24 hours of flu symptoms (up to 48 hours still confers benefits). For
the new suspension form: children as young as one year old may take
30–75 mg twice a day for 5 days.

Prophylaxis: 75 mg once daily for six weeks during local disease activity was
effective in one study.

Zanamivir: Treatment of adults or children more than 7 years old: Two doses
are used on the first day that this medicine is started. Take the first dose
once you get the medicine, then wait at least two hours and inhale the second dose. Subsequently, take two inhalations (5 mg each, total 10 mg)
inhaled twice a day (12 hours apart) for a total of 5 days.

**Note: Actual dose and schedule must be determined for each patient
individually.**

Conditions Requiring Dosing Adjustments

Liver Function: No dosing changes currently thought to be needed.

Kidney Function: Oseltamivir: Must be carefully adjusted in people with kidney problems. Those with creatinine clearances of less than 30 ml/min should receive 75 mg daily for five days. Those with clearances less than 10 ml/min have not been studied and can not be recommended.

Zanamivir: This medicine is absorbed into the body (systemically) to a limited extent—therefore even though it is primarily removed by the kidneys, dosing changes probably are not needed.

▷ **Dosing Instructions:** May be taken with or following meals. Can open the oseltamivir capsule to take it. The new oseltamivir suspension should be shaken well before dosing and given using the dosing syringe to measure the correct dose. Zanamivir is used with a device called a Diskhaler. Make sure you understand how to use this product. If your symptoms worsen or do not improve, call your doctor. If you forget a dose: Take or use the missed dose as soon as you remember it, unless it's nearly time for your next dose—if that is the case, skip the missed dose and take the next dose right on schedule. DO NOT double doses. Talk with your doctor if you find yourself missing doses.

Usual Duration of Use: Best results come from starting oseltamivir or zanamivir within a day of flu symptoms, but benefits are gained if started within 48 hours. Use as prescribed for five days is REQUIRED to get results. During influenza epidemics (for example, if flu vaccine is NOT available), oseltamivir was given for 6 weeks in one trial.

Typical Treatment Goals and Measurements (Outcomes and Markers)
Influenza: The general goal is to ease the severity of the flu (lessening of muscle aches, headache, vomiting, sore throat, fever and others). Prophylactic use of oseltamivir or zanamivir (investigational) seeks to avoid or prevent a "full blown" case of the flu if possible. **If you would like a copy of the ACIP recommendations, call 1-888-232-3228.**

▷ **These Drugs Should Not Be Taken If**
- you have had an allergic reaction to them previously.

▷ **Inform Your Physician Before Taking This Drug If**
- you have a history of kidney impairment (oseltamivir).
- you have a compromised immune system.
- you have severe or decompensated ongoing and obstructive lung disease (COPD) or asthma (zanamivir).
- you are pregnant (oseltamivir and zanamivir).

Possible Side Effects (natural, expected and unavoidable drug actions)
Not defined.

▷ **Possible Adverse Effects** (unusual, unexpected and infrequent reactions)
If any of the following develop, consult your physician promptly for guidance.
Mild Adverse Effects
Allergic reaction: Not defined.
Headache, nervousness, irritability, inability to concentrate, insomnia—rare to infrequent (oseltamivir).
Unsteadiness, dizziness—infrequent (oseltamivir).
Loss of appetite, nausea, vomiting—infrequent to frequent (oseltamivir).
Serious Adverse Effects
Not defined (oseltamivir).
Bronchospasm/respiratory distress—case report for zanamivir.

▷ **Possible Effects on Sexual Function:** None reported.

Adverse Effects That May Mimic Natural Diseases or Disorders
Not defined.

Natural Diseases or Disorders That May Be Activated by These Drugs
None reported for oseltamivir. Underlying respiratory disease such as COPD or asthma may be associated with an increased risk of bronchospasm or decline in lung function.

Possible Effects on Laboratory Tests
Not defined.

CAUTION
1. There may be a relative shortage of flu vaccine for the 2001–2002 flu season. These medicines may be very helpful for high-risk patients who are unable to prevent the flu with a shot and need to decrease the amount of time that they have the flu and also to decrease adverse outcomes from the flu.
2. Zanamivir may not work in COPD and can pose a safety risk in asthmatics.

Precautions for Use
By Infants and Children: Safety and effectiveness for those under 13 (oseltamivir) or under 7 (zanamivir) not established.
By Those Over 60 Years of Age: Special considerations not defined at present.

▷ **Advisability of Use During Pregnancy**
Pregnancy Category: C (oseltamivir), C (zanamivir). See Pregnancy Risk Categories at the back of this book.
Human studies: Adequate studies of pregnant women (both drugs) are not available. Ask your doctor for help.

Advisability of Use If Breast-Feeding
Presence of this drug in breast milk: Yes for oseltamivir; unknown for zanamivir.
Talk to your doctor about this benefit-to-risk decision.

Habit-Forming Potential: None.

Effects of Overdose: Single doses of roughly 1,000 mg of oseltamivir have resulted in vomiting. No data for zanamivir. Supportive care and contact of a poison control center are indicated for both medicines.

Possible Effects of Long-Term Use: Not defined.

Suggested Periodic Examinations While Taking This Drug (at physician's discretion)
Rapid influenza test.

▷ **While Taking This Drug, Observe the Following**
Foods: No restrictions.
Herbal Medicines or Minerals: Echinacea: Some patients use echinacea to attempt to boost their immune systems. Unfortunately, use of echinacea is not recommended in people with damaged immune systems. This herb may also actually weaken any immune system if it is used too often or for too long a time.
Beverages: No restrictions. May be taken with milk.
▷ *Alcohol:* No interactions expected.
Tobacco Smoking: No interactions expected, but smoking may further irritate airways. I advise everyone to quit smoking.

Marijuana Smoking: Added dizziness (oseltamivir).

▷ *Other Drugs*

Oseltamivir *taken concurrently* with

• Probenecid (various) may increase blood levels of oseltamivir, but adverse effects are not defined.

Author's Note: Zanamivir does not appear to have any clinically significant drug interactions, but has not been studied in conjunction with other inhaled medicines.

▷ *Driving, Hazardous Activities:* Oseltamivir may cause dizziness. Avoid hazardous activities until the extent of this effect is known.

Aviation Note: The use of this drug *may be a disqualification* for piloting. Consult a designated Aviation Medical Examiner.

Exposure to Sun: No restrictions.

NIACIN (NI a sin)

Other Names: Nicotinic acid, vitamin B3

Introduced: 1937   **Class:** Anticholesterol,   vasodilator   **Prescription:** USA: tablets and liquid: No; capsules: Yes   **Controlled Drug:** USA: No; Canada: No   **Available as Generic:**   USA: Yes; Canada: Yes

Brand Names: ✤Antivert [CD], Endur-Acin, Niac, Niacels, Niacin SR, Niacin TR, Niacor, Niacor-B, Nia-Bid, Niaplus, Niaspan, Nicobid, Nico-400, Nicolar, Nicotinex, ✤Novoniacin, SK-Niacin, Slo-Niacin, Span-Niacin-150, Tega-Span, Tri-B3

BENEFITS versus RISKS	
Possible Benefits	*Possible Risks*
EFFECTIVE REDUCTION OF TOTAL CHOLESTEROL, LOW-DENSITY CHOLESTEROL AND TRIGLYCERIDES IN TYPES II, III, IV AND V CHOLESTEROL DISORDERS	Activation of peptic ulcer Drug-induced hepatitis Aggravation of diabetes or gout
Specific prevention and treatment of pellagra (niacin-deficiency disease)	

▷ **Principal Uses**

As a Single Drug Product: Uses currently included in FDA-approved labeling: Treats (1) certain patterns of abnormally high blood levels of cholesterol and triglycerides; (2) pellagra, a niacin (vitamin B₃) deficiency disorder characterized by dementia, dermatitis and diarrhea; (3) Hartnup disease.

Other (unlabeled) generally accepted uses: (1) Therapy of certain types of vertigo and tinnitus (ringing in the ears); (2) may help decrease diarrhea in patients with cholera.

As a Combination Drug Product [CD]: In Canada this drug is combined with meclizine to enhance its effectiveness in the treatment of motion sickness and vertigo.

How This Drug Works: (1) May inhibit initial production of triglycerides and impair the conversion of fatty tissue to cholesterol and triglycerides.

(2) This drug corrects the specific deficiency of vitamin B₃ that is responsible for the symptoms of pellagra. (3) This drug causes direct dilation of peripheral blood vessels in the skin of the face and neck; for this reason it has been used to increase the blood flow to the inner ear in an attempt to relieve some types of vertigo and ringing in the ears. The effectiveness of this application is questionable.

Available Dosage Forms and Strengths

Capsules, prolonged action — 125 mg, 250 mg, 300 mg, 400 mg, 500 mg

Oral solution — 50 mg/5 ml

Tablets — 20 mg, 25 mg, 50 mg, 100 mg, 500 mg

Tablets, prolonged action — 150 mg, 250 mg, 500 mg, 750 mg, 1,000 mg

▷ **Usual Adult Dosage Ranges:** *For cholesterol disorders (immediate-release formulations):* Initially 100 mg three times daily. Dose may be increased in increments of 300 mg daily at intervals of 4 to 7 days as needed and tolerated. The usual ongoing dose is 1 to 2 g three times daily. Daily maximum is 6 g.

For cholesterol disorders (extended-release formulations): One 375 mg tablet at bedtime, which is increased as needed and tolerated at weekly intervals to 500, 750 and 1,000 mg daily. If further increases are needed, the dose is increased by 500 mg in four-week intervals to a maximum of 2,000 mg. This dose is given as two 1,000 mg tablets at bedtime.

For niacin deficiency: 10 to 20 mg daily.

For treatment of pellagra: 50 mg 3 to 10 times daily.

Note: Actual dose and schedule must be determined for each patient individually.

Conditions Requiring Dosing Adjustments

Liver Function: This drug is metabolized in the liver and is contraindicated in liver disease.

Kidney Function: Specific guidelines for adjustment of dosing are not available.

▷ **Dosing Instructions:** Take with or immediately following meals to prevent stomach irritation. Also take one-half of an adult's aspirin tablet or one children's aspirin tablet with each dose of niacin to help prevent facial flushing and itching. Dose should be increased very slowly over 2 to 3 months as needed. The prolonged-action form of niacin is preferable to improve tolerance. The regular tablet may be crushed, but the prolonged-action capsules and tablets should not be altered. If you forget a dose: Take the missed dose as soon as you remember it, unless it's nearly time for your next dose—if that is the case, skip the missed dose and take the next dose right on schedule. Talk with your doctor if you find yourself missing doses.

Usual Duration of Use: Use on a regular schedule for 3 to 5 weeks determines benefit in reducing levels of cholesterol and triglycerides. Long-term use (months to years) requires periodic physician evaluation.

Typical Treatment Goals and Measurements (Outcomes and Markers)

Cholesterol: The National Institutes of Health has released ATP III as part of the update to the National Cholesterol Education Program or NCEP. Key points in these new guidelines include acknowledging diabetes as one of the conditions that increases risk of heart disease, modifying risk factors and recommending routine testing for all of the cholesterol fractions (lipoprotein profile) versus total cholesterol alone. These new guidelines also recommend a desirable total cholesterol of 200 mg/dl as before, but change optimal LDL to 100 mg/dl, 130–159 mg/dl as borderline high, 160mg/dl as high and cite 190 mg/dl as very high. One other noteworthy change is that "good cholesterol" or HDL has been made more important. The "too low" measure for HDL has been increased to 40 mg/dl. Take your medicine and reach these new targets! Electron beam computed tomography (EBCT) is an important tool to use in conjunction with these laboratory studies. Findings show that even patients who meet cholesterol goals (particularly females over 55) can still be at significant cardiovascular risk. EBCT then defines that risk by giving a calcium score and a "virtual tour" of the coronary arteries.

▷ **This Drug Should Not Be Taken If**
  • you have had an allergic reaction to it previously.
  • you have active peptic ulcer disease or inflammatory bowel disease.
  • you have active liver disease.
  • you are bleeding from an artery.

▷ **Inform Your Physician Before Taking This Drug If**
  • you are prone to low blood pressure.
  • you have a heart rhythm disorder of any kind.
  • you have a history of peptic ulcer disease, inflammatory bowel disease, liver disease, jaundice or gallbladder disease.
  • you have diabetes or gout.

Possible Side Effects (natural, expected and unavoidable drug actions)
  Flushing, itching, tingling and feeling of warmth, usually in the face and neck. Sensitive individuals may experience orthostatic hypotension (see Glossary).

▷ **Possible Adverse Effects** (unusual, unexpected and infrequent reactions)
  If any of the following develop, consult your physician promptly for guidance.
  Mild Adverse Effects
  Allergic reactions: skin rash, itching, hives.
  Headache, dizziness, faintness, impaired vision—infrequent.
  Indigestion, nausea, vomiting, diarrhea—infrequent.
  Flushing and tingling—infrequent to frequent.
  Dryness of skin, grayish-black pigmentation of skin folds—infrequent.
  Gum pain—case reports.
  Serious Adverse Effects
  Drug-induced hepatitis with jaundice (see Glossary): yellow eyes and skin, dark-colored urine, light-colored stools—case reports.
  Worsening of diabetes and gout—possible.
  Development of heart rhythm disorders—case reports to infrequent.
  Myopathy or peptic ulcers—case reports.
  Vision changes (macular edema)—case reports.
  Abnormal blood sugar—possible.

▷ **Possible Effects on Sexual Function:** None reported.

▷ **Adverse Effects That May Mimic Natural Diseases or Disorders**
  Liver reactions may suggest viral hepatitis.

Natural Diseases or Disorders That May Be Activated by This Drug
  Latent diabetes, gout, inflammatory bowel disease or peptic ulcer.

Possible Effects on Laboratory Tests

Complete blood cell counts: decreased eosinophils and lymphocytes.

Blood total cholesterol, LDL cholesterol and triglyceride levels: decreased.

Blood HDL cholesterol level: increased.

Blood glucose level: increased.

Glucose tolerance test (GTT): decreased.

Blood uric acid level: increased.

Liver function tests: increased enzymes (ALT/GPT, AST/GOT, alkaline phosphatase) or bilirubin.

Urine sugar tests: inaccurate test results with Benedict's solution.

CAUTION

1. Large doses may cause increases in blood levels of sugar and uric acid. Diabetics or gout patients should monitor their status regularly.
2. Periodic measurements of blood cholesterol and triglyceride levels are essential for monitoring response and determining the need for changes in dose or medication.
3. Some reports indicate that the prolonged-action dose forms of niacin may be more likely to cause liver damage than the rapidly absorbed (crystalline) forms. Ask your doctor which is the most appropriate dose form and schedule for you.
4. Increased cholesterol should be treated to a specific goal or target. Women may have a better cholesterol lowering effect from this medicine than men. Talk with your doctor if the target cholesterol is not achieved within the target time frame.

Precautions for Use

By Infants and Children: Safety and effectiveness for use of large doses by those under 12 years of age have not been established.

By Those Over 60 Years of Age: Observe for the possible development of low blood pressure (light-headedness, dizziness, faintness) and heart rhythm disorders.

▷ ## Advisability of Use During Pregnancy

Pregnancy Category: A for doses used to treat high lipids, C for Niaspan. See Pregnancy Risk Categories at the back of this book.

Animal studies: Significant birth defects due to one form of this drug were found in chicks.

Human studies: Adequate studies of pregnant women are not available.

Use this drug only if clearly needed. Avoid completely during the first 3 months.

Advisability of Use If Breast-Feeding

Presence of this drug in breast milk: Yes.

Avoid drug or refrain from nursing (in cholesterol-lowering doses).

Habit-Forming Potential: None.

Effects of Overdose: Generalized flushing, nausea, vomiting, stomach cramps, diarrhea, weakness, fainting.

Possible Effects of Long-Term Use: Increased blood levels of sugar and uric acid; liver damage.

Suggested Periodic Examinations While Taking This Drug (at physician's discretion)

Measurements of blood levels of total cholesterol, HDL and LDL cholesterol fractions, triglycerides, sugar and uric acid.

Liver function tests.

▷ **While Taking This Drug, Observe the Following**
   Foods: Follow the low-cholesterol diet prescribed by your physician.
   Herbal Medicines or Minerals: The FDA has allowed one dietary supplement
      called Cholestin to continue to be sold. This preparation actually contains
      lovastatin, and since use of niacin with HMG-CoA inhibitors may increase
      risk of rhabdomyolysis or myopathy, the combination is NOT advised. No
      data exist from well-designed clinical studies about garlic and niacin and
      while the combination may be complementary, it can't presently be recom-
      mended. Additionally, garlic may inhibit blood-clotting (platelet) aggrega-
      tion—something to consider if you are already taking a platelet inhibitor.
      Soy products (milk, tofu, etc.) contain phytoestrogens that have led to an FDA-
      approved health claim for reducing risk of heart disease (if they have at least
      6.25 g of soy protein per serving). Use of soy products have been proven to
      lower cholesterol. Talk to your doctor to see if this makes sense for you.
   Beverages: No restrictions. May be taken with milk.
▷ *Alcohol:* Use with caution. Alcohol used with large doses of this drug may cause
      excessive lowering of blood pressure. There has been one case report of
      delirium.
   Tobacco Smoking: May increase risk of flushing and dizziness. I advise every-
      one to quit smoking.
▷ *Other Drugs*
   Niacin may *increase* the effects of
   • some antihypertensive drugs and cause excessive lowering of blood pressure.
   Niacin may *decrease* the effects of
   • antidiabetic drugs (insulin and oral antidiabetic drugs; see Drug Classes),
      by raising the level of blood sugar.
   • aspirin (various), which may decrease flushing but may also increase
      niacin blood levels; talk to your doctor.
   • probenecid (Benemid) and sulfinpyrazone (Anturane), by raising the level
      of blood uric acid.
   Niacin *taken concurrently* with
   • isoniazid (INH) may result in decreased niacin levels and require
      increased niacin dosing.
   • cholestyramine (Cholybar, Questran) may result in decreased niacin levels
      and require increased niacin dosing.
   • colestipol (Colestid) may result in decreased niacin levels and require
      increased niacin dosing.
   • lovastatin and other HMG-CoA-type cholesterol-lowering drugs (see Drug
      Classes) may result in reversible muscle problems (myopathy or rhab-
      domyolysis).
   • nicotine (particularly transdermal) may result in increased risk of flushing
      and dizziness.
▷ *Driving, Hazardous Activities:* This drug may cause dizziness and faintness.
      Restrict activities as necessary.
   Aviation Note: The use of this drug *may be a disqualification* for piloting. Con-
      sult a designated Aviation Medical Examiner.
   Exposure to Sun: No restrictions.
   Discontinuation: Do not stop this drug without your physician's knowledge and
      guidance. Abrupt withdrawal may be followed by excessive increase in
      blood cholesterol and triglyceride levels.

NICARDIPINE (ni KAR de peen)

Introduced: 1984   **Class:** Anti-anginal, antihypertensive, calcium channel blocker   **Prescription:** USA: Yes   **Controlled Drug:** USA: No; Canada: No   **Available as Generic:** USA: Yes

Brand Names: Cardene, Cardene SR

Controversies in Medicine: Medicines in this class have had many conflicting reports. The FDA has held hearings on the calcium channel blocker (CCB) class. Research at New York University found that nifedipine (a member of the same class) is a cause of reversible male infertility. CCBs are currently second-line agents for high blood pressure according to the JNC VI (see Glossary).

BENEFITS versus RISKS

Possible Benefits	*Possible Risks*
EFFECTIVE PREVENTION OF CLASSICAL ANGINA OF EFFORT	Increase in angina upon starting treatment
Second-line TREATMENT OF HYPERTENSION	Water retention, ankle swelling

---

▷ **Principal Uses**

As a Single Drug Product: Uses currently included in FDA-approved labeling: Treats (1) classical angina (due to atherosclerotic disease) or angina caused by coronary artery spasm; (2) mild to moderate high blood pressure.

Other (unlabeled) generally accepted uses: (1) Combination therapy in preventing repeat strokes; (2) may help refractory (not responding to nonsteroidal anti-inflammatory drugs) menstrual pain; (3) decreases frequency and severity of migraine attacks; (4) may halt some early atherosclerosis; (5) lowers postoperative hypertension; (6) may prevent vessel spasm in some kinds of blood vessel (vascular) surgery; (7) may treat premature labor; (8) decreases pain after shingles (herpes zoster); (9) eases Raynaud's phenomenon.

How This Drug Works: By blocking passage of calcium through certain cell walls (which is necessary to nerve and muscle function), this drug inhibits the contraction of coronary arteries and peripheral arterioles. As a result, it:

• promotes coronary artery dilation (anti-anginal effect).

• reduces the degree of contraction of peripheral arterial walls, lowering blood pressure. This further reduces heart workload and helps prevent angina.

Available Dosage Forms and Strengths

Capsules — 20 mg, 30 mg

Injection — 2.5 mg/ml

SR Capsules — 30 mg, 45 mg, 60 mg

▷ **Usual Adult Dosage Ranges:** *Chronic stable angina:* Immediate release forms: The starting dose is 20 mg taken three times a day. The dose can then be increased as needed and tolerated in 10 mg increases every three days or longer. The typical dose is 20–40 mg three times a day. *Hypertension:* Immediate-release—initially 20 mg three times daily, 6 to 8 hours apart. Dose may be increased gradually at 3-day intervals (as needed and tolerated) up to 40 mg three times daily. The total daily dose should not exceed 120 mg. Sustained-release—started at 30 mg twice daily and increased as needed and tolerated to 60 mg twice daily.

Note: Actual dose and schedule must be determined for each patient individually.

Conditions Requiring Dosing Adjustments

Liver Function: Starting dose is 20 mg twice a day. If the dose must be increased, it should be slowly advanced and taken twice a day.

Kidney Function: In moderate kidney failure, dosing starts at 20 mg twice daily. If needed, dose may be slowly increased. This drug may cause urine retention and is a benefit-to-risk decision in urine outflow problems.

▷ **Dosing Instructions:** May be taken with or following food to reduce stomach irritation, but not with a high-fat meal, as total amount that gets into your body (absorption) may be reduced by 20 to 30%. The capsule should be swallowed whole (not altered). If you forget a dose: Take the missed dose as soon as you remember it, unless it's nearly time for your next dose—if that is the case, skip the missed dose and take the next dose right on schedule. DO NOT double doses. Talk with your doctor if you find yourself missing doses.

Usual Duration of Use: Use on a regular schedule for 2 to 4 weeks determines this drug's benefit in reducing the frequency and severity of angina or controlling hypertension. For long-term use (months to years), the smallest effective dose should be used. Physician supervision and periodic evaluation are essential.

Typical Treatment Goals and Measurements (Outcomes and Markers)

Angina: Decrease in the severity and frequency of anginal attacks in patients who do not tolerate beta blockers. *Blood pressure:* The most recent treatment guidelines (JNC VI) actually define optimal blood pressure (BP) as less than 120/80 and high normal as 139/89. The American Diabetes Association has chosen a target of 130/80 as the blood pressure goal for people living with diabetes. Most clinicians try to achieve a BP that achieves the best balance of lower cardiovascular risk while avoiding the problem of too low a blood pressure. The goal and time frame (see peak benefits above) should be discussed with you when the prescription is written.

▷ **This Drug Should Not Be Taken If**
  • you have had an allergic reaction to it previously.
  • you have advanced aortic stenosis.

▷ **Inform Your Physician Before Taking This Drug If**
  • you have had an adverse reaction to any calcium channel blocker (see Drug Classes).
  • you currently take any form of digitalis or a beta-blocker drug (see Drug Classes).
  • you are taking any drugs that lower blood pressure.
  • you are taking cimetidine (Tagamet) or cyclosporine (Sandimmune).
  • you have a history of congestive heart failure, heart attack or stroke.
  • you have a history of circulation impairment to the fingers.
  • you have had a skin (Dermatologic) reaction to this medicine (tell your doctor as some initial skin reactions have progressed to more serious skin reactions such as exfoliative dermatitis.
  • you have Duchenne muscular dystrophy.

- you are subject to disturbances of heart rhythm.
- you have impaired liver or kidney function.

Possible Side Effects (natural, expected and unavoidable drug actions)
Rapid heart rate, swelling of the feet and ankles, flushing and sensation of warmth. Marked drop in blood pressure with fainting—rare.

▷ **Possible Adverse Effects** (unusual, unexpected and infrequent reactions)
If any of the following develop, consult your physician promptly for guidance.

Mild Adverse Effects
Allergic reaction: skin rash—rare.
Headache, dizziness, weakness, nervousness, insomnia or ringing in the ears (tinnitus); blurred vision, confusion, increased urination—rare to infrequent.
Palpitation, shortness of breath—rare.
Indigestion, nausea, vomiting, constipation—all rare.
Increased blood platelets—case reports.
Joint and muscle pain, cough—rare.
Abnormal growth (hyperplasia) of the gums—rare.

Serious Adverse Effects
Allergic reactions: initial skin reactions have progressed to exfoliative dermatitis or erythema multiforme in some cases.
Increased frequency or severity of angina when starting therapy or after an increase in dose—possible.
Difficult urination—rare.
Liver toxicity—rare.
Decreased white blood cell counts reported with medicines in the same class (agranulocytosis)—very rare.

▷ **Possible Effects on Sexual Function:** Impotence—rare.

▷ **Adverse Effects That May Mimic Natural Diseases or Disorders**
Flushing and warmth may resemble menopausal "hot flashes." Increased liver enzymes may resemble infectious hepatitis.

Possible Effects on Laboratory Tests
Liver function tests: elevated (rare).

CAUTION
1. If you are checking your own blood pressure, check it just before each dose and 1 to 2 hours after each dose to obtain an accurate picture of the drug's effect. The best results from any medicine for high blood pressure come from taking the medicine EXACTLY as prescribed.
2. Be sure to tell all health care providers who provide care for you that you take this drug. Note the use of this drug on a card placed in your purse or wallet.
3. You may use nitroglycerin and other nitrate drugs as needed to relieve acute episodes of angina pain. If your angina attacks are becoming more frequent or intense, call your doctor.

Precautions for Use
By Infants and Children: Safety and effectiveness for those under 18 years of age are not established.
By Those Over 60 Years of Age: Usually well tolerated, but watch for development of weakness, dizziness, fainting and falling. Take necessary precau-

tions to prevent injury. Report promptly any changes in your pattern of thirst and urination.

▷ **Advisability of Use During Pregnancy**

Pregnancy Category: C. See Pregnancy Risk Categories at the back of this book.

Animal studies: Embryo and fetal toxicity reported in small animals, but no birth defects due to this drug.

Human studies: Adequate studies of pregnant women are not available.

Avoid this drug during the first 3 months. Use during the final 6 months only if clearly needed. Ask your physician for guidance.

Advisability of Use If Breast-Feeding

Presence of this drug in breast milk: Probably yes.

Avoid drug or refrain from nursing.

Habit-Forming Potential: None.

Effects of Overdose: Weakness, light-headedness, fainting, fast pulse, low blood pressure, shortness of breath, flushed and warm skin, tremors.

Possible Effects of Long-Term Use: None reported.

Suggested Periodic Examinations While Taking This Drug (at physician's discretion)

Evaluations of heart function, including electrocardiograms.

Measurements of blood pressure in supine, sitting and standing positions.

▷ **While Taking This Drug, Observe the Following**

Foods: Food decreases the amount of this drug that is absorbed. DO NOT take this medicine with grapefruit or grapefruit juice. It is also prudent to avoid excessive salt intake.

Herbal Medicines or Minerals: Ginseng may increase blood pressure, blunting the benefits of this medicine. Hawthorn, saw palmetto, ma huang, goldenseal, yohimbe and licorice may also increase blood pressure. Calcium and garlic may help lower blood pressure. Indian snakeroot has a German Commission E monograph indication for hypertension—talk to your doctor. Eleuthero root and ephedra should be avoided by people living with hypertension. Talk with your doctor BEFORE adding any herbal medicine to nicardipine.

Beverages: DO NOT take this medicine with grapefruit or grapefruit juice. May be taken with water or milk.

▷ *Alcohol:* Use with caution until combined effects have been determined. Alcohol may exaggerate the drop in blood pressure experienced by some individuals.

Tobacco Smoking: Nicotine may reduce the effectiveness of this drug. I advise everyone to quit smoking.

Marijuana Smoking: Possibly causes reduced effectiveness of this drug; mild to moderate increase in angina; possible changes in electrocardiogram, confusing interpretation.

▷ *Other Drugs*

Nicardipine may *increase* the effects of

• cyclosporine (Sandimmune) and cause kidney toxicity.

Nicardipine *taken concurrently* with

• amiodarone (Cordarone) may result in cardiac arrest.

• beta-blocker drugs or digitalis preparations (see Drug Classes) may affect heart rate and rhythm adversely; careful monitoring by your physician is necessary if these drugs are taken concurrently.

- delavirdine (Rescriptor) and other medicines that inhibit cytochrome P450 3A4 may lead to increased nicardipine levels and toxicity.
- magnesium may cause worsening of neuromuscular blockade and further lowering of blood pressure.
- neuromuscular blocking agents (such as pancuronium-Pavulon, vecuronium-Norcuron, others) can result in increased severity of muscle blockade from nicardipine. Use of lower neuromuscular blocker doses is prudent.
- nonsteroidal anti-inflammatory agents (NSAIDs—see Drug Classes) may blunt the therapeutic effects of nicardipine.
- oral anticoagulants (warfarin, others) increase bleeding risk.
- phenytoin (Dilantin) or fosphenytoin (Cerebyx) may result in phenytoin or fosphenytoin toxicity or decreased efficacy of nicardipine.
- rifampin (Rifadin, others) has caused loss of control of blood pressure with some other calcium channel blockers; caution is advised if these medicines are combined.
- sirolimus (Rapamune) or tacrolimus (Prograf) may result in sirolimus or tacrolimus toxicity. The doses of the immunosuppressants may need to be reduced.

The following drugs may *increase* the effects of nicardipine:

- cimetidine (Tagamet).
- imidazole antifungals (ketoconazole [Nizoral]) or triazole antifungals (itraconazole [Sporanox] or fluconazole [Diflucan]). Dose reductions or discontinuation of the antifungal may be required.
- quinupristin/dalfopristin (Synercid) may result in nicardipine toxicity.
- ritonavir (Norvir) and other protease inhibitors.

▷ *Driving, Hazardous Activities:* Usually no restrictions. This drug may cause drowsiness or dizziness. Restrict activities as necessary.

Aviation Note: Coronary artery disease and hypertension *are disqualifications* for piloting. Consult a designated Aviation Medical Examiner.

Exposure to Sun: No restrictions.

Exposure to Heat: Caution is advised. Hot environments can exaggerate the blood-pressure-lowering effects of this drug. Observe for light-headedness or weakness.

Heavy Exercise or Exertion: This drug may improve your ability to be more active without resulting angina pain. Use caution and avoid excessive exercise that could impair heart function in the absence of warning pain.

Discontinuation: Do not stop this drug abruptly. Ask your doctor about gradual withdrawal. Watch for possible development of rebound angina.

NICOTINE (NIK oh teen)

Introduced: 1992, 1996, 1997   **Class:** Smoking cessation adjunct, nicotine replacement therapy   **Prescription:** USA: Both Nicorettes (2 mg and 4 mg) are now available without a prescription for those over 18 years old. Nicotine patches are FDA-approved for nonprescription use. The nicotine inhaler and nasal spray are only available with a prescription.   **Controlled Drug:** USA: No; Canada: No   **Available as Generic:** USA: Yes; Canada: Yes

Brand Names: Habitrol, Clear Nicoderm CQ, ✤Nicoderm, Nicorette, Nicorette DS, Nicotine Transdermal System, Nicotrol, Nicotrol Inhaler, Nicotrol NS, Prostep, Prostep Transdermal System

BENEFITS versus RISKS	
Possible Benefits	*Possible Risks*
EFFECTIVE REDUCTION OF NICOTINE CRAVING AND WITHDRAWAL EFFECTS WHEN USED ADJUNCTIVELY IN SMOKING-CESSATION TREATMENT PROGRAMS	Aggravation of existing angina, heart rhythm disorders, hypertension, insulin-dependent diabetes, peptic ulcer and vascular diseases Increased risk of abortion (if used during pregnancy)

▷ **Principal Uses**

As a Single Drug Product: Uses currently included in FDA-approved labeling: Nicotine chewing gum, nicotine transdermal systems, inhaler and nasal spray are used adjunctively in behavior modification programs to help cigarette smokers who wish to stop smoking.

Author's Note: The American Lung Association has an excellent resource called the "Quit Smoking Action Plan." If you are planning to stop smoking (and I hope that you are), call them at 1-800-LUNG-USA or find them at the web site listed in Table 17 at the back of this book. The new American Heart Association guidelines for primary and secondary prevention of cardiovascular disease once again tell people that smoking is a risk factor for heart attacks and that you should immediately STOP. Visit www.americanheart.org for more information.

Other (unlabeled) generally accepted uses: Gum and nasal spray have been used to increase nicotine levels in the blood and help ease sudden cravings.

How This Drug Works: By providing an alternate source of nicotine (for nicotine-dependent smokers), the appropriate use of these drug products can reduce nicotine craving and lessen smoking withdrawal effects, such as irritability, nervousness, headache, fatigue, sleep disturbances and drowsiness.

Available Dosage Forms and Strengths

Inhaler (per cartridge) — 10 mg

Nasal spray (10-ml bottle) — 10 mg/ml

Nicotine chewing gum tablets — 2 mg (nonprescription)

Nicorette (U.S., Canada) — 2 mg

Nicorette (Canada) — 4 mg

Nicorette DS (U.S., Canada) — 4 mg

Transdermal systems:

16-hour systems, U.S. only — 5 mg, 10 mg, 15 mg

24-hour systems — 7 mg (U.S., Canada), 11 mg (U.S.), 14 mg (U.S., Canada), 21 mg (U.S., Canada), 22 mg (U.S.)

How to Store

Store nicotine gum at room temperature and protect from light. Store nicotine patches at room temperature and be especially careful to avoid exposing the patches to temperatures greater than 86 degrees F (30 degrees C). Do not store unpouched. Once opened, patches should be used promptly because they may lose their strength.

▷ **Recommended Dosage Ranges** (Actual dose and schedule must be determined for each patient individually.)

Infants and Children: Avoid use completely in children. Avoid accidental exposure to patches.

18 to 60 Years of Age: For chewing gum tablets: Initially one piece every hour while awake (10 to 12 pieces daily); supplement with one additional piece if and when needed to control urge to smoke. Total daily dose should not exceed 30 pieces (60 mg).

For inhaler form: Dosing is divided into two parts (phases). At first, 6–16 cartridges a day for up to 12 weeks duration of use. Dosing is individualized to control smoking urges, excess nicotine or withdrawal. During the second phase, a quit date is set, patients are told to use the inhaler less often and the dose is gradually decreased. Maximum daily dose is six cartridges. If a particular patient is not able to quit smoking after 4 weeks, treatment should be stopped, and a "break" (therapeutic holiday) given before another attempt to stop is made.

For nasal spray: Two sprays, one in each nostril. Starting dose is usually two to four sprays each hour. Maximum is 5 doses per hour (5 mg) and 40 doses per day (40 mg or 80 sprays). It should be used for a maximum of 3 months.

For transdermal systems: Dose depends upon patient characteristics and product used:

For those weighing 100 lb or more, smoking 10 or more cigarettes daily and without cardiovascular disease: The 16-hour system (Nicotrol) is started with one 15 mg patch applied for 16 hours daily for 4 to 12 weeks. For those who have abstained from smoking, reduce dose to one 10-mg patch applied for 16 hours daily for the next 2 to 4 weeks and then to one 5-mg patch applied for 16 hours daily for the following 2 to 4 weeks. The 24-hour system (Habitrol, Nicoderm) is started with one 21-mg patch applied daily for 4 to 8 weeks. For those who have abstained from smoking, reduce dose to one 14-mg patch daily for the next 2 to 4 weeks and then to one 7-mg patch daily for the following 2 to 4 weeks. Prostep—initially one 22-mg patch applied daily for 4 to 8 weeks. For those who have abstained from smoking, reduce dose to one 11-mg patch daily for 2 to 4 weeks.

For those weighing less than 100 lb, smoking less than 10 cigarettes daily or with cardiovascular disease: The 24-hour system (Habitrol, Nicoderm) is started with one 14-mg patch applied daily for 4 to 8 weeks. For those who have abstained from smoking, reduce dose to one 7-mg patch daily for the next 2 to 4 weeks. Prostep—initially one 11-mg patch applied daily for 4 to 8 weeks.

Over 60 Years of Age: Same as 12 to 60 years of age in those without diseases that pose as risk factors (such as cardiovascular problems).

Conditions Requiring Dosing Adjustments

Liver Function: Lower starting doses are prudent in liver disease.

Kidney Function: Doses are decreased in severe kidney compromise.

Cardiovascular Disease: See above.

▷ **Dosing Instructions:** Carefully follow the manufacturer's directions provided with each product.

For chewing gum: Limit use to one piece of gum at a time. This product is much harder than typical chewing gum. Chew each piece slowly and intermittently for 30 minutes. A tingling of your gum tissue or peppery taste means the nicotine is being released. Try to gradually reduce the number of pieces chewed each day by using it only when there is an urge to smoke. When trying to quit smoking, always have the gum available.

For transdermal systems: Apply a new patch at the same time each day. Do not alter the patch in any way. Apply the patch to the upper arm or body where the skin is clean, dry and free of hair, oil, scars and irritation of any kind; alternate sites of application. Press the patch firmly in place for 10 seconds; ensure good contact throughout. Wash your hands when you have finished applying the patch. Replace patches that are dislodged by showering, bathing or swimming.

For spray: DO NOT swallow, inhale or sniff when spraying the spray. The nasal route may best mimic the effect of using a cigarette to deliver nicotine.

For the inhaler: Follow the patient package insert exactly. Make sure you understand how to use this product.

If you forget a dose: Take the missed dose as soon as you remember it, unless it's nearly time for your next dose—if that is the case, skip the missed dose and take the next dose right on schedule. DO NOT double doses. Talk with your doctor if you find yourself missing doses.

Usual Duration of Use: Use on a regular schedule for 2 to 3 months determines effectiveness in achieving lasting cessation of smoking. Nicotine chewing gum should not be used for more than 6 months; transdermal systems should not be used for more than 20 weeks. The nasal spray form should be used no longer than 3 months. The inhaler form should NOT be used for more than 6 months. Long-term use requires periodic physician evaluation of response and dose adjustment.

Typical Treatment Goals and Measurements (Outcomes and Markers)

Smoking cessation: The goal is to ease or eliminate signs or symptoms of tobacco withdrawal, encouraging patients to stop smoking. Replacing the nicotine that smokers previously received from tobacco products avoids the life-threatening by-products of tobacco smoke while replacing the chemical that a smoker has become addicted to. Once the replacement has occurred, the patch, nasal inhalation or inhaled nicotine dose can be gradually decreased, and then replacement stopped altogether.

Author's Note: There are NO DATA to show that smoking is good for you. Please make every effort to stop. I firmly believe that my father would be alive today if he had been able to stop smoking. A study in Iceland (Iceland has an abundance of genetic and family data) found that combining two methods of nicotine replacement (such as a patch and the spray) worked better than using a single method. The American Lung Association has a Quit Smoking Action Plan that can be very helpful. Find them on the web at www.lungusa.org.

Possible Advantages of These Drugs

Provides control and flexibility of gradual nicotine withdrawal for use in supervised smoking-cessation programs. Avoids the possible cancer causing "excipients" of cigarette smoke.

Currently a Drug of Choice

For people who are motivated to stop smoking. Since many forms are now available without a prescription, be sure to talk with your doctor or pharmacist about how to best use these medicines. Many pharmacists also offer programs to help you quit.

▷ **This Drug Should Not Be Taken If**
- you had an allergic reaction to any form of it previously or to any of the ingredients in the dosage form (read the label carefully).
- you have severe or uncontrolled or a pattern of worsening angina (physician's discretion)
- you keep smoking or using other tobacco products (yes, chewing tobacco or tobacco pouches count—in general if it is a product that has nicotine—it should be topped).
- you have uncontrolled, life-threatening heart rhythm disorders (physician's discretion).
- you have had a recent heart attack (physician's discretion).

▷ **Inform Your Physician Before Taking This Drug If**
- you have any form of angina (coronary heart disease).
- you have had a heart attack at any time.
- you are subject to heart rhythm disorders.
- you have insulin-dependent diabetes.
- you have hypertension (high blood pressure).
- you have hyperthyroidism (overactive thyroid function).
- you have a pheochromocytoma (adrenaline-producing tumor).
- you have a history of esophagitis or peptic ulcer disease.
- you have a history of Buerger's disease or Raynaud's phenomenon.
- you currently have any dental problems or skin disorders.
- you have a history of kidney or liver disease.
- you have an increase in cardiovascular effects while you are taking this medicine.
- you have already taken a 3-month course of the patch.
- you use birth control pills (oral contraceptives).
- you think you are pregnant or plan to become pregnant.
- you are unsure how much to take or how often to take this medicine.

Possible Side Effects (natural, expected and unavoidable drug actions)
Increased blood pressure.
For chewing gum: mouth or throat irritation; injury to teeth or dental repairs.
For transdermal systems: redness, itching or burning at site of application (mild and transient).
For nasal spray: runny nose, nasal irritation.
For inhaler: coughing and nose irritation—frequent.

▷ **Possible Adverse Effects** (unusual, unexpected and infrequent reactions)
If any of the following develop, consult your physician promptly for guidance.
Mild Adverse Effects
Allergic reactions: skin rash, hives, itching, local or generalized swellings.
Headache, light-headedness, dizziness, drowsiness, irritability, nervousness, insomnia, joint pain, muscle aches, abnormal dreams—possible to infrequent and some may be dose-related.
Rapid heartbeat, palpitation, increased sweating—infrequent to frequent, dose-related.

Increased or decreased appetite, nausea, dry mouth, indigestion, constipation or diarrhea—infrequent.

Serious Adverse Effects

Irregular heart rhythms, chest pain (angina), edema—infrequent.

Stroke—case report.

See "Effects of Overdose" below.

▷ **Possible Effects on Sexual Function:** There are some data questioning an effect on sperm, but a distinct demonstration of an effect is lacking.

Natural Diseases or Disorders That May Be Activated by This Drug

Latent angina, atrial fibrillation, hypertension, peptic ulcer disease, temporomandibular joint (TMJ) disorder (by chewing gum).

Possible Effects on Laboratory Tests

Free fatty acids (FFA blood level): increased.

Blood glucose: increased.

Prothrombin time (INR): decreased.

Urine screening test for drug abuse: no effect.

CAUTION

1. For these drug products to be safe and effective, it is mandatory that all smoking be stopped immediately at the beginning of drug treatment.

2. Extended use of chewing gum may cause damage to mouth tissues and teeth, loosen fillings, stick to dentures and initiate or aggravate TMJ dysfunction.

3. Smoking cessation and the use of these drug products can result in increased blood levels of insulin (in insulin-dependent diabetics); dose reduction of insulin may be necessary to prevent hypoglycemic reactions.

4. If you are taking any of the following drugs, consult your physician regarding the need to reduce their dose while participating in a smoking-cessation program: aminophylline, beta-blocker drugs, imipramine, oxazepam, oxtriphylline, pentazocine, prazosin, propoxyphene, theophylline.

5. If you are taking any of the following drugs, consult your physician regarding the need to increase their dose while participating in a smoking-cessation program: isoproterenol, phenylephrine.

6. Used patches should be folded in half with the adhesive sides sealed together; place them in the original pouch or aluminum foil and dispose of them promptly; keep out of reach of children and animals.

7. Use of antacids, such as Tums, prior to chewing nicotine gum can increase the amount of nicotine absorbed from the gum.

8. Habitrol patches have only been shown to be effective when they are part of a complete smoking-cessation program that includes counseling.

9. The Centers for Disease Control (CDC) has many excellent publications available to give you more information on stopping smoking. Call 1-800-232-1311 for more information

10. The possibility of becoming dependent on these replacement products also exists. The chance of this happening may be greater for the nasal spray than for the transdermal or "gum" products.

Precautions for Use

By Infants and Children: Safety and effectiveness for those under 12 years of age are not established for the gum, and for those under 18 not established for other forms.

By Those Over 60 Years of Age: Because of the increased possibility of cardio-vascular disorders in this age group, treatment should be cautiously started. Watch closely for adverse effects.

▷ **Advisability of Use During Pregnancy**

Pregnancy Category: For nicotine chewing gum: C. For nicotine transdermal systems, nasal spray and inhaler: D. See Pregnancy Risk Categories at the back of this book.

Animal studies: Impaired fertility found in mouse, rat and rabbit studies. Birth defects found in high-dose studies of mice.

Human studies: Adequate studies of pregnant women are not available, but it is known that cigarette smoking during pregnancy may cause low birth weight, increased risk of abortion and increased risk of newborn death.

The use of these drug products is not recommended during pregnancy.

Advisability of Use If Breast-Feeding

Presence of this drug in breast milk: Yes.

Avoid drug or refrain from nursing.

Habit-Forming Potential: The prolonged use of these drug products may per-petuate the physical dependence of nicotine-dependent smokers. Patches should have the lowest potential for dependence. Potential exists for abuse of nonprescription forms of this medicine.

Effects of Overdose: Nausea, vomiting, increased salivation, stomach cramps, diarrhea, headache, dizziness, impaired vision and hearing, weakness, confusion, fainting, difficult breathing, seizures.

Possible Effects of Long-Term Use: Perpetuation of nicotine dependence.

Suggested Periodic Examinations While Taking This Drug (at physician's dis-cretion)

Evaluation of patient's ability to abstain from smoking.

Evaluation of patient's blood pressure and heart function.

▷ **While Taking This Drug, Observe the Following**

Foods: Avoid any food with a nicotine content.

Herbal Medicines or Minerals: Using ephedra, ma huang, kola or similar prod-ucts may accentuate nervousness and anxiety people have when trying to quit smoking. On the other hand, valerian and kava kava may help ease tensions associated with smoking cessation. Talk to your doctor BEFORE combining any herbal medicine with nicotine.

Beverages: No restrictions.

▷ *Alcohol:* May cause an increase in cardiovascular effects.

Tobacco Smoking: Avoid all forms of tobacco completely.

Marijuana Smoking: Avoid completely.

▷ *Other Drugs*

Nicotine may *increase* the effects of

- adenosine.
- niacin (flushing and dizziness).

The following drugs may *increase* the effects of nicotine:
- antacids such as Tums used prior to chewing nicotine-containing gum— may increase the absorption of nicotine from the gum.
- cimetidine (Tagamet).
- lithium (Lithobid).
- ranitidine (Zantac).

Nicotine *taken concurrently* with
- niacin (Nicobid, others) can cause severe facial flushing.

▷ *Driving, Hazardous Activities:* This drug may cause dizziness or drowsiness. Restrict activities as necessary.

Aviation Note: The use of this drug *may be a disqualification* for piloting. Consult a designated Aviation Medical Examiner.

Exposure to Sun: No restrictions.

Exposure to Cold: Use caution until tolerance is determined. Cold environments may enhance the vasospastic action of nicotine.

Heavy Exercise or Exertion: Patients with angina, coronary artery disease or hypertension should use this drug with caution.

Special Storage Instructions: Store nicotine gum at room temperature and protect from light. Store nicotine patches at room temperature, and be especially careful to avoid exposing the patches to temperatures greater than 86 degrees F (30 degrees C). Do not store unpouched. Once opened, patches should be used promptly because they may lose their strength.

Discontinuation: As soon as a lasting cessation of smoking has been achieved, these drugs should be gradually reduced in dose and then discontinued. Continual use of the chewing gum or inhaler should not exceed 6 months, the nasal spray form no longer than 3 months and the transdermal system no more than 20 weeks.

NIFEDIPINE (ni FED i peen)

Introduced: 1972   **Class:** Anti-anginal, antihypertensive, calcium channel blocker   **Prescription:** USA: Yes   **Controlled Drug:** USA: No; Canada: No   **Available as Generic:** Yes

Brand Names: Adalat, Adalat CC, ✚Adalat FT, XL, ✚Adalat P.A., ✚Apo-Nifed, ✚Gen-Nifedipine, ✚Novo-Nifedin, ✚Nu-Nifed, Procardia, Procardia XL, ✚Scheinpharm Nifedipine XL

Controversies in Medicine: Medicines in this class have had many conflicting reports. The FDA has held hearings on the calcium channel blocker (CCB) class.

Research at New York University found that nifedipine (a member of the same class) is a cause of reversible male infertility. CCBs are currently second-line agents for high blood pressure according to the JNC VI (see Glossary).

BENEFITS versus RISKS

Possible Benefits	*Possible Risks*
EFFECTIVE PREVENTION OF CLASSICAL ANGINA OF EFFORT AND OTHER ANGINA TYPES	Rare increase in angina upon starting treatment
SECOND-LINE TREATMENT OF HYPERTENSION (sustained release form may confer increased benefits)	Rare precipitation of congestive heart failure
	Rare anemia and low white blood cell counts
	Very rare drug-induced hepatitis
	Fainting

▷ **Principal Uses**

As a Single Drug Product: Uses currently included in FDA-approved labeling: Treats (1) angina pectoris due to coronary artery spasm (Prinzmetal's variant angina) that occurs spontaneously and is not associated with exertion; (2) classical angina of effort (due to atherosclerotic disease of the coronary arteries) in people who have not responded to or cannot tolerate the nitrates and beta-blocker drugs customarily used to treat this disorder (sustained-release form); (3) mild to moderate hypertension (extended-release forms).

Author's Note: A retrospective chart review has found the immediate-release form of this medicine IS NOT recommended for use in treating hypertension, acute myocardial infarction (heart attack), hypertensive crisis and some forms of unstable angina.

Other (unlabeled) generally accepted uses: (1) Treats symptoms of Raynaud's phenomenon; (2) may stop some early atherosclerosis; (3) can have a role in treating pulmonary hypertension; (4) helps decrease risk of heart attack after coronary artery bypass grafting; (5) could have a role in some neurologically based pain disorders; (6) can help itching (urticaria) of unknown cause; (7) therapy of achalasia or esophageal spasm; (8) helps intractable hiccups; (9) helps amaurosis fugax; (10) has a role in helping abnormal reactions to cold (chilblains).

How This Drug Works: Blocks passage of calcium through certain cell walls (needed for nerve and muscle tissue function), slowing electrical activity through the heart and inhibits contraction of coronary arteries and peripheral arterioles. As a result:

- prevents spontaneous spasm of coronary arteries (Prinzmetal's angina).
- reduces heart rate and force during exertion, decreasing oxygen needs of heart muscle and reducing occurrence of effort-induced angina (classical angina pectoris).
- reduces the degree of contraction of peripheral arterial walls, lowering blood pressure. This further reduces the work of the heart during exertion and helps prevent angina.

Author's Note: One study found that nifedipine restored the function of the lining of blood vessels (endothelium).

Available Dosage Forms and Strengths

Capsules — 5 mg (Canada), 10 mg (U.S. and Canada), 20 mg (U.S.)

Tablets — 10 mg, 20 mg (Canada)

Tablets, extended release — 10 mg, 20 mg (Canada), 30 mg, 60 mg, 90 mg
(U.S.)

Tablets, sustained release — 30 mg, 60 mg, 90 mg

▷ **Recommended Dosage Ranges** (Actual dose and schedule must be determined for each patient individually.)

Infants and Children: Dose not established.

Adults up to 60 Years of Age: Chronic stable angina or vasospastic (Prinzmetal's) angina: Immediate-release form: Dosing is started with 10 mg three times a day. Most people respond to 10–20 mg three times a day. Change to extended-release forms can be accomplished on a same dose to same dose (mg to mg) basis. Extended-release form for high blood pressure: Initially 30 mg once daily. Dose may be increased gradually at 7- to 14-day intervals (as needed and tolerated) up to 60 mg. Maximum total daily dose should not exceed 90 mg.

Sublingual for hypertensive crisis: **The immediate-release form of this medicine IS NOT recommended for use in treating hypertension, acute myocardial infarction (heart attack), hypertensive crisis and some forms of unstable angina.**

Over 60 Years of Age: Same as for younger patients. **Nifedipine immediate-release use by those over 71 has been associated with almost a four-fold increase in risk for all-cause death when compared to ACE inhibitors, beta blockers or other calcium channel blockers.**

Conditions Requiring Dosing Adjustments

Liver Function: Lower doses are prudent in liver disease. This drug is also a rare cause of liver toxicity (allergic hepatitis) and should be used with caution. Also a potential cause of portal hypertension and should NOT be used by patients with portal hypertension.

Kidney Function: For patients with compromised kidneys, nifedipine is a benefit-to-risk decision, as it can lead to kidney toxicity.

▷ **Dosing Instructions:** May be taken with or following food to reduce stomach irritation. The capsule and the sustained-release tablet should be swallowed whole (not altered). If you forget a dose: Take the missed dose as soon as you remember it, unless it's nearly time for your next dose—if that is the case, skip the missed dose and take the next dose right on schedule. DON'T take two doses at the same time. Talk with your doctor if you find yourself missing doses.

Usual Duration of Use: Use on a regular schedule for 2 to 4 weeks determines effectiveness in reducing the frequency and severity of angina and in controlling hypertension. For long-term use (months to years), the smallest effective dose should be used. Supervision and periodic physician evaluation are essential.

Typical Treatment Goals and Measurements (Outcomes and Markers)

Blood pressure: The most recent treatment guidelines (JNC VI) actually define optimal blood pressure (BP) as less than 120/80 and high normal as 139/89. The American Diabetes Association has chosen a target of 130/80 as the blood pressure goal for people living with diabetes. Most clinicians try to achieve a BP that achieves the best balance of lower cardiovascular risk while avoiding the problem of too low a blood pressure. The goal and time frame (see peak benefits above) should be discussed with you when the prescription is written. Visit www.americanheart.org for the latest information on blood pressure.

Possible Advantages of This Drug

The sustained-release form of this drug permits effective once-a-day treatment for both angina and hypertension.

▷ **This Drug Should Not Be Taken If**

- you have had an allergic reaction to it previously.
- you have active liver disease.
- you are over 71 and have been prescribed the immediate-release form of nifedipine.
- you have low blood pressure—systolic pressure below 90—or you have had a heart attack in the last 4 weeks.
- you have significant narrowing of your aorta (aortic stenosis). Ask your doctor.

▷ **Inform Your Physician Before Taking This Drug If**

- you had an adverse response to any calcium channel blocker.
- you take any form of digitalis or a beta blocker (see Drug Classes).
- you are taking any drugs that lower blood pressure.
- you have a history of congestive heart failure, heart attack or stroke.
- you are subject to disturbances of heart rhythm.
- you have cardiomyopathy (nonobstructive) or aortic stenosis.
- you have impaired liver or kidney function.
- you have abnormal circulation to your fingers.
- you have atrial fibrillation.
- you develop a skin condition while taking this medicine.
- you have diabetes or Duchenne muscular dystrophy.
- you have a history of drug-induced liver damage.

Possible Side Effects (natural, expected and unavoidable drug actions)

Low blood pressure, rapid heart rate, swelling of the feet and ankles, flushing and sensation of warmth, sweating.

▷ **Possible Adverse Effects** (unusual, unexpected and infrequent reactions)

If any of the following develop, consult your physician promptly for guidance.

Mild Adverse Effects

Allergic reactions: skin rash, hives, itching, fever.

Headache, dizziness, weakness, nervousness, blurred vision, eye pain or swelling around eyes—infrequent.

Pedal edema—frequent.

Depression—rare.

Abnormal growth of the gums (gingival hyperplasia)—rare.

Taste disturbances—possible.

Ringing in the ears (tinnitus)—case reports.

Sleep disturbances or bedwetting—case reports.

Increased or decreased blood potassium—possible.

Palpitation, shortness of breath, wheezing, cough—infrequent.

Impaired sense of smell—possible.

Heartburn, nausea, taste disturbances, cramps, diarrhea—rare.

Tremors, muscle cramps—possible.

Serious Adverse Effects

Allergic reaction: drug-induced hepatitis—very rare; drug eruptions and erysipelaslike reactions and exfoliative dermatitis or erythema multiforme.

Idiosyncratic reactions: joint stiffness and inflammation.

Increased frequency or severity of angina on initiation of treatment or following an increase in dose.

Abnormal muscle movements (myoclonus)—case reports.

Kidney toxicity or pulmonary edema—case reports.

Bezoars—rare (seen with sustained-release forms).

Acute psychosis—case report.

Worsening of circulation to the fingers—possible.

Marked drop in blood pressure with fainting—possible.

Low white blood cells, platelets and hemoglobin—case reports.

▷ **Possible Effects on Sexual Function:** Altered timing and pattern of menstruation; excessive menstrual bleeding. Tenderness and swelling of male breast tissue (gynecomastia)—case reports.

▷ **Adverse Effects That May Mimic Natural Diseases or Disorders**

Allergic rash and swelling of the legs may resemble erysipelas. Drug-induced hepatitis may suggest viral hepatitis. Transient increases in liver function tests may suggest infectious hepatitis.

Possible Effects on Laboratory Tests

Bleeding time: increased.

Liver function tests: transient increases.

Blood total cholesterol level: no effect in those under 60 years old; decreased in those over 60 years old.

Blood HDL cholesterol level: no effect or increased.

Blood LDL and VLDL cholesterol levels: no effect.

Blood triglyceride levels: no effect or decreased.

CAUTION

1. Tell health care providers that you take this drug. Note the use of this drug on a card in your purse or wallet.

2. You may use nitroglycerin and other nitrate drugs as needed to relieve acute angina pain. If angina attacks become more frequent or intense, call your doctor.

Precautions for Use

By Infants and Children: Safety and effectiveness for those under 12 years of age are not established.

By Those Over 60 Years of Age: You may be more susceptible to the development of weakness, dizziness, fainting and falling. Take necessary precautions to prevent injury. Report promptly any changes in your pattern of thirst and urination.

▷ **Advisability of Use During Pregnancy**

Pregnancy Category: C. See Pregnancy Risk Categories at the back of this book.

Animal studies: Embryo and fetal deaths reported in mice, rats and rabbits; birth defects reported in rats.

Human studies: Adequate studies of pregnant women are not available.

Avoid this drug during the first 3 months. Use during the final 6 months only if clearly needed. Ask your physician for guidance.

Advisability of Use If Breast-Feeding
Presence of this drug in breast milk: Yes.
Avoid drug or refrain from nursing.

Habit-Forming Potential: None.

Effects of Overdose: Weakness, light-headedness, fainting, fast pulse, low blood pressure, shortness of breath, flushed and warm skin, tremors.

Possible Effects of Long-Term Use: None reported.

Suggested Periodic Examinations While Taking This Drug (at physician's discretion)
Evaluations of heart function, including electrocardiograms.
Measurements of blood pressure in supine, sitting and standing positions.

▷ **While Taking This Drug, Observe the Following**
Foods: Do not eat grapefruit for an hour after taking this medicine. It is also prudent to avoid excessive salt intake.

Herbal Medicines or Minerals: Ginseng may increase blood pressure, blunting the benefits of these medicines. Hawthorn, saw palmetto, ma huang, goldenseal, yohimbe and licorice may also increase blood pressure. Calcium and garlic may help lower blood pressure. Indian snakeroot has a German Commission E monograph indication for hypertension—talk to your doctor. Eleuthero root and ephedra should be avoided by people living with hypertension. St. John's wort and nifedipine can increase sun sensitivity. Caution is advised. Talk with your doctor BEFORE adding any herbal medicine to nifedipine.

Beverages: Grapefruit juice may greatly increase the absorption (bioavailability) of nifedipine and result in an exaggerated therapeutic effect. Water is the best liquid to take this medicine with. May be taken with milk.

▷ *Alcohol:* Use with caution. Alcohol may exaggerate the drop in blood pressure experienced by some people.

Tobacco Smoking: Nicotine may reduce the effectiveness of this drug. I advise everyone to quit smoking.

Marijuana Smoking: Possible reduced effectiveness of this drug; mild to moderate increase in angina; possible changes in electrocardiogram, confusing interpretation.

▷ *Other Drugs*
Nifedipine taken concurrently with
- amiodarone (Cordarone) may cause the heart to stop.
- beta-blocker drugs or digitalis preparations (see Drug Classes) may affect heart rate and rhythm adversely; careful monitoring by your physician is necessary if these drugs are taken concurrently.
- cyclosporine (Sandimmune) can lead to nifedipine toxicity.
- digoxin (Lanoxin) may lead to digoxin toxicity.
- diltiazem (Cardizem) may lead to nifedipine toxicity.
- magnesium can cause additive lowering of the blood pressure.
- oral anticoagulant drugs (see Drug Classes) may increase risk of bleeding.
- oral antidiabetic drugs (see Drug Classes) or insulin may result in loss of glucose control.
- phenytoin (Dilantin) or fosphenytoin (Cerebyx) can cause phenytoin or fosphenytoin toxicity.
- quinupristin/dalfopristin (Synercid) can cause nifedipine toxicity.
- rifampin (Rifadin) can decrease nifedipine's effectiveness.

- tacrolimus (Prograf) may lead to tacrolimus toxicity.
- theophylline can reduce the therapeutic benefits of nifedipine and may lead to theophylline toxicity as well.
- vincristine (Oncovin) can cause vincristine toxicity.

The following drugs may increase the effects of nifedipine:

- some antifungals (fluconazole, itraconazole and ketoconazole)—may increase nifedipine blood levels and lead to toxicity.
- cimetidine (Tagamet).
- quinidine (Quinaglute, others)—can lead to nifedipine toxicity as well as decreased quinidine effectiveness.
- ranitidine (Zantac).
- ritonavir (Norvir) and other protease inhibitors.

▷ *Driving, Hazardous Activities:* Usually no restrictions. This drug may cause drowsiness or dizziness. Restrict activities as necessary.

Aviation Note: Coronary artery disease *is a disqualification* for piloting. Consult a designated Aviation Medical Examiner.

Exposure to Sun: Caution—rare cases of phototoxicity have been reported.

Exposure to Heat: Caution is advised. Hot environments can exaggerate the blood pressure–lowering effects of this drug. Observe for light-headedness or weakness.

Heavy Exercise or Exertion: This drug may improve your ability to be more active without resulting angina pain. Use caution and avoid excessive exercise that could impair heart function in the absence of warning pain.

Discontinuation: Do not stop this drug abruptly. Consult your physician regarding gradual withdrawal. Observe for the possible development of rebound angina.

NISOLDIPINE (ni SOLD i peen)

Introduced: 1996 **Class:** Anti-anginal, antihypertensive, calcium channel blocker **Prescription:** USA: Yes **Controlled Drug:** USA: No; Canada: No **Available as Generic:** No

Brand Name: Sular

Author's Note: Information in this profile will be broadened in subsequent editions if data warrant.

NITROGLYCERIN (ni troh GLIS er in)

Introduced: 1847 **Class:** Anti-anginal, nitrates **Prescription:** USA: Yes **Controlled Drug:** USA: No; Canada: No **Available as Generic:** Yes

Brand Names: Deponit, Minitran Transdermal Delivery System, Nitro-Bid, Nitrocap TD, Nitrocine Timecaps, Nitrocine Transdermal, Nitrodisc, Nitro-Dur, Nitro-Dur II, Nitrogard, ♣Nitrogard-SR, Nitroglyn, Nitrol, Nitrolin, Nitrolingual Spray, ♣Nitrol TSAR Kit, Nitrong, ♣Nitrong SR, Nitroquick, Nitrospan, ♣Nitrostabilin, Nitrostat, Nitro Transdermal System, NTS Transdermal Patch, Transderm-Nitro, ♣Trates S.R., Tridil

BENEFITS versus RISKS	
Possible Benefits	**Possible Risks**
EFFECTIVE RELIEF AND PREVENTION OF ANGINA	Orthostatic hypotension with and without fainting
EFFECTIVE ADJUNCTIVE TREATMENT IN SELECTED CASES OF CONGESTIVE HEART FAILURE	Skin rash—rare
	Altered hemoglobin with large doses— very rare
	Low blood platelets—rare

▷ **Principal Uses**

As a Single Drug Product: Uses currently included in FDA-approved labeling: (1) Treats symptomatic coronary artery disease (rapid-action forms are used to relieve acute attacks of anginal pain; sustained-action forms prevent development of angina); (2) helps improve breathing difficulty caused by heart failure (left ventricle); (3) intravenous form used in surgery to control blood pressure; (4) relieves congestive heart failure after heart attacks.

Other (unlabeled) generally accepted uses: (1) May help ease spasms of the Oddi's sphincter; (2) topical use may help in impotence; (3) can help reduce the extent of heart damage if given following a heart attack (myocardial infarction); (4) helps relax cocaine-constricted heart arteries; (5) eases the pain of peripheral neuropathy; (6) may be of help in easing esophageal problems (achalasia); (7) when the anal sphincter does not work correctly, this drug can help reduce the muscle pressure and ease constipation; (8) nitroglycerin in combination with vasopressin may be of use in stopping bleeding esophageal varices; (9) can help loss of vision that has been caused by a clot in the retinal artery; (10) if ergot medications (see Drug Classes) have shut down circulation to the extremities, nitroglycerin can open up the circulation; (11) used to delay contractions in order to rotate an abnormally positioned fetus; (12) may help diabetics with nerve damage (diabetic neuropathy); (13) helps relax the uterus when the placenta has been retained; (14) relaxes the uterus in cases where a fetus's head is trapped or there is a second fetus.

How This Drug Works: Relaxes and dilates both arteries and veins. Beneficial effects in angina are due to (1) dilation of narrowed coronary arteries and (2) dilation of veins in the general circulation, with reduced volume and pressure of blood entering the heart. Net effects are improved blood supply to the heart and reduced work for the heart. Both actions reduce the frequency and severity of angina.

Available Dosage Forms and Strengths

Canisters, translingual spray — 13.8 g (200 doses), 0.4 mg per metered dose

Capsules, prolonged-action — 2.5 mg, 2.6 mg, 6.5 mg, 9 mg

Ointment — 2%

Tablets, buccal — 1 mg, 2 mg, 3 mg

Tablets, prolonged-action — 2.6 mg, 6.5 mg, 9 mg

Tablets, sublingual — 0.15 mg, 0.3 mg, 0.4 mg, 0.6 mg

Transdermal systems (all per 24 hours) — 2.5 mg, 5 mg, 7.5 mg, 10 mg, 15 mg

▷ **Usual Adult Dosage Ranges:** Translingual spray—one or two metered sprays (0.4 mg) under the tongue every 3 to 5 minutes, up to three doses within 15 minutes, to relieve acute angina. To prevent angina, one spray taken 5 to 10 minutes before exertion.

Sublingual tablets—0.15 to 0.6 mg (150 to 600 mcg) dissolved under tongue at 5-minute intervals to relieve acute angina. Up to three doses can be taken. One tablet can be taken 5–10 minutes BEFORE you participate in an activity that may cause angina in order to try to prevent an attack.

Prolonged-action tablets—2.5 mg at 6- to 8-hour intervals to prevent angina. Many clinicians give a 6- to 12-hour nitrate-free interval when using this dosage form.

Ointment—0.5 inch or 7.5 mg applied in a thin, even layer of uniform size to hairless skin at 3- to 4-hour intervals to prevent angina. A 10- to 12-hour ointment-free interval is recommended by some clinicians to avoid tolerance.

Buccal tablets—1 to 2 mg every 4 to 5 hours, placed between cheek and gum.

Transdermal patches—5-square-cm to 30-square-cm patch applied to hairless skin once every 24 hours (with a 10- to 12-hour nitrate-free interval to avoid tolerance) when used to prevent angina.

Note: Actual dose and schedule must be determined for each patient individually.

Author's Note: In order to avoid tolerance to the therapeutic effects of this medicine, a nitrate-free interval of 10–12 hours daily is recommended: 24-hour patches are removed after having been applied for 12 hours; dosing of ointment is interrupted for 12 hours a day; oral sustained-release formulations are dosed to give a 6- to 12-hour nitrate-free interval.

Conditions Requiring Dosing Adjustments

Liver Function: Specific dose adjustments in liver compromise are not defined.

Kidney Function: Specific guidelines for dosing changes are not available. This drug can discolor urine.

▷ **Dosing Instructions:** Dose forms to be swallowed are best taken when stomach is empty (1 hour before or 2 hours after eating) to obtain maximal blood levels. Tablets should not be crushed. Capsules may be opened, but contents should not be crushed or chewed before swallowing. If you forget a dose: Call your doctor for instructions as to what to do.

Usual Duration of Use: Use on a regular schedule for 3 to 5 days is often needed to determine effectiveness in preventing and relieving acute anginal attacks. Individual dose adjustments will be necessary for optimal results. Long-term use (months to years) requires physician supervision.

Typical Treatment Goals and Measurements (Outcomes and Markers)

Angina: The goal is to relieve chest pain with under the tongue (sublingual) forms or spray. If pain is NOT relieved, call your doctor and have someone take you to the hospital. For patch or prolonged action tablets, the frequency and severity of anginal attacks should decrease. Call your doctor if you gain a lowered severity and frequency of angina, and then start to lose that benefit.

▷ **This Drug Should Not Be Taken If**
- you have had an allergic reaction to it previously.
- you are severely anemic.
- you have had recent head trauma.

- you have had a heart attack and have an increased heart rate or increased blood pressure.
- you have pericarditis (intravenous form).
- you have hyperthyroidism.
- you have increased intraocular pressure.
- you have abnormal growth of the heart muscle in response to vascular disease (hypertrophic cardiomyopathy).
- you have closed-angle glaucoma (inadequately treated).

▷ **Inform Your Physician Before Taking This Drug If**
- you had an unfavorable response to other nitrates.
- you have low blood pressure.
- you have problems absorbing medicines (malabsorption syndromes) or excessive action of your stomach (gastric hypermotility).
- you have any form of glaucoma.
- you have an overactive thyroid or are pregnant.
- you have had recent bleeding or trauma to your head.

Possible Side Effects (natural, expected and unavoidable drug actions)
Flushing of face, headaches (50%), orthostatic hypotension (see Glossary), rapid heart rate, palpitation.

▷ **Possible Adverse Effects** (unusual, unexpected and infrequent reactions)
If any of the following develop, consult your physician promptly for guidance.
Mild Adverse Effects
Allergic reactions: skin rash.
Throbbing headaches (may be severe and persistent), dizziness, fainting—possible.
Nausea, vomiting, taste disorders—infrequent.
Serious Adverse Effects
Allergic reactions: severe skin reactions with peeling.
Idiosyncratic reaction: methemoglobinemia—case reports.
Abnormally slow heartbeat (bradycardia)—rare.
Low blood supply to the head (transient ischemic attacks)—case reports.
Increased intracranial pressure—rare.

▷ **Possible Effects on Sexual Function:** Correction of impotence (one report following sublingual use). Preventive use of nitroglycerin prior to sexual activity has been recommended to eliminate or reduce the risk of angina. Consult your physician for guidance.

▷ **Adverse Effects That May Mimic Natural Diseases or Disorders**
Hypotensive spells (sudden drops in blood pressure) due to this drug may be mistaken for late-onset epilepsy.

Possible Effects on Laboratory Tests
Blood platelet count: decreased—very rare.
Bleeding time: prolonged.

CAUTION
1. This drug can provoke migraine headaches in susceptible individuals.
2. Patients with impaired brain circulation (cerebral arteriosclerosis) have increased risk of transient ischemic attacks—periods of temporary speech impairment, paralysis, numbness, etc.
3. Tolerance to long-acting forms of nitrates will happen in most patients

after 24 hours of continuous use. A nitrate-free interval of 10 hours usually restores effectiveness.

4. Many over-the-counter (OTC) drug products for allergies, colds and coughs contain drugs that may counteract the desired effects of this drug. Ask your physician or pharmacist for help before using any such medications.

Precautions for Use

By Infants and Children: Limited usefulness and experience in this age group. Dose schedules are not established.

By Those Over 60 Years of Age: Begin treatment with small doses and increase dose cautiously as needed and tolerated. You may be more susceptible to the development of flushing, throbbing headache, dizziness, "blackout" spells, fainting and falling.

▷ **Advisability of Use During Pregnancy**

Pregnancy Category: C. See Pregnancy Risk Categories at the back of this book.
Animal studies: No information available.
Human studies: Adequate studies of pregnant women are not available.
Use this drug only if clearly needed. Ask your physician for guidance.

Advisability of Use If Breast-Feeding

Presence of this drug in breast milk: Unknown.
Watch nursing infant closely, and discontinue drug or nursing if adverse effects develop.

Habit-Forming Potential: None.

Effects of Overdose: Throbbing headache, dizziness, marked flushing, nausea, vomiting, abdominal cramps, confusion, delirium, paralysis, seizures, circulatory collapse.

Possible Effects of Long-Term Use: The development of tolerance (see Glossary) and the temporary loss of effectiveness.

Suggested Periodic Examinations While Taking This Drug (at physician's discretion)

Measurements of blood pressure and internal eye pressures.
Evaluation of hemoglobin.

▷ **While Taking This Drug, Observe the Following**

Foods: No restrictions.

Herbal Medicines or Minerals: Hawthorn and co-enzyme Q10 (co-Q10) can affect the way the heart works. BE CERTAIN to tell your doctor that you are taking or are considering taking these herbs if you are taking a nitrate.

Beverages: No restrictions. May be taken with milk.

▷ *Alcohol:* Avoid alcohol completely. This combination may result in severe lowering of blood pressure. There is a potential for collapse of the circulation and pumping effectiveness of the heart.

Tobacco Smoking: Nicotine can reduce the effectiveness of this drug. I advise everyone to quit smoking.

Marijuana Smoking: Possible reduced effectiveness of this drug; mild to moderate increase in angina; possible changes in the electrocardiogram, confusing interpretation.

▷ *Other Drugs*

Nitroglycerin *taken concurrently* with

• acetylcysteine (NAC) may reverse tolerance to the intravenous form of this medicine.

- alteplase (Activase) lessens the benefits of alteplase; nitroglycerin and alteplase combination should be avoided if possible.
- antihypertensive drugs may cause excessive lowering of blood pressure; careful dose adjustments may be necessary.
- dihydroergotamine or similar ergot medicines (see Drug Classes) may result in ergotamine toxicity.
- diltiazem (Cardizem) can result in abnormally low blood pressure when used with the sustained-release form of nitroglycerin.
- heparin can result in decreased therapeutic benefit of heparin.
- indomethacin (Indocin) can blunt the benefits of nitroglycerin.
- isosorbide dinitrate (Isordil) or mononitrate (Ismo) may result in decreased nitroglycerin therapeutic benefits.
- neuromuscular blocking agents (such as pancuronium-Pavulon, vecuronium-Norcuron, others) can result in increased severity of muscle blockade. Use of lower neuromuscular blocker doses is prudent.
- sildenafil (Viagra) may cause very low blood pressure—DO NOT COMBINE. The following drugs may *increase* the effects of nitroglycerin:
- aspirin in analgesic doses (500 mg or more) and perhaps other NSAIDs.

▷ *Driving, Hazardous Activities:* Usually no restrictions. This drug may cause dizziness or faintness. Restrict activities as necessary.

Aviation Note: Coronary artery disease *is a disqualification* for piloting. Consult a designated Aviation Medical Examiner.

Exposure to Sun: No restrictions.

Exposure to Heat: Hot environments can cause significant lowering of blood pressure.

Exposure to Cold: Cold environments can increase the need for this drug and limit its effectiveness.

Heavy Exercise or Exertion: This drug can increase your tolerance for exercise. Ask your doctor how much exercise is okay for you.

Special Storage Instructions: For sublingual tablets, to prevent loss of strength:
- keep tablets in the original glass container.
- do not transfer tablets to a plastic or metallic container (such as a pillbox).
- do not place absorbent cotton, paper (such as the prescription label) or other material inside the container.
- do not store other drugs in the same container.
- immediately close the container tightly after each use.
- store at room temperature.

Discontinuation: Do not stop this drug abruptly after long-term use. Best to lower the dose (of prolonged-action forms) slowly over 4 to 6 weeks. Watch for rebound angina.

NIZATIDINE (ni ZA te deen)

Please see the histamine (H2) blocking drug family profile.

NORFLOXACIN (nor FLOX a sin)

Please see the fluoroquinolone antibiotic family profile.

NORTRIPTYLINE (nor TRIP ti leen)

Introduced: 1963   **Class:** Antidepressant   **Prescription:** USA: Yes
Controlled Drug: USA: No; Canada: No   **Available as Generic:**   USA: Yes;
Canada: No
Brand Names: Aventyl, Pamelor

BENEFITS versus RISKS	
Possible Benefits	*Possible Risks*
EFFECTIVE RELIEF OF ENDOGENOUS DEPRESSION	ADVERSE BEHAVIORAL EFFECTS: confusion, disorientation, hallucinations, delusions
Possibly beneficial in other depressive disorders	CONVERSION OF DEPRESSION TO MANIA in manic-depressive (bipolar) disorders
Possibly beneficial in the management of some types of chronic, severe pain	Aggravation of schizophrenia Irregular heart rhythms Rare blood cell abnormalities

Author's Note: The information in this profile has been shortened to make room for more widely used medicines.

OFLOXACIN (oh FLOX a sin)

Please see the fluoroquinolone antibiotic family profile.

OLANZAPINE (oh LAN za pean)

Introduced: 1996   **Class:** Antipsychotic; tranquilizer, major; thienobenzo-diazepines; atypical antipsychotics   **Prescription:** USA: Yes   **Controlled Drug:**   USA: No; Canada: No   **Available as Generic:**   USA: No; Canada: No
Brand Name: Zyprexa, Zyprexa Zydis

BENEFITS versus RISKS	
Possible Benefits	*Possible Risks*
EFFECTIVE SHORT-TERM CONTROL OF ACUTE MENTAL DISORDERS: beneficial effects on thinking, mood and behavior	POSSIBLE TARDIVE DYSKINESIA (SERIOUS TOXIC BRAIN EFFECT WITH LONG-TERM USE)
DELIVERS BENEFITS IN EASING MANIA (IN BIPOLAR DISORDER) AS SOON AS IN THE FIRST WEEK OF TREATMENT	Orthostatic hypotension (see Glossary) Increased liver enzymes
Zyprexa Zydis form falls apart in the mouth, making it easier to take	
Relief of anxiety, agitation and tension	
Medicines in this class are probably drugs of choice in older adults.	

▷ **Principal Uses**

As a Single Drug Product: Uses currently included in FDA-approved labeling: (1) Helps manage thinking problems and other difficulties seen in psychosis; (2) treats mania in bipolar disorder (easing mania symptoms after only one week of treatment).

Other (unlabeled) generally accepted uses: (1) Works in marijuana (cannabis)-induced psychotic disorder.

How This Drug Works: This drug works as an antipsychotic by inhibiting the action of two primary nerve transmitters (dopamine and serotonin) in certain brain centers and acts to correct an imbalance of nerve impulse transmissions thought to be responsible for certain mental disorders. It also works at histamine, muscarinic, GABA, BZD and adrenergic sites. The mechanism of action in bipolar disorder is not fully known at present.

Available Dosage Forms and Strengths

Tablets — 2.5 mg, 5 mg, 7.5 mg,10 mg

Tablets, orally disintegrating (Zyprexa Zydis) — dosages pending

▷ **Recommended Dosage Ranges** (Actual dose and schedule must be determined for each patient individually.)

Infants and Children: Dose not established.

18 to 60 Years of Age: Psychosis: Dosing is started with 5 to 10 mg daily. If the 5-mg dose is used, the dose may be increased to a maximum of 10 mg as needed and tolerated. Dose changes should only be made after one week at a new dose.

Sudden (acute) mania: 10 to 15 mg once daily.

Author's Note: Gender data are now FDA-required for new approvals—it must be noted that the drug is removed (cleared) 30% slower in women than in men. Therefore effects (both desirable and undesirable) caused by the medicine may last longer in women (dose to dose) than in men.

Over 60 Years of Age: 5 mg of olanzapine is taken.

Conditions Requiring Dosing Adjustments

Liver Function: The drug is highly metabolized in the liver, and although the manufacturer does not have recommendations for dosing changes, smaller doses and close patient monitoring appear prudent.

Kidney Function: Dosing changes are not thought to be needed.

Seizure Disorders: Seizures happened in 0.9% of patients during clinical trials of olanzapine. Olanzapine should be used with caution by seizure patients. Dose decreases are not defined at present.

▷ **Dosing Instructions:** The tablet may be crushed and taken with food. It is best to take this medicine at the same time every day. If you forget a dose: Take the missed dose as soon as you remember it, unless it's nearly time for your next dose—if that is the case, skip the missed dose and take the next dose right on schedule. DO NOT double doses. Talk with your doctor if you find yourself missing doses.

Usual Duration of Use: Use on a regular schedule for at least 1 week is required to reach steady-state levels and hence determines effectiveness. Clinical benefits in mania of bipolar disorder may be seen in the first week of therapy. Clinical trials that led to FDA approval were conducted for 6 weeks. Use beyond 6 weeks requires physician supervision and was not studied in clinical trials. Studies are ongoing to evaluate longer use.

Typical Treatment Goals and Measurements (Outcomes and Markers)

Schizophrenia: The general goal: to ease the severity of symptoms in order to let the patient resume his or her usual activities. There should be lessened intrusion of abnormal thinking into more normal life.

Possible Advantages of This Drug Effective reversal of symptoms of psychosis while acting at different sites than previously available agents. Rapid onset in bipolar disorder. Medicines in this class are probably drugs of choice in older adults. Zyprexa Zydis form falls apart in the mouth making it easier to take.

▷ **This Drug Should Not Be Taken If**
  • you have had an allergic reaction to it previously.

▷ **Inform Your Physician Before Taking This Drug If**
  • you have a seizure disorder.
  • you have had neuroleptic malignant syndrome.
  • your liver is compromised.
  • you have constitutionally low blood pressure, take medicine to treat high blood pressure or have cardiovascular disease.
  • you have had narrow angle glaucoma.
  • you are pregnant.
  • you have severe liver disease.
  • you have a history of breast cancer.
  • you are taking any drug with sedative effects.
  • you tend to be constipated.
  • you plan to have surgery under general or spinal anesthesia in the near future.
  • you have problems swallowing.

Possible Side Effects (natural, expected and unavoidable drug actions)
  Orthostatic hypotension (see Glossary), drowsiness.

▷ **Possible Adverse Effects** (unusual, unexpected and infrequent reactions)
  If any of the following develop, consult your physician promptly for guidance.

  Mild Adverse Effects
  Allergic reactions: skin rash, itching—rare.
  Drowsiness, agitation, insomnia and dizziness—frequent.
  Headache, drowsiness—rare.
  Depression—rare.
  Dizziness—rare to infrequent.
  Somnolence—frequent.
  Prolonged QT interval—possible.
  Edema—infrequent.
  Weight gain, constipation—infrequent.

  Serious Adverse Effects
  Allergic reactions: hair loss—rare.
  Abnormal movements (appears to be dose-related)—infrequent.
  Drug-induced increased liver enzymes—rare.
  Low white blood cell count (neutropenia)—case reports.
  Difficulty swallowing (dysphagia)—case reports.
  Tardive dyskinesia—possible.
  Neuroleptic malignant syndrome—case reports.

Seizure—case report.

New onset diabetes mellitus—case reports.

▷ **Possible Effects on Sexual Function:** Case reports of extended and painful erections (priapism).

▷ **Adverse Effects That May Mimic Natural Diseases or Disorders**

Nervous system reactions may suggest true Parkinson's disease. Liver reactions may suggest viral hepatitis.

Possible Effects on Laboratory Tests

Prolactin levels: increased.

Liver function tests: increased liver enzymes (ALT/GPT, AST/GOT and alkaline phosphatase).

CAUTION

1. Other medicines (nonprescription or prescription) that can cause drowsiness or central nervous system effects may react unfavorably with this medicine. Talk with your doctor or pharmacist before combining any medicines.
2. Since this medicine can cause orthostatic hypotension, some high blood pressure (antihypertensive) medicines may have a greater than expected effect if taken with olanzapine.

Precautions for Use

By Infants and Children: Safety and effectiveness for those under 18 years of age are not established.

By Those Over 60 Years of Age: Lower starting doses should be taken; caution is advised regarding drowsiness, dizziness and orthostatic hypotension, since olanzapine can cause changes in the ability of the body to regulate changes in temperature and this regulation may be less intact in older patients to begin with. You may also be more susceptible to Parkinson-like reactions and/or tardive dyskinesia (see Glossary). Discuss early indications of these reactions with your doctor, as progression of these reactions may lead to symptoms that are not reversible.

▷ **Advisability of Use During Pregnancy**

Pregnancy Category: C. See Pregnancy Risk Categories at the back of this book.

Animal studies: Rat and mouse studies reveal increased mammary gland adenomas (when the animals were given 0.5 and 2 times the mg-per-square-meter human dose) respectively. Increased numbers of nonviable fetuses were seen in one rat study using nine times the maximum human dose.

Human studies: Adequate studies of pregnant women are not available.

Use of this drug is a benefit-to-risk decision. Ask your doctor for guidance.

Advisability of Use If Breast-Feeding

Presence of this drug in breast milk: Unknown in humans.

Avoid drug or refrain from nursing.

Habit-Forming Potential: None.

Effects of Overdose: Reports of 67 overdoses were made during clinical trials. The patient who took the largest dose had drowsiness and slurred speech.

Possible Effects of Long-Term Use: None defined as yet.

Suggested Periodic Examinations While Taking This Drug (at physician's discretion)

Liver function tests.

Careful inspection of the tongue for early evidence of fine, involuntary, wave-like movements that could be the beginning of tardive dyskinesia.

Sitting and standing blood pressure checks may be advisable when therapy is started, to assess orthostatic hypotension.

▷ **While Taking This Drug, Observe the Following**

Foods: No restrictions. Follow prescribed diet. See grapefruit warning below.

Herbal Medicines or Minerals: Using kola or ma huang may result in unacceptable central nervous system stimulation. Since part of the way ginseng works may be as a MAO inhibitor, do not combine ginseng with olanzapine. Valerian and kava kava may interact to increase drowsiness.

Beverages: Grapefruit juice may decrease metabolism of olanzapine and lead to toxicity. May be taken with milk or water.

▷ *Alcohol:* Avoid completely.

Tobacco Smoking: Olanzapine is removed from the body up to 40% faster in people who smoke compared to those who do not. Recommendations for dosing changes are not available. I advise everyone to quit smoking.

Marijuana Smoking: Expected to cause an increase in drowsiness; accentuation of orthostatic hypotension; increased risk of precipitating latent psychoses, confusing the interpretation of mental status and drug responses.

▷ *Other Drugs*

Olanzapine *taken concurrently* with

- activated charcoal will decrease absorption of olanzapine.(May be of use in overdoses.)
- any medicine that has central nervous system activity may result in additive effects.
- any medicine that can cause liver damage may result in additive liver problems.
- any sedative drugs (prescription and nonprescription) can cause excessive sedation.
- benzodiazepines (see Drug Classes) may magnify the orthostatic hypotension problem caused by olanzapine.
- carbamazepine (Tegretol) causes up to a 50% increase in removal of olanzapine from the body; dosing increases in olanzapine appear prudent.
- fluoroquinolone antibiotics, such as ciprofloxacin (Cipro) or norfloxacin (Noroxin), may lead to olanzapine toxicity.
- fluvoxamine (Luvox) may lead to olanzapine toxicity.
- lithium (Lithobid, others) may increase risk of serious nerve effects—extreme care should be taken and patients closely monitored for signs of toxicity and movement problems—especially if high doses of antipsychotic drugs and lithium are used. Call your doctor immediately if these signs or symptoms begin.
- medicines that *decrease* or inhibit cytochrome P450 1A2 or glucuronyl transferase enzymes may lead to olanzapine toxicity.

The following drugs may *decrease* the effects of olanzapine:

- medicines that increase (induce) cytochrome P450 1A2 or glucuronyl transferase enzymes may blunt olanzapine benefits.
- omeprazole (Prilosec).
- rifampin (Rifater, others).

▷ *Driving, Hazardous Activities:* This drug may cause drowsiness or dizziness. Restrict activities as necessary.

Aviation Note: The use of this drug *may be a disqualification* for piloting. Consult a designated Aviation Medical Examiner.

Exposure to Sun: No problems reported.

Exposure to Heat: This medicine can cause problems in regulating body temperature (core temperature homeostasis). If you work or are frequently in a hot environment, be careful to replace enough fluids to avoid dehydration.

Heavy Exercise or Exertion: Since this medicine may cause problems in temperature regulation, caution is advised.

Discontinuation: Do not stop this medicine without first talking to your doctor.

OLSALAZINE (ohl SAL a zeen)

Introduced: 1987   **Class:** Bowel anti-inflammatory   **Prescription:** USA: Yes   **Controlled Drug:** USA: No; Canada: No   **Available as Generic:** USA: No; Canada: No

Brand Name: Dipentum

BENEFITS versus RISKS	
Possible Benefits	*Possible Risks*
EFFECTIVE SUPPRESSION OF INFLAMMATORY BOWEL DISEASE	RARE BONE MARROW DEPRESSION (see Glossary) Drug-induced hepatitis Occasional aggravation of ulcerative colitis

▷ **Principal Uses**

As a Single Drug Product: Uses currently included in FDA-approved labeling: Used to maintain remission of chronic ulcerative colitis and proctitis.

Other (unlabeled) generally accepted uses: (1) Has a role in treatment of active ulcerative colitis; (2) works in collagenous colitis in adults.

How This Drug Works: This drug is actually two molecules of 5-aminosalicylic acid (ASA) joined together. In the body, it is converted to the active ASA and then suppresses the formation of prostaglandins (and related compounds), tissue substances that induce inflammation, tissue destruction and diarrhea—the main features of ulcerative colitis and proctitis.

Available Dosage Forms and Strengths

Capsules — 250 mg

Tablets (Canada only) — 500 mg

▷ **Recommended Dosage Ranges** (Actual dose and schedule must be determined for each patient individually.)

Infants and Children: Dose not established.

12 to 60 Years of Age: 500 mg twice daily, morning and evening.

Over 60 Years of Age: Same as 12 to 60 years of age.

Conditions Requiring Dosing Adjustments

Liver Function: No changes needed in liver disease, but since this drug can be toxic to the liver (granulomatous hepatitis), it should be used with caution by patients with liver problems.

Kidney Function: Some of the metabolites of olsalazine are eliminated by the kidneys. There is potential for kidney damage by one of these compounds, and the drug should be a benefit-to-risk decision by patients with compromised kidneys.

▷ **Dosing Instructions:** The capsule may be opened and taken with food, preferably with breakfast and dinner. If you forget a dose: Take the missed dose as soon as you remember it, unless it's nearly time for your next dose—if that is the case, skip the missed dose and take the next dose right on schedule. DON'T double doses. Talk with your doctor if you find yourself missing doses.

Usual Duration of Use: Use on a regular schedule for 1 to 3 weeks determines effectiveness in controlling the symptoms of ulcerative colitis. Ongoing treatment of up to two years has been successful in preventing relapse of ulcerative colitis. Long-term use (months to years) requires physician supervision.

Typical Treatment Goals and Measurements (Outcomes and Markers)

Ulcerative colitis: The general goal is to lower the frequency of stools, ease cramping, reduce amount of blood in the stools and stop fever. More involved exams will reveal an absence of bowel ulceration and easing of friability or granularity of the bowel itself. Use after acute cases have resolved seeks to prevent relapse of ulcerative colitis.

▷ **This Drug Should Not Be Taken If**
- you have had an allergic reaction to it previously.
- you have severely impaired kidney function.
- you are allergic to aspirin.

▷ **Inform Your Physician Before Taking This Drug If**
- you are allergic to aspirin (or other salicylates), mesalamine or sulfasalazine.
- you are allergic by nature: history of hay fever, asthma, hives, eczema.
- you have impaired kidney function.
- you have severe liver disease.
- you are currently taking sulfasalazine (Azulfidine).

Possible Side Effects (natural, expected and unavoidable drug actions)
None.

▷ **Possible Adverse Effects** (unusual, unexpected and infrequent reactions)
If any of the following develop, consult your physician promptly for guidance.

Mild Adverse Effects
Allergic reactions: skin rash, itching—rare.
Headache, drowsiness, depression, dizziness—rare.
Loss of appetite, indigestion, nausea, vomiting, stomach pain, diarrhea—rare to infrequent.
Paresthesias or blurred vision—rare.
Joint aches and pains—infrequent.

Serious Adverse Effects
Allergic reactions: dermatitis, hair loss—rare.
Bone marrow depression (see Glossary): fatigue, fever, sore throat, abnormal bleeding/bruising—case reports.
Drug-induced hepatitis (see Glossary), pericarditis, pancreatitis or kidney damage—rare.
Spasm of the bronchi of the lung—rare.

▷ **Possible Effects on Sexual Function:** Impotence, excessive menstrual flow—case reports.

Possible Effects on Laboratory Tests

Complete blood cell counts: decreased red cells, hemoglobin, white cells and platelets; increased eosinophils.

Liver function tests: increased liver enzymes (ALT/GPT, AST/GOT and alkaline phosphatase), increased bilirubin.

Urinalysis: red blood cells and protein present.

CAUTION
1. Report promptly any signs of infection or unusual bleeding or bruising.
2. Report promptly any indications of active or intensified ulcerative colitis: abdominal cramping, bloody diarrhea, fever.

Precautions for Use

By Infants and Children: Safety and effectiveness for those under 12 years of age are not established.

By Those Over 60 Years of Age: None.

▷ **Advisability of Use During Pregnancy**

Pregnancy Category: C. See Pregnancy Risk Categories at the back of this book.

Animal studies: Rat studies reveal toxic effects on the fetus, retarded bone development and impaired development of internal organs.

Human studies: Adequate studies of pregnant women are not available.

Use this drug only if clearly needed. Ask your physician for guidance.

Advisability of Use If Breast-Feeding

Presence of this drug in breast milk: Controversial, has caused diarrhea in some infants.

Avoid drug or refrain from nursing.

Habit-Forming Potential: None.

Effects of Overdose: Headache, dizziness, nausea, vomiting, abdominal cramping.

Possible Effects of Long-Term Use: Bone marrow depression (impaired production of blood cells).

Suggested Periodic Examinations While Taking This Drug (at physician's discretion)

Complete blood cell counts.

Liver function tests.

Kidney function tests.

Urinalysis.

▷ **While Taking This Drug, Observe the Following**

Foods: No restrictions. Follow prescribed diet.

Herbal Medicines or Minerals: Flaxseed, peppermint oil and psyllium husk have commission E monograph indications for irritable bowel syndrome. This is NOT the same as ulcerative colitis, and those products have not been studied in ulcerative colitis. Aloe, buckhorn berry or bark, cascara sagrada bark, rhubarb root and senna should not be taken by people living with ulcerative colitis.

Beverages: No restrictions. May be taken with milk.

▷ *Alcohol:* No interactions expected.

Tobacco Smoking: No interactions expected. I advise everyone to quit smoking.
▷ *Other Drugs*
  Olsalazine *taken concurrently* with
  • alendronate (Fosamax) may increase risk of GI upset.
  • low molecular weight heparins enoxaparin (Lovenox), Normiflo or Fragmin (see Drug Classes) may increase bleeding risk.
  • mercaptopurine (Purinethol) may lead to bone marrow depression.
  • varicella vaccine (Varivax) may result in an increased risk of Reye's syndrome; this drug should be avoided for 6 weeks after the vaccine is given.
  • warfarin (Coumadin) may increase INR; more frequent tests may be warranted if these medicines are combined.
▷ *Driving, Hazardous Activities:* This drug may cause drowsiness or dizziness. Restrict activities as necessary.
  Aviation Note: The use of this drug *may be a disqualification* for piloting. Consult a designated Aviation Medical Examiner.
  Exposure to Sun: Use caution—this drug can cause photosensitization (see Glossary).

OMEPRAZOLE (oh MEH pra zohl)

Introduced: 1986   **Class:** Proton pump inhibitor   **Prescription:** USA: Yes   **Controlled Drug:** USA: No; Canada: No   **Available as Generic:** USA: No; Canada: No
Brand Names: ❧Losec, Prilosec

BENEFITS versus RISKS	
Possible Benefits	*Possible Risks*
VERY EFFECTIVE TREATMENT OF CONDITIONS ASSOCIATED WITH EXCESSIVE PRODUCTION OF GASTRIC ACID: Zollinger-Ellison syndrome, mastocytosis, endocrine adenoma	Rare aplastic anemia Rare liver failure
VERY EFFECTIVE TREATMENT OF REFLUX ESOPHAGITIS, GASTRIC AND DUODENAL ULCERS	
EFFECTIVE IN COMBINATION WITH CLARITHROMYCIN and AMOXICILLIN in treatment of Helicobacter pylori infections	
ONCE DAILY DOSING ENHANCES COMPLIANCE	
Prevention of NSAID-induced ulcers	

▷ **Principal Uses**
  As a Single Drug Product: Uses currently included in FDA-approved labeling: (1) Inhibits stomach acid formation in acute and chronic gastritis, reflux esophagitis, gastroesophageal reflux disease, Zollinger-Ellison syndrome, mastocytosis, endocrine adenomas and active duodenal ulcer; (2)

approved for long-term use in erosive esophagitis; (3) approved for combination treatment (with clarithromycin [Biaxin]) in patients with positive Helicobacter pylori cultures (removes the bacteria in up to 92% of patients); (4) helps in the short-term treatment of active and benign stomach (gastric) ulcers; (5) part of a three-drug, 10-day regimen (omeprazole, amoxicillin and clarithromycin) to treat duodenal ulcers.

Other (unlabeled) generally accepted uses: (1) May have a role in treating severe stomach bleeding (hemorrhagic gastritis); (2) possible use in ulcerative colitis; (3) prevention of ulcers caused by NSAIDs; (4) could be of help in asthma; (5) could help hiccups resistant to other therapy (intractable).

How This Drug Works: Inhibits a specific enzyme system (proton pump H/K ATPase) in the stomach lining, stopping production of stomach acid and thereby (1) eliminates a principal cause of the condition under treatment and (2) creates an environment conducive to healing. Taking this medicine 15–30 minutes before the morning meal makes best use of the fact that this will allow the medicine to be at its peak just when the largest number of proton pumps are working.

Available Dosage Forms and Strengths

Capsules, delayed-release — 20 mg

▷ **Usual Adult Dosage Ranges:** *Reflux esophagitis:* 20 mg once daily 15–30 minutes before the morning meal for a duration of 4 to 8 weeks. Excessive stomach acid conditions: 60 mg once daily for as long as necessary. In extreme cases, doses of 120 mg three times a day have been used.

Gastric and duodenal ulcer: 20 mg once daily for 4 to 8 weeks.

Duodenal ulcer combination therapy (28-day regimen): Omeprazole 40 mg daily with clarithromycin 500 mg three times a day for days 1–14 and then omeprazole 20 mg daily for days 15–28.

Helicobacter pylori: Dual drug approach: 40 mg of omeprazole once a day combined with 500 mg of clarithromycin three times a day. Treatment is continued for two weeks. Triple drug approach: Omeprazole 20 mg twice a day or 40 mg once a day with clarithromycin 500 mg and amoxicillin 1,000 mg, all given twice a day for 10 days. Patients who have (present with) an ulcer when treatment is started also get omeprazole alone at 20 mg a day for another 18 days.

Note: Actual dose and schedule must be determined for each patient individually.

Conditions Requiring Dosing Adjustments

Liver Function: Patients should be monitored closely.

Kidney Function: Dose adjustments do not appear to be needed.

▷ **Dosing Instructions:** Take immediately before eating, preferably 15–30 minutes before the morning meal. The capsule should be swallowed whole without opening; the contents should not be crushed or chewed. This drug may be taken with antacids if they are needed to relieve stomach pain. If swallowing is a problem, the capsules CAN be opened and the intact granules mixed in a fruit juice (such as apple, cranberry, orange or grape—acidic fruit juices) or a small amount of applesauce just before you take it. If you forget a dose: Take the missed dose as soon as you remember it, unless it's nearly time for your next dose—if that is the case, skip the missed dose and take the next dose right on schedule. DO NOT double doses. Talk with your doctor if you find yourself missing doses.

Usual Duration of Use: Use on a regular schedule for 2 to 3 weeks determines benefit in suppressing stomach acid production. Long-term use (months to years) requires periodic physician evaluation of response.

Typical Treatment Goals and Measurements (Outcomes and Markers)

Ulcers: The role of *Helicobacter pylori* in ulcers is no longer questioned and a proton pump inhibitor is widely recognized as the standard for short-term treatment of stomach ulcers. When *H. pylori* is present, single medicine therapy is not recommended. Additionally, an antibiotic is often used with other agents. The goal is to heal the ulcer area and prevent reoccurrence of the ulceration. Sign and symptom relief as well as endoscopic examination help define success of treatment.

Possible Advantages of This Drug

Effectively inhibits acid secretion at all times: basal conditions (stomach empty and at rest) and following food, alcohol, smoking or other stimulants. More effective than histamine (H2) receptor blocking drugs in treating severe reflux esophagitis and refractory duodenal ulcer.

Currently a Drug of Choice

For the short-term treatment of severe reflux esophagitis and the long-term treatment of Zollinger-Ellison syndrome and erosive esophagitis. Part of a one-week regimen of choice (comparing outcomes) with clarithromycin and metronidazole for treating *H. pylori*.

▷ **This Drug Should Not Be Taken If**
- you have had an allergic reaction to it previously.
- you have a currently active bone marrow or blood cell disorder.

▷ **Inform Your Physician Before Taking This Drug If**
- you have a history of liver disease or impaired liver function.
- your history includes any bone marrow or blood cell disorder, especially a drug-induced one.
- you take any anticoagulant medication or diazepam (Valium) or phenytoin (Dilantin, etc.).

Possible Side Effects (natural, expected and unavoidable drug actions)

Acid in the stomach actually works to protect it from some bacterial infections. Since omeprazole is so effective in decreasing acid, it may increase the likelihood of infection by *Campylobacter*. This organism causes gastroenteritis. Symptoms may include mucous, loose stools and fever. Talk with your doctor if you start to develop these symptoms while taking omeprazole.

▷ **Possible Adverse Effects** (unusual, unexpected and infrequent reactions)

If any of the following develop, consult your physician promptly for guidance.

Mild Adverse Effects

Allergic reactions: skin rash—rare; itching.

Headache, dizziness, muscle pain or ringing in ears; drowsiness, paresthesias, weakness—rare to infrequent.

Indigestion, nausea, vomiting, diarrhea, constipation—rare to infrequent.

Serious Adverse Effects

Allergic reactions: rare allergic kidney damage (interstitial nephritis), rare anaphylactic reaction.

Bone marrow depression: fatigue, fever, sore throat, infections, abnormal bleeding/bruising—case reports.

Hemolytic anemia—case report.

Liver damage with jaundice (see Glossary)—case reports.

Low blood sugar—case report.

Chest pain or angina—case reports.

Half-facial pain—case reports.

Yeast infection (Candida) of the esophagus—possible.

Kidney inflammation (interstitial nephritis)—case reports.

Possible Effects on Sexual Function: Drug-induced male breast enlargement and tenderness (gynecomastia)—case reports.

Nocturnal erections—case report.

▷ **Adverse Effects That May Mimic Natural Diseases or Disorders**

Persistent infection or bruising may be bone marrow depression; blood counts are advisable.

Liver reactions may suggest viral hepatitis.

Possible Effects on Laboratory Tests

Complete blood cell counts: decreased red cells, hemoglobin, white cells and platelets.

Blood glucose level: decreased.

Liver function tests: increased liver enzymes (ALT/GPT, AST/GOT and alkaline phosphatase), increased bilirubin.

CAUTION

1. Take this drug for exactly as long as your doctor prescribed. Do not extend its use without your physician's guidance.
2. Report promptly any indications of infection.
3. Tell your doctor if you plan to take any other medications (prescription or over-the-counter) while taking omeprazole.
4. Acid in the stomach actually works to protect it from some bacterial infections. Since omeprazole is so effective in decreasing acid, it may increase the likelihood of infection by Campylobacter. This organism causes gastroenteritis. Symptoms may include mucus, loose stools and fever. Talk with your doctor if you start to develop these symptoms while taking omeprazole.
5. Although this drug effectively treats ulcers, it does not preclude the possibility of cancer of the stomach.

Precautions for Use

By Infants and Children: Safety and effectiveness for those under 12 years of age are not established.

By Those Over 60 Years of Age: Slower elimination of this drug makes it possible to achieve satisfactory response with smaller doses; this reduces the risk of adverse effects. Limit the daily dose to 20 mg if possible.

▷ **Advisability of Use During Pregnancy**

Pregnancy Category: C. See Pregnancy Risk Categories at the back of this book.

Animal studies: No drug-induced birth defects found in rats; drug-induced embryo and fetal toxicity were demonstrated in rats and rabbits.

Human studies: Adequate studies of pregnant women are not available.

Avoid use if possible. Use only if clearly necessary and for the shortest possible time.

Advisability of Use If Breast-Feeding
    Presence of this drug in breast milk: Yes.
    Avoid drug or refrain from nursing.

Habit-Forming Potential: None.

Effects of Overdose: Possible drowsiness, dizziness, lethargy, abdominal pain, nausea.

Possible Effects of Long-Term Use: Some long-term (2-year) studies in rats revealed the development of drug-induced carcinoid tumors in the stomach. To date, long-term use of this drug (more than 5 years) in humans has not revealed any drug-induced tumor potential. Pending more studies of long-term human use, it is advisable to limit the use of this drug to the shortest duration possible.

Suggested Periodic Examinations While Taking This Drug (at physician's discretion)
    Complete blood cell counts.

▷ **While Taking This Drug, Observe the Following**
    Foods: Follow your doctor's advice.
    Herbal Medicines or Minerals: Kola and ma huang may increase stomach acid, blunting the benefits of this medicine. Black cohosh root, ginkgo and squill are contraindicated in gastrointestinal disturbances. Licorice root has a German Commission E monograph indication for gastrointestinal ulcers, but use with proton pump inhibitors has not been studied. Talk to your doctor BEFORE adding any herbals to this medicine.
    Beverages: No restrictions. May be taken with milk.
▷   *Alcohol:* No interactions expected, but alcohol is best avoided; it stimulates the secretion of stomach acid.
    Tobacco Smoking: Smoking may stimulate the secretion of stomach acid. I advise everyone to quit smoking.
▷   *Other Drugs*
    Omeprazole may *increase* the effects of
    • anticoagulants (warfarin, etc.) and increase the risk of bleeding.
    • benzodiazepines [some such as diazepam] (see Drug Classes).
    • carbamazepine (Tegretol).
    • cilostazol (Pletal) by increasing an active metabolite called 3,4-dehydro cilostazol because of its action in inhibiting cytochrome P450 2C19. A lower dose of cilostazol and careful patient follow-up are prudent if these medicines must be combined.
    • clonazepam (Klonopin) and some other benzodiazepines (see Drug Classes) and lead to benzodiazepine toxicity.
    • cyclosporine (Sandimmune), by increasing its level (decreased levels also reported).
    • diazepam (Valium) and cause excessive sedation.
    • digoxin (Lanoxin) and lead to toxicity.
    • disulfiram (Antabuse).
    • fluvastatin (Lescol).
    • methotrexate (Rheumatrex).
    • phenytoin (Dilantin, etc.) or fosphenytoin (Cerebyx) and cause phenytoin or fosphenytoin toxicity.
    • warfarin (Coumadin) and lead to bleeding; more frequent INR (prothrom-

bin time or protime) testing is needed. Warfarin doses should be adjusted according to laboratory results.

Omeprazole may *decrease* the effects of
- ampicillin (various).
- iron preparations.
- itraconazole (Sporanox).
- ketoconazole (Nizoral).
- olanzapine (Zyprexa).
- ritonavir (Norvir)—may also increase omeprazole effects.
- trovafloxacin (Trovan).

▷ *Driving, Hazardous Activities:* This drug may cause drowsiness and dizziness. Limit activities as necessary.

Aviation Note: The use of this drug *may be a disqualification* for piloting. Consult a designated Aviation Medical Examiner.

Exposure to Sun: No restrictions.

Discontinuation: The duration of use will vary according to the condition under treatment and individual patient response. Premature discontinuation could result in incomplete healing or prompt recurrence of symptoms.

ONDANSETRON (on DAN sa tron)

Introduced: 1993　　**Class:** Antiemetic, 5-HT3 antagonist　　**Prescription:** USA: Yes　　**Controlled Drug:** USA: No; Canada: No　　**Available as Generic:** USA: No; Canada: No

Brand Names: Zofran, Zofran ODT, Zofran Oral Solution

BENEFITS versus RISKS	
Possible Benefits	*Possible Risks*
EFFECTIVE ORAL TREATMENT AND RELIEF OR PREVENTION OF SEVERE VOMITING	Bronchospasm Grand mal seizures Liver toxicity Heart rate and rhythm changes Low potassium (All rare)

▷ **Principal Uses**

As a Single Drug Product: Uses currently included in FDA-approved labeling: (1) Prevention of nausea and vomiting associated with initial and repeat courses of chemotherapy; (2) treatment or prevention of postoperative nausea and vomiting; (3) prevention or treatment of emesis (vomiting) caused by radiation therapy.

Other (unlabeled) generally accepted uses: (1) Helps patients keep from vomiting medicines used to treat drug overdoses; (2) may have a role in treating schizophrenia; (3) some data reducing the number of panic attacks; (4) eases some tremor cases.

How This Drug Works: Ondansetron antagonizes 5-HT3 receptors. It appears to block vomiting by blocking serotonin (a chemical causing vomiting) at 5-HT3 receptors.

Available Dosage Forms and Strengths
> Intravenous — 2 mg/ml
> Oral solution — 4 mg/5 ml
>> Tablets — 4 mg, 8 mg, 24 mg
> Tablets, ODT — 4 mg, 8 mg

▷ **Recommended Dosage Ranges** (Actual dose and schedule must be determined for each patient individually.)

Infants and Children: Little information is available regarding use in those less than 3 years old.

4 to 11 Years of Age: Vomiting from chemotherapy—one 4-mg tablet or 5 ml of the oral solution is given three times by mouth daily. The method and frequency are then the same as for adults.

12 to 60 Years of Age: One 8-mg tablet (tablet or ODT tablet) or 10 ml of the oral solution taken three times a day. The first dose should be taken 30 minutes before the start of the emetogenic chemotherapy. Subsequent doses should be taken 8 hours after the first dose. Further doses of 8 mg every 12 hours are taken for 1–2 days after chemotherapy is finished.

Vomiting from radiation therapy—8 mg three times a day. Doses are started 1–2 hours BEFORE radiation treatment. Doses after radiation are given every 8 hours for 1–2 days.

Postoperative nausea and vomiting—one 16-mg dose one hour before anesthesia is given.

Over 60 Years of Age: Same as 12 to 60 years of age.

Conditions Requiring Dosing Adjustments

Liver Function: Maximum dose for people with severe liver failure is 8 mg per day.

Kidney Function: Studies have not been conducted on patients with impaired kidneys. The decision to use ondansetron must be made by your physician. Only 5 to 10% of the drug is removed unchanged by the kidneys. Based on this small involvement of the kidneys, no changes are expected to be needed with short-term use.

▷ **Dosing Instructions:** May be taken on an empty stomach. DO NOT push the ODT form through the blister pack—simply peel back the foil before you take it. If you forget a dose: Take the missed dose as soon as you remember it, unless it's nearly time for your next dose—if that is the case, skip the missed dose and take the next dose right on schedule. DO NOT double doses. Talk with your doctor if you find yourself missing doses.

Usual Duration of Use: Since chemotherapy can cause vomiting long after it has been given, continual use on a regular schedule for 3 days is usually necessary.

Typical Treatment Goals and Measurements (Outcomes and Markers)

Vomiting: The goal is to prevent or at least to decrease vomiting (emesis) frequency, amount or severity.

Possible Advantages of This Drug

Effective oral prevention of severe vomiting caused by some kinds of chemotherapy that have been poorly controlled by earlier agents. Orally disintegrating tablets (ODT) form dissolves in a few seconds on the tongue WITHOUT water.

Currently a Drug of Choice
> For control of vomiting secondary to emetogenic (likely to cause vomiting) cancer chemotherapy.

▷ **This Drug Should Not Be Taken If**
- you had an allergic reaction to it previously.

▷ **Inform Your Physician Before Taking This Drug If**
- you have a history of liver disease.
- you have a history of kidney disease.
- you have a history of alcoholism.
- you have a history of PKU.
- you are unsure how much to take or how often to take it.

Possible Side Effects (natural, expected and unavoidable drug actions)
> Constipation, sedation.

▷ **Possible Adverse Effects** (unusual, unexpected and infrequent reactions)
> **If any of the following develop, consult your physician promptly for guidance.**

Mild Adverse Effects
Allergic reactions: skin rash—rare.
Headache—frequent.
Dizziness and light-headedness, constipation, diarrhea, dry mouth—infrequent.

Serious Adverse Effects
Allergic reactions: anaphylaxis—rare.
Extrapyramidal reactions (abnormal body movements) or seizures (intravenous form)—case reports.
Bronchospasm—rare.
Liver failure—one case report in a patient with hepatitis B.
Angina, tachycardia, arrhythmias—all rare.
Hypokalemia (low potassium)—rare.

▷ **Possible Effects on Sexual Function:** None reported.

Possible Delayed Adverse Effects: None reported.

▷ **Adverse Effects That May Mimic Natural Diseases or Disorders**
> Changes in liver enzymes may mimic hepatitis, but specific antibodies will not be present. Bronchospasm may mimic asthma.

Natural Diseases or Disorders That May Be Activated by This Drug
> Epilepsy, asthma.

Possible Effects on Laboratory Tests
> Liver function tests: Transient increases in SGPT, SGOT and bilirubin.

CAUTION
1. Even though you do not feel an urge to vomit, continue ondansetron for the prescribed length of therapy. The vomit-causing effect of cancer chemotherapy or radiation therapy continues after the medicine or radiation has been given.
2. The ODT form contains phenylalanine.

Precautions for Use
By Infants and Children: Safety and effectiveness for those under 3 years of age are not established.
By Those Over 60 Years of Age: Same as for general adult population.

▷ **Advisability of Use During Pregnancy**

Pregnancy Category: B. See Pregnancy Risk Categories at the back of this book.

Animal studies: Drug and its metabolites pass into the milk. No adverse effects on gestation, postnatal development or reproductive performance have been observed in rats.

Human studies: Adequate studies of pregnant women are not available. Ask your physician for guidance.

Advisability of Use If Breast-Feeding

Presence of this drug in breast milk: This medicine is excreted in the milk of rats; human data is not available.

Caution should be used if this medicine is to be used by nursing mothers.

Habit-Forming Potential: None.

Effects of Overdose: Doses 10 times greater than recommended have not resulted in illness.

Possible Effects of Long-Term Use: Not indicated for long-term use.

Suggested Periodic Examinations While Taking This Drug (at physician's discretion)

Observe for vomiting occurrence and frequency.

▷ **While Taking This Drug, Observe the Following**

Foods: No restrictions.

Herbal Medicines or Minerals: Since St. John's wort may act to increase serotonin, the combination is not advised. Since part of the way ginseng works may be as a MAO inhibitor, do not combine ginseng with ondansetron.

Beverages: No restrictions.

▷ *Alcohol:* Additive sedation and potential additive urge to vomit if alcohol is taken in large doses. Alcohol abuse that has led to liver problems may limit the total dose that can be taken.

Tobacco Smoking: No direct clinical interactions; I advise everyone to quit smoking.

Marijuana Smoking: May induce additive sedation and provide additive antiemetic effects.

▷ *Other Drugs*

The following drugs may increase the effects of ondansetron:

• allopurinol (Zyloprim).
• cimetidine (Tagamet).
• disulfiram (Antabuse).
• fluconazole (Diflucan).
• isoniazid (Nydrazid).
• macrolide antibiotics (erythromycin, azithromycin, clarithromycin, dirithromycin).
• metronidazole (Flagyl).
• monoamine oxidase (MAO) inhibitor antidepressants (Nardil).
• ritonavir (Norvir) and perhaps other protease inhibitors (see Drug Classes).

The following drugs may decrease the effects of ondansetron:

• barbiturates.
• carbamazepine (Tegretol).
• phenylbutazone (Butazolidin, Azolid).
• phenytoin (Dilantin).

- rifabutin (Mycobutin).
- rifampin (Rifadin)
- tolbutamide (Orinase).

▷ *Driving, Hazardous Activities:* This drug may cause drowsiness and dizziness. Restrict activities as necessary.

Aviation Note: The use of this drug **may be a disqualification** for piloting. Consult a designated Aviation Medical Examiner.

Exposure to Sun: No restrictions.

Special Storage Instructions: Keep at room temperature. Avoid exposing this medicine to extreme humidity.

Discontinuation: Ondansetron may be stopped after you've completed the prescribed course (usually 3 days) of therapy.

ORAL CONTRACEPTIVES (or al kon tra SEP tivs)

Other Names: Estrogens/progestins, OCs, birth control pills

Introduced: 1956   **Class:** Female sex hormones   **Prescription:** USA: Yes   **Controlled Drug:** USA: No; Canada: No   **Available as Generic:** USA: Yes, in some forms; Canada: No

Brand Names: Alesse, Brevicon, Cyclessa, Demulen, Desogen, Enovid, Estrostep FE, Genora, Gestodene, Jenest 28, Levlen, Levlite, Levora, Loestrin, Low-Ogestrel, Lo/Ovral, Micronor,* ♣Minestrin 1/20, Min-Ovral, Mircette, Modicon, Necon, NEE, Nelova, Nelova 1/50 M, Nelova 10/11, Norcept-E 1/35, Nordette, Norethin 1/35E, Norethin 1/50M, Norinyl, Norlestrin, Nor-Q.D.*, Ortho-Cept 21, Ortho Cyclen, Ortho-Novum 777, Ortho Tri-Cyclen, Ovcon, Ovral, Ovrette*, Preven, ♣Synphasic, Tri-Levlen, Tri-Norinyl, Triphasil, Triquilar, Trivora, Zovia

BENEFITS versus RISKS	
Possible Benefits	*Possible Risks*
HIGHLY EFFECTIVE FOR CONTRACEPTIVE PROTECTION	SERIOUS, LIFE-THREATENING THROMBOEMBOLIC DISORDERS in susceptible individuals
Moderately effective as adjunctive treatment in management of excessive menses and endometriosis	Hypertension
	Fluid retention
Helps decrease the risk of ovarian cancer while the pill is being taken	Intensification of migrainelike headaches and fibrocystic breast changes
Some forms decrease acne (especially Estrostep, Ortho Tri-Cyclen and Alesse)	Accelerated growth of uterine fibroid tumors
	Drug-induced hepatitis with jaundice
	Benign liver tumors—rare

▷ **Principal Uses**

As a Single Drug Product: Uses currently included in FDA-approved labeling: (1) Prevention of conception—the "Mini-Pill" contains only one component, a progestin; this has been shown to be slightly less effective than the combi-

*"Mini-Pill" type, containing progestin only.

nation of estrogen and progestin in preventing pregnancy; (2) used in cases where women do not make enough hormones (female hypogonadism); (3) helps decrease excessive blood flow at menstruation (hypermenorrhea); (4) of use in endometriosis as the combination mestranol and norethynodrel; (5) Estrostep and Ortho Tri-Cyclen are approved to prevent acne.

Other (unlabeled) generally accepted uses: (1) May be of benefit in abnormal hair growth in women (hirsutism); (2) some combination forms can have a protective effect against osteoporosis; (3) Alesse has had an application accepted by the FDA for use in acne.

As a Combination Drug Product [CD]: Uses currently included in FDA-approved labeling: (1) Most oral contraceptives consist of a combination of an estrogen and a progestin; these products are the most effective form of medicinal contraception available; (2) they are sometimes used to treat menstrual irregularity, excessively heavy menstrual flow and endometriosis; (3) norgestimate and ethinyl estradiol combination product (Ortho Tri-Cyclen) is used to treat acne in females over 15.

Other (unlabeled) generally accepted uses: (1) Gestodene has been reported to inhibit certain breast cancer cell lines (clinical studies are needed); (2) may have a protective effect against osteoporosis; (3) triphasic oral contraceptives can help in the prevention or treatment of menopause symptoms; (4) may have a role in rheumatoid arthritis, but the data are conflicting; (5) sometimes used around the time of menopause (perimenopausally) to provide regularity of menstruation; (6) used to reduce LH surges in order to improve results from in vitro fertilization or embryo transfer; (7) used as emergency contraception or a morning-after pill (MAP)—while Preven is the only dedicated product for this use, Alesse, Ovral, Ovrette, Nordette, Levlen, Levlite, Levora, Lo/Ovral, Trivora and Tri-Levlen have FDA safe and effective ratings as emergency contraceptives.

Author's Note: Research linked the number of times a woman ovulates to increased risk of ovarian cancer. This finding was associated with a P-53 gene, which may account for as much as 50% of ovarian cancer. Since birth control pills decrease the number of times that women ovulate, they may have a role in helping prevent cancer in women found to carry the P-53 gene. Further research is required.

How These Drugs Work: When estrogen and progestin are taken in sufficient doses and on a regular basis, the blood and tissue levels of these hormones increase to resemble those that occur during pregnancy. This results in suppression of the two pituitary gland hormones that normally cause ovulation (the formation and release of an egg by the ovary). In addition, these drugs may (1) alter the cervical mucus so that it resists the passage of sperm and (2) alter the lining of the uterus so that it resists implantation of the egg (if ovulation occurs).

Available Dosage Forms and Strengths

Tablets: Several combinations of synthetic estrogens and progestins in varying strengths; see the package label of the brand prescribed.

▷ **Usual Adult Dosage Ranges:** For contraception: Start with the first tablet on the fifth day after the onset of menstruation. Follow with one tablet daily (taken at the same time each day) for 21 consecutive days. Resume treatment on the eighth day following the last tablet taken during the preceding cycle. The schedule is to take the drug daily for 3 weeks and to omit it for 1 week. For the Mini-Pill (progestin only), initiate treatment on the first day of menstruation and take one tablet daily, every day, throughout the year (no interruption). The Mircette brand uses 20 mcg of ethinyl estradiol and 150 mcg of dogesterel for 21 days. Two days of dummy (placebo) tablets are then taken and then five days of 10 mcg ethinyl estradiol.

Emergency contraception (MAP): This is a critical situation. Talk to your doctor to be certain that you understand the possible side effects (nausea, etc.) and other issues and medical follow-up required for this procedure.

Author's Note: Research is now being conducted using longer cycles for birth control pill dosing. One company is testing a product tentatively called Seasonale that is taken for 84 days—thereby allowing for one period every three months.

Note: Actual dose and schedule must be determined for each patient individually.

Conditions Requiring Dosing Adjustments

Liver Function: Should NOT be taken if you have liver disease.

Kidney Function: Oral contraceptives are not significantly eliminated by the kidneys.

▷ **Dosing Instructions:** Combination products versus biphasic or triphasic forms are started in ways specific to the product. Make certain that you understand this. The tablets may be crushed and taken with or after food to reduce stomach upset. To ensure regular (every day) use and uniform blood levels, it is best to take the tablet at the same time daily. If you forget a dose (varies with the birth control form): For triphasic forms (Tri-Leven, Tri-Norinyl or Triphasil): Take the missed dose as soon as you remember. If you only remember on the next day, take two pills for the next two days, then return to your regular schedule, but USE ANOTHER TYPE OF BIRTH CONTROL UNTIL YOUR PERIOD BEGINS. Call your doctor for help. If you miss three pills in a row, stop the remaining pills for the month, USE A DIFFERENT KIND OF BIRTH CONTROL UNTIL YOUR PERIOD STARTS, and call your doctor. Your doctor will advise you as to when to re-start (usually just the same as when you first started the pills) with a new dose pack. For other birth control pill forms, if you forget a dose, call your doctor for detailed instructions.

Possible Advantages of These Drugs

Effective control of conception. Mircette form may benefit women who have migraines the second week they are "off the pill." A study of 46,000 British women released in early 1999 showed that women who took the pill did not show any increased risk of cancer. These data are important because of the large number of women and also because they were studied for 25 years. A Swedish study showed that oral contraceptives may increase bone density in women who take the pill between the ages of 30 and 40.

Usual Duration of Use: According to individual needs and circumstances. Long-term use (months to years) requires physician supervision and evaluation every 6 months.

Typical Treatment Goals and Measurements (Outcomes and Markers)

Contraceptive: The goal is to avoid pregnancy. Serum pregnancy tests (you have to have blood drawn for this) are presently the most sensitive tests to rule out pregnancy.

▷ **These Drugs Should Not Be Taken If**
- you have had an allergic reaction to any dose form of it.
- you have a history of thrombophlebitis, embolism, heart attack or stroke.
- you have breast cancer.
- you have active liver disease, seriously impaired liver function or a history of liver tumor.
- you have diabetes and have developed circulatory disease.
- you have high blood pressure.
- you have not had any periods (amenorrhea).
- you have abnormal and unexplained vaginal bleeding.
- you have sickle cell disease.
- you are pregnant.

▷ **Inform Your Physician Before Taking These Drugs If**
- you have had an adverse reaction to any oral contraceptive.
- you have a history of cancer of the breast or reproductive organs.
- you have fibrocystic breast changes, uterine fibroid tumors, endometriosis, migrainelike headaches, epilepsy, asthma, elevated lipids, prolapse of the mitral valve of the heart, heart disease, high blood pressure, gallbladder disease, diabetes or porphyria.
- you are over 40. This was an age-related limit previously, but current thinking says that use of these medicines may be a benefit-to-risk decision.
- you have been prescribed an antibiotic (some antibiotics may blunt the benefits of oral contraceptives and REQUIRE use of an alternative birth control method).
- you are using St. John's wort for depression.
- you smoke tobacco on a regular basis.
- you plan to have surgery in the near future.

Possible Side Effects (natural, expected and unavoidable drug actions)
Fluid retention, weight gain, "breakthrough" bleeding (spotting in middle of menstrual cycle), altered menstrual pattern, lack of menstruation (during and following cessation of drug), increased susceptibility to yeast infection of the genital tissues. Tannish pigmentation of the face. Modest increases in blood pressure.

▷ **Possible Adverse Effects** (unusual, unexpected and infrequent reactions)
If any of the following develop, consult your physician promptly for guidance.

Mild Adverse Effects
Allergic reactions: skin rash, hives, itching.
Headache, nervous tension, irritability, accentuation of migraine headaches—infrequent to frequent.
Rise in blood pressure (in some people)—possible.
Nausea, perhaps with vomiting—frequent (related to estrogen) and may ease if taken with evening meals.
Reduced tolerance to contact lenses or impaired color vision: blue tinge to objects, blue halo around lights—possible.

Serious Adverse Effects
Allergic reactions: anaphylaxis, erythema multiforme and nodosum (skin reactions), loss of scalp hair.
Idiosyncratic reactions: joint and muscle pains.

Emotional depression—frequent.

Eye changes: optic neuritis, retinal thrombosis, altered curvature of the cornea, cataracts—possible.

Gallbladder disease, benign liver tumors, jaundice—case reports.

Ischemic colitis—case report.

Enlargement of uterine fibroid tumors—possible.

Abnormal glucose tolerance (hyperglycemia)—frequent in people with pregnancy (gestational) diabetes.

Thrombophlebitis (inflammation of a vein with formation of blood clot): pain or tenderness in thigh or leg, with or without swelling of foot or leg—increased risk, especially with high estrogen doses.

Drug-induced porphyria or worsening of systemic lupus erythematosus (SLE)—case reports.

Esophageal ulcers (especially if the medicine is taken lying down with no water)—case reports.

Stroke (blood clot in brain): headaches, blackout, sudden weakness or paralysis of any part of the body, severe dizziness, altered vision, slurred speech, inability to speak—possible increased risk (more probable in one study with high-dose estrogen formulations).

Heart attack (blood clot in coronary artery): sudden pain in chest, neck, jaw or arm; weakness; sweating; nausea—increased risk (not seen with low-dose estrogen products)—possible increased risk with use in women having cardiovascular risk factors, taking pills with more than 50 mcg of estrogen and in those who smoke.

Liver cancer—possible increased risk with long-term use.

▷ **Possible Effects on Sexual Function:** Altered character of menstruation; midcycle spotting—may be frequent.

Increased or decreased libido—possible.

Breast enlargement and tenderness with milk production—possible.

Absent menstruation and infertility (temporary) after discontinuation of drug.

Possible Delayed Adverse Effects: Estrogens taken during pregnancy can predispose the female child to the later development of cancer of the vagina or cervix following puberty. Nonpregnant use does not increase breast cancer.

▷ **Adverse Effects That May Mimic Natural Diseases or Disorders**

Liver reactions may suggest viral hepatitis. Increased blood pressure may mimic increased blood pressure from other causes.

Natural Diseases or Disorders That May Be Activated by These Drugs

Latent hypertension, diabetes mellitus, clotting factor disorders that favor blood clots, acute intermittent porphyria, lupus erythematosus-like syndrome.

Possible Effects on Laboratory Tests

Blood lupus erythematosus (LE) cells: positive.

Blood-clotting time or INR: decreased.

Blood amylase and lipase levels: increased (very rare pancreatitis).

Blood total cholesterol, HDL, LDL and VLDL cholesterol levels: usually no effects; some variability, depending upon estrogen and progestin content of preparation used.

Blood triglyceride levels: no effect to increased, depending upon estrogen and progestin content of preparation used.

Blood glucose level: increased.

Blood thyroid-stimulating hormone (TSH) level: no effect.

Blood thyroid hormone levels: T3 and T4 increased; free T4 either no effect or decreased.

Liver function tests: increased liver enzymes (ALT/GPT, AST/GOT, alkaline phosphatase) and bilirubin.

CAUTION

1. Serious adverse effects due to these drugs are a very low risk. However, any unusual development should be reported and evaluated promptly by your doctor.

2. Studies indicate that women over 30 years of age who smoke and use oral contraceptives are at significantly greater risk of having a serious cardiovascular event than are nonusers.

3. The risk of thromboembolism increases with the amount of estrogen in the product and the age of the user. Low-estrogen combinations are advised. One larger United Kingdom study failed to find a difference in risk of unknown cause venous thromboembolism when combination oral contraceptives containing less than 50 micrograms of ethinyl estradiol were used. Other data says that combining smoking, asthma history, history of blood clots, increased body mass index with high estrogen combining pills increases risks of thromboembolism.

4. It is advisable to stop these drugs 1 month prior to elective surgery to reduce the risk of postsurgical thromboembolism. If they can't be stopped, preventive use of anticoagulants may be prudent.

5. Investigate promptly any alteration or disturbance of vision that occurs during the use of these drugs.

6. Investigate promptly the nature of recurrent, persistent or severe headaches that develop while taking these drugs.

7. Observe for significant change of mood. Call your doctor if depression develops.

8. Certain commonly used drugs may reduce the effectiveness of oral contraceptives. Some of these are listed in the category of "Other Drugs" below.

9. Diarrhea lasting more than a few hours (and occurring during the days the drug is taken) can prevent adequate absorption of these drugs and impair their effectiveness as contraceptives.

10. If two consecutive menstrual periods are missed, ask your doctor if you should get a pregnancy test. Do not continue to use these drugs until you know whether you are pregnant.

11. **Many antibiotics may stop the effectiveness of birth control pills** (oral contraceptives). If your doctor prescribes an antibiotic, ask whether a different method of birth control is needed.

12. One researcher uses the acronym ACHES (A=abdominal pain, C=chest pain, H=headaches, E=eye problems and S=severe leg pain) to list signs of adverse effects that require a patient taking these medicines to call her doctor immediately.

13. One 8-year study found that women who used oral contraceptives IN THE PAST do not have an increased risk of cardiovascular disease.

▷ **Advisability of Use During Pregnancy**

Pregnancy Category: X. See Pregnancy Risk Categories at the back of this book.

Animal studies: Genital defects reported in mice and guinea pigs; cleft palate reported in rodents.

Human studies: Information from studies of pregnant women indicates that estrogens can masculinize the female fetus. In addition, limb defects and heart malformations have been reported. It is now known that estrogens taken during pregnancy can predispose the female child to the development of cancer of the vagina or cervix following puberty.

Avoid these drugs completely during entire pregnancy.

Advisability of Use If Breast-Feeding

Presence of these drugs in breast milk: Yes, in minute amounts (ethinyl estradiol or norethindrone). These drugs may suppress milk formation if started early after delivery.

Breast-feeding is considered to be safe during the use of oral contraceptives.

Habit-Forming Potential: None.

Effects of Overdose: Headache, drowsiness, nausea, vomiting, fluid retention, abnormal vaginal bleeding, breast enlargement and discomfort.

Possible Effects of Long-Term Use: High blood pressure, gallbladder disease with stones, accelerated growth of uterine fibroid tumors, absent menstruation and impaired fertility after discontinuation of drug.

Suggested Periodic Examinations While Taking These Drugs (at physician's discretion)

Regular (every 6 months) evaluation of the breasts and pelvic organs, including Pap smears.

Liver function tests as indicated.

▷ **While Taking These Drugs, Observe the Following**

Foods: Avoid excessive use of salt if fluid retention occurs. Excessive vitamin C may increase risk of contraceptive failure.

Herbal Medicines or Minerals: Black cohosh appears to work by (1) suppressing luteinizing hormone; (2) binding to estrogen receptors in the pituitary and inhibiting luteinizing hormone release and (3) binding to estrogen receptors in the pituitary. The net effect is that this herb eases symptoms of menopause, but little is known about long-term use or heart and bone protective effects. This herb may lower the effectiveness of birth control pills. Talk to your doctor before starting black cohosh if you are currently taking estrogen or an estrogen-containing product. Since St. John's wort and this drug may cause increased sun sensitivity, caution is advised. St. John's wort may blunt contraceptive effects and result in unwanted pregnancy.

Beverages: No specific restrictions, but caffeine will stay in the body (increased half-life) longer and caffeine consumption should decrease while patients are on the pill. May be taken with milk.

▷ *Alcohol:* No interactions expected.

Tobacco Smoking: Studies indicate that smoking—especially heavy smoking (15 or more cigarettes daily) while taking oral contraceptives significantly increases the risk of heart attack (coronary thrombosis). Heavy smoking should be considered a contraindication to the use of oral contraceptives. I advise everyone to quit smoking.

▷ *Other Drugs*

Oral contraceptives may ***increase*** the effects of

- alprazolam (Xanax) and other benzodiazepines (see Drug Classes).
- some benzodiazepines (see Drug Classes) and cause excessive sedation.
- cyclosporine (Sandimmune) and cause toxicity.
- metoprolol (Lopressor) and cause excessive beta-blocker effects.
- prednisolone and prednisone and other corticosteroids such as dexamethasone may lead to excessive cortisonelike effects.
- ropinirole (Requip).
- selegiline (Eldepryl, others), leading to increased selegiline adverse effects risk.
- tacrine (Cognex).
- theophyllines (Theo-Dur, others) and increase the risk of toxic effects.

Oral contraceptives ***taken concurrently*** with

- antibiotics (such as amoxicillin or ampicillin) can seriously impair effectiveness and allow pregnancy to occur.
- antidiabetic drugs (oral hypoglycemic agents) may cause unpredictable fluctuations of blood sugar.
- arginine (R-Gene intravenous) may result in falsely increased growth hormone levels during pituitary function testing. Results of the arginine test should be interpreted with caution.
- ascorbic acid (vitamin C) may result in increased levels of ethinyl estradiol and breakthrough bleeding if the vitamin C is stopped.
- atorvastatin (Lipitor) leading to increased ethinyl estradiol and norethindrone levels.
- efavirenz (Sustiva), leading to increased ethinyl estradiol levels.
- liothyronine (Thyrostat) may lower benefits from thyroid supplementation in people with a functional thyroid gland. Liothyronine dosing may need to be adjusted.
- tricyclic antidepressants (Elavil, Sinequan, others) may enhance their adverse effects and reduce their antidepressant effectiveness.
- troleandomycin (TAO) may increase occurrence of liver toxicity and jaundice.
- warfarin (Coumadin) may cause unpredictable alterations of prothrombin activity; more frequent INR (prothrombin time or protime) testing is needed, and warfarin dosing should be adjusted to laboratory test results.
- zolmitriptan (Zomig) or naratriptan (Amerge) may lead to "triptan" toxicity.

The following drugs may ***decrease*** the effects of oral contraceptives (and impair their effectiveness):

- barbiturates (phenobarbital, etc.; see Drug Classes).
- carbamazepine (Tegretol).
- fluconazole (Diflucan).
- griseofulvin (Fulvicin, etc.).
- nelfinavir (Viracept).
- nevirapine (Viramune).
- penicillins (ampicillin, penicillin V).

- phenytoin (Dilantin) or fosphenytoin (Cerebyx).
- pioglitazone (Actos) may possibly interact.
- primidone (Mysoline).
- rifampin (Rifadin, Rimactane).
- ritonavir (Norvir) and perhaps other protease inhibitors (see Drug Classes).
- tetracyclines (see Drug Classes).

▷ *Driving, Hazardous Activities:* Usually no restrictions. Consult your physician for assessment of individual risk and for guidance regarding specific restrictions.

Aviation Note: Usually no restrictions, but watch for the rare occurrence of disturbed vision and restrict activities accordingly. Consult a designated Aviation Medical Examiner.

Exposure to Sun: Use caution—these drugs can cause photosensitivity (see Glossary).

Discontinuation: Do not stop these drugs if "breakthrough" bleeding occurs. If spotting or bleeding continues, call your doctor. A higher-estrogen pill may be required. Remember: Omitting this drug for only 1 day may allow pregnancy to occur. It is best to avoid pregnancy for 3 to 6 months after stopping these drugs; aborted fetuses from women who became pregnant within 6 months after discontinuation reveal significantly increased chromosome abnormalities.

ORLISTAT (OAR li stat)

Introduced: 1999   **Class:** Weight loss agent, lipase inhibitor   **Prescription:** USA: Yes   **Controlled Drug:** USA: No; Canada: No   **Available as Generic:** USA: No; Canada: No
Brand Name: Xenical

BENEFITS versus RISKS	
Possible Benefits	*Possible Risks*
EFFECTIVE REDUCTION IN WEIGHT WHEN USED IN CONJUNCTION WITH A REDUCED-CALORIE DIET	Reduced absorption of fat-soluble vitamins (A, D, E, K) and beta carotene
HELPS REDUCE RISK FOR WEIGHT GAIN AFTER PREVIOUS WEIGHT LOSS	Fecal incontinence and flatulence
LOWERED TOTAL CHOLESTEROL	
DECREASED LOW DENSITY LIPOPROTEINS	
Possible beneficial decreases in blood pressure	

▷ **Principal Uses**

As a Single Drug Product: Uses currently included in FDA-approved labeling: (1) Reduces weight in patients with a body mass index (BMI) of 30 kg/square meter or greater or in those with a BMI of 27 kg/square meter with other risk factors (such as diabetes, high blood pressure or high blood lipids); (2) helps maintain weight loss in patients who have already lost weight.

Other (unlabeled) generally accepted uses: (1) May have a role in type 2 diabetes because weight loss was associated with better blood sugar control; (2) could have a role in some cases of elevated lipids (hyperlipidemia).

How This Drug Works: Inhibits the action of an enzyme called lipase (both in the stomach and pancreas), thereby inhibiting the absorption of fats. Since fats can account for a significant number of daily calories and orlistat blocks roughly 30% of fat absorption, use of orlistat over time leads to weight loss.

Available Dosage Forms and Strengths
Capsules — 120 mg

▷ **Usual Adult Dosage Ranges:** *Weight loss:* One capsule three times a day with each main meal that contains fat. If a meal is eaten that has no fat, the capsule should not be taken until the next meal that has fat in it. **Note: Actual dose and schedule must be determined for each patient individually.**

Conditions Requiring Dosing Adjustments
Liver Function: This medicine is poorly absorbed, and liver function is not expected to be a factor (removed in the stool). Since the liver IS involved in making clotting factors, possible decreased vitamin K absorption from orlistat may be an issue in patients with liver disease.
Kidney Function: **Minimally** absorbed into the body, and kidney function is not expected to be a factor.

▷ **Dosing Instructions:** This medicine may be taken up to an hour before a meal that contains fat. If you skip a meal or eat a meal without any fat in it, it is okay to skip that dose of orlistat. You should be eating a well-balanced, reduced-carbohydrate diet that has roughly 30% of its calories as fat. This medicine can lower the amount of fat-soluble vitamins (A, D, E, K) and beta carotene that can get into your body from your diet. Over time, this may lead to a deficiency. A multivitamin containing those nutrients is important and should be taken two hours before or after your dose of orlistat. If you forget a dose, but eat a fat-free meal—simply skip the dose you forgot. If you forget a dose and have taken a fatty meal, take the missed dose if it is within an hour of the time the dose should have been taken. If you remember the missed dose more than an hour after the meal, skip the missed dose and wait until your next meal to take this medicine. DO NOT double doses. Talk with your doctor if you find yourself missing doses.

Usual Duration of Use: Regular use is required to get the best results from this medicine. Results (as measured by stool fat) can be seen in as little as 24–48 hours. Measurable weight loss will be determined by the amount of exercise, metabolic rate, adherence to diet and other factors. Use of this medicine for more than two years has not been studied as yet. Long-term use (months to years) requires ongoing follow-up by your doctor.

Typical Treatment Goals and Measurements (Outcomes and Markers)
Weight loss: The goal is to lower body weight or maintain weight loss by preventing absorption of fat. Body weight, percent body fat and laboratory tests such as triglycerides, VLDL, LDL and HDL can be checked to assess successful combination treatment. In some initial clinical data, people

who took this medicine for two years lost an average of 4.5% of their starting body weight or about 4 kilograms. Be sure to talk to your doctor about the benefits of losing some weight and keeping it off versus crash or fad diets and weight yo-yo-ing.

Possible Advantages of This Drug

Works in a novel way compared to previously available medicines for weight loss. Does not have an effect on heart valves.

▷ **This Drug Should Not Be Taken If**

- you have had an allergic reaction to it previously.
- you have ongoing (chronic) malabsorption.
- you have a cause for obesity (such as hypothyroidism that should be treated) which would then obviate the need for orlistat.
- you have stagnation of bile in the small bile ducts in the liver (cholestasis).

▷ **Inform Your Physician Before Taking This Drug If**

- you have significant disease in your stomach or intestine (gastrointestinal or GI tract), especially diseases that make you prone to diarrhea.
- you do not understand that increasing fat in your diet may also increase GI adverse effects from this medicine.
- you have a history of low thyroid function (hypothyroidism).
- you have a known deficiency of vitamin A, D, E or K or a poor diet that would lead you to tend toward deficiency of those vitamins or of beta carotene.

Possible Side Effects (natural, expected and unavoidable drug actions)

Interference with normal fat digestion and absorption; reduced absorption of vitamins A, D, E and K as well as beta carotene.

▷ **Possible Adverse Effects** (unusual, unexpected and infrequent reactions)

If any of the following develop, consult your physician promptly for guidance.

Mild Adverse Effects

Allergic reactions: skin rash—possible.

Excessive gas (flatus) with or without fecal discharge—possible to frequent and can increase with higher amounts of fat in the diet.

Oily spotting of stool—may be frequent.

Nausea and soft or liquid stools—frequent.

(All of the above effects may decrease over time.)

Headache or dizziness—infrequent to frequent.

Edema—infrequent.

Serious Adverse Effects

Allergic reaction: not reported.

Lowering of vitamins A, D, E and K. Vitamin K lowering may lead to an increased bleeding tendency if not supplemented—possible.

In clinical trials, nine cases of breast neoplasm were reported in patients taking 120 mg three times daily and one case was reported in the placebo group. Causation by orlistat is questionable, as the cases were seen within 6 months of the start of the clinical trials and the drug is minimally absorbed.

▷ **Possible Effects on Sexual Function:** Menstrual irregularity—infrequent.

Natural Diseases or Disorders That May Be Activated by This Drug

Problems with patients who have cholestasis are possible.

Possible Effects on Laboratory Tests

INR (prothrombin time): possibly increased (impaired vitamin K absorption).

LDL and total cholesterol: decreased.

CAUTION

1. Since this medicine may interfere with absorption of fat-soluble vitamins and beta carotene, these compounds should be supplemented while you are taking orlistat and the vitamin dosing separated from orlistat doses by two hours.

2. Causes of obesity that are organic (such as low thyroid function or hypothyroidism) should be evaluated BEFORE orlistat is prescribed.

3. If you have a history of kidney stones made of calcium oxalate (nephrolithiasis), this medicine may worsen this problem.

4. Weight loss may improve how well blood sugar is controlled in people with diabetes—a beneficial effect. Oral hypoglycemic medicines (see Drug Classes) may have to be used in lower doses.

5. No data are available on the combination of orlistat with other weight loss agents, such as sibutramine (Meridia) or phentermine.

Precautions for Use

By Infants and Children: Safety and effectiveness for those under 16 years of age not established.

By Those Over 60 Years of Age: Studies in special populations were not conducted.

▷ **Advisability of Use During Pregnancy**

Pregnancy Category: B. See Pregnancy Risk Categories at the back of this book.

Animal studies: No embryotoxicity or teratogenicity in mice or rabbits.

Human studies: Adequate studies of pregnant women are not available. NOT recommended for use during pregnancy.

Advisability of Use If Breast-Feeding

Presence of this drug in breast milk: Unknown.

Stop nursing or don't take the medicine if breast-feeding is to be undertaken.

Habit-Forming Potential: None, but misuse of the medicine is possible (as in anorexia).

Effects of Overdose: Reports of single 800-mg doses have been studied in people of normal weight without any adverse effects. If a significant overdose of orlistat happens, the patient should be medically observed for at least 24 hours. It is expected that any systemic effects would be rapidly reversible.

Possible Effects of Long-Term Use: Deficiencies of vitamins A, D, E and K and beta carotene. Calcium deficiency, osteoporosis. Acidosis (excessive retention of chloride).

Suggested Periodic Examinations While Taking This Drug (at physician's discretion)

Measurements of blood levels of total cholesterol, low-density (LDL) cholesterol and high-density (HDL) cholesterol. Possible bone mineral density tests if vitamin D is not supplemented.

Blood levels of vitamins may be prudent to guide supplementation or need for supplementation.

▷ **While Taking This Drug, Observe the Following**

Foods: Follow your doctor's recommended diet and portion control. Avoid foods that have tended to cause gas (flatus) formation previously.

Herbal Medicines or Minerals: A variety of products that promise weight loss has been or is available. Some of these products have contained ma huang or other potentially dangerous ingredients. DO NOT combine any herbal weight loss product with orlistat. Talk to your doctor if you are considering any herbal weight loss product.

Nutritional Support: Ask your doctor about the need for supplements of vitamins A, D, E and K as well as beta carotene.

Beverages: No restrictions.

▷ *Alcohol:* No interactions expected, but remember, many alcoholic beverages deliver a lot of calories.

Tobacco Smoking: No interactions expected. I advise everyone to quit smoking.

▷ *Other Drugs*

Orlistat may *decrease* the effects of
- beta carotene; take 2 hours before or after orlistat.
- fat-soluble vitamins, such as vitamin A, D, E or K.

Orlistat *taken concurrently* with
- cyclosporine (Sandimmune, others) may (because of possible variation in cyclosporine levels with changes in diet) lead to changes in cyclosporine levels. Caution is advised, and study is needed.
- pravastatin (Pravachol) or other HMG-CoA reductase inhibitors may work well in further lowering cholesterol. Pravastatin levels may be increased by roughly 30%. Patients taking this combination should be followed more closely for possible adverse effects.
- warfarin (Coumadin, others) may (because of possible decreases in vitamin K over time) lead to increased warfarin effects; more frequent INR testing is prudent.

▷ *Driving, Hazardous Activities:* No restrictions.

Aviation Note: The use of this drug is usually not a disqualification for piloting. Consult a designated Aviation Medical Examiner.

Exposure to Sun: No reports of problems at present.

Discontinuation: The dose of any potentially toxic or narrow therapeutic-window drug (such as warfarin) taken concurrently must be changed appropriately if orlistat is stopped.

OXAPROZIN (OX a proh zin)

Please see the propionic acids (nonsteroidal anti-inflammatory drug) family profile.

OXICAMS (Nonsteroidal Anti-Inflammatory Drug Family)

Piroxicam   (peer OX i kam)

Introduced: 1978   **Class:** Mild analgesic, anti-inflammatory   **Prescription:** USA: Yes   **Controlled Drug:** USA: No; Canada: No   **Available as Generic:** Yes

Brand Names: ✤Alti-Piroxicam, ✤Apo-Piroxicam, ✤Brexidol, ✤Dom-Piroxicam, Feldene, ✤Med-Pirocam, ✤Novo-Pirocam, ✤Nu-Pirox

BENEFITS versus RISKS	
Possible Benefits	*Possible Risks*
EFFECTIVE RELIEF OF MILD TO MODERATE PAIN AND INFLAMMATION	Gastrointestinal pain, ulceration and bleeding
	Drug-induced hepatitis—rare
	Rare kidney damage
	Mild fluid retention
	Reduced white blood cell and platelet counts

▷ **Principal Uses**

As a Single Drug Product: Uses currently included in FDA-approved labeling: Relieves mild to moderately severe pain and inflammation associated with (1) rheumatoid arthritis and (2) osteoarthritis.

Other (unlabeled) generally accepted uses: (1) Treats the morning and evening pain associated with ankylosing spondylitis; (2) helps relieve the pain and inflammation of acute gout; (3) used to treat terminal cancer pain in combination with doxepin; (4) may have a role in easing temporal arteritis; (5) effective in painful menstruation (primary dysmenorrhea); (6) second-line therapy in acute gout (7) may help in preventing colon cancer.

How This Drug Works: This drug suppresses the formation of prostaglandins (and related compounds), chemicals involved in the production of inflammation and pain.

Available Dosage Forms and Strengths

Capsules—10 mg, 20 mg

Rectal suppository—10 mg, 20 mg

▷ **Usual Adult Dosage Ranges:** *As antiarthritic:* 20 mg once daily. Higher doses may not confer added benefits.

Dysmenorrhea: 40 mg (two tablets) in the morning for two days, then 20 mg a day until symptoms ease or menstruation ends. **Note: Actual dose and schedule must be determined for each patient individually.**

Conditions Requiring Dosing Adjustments

Liver Function: This drug should be used with caution and in decreased dose by patients with liver compromise.

Kidney Function: Piroxicam should be used with caution in renal compromise and kidney function followed closely.

▷ **Dosing Instructions:** Take with or following food to prevent stomach irritation. Take with a full glass of water and remain upright (do not lie down) for 30 minutes. The capsule may be opened. If you forget a dose: Take the missed dose as soon as you remember it, unless it's nearly time for your next dose—if that is the case, skip the missed dose and take the next dose right on schedule. DO NOT double doses. Talk with your doctor if you find yourself missing doses.

Usual Duration of Use: Use on a regular schedule for 2 weeks usually determines effectiveness in relieving the discomfort of arthritis. Long-term use (months to years) requires physician supervision and periodic evaluation.

Typical Treatment Goals and Measurements (Outcomes and Markers)

Pain: Most clinicians treating pain use a device called an algometer to check your pain. This looks like a small ruler, but lets the clinician better understand your pain. The goals of treatment then relate to where the level of pain started (for example, a rating of 7 on a zero to ten scale) and what the cause of the pain was. Pain medicines may also be used together (in combination) in order to get the best result or outcome. If your pain control is not acceptable to YOU (remember, in hospitals and outpatient settings, etc. pain control is a patient right) and if after a week of arthritis pain treatment, results are not acceptable, be sure to call your doctor as you may need a different medicine or combination.

Arthritis: Control of arthritis symptoms (pain, loss of mobility, decreased ability to accomplish activities of daily living) is paramount in returning patient quality of life and to checking the results (beneficial outcomes) from this medicine. See WOMAC in glossary for rheumatoid arthritis.

▷ **This Drug Should Not Be Taken If**
- you have had an allergic reaction to it previously.
- you are subject to asthma or nasal polyps caused by aspirin.
- you have active peptic ulcer disease or any form of gastrointestinal bleeding.
- you have a bleeding disorder or a blood cell disorder.
- you have active liver disease.
- you have severe impairment of kidney function.

▷ **Inform Your Physician Before Taking This Drug If**
- you are allergic to aspirin or to other aspirin substitutes.
- you have a history of peptic ulcer disease, regional enteritis or ulcerative colitis.
- you have a history of any type of bleeding disorder.
- you have impaired liver or kidney function.
- you develop signs or symptoms of pancreatitis while taking this medicine (talk with your doctor).
- you have high blood pressure or a history of heart failure.
- you take acetaminophen, aspirin or other aspirin substitutes, anticoagulants or oral antidiabetic drugs.
- you have an infection.
- you plan to have surgery of any type in the near future.

Possible Side Effects (natural, expected and unavoidable drug actions)
Fluid retention (weight gain, edema), prolongation of bleeding time.

▷ **Possible Adverse Effects** (unusual, unexpected and infrequent reactions)
If any of the following develop, consult your physician promptly for guidance.

Mild Adverse Effects
Allergic reactions: skin rash, itching, spontaneous bruising.
Headache, dizziness, hair loss, altered vision, ringing in ears, drowsiness, fatigue, paresthesias, inability to concentrate—rare to infrequent.
Indigestion, nausea, vomiting, abdominal pain, diarrhea—infrequent to frequent.

Serious Adverse Effects
Esophagitis or active peptic ulcer, stomach or intestinal bleeding—possible and more likely in elderly.
Drug-induced liver or kidney damage—rare to infrequent.
Serious skin damage (toxic epidermal necrolysis)—case reports.
Worsening of congestive heart failure—possible.
Pancreatitis—rare.

Enteropathy—possible.

Bone marrow depression (see Glossary): abnormal bleeding or bruising—case reports.

Blood-clotting problems—related to dose and half-life.

Increased blood potassium or decreased sodium—case reports.

▷ **Possible Effects on Sexual Function:** None reported.

Possible Delayed Adverse Effects: Mild anemia due to "silent" blood loss from the stomach.

▷ **Adverse Effects That May Mimic Natural Diseases or Disorders**
Liver reaction may suggest viral hepatitis.

Natural Diseases or Disorders That May Be Activated by This Drug
Peptic ulcer disease, ulcerative colitis. This drug may hide symptoms of gout.

Possible Effects on Laboratory Tests
Red blood cell count and hemoglobin level: decreased.

Bleeding time: increased.

Blood uric acid level: increased.

Liver function tests: increased liver enzymes (ALT/GPT, AST/GOT and alkaline phosphatase), increased bilirubin.

Kidney function tests: blood creatinine and urea nitrogen (BUN) levels increased; urine analysis positive for red blood cells, casts and increased protein content (kidney damage).

Fecal occult blood test: positive.

CAUTION
1. The smallest effective dose should always be used.
2. This drug may hide early signs of infection. Tell your doctor if you think you are developing an infection.
3. Congestive heart failure in elderly patients may be unmasked or worsened. Risk appears to increase with use of higher doses.

Precautions for Use
By Infants and Children: Indications and dose recommendations for those under 12 years of age are not established.

By Those Over 60 Years of Age: Small doses are advisable until tolerance is determined. Observe for any indications of liver or kidney toxicity, fluid retention, dizziness, confusion, impaired memory, stomach bleeding or constipation. People in this age group are often more likely to have stomach problems from the medicine itself. Existing congestive heart failure may be worsened.

▷ **Advisability of Use During Pregnancy**
Pregnancy Category: B. D in the final 3 months of pregnancy. See Pregnancy Risk Categories at the back of this book.

Animal studies: No birth defects reported due to this drug.

Human studies: Adequate studies of pregnant women are not available.

The manufacturer does not recommend the use of this drug during pregnancy.

Advisability of Use If Breast-Feeding
Presence of this drug in breast milk: Yes.

Avoid drug or refrain from nursing.

Habit-Forming Potential: None.

Effects of Overdose: Possible drowsiness, dizziness, ringing in the ears, nausea, vomiting, indigestion.

Possible Effects of Long-Term Use: Development of anemia due to "silent" bleeding from the gastrointestinal tract.

Suggested Periodic Examinations While Taking This Drug (at physician's discretion)

Complete blood cell counts.

Liver and kidney function tests.

Complete eye examinations if vision is altered in any way.

Hearing examinations if ringing in the ears or hearing loss develops.

▷ **While Taking This Drug, Observe the Following**

Foods: No restrictions. No data from objective studies are available for combination use of this medicine and glucosamine. Talk to your doctor about possible combination.

Herbal Medicines or Minerals: Since St. John's wort and this drug may cause increased sun sensitivity, caution is advised. Ginseng, ginkgo, alfalfa, clove oil, feverfew, cinchona bark and garlic may also change clotting, so combining those herbals with these medicines is not recommended. Talk to your doctor BEFORE combining any medicines. NSAIDs may decrease feverfew effects. Hay flower, mistletoe herb and white mustard seed carry German Commission E monograph indications for arthritis but have not been tested in combination with this medicine. Talk to your doctor BEFORE adding any herbal to piroxicam.

Beverages: No restrictions. May be taken with milk.

▷ *Alcohol:* Use with caution. Both alcohol and piroxicam can irritate the stomach lining and can increase the risk of stomach ulceration and/or bleeding.

Tobacco Smoking: No interactions expected. I advise everyone to quit smoking.

▷ *Other Drugs*

Piroxicam may ***increase*** the effects of

- acetaminophen (Tylenol, etc.) and increase the risk of kidney damage; avoid prolonged use of this combination.
- adrenocortical steroids (see Drug Classes) and may result in additive stomach irritation.
- anticoagulants (Coumadin, etc.) and increase the risk of bleeding; more frequent INR (prothrombin time or protime) testing is needed, and dosing should then be adjusted accordingly. Low-molecular-weight heparins (see Drug Classes) combined with this medicine increase risk of hematoma.
- beta blockers (atenolol and others)—can decrease the effectiveness of the beta blocker.
- cyclosporine (Sandimmune) may increase seizure risk.
- enoxaparin (lovenox) and may increase bleeding risk.
- lithium (Lithobid, others) and can lead to lithium toxicity.
- methotrexate (Mexate) and may lead to methotrexate toxicity.

Piroxicam ***taken concurrently*** with

- antihypertensives such as thiazides (see Drug Classes), loop diuretics and others (ACE inhibitors) will blunt their therapeutic benefits.
- cholestyramine (Questran) may blunt piroxicam effectiveness.
- diuretics (see Drug Classes) may blunt diuretic benefits.
- ofloxacin (Floxin) and other quinolones such as levofloxacin (Levaquin) may increase seizure risk.
- oral hypoglycemics (see sulfonylureas) may increase risk of low blood sugar.

- ritonavir (Norvir) and perhaps other protease inhibitors (see Drug Classes) can lead to toxicity.
- tacrolimus (Prograf) may increase risk of kidney failure.

Piroxicam *taken concurrently* with the following drugs may increase bleeding risk. Avoid these:
- aspirin or other NSAIDs.
- dipyridamole (Persantine).
- indomethacin (Indocin).
- sulfinpyrazone (Anturane).
- valproic acid (Depakene).

▷ *Driving, Hazardous Activities:* This drug may cause drowsiness or dizziness. Restrict activities as necessary.

Aviation Note: The use of this drug *may be a disqualification* for piloting. Consult a designated Aviation Medical Examiner.

Exposure to Sun: This drug may cause photosensitivity (see Glossary). Use caution.

OXTRIPHYLLINE (ox TRY fi lin)

Other Names: Choline theophyllinate, theophylline cholinate

Introduced: 1965   **Class:** Antiasthmatic, bronchodilator, xanthines   **Prescription:**   USA: Yes

Controlled Drug: USA: No; Canada: No   **Available as Generic:**   Yes

Brand Names: ✤Apo-Oxtriphylline, Choledyl, Choledyl Delayed-Release, Choledyl SA, ✤Novotriphyl

Author's Note: This medicine is converted to 64% theophylline by the body. See the theophylline profile for further information.

OXYCODONE (ox ee KOH dohn)

Introduced: 1950   **Class:** Analgesic, strong; opioids   **Prescription:** USA: Yes   **Controlled Drug:**   USA: C-II*; Canada: No   **Available as Generic:**   USA: Yes; Canada: No

Brand Names: ✤Endocet [CD], ✤Endodan [CD], ✤Oxycocet [CD], ✤Oxycodan [CD], OxyContin, Percocet [CD], ✤Percocet-Demi [CD], Percodan [CD], Percodan-Demi [CD], Roxicet, Roxicodone, Roxilox, Roxiprin [CD], SK-Oxycodone, ✤Supeudol, Tylox [CD]

BENEFITS versus RISKS	
Possible Benefits	*Possible Risks*
EFFECTIVE RELIEF OF MODERATE TO SEVERE PAIN	POTENTIAL FOR HABIT FORMATION (DEPENDENCE)
	Sedative effects
	Mild allergic reactions—infrequent
	Nausea, constipation

*See Schedules of Controlled Drugs at the back of this book.

▷ **Principal Uses**

As a Single Drug Product: Uses currently included in FDA-approved labeling: (1) Used in tablet and suppository form (Canada) to relieve moderate to severe pain; (2) OxyContin form is approved for use appropriate to a schedule II narcotic to treat people in moderate to severe pain who are expected to require continuous opioids for an extended time. An important factor to be considered for OxyContin use is the severity of the pain that a patient is facing.

Other (unlabeled) generally accepted uses: None.

As a Combination Drug Product [CD]: Oxycodone is available in combinations with acetaminophen and with aspirin. These milder pain relievers are added to enhance the analgesic effect and reduce fever when present.

Author's Note: The FDA and Purdue Pharmaceuticals have worked together to strengthen warnings for OxyContin because of continuing reports of abuse and diversion of this medicine. A "Dear Healthcare Professional" letter has been sent out that explains the strengthening of the labeling including proper prescribing information and also highlights the problems associated with abuse and diversion of OxyContin. An important factor that MUST be considered when OxyContin is prescribed is the severity of the pain that is being treated, not simply the disease that is the root cause of the painful symptoms. The company has also responsibly undertaken a "Profiles in Pain Management" series in the *Pharmacy Today* journal of the American Pharmaceutical Association to increase awareness of prescription medication abuse. Because ALL opioids are subject to abuse, the FDA is also encouraging all makers of opioids sold in the US to voluntarily review and revise product labeling as needed to help ensure adequate warnings and precautions regarding risks of abuse, misuse and diversion are presented and that responsible prescribing practices are promoted. A MedWatch safety summary is available at www.fda.gov/ medwatch/safety/2001/safety01.htm#oxycon.

How This Drug Works: Acting primarily as a depressant of certain brain functions (by attaching to specific receptors), this drug suppresses pain perception and calms the emotional response to pain.

Available Dosage Forms and Strengths

Solution — 5 mg/5 ml

Suppositories — 10 mg, 20 mg (Canada)

Tablets — 5 mg, 10 mg (Canada)

Tablets — 2.44 mg, 4.88 mg (in combination drugs)

Tablets, controlled-release — 10 mg, 20 mg, 40 mg, 80 mg

▷ **Usual Adult Dosage Ranges:** Percodan is taken as one tablet (5 mg) every 6 hours. Current pain theory says that pain medicines should be scheduled—for example, given every 6 hours. The outdated "wait until it hurts" or PRN method tended to result in suffering. May be increased to 10 mg every 4 hours if needed for severe pain. The total daily dose should not exceed 60 mg.

The new Percocet (oxycodone and acetaminophen combination) tablets are now available in four strengths (2.5/325, 5/325, 7.5/500 and 10/650). These strengths represent the amount of oxycodone followed by the amount of acetaminophen. Make sure you understand how much and how often to take this medicine.

OxyContin is taken every 12 hours and is a sustained-release formulation. This product has an 80-mg strength that is used for increasing (escalating) pain in people who have been taking opioids and have become tolerant. Some clinicians use a rescue dose of the immediate-release forms of oxycodone to manage breakthrough pain and then add a percentage of the total daily rescue dosage used back to the extended-release formulation. New labeling for this form of oxycodone is meant to decrease the chance that OxyContin could be prescribed inappropriately for pain of lesser severity than the approved use or for other disorders or conditions inappropriate for a schedule II narcotic.

Note: Actual dose and schedule must be determined for each patient individually.

Conditions Requiring Dosing Adjustments

Liver Function: Dose adjustments should be empirically made in liver failure.

Kidney Function: Dose adjustment does not appear to be needed. Some combination products contain aspirin, which may be contraindicated in kidney failure.

▷ **Dosing Instructions:** The immediate-release tablets may be crushed and taken with or following food to reduce stomach upset or nausea. If you forget a dose: Take the missed dose as soon as you remember it, unless it's nearly time for your next dose—if that is the case, skip the missed dose and take the next dose right on schedule. DO NOT double doses. Talk with your doctor if you find yourself missing doses.

Author's Note: Current pain treatment theory calls for timed or scheduled dosing. This tends to prevent pain, rather than allowing pain to recur and then having to be treated. Some clinicians will use timed dosing immediately after surgery and then revert to as-needed dosing once the most severe period of pain has passed. Pain is now the fifth vital sign.

Usual Duration of Use: As long as significant pain is present and as required to control pain. Continual use should not exceed 5 to 7 days without interruption and reassessment of need.

Typical Treatment Goals and Measurements (Outcomes and Markers)

Pain: Most clinicians treating pain use a device called an algometer to check your pain. This looks like a small ruler, but lets the clinician better understand your pain. The goals of treatment then relate to where the level of pain started (for example, a rating of 7 on a zero to ten scale) and what the cause of the pain was. Pain medicines may also be used together (in combination) in order to get the best result or outcome. If your pain control is not acceptable to YOU (remember, in hospitals and outpatient settings, etc. pain control is a patient right and the fifth vital sign) and if after a reasonable attempt with good adherence, results are not acceptable, be sure to call your doctor. You may need a different dose, different medicine or combination.

▷ **This Drug Should Not Be Taken If**
- you had an allergic reaction to it previously.
- you are having an acute attack of asthma.
- Patients allergic to aspirin should not be given Percodan.

▷ **Inform Your Physician Before Taking This Drug If**
- you had an unfavorable reaction to any narcotic drug or are prone to constipation.
- you have had a head injury with increased pressure (intracranial) in the head.
- you have a history of drug abuse or alcoholism.
- you have chronic lung disease with impaired breathing.
- you have impaired liver or kidney function.
- you have gallbladder disease, a seizure disorder or an underactive thyroid gland.
- you have difficulty emptying the urinary bladder.
- you are taking any other drugs that have a sedative effect.
- you plan to have surgery under general anesthesia in the near future.

Possible Side Effects (natural, expected and unavoidable drug actions)
Drowsiness, light-headedness, dry mouth, urinary retention, constipation.

▷ **Possible Adverse Effects** (unusual, unexpected and infrequent reactions)
If any of the following develop, consult your physician promptly for guidance.

Mild Adverse Effects
Allergic reactions: skin rash, hives, itching.
Idiosyncratic reactions: skin rash and itching when combined with dairy products (milk or cheese).
Dizziness, sensation of drunkenness, depression, blurred or double vision—dose-related.
Nausea, vomiting—may be dose related.

Serious Adverse Effects
Impaired breathing: use with caution in chronic lung disease—variable and can be dose related.
Abnormal body movements, if the drug is abruptly stopped.

▷ **Possible Effects on Sexual Function:** Blunted sexual responses—case reports.

Possible Effects on Laboratory Tests
Urine screening tests for drug abuse: test result may be falsely **positive;** confirmatory test result may be **negative.** (Test results depend upon amount of drug taken and testing method used.)

CAUTION
1. If you have been prescribed Percocet, please be aware that there are now four strengths. Make certain that you understand how much to take. The strengths (oxycodone/acetaminophen) may be confusing. For example, it may be tempting for some prescribers to shorten Percocet 5/325 to Percocet-5. This kind of name change could lead to an impression that five tablets are to be taken instead of a correct one-tablet dose. Talk to your doctor and make sure you understand how much and how often you are to take this medicine!
2. If you have asthma, chronic bronchitis or emphysema, excessive use of this drug may cause significant respiratory difficulty, thickening of bronchial secretions and suppression of coughing.
3. If you have been taking an oxycodone form on an ongoing basis, slow tapering rather than sudden discontinuation is prudent.
4. The concurrent use of this drug with atropinelike drugs can increase the risk of urinary retention and reduced intestinal function.

5. Constipation can be a serious problem, particularly in older patients (as bowel function tends to slow down). Many clinicians prescribe a medicine to promote bowel movements at the same time that oxycodone is prescribed.

6. The FDA and the maker of OxyContin have worked together to strengthen warnings and precautions section of the OxyContin labeling (not available at the time of this writing). It would be prudent to discuss these changes with your doctor.

7. Do not take this drug following acute head injury.

8. Females will generally have a 25% higher oxycodone blood (plasma) level than males when weight is considered (on a body weight adjusted basis).

Precautions for Use

By Infants and Children: Do not use this drug in children under 2 years of age because of their vulnerability to life-threatening respiratory depression.

By Those Over 60 Years of Age: Small starting doses and short-term therapy are indicated. There may be increased susceptibility to the development of drowsiness, dizziness, unsteadiness, falling, urinary retention and constipation (may lead to fecal impaction).

▷ **Advisability of Use During Pregnancy**

Pregnancy Category: B. See Pregnancy Risk Categories at the back of this book.

Animal studies: No information available.

Human studies: Adequate studies of pregnant women are not available. Oxycodone taken repeatedly during the final few weeks before delivery may cause withdrawal symptoms in the newborn.

Use only if clearly needed and in small, infrequent doses.

Advisability of Use If Breast-Feeding

Presence of this drug in breast milk: Yes.

Avoid drug or refrain from nursing.

Habit-Forming Potential: Psychological and/or physical dependence can develop. The FDA and the maker of OxyContin have taken expanded steps to enhance prescriber awareness of possible diversion and abuse of OxyContin.

Effects of Overdose: Drowsiness, restlessness, agitation, nausea, vomiting, dry mouth, vertigo, weakness, lethargy, stupor, coma, seizures.

Possible Effects of Long-Term Use: Psychological and physical dependence, chronic constipation.

Suggested Periodic Examinations While Taking This Drug (at physician's discretion)

None.

▷ **While Taking This Drug, Observe the Following**

Foods: No restrictions.

Herbal Medicines or Minerals: Kava kava and valerian may worsen drowsiness. Caution is advised. St. John's wort can change (inducing or increasing) P450 enzymes, blunting the effects of oxycodone. Talk to your doctor BEFORE you combine any herbal medicines with oxycodone.

Beverages: No restrictions. May be taken with milk.

▷ *Alcohol:* Oxycodone can intensify the intoxicating effects of alcohol, and alcohol can intensify the depressant effects of oxycodone on brain function, breathing and circulation. Combined use is best avoided.

Tobacco Smoking: No interactions expected. I advise everyone to quit smoking.

Marijuana Smoking: Increase in drowsiness and pain relief; impairment of mental and physical performance.

▷ *Other Drugs*

Oxycodone may *increase* the effects of
- atropinelike drugs and increase the risk of constipation and urinary retention.
- other drugs with sedative effects (see Drug Classes for benzodiazepines, tricyclic antidepressants, antihistamines, MAO inhibitors, phenothiazines and opioid drugs [narcotics]).

Oxycodone *taken concurrently* with
- naltrexone (ReVia) may lead to withdrawal symptoms.
- rifabutin (Rifater, others) may blunt oxycodone benefits.
- ritonavir (Norvir) and perhaps other protease inhibitors (see Drug Classes) may lead to toxicity.
- sertraline (Zoloft) resulted in a serotonin syndrome in one case report. Caution is advised.
- tramadol (Ultram) may increase risk of adverse effects.

▷ *Driving, Hazardous Activities:* This drug can impair mental alertness, judgment, reaction time and physical coordination. Avoid hazardous activities accordingly.

Aviation Note: The use of this drug *is a disqualification* for piloting. Consult a designated Aviation Medical Examiner.

Exposure to Sun: No restrictions.

Discontinuation: It is best to limit this drug to short-term use. If extended use is needed, discontinuation should be gradual to minimize possible effects of withdrawal.

PANTOPRAZOLE (pan TOE prah sole)

Introduced: 2000   **Class:** Antiulcer, proton pump inhibitor   **Prescription:** USA: Yes   **Controlled Drug:** USA: No; Canada: No   **Available as Generic:** USA: No; Canada: No

Brand Name: Protonix

Author's Note: Information in this profile will be broadened if further data on this medicine warrants inclusion.

PAROXETINE (pa ROCKS a teen)

Introduced: 1993   **Class:** Antidepressant, other   **Prescription:** USA: Yes   **Controlled Drug:** USA: No; Canada: No   **Available as Generic:** USA: No; Canada: No

Brand Name: Paxil

BENEFITS versus RISKS	
Possible Benefits	*Possible Risks*
EFFECTIVE CONTROL OF DEPRESSION	Withdrawal symptoms
CONTROL OF SOCIAL ANXIETY DISORDER	Abnormal ejaculation in males
EFFECTIVE USE IN PANIC ATTACKS IN CHILDREN	
HELPS CONTROL OBSESSIVE COMPULSIVE DISORDER	
Fewer adverse effects than tricyclic antidepressants	
May help premature ejaculation	
Useful in some pain syndromes	

▷ **Principal Uses**

As a Single Drug Product: Uses currently included in FDA-approved labeling: (1) Treatment of depression; (2) helps control obsessive-compulsive disorder; (3) helps control panic attacks (panic disorder) in adults; (4) control of social anxiety disorder; (5) eases social phobia.

Other (unlabeled) generally accepted uses: (1) Can have a role in diabetic nerve pain (neuropathy); (2) helps long-standing (chronic) daily headaches; (3) can help premature ejaculation; (4) appears to have a role in helping prevent panic attacks in children.

How This Drug Works: Inhibits uptake of serotonin. When more of this chemical is available in the brain, a positive impact on thinking results. Because the specific cause of panic attacks is not known, how this medicine works to prevent panic attacks has not been identified.

Available Dosage Forms and Strengths

Tablets, controlled release — 12.5 mg, 25 mg

Tablets, immediate release — 10 mg, 20 mg, 30 mg and 40 mg

Oral suspension — 10 mg/5 ml

▷ **Recommended Dose Ranges** (Actual dose and schedule must be determined for each patient individually.)

Infants and Children: Some clinicians have used 5 to 10 mg per day in children with panic disorder (or 0.25 to 0.5 mg per kg per day).

18 to 60 Years of Age: Depression: Immediate-release form: The usual starting dose is 20 mg, taken in the morning. Dose can then be increased as needed and tolerated in 10-mg intervals to a maximum of 50 mg daily.

Depression: Controlled-release form: Started with 25 milligrams (mg) daily. If patient response does not meet physician goals, the dose may be increased by 12.5 mg daily (at intervals of 7 days or more). The maximum recommended dose is 62.5 mg daily.

Obsessive-compulsive disorder (immediate-release form): Started with 20 mg daily with increases as in depression to a usual benefit at 40 mg per day. Maximum dose is 60 mg daily.

Panic disorder: Dosing is started with 10 mg per day, and doses are increased (at weekly intervals) as needed and tolerated to the usual dose of 40 mg a day. Daily maximum is 60 mg.

Social anxiety disorder: 20 mg daily.

Over 60 Years of Age: The starting dose in this population is 10 mg daily. The maximum dose is 40 mg daily.

Conditions Requiring Dosing Adjustments

Liver Function: Starting dose is 10 mg, and the maximum dose is 40 mg daily. Drug levels may be needed.

Kidney Function: Same starting dose and maximum dose as in liver compromise.

▷ **Dosing Instructions:** The absorption of this medicine is not changed by food. If you forget a dose: Take the missed dose as soon as you remember it, unless it's nearly time for your next dose—if that is the case, skip the missed dose and take the next dose right on schedule. DO NOT double doses. Talk with your doctor if you find yourself missing doses.

Usual Duration of Use: Continual use on a regular schedule for 14 days is usually necessary to determine this drug's effectiveness in treating depression. Long-term use (months to years) requires periodic evaluation of response and dose adjustment by your doctor.

Typical Treatment Goals and Measurements (Outcomes and Markers)

Depression: The general goal: to at least help lessen the degree and severity of depression, letting patients return to their daily lives. Specific measures of depression involve testing or inventories and can be valuable in helping check benefits from this medicine. The Hamilton depression scale is widely used to assess depression. In any case the ability of the patient to return to normal activities or not have them interrupted is a hallmark of successful treatment.

Panic: Goals for panic tend to be more vague and subjective than hypertension or cholesterol. Frequently, the patient (in conjunction with physician assessment) will largely decide if panic has been successfully controlled. Decreased number of trips to the hospital or ER visits may also be a useful measure. The ability of the patient to return to normal activities is a hallmark of successful treatment.

Possible Advantages of This Drug

Fewer side effects than tricyclic antidepressants. May be a drug of choice in people with heart disease who are also depressed. Since a large National Cancer Institute study found that those who suffer depression for 6 years or more have a generally increased risk of cancer, one benefit of effective treatment of depression with this drug may be a generally reduced risk of cancer. This was the first medicine approved to treat social anxiety disorder.

▷ **This Drug Should Not Be Taken If**
  • you had an allergic reaction to it previously.
  • you have taken a MAO inhibitor (see Drug Classes) in the last 14 days.

▷ **Inform Your Physician Before Taking This Drug If**
  • you are pregnant or breast-feeding.
  • you have a history of mania or seizures.
  • you take diuretics or typically drink little water.
  • you have a history of liver or kidney disease.
  • you take prescription or nonprescription medicines not discussed with your doctor when paroxetine was prescribed.

Possible Side Effects (natural, expected and unavoidable drug actions)

Lowered blood pressure and fainting upon standing (postural hypotension). Sedation. Nausea (up to 27%). Often decreases in 3 weeks. May require ondansetron or a lower paroxetine dose.

▷ **Possible Adverse Effects** (unusual, unexpected and infrequent reactions)

If any of the following develop, consult your physician promptly for guidance.

Mild Adverse Effects

Allergic reactions: skin rash and itching.

Headache, nervousness or insomnia—infrequent to frequent.

Palpitations—infrequent.

Teeth grinding (bruxism)—case report.

Loss of appetite, nausea, taste disorders or constipation—infrequent to frequent.

Tingling of the hands (paresthesias)—infrequent.

Sweating—frequent.

Dizziness, blurred vision—infrequent to frequent.

Serious Adverse Effects

Allergic reactions: not reported.

Idiosyncratic reactions: bruising and excessive menstrual bleeding—case report (reversed with vitamin C).

Abnormal movements or positioning of the mouth or face—infrequent.

Abnormal urination (SIADH)—case report.

Seizures—rare.

Liver toxicity—rare and of questionable causation.

▷ **Possible Effects on Sexual Function:** Galactorrhea. USED TO TREAT premature ejaculation.

Abnormal ejaculation—infrequent to frequent.

Inability to achieve orgasm, impotence or sexual dysfunction—infrequent.

Prolonged and painful erection (priapism)—rare.

Possible Delayed Adverse Effects: None reported.

▷ **Adverse Effects That May Mimic Natural Diseases or Disorders**

Increased liver enzymes may mimic early hepatitis.

Natural Diseases or Disorders That May Be Activated by This Drug

None reported.

Possible Effects on Laboratory Tests

Liver function tests: increased.

CAUTION

1. Take this medicine as prescribed, and do not stop taking it without talking with your doctor.

Precautions for Use

By Infants and Children: Safety and effectiveness for use by those under 18 years of age have not been established.

By Those Over 60 Years of Age: Lower starting and maximum doses are indicated.

▷ **Advisability of Use During Pregnancy**

Pregnancy Category: C. See Pregnancy Risk Categories at the back of this book.

Animal studies: Reproduction studies in rabbits or rats using doses of up to 10 times the typical human dose have not revealed any fetal changes.

Human studies: Information from adequate studies of pregnant women is not available.

Ask your doctor for guidance.

Advisability of Use If Breast-Feeding

Presence of this drug in breast milk: Yes, in small amounts.

Ask your doctor for guidance.

Habit-Forming Potential: None, but a withdrawal syndrome characterized by dizziness, confusion, sweating and tremor has been described.

Effects of Overdose: Confusion, heart rhythm changes, seizures.

Possible Effects of Long-Term Use: Not defined.

Suggested Periodic Examinations While Taking This Drug (at physician's discretion)

Liver function tests.

▷ **While Taking This Drug, Observe the Following**

Foods: No restrictions. Vitamin C reversed abnormal bruising and increased menstrual bleeding in one patient.

Herbal Medicines or Minerals: Since paroxetine and St. John's wort may act to increase serotonin, the combination is not advised. Since part of the way ginseng and gingko work may be as a MAO inhibitor, it may be ill advised to combine ginseng and ginkgo with paroxetine. Ma huang, yohimbe, Indian snakeroot and kava kava are also best avoided while taking this medicine.

Beverages: No restrictions.

▷ *Alcohol:* The manufacturer recommends avoiding alcohol while taking this medicine.

Tobacco Smoking: No interactions expected. I advise everyone to quit smoking.

Marijuana Smoking: Additive sedation.

▷ *Other Drugs*

Paroxetine may *increase* the effects of

- benzodiazepines (see Drug Classes).
- buspirone (Buspar).
- desipramine (and potentially other tricyclic antidepressants: see Drug Classes).
- dofetilide (Tikosyn) by increasing blood levels. Checks of patient clinical status and dosing changes are appropriate.
- flecainide (Tambocor) because paroxetine inhibits an enzyme system needed to remove flecainide. More frequent flecainide blood levels are prudent.
- galantamine (Reminyl) because paroxetine inhibits an enzyme system needed to remove galantamine. Caution, careful patient monitoring and possible dose decreases of galantamine may be prudent.
- haloperidol (Haldol), because paroxetine blocks an enzyme system needed to remove haloperidol.
- labetalol (Normodyne), and perhaps other beta blockers (see Drug Classes), because paroxetine inhibits an enzyme system needed to remove labetalol.
- minimally sedating antihistamines (astemizole and terfenadine), because paroxetine may inhibit some liver systems that usually remove them from the body. This effect has not been documented but is theoretically possible.

Paroxetine *taken concurrently* with

- activated charcoal will reduce absorption of paroxetine.
- astemizole (Hismanal) now removed from the US market may lead to heart toxicity—DO NOT COMBINE.
- dextromethorphan (the DM ingredient in many cough suppressants) may lead to serotonin syndrome—DO NOT COMBINE.
- digoxin (Lanoxin) may lead to lowered digoxin levels. More frequent digoxin levels are prudent.
- fenfluramine (Pondimin) may cause toxicity (serotonin syndrome).
- lithium (Lithobid, others) may lead to increased adverse effects.
- MAO inhibitors (see Drug Classes) may result in a fatal serotonin syndrome. Do not combine these medicines.
- naratriptan (Amerge) and other triptan-type medicines may lead to loss of coordination and changes in reflexes.
- phenytoin (Dilantin) or fosphenytoin (Cerebyx) may result in decreased paroxetine blood levels and lessening of therapeutic benefits. Dose increases may be needed.
- quinidine (Quinaglute, others) may result in increased paroxetine levels and toxicity; decreased paroxetine doses may be needed.
- risperidone (Risperdal) may lead to serotonin syndrome.
- ritonavir (Norvir) may lead to paroxetine toxicity.
- sibutramine (Meridia) increases risk of serotonin syndrome.
- sumatriptan (Imitrex) and other triptan type medicines can lead to hyper-reflexia and poor coordination—the combination may not be advisable and if combination is required, careful patient follow up is very important.
- tramadol (Ultram) may lead to increased risk of seizures—DO NOT COMBINE.
- tryptophan may result in sweating, nausea and dizziness.
- venlafaxine (Effexor) can increase risk of serious serotonin syndrome.
- warfarin (Coumadin) may result in bleeding; more frequent INR (prothrombin time or protime) testing is recommended. Warfarin doses should be adjusted based on laboratory results.

The following drug may **increase** the effects of paroxetine:

- cimetidine (Tagamet).

Driving, Hazardous Activities: This drug may frequently cause sedation. Restrict activities as necessary.

Aviation Note: The use of this drug *is a disqualification* for piloting. Consult a designated Aviation Medical Examiner.

Exposure to Sun: No specific restrictions.

Exposure to Heat: This medicine can cause excessive sweating. If you work or are frequently in a hot environment, be careful to replace enough fluids to avoid dehydration.

Heavy Exercise or Exertion: Since this medicine may cause excessive sweating, be careful to replace lost fluids.

Occurrence of Unrelated Illness: Fevers may cause more severe dehydration.

Discontinuation: Do not stop this medicine without talking with your doctor. For patients taking more than 40 mg a day or who have been taking this medicine for an extended period of time, gradual dosing decreases (tapering) over several days is recommended.

PENBUTOLOL (pen BYU toh lohl)

Introduced: 1976   **Class:** Antihypertensive, beta-adrenergic blocker   **Prescription:** USA: Yes   **Controlled Drug:** USA: No; Canada: No   **Available as Generic:** Yes

Brand Name: Levatol

BENEFITS versus RISKS	
Possible Benefits	*Possible Risks*
EFFECTIVE, WELL-TOLERATED ANTIHYPERTENSIVE IN MILD TO MODERATE HIGH BLOOD PRESSURE	CONGESTIVE HEART FAILURE in advanced heart disease
	Worsening of angina in coronary heart disease (abrupt withdrawal)
	Masking of low blood sugar (hypoglycemia) in drug-treated diabetes
	Provocation of asthma (in asthmatics)

▷ **Principal Uses**

    As a Single Drug Product: Uses currently included in FDA-approved labeling: Treats mild to moderate high blood pressure; used alone or combined with other antihypertensive drugs.

    Other (unlabeled) generally accepted uses: (1) May help curb aggressive behavior; (2) can help decrease the frequency and severity of angina attacks; (3) may help decrease death from heart attack (myocardial infarction); (4) supportive role in panic attacks; (5) limited studies support penbutolol use in glaucoma. Large studies are needed.

How This Drug Works: Blocks certain actions of the sympathetic nervous system and:

- reduces heart rate and contraction force, lowering the pressure of the blood leaving the heart.
- reduces the degree of blood vessel wall contraction, resulting in lower blood pressure.

Available Dosage Forms and Strengths

    Tablets — 20 mg

▷ **Usual Adult Dosage Ranges:** *Hypertension*: Initially 20 mg once daily. The dose may be increased gradually by 10 mg/day at intervals of 2 weeks as needed and tolerated, up to 80 mg/day. Higher doses have been tolerated, but do not give greater efficacy. Twenty to 40 mg daily is a common ongoing dose. Daily maximum is 80 mg.

Note: Actual dose and schedule must be determined for each patient individually.

Conditions Requiring Dosing Adjustments

    Liver Function: Dose adjustments should be considered in mild to moderate liver disease, but specific guidelines are not available.

    Kidney Function: No dosing changes are thought to be needed.

▷ **Dosing Instructions:** The tablet may be crushed and taken without regard to eating. Do not stop this drug abruptly. If you forget a dose: Take the missed dose as soon as you remember it, unless it's less than 8 hours before your next dose—if that is the case, skip the missed dose and take the next dose right on schedule. DO NOT double doses. Talk with your doctor if you find yourself missing doses.

Usual Duration of Use: Use on a regular schedule for up to 2 weeks determines the full effect in lowering blood pressure. Long-term use of this drug (months to years) will determine your blood pressure over time and response to an overall treatment program (weight reduction, salt restriction, smoking cessation, etc.).

Typical Treatment Goals and Measurements (Outcomes and Markers)

Blood pressure: The most recent treatment guidelines (JNC VI) actually define optimal blood pressure (BP) as less than 120/80 and high normal as 139/89. The American Diabetes Association has chosen a target of 130/80 as the blood pressure goal for people living with diabetes. Most clinicians try to achieve a BP that achieves the best balance of lower cardiovascular risk while avoiding the problem of too low a blood pressure. The goal and time frame (see peak benefits above) should be discussed with you when the prescription is written.

Possible Advantages of This Drug

Adequate control of blood pressure with a single daily dose. Causes less slowing of the heart rate than most other beta-blocker drugs.

▷ **This Drug Should Not Be Taken If**
- you have had an allergic reaction to it previously.
- you have heart failure (overt).
- you have an abnormally slow heart rate or a serious form of heart block.
- you have abnormal growth of the left side of the heart (left ventricular hypertrophy).
- you have bronchial asthma.

▷ **Inform Your Physician Before Taking This Drug If**
- you had problems from any beta blocker (see Drug Classes).
- you have a history of serious heart disease.
- you have a history of hay fever (allergic rhinitis), asthma, chronic bronchitis or emphysema.
- you have a history of overactive thyroid function (hyperthyroidism).
- you have a history of low blood sugar (hypoglycemia).
- you have impaired liver or kidney function.
- you have diabetes or myasthenia gravis.
- you have congestive heart failure.
- you have impaired circulation in the extremities (Raynaud's phenomenon, claudication pains in legs).
- you take any form of digitalis, quinidine or reserpine or any calcium-channel-blocker drug (see Drug Classes).
- you plan to have surgery under general anesthesia in the near future.

Possible Side Effects (natural, expected and unavoidable drug actions)

Lethargy and fatigability, cold extremities, slow heart rate, light-headedness in upright position (see orthostatic hypotension in Glossary).

▷ **Possible Adverse Effects** (unusual, unexpected and infrequent reactions)

If any of the following develop, consult your physician promptly for guidance.

Mild Adverse Effects

Allergic reactions: skin rash, itching, reversible hair loss.

Headache, dizziness, blurred vision, insomnia, abnormal dreams—infrequent.

Indigestion, nausea, vomiting, constipation, diarrhea—infrequent.

Joint and muscle discomfort—infrequent.

Serious Adverse Effects

Allergic reactions: anaphylactic reaction (see Glossary).

Mental depression, anxiety, disorientation, short-term memory loss, hallucinations—possible.

Carpal tunnel syndrome or aggravation of myasthenia gravis—case reports.

High blood sugar or low blood sugar in diabetics—possible.

Worsening of circulatory problems (with preexisting conditions, Raynaud's phenomenon)—possible.

Bronchospasm—rare.

Chest pain, shortness of breath, precipitation of congestive heart failure—possible.

Rebound hypertension—if abruptly stopped.

Induction of bronchial asthma—possible in asthmatics.

▷ **Possible Effects on Sexual Function:** Decreased libido and impotence—rare but dose-related.

Peyronie's disease (see Glossary)—rare.

▷ **Adverse Effects That May Mimic Natural Diseases or Disorders**

Reduced blood flow to extremities may resemble Raynaud's phenomenon (see Glossary).

Natural Diseases or Disorders That May Be Activated by This Drug

Raynaud's phenomenon, intermittent claudication, myasthenia gravis.

Possible Effects on Laboratory Tests

Uric acid, potassium or blood sugar: increased.

CAUTION

1. ***Do not stop this drug suddenly*** without calling your doctor. Carry a card saying you take this drug.
2. Ask your doctor or pharmacist **before** using nasal decongestants (cold medicines and nose drops). May cause sudden increases in blood pressure when taken with beta blockers.
3. Call your doctor if emotional depression starts.

Precautions for Use

By Infants and Children: Safety and effectiveness in infants or children not established.

By Those Over 60 Years of Age: High blood pressure should be reduced avoiding risks of too low a blood pressure. Small starting doses and frequent blood pressure checks are needed. Sudden, rapid and excessive reduction of blood pressure can predispose to stroke or heart attack. Observe for dizziness, unsteadiness, tendency to fall, confusion, hallucinations, depression or urinary frequency.

▷ **Advisability of Use During Pregnancy**

Pregnancy Category: C. See Pregnancy Risk Categories at the back of this book.

Animal studies: No birth defects due to this drug found in rat or rabbit studies.

Human studies: Adequate studies of pregnant women are not available.

Ask your physician for guidance.

Advisability of Use If Breast-Feeding
> Presence of this drug in breast milk: Controversial.
> Avoid drug or refrain from nursing.

Habit-Forming Potential: None.

Effects of Overdose: Weakness, slow pulse, low blood pressure, fainting, cold and sweaty skin, congestive heart failure, possible coma and convulsions.

Possible Effects of Long-Term Use: Reduced heart reserve and eventual heart failure in susceptible individuals with advanced heart disease.

Suggested Periodic Examinations While Taking This Drug (at physician's discretion)
> Measurements of blood pressure.
> Evaluation of heart function.
> Complete blood cell counts.

▷ **While Taking This Drug, Observe the Following**
> *Foods:* No restrictions. Avoid excessive salt intake.
>
> *Herbal Medicines or Minerals:* Ginseng or ma huang may increase blood pressure, blunting the benefits of this medicine. Hawthorn, saw palmetto and licorice may also cause increased blood pressure. Calcium and garlic may lower blood pressure. Use caution and work with your doctor to make sure blood pressure is not lowered too much. Indian snakeroot has a German Commission E monograph indication for hypertension—talk to your doctor. Eleuthero root and ephedra should be avoided by people living with hypertension.
>
> *Beverages:* No restrictions. May be taken with milk.

▷ *Alcohol:* Alcohol may exaggerate this drug's ability to lower blood pressure and may increase its mild sedative effect.

> *Tobacco Smoking:* Nicotine may reduce this drug's benefit in treating high blood pressure. I advise everyone to quit smoking.

▷ *Other Drugs*
> Penbutolol may *increase* the effects of
> - other antihypertensive drugs and cause excessive lowering of blood pressure; dose adjustments may be necessary.
> - reserpine (Ser-Ap-Es, etc.) and cause sedation, depression, slowing of the heart rate and lowering of blood pressure—this combination is best avoided.
> - verapamil (Calan, Isoptin) and cause excessive depression of heart function; monitor this combination closely.
>
> Penbutolol may *decrease* the effects of
> - epinephrine, resulting in decreased benefits when used to correct allergic reactions; slow heartbeat and elevated blood pressure may also occur.
>
> Penbutolol *taken concurrently* with
> - amiodarone (Cordarone) may result in sinus arrest or symptomatic bradycardia—DO NOT COMBINE.
> - clonidine (Catapres) requires close monitoring for rebound high blood pressure if clonidine is withdrawn while penbutolol is still being taken.
> - digoxin (Lanoxin) increases risk of heartbeat or heart block.
> - fluoxetine (Prozac) may cause very slow heartbeat (bradycardia) and excessive lowering of blood pressure.

- fluvoxamine (Luvox) may cause very slow heartbeat (bradycardia) and excessive lowering of blood pressure.
- insulin or oral hypoglycemic agents requires close monitoring to avoid undetected hypoglycemia (see Glossary).
- mibefradil (Posicor) may impair heart performance in people with poor left heart function or in the elderly.
- venlafaxine (Effexor) may result in increased risk of toxicity from penbutolol.
- zileuton (Zyflo) may seriously increase penbutolol concentrations leading to penbutolol toxicity.

The following drugs may *increase* the effects of penbutolol:
- birth control pills (oral contraceptives).
- methimazole (Tapazole).
- propylthiouracil (Propacil).
- ritonavir (Norvir) and perhaps other protease inhibitors (see Drug Classes).

The following drugs may *decrease* the effects of penbutolol:
- barbiturates (phenobarbital, etc.).
- indomethacin (Indocin) and possibly other "aspirin substitutes," or NSAIDs—may impair penbutolol's antihypertensive effect.
- rifampin (Rifadin, Rimactane).

▷ *Driving, Hazardous Activities:* Use caution until the full extent of fatigue, dizziness and blood pressure change has been determined.

Aviation Note: The use of this drug is *a disqualification* for piloting. Consult a designated Aviation Medical Examiner.

Exposure to Sun: No restrictions.

Exposure to Heat: Hot environments can lower blood pressure and exaggerate effects.

Exposure to Cold: Cold environments can worsen low circulation to the extremities. Elderly should be careful to prevent hypothermia (see Glossary).

Heavy Exercise or Exertion: Avoid exertion that produces light-headedness, excessive fatigue or muscle cramping. The use of this drug may intensify the hypertensive response to isometric exercise.

Occurrence of Unrelated Illness: Fever can lower blood pressure and require lower doses. Vomiting may interrupt the regular dose schedule. Ask your doctor for help.

Discontinuation: Best to avoid stopping this drug suddenly. If possible, slow dose reduction over 2 to 3 weeks is recommended.

PENICILLAMINE (pen i SIL a meen)

Introduced: 1963   **Class:** Antiarthritic   **Prescription:** USA: Yes
Controlled Drug: USA: No; Canada: No   **Available as Generic:** USA: No;
Canada: No
Brand Names: Cuprimine, Depen

BENEFITS versus RISKS

Possible Benefits	*Possible Risks*
EFFECTIVE TREATMENT OF WILSON'S DISEASE (COPPER TOXICITY)	SEVERE ALLERGIC REACTIONS BONE MARROW DEPRESSION
Effective treatment of cystinuria and cystine kidney stones	Drug-induced damage of lungs, liver, pancreas and kidneys
Partially effective treatment of rheumatoid arthritis and poisoning due to heavy metals: iron, lead, mercury and zinc	

▷ **Principal Uses**

As a Single Drug Product: Uses currently included in FDA-approved labeling: Treatment of (1) Wilson's disease (copper toxicity of brain, cornea, liver and kidneys); (2) severe rheumatoid arthritis that has failed to respond to less hazardous conventional treatment and also helps rheumatoid arthritis that presents with interstitial lung disease; (3) cystinuria and cystine stone formation (excessive amounts of cystine in the urine).

Other (unlabeled) generally accepted uses: (1) Treatment of heavy metal poisoning, especially due to lead and mercury; (2) may help increase survival in scleroderma; (3) eases progression of systemic sclerosis.

Author's Note: Due to proliferation of new medicines, this profile has been abbreviated in order to make room for more widely used medicines.

PENICILLIN ANTIBIOTIC FAMILY

Amoxicillin (a mox i SIL in) **Amoxicillin/Clavulanate** (a mox i SIL in/KLAV yu lan ayt) **Ampicillin** (am pi SIL in) **Bacampicillin** (bak am pi SIL in) **Cloxacillin** (klox a SIL in) **Penicillin VK** (pen i SIL in VEE KAY)

Introduced: 1969, 1982, 1961, 1979, 1962, 1953, respectively   **Class:** Antibiotics, penicillins   **Prescription:** USA: Yes   **Controlled Drug:** USA: No; Canada: No   **Available as Generic:** USA: Yes (all but amoxicillin/clavulanate); Canada: Yes

Brand Names: Amoxicillin: A-Cillin, Amoxil, ✿Apo-Amoxi, ✿Clavulin, Larotid, ✿Novamoxin, ✿Nu-Amoxi, Polymox, Prevpac [CD], Trimox, Wymox, Amoxicillin/Clavulanate: Amcill, Ampicillin: ✿Ampicin, ✿Ampicin PRB [CD], ✿Ampilean, ✿Apo-Ampi, Augmentin, ✿Clavulin, D-Amp, Faspak Ampicillin, 500 Kit [CD], ✿Novo-Ampicillin, Nu-Ampi, Omnipen, Omnipen Pediatric Drops, Pardec Capsules [CD], ✿Penbritin, Polycillin, Polycillin Pediatric Drops, Polycillin-PRB [CD], ✿Pondocillin, Principen, SK-Ampicillin, Totacillin, Bacampicillin: ✿Penglobe, Spectrobid, Cloxacillin: ✿Apo-Cloxi, ✿Bactopen, Cloxapen, ✿Novo-Cloxin, ✿Nu-Cloxi, ✿Orbenin, Tegopen, Penicillin VK: ✿Apo-Pen-VK, Beepen VK, Betapen-VK, Ledercillin VK, ✿Nadopen-V, ✿Novopen-VK, ✿Nu-Pen-VK, Penapar VK, Pen-V, ✿Pen-Vee, Pen-Vee K, Pfizerpen VK, ✿PVF, ✿PVF K, Robicillin VK, SK-Penicillin VK, Uticillin VK, V-Cillin K, ✿VC-K 500, Veetids, Win-Cillin

```
┌─────────────────────────────────────────────────────────────────────┐
│                      BENEFITS versus RISKS                          │
│        Possible Benefits              Possible Risks                │
│  EFFECTIVE TREATMENT OF         ALLERGIC REACTIONS, MILD TO         │
│    INFECTIONS DUE TO              SEVERE                            │
│    SUSCEPTIBLE                   Superinfections (yeast)            │
│    MICROORGANISMS               Drug-induced colitis—possible       │
│                                 Lowering of white blood cells       │
│                                   (amoxicillin/clavulanate, ampicillin,│
│                                   cloxacillin)                      │
│                                 Decreased kidney function          │
└─────────────────────────────────────────────────────────────────────┘
```

▷ **Principal Uses**

As a Single Drug Product: Uses currently included in FDA-approved labeling: (1) Used to treat responsive infections of the upper and lower respiratory tract, the middle ear (acute otitis media) (amoxicillin is a drug of choice) and the skin; (2) helps prevent rheumatic fever and bacterial endocarditis in people with valvular heart disease; (3) treats some Haemophilus influenzae infections (amoxicillin); (4) treats some genitourinary tract infections (amoxicillin/clavulanate, ampicillin, penicillin VK); (5) treats some cases of sinusitis; (6) ampicillin is used in combination to treat some kinds of septicemia and meningitis; (7) amoxicillin is approved in combination with other medicines (such as omeprazole) to treat some *Helicobacter pylori* infections; (8) some forms treat anthrax.

Other (unlabeled) generally accepted uses: (1) Combined therapy of animal bite wounds; (2) treats stage one Lyme disease in children (amoxicillin or penicillin VK); (3) therapy of Lyme disease in the central nervous system (penicillin VK); (4) can treat some dental abscesses (penicillin VK); (5) treats typhoid fever (amoxicillin); (6) prevention of bacterial endocarditis (amoxicillin); (7) treats biliary tract infections or chancroid (amoxicillin/clavulanate); (8) cloxacillin treats some bone infections if intravenous (IV) drugs are not tolerated.

As a Combination Drug Product [CD]: Amoxicillin and clavulanate are combined (Augmentin) to give the benefits of amoxicillin combined with the ability to treat more resistant bacteria (clavulanate). Amoxicillin is available combined with two drugs: clarithromycin and lansoprazole. Since refractory ulcers are often actually *Helicobacter pylori* infections, the combination works to kill the bacteria and lower acid production.

How These Drugs Work: Destroy susceptible infecting bacteria by damaging ability to make protective cell walls as they multiply and grow. Amoxicillin/clavulanate uses clavulanate blockage of enzymes to enable treatment of resistant bacteria. Bacampicillin is converted to ampicillin, giving peak blood levels three times higher than ampicillin. This allows bacampicillin dosing every 12 hours.

Available Dosage Forms and Strengths

Amoxicillin:

Capsules — 250 mg, 500 mg
Oral liquid — 3 g
Oral suspension — 50 mg/ml, 125 mg/ml, 250 mg/5 ml

Pediatric drops — 50 mg/ml

Tablets, chewable — 125 mg, 250 mg

Amoxicillin/clavulanate:

Oral suspension — 125 mg (amoxicillin) and 31.25 mg (clavulanate) per 5 ml; 250 mg (amoxicillin) and 62.5 mg (clavulanate) per 5 ml; 250 mg (amoxicillin) and 125 mg (clavulanate); 500 mg (amoxicillin) and 125 mg (clavulanate)

Pediatric formulation, twice daily — 200 mg (amoxicillin) and 28.6 mg(clavulanate) per 5 ml; 400 mg (amoxicillin) and 57.1 (clavulanate) per 5 ml

Tablets, chewable — 125 mg (amoxicillin) and 31.25 mg (clavulanate); 250 mg (amoxicillin) and 62.5 mg (clavulanate)

Tablets, chewable twice-daily formulation — 200 mg (amoxicillin) and 28.6 mg (clavulanate); 400 mg (amoxicillin) and 57.1 mg (clavulanate)

Ampicillin:

Capsules — 250 mg, 500 mg

Oral suspension — 100 mg/ml, 125 mg/ml, 250 mg/ml, 500 mg/5 ml

Pediatric drops — 100 mg/ml

Bacampicillin:

Oral suspension — 125 mg/5 ml

Tablets — 400 mg, 800 mg (800 mg in Canada only)

Cloxacillin:

Capsules — 250 mg, 500 mg

Oral suspension — 125 mg/5 ml

Oral liquid — 125 mg/5 ml

Penicillin VK:

Oral solution — 125 mg/5 ml, 250 mg/5 ml

Tablets — 125 mg, 250 mg, 500 mg

▷ **Recommended Dosage Ranges** (Actual dose and schedule must be determined for each patient individually for all of these medicines.)

Dose is based on how sensitive the infection-causing bacteria are, infection severity and patient response.

Penicillin VK: Dose range is 125 to 500 mg every 6 to 8 hours. For prevention of bacterial endocarditis: 2 g (2,000 mg) taken 1 hour before the procedure, followed by 1 g 6 hours later. Daily maximum is 7 g (7,000 mg).

Infants and Children:

Amoxicillin: Up to 6 kg of body mass—25 to 50 mg every 8 hours. 6 to 8 kg of body mass—50 to 100 mg every 8 hours. 8 to 20 kg of body mass—6.7 to

13.3 mg per kg of body mass every 8 hours. 20 kg of body mass and over—
same as 12 to 60 years of age. Note: See higher dosing in ear infection (otitis media) below.

Amoxicillin/clavulanate: Up to 40 kg of body mass—6.7 to 13.3 mg (amoxicillin) per kg of body mass, every 8 hours. 40 kg of body mass and over—
same as 12 to 60 years of age. 12-hour formula: For severe infections—45
mg amoxicillin per kg of body mass **per day** (divided into two doses given
every 12 hours). For less severe infections (as in skin infections)—25 mg
per kg of body mass **per day** (divided into two doses given every 12 hours).

Bacampicillin: 25 mg per kg of body mass per day is given, divided into two
equal doses every 12 hours, for respiratory infections.

Cloxacillin: Children weighing less than 44 lb (20 kg) receive 50 to 100 mg
per kg of body mass per day, divided into four doses. Children greater than
20 kg get the adult dose. Intravenous dosing may be required for severe
infections.

12 to 60 Years of Age:

Amoxicillin: Usual dose—250 to 500 mg every 8 hours. Daily maximum is 4.5
g. For gonorrhea—3 g, with 1 g of probenecid, taken as a single dose. For
Lyme disease—250 to 500 mg, three or four times a day, for 10 to 30 days;
dose and duration depends on severity of infection and response to treatment.

Author's Note: American Heart Association (AHA) guidelines for prevention of bacterial endocarditis in patients at risk suggest amoxicillin in an initial dose of 2 g BEFORE (check current guidelines for timing and best choices) oral or dental procedures. There is no recommendation for follow-up doses of antibiotics. Because of limits on how well amoxicillin gets into the middle ear and prevalence of penicillin-resistant *Strep pneumoniae* causing middle ear infections, some clinicians are using 80–90 mg per kg per day, divided into two or three equal doses (12 or 8 hours apart) in children with sudden onset (acute) otitis media with *S. pneumoniae*. Resistance patterns of bacteria are changing in many areas making other antibiotics medicines of choice depending on the specific resistance patterns and bacteria being treated.

Amoxicillin/clavulanate: Usual dose—250 to 500 mg (amoxicillin) every 8
hours. Daily maximum (of amoxicillin) is 4.5 g.

Ampicillin: 50 to 100 mg per kg of body mass per day divided into four doses
or 500 to 1,000 mg every 6 hours. Usual daily maximum is 6,000 mg daily.

Bacampicillin: For those with a body mass of 25 kg or more—400 to 800 mg
every 12 hours.

Cloxacillin: 250 to 500 mg every 6 hours. The maximum dose is 6,000 mg (6
g) every 24 hours.

Over 60 Years of Age: Amoxicillin: Same as 12 to 60 years of age.

Amoxicillin/clavulanate: Same as 12 to 60 years of age. Note: The above doses
refer to the amoxicillin component of amoxicillin/clavulanate. The 250-mg
regular tablet and the 250-mg chewable tablet contain different amounts
of clavulanate and are NOT interchangeable. See "Dose Forms" above.

Ampicillin: Drug is removed more slowly by patients in this age group, but
specific dose decreases are not defined.

Bacampicillin: Tests of kidney function should be obtained. Doses of 400 mg per day have been used in moderate kidney disease or decline (age-related decline in kidney function may be moderate).

Cloxacillin: No specific dosing changes are available.

Conditions Requiring Dosing Adjustments

Liver Function: Dose adjustments do not appear to be needed (amoxicillin, amoxicillin/clavulanate, ampicillin and penicillin VK). Caution is advised for bacampicillin use by these patients. The dose is decreased or time between doses increased for cloxacillin.

Kidney Function:

Amoxicillin, amoxicillin/clavulanate, ampicillin: Dosing interval **must** be adjusted in renal compromise.

Bacampicillin: The dose must be decreased to 400 mg per day in moderate kidney failure. In severe kidney failure, a dose of 400 mg every 36 hours is used.

Cloxacillin: Patients should be watched closely for adverse effects in severe kidney compromise.

Penicillin VK: For patients with severe kidney compromise, the usual dose is taken every 8 hours.

▷ **Dosing Instructions:** The tablet (amoxicillin, bacampicillin, penicillin VK) may be crushed (or amoxicillin and amoxicillin/clavulanate chew-tabs chewed) or the capsule (amoxicillin) opened and taken on an empty stomach or with food or milk (amoxicillin). Absorption may be slightly faster if taken when stomach is empty (penicillin VK). Ampicillin, bacampicillin and cloxacillin are best taken on an empty stomach. Oral suspension forms should be shaken well before measuring each dose. If you forget a dose: Take the missed dose as soon as you remember it, unless it's nearly time for your next dose—if that is the case, skip the missed dose and take the next dose right on schedule. If the dose missed was the first dose of the day, separate the remaining doses into evenly spaced intervals. DO NOT double doses. Talk with your doctor if you find yourself missing doses.

Usual Duration of Use: For all streptococcal infections—not less than 10 consecutive uninterrupted days to reduce risk of rheumatic fever or glomerulonephritis. For all other infections—as long as needed to eradicate the infection. Incomplete treatment may lead to serious resistance and dangerous infections.

Typical Treatment Goals and Measurements (Outcomes and Markers)

Infections: The most commonly used measures of serious infections are white blood cell counts and differentials (the kind of blood cells that occur most often in your blood), and temperature. Many clinicians look for positive changes in 24–48 hours. NEVER stop an antibiotic because you start to feel better. For many infections, a full 14 days is REQUIRED to kill the bacteria. The goals and time frame (see peak benefits above) should be discussed with you when the prescription is written.

▷ **These Drugs Should Not Be Taken If**
- you had an allergic reaction to them previously.
- you are certain you are allergic to any form of penicillin.

▷ **Inform Your Physician Before Taking These Drugs If**
- you suspect you may be allergic to penicillin or have a history of a previous "reaction."

- you are allergic to any cephalosporin antibiotic (Ancef, Ceclor, etc.—see Drug Classes).
- you are allergic by nature (hay fever, asthma, hives, eczema).
- you are unsure how much to take or how often.
- you have a history of liver or kidney disease.
- you have a history of low blood counts (amoxicillin/clavulanate, ampicillin, cloxacillin).

Possible Side Effects (natural, expected and unavoidable drug actions)

Superinfections (see Glossary), often due to yeast organisms or for some penicillins due to Clostridium difficile.

▷ **Possible Adverse Effects** (unusual, unexpected and infrequent reactions)

If any of the following develop, consult your physician promptly for guidance.

Mild Adverse Effects

Allergic reactions: skin rashes, hives, itching.

Irritations of mouth or tongue, "black tongue," nausea, vomiting, diarrhea, dizziness—rare to infrequent.

Serious Adverse Effects

Allergic reactions: anaphylactic reaction (see Glossary), severe skin reactions, drug fever, swollen painful joints, sore throat, abnormal bleeding or bruising.

Severe skin reactions (Stevens-Johnson syndrome, bullous pemphigoid)—case reports.

Drug-induced colitis—rare.

Hemolytic anemia—case reports (penicillin VK).

Drug-induced periarteritis nodosa, meningitis or porphyria—case reports (penicillin VK).

Abnormal liver or kidney changes—rare.

Drug-induced abnormal lowering of white blood cells—rare (amoxicillin/clavulanate, ampicillin, cloxacillin, penicillin VK).

▷ **Possible Effects on Sexual Function:** None reported except for case reports of a small decrease in sperm counts for ampicillin.

Possible Effects on Laboratory Tests

Complete blood counts: decreased red cells, hemoglobin, white cells (therapeutic effects of each antibiotic) and platelets (penicillin VK); increased eosinophils (allergic reactions).

INR (prothrombin time): occasionally increased (ampicillin, cloxacillin and penicillin VK).

Liver function tests: increased aspartate aminotransferase (AST/GOT) and bilirubin (cloxacillin and penicillin VK).

Coombs' test: may be positive with ampicillin or penicillin VK therapy.

CAUTION

1. If your infection does not respond in 24–48 hours (reduced symptoms, temperature, etc.), CALL YOUR DOCTOR.
2. Take the exact dose and the full course prescribed
3. These medicines DO NOT treat viral infections. Considerable controversy has erupted regarding inappropriate prescribing of antibiotics to treat viral infections. Some intelligent clinicians are writing contingency antibiotics where the differential diagnosis of a bacterial infection ver-

sus a viral infection is unclear. Demanding an antibiotic or expecting an antibiotic to treat a viral infection (except in the case of a secondary bacterial infection) is an inappropriate patient action in most cases and only serves to lead to emergence of bacterial resistance.

4. If these drugs must be used concurrently with antibiotics, such as erythromycin or tetracycline, take the penicillin first.

Precautions for Use

By Infants and Children: Watch children with allergies closely for evidence of a developing allergy to penicillin. These drugs (amoxicillin, penicillin VK) may cause diarrhea, which sometimes necessitates discontinuation. Up to 90% of patients with mononucleosis who take amoxicillin, amoxicillin/clavulanate or ampicillin get a rash.

By Those Over 60 Years of Age: Natural skin changes may predispose to prolonged itching in the genital and anal regions. Report such reactions promptly.

▷ Advisability of Use During Pregnancy

Pregnancy Category: B. See Pregnancy Risk Categories at the back of this book.

Animal studies: Birth defects of the limbs reported in mice (penicillin VK only). (Not confirmed in other studies.)

Human studies: Adequate studies of pregnant women indicate no increased risk of birth defects.

Ask your doctor for guidance, but these drugs are generally considered safe for use during any period of pregnancy.

Advisability of Use If Breast-Feeding

Presence of these drugs in breast milk: Yes.

The nursing infant may be sensitized to penicillin and be at risk for developing diarrhea or yeast infections. Talk with your doctor. Penicillins may be drugs of choice versus chloramphenicol or tetracyclines.

Habit-Forming Potential: None.

Effects of Overdose: Possible nausea, vomiting and/or diarrhea.

Possible Effects of Long-Term Use: Superinfections, often due to yeast organisms or Clostridium difficile.

Suggested Periodic Examinations While Taking These Drugs (at physician's discretion)

Complete blood cell counts.

Kidney function tests.

▷ While Taking These Drugs, Observe the Following

Foods: No restrictions, except ampicillin, bacampicillin and cloxacillin, which are best taken on an empty stomach.

Herbal Medicines or Minerals: Some patients use echinacea to attempt to boost their immune systems. Unfortunately, use of echinacea is not recommended in people with damaged immune systems. This herb may also actually weaken any immune system if it is used too often or for too long a time. Do NOT take mistletoe herb, oak bark or F.C. of marshmallow root and licorice.

Since St. John's wort and ampicillin may cause increased sun sensitivity, caution is advised.

Beverages: No restrictions (except as above). May be taken with milk.

▷ *Alcohol:* No interactions expected, but alcohol can blunt the immune response. It is best NOT to drink while you have an infection severe enough to require antibiotics.

Tobacco Smoking: No interactions expected. I advise everyone to quit smoking.

▷ *Other Drugs*

Penicillins *taken concurrently* with

- disulfiram (Antabuse) can cause a disulfiramlike reaction (see Glossary) (bacampicillin only); avoid the combination of these drugs.
- entacapone (Comtan) (and other medicines) are removed by the bile tract (biliary elimination), and medicines such as ampicillin that have been found to change removal by the bile as well as a process known as glucuronidation and/or intestinal beta glucuronidase may lead to an increased entacapone effect or adverse effects (such as movement disorders or diarrhea) in some patients. Closer patient follow-up and caution are prudent.
- live typhoid vaccine may blunt the vaccine response and benefits (amoxicillin and amoxicillin/clavulanate).
- methotrexate (Mexate) may increase risk of methotrexate toxicity (especially amoxicillin and oral penicillin).
- omeprazole (Prilosec) and other proton pump inhibitors (see Drug Classes) will decrease the amount of ampicillin that gets into the body because ampicillin requires an acid environment to optimally be absorbed.
- probenecid (Benemid) will increase and sustain blood levels. This interaction is often used to therapeutic advantage.

Ampicillin *taken concurrently* with

- allopurinol may increase the risk of rashes.
- atenolol can blunt the therapeutic benefits of atenolol.

Ampicillin, cloxacillin or penicillin VK *taken concurrently* with

- warfarin (Coumadin) may intensify the anticoagulant effect and increase risk of bleeding; more frequent INR (prothrombin time or protime) testing is needed.

Penicillins may *decrease* the effects of

- birth control pills (oral contraceptives) and impair their effectiveness in preventing pregnancy.

The following drugs may *decrease* the effects of penicillins:

- antacids, histamine (H2) blockers or proton pump inhibitors (see Drug Classes)—may reduce the absorption of penicillins.
- chloramphenicol (Chloromycetin).
- erythromycin (Erythrocin, E-Mycin, etc.).
- tetracyclines (Achromycin, Declomycin, Minocin, etc.: see Drug Classes).

▷ *Driving, Hazardous Activities:* Usually no restrictions. Be alert to the rare occurrence of dizziness and/or nausea and restrict activities accordingly.

Aviation Note: The use of these drugs *may be a disqualification* for piloting. Consult a designated Aviation Medical Examiner.

Exposure to Sun: Ampicillin may increase sensitivity to the sun. Use caution.

Special Storage Instructions: Oral solutions and pediatric drops (amoxicillin) should be refrigerated.

Observe the Following Expiration Times: Do not take the oral solution of these drugs if older than 7 days (cloxacillin is good for only 3 days) if kept at room temperature or 14 days when kept refrigerated.

PENTAZOCINE (pen TAZ oh seen)

Introduced: 1967   **Class:** Analgesic, strong   **Prescription:** USA: Yes
Controlled Drug: USA: C-IV*; Canada: No   **Available as Generic:** USA:
No; Canada: No
Brand Names: Talacen [CD], Talwin, Talwin Compound [CD], ♣Talwin Compound-50 [CD], Talwin Nx [CD]

BENEFITS versus RISKS	
Possible Benefits	*Possible Risks*
RELIEF OF MODERATE TO SEVERE PAIN	POTENTIAL FOR HABIT FORMATION (DEPENDENCE)
	Respiratory depression
	Sedative effects
	Mental and behavioral disturbances
	Low blood pressure, fainting
	Nausea, constipation

Author's Note: The information in this profile has been shortened to make room for more widely used medicines.

PENTOXIFYLLINE (pen tox I fi leen)

Other Name: Oxpentifylline
Introduced: 1972   **Class:** Blood flow agent, xanthines   **Prescription:**
USA: Yes   **Controlled Drug:** USA: No; Canada: No   **Available as Generic:**
No
Brand Name: Trental

BENEFITS versus RISKS	
Possible Benefits	*Possible Risks*
IMPROVED BLOOD FLOW IN PERIPHERAL ARTERIAL DISEASE	Reduced blood pressure, angina, abnormal heart rhythms
REDUCTION OF INTERMITTENT CLAUDICATION PAIN	Rare low blood counts and aplastic anemia
May help in some AIDS-related pain	Indigestion, nausea, vomiting
	Dizziness, flushing

Author's Note: A medicine called cilostazol (Pletal) was approved by the FDA to treat intermittent claudication. Information in this profile has been shortened to make room for more widely used medicines.

PERGOLIDE (PER go lide)

Introduced: 1980   Class: Anti-Parkinsonism, ergot derivative   **Prescription:** USA: Yes   **Controlled Drug:** USA: No; Canada: No   **Available as Generic:** USA: No
Brand Name: ♣Drax-Pergolide, Permax

*See Schedules of Controlled Drugs at the back of this book.

```
┌─────────────────────────────────────────────────────────────┐
│                   BENEFITS versus RISKS                       │
│     Possible Benefits              Possible Risks             │
│  ADDITIVE RELIEF OF SYMPTOMS    ABNORMAL INVOLUNTARY          │
│    OF PARKINSON'S DISEASE          MOVEMENTS                  │
│    WHEN USED CONCURRENTLY        HALLUCINATIONS               │
│    WITH LEVODOPA/CARBIDOPA       INITIAL FALL IN BLOOD        │
│  PERMITS A REDUCTION IN            PRESSURE/ORTHOSTATIC       │
│    SINEMET DOSE                    HYPOTENSION                │
│                                  Premature heart contractions │
│                                  (ventricular)                │
└─────────────────────────────────────────────────────────────┘
```

▷ **Principal Uses**

As a Single Drug Product: Uses currently included in FDA-approved labeling: As an adjunct to levodopa/carbidopa treatment of Parkinson's disease for people who experience intolerable abnormal movements (dyskinesia) and/or increasing "on-off" episodes due to levodopa. The addition of pergolide (1) permits reduction of the daily dose of levodopa with consequent lessening of dyskinesia and erratic drug response and (2) provides additional relief of Parkinsonian symptoms.

Other (unlabeled) generally accepted uses: (1) May have a role in helping reduce drug craving in cocaine withdrawal; (2) helps in some conditions where excess prolactin is made; (3) may be of use in acromegaly; (4) works to lower increased prolactin levels (as in some pituitary tumors).

How This Drug Works: By directly stimulating part of the brain (dopamine receptor sites in the corpus striatum), this drug helps to compensate for the deficiency of dopamine that is responsible for the rigidity, tremor and sluggish movement characteristic of Parkinson's disease.

Available Dosage Forms and Strengths

Tablets — 0.05 mg, 0.25 mg, 1 mg

▷ **Usual Adult Dosage Ranges:** *Parkinson's (in conjunction with levodopa plus carbidopa):* Starts at 0.05 mg daily (first 2 days); slowly increased by 0.1 mg daily or 0.15 mg every third day over the next 12 days. If needed and tolerated, daily dose may be increased by 0.25 mg every third day until best response. Total daily dose, 0.4 mg, should be divided into three equal portions taken at 6- to 8-hour intervals. Usual ongoing dose is 3 mg every 24 hours; do not exceed 5 mg every 24 hours.

During gradual start of pergolide, dose of levodopa/carbidopa (Sinemet) may be lowered by your doctor.

Note: Actual dose and schedule must be determined for each patient individually.

Typical Treatment Goals and Measurements (Outcomes and Markers)

Parkinson's disease: The general goal is to minimize symptoms (tremor, sluggish movements, analysis of walking or gait, etc.) to the fullest extent possible. Additionally, many neurologists use Hahn-Yahr scores and the time it takes to maximum amount of finger tapping as indicators of the benefits of this drug.

Conditions Requiring Dosing Adjustments

Liver Function: Used with caution in liver disease.
Kidney Function: Consideration should be given to empirical decreases in dose.

▷ **Dosing Instructions:** The tablet may be crushed and taken with food or milk to reduce stomach irritation. If you forget a dose: Take the missed dose as soon as you remember it, unless it's nearly time for your next dose—if that is the case, skip the missed dose and take the next dose right on schedule. DO NOT double doses. Talk with your doctor if you find yourself missing doses.

Usual Duration of Use: Regular use for 4 to 6 weeks reveals benefits controlling Parkinson's symptoms and permitting lower levodopa/carbidopa dose. Onset time for conditions involving excessive prolactin (hyperprolactinemia) will require a similar length of time to work. Long-term use requires follow-up with your doctor.

Possible Advantages of This Drug: May give more effective and uniform control of Parkinsonian symptoms and fewer adverse effects from levodopa therapy. More powerful (potent) and longer lasting than bromocriptine.

▷ **This Drug Should Not Be Taken If**
- you have had an allergic reaction to it previously.
- you have had a serious adverse effect from any ergot preparation.
- you have severe coronary artery disease or peripheral vascular disease.

▷ **Inform Your Physician Before Taking This Drug If**
- you have constitutionally low blood pressure.
- you are pregnant or breast-feeding your infant.
- you are taking any antihypertensive drugs or antipsychotic drugs (see Drug Classes).
- you have any degree of coronary artery disease, especially angina or a history of heart attack.
- you have any type of heart rhythm disorder.
- you have impaired liver or kidney function.
- you have a seizure disorder.

Possible Side Effects (natural, expected and unavoidable drug actions)
Weakness; chest pain (possibly anginal); peripheral edema; orthostatic hypotension (see Glossary)—infrequent.

▷ **Possible Adverse Effects** (unusual, unexpected and infrequent reactions)
If any of the following develop, consult your physician promptly for guidance.

Mild Adverse Effects
Allergic reactions: skin rash, facial swelling—rare.
Headache, dizziness, hallucinations, drowsiness, insomnia, anxiety, double vision—rare to infrequent.
Nasal congestion, shortness of breath, palpitation, fainting—rare to infrequent.
Altered taste, dry mouth, indigestion, nausea, vomiting, constipation, diarrhea—infrequent.

Serious Adverse Effects
Allergic reactions: none reported.
Idiosyncratic reactions: flu-like symptoms.
Abnormal involuntary movements (dyskinesia)—frequent.
Psychotic behavior—case reports.
Hallucinations (accounted for 7.8% of patient withdrawals from therapy; 13.8% occurrence).
Abnormal heartbeat (ventricular arrhythmias)—infrequent to frequent.
Anemia—rare.

▷ **Possible Effects on Sexual Function:** Infrequent reports of altered libido (increased or decreased), impotence, breast pain, priapism (see Glossary).

▷ **Adverse Effects That May Mimic Natural Diseases or Disorders**

Effects on mental function and behavior may resemble psychotic disorders.

Natural Diseases or Disorders That May Be Activated by This Drug

Coronary artery disease with anginal syndrome, heart rhythm disorders, Raynaud's phenomenon (see Glossary), seizure disorders.

Possible Effects on Laboratory Tests

Blood prolactin level: decreased (marked reduction).

CAUTION

1. May cause abnormal movements (dyskinesias), or intensify existing dyskinesias. Watch for tremors, twitching or abnormal involuntary movements of any kind. Report these promptly.
2. Low starting doses help prevent possibility of excessive drop in blood pressure. See dose routine outlined above.
3. Tell your doctor promptly if you become pregnant or plan pregnancy. This drug has been reported (rarely) to cause abortion and birth defects.
4. May lead to abnormal heart rhythms in people prone to arrhythmia.

Precautions for Use

By Infants and Children: This drug is not utilized by this age group.

By Those Over 60 Years of Age: Small initial doses are mandatory. Watch closely for any tendency to light-headedness or faintness, especially on arising from a lying or sitting position. You may be more susceptible to the development of impaired thinking, confusion, agitation, nightmares or hallucinations.

▷ **Advisability of Use During Pregnancy**

Pregnancy Category: B. See Pregnancy Risk Categories at the back of this book.

Animal studies: No birth defects due to this drug were found in mouse or rabbit studies.

Human studies: Adequate studies of pregnant women are not available. However, there are four reports of birth defects associated with the use of this drug and infrequent reports of abortion. Causal relationships have not been established, but prudence advises against the use of this drug during pregnancy. Consult your physician for guidance.

Advisability of Use If Breast-Feeding

Presence of this drug in breast milk: Unknown.

Avoid drug or refrain from nursing.

Habit-Forming Potential: None.

Effects of Overdose: Nausea, vomiting, palpitations, low blood pressure, agitation, severe involuntary movements, hallucinations, seizures.

Possible Effects of Long-Term Use: Increased risk of developing dyskinesias.

Suggested Periodic Examinations While Taking This Drug (at physician's discretion)

Regular evaluation of drug response.

Heart function and blood pressure status.

▷ **While Taking This Drug, Observe the Following**

Foods: No restrictions.

Herbal Medicines or Minerals: Calcium and garlic may lower blood pressure. Since this medicine may also lower blood pressure, talk to your doctor BEFORE you add garlic or additional amounts of calcium to your diet.

Calabar bean (chop nut, Fabia, ordeal nut, others) is unsafe when taken by mouth (physostigmine is the active ingredient) and should never be taken by people with Parkinson's disease. Octacosanol (a cousin of vitamin E) can worsen movement problems and should also be avoided.

Beverages: No restrictions. May be taken with milk.

▷ *Alcohol:* Alcohol can exaggerate the blood-pressure-lowering and sedative effects of this drug.

Tobacco Smoking: No interactions expected. I advise everyone to quit smoking.

▷ *Other Drugs*

Pergolide *taken concurrently* with
- antihypertensive drugs (and other drugs that can lower blood pressure) requires careful monitoring for excessive drops in pressure (lisinopril case report); dose changes may be needed.

The following drugs may *decrease* the effects of pergolide and diminish its effectiveness:
- chlorprothixene (Taractan).
- haloperidol (Haldol).
- metoclopramide (Reglan).
- phenothiazines (see Drug Classes).
- thiothixene (Navane).

▷ *Driving, Hazardous Activities:* This drug may cause dizziness, drowsiness, impaired coordination or fainting. Restrict activities as necessary.

Aviation Note: The use of this drug *is a disqualification* for piloting. Consult a designated Aviation Medical Examiner.

Exposure to Sun: No restrictions.

Exposure to Heat: Use caution until the combined effects have been determined. Hot environments can cause lowering of blood pressure.

Discontinuation: **Do not stop this drug abruptly**. Sudden withdrawal can cause confusion, paranoid thinking and severe hallucinations. Consult your physician regarding a schedule for gradual withdrawal.

PERPHENAZINE (per FEN a zeen)

Introduced: 1957   **Class:** Tranquilizer, major; phenothiazines   **Prescription:** USA: Yes   **Controlled Drug:** USA: No; Canada: No   **Available as Generic:** USA: Yes; Canada: Yes

Brand Names: ✤Apo-Perphenazine, ✤Elavil Plus [CD], ✤Entrafon, Etrafon [CD], Etrafon-A [CD], Etrafon Forte [CD], ✤Phenazine, ✤PMS-Levazine, ✤PMS-Perphenazine, Triavil [CD], Trilafon

BENEFITS versus RISKS	
Possible Benefits	*Possible Risks*
EFFECTIVE CONTROL OF ACUTE MENTAL DISORDERS	SERIOUS TOXIC EFFECTS ON BRAIN WITH LONG-TERM USE
Beneficial effects on thinking, mood and behavior	Liver damage with jaundice
Relief of anxiety and tension	Blood cell disorders: hemolytic anemia, abnormally low white blood cell and platelet counts
Moderately effective control of nausea and vomiting	

▷ **Principal Uses**

As a Single Drug Product: Uses currently included in FDA-approved labeling: (1) Treats acute and chronic psychotic disorders: agitated depression, schizophrenia and similar mental dysfunction; (2) used as a tranquilizer to help agitated and disruptive behavior; (3) severe nausea and vomiting treatment; (4) used to prevent vomiting from cisplatin; (5) eases vertigo.

Other (unlabeled) generally accepted uses: (1) Can ease tremors caused by tricyclic antidepressants.

As a Combination Drug Product [CD]: Available combined with amitriptyline. In some severe agitated depression, combining an antipsychotic drug and an antidepressant will be more effective than either drug used alone.

Author's Note: Information in this profile has been shortened to make room for more widely used medicines.

PHENELZINE (FEN el zeen)

Introduced: 1961   **Class:** Antidepressant, MAO type A inhibitor   **Prescription:** USA: Yes   **Controlled Drug:** USA: No; Canada: No   **Available as Generic:** No
Brand Name: Nardil

BENEFITS versus RISKS	
Possible Benefits	*Possible Risks*
EFFECTIVE RELIEF OF REACTIVE, NEUROTIC, ATYPICAL DEPRESSIONS WITH ASSOCIATED ANXIETY OR PHOBIA	DANGEROUS INTERACTIONS WITH MANY DRUGS AND FOODS CONDUCIVE TO HYPERTENSIVE CRISIS
Beneficial in some depressions that are not responsive to other treatments	DISORDERED HEART RATE AND RHYTHM
	Drug-induced hepatitis—rare
	Mental changes: agitation, confusion, impaired memory, hypomania

Author's Note: Since other medicines are more widely used, the information in this profile has been shortened.

PHENOBARBITAL (fee noh BAR bi tawl)

Other Name: Phenobarbitone
Introduced: 1912   **Class:** Sedative, anticonvulsant, barbiturates   **Prescription:** USA: Yes   **Controlled Drug:** USA: C-IV*; Canada: Yes   **Available as Generic:** Yes
Brand Names: Aasquel, Alised, Alubelap [CD], Aminodrox-Forte, Antispasmodic [CD], Azpan, Barbidonna [CD], Barbidonna Elixir [CD], Barbita, Belap, Belladenal [CD], Belladenal-S [CD], ✦Belladenal Spacetabs [CD], ✦Bellergal [CD], Bellergal-S [CD], ✦Bellergal Spacetabs [CD], Bronchotabs [CD], Bronkolixir [CD], ✦Cafergot-PB, Chardonna-2 [CD], Daricon PB, ✦Di-

*See Schedules of Controlled Drugs at the back of this book.

clophen [CD], Dilantin w/Phenobarbital [CD], Donna-Sed, Donnatal [CD], Donphen, Ergobel [CD], Eskabarb, Eskaphen B [CD], Floramine, ✤Gardenal, Hybephen [CD], Hypnaldyne [CD], Isuprel Compound [CD], Kinesed [CD], Luminal, Mudrane GG Elixir and Tablets [CD], Mudrane Tablets [CD], Neospect, ✤Neuro-Spasex [CD], ✤Neuro-Trasentin [CD], ✤Neuro-Trasentin Forte [CD], Novalene, Phedral [CD], ✤Phenaphen Capsules [CD], ✤ Phenaphen No. 2, 3, 4 [CD], Phenergan w/Codeine [CD], Phyldrox, Quadrinal [CD], Relaxadron, SBP [CD], Scodonnar [CD], Sedacord [CD], SK-Phenobarbital, Solfoton, Spasquid [CD], Spazcaps, Tedral Preparations [CD], T.E.P. [CD], Thalfed [CD], Theocardone, Theocord [CD], Theolixer, Vitaphen

---

BENEFITS versus RISKS

Possible Benefits	*Possible Risks*
EFFECTIVE CONTROL OF TONIC-CLONIC SEIZURES AND ALL TYPES OF PARTIAL SEIZURES	POTENTIAL FOR DEPENDENCE LIFE-THREATENING TOXICITY WITH OVERDOSE
EFFECTIVE CONTROL OF FEBRILE SEIZURES OF CHILDHOOD	Drug-induced hepatitis or decreased kidney function
Effective relief of anxiety and nervous tension	Blood cell disorders: abnormally low red cell, white cell and platelet counts

---

▷ **Principal Uses**

As a Single Drug Product: Uses currently included in FDA-approved labeling: (1) Used as a mild sedative; (2) used as an anticonvulsant to control grand mal epilepsy and all types of partial seizures, including febrile seizures of childhood; (3) used as a sedative, yet newer agents carry fewer drug interactions or effects on sleep cycles.

Other (unlabeled) generally accepted uses: (1) May be helpful in detoxification of sedative-hypnotic addiction; (2) can help control seizures found in cerebral malaria; (3) eases neonatal seizures; (4) may have a role in treating pain syndromes.

As a Combination Drug Product [CD]: This drug is available in many combinations with derivatives of belladonna, an antispasmodic commonly used to treat functional disorders of the gastrointestinal tract. It is also available in combination with bronchodilators for the treatment of asthma and with ergotamine for the treatment of headaches.

How This Drug Works: Impedes transfer of sodium and potassium across cells and selectively blocks nerve impulses. This can give a sedative effect or suppress nerve impulses that cause seizures

Author's Note: Information in this profile has been shortened to make room for more widely used medicines.

PHENYTOIN (FEN i toh in)

Other Name: Diphenylhydantoin

Introduced: 1938   **Class:** Anticonvulsant, hydantoins, pain syndrome modifier   **Prescription:** USA: Yes   **Controlled Drug:** USA: No; Canada: No
Available as Generic: USA: Yes; Canada: Yes

Brand Names: Dilantin, Dilantin Infatabs, Dilantin w/Phenobarbital [CD], Di-Phen, Diphenylan, Ekko JR, Ekko SR, Ekko Three, ✹Mebroin [CD], ✹ Phelantin

BENEFITS versus RISKS	
Possible Benefits	*Possible Risks*
EFFECTIVE CONTROL OF TONIC-CLONIC (GRAND MAL), PSYCHOMOTOR (TEMPORAL LOBE), MYOCLONIC and FOCAL SEIZURE	VERY NARROW TREATMENT MARGIN
	POSSIBLE BIRTH DEFECTS
	Overgrowth of gums
	Excessive hair growth
May have a role used as a powder helping heal wounds (diabetic wounds and pressure or bed sores)	Blood cell disorders: impaired production of all blood cells
	Drug-induced hepatitis or nephritis

▷ **Principal Uses**

As a Single Drug Product: Uses currently included in FDA-approved labeling: As an antiepileptic drug to control grand mal, psychomotor, myoclonic and focal seizures. It can also be used to control seizures following brain surgery. Other (unlabeled) generally accepted uses: (1) Used to initiate treatment of trigeminal neuralgia—it is sometimes effective in relieving the severe facial pain of this disorder; (2) used in chronic pain syndromes; (3) may have a role (as an applied powder) in helping heal wounds (such as bed sores and diabetic wounds); (4) effective in eclampsia or pre-eclampsia.

As a Combination Drug Product [CD]: This drug is available in combination with phenobarbital, another effective anticonvulsant. Some seizure disorders require the combined actions of these two drugs for effective control.

How This Drug Works: By promoting the loss of sodium from nerve fibers, this drug lowers and stabilizes their excitability and thereby inhibits the repetitious spread of electrical impulses along nerve pathways. This action may prevent seizures altogether or it may reduce their frequency and severity. In helping wound healing it probably works in a similar way as the adverse effect of causing excessive gum growth. Phenytoin appears to promote fibroblast growth leading to collagen, etc.

Available Dosage Forms and Strengths

Capsules, extended — 30 mg, 100 mg
Capsules, prompt — 30 mg, 100 mg
Injection — 50 mg/ml
Kapseals — 30 mg, 100 mg
Oral suspension — 30 mg/5 ml, 125 mg/5 ml
Tablets, chewable — 50 mg

▷ **Usual Adult Dosage Ranges:** *Seizures*: Initially (prompt or extended form) 100 mg three times a day. Dose may be increased cautiously by 100 mg/week as needed and tolerated. Once the optimal maintenance dose has been identified, the total daily dose may be taken as a single dose every 24 hours if Dilantin capsules are used. No other formulation is approved for once-a-day use. The total daily dose should not exceed 600 mg. In wound healing, some clinicians have used a phenytoin capsule content mixed with sterile saline using sterile technique. A sterile gauze pad is then soaked in the mixture and the gauze applied to the wound. Others have applied phenytoin powder USP directly to the wound once a day and than have covered the wound with a sterile dressing. This is not an FDA-approved use and standardized protocols and research are needed. **Note: Actual dose and schedule must be determined for each patient individually.**

Conditions Requiring Dosing Adjustments

Liver Function: The ongoing dose should be decreased based on blood levels.

Kidney Function: The dose or dosing interval must be decreased in moderate kidney failure.

Obesity: The way this medicine is distributed (volume of distribution) changes with increasing body fat. Loading doses must be calculated based on ideal body weight. The product of 1.33 times actual weight divided by the ideal weight is then added to the original number to decide the final loading dose.

▷ **Dosing Instructions:** May be taken with or after food to reduce stomach irritation. The capsule may be opened, and the tablet may be crushed. If you forget a dose: Take the missed dose as soon as you remember it, unless it's nearly time for your next dose—if that is the case, skip the missed dose and take the next dose right on schedule. DO NOT double doses unless your doctor tells you to do that. If you miss two doses or more in a row, call your doctor.

Usual Duration of Use: Use on a regular schedule for 2 to 3 weeks usually determines benefit in reducing frequency and severity of seizures. Optimal control will require careful dose adjustments over a period of several months. Long-term use (months to years) requires ongoing physician supervision.

Typical Treatment Goals and Measurements (Outcomes and Markers)

Seizures: The general goal for this medicine is effective seizure control. Neurologists tend to define "effective" on a case-by-case basis depending on the seizure type and patient factors. If seizure control is not effective, it's not unusual to use combination treatment. For this medicine, a balance must be struck between too little medicine and too much medicine. Blood levels are used to make certain that the blood level is in the right range.

▷ **This Drug Should Not Be Taken If**
- you have had an allergic reaction to this drug or other hydantoin drugs previously.
- you have sinus bradycardia or serious heart block.

▷ **Inform Your Physician Before Taking This Drug If**
- you are taking any other drugs at this time.
- you have a history of liver disease or impaired liver function.
- you have a history of alcohol abuse. Alcohol can change blood levels of this medicine.
- you have low blood pressure, diabetes or any type of heart disease.
- you are pregnant or planning pregnancy.
- you plan to have surgery under general anesthesia in the near future.

Possible Side Effects (natural, expected and unavoidable drug actions)

Mild fatigue, sluggishness and drowsiness (in sensitive individuals).

Pink to red to brown coloration of urine (of no significance).

▷ **Possible Adverse Effects** (unusual, unexpected and infrequent reactions)

If any of the following develop, consult your physician promptly for guidance.

Mild Adverse Effects

Allergic reactions: skin rashes, hives, drug fever (see Glossary).

Headache, dizziness, nervousness, insomnia, muscle twitching—infrequent.

Nausea, vomiting, constipation—infrequent.

Bedwetting—case reports.

Abnormal eye movements—dose-related.

Low blood calcium (and potential osteoporosis) and elevated blood sugar—
possible.

Overgrowth of gum tissues—most common in children.

Excessive growth of body hair—most common in young girls.

Serious Adverse Effects

Allergic reactions: drug-induced hepatitis, with or without jaundice (see
Glossary).

Drug-induced nephritis, with acute kidney failure.

Severe skin reactions (toxic epidermal necrolysis, Stevens-Johnson syndrome or erythema multiforme).

Myocarditis, generalized enlargement of lymph glands (pseudolymphoma)—
case reports.

Idiosyncratic reactions: hemolytic anemia (see Glossary).

Acute psychotic episodes—case reports.

Mental confusion, unsteadiness, double vision, jerky eye movements, slurred
speech—possible.

Drug-induced seizures—possible.

Blood-clotting disorders in infants of mothers maintained on phenytoin—rare.

Bone marrow depression (see Glossary): weakness, fever, sore throat, bleeding or bruising—case reports.

Drug-induced periarteritis nodosa, low thyroid function or myasthenia
gravis—case reports.

Tardive dyskinesia or porphyria—case reports.

Abnormal IgA (increased risk of respiratory infections)—possible.

Peripheral nerve damage (neuropathy) or muscle damage (myopathy)—case
reports.

Serious heart rhythm problems—with rapid intravenous use.

Elevated blood sugar, due to inhibition of insulin release—possible.

▷ **Possible Effects on Sexual Function:** Decreased libido and/or impotence—
infrequent.

Swelling and tenderness of male breast tissue (gynecomastia) or Peyronie's
disease (see Glossary)—rare.

Decreased effectiveness of oral contraceptives.

▷ **Adverse Effects That May Mimic Natural Diseases or Disorders**

Drug-induced hepatitis may suggest viral hepatitis. Skin reactions may
resemble lupus erythematosus.

Natural Diseases or Disorders That May Be Activated by This Drug

Latent diabetes, porphyria, systemic lupus erythematosus, low bone mineral
density predisposing to osteoporosis.

Possible Effects on Laboratory Tests

Complete blood cell counts: decreased red cells, hemoglobin, white cells and
platelets; increased eosinophils (allergic reaction).

Blood lupus erythematosus (LE) cells: positive.

Prothrombin time: increased (when phenytoin is taken concurrently with warfarin).

Blood calcium level: decreased.

Blood total cholesterol, LDL and VLDL cholesterol levels: no effects.

Blood HDL cholesterol level: increased.

Blood triglyceride levels: no effect.

Blood glucose level: increased.

Blood thyroid hormone levels: T3, T4 and free T4 increased.

Liver function tests: increased liver enzymes (ALT/GPT, AST/GOT, alkaline phosphatase) and bilirubin.

CAUTION

1. Some brand-name capsules of this drug have a significantly longer duration of action than generic-name capsules of the same strength. To assure a correct dosing schedule, it is necessary to distinguish between "prompt"-action and "extended"-action capsules. Do not substitute one for the other without your physician's knowledge and guidance.

2. When used for the treatment of epilepsy, *this drug must not be stopped abruptly.*

3. Periodic blood levels of this drug are essential to get the right dose (see "Therapeutic Drug Monitoring" in Section One).

4. Use of phenytoin in wound healing has some early data, but requires further research and standardization of protocols.

5. Take this medicine EXACTLY as prescribed and at the same time each day.

6. Shake the suspension form of this drug thoroughly before measuring the dose. Use a standard measuring device to assure that the dose is accurate.

7. Side effects and mild adverse effects are usually most apparent during the first several days of treatment and often subside with continued use

8. It may be necessary to take folic acid to prevent anemia. Talk with your doctor about this.

9. Case reports have been made about atypical allergy (cross-sensitivity) between phenytoin and carbamazepine (Tegretol, others). Talk to your doctor if you are allergic to phenytoin.

10. This medicine has an unusual pathway for removal that can fill up (become saturated) and stop working. This means that a small change in dose may give a huge change in blood levels. Make certain you know exactly how much phenytoin your doctor wants you to take.

11. Carry personal identification card that says you are taking this drug.

Precautions for Use

By Infants and Children: Elimination of this drug varies widely with age. Periodic measurement of blood levels is essential for all ages. Some children will require more than one dose daily for good control.

Observe for early indications of drug toxicity: jerky eye movements, unsteadiness in stance and gait, slurred speech, abnormal involuntary movements of the extremities and odd behavior.

By Those Over 60 Years of Age: You may be more sensitive to all of the actions of this drug and require smaller doses. Observe closely for any indications of early toxicity: drowsiness, fatigue, confusion, unsteadiness, disturbances of vision, slurred speech, muscle twitching.

▷ **Advisability of Use During Pregnancy**

Pregnancy Category: D. See Pregnancy Risk Categories at the back of this book.

Animal studies: Cleft lip and palate, skeletal and visceral defects in mice and rats.

Human studies: Available information is conflicting. Some studies suggest a small but significant increase in birth defects. The incidence of birth defects in children of epileptics not taking anticonvulsant drugs is 3.2%; incidence increases to 6.4% with anticonvulsant use in pregnancy. The "fetal hydantoin syndrome" in infants exposed to phenytoin during pregnancy shows birth defects of skull, face and limbs; deficient growth and development; and subnormal intelligence. Other effects on the infant include reduction in blood-clotting factors that predispose it to severe bruising and hemorrhage.

Discuss the benefits and risks of using this drug during pregnancy with your doctor. It is advisable to use the smallest maintenance dose that will control seizures. In addition, you should take vitamin K during the final month of pregnancy to prevent a deficiency of fetal blood-clotting factors.

Advisability of Use If Breast-Feeding

Presence of this drug in breast milk: Yes, in trace amounts.

Monitor nursing infant closely, and discontinue drug or nursing if adverse effects develop.

Habit-Forming Potential: None.

Effects of Overdose: Drowsiness, jerky eye movements, hand tremor, unsteadiness, slurred speech, hallucinations, delusions, nausea, vomiting, stupor progressing to coma.

Possible Effects of Long-Term Use: Low blood calcium resulting in rickets or osteomalacia; megaloblastic anemia; peripheral neuropathy (see Glossary); schizophreniclike psychosis. Lymphosarcoma, malignant lymphoma and leukemia have been associated with long-term use; a cause-and-effect relationship (see Glossary) has not been established.

Suggested Periodic Examinations While Taking This Drug (at physician's discretion)

Monitoring of blood phenytoin levels to guide dose. Time to sample blood for phenytoin level: just before next dose. Recommended therapeutic range: 10 to 20 ng/ml.

Complete blood cell counts.

Liver function tests.

Measurements of the following blood levels: glucose, calcium, phosphorus, folic acid, vitamin B_{12}.

Bone mineral density testing (DEXA) to check risk for osteoporosis and fracture.

▷ **While Taking This Drug, Observe the Following**

Foods: No restrictions.

Herbal Medicines or Minerals: Using kola or ma huang may result in unacceptable central nervous system stimulation. Valerian and kava kava may interact to increase drowsiness. St. John's wort may also cause increased sun sensitivity—caution is advised. Increased calcium and vitamin D are prudent.

Nutritional Support: Supplements of folic acid, calcium, vitamin D and vitamin K may be necessary.

Beverages: No restrictions. May be taken with milk.

▷ *Alcohol:* Use extreme caution. Alcohol (in large quantities or with continual use) may reduce this drug's effectiveness in preventing seizures.

Tobacco Smoking: No interactions expected. I advise everyone to quit smoking.

▷ *Other Drugs*

Phenytoin may *decrease* the effects of
- acetaminophen (Tylenol, others).
- acyclovir (Zovirax).
- atorvastatin (Lipitor) and simvastatin (Zocor) probably by increasing liver enzymes (cytochrome P450 3A4) which are partly involved in removing atorvastatin. More frequent checks of progress toward cholesterol goals are prudent if these medicines must be combined.
- bupropion (Wellbutrin).
- cholecalciferol (vitamin D).
- clofibrate (Atromid-S).
- clozapine (Clozaril).
- conjugated estrogens (Premarin).
- cortisonelike drugs (see Drug Classes).
- cyclosporine (Sandimmune).
- disopyramide (Norpace).
- donepezil (Aricept).
- doxycycline (Vibramycin, etc.).
- itraconazole (Sporanox) and other antifungals using the same liver removal system.
- levodopa (Larodopa, Sinemet).
- levothyroxine (Synthroid, others).
- meperidine (Demerol).
- methadone (Dolophine).
- mexiletine (Mexitil).
- miconazole (Monistat, Micatin, others).
- neuromuscular blocking agents (such as pancuronium-Pavulon or vecuronium-Norcuron).
- oral antidiabetic drugs (see Drug Classes).
- oral contraceptives (birth control pills).
- paclitaxel (Taxol).
- paroxetine (Paxil).
- quetiapine (Seroquel).
- quinidine (Quinaglute, etc.).
- ritonavir (Norvir) and perhaps other protease inhibitors (see Drug Classes).
- sirolimus (Rapamune) and tacrolimus (Prograf).
- triamcinolone.

Phenytoin *taken concurrently* with
- acetazolamide (Diamox) may lead to bone problems (osteomalacia).
- carbamazepine (Tegretol) may result in increased or decreased levels of phenytoin.
- chlordiazepoxide (Librium, and perhaps other benzodiazepines) may increase or decrease phenytoin levels; levels should be obtained more frequently if these drugs are combined.

- ciprofloxacin (Cipro) may increase or decrease phenytoin levels. Check phenytoin levels more frequently.
- dopamine will result in very low blood pressure.
- flu shots (influenza vaccine) may change phenytoin levels.
- ketorolac (Toradol) may result in seizures—DO NOT COMBINE these medicines.
- oral anticoagulants (Coumadin, etc.) can either increase or decrease the anticoagulant effect; monitor this combination very closely with INR (serial prothrombin) testing.
- primidone (Mysoline) may alter primidone actions and enhance its toxicity.
- theophyllines (Aminophyllin, Theo-Dur, etc.) may cause a decrease in the effectiveness of both drugs.
- valproic acid (Depakene) may result in altered phenytoin or valproic acid levels; increased blood level testing of both medicines is needed if these medicines are to be combined.
- warfarin (Coumadin) may lead to initial increased bleeding risk and subsequent decrease in anticoagulation; more frequent INR (prothrombin time or protime) testing is needed. Warfarin doses should be adjusted to results.

The following drugs may *increase* the effects of phenytoin:
- amiodarone (Cordarone).
- chloramphenicol (Chloromycetin).
- chlorpheniramine.
- cimetidine (Tagamet).
- clopidogrel (Plavix)—extent unknown—yet clopidogrel inhibits cytochrome P450 2C9 which helps remove phenytoin from the body. More frequent checks of phenytoin levels are prudent if these medicines are combined.
- cotrimoxazole (Bactrim).
- diltiazem (Cardizem).
- disulfiram (Antabuse).
- felbamate (Felbatol).
- fluconazole (Diflucan).
- fluoxetine (Prozac).
- fluvoxamine (Luvox).
- gabapentin (Neurontin).
- ibuprofen and perhaps other NSAIDs.
- isoniazid (INH, Niconyl, etc.).
- nefazodone (Serzone).
- nifedipine (Adalat).
- omeprazole (Prilosec).
- phenacemide (Phenurone).
- S-Liposomal doxorubicin.
- sertraline (Zoloft).
- sulfonamides (see Drug Classes).
- trazodone (Desyrel).
- tricyclic antidepressants (see Drug Classes).
- trimethoprim (Proloprim, Trimpex).
- valproic acid (Depakene).

- venlafaxine (Effexor).
- zotepine (Nipolept).

The following drugs may *decrease* the effects of phenytoin:
- antacids (various)—separate doses by two hours.
- bleomycin (Blenoxane).
- carmustine (BiCNU).
- cisplatin (Platinol).
- diazoxide (Proglycem, Hyperstat).
- folic acid (various).
- methotrexate (Mexate).
- rifampin (Rifadin).
- vinblastinc (Vclban).

▷ *Driving, Hazardous Activities:* This drug may impair mental alertness, vision and coordination. Restrict activities as necessary.

Aviation Note: The use of this drug *is a disqualification* for piloting. Consult a designated Aviation Medical Examiner.

Exposure to Sun: Use caution—this drug may cause photosensitivity (see Glossary).

Occurrence of Unrelated Illness: Intercurrent infections may slow the elimination of this drug and increase the risk of toxicity, due to higher blood levels.

*Discontinuation: **This drug must not be discontinued abruptly.*** Sudden withdrawal can precipitate severe and repeated seizures. If this drug is to be discontinued, gradual reduction in dose should be made over a period of 3 months. Total drug withdrawal may be attempted after a period of 3 to 4 years without a seizure. However, seizures are likely to recur in 40% of adults and in 20–30% of children.

PILOCARPINE (pi loh KAR peen)

Introduced: 1875   **Class:** Antiglaucoma   **Prescription:** USA: Yes
Controlled Drug: USA: No; Canada: No   **Available as Generic:**   Yes
Brand Names: Adsorbocarpine, Akarpine, Almocarpine, E-Pilo Preparations [CD], I-Pilopine, Isopto Carpine, ✤Minims, ✤Miocarpine, Ocusert Pilo-20, Ocusert Pilo-40, PE Preparations [CD], Pilagan, Pilocar, Pilopine HS, Piloptic-1, Piloptic-2, Pilosyst 20/40, Salagen, ✤Spersacarpine

BENEFITS versus RISKS	
Possible Benefits	*Possible Risks*
EFFECTIVE REDUCTION OF INTERNAL EYE PRESSURE FOR CONTROL OF ACUTE AND CHRONIC GLAUCOMA	Mild side effects with systemic absorption Minor eye discomfort Altered vision

▷ **Principal Uses**

As a Single Drug Product: Uses currently included in FDA-approved labeling: (1) Used to manage all types of glaucoma (selection of the appropriate dose form and strength must be carefully individualized); (2) can help in dry mouth (xerostomia) even after radiation therapy; (3) eases symptoms in Sjögren's syndrome.

Other (unlabeled) generally accepted uses: (1) Treatment of Adie syndrome; (2) can help before laser surgery in order to prevent excessive increases in eye (intraocular) pressure after surgery.

As a Combination Drug Product [CD]: This drug is combined with epinephrine (in eyedrop solutions) to utilize the actions of both drugs in lowering internal eye pressure. The opposite effects of these two drugs on the size of the pupil (pilocarpine constricts, epinephrine dilates) provides a balance that prevents excessive constriction or dilation.

How This Drug Works: By directly stimulating constriction of the pupil, this drug enlarges the outflow canal in the anterior chamber of the eye and promotes the drainage of excess fluid (aqueous humor), thus lowering the internal eye pressure.

Available Dosage Forms and Strengths

Eyedrop solutions — 0.25%, 0.5%, 1%, 2%, 3%, 4%, 5%, 6%

Gel — 4%

Ocuserts — 20 mcg, 40 mcg

Tablets — 5 mg

▷ **Usual Adult Dosage Ranges:** *For open-angle glaucoma*: Eyedrop solutions—one drop of a 1% to 2% solution three to four times daily (every 6–8 hours). Eye gel—apply 0.5-inch strip of gel into the eye once daily at bedtime. Ocusert—insert one into affected eye and replace every 7 days with a new one.

Note: Actual dose and dosing schedule must be determined for each patient individually.

Conditions Requiring Dosing Adjustments

Liver Function: The specific elimination of this drug is unclear.

Kidney Function: The elimination of this drug has yet to be defined.

▷ **Dosing Instructions:** To avoid excessive absorption into the body, press finger against inner corner of the eye (to close off the tear duct) during and for 2 minutes following instillation of the eyedrop. Place the gel and the Ocusert in the eye at bedtime. If you forget a dose: Use the missed dose as soon as you remember it, unless it's nearly time for your next dose—if that is the case, skip the missed dose and take the next dose right on schedule. DO NOT double doses. Talk with your doctor if you find yourself missing doses. Adherence to medicines is critical to results.

Usual Duration of Use: Use on a regular schedule for 1 to 2 weeks usually determines this drug's effectiveness in controlling internal eye pressure. Long-term use (months to years) requires physician supervision and follow up.

Typical Treatment Goals and Measurements (Outcomes and Markers)

Glaucoma: Ophthalmologists measure intraocular pressure (IOP), and then check IOP lowering once this medicine is started. The chamber angle can be checked prior to treatment.

Currently a "Drug of Choice"

For primary open-angle glaucoma (along with timolol and dipivefrin) especially in people over 50 years old.

▷ **This Drug Should Not Be Taken If**
- you have had an allergic reaction to it previously.
- you have acute iritis.
- you have active bronchial asthma and are using the tablet form.

▷ **Inform Your Physician Before Taking This Drug If**
  • you have a history of bronchial asthma.
  • you have a history of acute iritis.
  • you have significant heart disease, kidney or liver disease.
  • your thyroid is overactive (hyperthyroidism).
  • you have chronic obstructive pulmonary disease.
  • you have gallstones.
  • you are trying to have a baby.

Possible Side Effects (natural, expected and unavoidable drug actions)
  Temporary impairment of vision, usually lasting 2 to 3 hours following instillation of drops. Burning of the eyes and trouble seeing at night—frequent.

▷ **Possible Adverse Effects** (unusual, unexpected and infrequent reactions)
  If any of the following develop, consult your physician promptly for guidance.
  Mild Adverse Effects
  Allergic reactions: itching of the eyes, eyelid itching and/or swelling.
  Headache, heart palpitation, tremors—infrequent.
  Sweating—frequent.
  Nausea—case reports.
  Serious Adverse Effects
  Provocation of acute asthma in susceptible individuals.
  Mental status changes (memory loss, confusion)—case reports.
  Atrioventricular block (abnormal heart conduction)—case reports.
  Retinal detachment—possible.

▷ **Possible Effects on Sexual Function:** None reported.

Possible Effects on Laboratory Tests
  Red blood cell and white blood cell counts: increased.

Precautions for Use
  By Those Over 60 Years of Age: Maintain personal cleanliness to prevent eye infections. Report promptly any indication of eye infection.

▷ **Advisability of Use During Pregnancy**
  Pregnancy Category: C. See Pregnancy Risk Categories at the back of this book.
  Animal studies: Significant birth defects due to this drug reported in rats.
  Human studies: Adequate studies of pregnant women are not available. Limit use to the smallest effective dose. Minimize systemic absorption (see "Dosing Instructions" above).

Advisability of Use If Breast-Feeding
  Presence of this drug in breast milk: May be present in small amounts.
  Monitor nursing infant closely, and discontinue drug or nursing if adverse effects develop.

Habit-Forming Potential: None.

Effects of Overdose: Flushing of face, increased flow of saliva, sweating. If solution is swallowed: nausea, vomiting, diarrhea, profuse sweating, rapid pulse, difficult breathing, loss of consciousness.

Possible Effects of Long-Term Use: Development of tolerance (see Glossary), temporary loss of effectiveness.

Suggested Periodic Examinations While Taking This Drug (at physician's discretion)

Measurement of internal eye pressure on a regular basis.

Examination of eyes for development of cataracts.

▷ **While Taking This Drug, Observe the Following**

Foods: No restrictions.

Herbal Medicines or Minerals: St. John's wort may also cause increased sun sensitivity—caution is advised. Scopolia root has glaucoma as a possible side effect. DO NOT COMBINE. Henbane, ephedra and belladonna should also be avoided.

Beverages: No restrictions.

▷ *Alcohol:* Use caution. If this drug is absorbed, it may prolong the effect of alcohol on the brain.

Tobacco Smoking: No interactions expected. I advise everyone to quit smoking.

Marijuana Smoking: Sustained additional decrease in internal eye pressure.

▷ *Other Drugs*

The following drugs may *decrease* the effects of pilocarpine:

• atropine and drugs with atropinelike actions (see Drug Classes).

Pilocarpine *taken concurrently* with

• dipivefrin (Propine) may result in increased myopia and blurred vision.

• epinephrine (various) will result in increased myopia.

• latanoprost (Xalatan) may decrease latanoprost effectiveness. The bedtime dose of pilocarpine should be given an hour after the latanoprost dose.

• sulfacetamide (Sulamyd) may lead to pilocarpine precipitation. Separate these drugs by 20 minutes.

• timolol can produce additive effects in treating glaucoma.

▷ *Driving, Hazardous Activities:* This drug may impair your ability to focus your vision properly. Restrict activities as necessary.

Aviation Note: The use of this drug *may be a disqualification* for piloting. Consult a designated Aviation Medical Examiner.

Exposure to Sun: This medicine may make you very sensitive to the sun. Wear sunglasses.

Discontinuation: Do not stop regular use of this drug without consulting your physician. Periodic discontinuation and temporary substitution of another drug may be necessary to preserve its effectiveness in treating glaucoma.

PINDOLOL (PIN doh lohl)

Introduced: 1972   **Class:** Antihypertensive, beta-adrenergic blocker   **Prescription:** USA: Yes   **Controlled Drug:** USA: No; Canada: No   **Available as Generic:** Yes

Brand Names: ✤Apo-Pindol, ✤Dom-Pindolol, ✤Novo-Pindol, ✤Nu-Pindol, ✤Syn-Pindolol, ✤Viskazide [CD], Visken

```
┌─────────────────────────────────────────────────────────────────────┐
│                     BENEFITS versus RISKS                            │
│     Possible Benefits              Possible Risks                    │
│  EFFECTIVE, WELL-TOLERATED      CONGESTIVE HEART FAILURE IN           │
│    ANTIHYPERTENSIVE IN            ADVANCED HEART DISEASE              │
│    MILD TO MODERATE HIGH        Worsening of angina in coronary heart │
│    BLOOD PRESSURE                 disease (abrupt withdrawal)         │
│  EFFECTIVE PREVENTION OF        Masking of low blood sugar            │
│    ANGINA                         (hypoglycemia) in drug-treated      │
│                                   diabetes                           │
│                                 Provocation of asthma (with high     │
│                                   doses in asthmatics)               │
└─────────────────────────────────────────────────────────────────────┘
```

▷ **Principal Uses**

    As a Single Drug Product: Uses currently included in FDA-approved labeling: Treats mild to moderate high blood pressure, alone or with other drugs.

    Other (unlabeled) generally accepted uses: (1) May be of benefit in helping control aggressive behavior; (2) can help prevent migraine headaches; (3) combination therapy with digoxin may be effective in limiting some abnormal heart rhythms (atrial fibrillation); (4) can be of benefit in some kinds of anxiety; (5) decreases sympathetic output in hyperthyroidism; (5) helps prevent angina.

    As a Combination Drug Product [CD]: This drug is available in combination with hydrochlorothiazide (in Canada). The addition of a thiazide diuretic to this beta-blocker drug enhances its effectiveness as an antihypertensive.

How This Drug Works: Blocks certain actions of the sympathetic nervous system:
- reducing rate and contraction force of the heart, thus lowering ejection pressure of blood leaving the heart
- reducing degree of contraction of blood vessel walls, lowering blood pressure.

Available Dosage Forms and Strengths

        Tablets — 5 mg, 10 mg

    Tablets (Canada) — 15 mg

▷ **Usual Adult Dosage Ranges:** *Hypertension*: Starts with 5 mg twice daily (12 hours apart). The dose may be increased gradually by 10 mg/day at intervals of 3 to 4 weeks as needed and tolerated, up to 60 mg/day. For maintenance, 5 to 10 mg two or three times daily is often effective. The total daily dose should not exceed 60 mg. *Angina prevention*: Starting dose is 2.5 to 5 mg. This starting dose can then be increased as needed and tolerated over several weeks. **Note: Actual dose and schedule must be determined for each patient individually.**

Conditions Requiring Dosing Adjustments

    Liver Function: Dose should be decreased for patients with severe liver disease and for those with combined liver and kidney disease.

    Kidney Function: Dose should be decreased if urine output is seriously lowered.

▷ **Dosing Instructions:** The tablet may be crushed and taken without regard to eating. Do not stop this drug abruptly. If you forget a dose: Take the missed dose as soon as you remember it, unless it's 4 hours or less until your next scheduled dose—if that is the case, skip the missed dose and take the next dose right on schedule. DO NOT double doses. Talk with your doctor if you find yourself missing doses.

Usual Duration of Use: Use on a regular schedule for 2 to 3 weeks usually determines effectiveness in lowering blood pressure. The long-term use of this drug (months to years) will be determined by the course of your blood pressure over time and your response to an overall treatment program (weight reduction, salt restriction, smoking cessation, etc.). See your doctor on a regular basis. Reaching and maintaining goal blood pressure is critical to long term health.

Typical Treatment Goals and Measurements (Outcomes and Markers)

Blood pressure: The most recent treatment guidelines (JNC VI) actually define optimal blood pressure (BP) as less than 120/80 and high normal as 139/89. The American Diabetes Association has chosen a target of 130/80 as the blood pressure goal for people living with diabetes. Most clinicians try to achieve a BP that achieves the best balance of lower cardiovascular risk while avoiding the problem of too low a blood pressure. The goal and time frame (see peak benefits above) should be discussed with you when the prescription is written.

Possible Advantages of This Drug

Causes less slowing of the heart rate than most other beta-blocker drugs.

Currently a "Drug of Choice"

For starting treatment of hypertension (diuretics such as hydrochlorothiazide are the other class) with a single drug.

▷ **This Drug Should Not Be Taken If**

- you have bronchial asthma.
- you have had an allergic reaction to it previously.
- you have congestive heart failure.
- you have an abnormally slow heart rate or a serious form of heart block.
- you are taking, or have taken within the past 14 days, any monoamine oxidase (MAO) type A inhibitor (see Drug Classes).

▷ **Inform Your Physician Before Taking This Drug If**

- you had an adverse reaction to any beta blocker (see Drug Classes).
- you have a history of serious heart disease.
- you have a history of hay fever (allergic rhinitis), asthma, chronic bronchitis or emphysema.
- you have a history of overactive thyroid function (hyperthyroidism).
- you have a history of low blood sugar (hypoglycemia) or diabetes.
- you have impaired liver or kidney function.
- you have diabetes or myasthenia gravis.
- you take digitalis, quinidine or reserpine or any calcium-channel-blocker drug (see Drug Classes).
- you have bad circulation to your legs or arms (peripheral vascular disease).
- you plan to have surgery under general anesthesia in the near future.

Possible Side Effects (natural, expected and unavoidable drug actions)

Lethargy and fatigability, cold extremities, slow heart rate, light-headedness in upright position (see orthostatic hypotension in Glossary).

▷ **Possible Adverse Effects** (unusual, unexpected and infrequent reactions)

If any of the following develop, consult your physician promptly for guidance.

Mild Adverse Effects

Allergic reactions: skin rash, itching.

Headache, dizziness, insomnia, abnormal dreams, fainting—infrequent.

Indigestion, nausea, vomiting, constipation, diarrhea—infrequent.

Joint and muscle discomfort, tremor, fluid retention (edema)—infrequent.

Serious Adverse Effects

Allergic reactions: typical reactions to known allergens (such as bee stings) may be exaggerated.

Mental depression, anxiety—infrequent.

Chest pain, shortness of breath—possible.

Induction of bronchial asthma—in asthmatic individuals.

Abnormally slow heartbeat or congestive heart failure—possible to infrequent.

Drug-induced systemic lupus erythematosus or myasthenia gravis—case reports.

Worsening of poor circulation to the arms or legs (intermittent claudication)—possible.

Carpal tunnel syndrome—reported with other beta blockers.

▷ **Possible Effects on Sexual Function:** Decreased libido or impaired erection—infrequent.

Possible Effects on Laboratory Tests

Blood lupus erythematosus (LE) cells: positive (one case of drug-induced LE).

Blood total cholesterol level: decreased (with long-term use).

Blood HDL cholesterol level: increased.

Blood LDL and VLDL cholesterol levels: no effects.

Blood triglyceride levels: no effects.

Glucose tolerance test (GTT): decreased or increased.

Liver function tests: slightly increased liver enzymes (ALT/GPT and AST/GOT) possible.

CAUTION

1. ***Do not stop this drug suddenly*** without the knowledge and help of your doctor. Carry a card that says you are taking this drug.

2. Ask your doctor or pharmacist before using nasal decongestants, which are usually present in over-the-counter cold preparations and nose drops. These can cause sudden increases in blood pressure when taken concurrently with beta blocker drugs.

3. Report the development of any tendency to emotional depression.

Precautions for Use

By Infants and Children: Safety and effectiveness for those under 12 years of age are not established. If this drug is used, however, observe for the development of low blood sugar (hypoglycemia) during periods of reduced food intake.

By Those Over 60 Years of Age: Unacceptably high blood pressure should be reduced without creating the risks associated with excessively low blood pressure. Small starting doses and frequent blood pressure checks are indicated. Sudden, rapid and excessive reduction of blood pressure can predispose to stroke or heart attack. Watch for dizziness, unsteadiness, tendency to fall, confusion, hallucinations, depression or urinary frequency.

▷ **Advisability of Use During Pregnancy**

Pregnancy Category: B. See Pregnancy Risk Categories at the back of this book.

Animal studies: No significant increase in birth defects due to this drug.

Human studies: Adequate studies of pregnant women not available, but there are some reports of lower growth and fetal problems. Ask your physician for guidance.

Advisability of Use If Breast-Feeding

Presence of this drug in breast milk: Yes.

Avoid drug or refrain from nursing.

Habit-Forming Potential: None.

Effects of Overdose: Weakness, slow pulse, low blood pressure, fainting, cold and sweaty skin, congestive heart failure, possible coma and convulsions.

Possible Effects of Long-Term Use: Reduced heart reserve and eventual heart failure in susceptible individuals with advanced heart disease.

Suggested Periodic Examinations While Taking This Drug (at physician's discretion)

Measurements of blood pressure.

Evaluation of heart function.

▷ **While Taking This Drug, Observe the Following**

Foods: No restrictions. Avoid excessive salt intake.

Herbal Medicines or Minerals: Ginseng may increase blood pressure, blunting the benefits of these medicines. Hawthorn, saw palmetto, ma huang, goldenseal, yohimbe and licorice may also increase blood pressure. Calcium and garlic may help lower blood pressure. Indian snakeroot has a German Commission E monograph indication for hypertension—talk to your doctor. Eleuthero root and ephedra should be avoided by people living with hypertension.

Beverages: No restrictions. May be taken with milk.

▷   *Alcohol:* Use with caution. Alcohol may exaggerate lowering of blood pressure or increase mild sedative effect.

Tobacco Smoking: Nicotine may reduce this drug's effectiveness. I advise everyone to quit smoking.

▷   *Other Drugs*

Pindolol may *increase* the effects of

- other antihypertensive drugs and cause excessive lowering of blood pressure; dose adjustments may be necessary.
- digoxin (Lanoxin) on the heart conduction system, leading to AV block and possible digoxin toxicity as well.
- reserpine (Ser-Ap-Es, etc.) and cause sedation, depression, slowing of the heart rate and lowering of blood pressure.
- verapamil (Calan, Isoptin) and cause excessive depression of heart function; monitor this combination closely.

Pindolol *taken concurrently* with

- amiodarone (Cordarone) may cause extremely slow heartbeats and risk of sinus arrest.
- clonidine (Catapres) requires close monitoring for rebound high blood pressure if clonidine is withdrawn while pindolol is still being taken.

- epinephrine (various) will result in a large increase in blood pressure and reflex increase in heart rate (tachycardia).
- fentanyl (various) can lead to severe decreases in blood pressure. Extreme caution and dose adjustments are warranted if these medicines must be combined.
- fluoxetine (Prozac) may result in increased risk of pindolol toxicity.
- fluvoxamine (Luvox) may result in increased risk of pindolol toxicity.
- insulin requires close monitoring to avoid undetected hypoglycemia (see Glossary).
- oral antidiabetic drugs (see Drug Classes) can result in slowed recovery from low blood sugar.
- phenylpropanolamine (various) may result in severe increases in blood pressure—avoid this combination.
- venlafaxine (Effexor) may result in beta-blocker or venlafaxine toxicity—avoid this combination if possible or use decreased doses of both medicines.

The following drugs may *increase* the effects of pindolol:
- cimetidine (Tagamet).
- methimazole (Tapazole).
- oral contraceptives.
- propylthiouracil (Propacil).
- ritonavir (Norvir) and perhaps other protease inhibitors (see Drug Classes).
- zileuton (Zyflo), close patient monitoring is prudent and dose adjustments may be required.

The following drugs may *decrease* the effects of pindolol:
- barbiturates (phenobarbital, etc.).
- indomethacin (Indocin) and possibly other NSAIDs—may impair pindolol's antihypertensive effect.
- rifampin (Rifadin, Rimactane).
- theophylline (Theo-Dur, others).

▷ *Driving, Hazardous Activities:* Use caution until the full extent of fatigue, dizziness and blood pressure change have been determined.

Aviation Note: The use of this drug *is a disqualification* for piloting. Consult a designated Aviation Medical Examiner.

Exposure to Sun: No restrictions.

Exposure to Heat: Caution is advised. Hot environments can lower blood pressure and exaggerate the effects of this drug.

Exposure to Cold: Caution is advised. Cold environments can enhance the circulatory deficiency in the extremities that may occur with this drug. The elderly should take precautions to prevent hypothermia (see Glossary).

Heavy Exercise or Exertion: It is advisable to avoid exertion that produces light-headedness, excessive fatigue or muscle cramping. The use of this drug may intensify the hypertensive response to isometric exercise.

Occurrence of Unrelated Illness: Fever can lower blood pressure and require adjustment of dose. Nausea or vomiting may interrupt regular doses. Ask your doctor for help.

Discontinuation: It is advisable to avoid sudden discontinuation of this drug in all situations. If possible, gradual reduction of dose over a period of 2 to 3 weeks is recommended. Ask your physician for specific guidance.

PIRBUTEROL (peer BYU ter ohl)

Introduced: 1983   **Class:** Antiasthmatic, bronchodilator   **Prescription:**
USA: Yes   **Controlled Drug:** USA: No; Canada: No   **Available as Generic:**
No

Brand Name: Maxair

<table>
<tr><td colspan="2" align="center">BENEFITS versus RISKS</td></tr>
<tr><td align="center">Possible Benefits</td><td align="center">Possible Risks</td></tr>
<tr><td>VERY EFFECTIVE RELIEF OF
  BRONCHOSPASM</td><td>Increased blood pressure
Nervousness
Fine hand tremor
Irregular heart rhythm (with
  excessive use)</td></tr>
</table>

▷ **Principal Uses**

As a Single Drug Product: Uses currently included in FDA-approved labeling: (1) Relieves acute attacks of bronchial asthma; (2) reduces the frequency and severity of chronic, recurrent asthmatic attacks (prevention); (3) relieves reversible bronchospasm seen in chronic bronchitis, bronchiectasis and emphysema.

Other (unlabeled) generally accepted uses: None at present.

How This Drug Works: By increasing the production of cyclic AMP, this drug relaxes constricted bronchial muscles to relieve asthmatic wheezing.

Available Dosage Forms and Strengths

Aerosol (in canisters of 300 inhalations) — 200 mcg per actuation

▷ **Usual Adult Dosage Range (or children over 12):** Inhaler: Two inhalations (400 mcg) every 4 to 6 hours. **Do not exceed** 12 inhalations (2,400 mcg) every 24 hours. Some patients may get benefits from one inhalation every 4 to 6 hours. **Note: Actual dose and schedule must be determined for each patient individually.**

Conditions Requiring Dosing Adjustments

Liver Function: Used with caution by patients with liver disease who use it often.

Kidney Function: No dose adjustments thought to be needed.

▷ **Dosing Instructions:** Carefully follow the "Patient's Instructions for Use" provided with the inhaler. Do not overuse. If you forget a dose: Use the missed dose as soon as you remember it, unless it's nearly time for your next dose—if that is the case, skip the missed dose and take the next dose right on schedule. DO NOT double doses. Talk with your doctor if you find yourself missing doses.

Usual Duration of Use: According to individual requirements. Do not use beyond the time necessary to terminate episodes of asthma.

Typical Treatment Goals and Measurements (Outcomes and Markers)

Asthma: Short-acting beta agonists like albuterol are used to prevent or treat reversible spasms of the bronchial tubes. The peak effect happens 1 to 2 hours after dosing. Some pulmonologists use arterial blood gases in extreme cases. FEV-1 in mild to moderate cases is important for checking response. Clinical symptoms such as chest tightening and wheezing should also ease. If the usual benefit is not realized, call your doctor.

Possible Advantages of This Drug

Has a more rapid onset of action and a longer duration of effect than most other drugs of this class.

▷ **This Drug Should Not Be Taken If**

- you have had an allergic reaction to it previously.
- you currently have an irregular heart rhythm.
- you are taking, or have taken within the past 2 weeks, any monoamine oxidase (MAO) type A inhibitor (see Drug Classes).

▷ **Inform Your Physician Before Taking This Drug If**

- you have any type of heart or circulatory disorder, especially high blood pressure, coronary heart disease or heart rhythm abnormality.
- you have diabetes or an excessively active thyroid gland (hyperthyroidism).
- you have any type of seizure disorder.
- you are taking any form of digitalis or any stimulant drug.

Possible Side Effects (natural, expected and unavoidable drug actions)

Aerosol—dryness or irritation of mouth or throat, altered taste. Cough.

▷ **Possible Adverse Effects** (unusual, unexpected and infrequent reactions)

If any of the following develop, consult your physician promptly for guidance.

Mild Adverse Effects

Allergic reactions: skin rash, itching—rare.

Headache, dizziness, nervousness, fine tremor of hands—infrequent.

Palpitations, rapid heart rate, chest pain, cough—rare to infrequent.

Nausea, diarrhea, taste disorders—rare.

Serious Adverse Effects

Irregular heart rhythm, increased blood pressure—possible.

Paradoxical spasm of the bronchi—possible.

▷ **Possible Effects on Sexual Function:** None reported.

Natural Diseases or Disorders That May Be Activated by This Drug

Latent coronary artery disease, diabetes, epilepsy or high blood pressure.

Possible Effects on Laboratory Tests

None reported.

CAUTION

1. Combined use of this drug by inhalation with beclomethasone aerosol (Beclovent, Vanceril) may increase the risk of toxicity due to fluorocarbon propellants (fluorocarbons are being phased out). It is advisable to use pirbuterol aerosol 20 to 30 minutes before beclomethasone aerosol. This will reduce the risk of toxicity and help beclomethasone reach the lung.
2. Excessive or prolonged use of this drug by inhalation can reduce its effectiveness (tolerance) and cause serious heart rhythm disturbances, including cardiac arrest.

Precautions for Use

By Infants and Children: Safety and effectiveness of use in children under 12 years of age have not been established.

By Those Over 60 Years of Age: Avoid excessive and continual use. If acute asthma is not relieved promptly, other drugs may be needed. Watch for nervousness, palpitations, irregular heart rhythm and muscle tremors.

▷ **Advisability of Use During Pregnancy**

Pregnancy Category: C. See Pregnancy Risk Categories at the back of this book.

Animal studies: High-dose studies in rabbits revealed abortion and increased fetal deaths. Studies in rats and rabbits found no drug-associated birth defects.

Human studies: Adequate studies of pregnant women are not available. Avoid use during first 3 months if possible.

Advisability of Use If Breast-Feeding

Presence of this drug in breast milk: Unknown.

Avoid drug or refrain from nursing.

Habit-Forming Potential: None. Tolerance to beneficial effects has been reported.

Effects of Overdose: Nervousness, palpitation, rapid heart rate, sweating, headache, tremor, vomiting, chest pain.

Possible Effects of Long-Term Use: Loss of effectiveness (tolerance).

Suggested Periodic Examinations While Taking This Drug (at physician's discretion)

Blood pressure measurements.

Evaluation of heart status.

▷ **While Taking This Drug, Observe the Following**

Foods: No restrictions.

Herbal Medicines or Minerals: Using St. John's wort, ma huang, ephedrine-like compounds or kola while taking this medicine may result in unacceptable central nervous system stimulation. Fir or pine needle oil should NOT be used by asthmatics. Ephedra alone does carry a German Commission E monograph indication for asthma treatment. If you are allergic to plants in the Asteraceae family (aster, chrysanthemum, daisy or ragweed), you may also be allergic to echinacea, chamomile, feverfew and St. John's wort. Since part of the way that ginseng works may be as a MAO inhibitor, DO NOT combine with pirbuterol.

Beverages: Avoid excessive use of caffeine-containing beverages—coffee, tea, cola, chocolate.

▷ *Alcohol:* No interactions expected.

Tobacco Smoking: No interactions expected. I advise everyone to quit smoking.

▷ *Other Drugs*

Pirbuterol **taken concurrently** with

- albuterol (Proventil, Ventolin) may result in adverse effects on the heart.
- monoamine oxidase (MAO) type A inhibitors may cause excessive increase in blood pressure and undesirable heart stimulation.
- phenothiazines (see Drug Classes) may result in blunting of the therapeutic effects of pirbuterol.

▷ *Driving, Hazardous Activities:* Use caution if excessive nervousness or dizziness occurs.

Aviation Note: The use of this drug **is a disqualification** for piloting. Consult a designated Aviation Medical Examiner.

Exposure to Sun: No restrictions.

Heavy Exercise or Exertion: Use caution—excessive exercise can induce asthma in sensitive individuals.

PIROXICAM (peer OX i kam)

Please see the oxicam (nonsteroidal anti-inflammatory drug) family profile.

PNEUMOCOCCAL CONJUGATE VACCINE (NEW mo kok uhl)

Other Name: Pneumonia vaccine
Introduced: Presently this is a specific formulation to help confer immunity to seven kinds (4, 6B, 9V, 14, 18C, 19F and 23F) of bacteria called pneumococcus
Class: Antibacterial vaccine   **Prescription:** USA: Yes   **Controlled Drug:**   USA: No; Canada: No   **Available as Generic:**   USA: No; Canada: No
Brand Names: Prevnar

BENEFITS versus RISKS	
Possible Benefits	*Possible Risks*
PREVENTION OF DISEASE CAUSED BY THE MOST SERIOUS OR PREVALENT STRAINS OF STREPTOCOCCUS PNEUMONIA	Lowered platelets Hypersensitivity Fever
PREVENTION OF PNEUMOCOCCAL MENINGITIS	
PREVENTION OF BACTEREMIC PNEUMONIA CAUSED BY STREPTOCOCCUS	
Possible prevention (less effectively than it prevents meningitis or pneumonia) of ear infection (otitis media)	
Possible cross-protection from other similar bacterial strains	

Author's Note: There is a Vaccine Adverse Event Reporting System (VAERS). The toll-free number is 1-800-822-7967. The information in this profile will be broadened as more data becomes available.

PRAMIPEXOLE (PRAM ih pex ohl)

Other Name: None
Introduced: 1997   **Class:**   Antiparkinsonian, dopamine receptor agonist
Prescription: USA: Yes   **Controlled Drug:** USA: No; Canada: No   **Available as Generic:**   USA: No; Canada: No
Brand Names: Mirapex

```
┌─────────────────────────────────────────────────────────────┐
│                   BENEFITS versus RISKS                       │
│        Possible Benefits              Possible Risks          │
│  EFFECTIVE SYMPTOM RELIEF IN     Movement disorders           │
│    IDIOPATHIC PARKINSON'S        Hallucinations               │
│    DISEASE                       Somnolence                   │
│  BINDS SEVEN TIMES MORE          Postural hypotension         │
│    AGGRESSIVELY TO D3                                         │
│    RECEPTORS THAN TO D2                                       │
│    RECEPTORS                                                  │
│  SOME EARLY DATA FROM CELLS                                  │
│    OUTSIDE THE BODY FOUND                                    │
│    THAT PRAMIPEXOLE MAY                                      │
│    PROTECT AGAINST DISEASE                                   │
│    PROGRESSION                                               │
│  May be an alternative therapy for                          │
│    restless leg syndrome when                               │
│    other medicines like carbidopa/                          │
│    levodopa have not worked                                 │
└─────────────────────────────────────────────────────────────┘
```

▷ **Principal Uses**

As a Single Drug Product: Uses currently included in FDA-approved labeling: Treats major types of Parkinson's disease: paralysis agitans ("shaking palsy" of unknown cause), the type that follows encephalitis and parkinsonism that develops with aging (associated with hardening of the brain arteries).

Other (unlabeled) generally accepted uses: (1) May have a limited role in restless leg syndrome; (2) can improve depression.

As a Combination Drug Product [CD]: Not available.

How This Drug Works: This drug acts as a dopamine receptor activator (agonist). This drug is also unique in that it has a strong affinity for a specific receptor (D3).

Available Dosage Forms and Strengths

Tablets — 0.125 mg, 0.25 mg, 0.5 mg, 1 mg and 1.5 mg

Author's Note: Information in this profile will be broadened once further information is available.

PRAVASTATIN (pra vah STA tin)

Introduced: 1986   **Class:** Cholesterol-lowering agent, HMG-CoA reductase inhibitor   **Prescription:** USA: Yes   **Controlled Drug:** USA: No; Canada: No   **Available as Generic:** USA: No; Canada: No

Brand Names: ✢Lin-Pravastatin, Pravachol

```
┌─────────────────────────────────────────────────────────────────────────┐
│                        BENEFITS versus RISKS                              │
│          Possible Benefits                      Possible Risks            │
│  REDUCES RISK OF STROKES              Drug-induced hepatitis              │
│  EFFECTIVE REDUCTION OF               Drug-induced myositis (muscle       │
│    TOTAL BLOOD CHOLESTEROL              inflammation)                      │
│    AND LDL CHOLESTEROL                Decreased co-enzyme Q10              │
│  EFFECTIVE REDUCTION IN THE                                               │
│    NUMBER OF FIRST-TIME AND                                               │
│    REPEAT HEART ATTACKS                                                    │
│    (PRIMARY AND SECONDARY                                                  │
│    PREVENTION)                                                             │
│  REDUCTION IN THE NUMBER OF                                               │
│    PATIENT DEATHS                                                          │
│  SLOWS PROGRESSION OF                                                      │
│    ATHEROSCLEROSIS                                                         │
│  REDUCES RISK OF TRANSIENT                                                 │
│    ISCHEMIC ATTACKS (TIAs)                                                 │
│  LOWERS APOLIPOPROTEIN B                                                   │
│  INCREASES HDL-C IN PEOPLE                                                 │
│    WITH HETEROZYGOUS FAMILIAL                                              │
│    AND NONFAMIAL PRIMARY                                                   │
│    HYPERCHOLESTEROLEMIA                                                    │
│    AND MIXED DYSLIPIDEMIA                                                  │
│    (FREDERICKSON TYPES 2a                                                  │
│    AND 2b)                                                                 │
│  May have a role in preventing                                            │
│    development of type 2 diabetes in                                       │
│    men                                                                     │
│  May have a role in preventing                                            │
│    osteoporosis                                                           │
└─────────────────────────────────────────────────────────────────────────┘
```

▷ **Principal Uses**

As a Single Drug Product: Uses currently included in FDA-approved labeling: (1) Treats abnormally high total blood cholesterol levels (in people with types IIa and IIb hypercholesterolemia) due to increased low-density lipoprotein (LDL) cholesterol (used with a cholesterol-lowering diet after an adequate trial of nondrug methods has failed); (2) helps prevent a first heart attack and reduces death from cardiovascular disease in people with increased blood cholesterol levels at risk of a first heart attack and also serves to help prevent a repeat heart attack; (3) slows progression and in some cases makes small reversals in coronary artery disease (atherosclerosis); (4) used to decrease triglycerides in mixed lipidemias; (5) reduces risk of strokes or transient ischemic attacks (TIAs)—the CARE trial of 4,159 patients found that strokes were lowered by 32%; (6) approved to increase HDL-C in patients with heterozygous familial and nonfamilial primary hypercholesterolemia and mixed dyslipidemia; (7) lowers apolipoprotein B.

Other (unlabeled) generally accepted uses: (1) Reduces temporary blood flow (to the heart) problems (myocardial ischemia) when combined with other therapies; (2) may have a role in decreasing development of type two diabetes in men; (3) may have a role in reducing development of osteoporosis.

How This Drug Works: This drug blocks the liver enzyme that starts production of cholesterol. Its principal action is the reduction of low-density lipoproteins (LDL), the fraction of total blood cholesterol that is thought to increase the risk of coronary heart disease. This drug also increases the level of high-density lipoproteins (HDL), the cholesterol fraction that is thought to reduce the risk of heart disease.

Available Dosage Forms and Strengths

Tablets — 10 mg, 20 mg, 40 mg

▷ **Recommended Dose Ranges** (Actual dose and schedule must be determined for each patient individually.)

Infants and Children: Under 2 years of age—do not use this drug. 2 to 18 years of age—dose not established.

18 to 60 Years of Age: Hypercholesterolemia: Initially 10 to 20 mg daily, taken at bedtime. Ongoing or maintenance dose is 10 to 20 mg daily and is adjusted as needed and tolerated at intervals of 4 weeks. In primary (40 mg in the evening in the West of Scotland Study) or secondary prevention (40 mg in the evening in the Cholesterol and Recurrent Events Study) of cardiovascular problems (events): 40 mg taken in the evening lowered the risk of cardiovascular mortality as well as risk of another heart attack.

Over 60 Years of Age: Starting dose for those with kidney or liver compromise is 10 mg daily. A geriatric use subsection has been added to the Precautions of FDA-sanctioned labeling. It is unavailable at the time of this writing.

Conditions Requiring Dosing Adjustments

Liver Function: Used with caution by patients with liver disease. Starting dose is decreased to 10 mg per day. Pravastatin should not be used in sudden (acute) liver disease.

Kidney Function: Those with significant kidney disease take a starting dose of 10 mg per day. Used with caution in kidney compromise.

▷ **Dosing Instructions:** The tablet may be crushed and can be taken without regard to eating. New labeling says that it can be taken at any time. Previously, it was preferably taken at bedtime. (Highest rates of cholesterol production occur between midnight and 5 a.m.) If you forget a dose: Take the missed dose as soon as you remember it, unless it's nearly time for your next dose—if that is the case, skip the missed dose and take the next dose right on schedule. DO NOT double doses. Talk with your doctor if you find yourself missing doses.

Usual Duration of Use: Use on a regular schedule for 4 to 6 weeks usually determines effectiveness in reducing blood levels of total and LDL-C cholesterol. Long-term use (months to years) requires periodic physician evaluation. It is critical to take this medicine as directed to take control of an ongoing condition such as increased cholesterol, stroke risk or heart attack risk.

Typical Treatment Goals and Measurements (Outcomes and Markers)

Cholesterol: The National Institutes of Health has released ATP III as part of the update to the National Cholesterol Education Program or NCEP. Key points in these new guidelines include acknowledging diabetes as one of the conditions that increases risk of heart disease, modifying risk factors and recommending routine testing for all of the cholesterol fractions (lipoprotein profile) versus total cholesterol alone. These new guidelines also recommend a desirable total cholesterol of 200 mg/dl as before, but change optimal LDL to 100 mg/dl, 130–159 mg/dl as borderline high, 160mg/dl as high and cite 190 mg/dl as very high. One other noteworthy change is that "good cholesterol" or HDL has been made more important. The "too low" measure for HDL has been increased to 40 mg/dl. Take your medicine and reach these new targets! Electron beam computed tomography (EBCT) is an important tool to use in conjunction with these laboratory studies. Findings show that even patients who meet cholesterol goals (particularly females over 55) can still be at significant cardiovascular risk. EBCT then defines that risk by giving a calcium score and a "virtual tour" of the coronary arteries.

Possible Advantages of This Drug

Several studies show that drugs of this class (HMG-CoA reductase inhibitors) are more effective and better tolerated than other drugs currently available for reducing total and LDL-C cholesterol. This medicine is proven to increase HDL, has growing bone health and diabetes data and works in primary and secondary heart (coronary) events.

▷ ### This Drug Should Not Be Taken If
- you have had an allergic reaction to it previously.
- you have an unexplained and ongoing increase in liver function tests.
- you have active liver disease.
- you are pregnant or breast-feeding your infant.

▷ ### Inform Your Physician Before Taking This Drug If
- you have previously taken and have not tolerated any other drugs in this class: lovastatin (Mevacor), simvastatin (Zocor).
- you have a history of liver disease or impaired liver function.
- you are not using any method of birth control or you are planning pregnancy.
- you regularly consume substantial amounts of alcohol.
- you have kidney disease.
- you have cataracts or impaired vision.
- you get unexplained muscle weakness, pain or tenderness.
- you have any type of chronic muscular disorder.
- you plan to have major surgery in the near future.

Possible Side Effects (natural, expected and unavoidable drug actions)

Development of abnormal liver tests without symptoms.
Decreased co-enzyme Q10 (co-Q10 or ubiquinone) levels.

▷ ### Possible Adverse Effects (unusual, unexpected and infrequent reactions)

If any of the following develop, consult your physician promptly for guidance.

Mild Adverse Effects
Allergic reactions: skin rash, itching—rare.
Headache, dizziness, depression—case reports to rare.
Flu-like syndrome, cough—case reports.
Indigestion, stomach pain, nausea, excessive gas, constipation, diarrhea—rare to infrequent.
Muscle cramps and/or pain—rare.

Serious Adverse Effects
Allergic reactions: rash (lichenoid dermatitis).
Porphyria cutanea tarda (PCT)—case reports.

Marked and persistent abnormal liver function tests with focal hepatitis (without jaundice)—rare.

Acute myositis (muscle pain and tenderness) during long-term use—case reports.

Rhabdomyolysis—rare and more likely if combined with fibrates.

Low white blood cells (leukopenia)—rare and questionable causation.

Neuropathy—case report.

▷ **Possible Effects on Sexual Function:** Impotence—questionable causation with medicines that lower cholesterol.

Possible Delayed Adverse Effects: Increased liver enzymes, decreased co-Q10.

Natural Diseases or Disorders That May Be Activated by This Drug
Latent liver disease.

Possible Effects on Laboratory Tests
Blood alanine aminotransferase (ALT) enzyme level: increased (with higher doses of drug).

Blood total cholesterol, LDL cholesterol and triglyceride levels: decreased.

Blood HDL cholesterol level: increased.

CAUTION
1. If pregnancy occurs while taking this drug, discontinue the drug immediately and consult your physician.
2. Report promptly any development of muscle pain or tenderness, especially if accompanied by fever or malaise.
3. Report promptly the development of altered or impaired vision so that appropriate evaluation can be made.
4. If CPK levels become markedly elevated, this medicine should be stopped.
5. A geriatric use subsection has been added to the Precaution section of FDA-sanctioned labeling for this product. Exact labeling is unavailable at the time of this writing.

Precautions for Use
By Infants and Children: Safety and effectiveness for those under 18 years of age are not established.

By Those Over 60 Years of Age: Tell your doctor about any personal or family history of cataracts. Comply with all recommendations regarding periodic eye examinations. Report promptly any alterations in vision. 10 mg starting dose is prudent.

▷ **Advisability of Use During Pregnancy**
Pregnancy Category: X. See Pregnancy Risk Categories at the back of this book.

Animal studies: Mouse and rat studies reveal skeletal birth defects due to a closely related drug of this class.

Human studies: Adequate studies of pregnant women are not available.

This drug should be avoided during entire pregnancy.

Advisability of Use If Breast-Feeding
Presence of this drug in breast milk: Yes, in small amounts.

Avoid drug or refrain from nursing.

Habit-Forming Potential: None.

Effects of Overdose: Increased indigestion, stomach distress, nausea, diarrhea.

Possible Effects of Long-Term Use: Abnormal liver function with focal hepatitis.

Suggested Periodic Examinations While Taking This Drug (at physician's discretion)

Blood cholesterol studies: total cholesterol, HDL and LDL fractions.

Liver function tests before treatment, at 12 weeks of treatment (and after a dose is increased) and then every 6 months if the 12-week tests are normal. **This is new labeling and pravastatin was the first HMG-CoA reductase inhibitor to receive labeling from the FDA for less-frequent liver testing.** Complete eye examination at beginning of treatment and at any time that significant change in vision occurs. Ask your doctor for guidance.

Author's Note: A related medicine called cerivastatin (Baycol) was removed from the market because of liver changes. It is unknown at the time of this writing if the FDA will review similar medicines and ask for more frequent checks of liver function.

Bone mineral density tests (DEXA, PDEXA or ultrasound) will help show retention of bone mineral density (a new possible beneficial effect).

Electron beam computed tomography can help predict silent ischemia and other problems with blood vessels that supply the heart itself. This also may help define the results (outcomes) you are getting from this medicine.

▷ **While Taking This Drug, Observe the Following**

Foods: Follow a standard low-cholesterol diet.

Herbal Medicines or Minerals: No data exist from well-designed clinical studies about garlic and pravastatin combinations and they cannot presently be recommended. Additionally, garlic may inhibit blood-clotting (platelet) aggregation—something to consider if you are already taking a platelet inhibitor. The FDA has allowed one dietary supplement called Cholestin to continue to be sold. This preparation actually contains lovastatin. Since use of two HMG-CoA inhibitors may increase risk of rhabdomyolysis or myopathy, the combination is NOT advised.

Use of plant stanol ester products (Benecol) with this medicine can help further lower total and LDL cholesterol. Soy (milk, tofu, etc.) contains phytoestrogens, which has led to an FDA-approved health claim for reducing risk of heart disease (if there is at least 6.25 g of soy protein per serving). Substituting soy for some of the meat in your diet can also help lower cholesterol. Because pravastatin like other medicines in this drug class can deplete co-Q10, supplementation may be needed. One report of type 2 diabetics with low co-Q10 found beneficial effects from supplementation.

Beverages: No restrictions. May be taken with milk.

▷ *Alcohol:* No interactions expected. Use sparingly.

Tobacco Smoking: No interactions expected. I advise everyone to quit smoking.

▷ *Other Drugs*

Pravastatin *taken concurrently* with

- amprenavir (Agenerase) and ritonavir (Norvir) and perhaps other protease inhibitors may increase cerivastatin levels and the risk of muscle damage (myopathy).
- clofibrate (Atromid-S) has been associated with muscle damage (rhabdomyolysis).
- cyclosporine (Sandimmune) increases the risk for myopathy.
- erythromycin (various) may increase muscle damage risk.

- fluconazole (Diflucan) or itraconazole (Sporanox) or ketoconazole (Nizoral) will increase risk of myopathy. Extreme caution is advised.
- gemfibrozil (Lopid) may alter the absorption and excretion of pravastatin and may also increase risk of muscle damage (rhabdomyolysis); these drugs should not be taken concurrently.
- niacin (various) may increase muscle damage risk.
- quinupristin/dalfopristin (Synercid) may increase the risk for myopathy by increasing cerivastatin blood levels.
- warfarin (Coumadin) can increase the risk of bleeding; more frequent INR (prothrombin time or protime) testing is indicated. Ongoing warfarin doses should be based on laboratory results.

The following drug may **decrease** the effects of pravastatin:
- cholestyramine (Questran)—may reduce absorption of pravastatin; take pravastatin 1 hour before or 4 hours after cholestyramine.

▷ *Driving, Hazardous Activities:* This drug may cause dizziness. Restrict activities as necessary.

Aviation Note: The use of this drug **may be a disqualification** for piloting. Consult a designated Aviation Medical Examiner.

Exposure to Sun: No restrictions.

Discontinuation: Do not stop this drug without your doctor's knowledge and help. There may be a significant increase in blood cholesterol levels following discontinuation of this drug.

PRAZOSIN (PRA zoh sin)

Introduced: 1970   **Class:** Antihypertensive   **Prescription:** USA: Yes
Controlled Drug: USA: No; Canada: No   **Available as Generic:** Yes
Brand Names: ✿Apo-Prazo, Minipres, Minizide [CD], ✿Novo-Prazin, ✿Nu-Prazo

BENEFITS versus RISKS	
Possible Benefits	*Possible Risks*
EFFECTIVE INITIAL THERAPY FOR MILD TO MODERATE HYPERTENSION	"First-dose" drop in blood pressure with fainting
EFFECTIVE ANTIHYPERTENSIVE IN MODERATE TO SEVERE HYPERTENSION	May cause increased heart rate (paroxysmal tachycardia)
EFFECTIVE CONTROL OF HYPERTENSION IN PHEOCHROMOCYTOMA	
HELPS URINE FLOW IN BENIGN PROSTATIC HYPERPLASIA	
Effective in presence of impaired kidney function	

Author's Note: Data from the ALLHAT trial found that alpha blockers such as this medicine are not drugs of first choice in high blood pressure. Information in this profile has been shortened for more widely used medicines.

PREDNISOLONE (pred NIS oh lohn)

Introduced: 1955   **Class:** Cortisonelike drugs   **Prescription:** USA: Yes
Controlled Drug: USA: No; Canada: No   **Available as Generic:** USA: Yes; Canada: Yes

Brand Names: A&D w/Prednisolone [CD], ✽Ak-Cide [CD], ✽Ak-Pred, ✽Ak-Tate, Blephamide, Cortalone, Delta-Cortef, Duapred, Econopred Ophthalmic, Fernisolone-P, Hydelta-TBA, Hydeltrasol, ✽Inflamase, ✽Inflamase Forte, Isopto Cetapred [CD], Key-Pred, Meticortelone, Meti-Derm, Metimyd [CD], Metreton, ✽Minims Prednisolone, Mydrapred, Niscort, Nor-Pred, ✽Nova-Pred, ✽Novoprednisolone, Ophtho-Tate, Optimyd [CD], Otobione [CD], Pediaject, Pediapred, Polypred, Predcor, ✽Pred Forte, Pred-G [CD], ✽Pred Mild, Prelone, PSP-IV, Savacort, Sterane, TBA Pred, ✽Vasocidin [CD]

BENEFITS versus RISKS	
Possible Benefits	*Possible Risks*
EFFECTIVE RELIEF OF SYMPTOMS IN A WIDE VARIETY OF INFLAMMATORY AND ALLERGIC DISORDERS	Use exceeding 2 weeks is associated with many possible adverse effects:
	ALTERED MOOD AND PERSONALITY
EFFECTIVE IMMUNOSUPPRESSION IN SELECTED BENIGN AND MALIGNANT DISORDERS	CATARACTS, GLAUCOMA HYPERTENSION OSTEOPOROSIS
Prevention of rejection in organ transplantation	ASEPTIC BONE NECROSIS INCREASED SUSCEPTIBILITY TO INFECTIONS

Author's Note: Adverse effects from ophthalmic use are much more limited and more rare than those from systemic use.

▷ **Principal Uses**

As a Single Drug Product: Uses currently included in FDA-approved labeling: (1) Used in the treatment of a wide variety of allergic and inflammatory conditions—it is used most commonly in the management of serious skin disorders, asthma, regional enteritis, ulcerative colitis and all types of major rheumatic disorders including bursitis, tendonitis, most forms of arthritis and inflammatory eye conditions; (2) used as part of combination therapy in lymphoma; (3) used in some kinds of adrenal insufficiencies; (4) used to help tuberculosis patients who also have inflammation around the heart without fluid buildup; (5) eases symptoms in ulcerative colitis.

Other (unlabeled) generally accepted uses: (1) Used as part of combination therapy in acute leukemias (lymphoblastic, lymphocytic and myelogenous); (2) may have a role in combination therapy of breast cancer; (3) can help relieve the muscle pain of familial Mediterranean fever; (4) part of a combination therapy in treating abnormal liver tumors (hemangiomas); (5) can help subfertile men decrease seminal antibodies and become fertile; (6) helps people who have drug-induced lowering of white blood cells recover; (7) treats anaphylactic reactions of unknown cause; (8) treats thrombocytopenic purpura of unknown cause; (9) eases symptoms in myasthenia gravis; (10) can help reflex sympathetic dystrophy.

How This Drug Works: Not fully established. It is thought that this drug's anti-inflammatory effect is due to its ability to inhibit the normal defensive functions of certain white blood cells. Its immunosuppressant effect is attributed to a reduced production of lymphocytes and antibodies.

Available Dosage Forms and Strengths

> Eye ointment — 0.6%
> Eye suspension — 0.5%, 1%
> Oral liquid — 6.7 mg/5 ml
> Syrup — 15 mg/5 ml
> Tablets — 5 mg

▷ **Usual Adult Dosage Ranges:** 5 to 60 mg daily as a single dose or in divided doses (some patients are put on alternate-day schedules). Once an adequate response is achieved, the dose should be decreased to the lowest effective dose. Ophthalmic drops—one to two drops is instilled into the eye sac (conjunctival sac) every 3 to 12 hours. Dosing may be increased to every hour in severe cases. **Note: Actual dose and schedule must be determined for each patient individually.**

Typical Treatment Goals and Measurements (Outcomes and Markers)

Inflammation: The general goal is to relieve the swelling and the inflammatory response. Use in asthma should help decrease the frequency and severity of acute attacks. Some clinicians use decreased frequency of rescue inhaler use as a measure of success. Improvement in lung (pulmonary function) testing also helps define results in asthma. Lastly, clinical signs and symptoms such as wheezing, tightness in the chest and exercise tolerance should all move in favorable directions.

Conditions Requiring Dosing Adjustments

Liver Function: Dosing adjustments do not appear to be needed in liver compromise.

Kidney Function: Dosing adjustments in renal compromise do not appear to be needed. This drug can cause proteinuria. It is a benefit-to-risk decision for kidney compromise (nephropathy) patients who tend to lose protein.

▷ **Dosing Instructions:** The tablet may be crushed and taken with or following food to prevent stomach irritation, preferably in the morning. Suspensions should be gently mixed before using. If you forget a dose: Call your doctor for instructions.

Usual Duration of Use: For acute disorders: 4 to 10 days. For chronic disorders: according to individual requirements. Use only for time needed to relieve symptoms in acute self-limiting conditions or the time required to stabilize a chronic condition and permit gradual withdrawal. Because of its intermediate duration of action, this drug is appropriate for alternate-day dosing for many forms. See your doctor regularly.

Author's Note: The information categories provided in this profile are appropriate for prednisolone. For specific information that is normally found in those categories that have been omitted from this profile, see the following profile of prednisone. Prednisolone is a

derivative of prednisone; all significant actions and effects are shared by both drugs.

PREDNISONE (PRED ni sohn)

Introduced: 1955   **Class:** Cortisonelike drugs   **Prescription:** USA: Yes
Controlled Drug: USA: No; Canada: No   **Available as Generic:** USA: Yes; Canada: Yes

Brand Names: ❦Apo-Prednisone, Aspred C [CD], Deltasone, Liquid Pred, Meti-corten, ❦Metreton [CD], ❦Novoprednisone, Orasone, Panasol-S, Paracort, Prednicen-M, Prednisone Intensol, SK-Prednisone, Sterapred, Sterapred-DS, ❦Winpred

BENEFITS versus RISKS	
Possible Benefits	*Possible Risks*
EFFECTIVE RELIEF OF SYMPTOMS IN A WIDE VARIETY OF INFLAMMATORY AND ALLERGIC DISORDERS	Use exceeding 2 weeks is associated with many possible adverse effects:
	ALTERED MOOD AND PERSONALITY
EFFECTIVE IMMUNOSUPPRESSION IN SELECTED BENIGN AND MALIGNANT DISORDERS	CATARACTS, GLAUCOMA HYPERTENSION OSTEOPOROSIS
Prevention of rejection in organ transplantation	ASEPTIC BONE NECROSIS INCREASED SUSCEPTIBILITY TO INFECTIONS

▷ **Principal Uses**

  As a Single Drug Product: Uses currently included in FDA-approved labeling: (1) Treats a wide variety of allergic and inflammatory conditions—it is used most commonly in the management of serious skin disorders, asthma, gout, lupus erythematosus, regional enteritis, ulcerative colitis, nephrotic syndrome and all types of major rheumatic disorders including bursitis, tendonitis and most forms of arthritis; (2) used as part of combination therapy of lymphoma; (3) helps address adrenal insufficiency; (4) used as part of combination therapy of several kinds of leukemia; (5) used in kidney transplant patients; (6) helps patients recover from symptoms of multiple sclerosis.

  Other (unlabeled) generally accepted uses: (1) Used in combination therapy of acute (lymphoblastic, lymphocytic and myelogenous) leukemias; (2) combination therapy of breast cancer; (3) may be helpful in therapy of familial Mediterranean fever; (4) used with other medications to treat liver tumors (hemangiomas); (5) may help subfertile men decrease seminal antibodies and become fertile; (6) helps prevent early lung deterioration in children with AIDS; (7) eases symptoms in alcoholics who have hepatitis and encephalopathy; (8) used in some chronic pain syndromes.

How This Drug Works: Anti-inflammatory effect is due to its ability to inhibit normal defensive functions of certain white blood cells. Its immunosuppressant effect is due to a reduced production of lymphocytes and antibodies.

Available Dosage Forms and Strengths
Oral solution — 5 mg/5 ml
> Syrup — 5 mg/5 ml (5% alcohol)
> Tablets — 1 mg, 2.5 mg, 5 mg, 10 mg, 20 mg, 25 mg, 50 mg

▷ **Usual Adult Dosage Ranges:** Five to 60 mg daily as a single dose or in divided doses depending on the condition being treated. With myasthenia gravis, patients not responding to 100 mg will not respond to higher doses. Once initial inflammation has eased, the dose should be gradually lowered to the lowest effective dose for the condition being treated.

Note: Actual dose and schedule must be determined for each patient individually.

Conditions Requiring Dosing Adjustments
Liver Function: No dosing changes needed.

Kidney Function: Dosing adjustments in kidney disease do not appear to be needed. May cause proteinuria. Use is a benefit-to-risk decision for patients with protein-losing kidney disease (nephropathy).

▷ **Dosing Instructions:** The tablet may be crushed and taken with or following food to prevent stomach irritation, preferably in the morning. If you forget a dose: Call your doctor for instructions. Be sure to check with your doctor BEFORE getting any vaccines.

Usual Duration of Use: For acute disorders: 4 to 10 days. For chronic disorders: according to individual requirements. Use should not exceed time needed for symptomatic relief in acute self-limiting conditions or time required to stabilize a chronic condition and permit gradual withdrawal. Intermediate duration of action allows alternate-day dosing. See your doctor regularly.

Typical Treatment Goals and Measurements (Outcomes and Markers)
Inflammation: The general goal is to relieve the swelling and the inflammatory response. Use in asthma should help decrease the frequency and severity of acute attacks. Some clinicians use decreased frequency of rescue inhaler use as a measure of success. Improvement in lung (pulmonary function) testing also helps define results in asthma. Lastly, clinical signs and symptoms such as wheezing, tightness in the chest and exercise tolerance should all move in favorable directions if asthma is being treated.

▷ **This Drug Should Not Be Taken If**
- you had an allergic reaction to it previously.
- you have active peptic ulcer disease.
- you have an active herpes simplex virus eye infection.
- you have active tuberculosis.
- you have a fungal infection in a large area inside your body (systemic fungal infection).

▷ **Inform Your Physician Before Taking This Drug If**
- you have had an adverse reaction to any cortisonelike drug.
- you have a history of peptic ulcer disease, thrombophlebitis or tuberculosis.
- you have diabetes, kidney failure, glaucoma, high blood pressure, deficient thyroid function or myasthenia gravis.
- you have osteoporosis.

- you have been exposed to any viral illness, such as measles or chicken pox. (Cases may be severe if you are taking this medicine.)
- you are prone to depression.
- you have diverticulitis.
- you plan to have surgery of any kind in the near future.

Possible Side Effects (natural, expected and unavoidable drug actions)

Increased appetite, weight gain, retention of salt and water leading to increased blood pressure, excretion of potassium, increased susceptibility to infection. Mild euphoria.

▷ **Possible Adverse Effects** (unusual, unexpected and infrequent reactions)

If any of the following develop, consult your physician promptly for guidance.

Mild Adverse Effects

Allergic reaction: skin rash.

Headache, dizziness, insomnia—infrequent.

Acid indigestion, abdominal distention—infrequent.

Patchy blue areas on the great toe (blue toe syndrome)—case reports.

Muscle cramping and weakness—possible.

Elevated intracranial pressure (pseudotumor cerebri)—infrequent.

Acne, excessive growth of facial hair—frequent.

Serious Adverse Effects

Serious mental or emotional disturbances—case reports.

Reactivation of latent tuberculosis—possible in those with past tuberculosis.

Development of peptic ulcer—possible and more likely in those with previous ulcers.

Development of inflammation of the pancreas—rare.

Thrombophlebitis (inflammation of a vein with the formation of blood clot): pain or tenderness in thigh or leg, with or without swelling of the foot, ankle or leg—rare.

Increased intraocular (inner eye) pressure, glaucoma or cataracts—infrequent.

Kaposi's sarcoma—case reports.

Growth retardation—possible in children with long-term use.

Cushing's syndrome—possible with long-term use.

Necrosis of bone (osteonecrosis, avascular necrosis or aseptic necrosis)—case reports.

Osteoporosis—possible with long-term use.

Superinfections—possible.

Inflammation or wasting of muscle (myositis or myopathy)—infrequent.

Increased blood sugar—possible and may be dose-related.

Drug-induced porphyria or seizures—case reports.

Pulmonary embolism (movement of a blood clot to the lung): sudden shortness of breath, pain in the chest, coughing, bloody sputum—increased risk.

▷ **Possible Effects on Sexual Function:** Altered timing and pattern of menstruation. Correction of male infertility when due to autoantibodies that suppress sperm activity.

▷ **Adverse Effects That May Mimic Natural Diseases or Disorders**

Pattern of symptoms and signs resembling Cushing's syndrome.

Natural Diseases or Disorders That May Be Activated by This Drug
Latent diabetes, glaucoma, peptic ulcer disease, tuberculosis.

Possible Effects on Laboratory Tests
Complete blood cell counts: decreased eosinophils, lymphocytes and platelets.
Blood amylase level: increased (possible pancreatitis).
Blood total cholesterol and HDL cholesterol levels: increased.
Blood LDL cholesterol level: no effect.
Blood triglyceride levels: no significant effect.
Blood glucose level: increased.
Glucose tolerance test (GTT): decreased.
Blood potassium or testosterone level: decreased.
Blood thyroid hormone (T3): decreased.
Blood uric acid level: increased.
Urine sugar tests: no effect with Tes-Tape; false low result with Clinistix and Diastix.
Fecal occult blood test: positive (if gastrointestinal bleeding).

CAUTION
1. If therapy exceeds 1 week, carry an identification card noting that you are taking this drug.
2. Do not stop this drug abruptly after long-term use.
3. If vaccination against measles, rabies, smallpox or yellow fever is required, discontinue this drug 72 hours before vaccination and do not resume it for at least 14 days after vaccination.

Precautions for Use
By Infants and Children: Avoid prolonged use if possible. During long-term use, observe for suppression of normal growth and the possibility of increased intracranial pressure. Following long-term use, the child may be at risk for adrenal gland deficiency during stress for as long as 18 months after cessation of this drug.

By Those Over 60 Years of Age: Cortisonelike drugs should only be used when the disorder under treatment is unresponsive to adequate trials of unrelated drugs. Avoid the prolonged use of this drug. Continual use (even in small doses) can increase severity of diabetes, enhance fluid retention, raise blood pressure, weaken resistance to infection, induce stomach ulcer and accelerate development of cataract and osteoporosis.

▷ **Advisability of Use During Pregnancy**
Pregnancy Category: B. See Pregnancy Risk Categories at the back of this book.
Animal studies: Birth defects reported in mice, rats and rabbits.
Human studies: Adequate studies of pregnant women are not available.
Avoid completely during the first 3 months. Limit use during the final 6 months as much as possible. If used, examine infant for possible deficiency of adrenal gland function.

Advisability of Use If Breast-Feeding
Presence of this drug in breast milk: Yes, but amounts received via breast milk are generally less than 0.1% of a therapeutic dose.
Talk to your doctor. Prednisolone or prednisone may be drugs of choice in women who wish to breast-feed while taking one of those medicines for one of its indicated uses.

Habit-Forming Potential: Long-term use of this drug may produce a state of functional dependence (see Glossary). In therapy of asthma and rheumatoid arthritis, it is advisable to keep the dose as small as possible and attempt drug withdrawal after periods of reasonable improvement. Such procedures may reduce the degree of "steroid rebound"—the return of symptoms as the drug is withdrawn.

Effects of Overdose: Fatigue, muscle weakness, stomach irritation, acid indigestion, excessive sweating, facial flushing, fluid retention, swelling of extremities, increased blood pressure.

Possible Effects of Long-Term Use: Increased blood sugar (possible diabetes), increased fat deposits on the trunk of the body ("buffalo hump"), rounding of the face ("moon face"), thinning and fragility of skin, loss of texture and strength of bones (osteoporosis, aseptic necrosis), cataracts, glaucoma, retarded growth and development in children.

Suggested Periodic Examinations While Taking This Drug (at physician's discretion)

Measurements of blood pressure, blood sugar and potassium levels.

Complete eye examinations at regular intervals.

Chest X ray if history of tuberculosis.

Bone mineral density testing (DEXA) to check for osteoporosis. Check of bone status relative to osteonecrosis.

Determination of the rate of development of the growing child to detect retardation of normal growth.

▷ **While Taking This Drug, Observe the Following**

Foods: No interactions expected. Ask your doctor about restricting salt or eating potassium-rich foods. During long-term use, it is best to eat a high-protein diet.

Herbal Medicines or Minerals: Hawthorn, ginger, garlic, ma huang, ginseng and nettle may change blood sugar. Since dexamethasone may also change blood sugar control, caution is advised.

Fir or pine needle oil should NOT be used by asthmatics. Ephedra alone does carry a German Commission E monograph indication for asthma treatment. If you are allergic to plants in the Asteraceae family (aster, chrysanthemum, daisy or ragweed), you may also be allergic to echinacea, chamomile, feverfew and St. John's wort.

During long-term use, take a vitamin D supplement and increase calcium. During wound repair, take a zinc supplement. Potassium loss may need to be replaced. Ask your doctor if glucosamine makes sense for you. Talk to your doctor BEFORE adding any herbal to any other medicines that you already take.

Beverages: No restrictions. Drink all forms of milk liberally.

▷ *Alcohol:* Use caution if you are prone to peptic ulcers. Talk to your doctor to get their approval of drinking beer, wine or other liquor while taking this medicine.

Tobacco Smoking: Nicotine increases the blood levels of naturally produced cortisone. I advise everyone to quit smoking.

Marijuana Smoking: May cause additional impairment of immunity.

▷   *Other Drugs*

Prednisone may ***decrease*** the effects of
- insulin (various), requiring dosing changes of insulin.
- isoniazid (INH, Niconyl, etc.).
- salicylates (aspirin, sodium salicylate, etc.) and also increases the risk of stomach irritation.
- vaccines (such as flu vaccine), by blunting the immune response to them.

Prednisone ***taken concurrently*** with
- amphotericin B (Abelcet, Fungizone) may result in additive potassium loss.
- asparaginase (Elspar) may result in increased risk of toxicity if given with or before prednisone. Asparaginase dosing should be accomplished after prednisone dosing.
- birth control pills (oral contraceptives) will prolong the prednisone effect.
- clarithromycin (Biaxin) may lead to psychotic symptoms (one case report). Patients must be closely watched if these medicines are combined.
- cyclosporine (Sandimmune) can cause increased cyclosporine levels and increased prednisone levels. Dose decreases may be needed for both drugs.
- foscarnet (Foscavir) may result in additive potassium loss.
- ketoconazole (Nizoral) will lessen the therapeutic benefits of ketoconazole.
- loop diuretics (furosemide [Lasix], bumetanide [Bumex]) may blunt their effects.
- macrolide antibiotics (erythromycin, troleandomycin and perhaps others) can lead to prednisone toxicity.
- montelukast (Singulair) resulted in severe edema (peripheral) in one case report. Caution and close patient monitoring are prudent if these medicines must be combined.
- neuromuscular blocking agents (such as pancuronium-Pavulon, vecuronium-Norcuron, others) can result in increased risk and or severity of muscle problems (myopathy and flaccid paralysis) and can also antagonize blockade from these medicines. Caution and unparalyzed periods are prudent.
- NSAIDs may result in additive stomach and intestinal irritation.
- oral anticoagulants may either increase or decrease their effectiveness; consult your physician regarding the need for prothrombin time testing and dose adjustment.
- oral antidiabetic drugs (see Drug Classes) or insulin may result in loss of glucose control.
- ritonavir (Norvir) and perhaps other protease inhibitors (see Drug Classes) may lead to toxicity.
- theophylline (Theo-Dur, others) may result in variable responses to this medicine. Increased frequency of theophylline level testing is recommended.
- thiazide diuretics (see Drug Classes) or loop diuretics may result in additive potassium loss.
- vaccines (flu, pneumococcal, varicella and others) may result in blunted response to the vaccine and decreased preventive benefits.

The following drugs may ***decrease*** the effects of prednisone:
- antacids—may reduce its absorption.
- barbiturates (Amytal, Butisol, phenobarbital, etc.).
- carbamazepine (Tegretol).

- phenytoin (Dilantin, etc.) and fosphenytoin (Cerebyx).
- primidone (Mysoline).
- rifampin (Rifadin, Rimactane, etc.).

▷ *Driving, Hazardous Activities:* Usually no restrictions. Be alert to the rare occurrence of dizziness.

Aviation Note: The use of this drug *may be a disqualification* for piloting. Consult a designated Aviation Medical Examiner.

Exposure to Sun: No restrictions.

Occurrence of Unrelated Illness: This drug may decrease resistance to infection. Tell your doctor if you develop an infection of any kind. It may also reduce your ability to respond to the stress of acute illness, injury or surgery. Keep your doctor informed of any changes in health.

Discontinuation: After long-term use, do not stop prednisone abruptly. For 2 years after stopping this drug, it is essential in the event of illness, injury or surgery that you tell medical personnel that you have used this drug.

PRIMIDONE (PRI mi dohn)

Introduced: 1953   **Class:** Anticonvulsant   **Prescription:** USA: Yes
Controlled Drug: USA: No; Canada: No   **Available as Generic:** USA: Yes; Canada: Yes
Brand Names: ❧Apo-Primidone, Myidone, Mysoline, ❧PMS-Primidone, ❧Sertan

BENEFITS versus RISKS	
Possible Benefits	*Possible Risks*

EFFECTIVE CONTROL OF TONIC-CLONIC (GRAND MAL) AND ALL TYPES OF PARTIAL SEIZURES	Allergic skin reactions
	Rare blood cell disorders:
	  megaloblastic anemia, deficient
	  white blood cells and platelets

▷ **Principal Uses**

As a Single Drug Product: Uses currently included in FDA-approved labeling: This drug is used exclusively to control generalized grand mal seizures and all types of partial seizures. It can be used to supplement the anticonvulsant action of phenytoin.

Other (unlabeled) generally accepted uses: (1) May have a minor role in helping in therapy of orthostatic tremor; (2) can help ringing in the ears (tinnitus).

How This Drug Works: Reduces and stabilizes the excitability of nerve fibers and inhibits the repetitive spread of electrical impulses along nerve pathways. This action may prevent seizures altogether or it may reduce their frequency and severity. (Part of this drug's action is attributable to phenobarbital, one of its conversion products in the body.)

Available Dosage Forms and Strengths

Oral suspensions — 250 mg/5 ml
Tablets — 50 mg, 125 mg, 250 mg
Tablets, chewable — 125 mg

▷ **Usual Adult Dosage Ranges:** Initially 100 mg every 24 hours as a single dose at bedtime for 3 days; 100 to 125 mg twice a day for days 4–6; 100 to 125 mg three times a day for days 7–9 and an ongoing (maintenance) dose of 250 mg three times a day, 8 hours apart. Daily maximum is 2,000 mg. *Note: Actual dose and schedule must be determined for each patient individually.*

Conditions Requiring Dosing Adjustments

Liver Function: The dose must be decreased and blood levels obtained more frequently for patients with liver compromise.

Kidney Function: For patients with mild to moderate kidney failure, the usual dose can be taken every 8 hours. Patients with moderate to severe kidney failure can take the usual dose every 8–12 hours. Patients with severe kidney failure should take the usual dose every 12–24 hours. Primidone should be used with caution in renal compromise, as it can be a cause of crystalluria.

▷ **Dosing Instructions:** The tablet may be crushed and taken with or following food to reduce stomach irritation. Shake the suspension well before measuring the dose. If you forget a dose: Take the missed dose as soon as you remember it, unless it's nearly time for your next dose—if that is the case, skip the missed dose and take the next dose right on schedule. DO NOT double doses. Talk with your doctor if you find yourself missing doses.

Usual Duration of Use: Use on a regular schedule for 2 to 4 weeks usually determines effectiveness in reducing the frequency and severity of seizures. Long-term use (months to years) requires physician supervision.

Typical Treatment Goals and Measurements (Outcomes and Markers)

Seizures: The general goal for this medicine is effective seizure control. Neurologists tend to define "effective" on a case-by-case basis depending on the seizure type and patient factors. If seizure control is not effective with an initial choice, it's not unusual to use a second-line agent or combination treatment.

▷ **This Drug Should Not Be Taken If**
- you have had an allergic reaction to it previously.
- you are allergic to phenobarbital.
- you have a history of porphyria.

▷ **Inform Your Physician Before Taking This Drug If**
- you have had an allergic or idiosyncratic reaction to any barbiturate drug in the past.
- you have a family history of intermittent porphyria.
- you have impaired liver, kidney or thyroid gland function.
- you have asthma, emphysema or myasthenia gravis.
- you are pregnant or planning pregnancy.
- you plan to have surgery under general anesthesia in the near future.

Possible Side Effects (natural, expected and unavoidable drug actions)
Drowsiness, impaired concentration, mental and physical sluggishness.

▷ **Possible Adverse Effects** (unusual, unexpected and infrequent reactions)
If any of the following develop, consult your physician promptly for guidance.

Mild Adverse Effects
Allergic reactions: skin rashes, hives, localized swelling.
"Hangover" effect, dizziness, unsteadiness, impaired vision, double vision,

fatigue, emotional disturbances—more likely during first 3 months, may ease with time.

Low blood pressure, faintness—possible.

Shoulder pain, joint pain—possible with longer-term therapy.

Nausea, vomiting, thirst, increased urine volume—rare to infrequent.

Serious Adverse Effects

Allergic reactions: swelling of lymph glands.

Idiosyncratic reactions: paradoxical anxiety, seizures, agitation, restlessness, rage.

Visual or auditory hallucinations—rare.

Drug-induced porphyria, systemic lupus erythematosus or low thyroid gland function (hypothyroidism)—case reports.

Blood cell disorders: megaloblastic anemia, low white blood cells or platelets—case reports.

Drug-induced kidney problems (crystalluria)—case report.

▷ **Possible Effects on Sexual Function:** Decreased libido and/or impotence—case reports.

Decreased effectiveness of oral contraceptives.

▷ **Adverse Effects That May Mimic Natural Diseases or Disorders**

Allergic swelling of lymph glands may suggest a naturally occurring lymphoma.

Natural Diseases or Disorders That May Be Activated by This Drug

Acute intermittent and/or cutaneous porphyria (see Glossary). Systemic lupus erythematosus.

Possible Effects on Laboratory Tests

Complete blood cell counts: decreased red cells, hemoglobin, white cells and platelets; increased eosinophils.

Blood lupus erythematosus cells: positive.

Prothrombin time: decreased (when taken concurrently with warfarin).

Urine screening tests for drug abuse: may be **positive** for phenobarbital (a normal derivative of this drug). Test results depend upon amount of drug taken and testing method.

CAUTION

1. This drug must not be stopped abruptly.
2. A wide variation of drug action from person to person requires careful individualization of dose.
3. Regularity of drug use is essential for the successful management of seizure disorders. Take your medication at the same time each day.
4. Side effects and mild adverse effects are usually most apparent during the first several weeks of treatment and often subside with continued use.
5. It may be necessary to take folic acid to prevent anemia while taking this drug. Consult your physician.
6. It is advisable to carry a card of personal identification with a notation that you are taking this drug.

Precautions for Use

By Infants and Children: This drug should be used with caution in children. Paradoxical hyperactivity is possible. Puberty changes characteristically slow phenobarbital metabolism, permitting gradual accumulation. Measurements of blood levels in young adolescents can detect rising concentrations of this drug that could lead to toxicity (see "Therapeutic Drug Monitoring" in Section One).

By Those Over 60 Years of Age: It is advisable for the elderly to avoid all barbiturates if possible. If use of this drug is attempted, small starting doses are indicated. Watch for confusion, delirium, agitation or paradoxical excitement. This drug may be conducive to hypothermia (see Glossary).

▷ **Advisability of Use During Pregnancy**

Pregnancy Category: D. See Pregnancy Risk Categories at the back of this book.

Animal studies: Birth defects due to this drug reported in mice.

Human studies: Adequate studies of pregnant women are not available, but recent reports suggest a possible association between the use of this drug during the first 3 months of pregnancy and the development of birth defects in the fetus.

Discuss with your physician the advantages and possible disadvantages of using this drug during pregnancy. If it is used, determine the smallest maintenance dose that will prevent seizures. The newborn infants of mothers who take this drug during pregnancy may develop abnormal bleeding or bruising due to the deficiency of certain blood-clotting factors in the blood. Consult your physician regarding the need to take vitamin K during the final month of pregnancy.

Advisability of Use If Breast-Feeding

Presence of this drug in breast milk: Yes.

Monitor nursing infant closely, and discontinue drug or nursing if adverse effects develop.

Habit-Forming Potential: None.

Effects of Overdose: Drowsiness, jerky eye movements, blurred vision, staggering gait, incoordination, slurred speech, stupor progressing to coma.

Possible Effects of Long-Term Use: Enlargement of lymph glands; enlargement of thyroid gland. Megaloblastic anemia due to folic acid deficiency. Reduced blood levels of calcium and phosphorus, leading to rickets in children and loss of bone texture (osteomalacia) in adults.

Suggested Periodic Examinations While Taking This Drug (at physician's discretion)

Complete blood cell counts.

Measurements of blood levels of calcium and phosphorus.

Evaluation of lymph and thyroid glands.

Skeletal X-ray examinations for bone demineralization during long-term use.

▷ **While Taking This Drug, Observe the Following**

Foods: No restrictions.

Herbal Medicines or Minerals: Valerian and kava kava may interact to increase drowsiness. Using kola or ma huang may result in unacceptable central nervous system stimulation. Increased calcium and vitamin D are prudent.

Nutritional Support: Talk with your doctor about calcium, vitamin D and K and folic acid supplements.

Beverages: No restrictions. May be taken with milk or fruit juice.

▷ *Alcohol:* Avoid completely. Alcohol can greatly increase the sedative and depressant effects of this drug on brain function.

Tobacco Smoking: May enhance the sedative effects of this drug. I advise everyone to quit smoking.

▷ *Other Drugs*

Note: 15% of primidone is converted to phenobarbital in the body. As such,
phenobarbital possible interactions with other drugs are included for com-
pleteness.

Phenobarbital may *increase* the effects of
- all other drugs with sedative effects and cause excessive sedation.

Phenobarbital may *decrease* the effects of
- anticoagulants (Coumadin, etc.) and require dose adjustments based on
  more frequent INR (prothrombin time or protime) testing.
- certain beta blockers (Inderal, Lopressor) and reduce their effectiveness.
- birth control pills (oral contraceptives) and reduce their effectiveness in
  preventing pregnancy.
- bupropion (Wellbutrin).
- carbamazepine (Tegretol).
- cortisonelike drugs (see Drug Classes).
- cyclosporine (Sandimmune).
- delavirdine (Rescriptor).
- diltiazem (Cardizem).
- disopyramide (Norpace).
- donepezil (Aricept).
- doxycycline (Vibramycin).
- felodipine (Plendil).
- griseofulvin (Fulvicin, etc.).
- indinavir (Crixivan) and perhaps other protease inhibitors (see Drug
  Classes).
- lamotrigine (Lamictal).
- levonorgestrel (Norplant), requiring alternative birth control.
- metoprolol (Lopressor, others).
- montelukast (Singulair).
- nimodipine (Nimotop).
- quinidine (Quinaglute, etc.) and reduce its effectiveness.
- paroxetine (Paxil).
- propafenone (Rythmol).
- propranolol (Inderal).
- serolimus (Rapamune) or tacrolimus (Prograf).
- ritonavir (Norvir).
- theophyllines (Aminophyllin, Theo-Dur, etc.) and reduce their antiasthmatic effectiveness.
- tretinoin (Vesanoid).
- tricyclic antidepressants (see Drug Classes).
- verapamil (Calan) and reduce its effectiveness.
- venlafaxine (Effexor).
- warfarin (Coumadin) and increase risk of clots.

Phenobarbital *taken concurrently* with
- chloramphenicol (Chloromycetin) may result in decreased chloramphenicol benefits and phenobarbital toxicity—these drugs are NOT to be combined.
- clonazepam (Klonopin) may lead to more severe side effects than use with

phenytoin or carbamazepine. This combination would not be a first-line combination.

- colestipol (Colestid) and other cholesterol-lowering resins may bind phenobarbital and limit absorption.
- influenza vaccine may cause phenobarbital toxicity.
- itraconazole (and perhaps other antifungals) may decrease the antifungal effect of itraconazole.
- monoamine oxidase (MAO) inhibitors (see Drug Classes) may lead to excessive lethargy and difficulty talking.
- phenytoin (Dilantin) or fosphenytoin (Cerebyx) may alter phenytoin blood levels: a high phenobarbital level will increase the phenytoin level; a low phenobarbital level will decrease the phenytoin level. Periodic determination of blood levels of both drugs is advised.

The following drugs may *increase* the effects of phenobarbital:

- ascorbic acid (vitamin C).
- felbamate (Felbatol).
- valproic acid (Depakene).
- zotepine (Nipolept).

▷ *Driving, Hazardous Activities:* This drug may cause drowsiness and dizziness; it can also impair mental alertness, vision and physical coordination. Restrict activities as necessary.

Aviation Note: The use of this drug *is a disqualification* for piloting. Consult a designated Aviation Medical Examiner.

Exposure to Sun: No restrictions.

Occurrence of Unrelated Illness: Notify your physician of any illness or injury that prevents the use of this drug according to your regular dose schedule.

Discontinuation: **Do not stop this drug without your physician's knowledge and approval**. Sudden withdrawal of any anticonvulsant drug can cause severe and repeated seizures.

PROBENECID (proh BEN e sid)

Introduced: 1951   **Class:** Antigout   **Prescription:** USA: Yes   **Controlled Drug:**   USA: No; Canada: No   **Available as Generic:**   USA: Yes; Canada: No

Brand Names: ♣Ampicin PRB [CD], Benemid, ♣Benuryl, Colabid [CD], Col-Benemid [CD], Polycillin-PRB [CD], Probalan, Probampacin [CD], Proben-C [CD], ♣Pro-Biosan 500 Kit [CD], SK-Probenecid

BENEFITS versus RISKS	
Possible Benefits	*Possible Risks*
EFFECTIVE LONG-TERM PREVENTION OF ACUTE ATTACKS OF GOUT	Formation of uric acid kidney stones
	Bone marrow depression (aplastic anemia)
Useful adjunct to penicillin therapy (to achieve high blood and tissue levels of penicillin)	Drug-induced liver and kidney damage

▷ **Principal Uses**

As a Single Drug Product: Uses currently included in FDA-approved labeling: (1) Used in helping maintain penicillin levels in therapy of gonorrhea; (2) helps decrease elevated uric acid levels caused by thiazide diuretics; (3) helps prevent gout.

Other (unlabeled) generally accepted uses: (1) May have a role in preventing kidney toxicity in cisplatin chemotherapy; (2) adjunctive use in maintaining effective antibiotic levels in treatment of syphilis; (3) may prevent kidney damage from some kinds of nephrotoxic drugs (such as Vistide for HIV).

As a Combination Drug Product [CD]: This drug is available in combination with colchicine, a drug often used for the treatment of acute gout. Each drug works in a different way; when used in combination they provide both relief of the acute gout and some measure of protection from recurrence of acute attacks.

How This Drug Works: Works in the kidney (tubular systems) to increase uric acid excretion in the urine; this drug reduces the levels of uric acid in the blood and body tissues. It also works in the kidney to decrease the amount of penicillin excreted in the urine, prolongs the presence of penicillin in the blood and helps achieve higher concentrations in body tissues.

Available Dosage Forms and Strengths

Tablets — 500 mg

▷ **Usual Adult Dosage Ranges:** *Anti-gout*: Initially 250 mg twice a day for 1 week and then 500 mg twice a day. *Adjunct to penicillin therapy*: 500 mg four times a day. **Note: Actual dose and schedule must be determined for each patient individually.**

Conditions Requiring Dosing Adjustments

Liver Function: Specific guidelines for dose adjustment in liver compromise are not available. This drug should be used with caution.

Kidney Function: Patients with kidney failure (creatinine clearance less than 30 ml/min) should not use this drug, as the effectiveness is questionable. Those with moderate kidney failure may still benefit from this medicine, and dose increases (as needed and tolerated) in 500-mg steps up to 2,000 mg a day in equally divided doses may be required.

▷ **Dosing Instructions:** The tablet may be crushed and taken with or following food to reduce stomach irritation. Drink 2.5 to 3 quarts of liquids daily. If you forget a dose: Take the missed dose as soon as you remember it, unless it's nearly time for your next dose—if that is the case, skip the missed dose and take the next dose right on schedule. DO NOT double doses. Talk with your doctor if you find yourself missing doses as there are many strategies to help.

Usual Duration of Use: Use on a regular schedule for several months usually determines effectiveness in preventing acute attacks of gout. Long-term use (months to years) requires supervision and periodic evaluation by your physician.

Typical Treatment Goals and Measurements (Outcomes and Markers)

Uric acid: Blood uric acid levels often decrease in 48 to 72 hours and may reach normal range in 1 to 3 weeks. Attacks of gout should become shorter and lessen in severity over time.

▷ **This Drug Should Not Be Taken If**
  - you have had an allergic reaction to it previously.
  - you have active liver disease.
  - you have acute kidney failure or kidney stones made of uric acid.
  - you are less than 2 years old.
  - you have an active blood cell or bone marrow disorder.
  - you are having an attack of acute gout at the present time.

▷ **Inform Your Physician Before Taking This Drug If**
  - you have a history of kidney disease or kidney stones.
  - you have a history of liver disease or impaired liver function.
  - you have a history of peptic ulcer disease.
  - you have a history of a blood cell or bone marrow disorder.
  - you are taking any drug product that contains aspirin or aspirinlike drugs.

Possible Side Effects (natural, expected and unavoidable drug actions)
  Development of kidney stones (composed of uric acid)—this is preventable.
  Consult your physician regarding the use of sodium bicarbonate (or other
  urine alkalizer) to prevent stone formation.

▷ **Possible Adverse Effects** (unusual, unexpected and infrequent reactions)
  **If any of the following develop, consult your physician promptly for
  guidance.**
  Mild Adverse Effects
  Allergic reactions: skin rash, itching, drug fever (see Glossary).
  Headache, dizziness, flushing of face—infrequent.
  Reduced appetite, sore gums, nausea, vomiting—possible to infrequent.
  Serious Adverse Effects
  Allergic reactions: anaphylactic reaction (see Glossary).
  Idiosyncratic reactions: hemolytic anemia (see Glossary).
  Bone marrow depression (see Glossary): fatigue, sore throat, bleeding/bruis-
  ing—case reports.
  Drug-induced liver damage with jaundice (see Glossary) or porphyria—case
  reports.
  Fluid in the retina (retinal edema)—case reports.
  Drug-induced kidney damage: marked fluid retention, reduced urine forma-
  tion—case reports.

▷ **Possible Effects on Sexual Function:** None reported.

▷ **Adverse Effects That May Mimic Natural Diseases or Disorders**
  Liver reactions may suggest viral hepatitis. Kidney reactions may suggest
  nephrosis.

Possible Effects on Laboratory Tests
  Complete blood cell counts: decreased red cells, hemoglobin, white cells and
  platelets.
  INR (prothrombin time): increased (when taken concurrently with war-
  farin).
  Blood glucose level and uric acid level: decreased.
  Blood urea nitrogen (BUN) level: increased (kidney damage).
  Liver function tests: increased enzymes (ALT/GPT, AST/GOT, alkaline phos-
  phatase) or bilirubin.
  Urine sugar tests: false positive with Benedict's solution and Clinitest.

CAUTION
1. This drug should not be started until 2 to 3 weeks after an acute attack of gout has subsided.
2. This drug may increase the frequency of acute attacks of gout during the first few months of treatment. Concurrent use of colchicine is advised to prevent acute attacks.
3. Aspirin (and aspirin-containing drug products) can reduce the effectiveness of this drug. Use acetaminophen or a nonaspirin analgesic for pain relief as needed.

Precautions for Use
By Infants and Children: Safety and effectiveness for those under 2 years of age are not established.
By Those Over 60 Years of Age: The natural decline in kidney function that occurs after 60 may require adjustment of your dose. You may be more susceptible to the serious adverse effects of this drug. Report any unusual symptoms promptly for evaluation.

▷ **Advisability of Use During Pregnancy**
Pregnancy Category: B. See Pregnancy Risk Categories at the back of this book.
Animal studies: No information available.
Human studies: Adequate studies of pregnant women are not available.
This drug has been used during pregnancy with no reports of birth defects or adverse effects on the fetus. Ask your physician for guidance.

Advisability of Use If Breast-Feeding
Presence of this drug in breast milk: Unknown.
Avoid drug or refrain from nursing.

Habit-Forming Potential: None.

Effects of Overdose: Stomach irritation, nausea, vomiting, nervous agitation, delirium, seizures, coma.

Possible Effects of Long-Term Use: Formation of kidney stones. Kidney damage in sensitive individuals.

Suggested Periodic Examinations While Taking This Drug (at physician's discretion)
Complete blood cell counts.
Blood uric acid.
Liver and kidney function tests.

▷ **While Taking This Drug, Observe the Following**
Foods: Follow your physician's advice regarding the need for a low-purine diet.
Herbal Medicines or Minerals: Acerola is high in vitamin C. Inosine, like acerola, may increase uric acid levels. Aspen should be avoided in gout. Lipase may worsen gout. Goutweed (aegopodium podagraria) does not have enough data to assess effectiveness.
Beverages: A large intake of coffee, tea or cola beverages may reduce the effectiveness of treatment.
▷ *Alcohol:* No interactions expected, but large amounts of alcohol can raise the blood uric acid level and reduce the effectiveness of treatment.
Tobacco Smoking: No interactions expected. I advise everyone to quit smoking.

▷ *Other Drugs*

Probenecid may *increase* the effects of
- acetaminophen (Tylenol), increasing risk of toxicity.
- acyclovir (Zovirax) and result in toxicity unless doses are reduced.
- ciprofloxacin (Cipro) and gatifloxacin (Tequin), increasing toxicity risk.
- clofibrate (Atromid-S).
- dyphylline (Neothylline).
- entacapone (Comtan).
- ketoprofen and perhaps other NSAIDs (see Drug Classes).
- ketorolac (Toradol) and increase toxicity risk.
- methotrexate (Mexate) and increase its toxicity.
- midazolam (Versed) and increase CNS depression.
- oral antidiabetic agents (see Drug Classes).
- oseltamivir (Tamiflu).
- thiopental (Pentothal) and prolong its anesthetic effect.
- valacyclovir (Valtrex) and result in toxicity unless doses are reduced.
- zalcitabine (Hivid).
- zidovudine (Retrovir) and increase toxicity risk.

Probenecid *taken concurrently* with
- allopurinol (Zyloprim) may result in extended allopurinol half-life.
- cephalosporins (see Drug Classes) may cause a doubling of antibiotic levels. Caution must be used to avoid toxicity.
- dapsone may cause up to a 50% increased dapsone level and result in toxicity unless dapsone doses are decreased.
- penicillins (see Drug Classes) may cause a threefold to fivefold increase in penicillin blood levels, greatly increasing the effectiveness of each penicillin dose.
- rifampin (Rifadin, others) may result in increased blood levels of rifampin.
- ritonavir (Norvir) may lead to changes in probenecid blood levels.

The following drugs may *decrease* the effects of probenecid:
- aspirin and other salicylates—may reduce its effectiveness in promoting the excretion of uric acid.
- bismuth subsalicylate (Pepto-Bismol, others).

▷ *Driving, Hazardous Activities:* This drug may cause dizziness. Restrict activities as necessary.

Aviation Note: The use of this drug *may be a disqualification* for piloting. Consult a designated Aviation Medical Examiner.

Exposure to Sun: No restrictions.

Discontinuation: Do not stop this drug without consulting your physician.

PROCAINAMIDE (proh KAYN a mide)

Introduced: 1950   **Class:** Antiarrhythmic   **Prescription:** USA: Yes
Controlled Drug: USA: No; Canada: No   **Available as Generic:** USA: Yes; Canada: No
Brand Names: ✤Apo-Procainamide, Procamide SR, Procanbid, Procan SR (no longer manufactured), Promine, Pronestyl, Pronestyl-SR, Rhythmin

---

BENEFITS versus RISKS

Possible Benefits	*Possible Risks*
EFFECTIVE TREATMENT OF SELECTED HEART RHYTHM DISORDERS	NARROW TREATMENT RANGE CAUSES SYSTEMIC LUPUS ERYTHEMATOSUS SYNDROME Provocation of abnormal heart rhythms Blood cell disorders: insufficient white blood cells and platelets

---

▷ **Principal Uses**

As a Single Drug Product: Uses currently included in FDA-approved labeling: Used to abolish and prevent the recurrence of premature beats arising in the ventricles (lower chambers) of the heart.

Other (unlabeled) generally accepted uses: (1) Used to treat and prevent atrial fibrillation, atrial flutter and abnormally rapid heart rates (tachycardia) that originate in the atria or the ventricles; (2) helps treat myotonia and improve breathing in myotonic dystrophy.

How This Drug Works: By slowing the activity of the pacemaker and delaying the transmission of electrical impulses through the conduction system and muscle of the heart, this drug assists in restoring normal heart rate and rhythm.

Available Dosage Forms and Strengths

Capsules — 250 mg, 375 mg, 500 mg

Injections — 100 mg/ml, 500 mg/ml

Tablets — 250 mg, 375 mg, 500 mg

Tablets, prolonged action — 250 mg, 500 mg, 750 mg, 1,000 mg

▷ **Usual Adult Dosage Ranges:** Dose varies according to indication. Starting dose is up to 50 mg per kg of body mass per day of the immediate-release form. This calculated dose is then divided into equal doses and is taken every 3, 4 or 6 hours. The ongoing daily dose should be adjusted to individual patient response and blood levels. People over 50 years old may get an acceptable clinical response and blood level from a lower dose. The sustained-release form is usually started in younger patients who do not have kidney problems at 50 mg per kg of body mass per day. This calculated dose is divided into equal doses and is taken every 6 to 12 hours, depending on patient response and blood levels. The Procanbid form is a true twice-a-day dosage form given every 12 hours. The prior Procan-SR was taken four times daily (QID). **Note: Actual dose and schedule must be determined for each patient individually.**

Author's Note: Information in this profile has been shortened to make room for more widely used medicines.

PROCHLORPERAZINE (proh klor PER a zeen)

Introduced: 1956   **Class:** Antipsychotic, antiemetic, phenothiazines   **Prescription:** USA: Yes   **Controlled Drug:** USA: No; Canada: No   **Available as Generic:** USA: Yes; Canada: Yes

Brand Names: ✦Combid [CD], Compazine, Eskatrol, ✦PMS-Prochlorperazine, Pro-Iso, ✦Stemetil, Ultrazine [CD]

```
┌─────────────────────────────────────────────────────────────────────┐
│                       BENEFITS versus RISKS                          │
│        Possible Benefits                    Possible Risks           │
│ EFFECTIVE CONTROL OF ACUTE        SERIOUS TOXIC EFFECTS ON            │
│   MENTAL DISORDERS, NAUSEA          BRAIN WITH LONG-TERM USE          │
│   AND VOMITING                    Liver damage with jaundice          │
│ Relief of anxiety and nervous tension   Blood cell disorders: abnormally low │
│                                     white cell and platelet counts   │
└─────────────────────────────────────────────────────────────────────┘
```

▷ **Principal Uses**

As a Single Drug Product: Uses currently included in FDA-approved labeling: (1) Relieves severe nausea and vomiting; (2) may be used to treat schizophrenia; (3) helps prevent motion sickness.

Other (unlabeled) generally accepted uses: (1) Sometimes used to increase the effects of anesthesia; (2) may be of use in treating Ménière's disease (for nausea and vomiting).

How This Drug Works: By inhibiting the action of dopamine, this drug acts to correct an imbalance of nerve impulse transmissions that is thought to be responsible for certain mental disorders. By blocking dopamine in the brain's chemoreceptor trigger zone, this drug prevents stimulation of the vomiting center.

Available Dosage Forms and Strengths

Capsules, prolonged action — 10 mg, 15 mg, 30 mg

Injection — 5 mg/ml

Suppositories — 2.5 mg, 5 mg, 25 mg

Syrup — 5 mg/5 ml

Tablets — 5 mg, 10 mg, 25 mg

▷ **Usual Adult Dosage Ranges:** *For nausea and vomiting*: 5 to 10 mg three or four times daily. The sustained-release form can be taken as 15 mg when you wake up in the morning or 10 mg of the sustained-release form every 12 hours.

For moderate to severe psychotic problems: Initially 10 mg of the immediate-release form every 6 to 8 hours. If needed and tolerated, dose may be increased by 5 mg at intervals of 3 to 4 days. Usual range is 50 to 75 mg daily. The total daily dose should not exceed 150 mg.

Note: Actual dose and dosing schedule must be determined for each patient individually.

Conditions Requiring Dosing Adjustments

Liver Function: This drug should be used with caution by patients with liver compromise. Specific guidelines for dose adjustment are not available.

Kidney Function: Specific guidelines for adjustment of doses are not available.

▷ **Dosing Instructions:** The tablets may be crushed and taken with or following food to reduce stomach irritation. Prolonged-action capsules should be swallowed whole without alteration. If you forget a dose: and you take several doses a day, take the missed dose as soon as you remember it, unless your next dose is due in about an hour—if that is the case, skip the missed dose and take the next dose right on schedule. If you only take one dose a day, take the missed dose as soon as you remember it, unless it's almost time for your next dose—then skip the dose you forgot and take the next dose on schedule. Talk with your doctor if you find yourself missing doses.

Usual Duration of Use: Use on a regular schedule for 12 to 24 hours usually determines effectiveness in controlling nausea and vomiting. If used for severe anxiety-tension states or acute psychotic behavior, a trial of several weeks is usually necessary to determine effectiveness. If not significantly beneficial within 6 weeks, it should be stopped. Consult your physician on a regular basis.

Typical Treatment Goals and Measurements (Outcomes and Markers)

Vomiting: The goal is to prevent or at least to decrease vomiting (emesis) frequency, amount or severity.

▷ **This Drug Should Not Be Taken If**
- you have had an allergic reaction to it previously.
- you have active liver disease.
- you have signs that are indicative of Reye's syndrome.
- you have extremely low blood pressure.
- you have cancer of the breast.
- this drug was prescribed for a child who is less than 2 years old or who weighs less than 20 lb.
- you have a current blood cell or bone marrow disorder.

▷ **Inform Your Physician Before Taking This Drug If**
- you are allergic or abnormally sensitive to any phenothiazine drug (see Drug Classes).
- you have impaired liver or kidney function.
- you have any type of seizure disorder.
- you have bone marrow depression or a history of blood diseases or ulcers.
- you have diabetes, glaucoma or heart disease.
- you have prostate trouble (prostatic hypertrophy).
- you are pregnant.
- you have had neuroleptic malignant syndrome or lupus erythematosus.
- you are taking any drug with sedative effects.
- you plan to have surgery under general or spinal anesthesia in the near future.

Possible Side Effects (natural, expected and unavoidable drug actions)

Drowsiness (usually during the first 2 weeks), orthostatic hypotension (see Glossary), blurred vision, dry mouth, nasal congestion, constipation, impaired urination. Pink or purple coloration of urine—of no significance.

▷ **Possible Adverse Effects** (unusual, unexpected and infrequent reactions)

If any of the following develop, consult your physician promptly for guidance.

Mild Adverse Effects

Allergic reactions: skin rash, hives, low-grade fever.

Lowering of body temperature, especially in the elderly (see hypothermia in Glossary)—possible.

Increased appetite and weight gain—possible.

Increased blood pressure—infrequent.

Dizziness, weakness—frequent.

Agitation, insomnia, impaired day and night vision—infrequent.

Chronic constipation, fecal impaction, incontinence—infrequent.

Serious Adverse Effects

Allergic reactions: hepatitis with jaundice (see Glossary), usually between second and fourth week; high fever; asthma; anaphylactic reaction (see Glossary).

Idiosyncratic reactions: toxic dermatitis, Stevens-Johnson syndrome.

Neuroleptic malignant syndrome (see Glossary).

Liver toxicity or porphyria—case reports.

Abnormal eye positioning (oculogyric crisis)—case reports.

Depression, disorientation, seizures—case reports.

Abnormally high blood pressure—rare.

Disturbances of heart rhythm, rapid heart rate—rare.

Bone marrow depression (see Glossary)—case reports.

Parkinson-like disorders (see Glossary); muscle spasms of face, jaw, neck, back, extremities; slowed movements, muscle rigidity, tremors; tardive dyskinesias (see Glossary)—case reports.

▷ **Possible Effects on Sexual Function:** Altered timing and pattern of menstruation.

Female breast enlargement with milk production—case reports.

Causes false-positive pregnancy test result.

Male breast enlargement and tenderness (gynecomastia), inhibited ejaculation or priapism (see Glossary)—case reports.

▷ **Adverse Effects That May Mimic Natural Diseases or Disorders**

Nervous system reactions may suggest Parkinson's disease. Liver reactions may suggest viral hepatitis. Reactions resembling systemic lupus erythematosus can occur.

Natural Diseases or Disorders That May Be Activated by This Drug

Latent epilepsy, glaucoma, diabetes mellitus, prostatism (see Glossary).

Possible Effects on Laboratory Tests

White blood cell count: decreased.

Liver function tests: increased enzymes (ALT/GPT, AST/GOT, alkaline phosphatase) or bilirubin.

CAUTION

1. Many over-the-counter medications (see Glossary) for allergies, colds and coughs contain drugs that can interact unfavorably with this drug. Ask your doctor or pharmacist for help before using any such medications.
2. Aluminum- or magnesium-containing antacids can limit absorption of this drug and reduce its effectiveness.
3. Obtain prompt evaluation of any change or disturbance of vision.

Precautions for Use

By Infants and Children: Do not use this drug in infants under 2 years of age or in children of any age with symptoms suggestive of Reye's syndrome (see Glossary). Children with acute illnesses ("flu-like" infections, measles, chicken pox, etc.) are very susceptible to adverse effects when this drug is given to control nausea and vomiting.

By Those Over 60 Years of Age: Small starting doses are advisable. You may be more susceptible to drowsiness, lethargy, constipation, lowering of body temperature (hypothermia) and orthostatic hypotension (see Glossary).

This drug can worsen existing prostatism (see Glossary). You may also be more susceptible to the development of Parkinson-like reactions and/or tardive dyskinesia (see discussion of these terms in Glossary). These reactions must be recognized early, because they may become unresponsive to treatment and irreversible.

▷ **Advisability of Use During Pregnancy**

Pregnancy Category: C. See Pregnancy Risk Categories at the back of this book.

Animal studies: Cleft palate reported in mouse and rat studies.

Human studies: No increase in birth defects reported in 2,023 exposures. Information from adequate studies of pregnant women is not available.

Limit use to small and infrequent doses. Avoid drug during the final month because of possible effects on the newborn infant.

Advisability of Use If Breast-Feeding

Presence of this drug in breast milk: Yes, in small amounts.

Stop nursing or change to a different medicine. Talk to your doctor before making any medicine changes.

Habit-Forming Potential: None, but it has been used in combination with pentazocine as a heroin substitute by drug abusers.

Effects of Overdose: Marked drowsiness, weakness, tremor, agitation, unsteadiness, deep sleep, coma, convulsions.

Possible Effects of Long-Term Use: Tardive dyskinesias. Eye changes—opacities in cornea or lens, retinal pigmentation.

Suggested Periodic Examinations While Taking This Drug (at physician's discretion)

Complete blood cell counts, especially between the 4th and 10th weeks of treatment.

Liver function tests.

Electrocardiograms.

Complete eye examinations—eye structures and vision.

Careful inspection of the tongue for early evidence of fine, involuntary, wavelike movements that could indicate the beginning of tardive dyskinesia.

▷ **While Taking This Drug, Observe the Following**

Foods: No restrictions. Vitamin C in high doses may lower therapeutic benefits.

Herbal Medicines or Minerals: Kava and valerian may worsen drowsiness. Caution is advised. Since part of the way that ginseng works may be as a MAO inhibitor, the combination is NOT advisable. Both prochlorperazine and St. John's wort may lead to increased sun sensitivity—CAUTION IS ADVISED.

Nutritional Support: A riboflavin (vitamin B_2) supplement should be taken with long-term use.

Beverages: No restrictions. May be taken with milk.

▷ *Alcohol:* Avoid completely. Alcohol can increase phenothiazine sedation and accentuate depressant effects on brain function and blood pressure. Phenothiazines can increase intoxicating effects of alcohol.

Tobacco Smoking: Possible reduction of drowsiness from drug. I advise everyone to quit smoking.

Marijuana Smoking: Moderate increase in drowsiness; accentuation of orthostatic hypotension; increased risk of precipitating latent psychoses, confusing the interpretation of mental status and drug responses.

▷   *Other Drugs*

Prochlorperazine may *increase* the effects of
- all atropinelike drugs and cause nervous system toxicity.
- cisapride (Propulsid), increasing risk of dangerous heart rhythms.
- gatifloxacin (Tequin), grepafloxacin (Raxar), moxifloxacin (Avelox) or sparfloxacin (Zagam), increasing risk of abnormal heartbeats.
- all sedative drugs, especially meperidine (Demerol), and cause excessive sedation.

Prochlorperazine may **decrease** the effects of
- guanethidine (Ismelin, Esimil) and reduce its effectiveness in lowering blood pressure.

Prochlorperazine *taken concurrently* with
- dofetilide (Tikosyn), increases risk of abnormal heartbeats.
- lithium (Lithobid, others) may lead to movement disorders and brain damage.
- MAO inhibitors (see Drug Classes) may result in increased risk of abnormal body movements (extrapyramidal reactions).
- oral antidiabetic drugs (see Drug Classes) may blunt their therapeutic benefits.
- phenytoin (Dilantin, others) or fosphenytoin (Cerebyx) may have variable effects on phenytoin blood levels; more frequent blood levels are prudent if these drugs are combined.
- propranolol (Inderal) may cause increased effects of both drugs; monitor drug effects closely and adjust doses as necessary.
- ritonavir (Norvir) may lead to prochlorperazine toxicity.
- sparfloxacin (Zagam) may increase risk of abnormal heartbeats.
- tramadol (Ultram) may increase seizure risk.
- zotepine (Nipolept) may increase seizure risk.

The following drugs may decrease the effects of prochlorperazine:
- antacids containing aluminum and/or magnesium.
- benztropine (Cogentin).
- trihexyphenidyl (Artane).

▷   *Driving, Hazardous Activities:* This drug can impair mental alertness, judgment and physical coordination. Avoid hazardous activities.

Aviation Note: The use of this drug *is a disqualification* for piloting. Consult a designated Aviation Medical Examiner.

Exposure to Sun: Use caution until sensitivity has been determined. Some phenothiazines can cause photosensitivity (see Glossary).

Exposure to Heat: Use caution and avoid excessive heat as much as possible. This drug may impair the regulation of body temperature and increase the risk of heatstroke.

Exposure to Cold: Use caution and dress warmly. This drug can increase the risk of hypothermia in the elderly.

Discontinuation: After long-term use, do not stop this drug suddenly. Gradual withdrawal over 2 to 3 weeks under physician supervision is recommended.

PROPAFENONE (pro PAAF in own)

Introduced: 1998   **Class:** Antiarrhythmic (1C)   **Prescription:** USA:
Yes   **Controlled Drug:** USA: No; Canada: No   **Available as Generic:** No
Brand Name: Rythmol

BENEFITS versus RISKS

Possible Benefits	*Possible Risks*
EFFECTIVE TREATMENT IN SELECTED HEART RHYTHM DISORDERS	NARROW TREATMENT RANGE
	May worsen some arrhythmias
	Rare liver injury, reduced white blood cell count or positive ANA
BENEFICIAL IN LIFE-THREATENING VENTRICULAR ARRHYTHMIAS	

▷ **Principal Uses**

As a Single Drug Product: Uses currently included in FDA-approved labeling:
(1) Helps correct abnormal heartbeats (symptomatic paroxysmal atrial fibrillation or PAF or symptomatic paroxysmal supraventricular tachycardia
or PSVT) in people who do not have structural heart disease; (2) treats life-
threatening ventricular arrhythmias (such as sustained ventricular tachycardia).

Other (unlabeled) generally accepted uses: (1) Treats a variety of abnormal
heartbeats not arising from the ventricles (such as supraventricular tachycardia, Wolff-Parkinson-White syndrome and atrial flutter or fibrillation);
(2) helps correct or prevent ventricular arrhythmias that are started
(induced) by exercise.

How This Drug Works: Slows transmission of electrical impulses in the heart,
restoring normal heart rate and rhythm in selected types of arrhythmia.
(Class 1C agent that blocks the fast sodium current in Purkinje fibers and
heart muscle and slows the rate of increase of Phase 0 of the action
potential.)

Available Dosage Forms and Strengths

Tablets, coated — 150 mg, 225 mg, 300 mg

▷ **Usual Adult Dosage Ranges:** *Arrhythmia*: Dosing is started with 150 mg every 8
hours (450 mg daily). Dosing can then be increased (every 3 to 4 days), as
needed and tolerated to 225 mg every eight hours or 300 mg every eight
hours (900 mg daily). If the heartbeat changes (QRS widens) or if there is
second- or third-degree heart (atrioventricular) block, consideration
should be given to lowering the dose. Testing blood levels is advised even
though they have not related well to clinical effects.

Recently started (onset) atrial fibrillation: One loading dose by mouth of 600
mg often works. Some clinicians have used 150 mg every 4 hours to convert this kind of atrial fibrillation to normal sinus rhythm in 48 hours (for
patients who do not have cardiovascular decompensation). **Note: Actual
dose and schedule must be determined for each patient individually.**

Conditions Requiring Dosing Adjustments

Liver Function: The dose should be decreased by 20 to 30 percent, and blood
levels should be checked more frequently.

Kidney Function: Only one percent of this drug is removed by the kidneys. More frequent check of blood levels is prudent.

▷ **Dosing Instructions:** The tablet may be opened and taken with food or milk to reduce stomach upset. Take at the same times each day to obtain uniform results (even blood levels). If you forget a dose: Take the missed dose as soon as you remember it, unless you are more than four hours late—if that is the case, skip the missed dose and take the next dose right on schedule. DO NOT double doses. Talk with your doctor if you find yourself missing doses. Adherence—taking your medicine right on time and in the right dose is very important!

Usual Duration of Use: Use on a regular schedule determines effectiveness in correcting or preventing responsive rhythm disorders. If effective, use will often be ongoing. The time it takes to reach its peak effect can vary from patient to patient and may require dosing adjustments. Long-term use requires physician supervision. Use in stopping (aborting) recent onset atrial fibrillation may produce immediate results.

Typical Treatment Goals and Measurements (Outcomes and Markers)

Abnormal heartbeats: The general goal is to return the heart to a normal rhythm or at least to markedly reduce the occurrence of abnormal heartbeats. In life-threatening arrhythmias, the goal is to abort the abnormal beats and return the pattern to normal. Success at ongoing suppression may involve ambulatory checks of heart rate and rhythm for a day (such as in Holter monitoring). This kind of testing involves placement of adhesive backed temporary electrodes on the skin in several positions around the heart. A small heart rate and rhythm (EKG or ECG) recording device is carried around via a shoulder strap and records what the heart is doing over 24 hours. Once the recording is made, a scanning machine reviews the record, tallies abnormal heart beats or rhythms and gives a close and extended look at how the heart is reacting or benefiting from the medicines that the patient is taking. Repeat measurements can be made if doses are changes to check the success at keeping the heart in normal sinus rhythm!

▷ **This Drug Should Not Be Taken If**
- you have had an allergic reaction to it previously.
- your electrolytes are out of balance (talk to your doctor).
- you have second- or third-degree heart block (determined by electrocardiogram), uncorrected by a pacemaker.
- you have congestive heart failure that is not controlled.
- your bronchi are subject to spasm (bronchospasm).
- you have an excessively slow heartbeat (bradycardia).

▷ **Inform Your Physician Before Taking This Drug If**
- you had adverse reactions to other antiarrhythmic drugs.
- you have a seizure disorder.
- you have a history of heart disease of any kind, especially "heart block" or heart failure AND YOU DO NOT HAVE A PACEMAKER.
- you have impaired liver function.
- you have had an antinuclear antibody (ANA) test and the result (titer) was elevated.
- you have difficulty making sperm (spermatogenesis).

- you are prone to low blood pressure.
- you take digitalis, a potassium supplement or any diuretic drug that can cause potassium loss (ask your doctor).

Possible Side Effects (natural, expected and unavoidable drug actions)
Dizziness (may be frequent), unpleasant taste.

▷ **Possible Adverse Effects** (unusual, unexpected and infrequent reactions)
If any of the following develop, consult your physician promptly for guidance.

Mild Adverse Effects
Allergic reaction: skin rash.
Fatigue, sleep problems, headache, tremor—rare to infrequent.
Drug-induced fever—case report.
Cough or wheezing—case report.
Hair loss (alopecia)—rare.
Loss of appetite, nausea, vomiting, constipation, diarrhea, abdominal pain—rare to infrequent.

Serious Adverse Effects
Allergic reactions: anaphylaxis—case report.
Idiosyncratic reactions: not reported.
Peripheral neuropathy—case report.
Seizure—case report.
Drug-induced heart rhythm disorders: shortness of breath, palpitations, chest pain, swelling, ventricular fibrillation—infrequent.
Lowered sodium and increased urination (SIADH)—case reports.
Systemic lupus erythematosus—case report.
Liver damage with jaundice (see Glossary)—case reports (may happen after 2–4 weeks or after prolonged therapy).
Low white blood cell or platelet counts: fever, sore throat, abnormal bleeding/bruising-case reports.

▷ **Possible Effects on Sexual Function:**
Decreased sperm formation—possible.
Impotence—rare.

▷ **Adverse Effects That May Mimic Natural Diseases or Disorders**
Liver toxicity may suggest viral hepatitis.

Natural Diseases or Disorders That May Be Activated by This Drug
Latent epilepsy.

Possible Effects on Laboratory Tests
Blood white cell and platelet counts: decreased.
Liver function tests: increased liver enzymes (ALT/GPT, AST/GOT)—rare.
ANA titer: possibly increasing.

CAUTION
1. Thorough evaluation of your heart function (including electrocardiograms) is necessary prior to using this drug.
2. Periodic evaluation of your heart function is needed to determine your response to this drug. Some individuals may experience worsening of their heart rhythm disorder and/or deterioration of heart function. Close monitoring of heart rate, rhythm and overall performance is essential.
3. Dose must be adjusted carefully for each person. Do not change your dose without talking to your doctor.

4. Do not take any other antiarrhythmic drug while taking this drug unless you are directed to do so by your physician.
5. Carry a card in your purse or wallet saying that you take this drug. Tell health care providers that you take it.
6. In roughly 10% of patients and in people who also take quinidine, propafenone removal (metabolism) is slower than in other patients. Lower doses and more frequent blood level checks are prudent.
7. Removal of this drug from the body happens in a way that can become filled up (saturable biotransformation). This means that a small dose change may result in a larger than normally expected increase in blood level. If dosing is changed, a recheck of blood levels is prudent.
8. In a study called CAST (Cardiac Arrhythmia Suppression Trial), medicines similar to propafenone (Class 1C) used in patients who had a heart attack (MI) more than 6 days after the heart attack in treating non-life-threatening ventricular arrhythmias were found to actually lead to an increased risk of reversed cardiac arrest or death.
9. If an ANA titer is checked and persists or worsens, consideration must be given to stopping this medicine.
10. This medicine has NOT been evaluated for use in ongoing or chronic atrial fibrillation.

Precautions for Use
By Infants and Children: Safety and effectiveness have not been established.
By Those Over 60 Years of Age: Reduced liver function may require reduction in dose. Lower doses and slower increases (if required) in doses are prudent. Watch carefully for light-headedness, dizziness, unsteadiness and tendency to fall. One study reported use of one 600-mg loading dose of propafenone as effective for treating atrial fibrillation that has recently started.

▷ **Advisability of Use During Pregnancy**
Pregnancy Category: C. See Pregnancy Risk Categories at the back of this book.
Animal studies: No birth defects reported in mice, rats or rabbits, but an increased rate of fetal resorption was found.
Human studies: Adequate studies of pregnant women are not available.
Avoid during first 3 months. Use this drug only if clearly needed. Ask your physician for guidance.

Advisability of Use If Breast-Feeding
Presence of this drug in breast milk: Probably Yes.
This is a benefit-to-risk decision to be discussed with your doctor.

Habit-Forming Potential: None.

Effects of Overdose: Marked drop in blood pressure, abnormal heart rhythms, slow heartbeat, seizures.

Possible Effects of Long-Term Use: Liver function tests may increase.

Suggested Periodic Examinations While Taking This Drug (at physician's discretion)
Electrocardiograms.
Complete blood cell counts.
Liver function tests.
Blood levels.
ANA titer.

▷ **While Taking This Drug, Observe the Following**

Foods: No restrictions. Ask your physician about the need for salt restriction.

Herbal Medicines or Minerals: Kola, St. John's wort, ma huang and yohimbe may cause additive heart rate or rhythm problems. These are not advisable if you have heart rhythm difficulties. Using St. John's wort, ma huang, ephedra or kola while taking this medicine may result in unacceptable heart stimulation. Belladonna, henbane, scopolia, pheasant's eye extract or lily of the valley or squill powdered extracts should NOT be taken if you have abnormal heart rhythms.

Beverages: Caffeine may have an effect on heart rate and may not be desirable. Talk to your doctor about caffeine. Can be taken with milk.

▷ *Alcohol:* Use caution. Alcohol can increase the blood-pressure-lowering effects of this drug.

Tobacco Smoking: Nicotine may irritate the heart, reducing drug effectiveness. I advise everyone to quit smoking.

▷ *Other Drugs*

Propafenone may *increase* the effects of
- amitriptyline (Elavil, others) and perhaps other tricyclic antidepressants.
- antihypertensive drugs and cause excessive lowering of blood pressure.
- beta blockers (such as metoprolol or propranolol: see Drug Classes).
- cyclosporine (Sandimmune), leading to toxicity.
- quinidine (Quinaglute, various).
- theophylline (Theo-Dur, others), leading to theophylline toxicity and seizures.
- warfarin (Coumadin, others); more frequent INR tests and dose adjustments are needed.

Propafenone *taken concurrently* with
- amiodarone (Cordarone) may lead to excessive propafenone levels and toxicity; reduced doses may be required.
- bupropion (Zyban, Wellbutrin) increases propafenone levels and can cause toxicity.
- digoxin (Lanoxin, others) increases digoxin levels and can cause toxicity.
- dofetilide (Tikosyn) increases QTc interval and can lead to abnormal heart rhythms or cardiac arrest. Combination should be avoided.
- drugs that inhibit or are removed by CYP 2D6 (talk to your doctor) may increase propafenone effects.
- fluoxetine (Prozac) may lead to increased propafenone blood levels and toxicity if doses are not adjusted.
- paroxetine (Paxil) may lead to increased propafenone blood levels and toxicity if doses are not adjusted.
- quinidine (Quinaglute) may increase propafenone levels and lead to toxicity if doses are not adjusted.
- ritonavir (Norvir) and perhaps other protease inhibitors (see Drug Classes) may lead to propafenone toxicity.
- sertraline (Zoloft) may lead to propafenone toxicity.

The following drugs may *decrease* the effects of propafenone:
- carbamazepine (Tegretol).
- phenobarbital (various).
- rifampin (Rifadin, Rimactane).

▷ *Driving, Hazardous Activities:* This drug may cause weakness, dizziness or blurred vision. Restrict activities as necessary.

Aviation Note: The use of this drug *may be a disqualification* for piloting. Consult a designated Aviation Medical Examiner.

Exposure to Sun: No restrictions.

Occurrence of Unrelated Illness: Vomiting, diarrhea or dehydration can affect this drug's action adversely. Report such developments promptly.

Discontinuation: Should not be stopped abruptly after long-term use. Ask your doctor about slowly reducing the dose.

PROPIONIC ACID (NONSTEROIDAL ANTI-INFLAMMATORY DRUG) FAMILY

Fenoprofen (FEN oh proh fen) **Flurbiprofen** (flur BI proh fen) **Ibuprofen** (common: I byu PROH fen; correct: i BYU proh fen) **Ketoprofen** (kee toh PROH fen) **Naproxen** (na PROX in) **Oxaprozin** (OX a proh zin)

Introduced: 1976, 1977, 1974, 1973, 1974, 1992, respectively   **Class:** Analgesic, mild; NSAIDs   **Prescription:** USA: Varies   **Controlled Drug:** USA: No; Canada: No   **Available as Generic:** Yes

Brand Names: Fenoprofen: Nalfon, Flurbiprofen: Ansaid, ✦Apo-Flurbiprofen, ✦Froben, ✦Froben-SR, Novo-Flurbiprofen, Ocufen, Ibuprofen: Aches-N-Pain, Actiprofen, Advil, Advil Migraine, ✦Amersol, ✦Apo-Ibuprofen, Arthritis Foundation Pain Reliever/Fever Reducer, Bayer Select, Children's Advil, Children's Motrin, Children's Motrin Drops (nonprescription), Children's Motrin Suspension (nonprescription), CoAdvil [CD], Dimetapp Sinus [CD], Dologesic, Dristan Sinus, Excedrin IB, Genpril, Guildprofen, Haltran, Ibu, Ibuprohm, Junior Strength Motrin Caplets (nonprescription), Medipren, Medi-Profen, Midol IB, Motrin, Motrin IB, ✦Novo-Profen, Nuprin, PediaProfen, Profen-IB, Rufen, Superior Pain Medicine, Supreme Pain Medicine, Tab-Profen, Ketoprofen: Actron (12.5 mg nonprescription), ✦Apo-Keto, ✦Apo-Keto E, Orudis, Orudis E-50, Orudis E-100, Orudis KT (nonprescription), Orudis SR, Oruvail, Oruvail ER, ✦Oruvail SR, ✦Rhodis, ✦Rhodis EC, ✦Rhodis EC Suppository, Naproxen: Aleve (220 mg nonprescription), Anaprox, Anaprox DS, ✦Apo-Naproxen, Naprelan, Naprelan Once Daily, Naprosyn, ✦Naxen, Neo-Prox, ✦Novo-Naprox, ✦Nu-Naprox, ✦Synflex, Oxaprozin: Daypro

BENEFITS versus RISKS	
Possible Benefits	*Possible Risks*
EFFECTIVE RELIEF OF MILD TO MODERATE PAIN AND INFLAMMATION	Gastrointestinal pain, ulceration, bleeding
EFFECTIVE RELIEF OF FEVER	Kidney damage
ADVIL MIGRAINE WORKS TO TREAT MIGRAINE HEADACHES	Fluid retention
	Bone marrow depression (except oxaprozin)
	Liver toxicity (naproxen, oxaprozin, ketoprofen and flurbiprofen)
	(All rare)

▷ **Principal Uses**

As a Single Drug Product: Uses currently included in FDA-approved labeling: (1) All six agents in this class treat rheumatoid and osteoarthritis; (2) naproxen is useful in treating bursitis, gout, dysmenorrhea (ketoprofen and ibuprofen are also approved for use in primary dysmenorrhea), pain, juvenile rheumatoid arthritis and tendonitis; (3) fenoprofen is the only agent approved to treat tennis elbow; (4) flurbiprofen ophthalmic is used to prevent intraoperative miosis; (5) Advil Migraine form treats migraine headaches.

Other (unlabeled) generally accepted uses: (1) Naproxen has been used to treat migraine and colds caused by rhinoviruses; (2) oxaprozin is useful in gout and tendonitis; (3) ketoprofen may have a role in temporal arteritis; (4) flurbiprofen has some support for therapy of periodontal disease; (5) fenoprofen has been used successfully in therapy of migraine; (6) ibuprofen treats interleukin-2 toxicity and chronic urticaria and can decrease IUD-associated bleeding; (7) all of the agents have been used for a variety of pains and fever; (8) ibuprofen has new data from a study of 148 infants with patent ductus arteriosus comparing it to indomethacin. The research concluded that benefits were similar, and ibuprofen caused less decreased urine (oliguria).

How These Drugs Work: They reduce levels of prostaglandins (and related compounds), chemicals involved in inflammation and pain.

Available Dosage Forms and Strengths

Fenoprofen:

Capsules — 200 mg, 300 mg, 600 mg
Tablets — 600 mg

Flurbiprofen:

Ophthalmic drops — 0.03%
Tablets — 50 mg, 100 mg

Ibuprofen:

Caplets — 200 mg
Oral suspension — 100 mg/5 ml
Tablets — 40 mg, 200 mg, 300 mg, 400 mg, 600 mg, 800 mg
Tablets, chewable — 50 mg, 100 mg

Ketoprofen:

Capsules — 50 mg, 75 mg, 100 mg, 150 mg
Suppositories (Canada) — 100 mg
Tablets, enteric (Canada) — 50 mg
Tablets (nonprescription) — 12.5 mg

Naproxen:

Caplets — 220 mg
Naprelan Once Daily — 375 mg, 500 mg
Oral suspension — 125 mg/5 ml
Rectal suppository (Canada) — 500 mg
Tablets — 125 mg, 250 mg, 275 mg, 375 mg, 500 mg, 550 mg
Tablets, controlled-release — 375 mg, 500 mg

Oxaprozin:

Caplets — 600 mg

▷ **Usual Adult Dosage Ranges:**

Fenoprofen: 300 to 600 mg three or four times daily. Daily maximum is 3,200 mg.

Flurbiprofen: 100 to 300 mg daily in two to four divided doses. The lowest effective dose should be used. Daily maximum is 300 mg.

Ibuprofen: 200 to 800 mg three or four times daily. Total daily dose should not exceed 3,200 mg.

Ketoprofen: 75 mg three times daily or 50 mg four times daily. Usual daily dose is 100 to 300 mg, divided into three or four doses. Daily maximum is 300 mg.

Naproxen: Gout—750 mg initially and then 250 mg every 8 hours until attack is relieved. Arthritis—250 mg, 375 mg or 500 mg twice daily, 12 hours apart. The sustained-release form (Naprelan) offers an intestinal-protective drug absorption system (IPDAS) and once-daily (two tablets once a day) dosing. Menstrual pain—500 mg initially and then 250 mg every 6 to 8 hours as needed. Maximum dose for pain is 1,375 mg.

Oxaprozin: 1,200 mg as a single daily dose in the morning. Daily maximum is 1,800 mg (or 26 mg per kg of body mass for patients with normal liver and kidney function).

Author's Note: Medicines in this class with available nonprescription forms usually have lower daily maximum doses. For example, Children's Motrin is approved for nonprescription use as temporary relief of minor aches and pains or reduction of fever in children 2 years of age and older. Adverse effects are also less common and fewer in number. Less than 11 kg of body mass and under 2 years old—consult your doctor; 2 to 3 years old and 11–15.9 kg of body mass—100 mg every 6 to 8 hours. Up to four doses may be given a day. Use should NOT go on for longer than 3 days. Please consult individual package labels or ask your pharmacist or doctor for dosing advice.

Note: Actual dose and dosing schedule must be determined for each patient individually.

Conditions Requiring Dosing Adjustments

Liver Function: All of these drugs are metabolized in the liver and therefore should be used with caution and consideration given to lower doses, by patients with liver compromise.

Kidney Function: These drugs share the risks common to most nonsteroidal anti-inflammatory drugs (NSAIDs). Some patients with kidney compromise are dependent on prostaglandins for kidney function. A benefit-to-risk decision must be made regarding the use of NSAIDs by these patients.

▷ **Dosing Instructions:** Take either on an empty stomach or with food or milk to prevent stomach irritation. Take with a full glass of water and remain upright (do not lie down) for 30 minutes. The tablets may be crushed and the capsules opened, except for ketoprofen tablets (should not be crushed or altered). If you forget a dose: Take the missed dose as soon as you remember it, unless it's nearly time for your next dose—if that is the case, skip the missed dose and take the next dose right on schedule. DO NOT double doses. Talk with your doctor if you find yourself missing doses.

Usual Duration of Use: Use on a regular schedule for 1 to 2 weeks usually determines effectiveness. Peak oxaprozin effect may take 6 weeks. Long-term use requires supervision and periodic physician evaluation. If you feel that you require a nonprescription form for more than occasional use, please talk to your doctor about an evaluation of the problem you are taking the nonprescription form for.

Typical Treatment Goals and Measurements (Outcomes and Markers)

Pain: Most clinicians treating pain use a device called an algometer to check your pain. This looks like a small ruler, but lets the clinician better understand your pain. The goals of treatment then relate to where the level of pain started (for example, a rating of seven on a zero to ten scale) and what the cause of the pain was. Pain medicines may also be used together (in combination) in order to get the best result or outcome. If your pain control is not acceptable to YOU (remember, in hospitals and outpatient settings, etc., pain control is a patient right) and if after a week of arthritis pain treatment, results are not acceptable, be sure to call your doctor —you may need a different medicine or combination.

Arthritis: Control of arthritis symptoms (pain, loss of mobility, decreased ability to accomplish activities of daily living, range of motion, etc.) is paramount in returning patient quality of life and to checking the results (beneficial outcomes) from these medicines. Clinicians use the WOMAC osteoarthritis index (see Glossary) to globally assess the health status of people living with osteoarthritis. Many arthritis management or pain centers use interdisciplinary teams (physicians from several specialties, nurses, physician's assistants, physical and occupational therapists, pharmacotherapists, psychotherapists, social workers and others) to get the best results. Laboratory measures of results for rheumatoid arthritis include decreases in chemicals released by the body (acute phase reactants) such as C-reactive protein. A more general test to roughly measure inflammation is a sed rate (erythrocyte sedimentation rate).

▷ **These Drugs Should Not Be Taken If**
- you have had an allergic reaction to them previously.
- you are subject to asthma or nasal polyps caused by aspirin.
- you have a bleeding disorder or a blood cell disorder.
- flurbiprofen ophthalmic drops should NOT be used by people with herpes simplex keratitis.
- you have severe impairment of kidney function (some cases).

▷ **Inform Your Physician Before Taking These Drugs If**
- you are allergic to aspirin or other aspirin substitutes.
- you have active peptic ulcer disease or any form of gastrointestinal bleeding.
- you have a history of peptic ulcer disease or any type of bleeding disorder.
- you have impaired liver or kidney function.
- you have high blood pressure or a history of heart failure.
- you are taking acetaminophen, aspirin or other aspirin substitutes or anticoagulants.

Possible Side Effects (natural, expected and unavoidable drug actions)

Fluid retention (weight gain); ringing in the ears. Pink, red, purple or rust coloration of urine (ibuprofen only).

▷ **Possible Adverse Effects** (unusual, unexpected and infrequent reactions)

If any of the following develop, consult your physician promptly for guidance.

Mild Adverse Effects

Allergic reactions: skin rash, hives, itching.

Headache, dizziness, altered or blurred vision, ringing in the ears, depression—infrequent.

Stinging or burning of the eyes with ophthalmic flurbiprofen drops—possible.

Sleep disturbances—infrequent (oxaprozin).

Mouth sores, indigestion, nausea, vomiting, constipation, diarrhea—infrequent.

Palpitations—rare (fenoprofen).

Serious Adverse Effects

Allergic reactions: anaphylactic reaction (see Glossary), severe skin reactions—rare.

Lung inflammation (naproxen—pneumonitis)—rare.

Idiosyncratic reactions: drug-induced meningitis with fever and coma—rare (ibuprofen and naproxen).

Active peptic ulcer, with or without bleeding—rare with 6 months use, infrequent after 1 year of use.

Inflammation of the colon—rare.

Porphyria—case reports (some drugs in this class).

Pancreatitis or lupus erythematosus—two case reports with naproxen.

Some medicines in this class may cause Parkinson-like symptoms in susceptible patients—case reports.

Worsening of congestive heart failure—possible.

Inflammation of the esophagus—probable if patients lie down soon after taking these medicines.

Liver damage with jaundice (see Glossary)—case reports.

Kidney damage with painful urination, bloody urine, reduced urine formation—possible.

Bone marrow depression (see Glossary): fatigue, sore throat, abnormal bleeding/bruising—case reports.

▷ **Possible Effects on Sexual Function:** Altered timing and pattern of menstruation (ibuprofen, ketoprofen and naproxen) and excessive menstrual bleeding (ibuprofen and ketoprofen)—case reports.

Male breast enlargement and tenderness—rare (ibuprofen).

Naproxen may rarely inhibit ejaculation.

Ketoprofen may rarely decrease libido.

Possible Delayed Adverse Effects: Mild anemia due to "silent" blood loss from the stomach.

▷ **Adverse Effects That May Mimic Natural Diseases or Disorders**

Liver reaction may suggest viral hepatitis.

Natural Diseases or Disorders That May Be Activated by These Drugs

Peptic ulcer disease, ulcerative colitis.

Possible Effects on Laboratory Tests

Erythrocyte sedimentation rate: decreased (a desired effect).

Complete blood cell counts: decreased red cells, hemoglobin, white cells and platelets.

Blood cholesterol or uric acid levels: increased.

Blood lithium level: increased.

Liver function tests: increased enzymes (ALT/GPT, AST/GOT, alkaline phosphatase) or bilirubin.

Kidney function tests: increased blood creatinine and urea nitrogen (BUN) levels.

Fecal occult blood test: positive.

CAUTION
1. Dose should always be limited to the smallest amount that produces reasonable improvement.
2. These drugs may mask early indications of infection. Inform your physician if you think you are developing an infection of any kind.
3. Congestive heart failure in elderly patients may be unmasked or worsened. Risk appears to increase with use of higher doses.

Precautions for Use

By Infants and Children: Safety and effectiveness for those under 12 years of age are not established.

By Those Over 60 Years of Age: Small doses are prudent until tolerance is determined. Watch for signs of liver or kidney toxicity, fluid retention, dizziness, confusion, impaired memory, stomach bleeding or constipation.

▷ **Advisability of Use During Pregnancy**

Pregnancy Category: B for ibuprofen, fenoprofen, flurbiprofen, ketoprofen and naproxen. C for oxaprozin. Ibuprofen and fenoprofen are FDA category D if used in the final 3 months (trimester) of pregnancy. The manufacturers of ketoprofen and flurbiprofen say that both medicines should be avoided in late pregnancy. See Pregnancy Risk Categories at the back of this book.

Animal studies: No birth defects reported in rats or rabbits.

Human studies: Adequate studies of pregnant women are not available.

Avoid these drugs during the final 3 months. Use during the first 6 months only if clearly needed. Ask your physician for guidance.

Advisability of Use If Breast-Feeding

Presence of these drugs in breast milk: Yes or expected.

Avoid drugs or refrain from nursing.

Habit-Forming Potential: None.

Effects of Overdose: Drowsiness, dizziness, ringing in the ears, nausea, vomiting, diarrhea, confusion, unsteadiness, stupor progressing to coma.

Possible Effects of Long-Term Use: Fluid retention.

Suggested Periodic Examinations While Taking These Drugs (at physician's discretion)

Complete blood cell counts.

Liver and kidney function tests.

Complete eye examinations if vision is altered in any way.

▷ **While Taking These Drugs, Observe the Following**

Foods: No restrictions.

Herbal Medicines or Minerals: Ginseng, ginkgo, alfalfa, clove oil, feverfew, cinchona bark and garlic may also change clotting, so combining those herbals with these medicines is not recommended. Talk to your doctor BEFORE combining any medicines. NSAIDs may decrease feverfew effects. Since St. John's wort and some of these medicines may increase sensitivity to the sun, CAUTION IS ADVISED. Hay flower, mistletoe herb and white mustard seed carry German Commission E monograph indications for arthritis.

Beverages: No restrictions. May be taken with milk.

▷ *Alcohol:* Use with caution. The irritant action of alcohol on the stomach lining, added to the irritant action of these drugs, can increase the risk of stomach ulceration and/or bleeding.

Tobacco Smoking: No interactions expected. I advise everyone to quit smoking.

▷ *Other Drugs*

These medicines may ***increase*** the effects of

- anticoagulants (Coumadin, etc.) and increase the risk of bleeding; more frequent INR (prothrombin time or protime) tests are needed, and ongoing doses should be adjusted to the laboratory test results.
- cyclosporine (Sandimmune), leading to toxicity.
- fosphenytoin (Cerebyx) or phenytoin (Dilantin) and may lead to increased risk of antiepileptic toxicity.
- lithium (Lithobid, others), by causing toxic lithium levels.
- methotrexate (Mexate, others) and result in major methotrexate toxicity with possible anemia, hemorrhage and blood infections.
- oral hypoglycemic agents (Sulfonylureas).

These medicines may ***decrease*** the effects of

- beta blockers (see Drug Classes), such as carteolol (Cartrol).
- diuretics (see Drug Classes), such as hydrochlorothiazide (Esidrix) and furosemide (Lasix).

These medicines ***taken concurrently*** with the following drugs may increase the risk of bleeding; avoid these combinations if possible and closely monitor patients for bleeding (PTT or PT may not fully estimate bleeding risk):

- aspirin.
- dipyridamole (Persantine).
- enoxaparin (Lovenox).
- indomethacin (Indocin).
- ketorolac (Toradol).
- low molecular weight heparins (Lovenox, others see Drug Classes).
- sulfinpyrazone (Anturane).
- valproic acid (Depakene).
- warfarin (Coumadin).

These medicines **taken concurrently** with

- ACE inhibitors (see Drug Classes) can worsen kidney diseases and blunt benefits.
- alendronate (Fosamax) can worsen stomach irritation. Caution is advised.
- histamine (H2) blockers (see Drug Classes) may increase toxicity from NSAIDs.
- ofloxacin (and perhaps other fluoroquinolones; see Drug Classes) may increase risk of seizures.
- ritonavir (Norvir) may lead to toxic propionic acid NSAID levels.
- tacrine (Cognex) led to delirium in a patient taking ibuprofen.
- tacrolimus (Prograf) poses a serious risk for kidney failure. This combination is not advisable.

▷ *Driving, Hazardous Activities:* These drugs may cause drowsiness or dizziness. Restrict activities as necessary.

Aviation Note: The use of these drugs *may be a disqualification* for piloting. Consult a designated Aviation Medical Examiner.

Exposure to Sun: Use caution until sensitivity is determined. Ibuprofen, ketoprofen, flurbiprofen and naproxen cause photosensitivity (see Glossary).

PROPRANOLOL (proh PRAN oh lohl)

Introduced: 1966   **Class:** Anti-anginal, antiarrhythmic, antihypertensive, antimigraine, beta blocker   **Prescription:** USA: Yes   **Controlled Drug:** USA: No; Canada: No   **Available as Generic:** Yes

Brand Names: ✤Apo-Propranolol, Betachron, ✤Detensol, Inderal, Inderal-LA, Inderide [CD], Inderide LA [CD], Ipran, ✤Novo-Pranol, ✤PMS Propranolol

---

BENEFITS versus RISKS

Possible Benefits	*Possible Risks*
EFFECTIVE, WELL-TOLERATED AS ANTI-ANGINAL DRUG IN EFFORT-INDUCED ANGINA; ANTIARRHYTHMIC DRUG IN CERTAIN HEART RHYTHM DISORDERS; ANTIHYPERTENSIVE DRUG IN MILD TO MODERATE HYPERTENSION	CONGESTIVE HEART FAILURE in advanced heart disease
	Worsening of angina in coronary heart disease (if drug is abruptly withdrawn)
	Masking of low blood sugar (hypoglycemia) in drug-treated diabetes
PREVENTION OF MIGRAINE HEADACHES	Provocation of asthma (in asthmatics)
REDUCES DEATH AND LOSS OF FUNCTION AFTER A HEART ATTACK	Depression
	Blood cell disorders: low white cell and platelet counts
Effective adjunct in the management of pheochromocytoma	

▷ **Principal Uses**

As a Single Drug Product: Uses currently included in FDA-approved labeling: (1) Treats several cardiovascular disorders: classical effort-induced angina, certain types of heart rhythm disturbance and high blood pressure; (2) also helps prevent repeat heart attacks (myocardial infarction); (3) reduces frequency and severity of migraine headaches; (4) decreases tremors in essential and action tremor.

Other (unlabeled) generally accepted uses: (1) Helps control physical signs of anxiety and nervous tension (as in stage fright); (2) helps control familial tremors and symptoms seen with markedly overactive thyroid function (thyrotoxicosis); (3) decreases abnormal abdominal fluid accumulation (ascites) in people with cirrhosis of the liver; (4) may have a role in combination therapy with metronidazole in resistant Giardia infections; (5) helps control headaches caused by cyclosporine (Sandimmune); (6) may be useful in certain kinds of pain, especially after amputations; (7) can help control panic attacks; (8) useful in helping decrease bleeding in patients with esophageal varices and liver cirrhosis; (9) helps fight symptoms in narcotic withdrawal cases.

As a Combination Drug Product [CD]: This drug is available in combination with hydrochlorothiazide for the treatment of hypertension. This combination product includes two drugs with different mechanisms of action; it is intended to provide greater effectiveness and convenience for long-term use.

How This Drug Works: Blocks certain actions of the sympathetic nervous system:
- reducing rate and contraction force of the heart, lowering the ejection pressure of the blood leaving the heart and reducing the oxygen requirement for heart function.
- reduces degree of contraction of blood vessel walls, lowering blood pressure.
- prolongs conduction time of nerve impulses through the heart, helping manage certain heart rhythm disorders.

Available Dosage Forms and Strengths

Capsules, prolonged action — 60 mg, 80 mg, 120 mg, 160 mg

Concentrate — 80 mg/ml

Injection — 1 mg/ml

Oral solution — 4 mg/ml, 8 mg/ml

Tablets — 10 mg, 20 mg, 40 mg, 60 mg, 80 mg, 90 mg, 120 mg

▷ **Usual Adult Dosage Ranges:**

Anti-anginal: Initially 10 mg three or four times a day; increase dose gradually every 3 to 7 days as needed and tolerated. The total daily dose should not exceed 400 mg.

Antiarrhythmic: 10 to 30 mg three or four times a day as needed and tolerated.

Antihypertensive: Initially 40 mg twice a day; increase dose gradually as needed and tolerated. The total daily dose should not exceed 640 mg.

Migraine headache prevention: Initially 20 mg four times a day; increase dose gradually as needed and tolerated. The total daily dose should not exceed 480 mg. Long-acting formulations offer the advantage of once-daily dosing for many patients.

> **Note: Actual dose and schedule must be determined for each patient individually.**

Conditions Requiring Dosing Adjustments

Liver Function: Used with caution by patients with liver disease. In general, lower starting doses and slower dose increases are indicated.

Kidney Function: This drug should be used with caution by people with combined kidney and liver compromise. Dose adjustments are not needed for people with compromised kidneys.

▷ **Dosing Instructions:** This drug is preferably taken 1 hour before eating to maximize absorption. The tablet may be crushed; to prevent harmless numbing effect, mix with soft food and swallow promptly. The prolonged-action capsules should be swallowed whole. Do not stop this drug abruptly. If you forget a dose: Take the missed dose as soon as you remember it, unless it's WITHIN 8 hours of your next dose for an extended release form or if your next dose is DUE in 4 hours for the immediate release forms—if that is the case, skip the missed dose and take the next dose right on schedule. DO NOT double doses. Talk with your doctor if you find yourself missing doses. There are some pager based reminder systems that can be of great help.

Usual Duration of Use: Use on a regular schedule for 10 to 14 days usually determines effectiveness in preventing angina, controlling heart rhythm disorders and lowering blood pressure. Peak benefits may be seen in 6 to 8 weeks. Long-term use is determined by your symptoms over time and response to the overall treatment program (weight reduction, salt restriction, smoking cessation, etc.). See your physician on a regular basis.

Typical Treatment Goals and Measurements (Outcomes and Markers)

Blood pressure: The most recent treatment guidelines (JNC VI) actually define optimal blood pressure (BP) as less than 120/80 and high normal as 139/89. The American Diabetes Association has chosen a target of 130/80 as the blood pressure goal for people living with diabetes. Most clinicians try to achieve a BP that achieves the best balance of lower cardiovascular risk while avoiding the problem of too low a blood pressure. The goal and time frame (see peak benefits above) should be discussed with you when the prescription is written.

Abnormal heartbeats: The general goal is to return the heart to a normal rhythm or at least to markedly reduce the occurrence of abnormal heartbeats. In life-threatening arrhythmias, the goal is to abort the abnormal beats and return the pattern to normal. Success at ongoing suppression may involve ambulatory checks of heart rate and rhythm for a day (such as in Holter monitoring). This kind of testing involves placement of adhesive backed temporary electrodes on the skin in several positions around the heart. A small heart rate and rhythm (EKG or ECG) recording device is carried around via a shoulder strap and records what the heart is doing over 24 hours. Once the recording is made, a scanning machine reviews the record, tallies abnormal heart beats or rhythms and gives a close and extended look at how the heart is reacting or benefiting from the medicines that the patient is taking. Repeat measurements can be made if doses are changes to check the success at keeping the heart in normal sinus rhythm!

Possible Advantage of This Drug

Has a clear benefit in reducing the chance of a second heart attack once a first heart attack has been diagnosed.

▷ **This Drug Should Not Be Taken If**

- you have bronchial asthma.
- you have had an allergic reaction to it previously.
- you have Prinzmetal's variant angina (coronary artery spasm).
- you have heart failure (overt).
- you have Raynaud's phenomenon.
- you have an abnormally slow heart rate (bradycardia) or a serious form of heart block (second or third degree AV block).
- you are taking, or have taken within the past 14 days, any monoamine oxidase (MAO) type A inhibitor (see Drug Classes).

▷ **Inform Your Physician Before Taking This Drug If**

- you had an adverse reaction to a beta blocker (see Drug Classes).
- you have a history of serious heart disease.
- you have a history of hay fever (allergic rhinitis), asthma, chronic bronchitis or emphysema.
- you have a history of overactive thyroid function (hyperthyroidism).

- you have a history of low blood sugar (hypoglycemia).
- you have impaired liver or kidney function.
- you are allergic to bee stings.
- you have diabetes or myasthenia gravis.
- you take digitalis, quinidine or reserpine or any calcium-channel-blocker drug (see Drug Classes).
- you plan to have surgery under general anesthesia in the near future.

Possible Side Effects (natural, expected and unavoidable drug actions)

Lethargy and fatigability, cold extremities, slow heart rate, light-headedness in upright position (see orthostatic hypotension in Glossary). Increased bowel movements.

▷ **Possible Adverse Effects** (unusual, unexpected and infrequent reactions)

If any of the following develop, consult your physician promptly for guidance.

Mild Adverse Effects

Allergic reactions: skin rash, temporary loss of hair, drug fever (see Glossary).

Joint pain—case reports.

Headache, dizziness, insomnia, vivid dreams—infrequent.

Indigestion, taste disorder, nausea, vomiting, diarrhea—infrequent.

Weight gain—possible.

Serious Adverse Effects

Allergic reactions: anaphylaxis. Reactions may be exaggerated if a patient is taking this medicine and is exposed to the allergen. For example, epinephrine use can result in epinephrine resistance and severe increases in blood pressure and a reactionary (reflex) slowing of the heart rate.

Idiosyncratic reactions: acute behavioral disturbances (disorientation, confusion, hallucinations, amnesia).

Paradoxical hypertension—case reports.

Mental depression, anxiety—case reports and dose-related.

Chest pain, shortness of breath, precipitation of congestive heart failure—possible.

Peripheral neuropathy or hyperthyroidism—rare.

Drug-induced systemic lupus erythematosus, myasthenia gravis or porphyria—case reports.

Kidney problems (interstitial nephritis)—rare.

Induction of bronchial asthma—in asthmatics.

May precipitate problems walking (intermittent claudication)—possible.

Blood cell disorders: abnormally low white blood cell or platelet counts—case reports.

Carpal tunnel syndrome—case reports.

▷ **Possible Effects on Sexual Function:** Decreased libido; impaired erection; impotence—infrequent (has the highest incidence of libido reduction and erectile impairment of all beta-blocker drugs).

Male infertility (inhibited sperm motility); Peyronie's disease (see Glossary)—possible.

▷ **Adverse Effects That May Mimic Natural Diseases or Disorders**

Reduced blood flow to extremities may resemble Raynaud's phenomenon (see Glossary).

Natural Diseases or Disorders That May Be Activated by This Drug

Prinzmetal's variant angina, Raynaud's phenomenon, intermittent claudication, myasthenia gravis (questionable).

Possible Effects on Laboratory Tests

White blood cell count: occasionally decreased.

Blood platelet count: increased or decreased.

Bleeding time: increased.

Blood total cholesterol, triglycerides or VLDL level: no effect in some; increased in others.

Blood HDL cholesterol level: no effect in some; decreased in others.

Blood LDL cholesterol level: no effect in some; increased and decreased in others.

Blood glucose level: no effect in some; increased or decreased in others.

Glucose tolerance test (GTT): decreased.

Blood thyroid hormone levels: T3—no effect in some, decreased in others; T4—increased; free T4—increased.

Blood uric acid level: no effect in some; increased in others.

Liver function tests: increased liver enzymes (ALT/GPT, AST/GOT and alkaline phosphatase); effects probably not due to liver damage.

CAUTION

1. ***Do not stop this drug suddenly*** without the knowledge and help of your doctor. Carry a notation that states you are taking this drug.
2. Ask your physician or pharmacist before using nasal decongestants, which are usually present in over-the-counter cold preparations and nose drops. These can cause sudden increases in blood pressure when taken concurrently with beta-blocker drugs.
3. Report the development of any tendency to emotional depression.

Precautions for Use

By Infants and Children: Safety and effectiveness for those under 12 years of age are not established, but if this drug is used, watch for low blood sugar (hypoglycemia) during periods of reduced food intake.

By Those Over 60 Years of Age: Unacceptably high blood pressure should be reduced without creating the risks associated with excessively low blood pressure. Therapy is started with small doses and blood pressure checked frequently. Sudden, rapid and excessive reduction of blood pressure can predispose to stroke or heart attack. Observe for dizziness, unsteadiness, tendency to fall, confusion, hallucinations, depression or urinary frequency.

▷ **Advisability of Use During Pregnancy**

Pregnancy Category: C. See Pregnancy Risk Categories at the back of this book.

Animal studies: No significant increase in birth defects due to this drug. Some toxic effects on embryo reported.

Human studies: Adequate studies of pregnant women are not available.

Avoid use of drug during the first 3 months if possible. Ask your physician for guidance.

Advisability of Use If Breast-Feeding

Presence of this drug in breast milk: Yes.

Monitor nursing infant closely, and discontinue drug or nursing if adverse effects develop.

Habit-Forming Potential: None.

Effects of Overdose: Weakness, slow pulse, low blood pressure, fainting, cold and sweaty skin, congestive heart failure, possible coma and convulsions.

Possible Effects of Long-Term Use: Reduced heart reserve and eventual heart failure in susceptible patients with advanced heart disease.

Suggested Periodic Examinations While Taking This Drug (at physician's discretion)

Complete blood cell counts.

Measurements of blood pressure.

Evaluation of heart function.

Liver function tests.

▷ **While Taking This Drug, Observe the Following**

Foods: Avoid excessive salt intake. Excessive fat intake can worsen existing cardiovascular disease. Talk to your doctor about a sensible diet.

Herbal Medicines or Minerals: Ginseng may increase blood pressure, blunting the benefits of this medicine. Hawthorn, saw palmetto, ma huang, goldenseal, yohimbe and licorice may also cause increased blood pressure. Calcium and garlic may help lower blood pressure. Use caution and work with your doctor to make sure blood pressure is not lowered too much. Indian snakeroot has a German Commission E monograph indication for hypertension—talk to your doctor. Eleuthero root and ephedra should be avoided by people living with hypertension.

Beverages: No restrictions. May be taken with milk.

▷ *Alcohol:* Use with caution. Alcohol may exaggerate this drug's ability to lower blood pressure and may increase its mild sedative effect.

Tobacco Smoking: Nicotine may reduce this drug's effectiveness in treating angina, heart rhythm disorders and high blood pressure. Smoking increases the rate of elimination of this drug. I advise everyone to quit smoking.

▷ *Other Drugs*

Propranolol may **increase** the effects of

• other antihypertensive drugs and cause excessive lowering of blood pressure; dose adjustments may be necessary.

• lidocaine (Xylocaine, etc.).

• quinidine (Quinaglute). Careful patient monitoring for heart failure, excessively low blood pressure and very slow heart rate is required.

• reserpine (Ser-Ap-Es, etc.) and cause sedation, depression, slowing of the heart rate and lowering of blood pressure.

• rizatriptan (Maxalt); a 5-mg starting dose and a maximum of 15 mg of rizatriptan should be used if these medicines are combined.

• verapamil (Calan, Isoptin) and cause excessive depression of heart function; monitor this combination closely.

• warfarin (Coumadin) and increase bleeding risk; more frequent INR (prothrombin time or protime) testing is needed. Warfarin dosing should be adjusted to laboratory results.

Propranolol may decrease the effects of

• albuterol (Proventil).

• theophyllines (Aminophyllin, Theo-Dur, etc.) and reduce their antiasthmatic effectiveness.

Propranolol taken concurrently with

• amiodarone (Cordarone) may result in abnormal heart rhythms and low pulse—these agents should not be combined.

- clonidine (Catapres) requires close monitoring for rebound high blood pressure if clonidine is withdrawn while propranolol is still being taken.
- cocaine may lead to heart attack.
- colestipol (Colestid) may decrease propranolol benefits.
- digoxin (Lanoxin) can result in severe slowing of the heart (bradycardia).
- epinephrine (Adrenalin, etc.) may cause marked rise in blood pressure and slowing of the heart rate.
- ergot derivatives (see Drug Classes) may lead to excessive blood vessel constriction and cold extremities (peripheral ischemia).
- fluoxetine (Prozac) may increase the risk of slow heartbeat and sedation.
- fluvoxamine (Luvox) may increase the risk of slow heartbeat and sedation.
- insulin requires close monitoring to avoid undetected hypoglycemia (see Glossary).
- methyldopa (various) can lead to an excessive blood pressure increase during stress.
- nefazodone (Serzone) may decrease propranolol benefits and lead to nefazodone toxicity.
- oral antidiabetic drugs (see Drug Classes) and cause slow recovery from any low blood sugar that may occur.
- quinidine (Quinaglute) can increase adverse effects without increased therapeutic benefits.
- sertraline (Zoloft) may lead to sudden chest pain.
- venlafaxine (Effexor) may result in increased risk of propranolol toxicity.
- X-ray contrast media such as diatrizoate results in up to an eightfold increase in risk of severe allergic (anaphylactic) drug reactions.
- zolmitriptan (Zomig) may increase risk of zolmitriptan adverse effects.
- zotepine (Nipolept) may increase risk of toxicity from both drugs.

The following drugs may *increase* the effects of propranolol:
- chlorpromazine (Thorazine, etc.).
- cimetidine (Tagamet).
- ciprofloxacin (Cipro).
- diltiazem (Cardizem).
- disopyramide (Norpace).
- furosemide or other diuretics.
- methimazole (Tapazole).
- metoclopramide (Reglan) (conventional immediate-release forms of propranolol).
- nicardipine (Cardene).
- propafenone (Rythmol) especially if doses of 150 mg a day or more of propafenone are used.
- propoxyphene (various).
- propylthiouracil (Propacil).
- ritonavir (Norvir) and perhaps other protease inhibitors (see Drug Classes).
- zileuton (Zyflo).

The following drugs may *decrease* the effects of propranolol:
- antacids.
- barbiturates (phenobarbital, etc.).
- indomethacin (Indocin) and possibly other "aspirin substitutes," or NSAIDs—may impair propranolol's antihypertensive effect.
- rifampin (Rifadin, Rimactane).

- sertraline (Zoloft) may increase risk of chest pain.
- simvastatin (Zocor) by decreasing the peak blood concentration.

▷ *Driving, Hazardous Activities:* Use caution until the full extent of drowsiness, lethargy and blood pressure change have been determined.

Aviation Note: The use of this drug *may be a disqualification* for piloting. Consult a designated Aviation Medical Examiner.

Exposure to Sun: No restrictions.

Exposure to Heat: Caution is advised. Hot environments can lower blood pressure and exaggerate the effects of this drug.

Exposure to Cold: Caution is advised. Cold environments can enhance the circulatory deficiency in the extremities that may occur with this drug. The elderly should take precautions to prevent hypothermia (see Glossary).

Heavy Exercise or Exertion: It is advisable to avoid exertion that produces lightheadedness, excessive fatigue or muscle cramping. The use of this drug may intensify the hypertensive response to isometric exercise.

Occurrence of Unrelated Illness: Fever can lower blood pressure and require adjustment of dose. Nausea or vomiting may interrupt the regular dose schedule. Ask your physician for guidance.

Discontinuation: Best to avoid sudden stopping of this drug, especially in coronary artery disease. If possible, a gradual reduction of dose over a period of 2 to 3 weeks is recommended. Ask your physician for specific guidance.

PROTEASE INHIBITOR FAMILY

Amprenavir (am PREN a veer) **Indinavir** (in DIN a veer) **Nelfinavir** (nel FIN a veer) **Ritonavir** (ri TOHN a veer) **Saquinavir** (sa KWIN a veer)

Introduced: 1999, 1996, 1997, 1996, 1995, respectively **Class:** Protease inhibitor, antiviral, anti-AIDS **Prescription:** USA: Yes **Controlled Drug:** USA: No; Canada: Yes **Available as Generic:** USA: No; Canada: No

Brand Names: Amprenavir: Agenerase, Indinavir: Crixivan, Nelfinavir: Viracept Ritonavir: Kaletra [CD], Norvir, Saquinavir: Fortovase, Invirase

---

BENEFITS versus RISKS

Possible Benefits	*Possible Risks*
INCREASED CD4 COUNTS	SERIOUS CHANGES IN INSULIN
DECREASED OPPORTUNISTIC	LEVELS TO KETOACIDOSIS
INFECTIONS	SERIOUS INCREASES IN
EFFECTIVE COMBINATION	CHOLESTEROL
THERAPY OF HIV	Increased liver function tests (not
MAY DECREASE HIV TO	reported for amprenavir)
UNDETECTABLE LEVELS WITH	Kidney stones (indinavir)
EARLY THERAPY	May have SERIOUS drug interactions
Novel primary resistance mutation	(see below)
pattern (amprenavir)	
Few overlapping secondary	
mutations (amprenavir)	

▷ **Principal Uses**

As a Single Drug Product: Uses currently included in FDA-approved labeling: Treatment of HIV infection when antiretroviral therapy is indicated, in combination with other antiretroviral agents.

Author's Note: The *Panel on Clinical Practices for Treatment of HIV Infection Report* says that the preferred regimen is two nucleoside analogs and one potent protease inhibitor. Single-agent therapy is not recommended. Indinavir received traditional FDA approval in 1998. The new antiretroviral therapy guidelines from NIAID take into account how easily the medicine treating IIIV can fit into a patient's life.

Other (unlabeled) generally accepted uses: Used in making HIV infection undetectable with combination therapy.

As a Combination Drug Product [CD]: Ritonavir is available combined with lopinavir (Kaletra). This combination works to use the blood level sustaining role of ritonavir and the mechanism of action of lopinavir. While we usually think of drug interactions as undesirable, low dose ritonavir in this combination inhibits the cytochrome P450 3A4 leading to increased and sustained lopinavir blood levels.

How These Drugs Work: They inhibit HIV reproduction (replication) by inhibiting an HIV enzyme (protease), which blocks the ability of the virus to make mature, infectious virus particles.

Available Dosage Forms and Strengths

Amprenavir:
　　　　Capsules — 50 mg, 150 mg
　　　Oral solution — 15 mg/ml
Indinavir:
　　　　Capsules — 200 mg, 400 mg
Nelfinavir:
　　　Oral powder — 50 mg/g
　　　　　Tablet — 250 mg
Ritonavir:
　　　　Capsule — 100 mg
　　　Oral solution — 80 mg/ml
　　Soft gel capsule — 100 mg
Ritonavir/lopinavir (Kaletra):
　　　　Capsule — 33.3 mg ritonavir and 133.3 mg lopinavir
　　　Oral solution — 20 mg/ml ritonavir and 80 mg/ml lopinavir
Saquinavir:
　　Gelcap (Fortovase) — 200 mg
　　Gelcap (Invirase) — 200 mg
Author's Note: This profile gives Fortovase data.

▷ **Recommended Dose Ranges** (Actual dose and schedule must be determined for each patient individually.)

18 to 60 Years of Age:
Amprenavir: 1,200 mg twice a day (in combination with other antiretrovirals).
Indinavir: 800 mg by mouth every 8 hours.
Nelfinavir: 750 mg every 8 hours.
Ritonavir: In order to help minimize adverse effects, ritonavir is started at

300 mg twice daily and then is increased by 100 mg twice daily at two- to three-day intervals. The desired "goal dose" is 600 mg twice daily. If ritonavir is taken with saquinavir, dose is reduced to 400 mg twice daily.

Ritonavir/lopinavir: three capsules or 5 ml of the oral solution twice a day with food.

Saquinavir: 1,200 mg three times daily.

Over 65 Years of Age: These drugs have not been specifically studied in those over 65.

Conditions Requiring Dosing Adjustments

Liver function:

Amprenavir: People with impaired liver function (Child-Pugh score of 5–8) require dosing adjustments. Those with this degree of compromise are given 450 mg twice daily and should be closely followed for possible adverse effects.

Indinavir: The dose should be decreased to 600 mg by mouth every 8 hours in mild to moderate liver failure.

Nelfinavir, ritonavir and saquinavir: Have not been studied in liver disease, but caution is advised as much of these drugs are removed by the liver.

Kidney function: Amprenavir, indinavir, nelfinavir, ritonavir and saquinavir: Dosing changes are not thought to be needed.

▷ **Dosing Instructions:** Indinavir is best taken on an empty stomach, but may be taken with a light snack, such as dry toast with jelly, apple juice or coffee. Nelfinavir, ritonavir and saquinavir should be taken with a meal or light snack. Ritonavir oral solution SHOULD NOT be refrigerated and should be shaken well BEFORE you take your dose. Amprenavir can be taken with or without food but SHOULD NOT be taken with a high-fat meal. IT IS CRITICAL THAT PROTEASE INHIBITOR DOSES NOT BE MISSED, as resistance to the medicine may develop. Since reports of altered blood sugar have been made, knowledge of signs and symptoms of high blood sugar or ketoacidosis and periodic checks of blood sugar appear prudent. If you forget a dose: Take the missed dose as soon as you remember it, unless it's nearly time for your next dose—if that is the case, skip the missed dose and take the next dose right on schedule. DO NOT double doses. Talk with your doctor if you find yourself missing doses. There are several excellent timers and even beeper-based systems to help you remember your medicine.

Usual Duration of Use: Use on a regular schedule for several months usually determines effectiveness in lowering the viral burden. The lowest level of viral burden, the 12-week level of viral burden and how consistently you take these medicines (adherence) are key factors in long-term results. Long-term use (months to years) requires periodic physician evaluation of response (viral burden and CD4).

Typical Treatment Goals and Measurements (Outcomes and Markers)

HIV: Goals for HIV treatment presently are maximum suppression of viral replication, maximum lowering of the amount of virus in your body (viral load or burden), and maximum patient survival. Markers of successful therapy include undetectable viral load, increased CD4 cells, absence of indicator or opportunistic infections (OIs) and in the case of the HIV positive patient, failure of the infection to progress to AIDS. If goals are not achieved in the time your doctor has set, typical strategies include intensification as well as phenotypic resistance testing of the virus itself. If goals are achieved and the viral load later rebounds despite excellent compliance, medication change (salvage therapy) is indicated.

Possible Advantages of These Drugs

These medicines are part of combination regimens (termed cocktails by television news) that can lower the amount of HIV in the body to nondetectable levels in many patients. Resistance to these medicines still occurs in a variety of ways. Amprenavir appeared to have a novel resistance pattern (codon 50V mutation that confers resistance), however, overlapping secondary resistance locations have become problematic. New dosing strategies and even a once-a-day protease inhibitor (see drug classes) are being studied. Regardless of the patient, it is not unusual for HIV treatment to have to be changed. PI containing regimens tend to offer reasonably durable virus suppression.

▷ **These Drugs Should Not Be Taken If**

- you had an allergic reaction to any dose form.
- you are taking cisapride, ergotamine or triazolam (see "Other Drugs" section).

▷ **Inform Your Physician Before Taking These Drugs If**

- you have diabetes or a history of blood sugar regulation problems.
- you are taking amprenavir and develop a rash.
- you are allergic to sulfonamide type medicines (amprenavir).
- you have elevated cholesterol or lipids.
- you have had kidney stones previously (indinavir especially).
- you have kidney or liver compromise.
- you have phenylketonuria (nelfinavir powder has 11.2 mg of phenylalanine in each gram).
- you are taking one of the medicines that interacts with a protease inhibitor and have not had a blood level check.
- you have had adverse reactions to other protease inhibitors.
- you are unsure how much to take or how often to take them.

Possible Side Effects (natural, expected and unavoidable drug actions)

Rare kidney stones (indinavir). Increased liver function tests.

▷ **Possible Adverse Effects** (unusual, unexpected and infrequent reactions)

If any of the following develop, consult your physician promptly for guidance.

Mild Adverse Effects

Allergic reactions: skin rash.

Headache (frequent with amprenavir) or dizziness—rare to infrequent.

Weakness—infrequent

Toe nail changes (ingrown)—possible.

Blurred vision—rare.

Chills, fever or sweating—rare to infrequent.

Nausea and vomiting or abdominal pain—infrequent to frequent.

Palpitations—rare.

Joint pain—rare.

Tingling around the mouth (paresthesias)—frequent for ritonavir and agenerase.

Lipodystrophy—possible

Author's Note: Current controversy as to possible lipid changes (lipodystrophy or LD) from protease inhibitors and/or nucleoside reverse transcriptase inhibitors involves presence of mild changes versus moderate to severe problems. The HOPS data found that risk of LD increases with increasing time on antiretrovirals and that LD increases with an increasing number of nondrug factors (age 40 or older, HIV infection 7 or more years, AIDS 2 or more years, hemophiliacs, nadir CD4 count less than 100 or less than 15 and time since nadir 3 or more years).

Diarrhea—infrequent to frequent (frequent with nelfinavir).

Serious Adverse Effects

Allergic reactions: life-threatening rash (Stevens-Johnson syndrome)—rare for amprenavir.

Anemia or spleen disorder—rare (indinavir, ritonavir and saquinavir).

Hemolytic anemia—case report for agenerase.

Kidney stones—infrequent (indinavir).

Changes in insulin levels (increased blood sugar [hyperglycemia]) or ketoacidosis—many case reports for the protease inhibitors.

Increased cholesterol—many case reports.

Fat redistribution (lipodystrophy)—possible (starts from 4–61 weeks and greatest risk appears to be with indinavir).

Increased risk of blood clots (thrombosis)—possible (indinavir only).

Increased bleeding risk in people with hemophilia (nelfinavir).

▷ **Possible Effects on Sexual Function:** Rare reports of premenstrual syndrome in some early studies with indinavir. Four cases of extended and excessive menstruation (hypermenorrhea) have been reported with ritonavir.

Possible Delayed Adverse Effects: Kidney stones (indinavir). Blood sugar problems (low blood sugar or ketoacidosis) or cholesterol changes. Fat redistribution. Ingrown toenails.

▷ **Adverse Effects That May Mimic Natural Diseases or Disorders**

Increased liver function tests may mimic hepatitis (not reported for amprenavir). Changes in insulin levels may mimic diabetes.

Possible Effects on Laboratory Tests

Liver function tests: increased (not reported for amprenavir).

Complete blood counts: decreased red blood cells and hematocrit.

Insulin levels: lowered.

Blood sugar (glucose): increased.

Cholesterol—may be significantly increased.

CAUTION

1. Serious increases in cholesterol (lipids) have been reported.
2. Serious increases in blood sugar has been reported in many case reports to date for protease inhibitors. This effect has been seen in early reports on average after 76 days of therapy, but has also been reported after as little as 4 days of treatment with protease inhibitors.
3. Make certain you know high blood sugar (hyperglycemia) and ketoacidosis signs and symptoms if you are taking this medicine. Blood sugar problems have been reported for protease inhibitors.
4. These medicines may decrease the amount of virus in your body, but the virus can still be spread to others through sexual contact or blood contamination.

5. Promptly report flank pain or blood in the urine; this could indicate a kidney stone.
6. Periodic measures of viral load and CD4 are critical to make certain that therapy is still working.
7. IT IS CRITICAL to take these medicines exactly as directed to get the best results.
8. Ritonavir (Norvir) has MANY drug interactions. Ask your pharmacist to check the most current list. Amprenavir also has some serious drug interactions. Doses of the protease inhibitor may need to be increased or decreased.
9. Fat redistribution should be reported to your doctor (one patient responded to ketoconazole treatment).
10. Amprenavir contains a significant amount of vitamin E. DO NOT USE vitamin E supplements while taking this medicine.

Precautions for Use
By Infants and Children:
> *Amprenavir:* Capsules: 4–12 years old or if 13–16 and weight is less than 50 kg—20 mg per kg twice daily or 15 mg per kg three times daily up to 2,400 mg. 13–16 years of age and weighing more than 50 kg—same as adult dose. Oral solution (NOT INTERCHANGEABLE WITH CAPSULES): 4–12 years old or if 13–16 and weight is less than 50 kg: 22.5 mg per kg twice daily or 17 mg per kg three times daily up to 2,800 mg.
>
> *Indinavir:* dosing in children is not clearly defined.
>
> *Nelfinavir:* 2–13 years old—One open-label study used 20–30 mg per kg per dose, which was taken three times daily with a meal or light snack.
>
> *Ritonavir:* Started at 250 mg per square meter and increased at 2- to 3-day intervals by 30 mg per square meter. The goal dose is 400 mg per square meter twice daily in combination with other antiretroviral agents (up to 600 mg twice daily).
>
> *Saquinavir:* Dosing in those less than 16 years old has not been defined.

By Those Over 65 Years of Age: Have not been studied in this age group.

▷ **Advisability of Use During Pregnancy**
> *Pregnancy Category:* Nelfinavir, ritonavir and saquinavir: B; Amprenavir, indinavir: C. See Pregnancy Risk Categories at the back of this book.
>
> *Animal studies:* Clinical doses in rats and rabbits have not revealed teratogenicity.
>
> *Human studies:* Adequate studies of pregnant women are not available.
>
> Ask your doctor for help.

Advisability of Use If Breast-Feeding
> Presence of this drug in breast milk: Yes in rats (amprenavir, indinavir); unknown (nelfinavir, ritonavir, saquinavir).
>
> Refrain from nursing if you are HIV-positive or are taking this drug. Breast milk may also transfer the AIDS virus from mother to infant.

Habit-Forming Potential: None.

Effects of Overdose:
> *Amprenavir:* No known antidote exists. If overdose occurs, the manufacturer suggests the patients should be treated according to the signs and symptoms they develop.
>
> *Indinavir:* No human data are available. Doses of 20 times the human dose in rats and 10 times the human dose in mice were not lethal for indinavir.

Ritonavir: Limited experience, with one case reporting paresthesias and another showing sudden kidney failure with eosinophilia.

Possible Effects of Long-Term Use: Resistance may develop. Lipodystrophy and blood sugar problems may occur

Suggested Periodic Examinations While Taking These Drugs (at physician's discretion)

Liver function tests.

Complete blood counts.

CD4 or viral load measurement.

Measurement of blood sugar (glucose), especially for those with prior blood sugar problems or patients who show signs or symptoms of hyperglycemia or ketoacidosis.

Measurement of cholesterol and fractions before starting therapy and periodically while taking these medicines.

▷ **While Taking These Drugs, Observe the Following**

Foods: If indinavir is taken with a meal high in fat, calories or protein, a 77% to 91% decrease in the total amount of drug absorbed has been reported. Amprenavir absorption is decreased if it is taken with a high-fat meal. The other medicines in this class are better absorbed if taken with food.

Herbal Medicines or Minerals: Some patients use echinacea to attempt to boost their immune systems. Unfortunately, use of echinacea is not recommended in people with damaged immune systems. This herb may also actually weaken any immune system if it is used too often or for too long a time.

Nutritional Support: Since amprenavir contains a significant amount of vitamin E, supplements or multivitamins high in vitamin E should be avoided.

Beverages: No restrictions.

▷ *Alcohol:* No interactions expected.

Tobacco Smoking: May blunt therapeutic benefits of ritonavir. I advise everyone to quit smoking.

▷ *Other Drugs*

These medicines *taken concurrently* with

- amiodarone (Cordarone) increase heart toxicity risk—DO NOT combine with ritonavir; if combined with indinavir, blood levels are required.
- antacids (various, didanosine also) may lead to lower blood levels of these medicines and poor antiviral effects; separate antacid dosing by at least an hour.
- astemizole (Hismanal) may cause serious toxicity—DO NOT COMBINE (astemizole now removed from the market).
- azole antifungals (itraconazole, ketoconazole, others) may lead to increased protease inhibitor levels and toxicity.
- bepridil (Vascor) may lead to serious toxicity—DO NOT COMBINE with these medicines.
- birth control pills (oral contraceptives) may lead to low birth control levels and pregnancy (ritonavir, saquinavir and amprenavir).
- bupropion (Wellbutrin) increase seizure risk with ritonavir—DO NOT COMBINE.
- carbamazepine (Tegretol) decrease protease inhibitor levels.
- cimetidine (Tagamet) may lead to cimetidine toxicity (ritonavir only).

- cisapride (Propulsid) may cause serious toxicity—DO NOT COMBINE.
- cyclosporine (Sandimmune) may lead to cyclosporine toxicity. Blood levels and dosing changes are prudent.
- delavirdine (Rescriptor) may lead to delavirdine toxicity.
- diazepam (Valium, others) may be increased by protease inhibitors to toxic levels—DO NOT COMBINE.
- didanosine (Videx) may blunt therapeutic benefits; separate doses by 1 hour.
- digoxin (Lanoxin, others) may increase digoxin levels; lower doses of digoxin and digoxin blood levels are needed.
- diltiazem (Cardizem) may lead to diltiazem toxicity (ritonavir and saquinavir, perhaps others).
- dofetilide (Tikosyn) may lead to dofetilide toxicity.
- ergot derivatives (see Drug Classes) may lead to toxicity—DO NOT COMBINE.
- felodipine (Plendil) may lead to felodipine toxicity.
- flecainide (Tambocor) SHOULD NOT be taken with ritonavir.
- fluvastatin (Lescol) and other HMG-CoA reductase inhibitors (see Drug Classes) removed by liver CYP3A4 (atorvastatin, lovastatin, pravastatin and simvastatin) may lead to HMG-CoA toxicity. Cerivastatin (Baycol) is also removed by CYP3A4, but it is equally removed by CYP2C8 and may be a safer alternative.
- fluvoxamine (Luvox) may lead to fluvoxamine toxicity (ritonavir, perhaps others).
- gemfibrozil (Lopid) may increase gemfibrozil levels (ritonavir); patients who show signs of gemfibrozil toxicity should have gemfibrozil doses lowered.
- glimepiride (Amaryl), glipizide (Glucotrol) or glyburide (Glynase) may have blood levels changed (ritonavir); caution and possible oral hypoglycemic dosing changes are prudent.
- ibuprofen (Motrin, others) and other NSAIDs may lead to ibuprofen or other NSAID toxicity (ritonavir only)—caution is advised.
- isradipine (DynaCirc) may lead to isradipine toxicity.
- itraconazole (Sporanox) or ketoconazole (Nizoral) may cause protease inhibitor toxicity and doses of the protease inhibitor may need to be reduced. Combination with ritonavir may lead to itraconazole or ketoconazole toxicity.
- macrolide antibiotics (clarithromycin, erythromycin) may increase antibiotic levels; macrolide doses may need to be lowered (based on increased nausea/vomiting). Azithromycin may be the best macrolide to use if one is needed.
- medicines removed (metabolized) by CYP3A4 may increase blood levels greater than expected and increase risk of toxicity.
- methylenedioxymethamphetamine (MDMA or ecstasy) led to a serotonin reaction and death in one case report for ritonavir—DO NOT COMBINE.
- midazolam (Versed) may cause serious toxicity—DO NOT COMBINE.
- narcotics such as morphine (MS Contin) or methadone (Dolophine) may lead to toxic narcotic levels.
- nevirapine (Viramune) may blunt therapeutic effects of indinavir—Caution and dosing changes are prudent.

- oral hypoglycemics (see Drug classes) may lead to excessive lowering of blood sugar (ritonavir only).
- other antiretrovirals may reduce viral load to nondetectable levels but may also interact (ritonavir lowers nelfinavir levels, while indinavir increases nelfinavir or saquinavir levels).
- other drugs that are toxic to the liver may result in additive toxicity (except amprenavir).
- other drugs that can lead to kidney stones may result in additive risk with indinavir.
- paclitaxel (Taxol) may lead to paclitaxel toxicity (ritonavir).
- phenytoin (Dilantin) or fosphenytoin (Cerebyx) may lower protease benefits.
- propafenone (Rythmol) should NOT be taken with ritonavir and may be contraindicated with other protease inhibitors.
- quinidine (Quinaglute, others) should NOT be taken with ritonavir, nelfinavir. Other protease inhibitors may increase quinidine blood levels, and more frequent quinidine levels are prudent. Indinavir is considered to be safe to give with quinidine.
- rifabutin (Mycobutin) may increase rifabutin and decrease indinavir levels; half the usual dose of rifabutin is used if these drugs are combined.
- rifampin (Rifater, others) may cause loss of indinavir and amprenavir benefits—DO NOT COMBINE.
- saquinavir (Fortovase) (and ritonavir) may lead to increased saquinavir levels and possible toxicity unless doses are reduced.
- sirolimus (Rapamune) may cause sirolimus or tacrolimus (Prograf) with ritonavir may lead to toxicity.
- sildenafil (Viagra) may lead to excessive blood levels of sildenafil and possible toxicity (amprenavir, ritonavir and saquinavir).
- tramadol (Ultram) may lead to tramadol toxicity; reduced tramadol doses are mandatory if these medicines are combined.
- triazolam (Halcion) and perhaps other benzodiazepines may cause serious toxicity.
- tricyclic antidepressants (see Drug Classes) should have blood levels checked.
- venlafaxine (Effexor) may increase risk of venlafaxine toxicity when combined with some PIs.
- warfarin (Coumadin) may increase risk of bleeding (amprenavir, ritonavir and nelfinavir only); frequent INR checks are prudent.
- zolpidem (Ambien) may produce toxic zolpidem levels (if combined with ritonavir)—DO NOT COMBINE.

▷ *Driving, Hazardous Activities:* Some of these drugs may rarely cause sleepiness. Restrict activities as necessary.

Aviation Note: The use of these drugs *may be a disqualification* for piloting. Consult a designated Aviation Medical Examiner.

Exposure to Sun: No restrictions.

Special Storage Instructions: The new ritonavir soft gelatin capsules DO NOT require refrigeration if they are stored below 77 degrees Fahrenheit.

Discontinuation: Do not stop these drugs without your doctor's knowledge and guidance.

PROTRIPTYLINE (proh TRIP ti leen)

Introduced: 1966   **Class:** Antidepressant   **Prescription:** USA: Yes
Controlled Drug: USA: No; Canada: No   **Available as Generic:** USA: Yes;
Canada: No
Brand Names: ♣Triptil, Vivactil

BENEFITS versus RISKS	
Possible Benefits	*Possible Risks*
EFFECTIVE RELIEF OF MAJOR ENDOGENOUS DEPRESSIONS	ADVERSE BEHAVIORAL EFFECTS: confusion, disorientation, hallucinations, delusions
HELPS MANAGE OTHER DEPRESSIVE DISORDERS	CONVERSION OF DEPRESSION TO MANIA in manic-depressive (bipolar) disorders
Beneficial in management of narcolepsy/cataplexy syndrome	Aggravation of schizophrenia
	Irregular heart rhythms
	Blood cell abnormalities

▷ **Principal Uses**
   As a Single Drug Product: Uses currently included in FDA-approved labeling:
      Relieves symptoms associated with major spontaneous (endogenous)
      depression, depressed bipolar disorder and mixed bipolar disorder.
      Other (unlabeled) generally accepted uses: (1) Treatment of sleep disorders
      such as apnea, hypersomnia and impaired morning arousal; (2) may have
      a role in treating glaucoma; (3) used in combination with methylphenidate
      or amphetamines in treating narcolepsy.
**Author's Note: The information in this profile has been shortened to make
room for more widely used medicines.**

PYRAZINAMIDE (peer a ZIN a mide)

Introduced: 1968   **Class:** Anti-infective, antituberculosis   **Prescription:**
USA: Yes   **Controlled Drug:** USA: No; Canada: No   **Available as Generic:**
USA: Yes; Canada: No
Brand Names: ♣PMS Pyrazinamide, Rifater [CD], ♣Tebrazid

BENEFITS versus RISKS	
Possible Benefits	*Possible Risks*
EFFECTIVE ADJUNCTIVE TREATMENT OF TUBERCULOSIS	DRUG-INDUCED HEPATITIS—rare
	Activation of gouty arthritis and porphyria
	Decreased platelets and hemoglobin

▷ **Principal Uses**
   As a Single Drug Product: Uses currently included in FDA-approved labeling:
      Treatment of active tuberculosis, in combination with other antitubercular
      drugs.

Other (unlabeled) generally accepted uses: (1) Combination therapy of Mycobacterium xenopi infections; (2) combination therapy of resistant tuberculosis; (3) combination therapy of tuberculosis in AIDS.

As a Combination Drug Product [CD]: This medicine is combined with other antituberculosis medicines (isoniazid and rifampin) in order to attack tuberculosis with combination treatment in a single-dose form. This undoubtedly helps adherence!

How This Drug Works: This drug is ideal for killing tuberculosis organisms that are in acid environments, such as in some kinds of white blood (macrophages) cells.

Available Dosage Forms and Strengths

Tablets — 500 mg

Tablets — 300 mg pyrazinamide, 50 mg isoniazid and 120 mg of rifampin (Rifater brand)

▷ **Recommended Dosage Ranges** (Actual dose and schedule must be determined for each patient individually.)

Infants and Children: 7.5 to 15 mg per kg of body mass, twice daily; or 15 to 30 mg per kg of body mass, once daily. Total daily dose should not exceed 1.5 g.

12 to 60 Years of Age: For tuberculosis—15 to 30 mg per kg of body mass (up to a maximum of 2,000 mg) daily. Some patients do better with twice-weekly dosing with 50 to 70 mg per kg of body mass (up to 4,000 mg).

Author's Note: Because of the current resistant tuberculosis problem, most clinicians start all patients on a four-drug regimen for 8 weeks (until laboratory culture results are available). Treatment of this widespread resistant organism should be based on local resistance trends and individual patient organisms and typically continues for 6 months.

Over 60 Years of Age: Same as 12 to 60 years of age.

Conditions Requiring Dosing Adjustments

Liver Function: This drug should be used with caution and in decreased doses by patients with liver compromise. Contraindicated in patients with severe liver dysfunction.

Kidney Function: For patients with end-stage renal failure, the dose must be adjusted. One researcher recommends 60 mg per kg of body mass, twice weekly. The dose of pyrazinamide should be given at least 24 hours before any given dialysis session. Patients should be closely monitored.

▷ **Dosing Instructions:** The tablet may be crushed and taken with or following food to reduce stomach irritation. Take the full course prescribed. This drug should be taken concurrently with other antitubercular drugs to prevent the development of drug-resistant strains of tuberculosis bacteria. The Rifater product accomplishes triple therapy in a single pill. If you forget a dose: Take the missed dose as soon as you remember it, unless it's nearly time for your next dose—if that is the case, skip the missed dose and take the next dose right on schedule. DO NOT take two doses at the same time. Talk with your doctor if you find yourself missing doses. IT IS CRITICAL to take this medicine exactly as prescribed.

Usual Duration of Use: Use on a regular schedule for 2 months usually determines effectiveness in controlling active tuberculosis. Long-term use of antitubercular drugs (6 months is typical) requires periodic physician evaluation.

Typical Treatment Goals and Measurements (Outcomes and Markers)

Infections: The most commonly used measures of serious infections are white blood cell counts and differentials (the kind of blood cells that occur most often in your blood), and temperature. While clinicians look for positive changes in 24–48 hours in typical infections, this kind of infection REQUIRES long-term treatment to kill it. NEVER stop an antibiotic because you start to feel better. The goals and time frame (see peak benefits above) should be discussed with you when the prescription is written. Months of treatment are usually required to kill this resistant organism.

Possible Advantages of This Drug

May reduce the period of drug treatment from 9 months down to 6 months in responsive infections.

▷ ### This Drug Should Not Be Taken If

- you have had an allergic reaction to it previously.
- you have permanent liver damage with impaired function.
- you have active gout.
- you have active peptic ulcer disease.

▷ ### Inform Your Physician Before Taking This Drug If

- you have had an allergic reaction to ethionamide, isoniazid or niacin (nicotinic acid).
- you have a history of liver disease.
- you have a history of peptic ulcer or porphyria.
- you tried to take medicines for tuberculosis before, but did not complete the prescribed therapy.
- you have gout or diabetes.
- you have impaired kidney function.

Possible Side Effects (natural, expected and unavoidable drug actions)

Increased blood uric acid levels. Fever.

▷ ### Possible Adverse Effects (unusual, unexpected and infrequent reactions)

If any of the following develop, consult your physician promptly for guidance.

Mild Adverse Effects

Allergic reactions: skin rash, itching, fever.

Loss of appetite, mild nausea, vomiting—frequent.

Joint pain—frequent.

Acne—rare.

Serious Adverse Effects

Idiosyncratic reactions: Rare sideroblastic anemia.

Decreased blood platelets—rare.

Seizures—rare.

Drug-induced porphyria or pellagra—case reports.

Kidney problems (interstitial nephritis)—case reports.

Drug-induced hepatitis, with and without jaundice (see Glossary)—case reports.

Gouty arthritis, due to increased blood uric acid levels—possible.

▷ ### Possible Effects on Sexual Function: None reported other than rare reports of painful urination.

▷ ### Adverse Effects That May Mimic Natural Diseases or Disorders

Drug-induced hepatitis may suggest viral hepatitis.

Natural Diseases or Disorders That May Be Activated by This Drug
Gout, peptic ulcer, porphyria.

Possible Effects on Laboratory Tests
Complete blood cell counts: decreased red cells, hemoglobin and platelets.
INR (prothrombin time): increased.
Blood sugar: tight control may become more difficult.
Blood uric acid level: increased.
Liver function tests: increased enzymes (ALT/GPT, AST/GOT, alkaline phosphatase) or bilirubin.
Urine ketone tests: false-positive test result with Acetest and Ketostix.

CAUTION
1. When this drug is used alone, tuberculosis bacteria rapidly develop resistance to it. To be effective, this drug must be used in combination with other effective antitubercular drugs, such as isoniazid and rifampin. The CDC states that the rifampin combination requires frequent liver tests.
2. This drug may interfere with control of diabetes.

Precautions for Use
By Infants and Children: Safety and effectiveness for those under 12 years of age are not established. The rare occurrence of drug-related seizure has been reported in a 2-year-old child.
By Those Over 60 Years of Age: No specific information available.

▷ **Advisability of Use During Pregnancy**
Pregnancy Category: C. See Pregnancy Risk Categories at the back of this book.
Animal studies: No information available.
Human studies: Adequate studies of pregnant women are not available.
Use this drug only if clearly needed. Ask your physician for guidance.

Advisability of Use If Breast-Feeding
Presence of this drug in breast milk: Yes.
Avoid drug or refrain from nursing.

Habit-Forming Potential: None.

Effects of Overdose: Nausea, vomiting, malaise.

Possible Effects of Long-Term Use: Liver damage.

Suggested Periodic Examinations While Taking This Drug (at physician's discretion)
Complete blood cell counts.
Liver function tests.
Uric acid blood levels.

▷ **While Taking This Drug, Observe the Following**
Foods: No restrictions.
Herbal Medicines or Minerals: Some patients use echinacea to attempt to boost their immune systems. Unfortunately, use of echinacea is not recommended in people with damaged immune systems. This herb may also actually weaken any immune system if it is used too often or for too long a time. Do NOT take mistletoe herb, oak bark or F.C. of marshmallow root, woody nightshade stem or licorice. Since St. John's wort and pyrazinamide may cause increased sun sensitivity, caution is advised.
Beverages: No restrictions. May be taken with milk.
▷ *Alcohol:* Use sparingly to minimize liver toxicity.

Tobacco Smoking: No interactions expected. I advise everyone to quit smoking.
▷ *Other Drugs*
Pyrazinamide may *decrease* the effects of
- allopurinol (Zyloprim).
- BCG vaccine.
- cyclosporine (Sandimmune).
- probenecid (Benemid).
- sulfinpyrazone (Anturane).

Pyrazinamide *taken concurrently* with
- phenytoin (Dilantin) or fosphenytoin (Cerebyx) may lead to phenytoin or fosphenytoin toxicity.
- zidovudine (AZT) may lead to low pyrazinamide levels. Dosing changes may be needed.

▷ *Driving, Hazardous Activities:* No restrictions.
Aviation Note: The use of this drug is probably not a disqualification for piloting. Consult a designated Aviation Medical Examiner.
Exposure to Sun: Use caution—this drug may cause photosensitivity (see Glossary).
Discontinuation: If tolerated, this drug is usually taken for a minimum of 2 months. Do not stop it without your physician's knowledge and guidance.

PYRIDOSTIGMINE (peer id oh STIG meen)

Introduced: 1962   **Class:** Antimyasthenic   **Prescription:** USA: Yes
Controlled Drug: USA: No; Canada: No   **Available as Generic:** USA: No; Canada: No
Brand Names: ✸Anaplex SR, Mestinon, Mestinon-SR, Mestinon Timespan, Regonol

BENEFITS versus RISKS	
Possible Benefits	*Possible Risks*
MODERATELY EFFECTIVE TREATMENT OF OCULAR AND MILD FORMS OF MYASTHENIA GRAVIS (symptomatic relief of muscle weakness) PRETREATMENT ADJUNCT IN WARTIME WHEN NERVE AGENT EXPOSURE IS POSSIBLE	Cholinergic crisis (overdose): excessive salivation, nausea, vomiting, stomach cramps, diarrhea, shortness of breath (asthmalike wheezing), excessive weakness

▷ **Principal Uses**
As a Single Drug Product: Uses currently included in FDA-approved labeling:
(1) Used to treat the ocular and milder forms of myasthenia gravis by providing temporary relief of muscle weakness and fatigability (most useful in long-term treatment when there is little or no swallowing difficulty); (2) used to reverse muscle relaxants.
Other (unlabeled) generally accepted uses: (1) Combination therapy in chronic pain; (2) may help in combination therapy of Huntington's chorea and Lambert-Eaton syndrome; (3) adjunctive use with scopolamine to prevent

side effects of scopolamine in treating motion sickness; (4) used in war zones to treat the effects of nerve gas; (5) may have a role in treating nonepidemic parotitis.

How This Drug Works: This drug inhibits cholinesterase, the enzyme that destroys acetylcholine. This results in higher levels of acetylcholine, the nerve transmitter that facilitates the stimulation of muscular activity. The net effects are increased muscle strength and endurance.

Available Dosage Forms and Strengths

Syrup — 60 mg/5 ml (5% alcohol)

Tablets — 30 mg, 60 mg

Tablets, prolonged action — 180 mg

▷ **Usual Adult Dosage Ranges:** *Myasthenia gravis*: Initially 1 to 6 normal-release tablets, spaced throughout the day when maximum strength is needed. Maintenance varies with the severity of the disease—1 to 3 extended-release tablets once or twice a day. If twice-daily extended-release doses are needed, they should be separated by 6 hours. Some patients may need to supplement the extended-release tablets with the 30-mg, immediate-release tablets or the syrup in order to best control symptoms.

Nerve gas or agent protection: 30 mg every 8 hours when the threat of a nerve agent attack is present. Pralidoxime (600 mg) and atropine citrate (2 mg) are also given injected into a muscle if there actually is nerve gas exposure. **Note: Actual dose and schedule must be determined for each patient individually.**

Conditions Requiring Dosing Adjustments

Liver Function: No dosing changes are defined in liver compromise.

Kidney Function: This drug is primarily eliminated in the urine, but specific guidelines for dose adjustments in renal compromise are not available.

▷ **Dosing Instructions:** Take with food or milk to reduce the intensity of side effects. Larger portions of the daily maintenance dose should be timed according to the pattern of fatigue and weakness. The syrup will permit a finer adjustment of dose. The regular tablet may be crushed. Mestinon sustained-release tablets can be cut in half. These tablets may NOT be crushed or cut into four pieces, as that would change the way that the drug is released. If you forget a dose: Take the missed dose as soon as you remember it, unless it's nearly time for your next dose—if that is the case, skip the missed dose and take the next dose right on schedule. DO NOT double doses. Talk with your doctor if you find yourself missing doses.

Usual Duration of Use: Use on a regular schedule (with dose adjustment) for 10 to 14 days usually determines effectiveness in relieving myasthenia symptoms. Long-term use (months to years) requires periodic physician evaluation.

Typical Treatment Goals and Measurements (Outcomes and Markers)

Myasthenia gravis: The general goal is to increase muscle strength while avoiding nicotinic or muscarinic effects (diarrhea, salivation, nausea and vomiting). Immediate release-form dosing is timed to correspond to fatigue or weakness.

▷ **This Drug Should Not Be Taken If**

- you are known to be allergic to bromide compounds.
- you have a urinary obstruction or mechanical intestinal obstruction.

▷ **Inform Your Physician Before Taking This Drug If**
- you have heart rhythm disorders or bronchial asthma.
- you are sensitive to bromides.
- you have recurrent urinary tract infections.
- you have prostatism (see Glossary).
- you will have surgery with general anesthesia.

Possible Side Effects (natural, expected and unavoidable drug actions)
Small pupils (miosis), watering of eyes, slow pulse, excessive salivation, nausea, vomiting, stomach cramps, diarrhea, urge to urinate, increased sweating, increased bronchial secretions.

▷ **Possible Adverse Effects** (unusual, unexpected and infrequent reactions)
If any of the following develop, consult your physician promptly for guidance.
Mild Adverse Effects
Allergic reactions: skin rash.
Nervousness, anxiety, unsteadiness, muscle cramps or twitching—infrequent.
Loss of scalp hair (alopecia)—case report.
Serious Adverse Effects
Confusion, slurred speech, seizures, difficult breathing (asthmatic wheezing).
Increased muscle weakness or paralysis—case report.
Psychosis—rare.
Excessive vomiting or diarrhea may cause low potassium levels (hypokalemia). This accentuates muscle weakness.

▷ **Possible Effects on Sexual Function:** None reported.

▷ **Adverse Effects That May Mimic Natural Diseases or Disorders**
Seizures may suggest the possibility of epilepsy.

Natural Diseases or Disorders That May Be Activated by This Drug
Latent bronchial asthma.

Possible Effects on Laboratory Tests: None reported.

CAUTION
1. Some drugs block this drug, reducing effectiveness in treating myasthenia gravis (see "Other Drugs" below). Ask your doctor before starting any other medicine.
2. Variations in response may occur from time to time. Because generalized muscle weakness is a major symptom of both myasthenia crisis (underdose) and cholinergic crisis (overdose), it may be difficult to recognize the correct cause. As a rule, weakness that starts an hour after taking this drug probably represents overdose; weakness that begins 3 or more hours after taking this drug is probably due to underdose. Watch these relationships and tell your doctor.
3. During long-term use, watch for development of resistance to the therapeutic action (loss of effect). Ask your doctor if the drug should be stopped for a few days to see if response can be restored.

Precautions for Use
By Infants and Children: The syrup form of this drug permits greater precision of dose adjustment and ease of administration in this age group. Neonates have received 5 mg every 4 to 6 hours. Since this is often self-limiting in neonates, the medicine can frequently be tapered and stopped.

By Those Over 60 Years of Age: The natural decline of kidney function with aging may require smaller doses to prevent accumulation of this drug to toxic levels.

▷ **Advisability of Use During Pregnancy**

Pregnancy Category: C. See Pregnancy Risk Categories at the back of this book.

Animal studies: No information available.

Human studies: Adequate studies of pregnant women are not available.

There are no reports of birth defects due to the use of this drug during pregnancy. However, there are reports of significant muscular weakness in newborn infants whose mothers had taken this drug during pregnancy.

Ask your physician for guidance.

Advisability of Use If Breast-Feeding

Presence of this drug in breast milk: Yes, as roughly 0.01% of the mother's dose.

Monitor nursing infant closely, and discontinue drug or nursing if adverse effects develop.

Habit-Forming Potential: None.

Effects of Overdose: Generalized muscular weakness, blurred vision, very small pupils, slow heart rate, difficult breathing (wheezing), excessive salivation, nausea, vomiting, stomach cramps, diarrhea, muscle cramps or twitching. This syndrome constitutes the cholinergic crisis.

Possible Effects of Long-Term Use: Development of tolerance (see Glossary) with loss of therapeutic effectiveness.

Suggested Periodic Examinations While Taking This Drug (at physician's discretion)

Assessment of drug effectiveness and dose schedule for optimal therapeutic results.

▷ **While Taking This Drug, Observe the Following**

Foods: No restrictions.

Herbal Medicines or Minerals: Echinacea pallida root or purpurea herb as well as woody nightshade stem or belladonna should be avoided.

Beverages: No restrictions. May be taken with milk.

▷ *Alcohol:* Use caution until the combined effects are determined. Weakness and unsteadiness may be accentuated.

Tobacco Smoking: No interactions expected. I advise everyone to quit smoking.

▷ *Other Drugs*

Pyridostigmine *taken concurrently* with

• disopyramide (Norpace) may ease undesirable anticholinergic effects (problems urinating, decreased sweating, etc.).

• succinylcholine (various) may increase muscular problems (neuromuscular blockade). This combination should usually be avoided in patients taking pyridostigmine.

The following drugs may *decrease* the effects of pyridostigmine:

• adrenocortical steroids (see Drug Classes).

• atropine (belladonna).

• clindamycin (Cleocin).

• guanadrel (Hylorel).

• guanethidine (Esimil, Ismelin).

- procainamide (Procan SR, Pronestyl).
- quinidine (Cardioquin, Duraquin, etc.).
- quinine (Quinamm).

▷ *Driving, Hazardous Activities:* This drug may cause blurred vision, confusion or generalized weakness. Restrict activities as necessary.

Aviation Note: The use of this drug **is a disqualification** for piloting. Consult a designated Aviation Medical Examiner.

Exposure to Sun: No restrictions.

Exposure to Heat: Use caution—this drug may cause excessive sweating and increased weakness.

Exposure to Environmental Chemicals: Avoid excessive exposure (inhalation, skin contamination) to the insecticides Baygon, Diazinon and Sevin. These can worsen potential drug toxicity.

Discontinuation: Do not stop this drug abruptly without your doctor's knowledge and guidance.

QUAZEPAM (KWAH zee pam)

Introduced: 1982   **Class:** Hypnotic, benzodiazepines   **Prescription:** USA: Yes   **Controlled Drug:** USA: C-IV*   **Available as Generic:** USA: No
Brand Names: Doral, Dormalin
Author's Note: The National Institute of Mental Health has an informatio page on anxiety. It can be found on the World Wide Web (www.nimh.nih. gov/anxiety). The information in this profile has been abbreviated to make room for more widely used medicines.

QUINAPRIL (KWIN a pril)

Introduced: 1984   **Class:** Antihypertensive, ACE inhibitor
Please see the angiotensin converting enzyme (ACE) inhibitor family profile.

QUINIDINE (KWIN i deen)

Introduced: 1918   **Class:** Antiarrhythmic   **Prescription:** USA: Yes
Controlled Drug: USA: No; Canada: No   **Available as Generic:** Yes
Brand Names: ✿Apo-Quinidine, ✿Biquin Durules, Cardioquin, Cin-Quin, Duraquin, ✿Natisedine, ✿Novo-Quinidin, Quinaglute Dura-Tabs, ✿ Quinate, Quinatime, Quinidex Extentabs, ✿Quinobarb [CD]†, Quinora, Quin-Release, SK-Quinidine Sulfate

*See Schedules of Controlled Drugs at the back of this book.
†Quinobarb contains phenylethylbarbiturate, a sedative of the barbiturate family.

```
┌─────────────────────────────────────────────────────────────────┐
│                      BENEFITS versus RISKS                        │
│        Possible Benefits              Possible Risks              │
│   EFFECTIVE TREATMENT OF        NARROW TREATMENT RANGE            │
│     SELECTED HEART RHYTHM       FREQUENT ADVERSE EFFECTS          │
│     DISORDERS                   NUMEROUS ALLERGIC AND             │
│                                   IDIOSYNCRATIC REACTIONS         │
│                                 Dose-related toxicity             │
│                                 Provocation of abnormal heart     │
│                                   rhythms                         │
│                                 Abnormally low blood platelet count│
│                                 Hemolytic anemia                  │
│                                 Kidney or liver toxicity          │
└─────────────────────────────────────────────────────────────────┘
```

▷ **Principal Uses**

As a Single Drug Product: Uses currently included in FDA-approved labeling: (1) Helps control the following types of abnormal heart rhythm: atrial fibrillation and flutter, paroxysmal atrial tachycardia, paroxysmal ventricular tachycardia, premature atrial and ventricular contractions; (2) intravenous treatment of malaria in people who cannot take medicine by mouth.

Other (unlabeled) generally accepted uses: None.

As a Combination Drug Product [CD]: This drug is available (in Canada) in combination with a barbiturate, a mild sedative that is added to allay the anxiety and nervous tension that often accompany heart rhythm disorders.

How This Drug Works: Slows activity of the heart pacemaker and delays electrical impulses through the heart conduction system, restoring normal heart rate and rhythm.

Available Dosage Forms and Strengths

>   Capsules — 200 mg, 300 mg
>   Injections — 80 mg/ml, 200 mg/ml
>   Tablets — 100 mg, 200 mg, 275 mg, 300 mg
>   Tablets, prolonged action — 250 mg, 300 mg, 324 mg, 330 mg

▷ **Usual Adult Dosage Ranges:** *Premature atrial or ventricular contractions*: Quinidine sulfate immediate-release—200 to 400 mg every 4 to 6 hours. Quinidine sulfate extended-release (Quinidex Extentabs)—300 to 600 mg every 8–12 hours. Quinidine gluconate—324 mg to 648 mg or 1–2 tablets every 8–12 hours.

Paroxysmal atrial tachycardia: 400 to 600 mg every 2 to 3 hours until paroxysm is terminated.

Atrial flutter: Digitalize first; then individualize dose schedule as appropriate.

Atrial fibrillation: Digitalize first; then try 200 mg every 2 to 3 hours for five to eight doses; increase dose daily until normal rhythm is restored or toxic effects develop.

Maintenance schedule: 200 to 300 mg three or four times daily. Total daily dose should not exceed 4,000 mg.

Note: Actual dose and schedule must be determined for each patient individually.

Conditions Requiring Dosing Adjustments

Liver Function: This drug is extensively metabolized in the liver. Blood levels should be obtained to guide dosing. A larger loading dose and a 50% decreased maintenance dose may be indicated.

Kidney Function: Blood levels should be obtained and used to guide dosing. Quinidine should be used with **CAUTION** in renal compromise.

▷ **Dosing Instructions:** This drug is preferably taken on an empty stomach to achieve high blood levels rapidly. However, it may be taken with or following food to reduce stomach irritation. The regular tablets may be crushed and the capsules opened. Prolonged-action forms should be swallowed whole without alteration. If you forget a dose: Take the missed dose as soon as you remember it, unless you've missed your dose by 2 hours for immediate-release forms or 4 hours for sustained-release forms—if that is the case, skip the missed dose and take the next dose right on schedule. Call your doctor if you've missed more than two doses. Talk with your doctor if you find yourself missing doses. There are a variety of reminder pill boxes or even beeper systems to help.

Usual Duration of Use: Use on a regular schedule for 2 to 4 days usually determines effectiveness in correcting or preventing responsive abnormal rhythms. Long-term use (months to years) requires physician supervision and periodic evaluation and blood levels.

Typical Treatment Goals and Measurements (Outcomes and Markers)

Abnormal heartbeats: The general goal is to return the heart to a normal rhythm or at least to markedly reduce the occurrence of abnormal heartbeats. In life-threatening arrhythmias, the goal is to abort the abnormal beats and return the pattern to normal. Success at ongoing suppression may involve ambulatory checks of heart rate and rhythm for a day (such as in Holter monitoring). This kind of testing involves placement of adhesive backed temporary electrodes on the skin in several positions around the heart. A small heart rate and rhythm (EKG or ECG) recording device is carried around via a shoulder strap and records what the heart is doing over 24 hours. Once the recording is made, a scanning machine reviews the record, tallies abnormal heart beats or rhythms and gives a close and extended look at how the heart is reacting or benefiting from the medicines that the patient is taking. Repeat measurements can be made if doses are changes to check the success at keeping the heart at normal sinus rhythm!

▷ **This Drug Should Not Be Taken If**
- you have had an allergic or idiosyncratic reaction to it previously.
- you currently have an acute infection of any kind.
- you have taken too much digoxin (digoxin toxicity).
- you have myasthenia gravis or kidney disease.
- you have an AV block (complete) and do not have an artificial pacemaker or you have conduction problems in the ventricles (intraventricular conduction defects).
- you have abnormal heart rhythms caused by an escape mechanism (ask your specialist).

▷ **Inform Your Physician Before Taking This Drug If**
- you have coronary artery disease or sick sinus syndrome.
- you have a history of excessive thyroid function (hyperthyroidism).
- you usually have very low blood pressure.
- you have had a deficiency of blood platelets in the past from any cause.

- your blood chemistry (electrolyte content) is not in balance.
- you are now taking, or have taken recently, any digitalis preparation (digitoxin, digoxin, etc.).
- you will have surgery with general anesthesia.
- you have a history of passing out (syncopal episodes).
- you have acute rheumatic fever or subacute bacterial endocarditis (SBE).

Possible Side Effects (natural, expected and unavoidable drug actions)

Drop in blood pressure, may be marked in some patients and cause passing out (syncope).

▷ **Possible Adverse Effects** (unusual, unexpected and infrequent reactions)

If any of the following develop, consult your physician promptly for guidance.

Mild Adverse Effects

Allergic reactions: skin rash, hives, itching, drug fever—rare.

Irritation of the esophagus (esophagitis)—possible.

Nausea, vomiting, diarrhea—infrequent.

Serious Adverse Effects

Allergic reactions: severe skin reactions, hemolytic anemia (see Glossary), joint and muscle pains, anaphylactic reaction (see Glossary), reduced blood platelet count, drug-induced hepatitis (see Glossary).

Idiosyncratic reactions: skin rash, fast heart rate, delirium, difficult breathing.

Dose-related toxicity (cinchonism): blurred vision, ringing ears, hearing loss, heart arrest.

Drug-induced myasthenia gravis, systemic lupus erythematosus (SLE) or carpal tunnel syndrome—case reports.

Swelling of the lymph glands in the inguinal area (lymphadenopathy)—case report.

Kidney toxicity—case reports.

Heart conduction abnormalities—case reports.

Optic neuritis, impaired vision—case report.

Abnormally low white blood cell count: fever, sore throat, infections—case reports.

Abnormally low platelet count—case reports.

▷ **Possible Effects on Sexual Function:** None reported.

▷ **Adverse Effects That May Mimic Natural Diseases or Disorders**

Drug-induced hepatitis may suggest viral hepatitis.

Natural Diseases or Disorders That May Be Activated by This Drug

Systemic lupus erythematosus, myasthenia gravis, psoriasis (in sensitive people).

Possible Effects on Laboratory Tests

Complete blood cell counts: decreased red cells, hemoglobin, white cells and platelets; increased eosinophils (allergic reaction); marked increase of white blood cells in association with "quinidine fever"—very rare.

Antinuclear antibodies (ANA): positive.

INR (protime): increased (when *taken concurrently* with warfarin).

Liver function tests: increased enzymes (ALT/GPT, AST/GOT, alkaline phosphatase) or bilirubin.

CAUTION

1. Dose adjustments must be based upon individual reaction.
2. Dosing schedules differ for the various salt forms. For example, quini-

dine sulfate (83% anhydrous quinidine) is not the same as quinidine gluconate (62% anhydrous quinidine) or quinidine polygalacturonate (60% anhydrous quinidine). MAKE CERTAIN that any refill prescriptions contain the correct medicine.

3. It is prudent to carry a card saying that you take this drug in case of an accident.

Precautions for Use
By Infants and Children: A test for drug idiosyncrasy should be made before starting treatment with this drug. If there is no beneficial response after 3 days of adequate dose, this drug should be discontinued.

By Those Over 60 Years of Age: Small doses are mandatory until your individual response has been determined. Observe for the development of light-headedness, dizziness, weakness or sense of impending faint. Use *CAUTION* to prevent falls.

▷ ### Advisability of Use During Pregnancy
Pregnancy Category: C. See Pregnancy Risk Categories at the back of this book.
Animal studies: No information available.
Human studies: Adequate studies of pregnant women are not available. No birth defects have been reported following use of this drug during pregnancy. Use this drug only if clearly needed.

Advisability of Use If Breast-Feeding
Presence of this drug in breast milk: Yes.
Avoid drug or refrain from nursing.

Habit-Forming Potential: None.

Effects of Overdose: Nausea, vomiting, ringing in the ears, headache, jerky eye movements, double vision, altered color vision, confusion, delirium, hot skin, seizures, coma.

Possible Effects of Long-Term Use: None reported.

Suggested Periodic Examinations While Taking This Drug (at physician's discretion)
Complete blood cell counts.
Electrocardiograms.
Blood levels.

▷ ### While Taking This Drug, Observe the Following
Foods: No restrictions.
Herbal Medicines or Minerals: Kola, St. John's wort, ma huang and yohimbe may cause additive heart rate or rhythm problems. These are not advisable if you have heart rhythm difficulties. Using St. John's wort, ma huang, ephedra or kola while taking this medicine may result in unacceptable heart stimulation. Belladonna, henbane, scopolia, pheasant's eye extract or lily of the valley or squill powdered extracts should NOT be taken if you have abnormal heart rhythms. Since St. John's wort and quinidine may increase sun sensitivity, the combination is NOT advised.
Beverages: No restrictions. May be taken with milk.
▷ *Alcohol:* Use caution—alcohol may enhance the blood-pressure-lowering effects of this drug.
Tobacco Smoking: Nicotine can increase irritability of the heart and aggravate rhythm disorders. Avoid all forms of tobacco.

▷   *Other Drugs*

Quinidine *taken concurrently* with

- aspirin may prolong the bleeding time.
- beta blockers may result in additive and undesirable beta-blockade; lower starting doses may be needed for both medicines.
- cisapride (Propulsid) may lead to serious heart rhythm problems—DO NOT COMBINE.
- codeine may blunt the effectiveness of codeine.
- dextromethorphan (the DM in many cough preparations) can lead to dextromethorphan toxicity—DO NOT COMBINE.
- dofetilide (Tikosyn) may lead to serious heart rhythm problems—DO NOT COMBINE. Prudent to wait roughly five (4.32 half-lives) after stopping a prior class-one antiarrhythmic or other QTc prolonging drug before starting dofetilide.
- fluoxetine (Prozac) may lead to quinidine or fluoxetine toxicity.
- gatifloxacin (Tequin), grepafloxacin (Raxar), moxifloxacin (Avelox) or sparfloxacin (Zagam) may lead to abnormal heartbeats.
- magnesium containing antacids (various) may lead to excessive accumulation of quinidine and quinidine toxicity. More frequent checks of blood levels are prudent if these medicines must be combined.
- metformin (Glucophage) may increase risk of lactic acidosis.
- neuromuscular blocking agents (such as pancuronium-Pavulon, vecuronium-Norcuron, others) can result in increased severity of muscle blockade. Use of lower neuromuscular blocker doses is prudent.
- nisoldipine (Sular) may blunt nisoldipine benefits.
- tramadol (Ultram) may lead to tramadol toxicity.
- tricyclic antidepressants (see Drug Classes) may result in antidepressant toxicity.
- venlafaxine (Effexor) may result in venlafaxine toxicity.

Quinidine may *increase* the effects of

- anticoagulants (Coumadin, etc.) and increase the risk of bleeding; more frequent INR (prothrombin time or protime) testing is needed.
- digitoxin and digoxin (Lanoxin) and cause digitalis toxicity.
- disopyramide (Norpace).
- metformin (Glucophage).
- propafenone (Rythmol) may lead to propafenone toxicity. Careful patient follow up is critical as propafenone dosing adjustments may be required.
- tricyclic antidepressants (amitriptyline, doxepin).
- warfarin (Coumadin) and may result in coagulation changes (inconsistent effect). More frequent INR checks are prudent.

The following drugs may *increase* the effects of quinidine:

- amiodarone (Cordarone). The quinidine dose should be about half the usually recommended dose for patients who are already taking amiodarone and a decision has been made to switch from amiodarone to quinidine. If combination treatment is thought to be required, careful checks of dosing and cautious checks of blood levels are needed to avoid development of atypical quick heart rates in the ventricles (such as torsades de pointes).
- cimetidine (Tagamet).
- delavirdine (Rescriptor).

- diclofenac (Voltaren).
- diltiazem (Cardizem).
- erythromycin (various).
- itraconazole (Sporanox).
- ketoconazole (Nizoral).
- quinupristin/dalfopristin (Synercid) may lead to serious heart rhythm problems—extremely careful quinidine level follow up and careful patient monitoring are critical if these medicines must be combined.
- ritonavir (Norvir), nelfinavir (Viracept) and perhaps other protease inhibitors (see Drug Classes)—Do not combine.
- sertraline (Zoloft).
- verapamil (Verelan).

The following drugs may **_decrease_** the effects of quinidine:
- barbiturates (phenobarbital, etc.).
- phenytoin (Dilantin) or fosphenytoin (Cerebyx).
- rifabutin (Mycobutin).
- rifampin (Rifadin, Rimactane).
- sucralfate (Carafate).

▷ *Driving, Hazardous Activities:* This drug may cause dizziness and alter vision. Restrict activities as necessary.

Aviation Note: The use of this drug **_may be a disqualification_** for piloting. Consult a designated Aviation Medical Examiner.

Exposure to Sun: Use caution—this drug may cause photosensitivity (see Glossary).

RALOXIFENE (rah LOX i feen)

Introduced: 1997   **Class:** Antiestrogen, selective estrogen receptor inhibitor (SERM), anti-osteoporosis   **Prescription:** USA: Yes   **Controlled Drug:** USA: No; Canada: No   **Available as Generic:** No
Brand Name: Evista

BENEFITS versus RISKS	
Possible Benefits	*Possible Risks*
EFFECTIVE PREVENTION OF POSTMENOPAUSAL OSTEOPOROSIS	Changes in blood clotting
EFFECTIVE TREATMENT OF POSTMENOPAUSAL OSTEOPOROSIS	Hot flashes (flushes)
DECREASES RISK OF NEW VERTEBRAL FRACTURES	Weight gain
REDUCED LDL CHOLESTEROL	
Possible benefits on heart health	
Possible benefits in preventing breast cancer (being studied in the STAR trial)	

▷ **Principal Uses**

As a Single Drug Product: Uses currently included in FDA-approved labeling: (1) Helps prevent osteoporosis in women after menopause; (2) treats osteoporosis after menopause.

Other (unlabeled) generally accepted uses: (1) Because of LDL and homocysteine lowering, may have a role in maintaining heart (cardiovascular) health; (2) may have a role in preventing breast cancer (one study found a 76% lower risk of breast cancer in a group of women who took this drug for 3 years [MORE trial], and is now being studied in the STAR trial).

Author's Note: Tamoxifen reduced breast cancer rates by almost half in a very large (13,388 patients) cancer prevention study performed by the National Cancer Institute over 6 years. The FDA has launched a new oncology tools website. Visit this at www.fda.gov/cder/cancer. There is a listing of cancer medicine trials on the World Wide Web at http://cancertrials.nci.nih.gov. The STAR (Study of Tamoxifen and Raloxifene) trial is underway. This is a National Cancer Institute study evaluating 20,000 women who are at risk for breast cancer. They will be given either 20 mg per day of tamoxifen or 60 mg of raloxifene each day for five years. For more information, you can reach the National Cancer Institute at 1-800-422-6237.

How This Drug Works: Works similar to estrogen itself on the bone (increasing bone density) and on LDL cholesterol (lowering it). Because of this, some people in the news media call raloxifene a designer estrogen. May block use (uptake) of estrogen (estradiol) and remove one stimulus for breast cancer.

Available Dosage Forms and Strengths

Tablets — 60 mg

▷ **Usual Adult Dosage Ranges:**

Prevention of postmenopausal osteoporosis: 60 mg once daily.
Treatment of postmenopausal osteoporosis: 60 mg once daily.
Note: Actual dose and schedule must be determined for each patient individually.

Conditions Requiring Dosing Adjustments

Liver Function: Extensively changed (metabolized) in the liver. Dose decreases appear prudent, but drug use not studied in this population.
Kidney Function: Not studied in people with kidney disease or compromise.

▷ **Dosing Instructions:** The tablet may be crushed and taken without regard to food. If you forget a dose: Take the missed dose as soon as you remember it, unless it's nearly time for your next dose—if that is the case, skip the missed dose and take the next dose right on schedule. Talk with your doctor if you find yourself missing doses. There are beeper-based systems to help you. If a switch is being made from estrogen to raloxifene, some clinicians taper estrogen over at least a month to help decrease the chance of sudden menopause symptoms. It may also be best to have stopped taking estrogen for a month before starting raloxifene—this approach will allow any raloxifene related problems to be clearly identified.

Usual Duration of Use: Use in clinical trials compared two years of raloxifene use to calcium use alone and a three year trial is ongoing. These trials used measures of bone mineral density (BMD) to check the benefits of this drug. It appears prudent to check BMD before starting this medicine and then to recheck markers of bone turnover (such as N-telopeptides) and BMD once the medicine has been started to make sure that it is working. Long-term use requires physician supervision.

Typical Treatment Goals and Measurements (Outcomes and Markers)

Bone mineral density: The general goal is to at least prevent further bone loss, and ideally, increase bone mineral density or BMD. Results can be checked by a lab test (N-telopeptide) and repeat DEXA, PDEXA or ultrasound. The overall goal is to decrease fracture risk.

Possible Advantages of This Drug

Effective treatment of osteoporosis. May also confer some heart (cardioprotective) benefits as well as possible prevention of breast cancer with a single medicine.

▷ **This Drug Should Not Be Taken If**
- you had a serious allergic or adverse reaction to it before.
- you have a history of blood clots (clot in the retinal vein, DVT or pulmonary embolism [PE]).
- you are pregnant.

▷ **Inform Your Physician Before Taking This Drug If**
- you are taking estrogen (not studied with this drug).
- you have a history of thrombophlebitis or pulmonary embolism.
- you have impaired liver function.
- you plan to have surgery or will be immobilized (prolonged rest in bed) in the near future.
- you have an active malignancy (benefit-to-risk decision).
- your diet is low in calcium or vitamin D (smart to take a supplement if your diet is deficient).

Possible Side Effects (natural, expected and unavoidable drug actions)

Hot flashes—may be frequent.

▷ **Possible Adverse Effects** (unusual, unexpected and infrequent reactions)

If any of the following develop, consult your physician promptly for guidance.

Mild Adverse Effects

Allergic reactions: skin rash.

Insomnia, migraine or depression—infrequent.

Weight gain—infrequent.

Indigestion (dyspepsia), nausea or vomiting—infrequent.

Cough, sinusitis or pharyngitis—infrequent.

Joint or muscle pain—infrequent.

Swelling of the ankles or wrists (edema)—infrequent.

Serious Adverse Effects

Increased uterine cancer risk was found in mice and rats. How this applies to humans is not known.

Chest pain—infrequent.

Liver toxicity—case report.

Blood clots (thromboembolism)—twofold increased risk of lung (PE) and 3.4-fold increased risk of clots in veins (venous thromboembolism).

▷ **Possible Effects on Sexual Function:** None reported.

Possible Effects on Laboratory Tests

Markers of bone turnover (bone specific alkaline phosphatase): decreased.

Bone mineral density: increased.

LDL cholesterol: decreased (a positive result).

HDL: increased (a positive result).

Liver function tests: may be increased (questionable cause).

CAUTION

1. Calcium supplements should be added to your diet if your diet does not include enough calcium. Talk to your doctor about the need for vitamin D.
2. Research has not been done combining this medicine with estrogen.
3. Ask your doctor about how to decrease risk factors for osteoporosis. Also ask about an exercise program appropriate to your degree of bone loss.
4. One researcher questioned mouse and rat data that showed raloxifene causing cancer of the ovaries in those animals. The manufacturer said that cancer in rodents did not correspond to risk of cancer in humans.
5. This drug has not been studied for use in men.
6. A head-to-head trial of tamoxifen and raloxifene has started to look at benefits and risks of use in preventing breast cancer (STAR trial).
7. Data are available (MORE trial) that show that this medicine can help prevent fractures in the spine (vertebral fractures). At the time of this writing, there are no data to show that this medicine prevents fractures of the hip.
8. This medicine may increase risk of blood clots, and therefore use is a benefit-to-risk decision in patients with active malignancies (which may also increase blood clots).

▷ **Advisability of Use During Pregnancy**

Pregnancy Category: X. See Pregnancy Risk Categories at the back of this book.

Human studies: Studies of pregnant women will not be done. This drug should NOT be used during pregnancy.

Advisability of Use If Breast-Feeding

Presence of this drug in breast milk: Unknown.

Avoid drug or refrain from nursing.

Habit-Forming Potential: None.

Effects of Overdose: An accidental dose of 600 mg was tolerated in clinical trials.

Possible Effects of Long-Term Use: Increased bone mineral density.

Suggested Periodic Examinations While Taking This Drug (at physician's discretion)

Bone mineral density testing.

Laboratory tests of bone turnover.

Periodic liver function tests.

Check for blood clots.

Must have regular gynecological examinations.

▷ **While Taking This Drug, Observe the Following**

Foods: No restrictions.

Herbal Medicines or Minerals: Make certain that you are getting adequate calcium in your diet if you have osteoporosis or thin bones (osteopenia). The average American diet has about 200–400 mg. Most people need 1,000 to 1,500 mg per day. Effervescent calcium (resulting in a solution) may be absorbed more rapidly than other forms of calcium and can help prevent osteoporosis. Vitamin D and adequate sunlight are also needed. Soy or other plant-derived phytoestrogens may work to complement raloxifene, but have not been studied together with raloxifene. Ipriflavone is a synthetic flavonoid currently investigational for osteoporosis (which both inhibits bone resorption by reducing osteoclast recruitment and encourages osteoblast function). Combined use once again has not been studied in osteoporosis used with raloxifene. Some breast cancer patients are taking mistletoe (Iscador, others). This herbal is available by prescription in Europe and may work to stimulate the immune system, but there are no combined raloxifene trials.

Beverages: Watch intake of phosphorous from soda. May be taken with milk.

▷ *Alcohol:* No interactions expected, but some clinicians count alcohol as something that slows the cells that make bone.

Tobacco Smoking: No interactions expected. I advise everyone to quit smoking.

▷ *Other Drugs*

The following drugs may ***decrease*** the effects of raloxifene:
- ampicillin (Polycillin, Principen).
- ampicillin/sulbactam (Unasyn).
- cholestyramine (Questran).
- corticosteroids such as prednisone (Deltasone, others), as long-term use of those medicines can lead to osteoporosis.

Raloxifene ***taken concurrently*** with
- other highly protein bound medicines, such as diazepam (Valium), indomethacin (Indocin), naproxen (Naprosyn) or others, should be done only with great caution.
- warfarin (Coumadin) may lower benefits of warfarin; increased frequency of INR (prothrombin time or protime) testing is needed.

▷ *Driving, Hazardous Activities:* No restrictions thought to be needed.

Aviation Note: The use of this drug ***is probably not a disqualification for piloting.*** Consult a designated Aviation Medical Examiner.

Exposure to Sun: No restrictions.

RAMIPRIL (ra MI pril)

Introduced: 1985   **Class:** Antihypertensive, ACE inhibitor

Please see the angiotensin converting enzyme (ACE) inhibitor family profile.

RANITIDINE (ra NI te deen)

Author's Note: ALL of the four available histamine (H2) receptor blocking drugs are now available without prescription. See the histamine (H2) blocking drug family profile.

REPAGLINIDE (ra PAG lyn ide)

Introduced: 1998   **Class:** Antidiabetic, meglitinides   **Prescription:** USA: Yes   **Controlled Drug:** USA: No; Canada: No   **Available as Generic:** No
Brand Name: ❧Gluconorm, Prandin

```
┌─────────────────────────────────────────────────────────────────┐
│                      BENEFITS versus RISKS                        │
│        Possible Benefits               Possible Risks             │
│ HELPS REGULATE BLOOD SUGAR      Hypoglycemia (less common than    │
│   IN TYPE 2 DIABETES (adjunctive   sulfonylureas)                 │
│   to appropriate diet and weight  Possible increased risk of heart│
│   control)                          (cardiovascular) problems (based on│
│ MAY BE COMBINED WITH                a 1970 UGDP study)            │
│   METFORMIN IF BLOOD SUGAR                                         │
│   CONTROL IS NOT ACCEPTABLE                                        │
│ Absorbed well and cleared quickly                                 │
│   from the blood                                                  │
└─────────────────────────────────────────────────────────────────┘
```

▷ **Principal Uses**

 As a Single Drug Product: Uses currently included in FDA-approved labeling: (1) Type 2 diabetes mellitus (adult, maturity-onset) that does not require insulin but can't be adequately controlled by diet alone; (2) combination treatment with metformin in people who do not have an adequate blood sugar response from repaglinide alone.

 Other (unlabeled) generally accepted uses: None.

How This Drug Works: Stimulates secretion of insulin (closes ATP-sensitive potassium channels in beta cells).

Available Dosage Forms and Strengths

 Tablets — 0.5 mg, 1 mg, 2 mg

▷ **Usual Adult Dosage Ranges:** *People with a hemoglobin A1C (HGB A1C or glyco-sylated hemoglobin) less than 8% or who have not been treated:* 0.5 mg before meals.

 Previously treated patients or those with HGB A1C more than 8%: One to two mg is given before meals. Adjustments should be made based on ongoing blood sugar and HGB A1C at 7 day (or more) intervals. Maximum daily dose is 16 mg.

 Note: Actual dose and schedule must be determined for each patient individually.

Conditions Requiring Dosing Adjustments

 Liver Function: Blood levels are higher and stay longer in moderate to severe liver failure. Decreased doses and more frequent finger stick blood sugar testing is prudent.

 Kidney Function: The same starting dose is used in kidney disease or compromise. Any subsequent dose increases should be made cautiously.

▷ **Dosing Instructions:** Hypoglycemia is the most common adverse effect of this medicine. Make sure you know the signs and symptoms of low blood sugar (weakness, drowsiness, confusion, etc.). Keep some glucose tablets nearby in case you develop hypoglycemia. It is important to take this medicine before meals. You can take it up to 30 minutes before a meal. If you skip a meal, then skip the dose of repaglinide. On occasions where you have an extra meal, take an extra dose of this medicine before that meal. If a dose adjustment is made, one week should pass before another dose change is made. The tablet may be crushed. If you forget a dose: Skip the missed dose and take the next dose right on schedule. DO NOT double doses. Talk with your doctor if you find yourself missing doses.

Usual Duration of Use: Use on a regular schedule for 1 to 2 weeks determines effectiveness in controlling diabetes. Checking blood sugar by finger stick is the best way to make sure you are getting the best results from this medicine. Some patients will have control of their blood sugar for a while and then the medicine will not continue to work and will need to be changed. Diabetes is now recognized as a risk factor for cardiovascular disease. Take control of your blood sugar and help your heart.

Typical Treatment Goals and Measurements (Outcomes and Markers)

Blood sugar: The general goal for blood sugar is to return it to the usual "normal" range (generally 80–120 mg/dl), while avoiding risks of excessively low blood sugar. One study (UKPDS) used a fasting plasma sugar (glucose) of less than 108 mg/dl.

Fructosamine and glycosylated hemoglobin: Fructosamine levels (a measure of the past two to three weeks of blood sugar control) should be less than or equal to 310 micromoles per liter. Glycosylated hemoglobin or hemoglobin A1C (a measure of the past 2–3 months of blood sugar control) should be less than or equal to 7.0%.

▷ **This Drug Should Not Be Taken If**
- you have had an allergic reaction to it previously.
- you have diabetic ketoacidosis.
- you are pregnant.
- you have the kind of diabetes that requires insulin.

▷ **Inform Your Physician Before Taking This Drug If**
- your blood sugar begins to drift up. This may be a sign of secondary failure and require a change in medicine.
- you do not know how to recognize or treat hypoglycemia (see Glossary).
- you have a history of congestive heart failure, cirrhosis of the liver or hypothyroidism.
- you have an infection or a fever—insulin may be required.

Possible Side Effects (natural, expected and unavoidable drug actions)

If drug dose is excessive or food intake is delayed or inadequate, abnormally low blood sugar (hypoglycemia) will occur as a predictable drug effect.

▷ **Possible Adverse Effects** (unusual, unexpected and infrequent reactions)

If any of the following develop, consult your physician promptly for guidance.

Mild Adverse Effects

Allergic reactions: skin rash, hives, itching.

Headache, drowsiness, dizziness, fatigue—possible.

Nausea vomiting, diarrhea, heartburn—infrequent.

Serious Adverse Effects

Allergic reactions: not defined.

Idiosyncratic reactions: not reported.

Hypoglycemia—possible but less than sulfonylureas.

Cardiovascular mortality (based on an old study of a different medicine)—possible increased risk.

▷ **Possible Effects on Sexual Function:** None reported.

▷ **Adverse Effects That May Mimic Natural Diseases or Disorders**

Liver reactions may suggest viral hepatitis.

Possible Effects on Laboratory Tests

Blood glucose levels: decreased.

Glycated hemoglobin or protein: trending toward normal.

CAUTION

1. This drug is only part of diabetes management. Much of the damage from diabetes can be delayed or avoided if you keep your blood sugar in the normal range. Ask your doctor about a proper diet and regular exercise.
2. Over time, this drug may not work. Periodic follow-up examinations are necessary.
3. If you develop an infection, insulin may be required to control your blood sugar.

Precautions for Use

By Infants and Children: Safety and efficacy not defined.

By Those Over 65 Years of Age: No differences in pharmacokinetics in this age group in clinical trials. People with significant age-related declines in kidney function should be closely followed. If dose changes are required, they should be made more slowly than in those with normal kidneys.

▷ **Advisability of Use During Pregnancy**

Pregnancy Category: C. See Pregnancy Risk Categories at the back of this book.

Animal studies: No birth defects reported in rats and rabbits.

Human studies: Adequate studies of pregnant women are not available.

Uncontrolled blood sugar levels during pregnancy are associated with a higher incidence of birth defects, so many experts recommend insulin (instead of an oral agent) to control diabetes during the entire pregnancy.

Advisability of Use If Breast-Feeding

Presence of this drug in breast milk: Unknown.

Avoid drug or refrain from nursing.

Habit-Forming Potential: None.

Effects of Overdose: Symptoms of mild to severe hypoglycemia: headache, lightheadedness, faintness, nervousness, confusion, tremor, sweating, heart palpitation, weakness, hunger, nausea, vomiting, stupor progressing to coma.

Possible Effects of Long-Term Use: More normal hemoglobin A1C.

Suggested Periodic Examinations While Taking This Drug (at physician's discretion)

Periodic evaluation of heart and circulatory system.

Self-assessment of blood sugar is prudent as well as periodic glycosylated hemoglobin tests and/or fructosamine tests.

▷ **While Taking This Drug, Observe the Following**

Foods: Follow the diabetic diet prescribed by your physician.

Herbal Medicines or Minerals: Using chromium may change the way your body is able to use sugar. Some health food stores advocate vanadium as mimicking the actions of insulin, but possible toxicity and need for rigorous studies presently preclude recommending it.

DHEA may change sensitivity to insulin or insulin resistance. Hawthorn, ginger, garlic, ginseng and licorice, nettle and yohimbe may change blood sugar. Since this may require adjustment of hypoglycemic medicine dosing, talk to your doctor **BEFORE** combining any of these herbal medicines with this medicine. Echinacea pupurea (injectable) and blonde psyllium seed or husk should NOT be taken by people living with diabetes.

Beverages: As directed in the diabetic diet. May be taken with milk.

▷ *Alcohol:* Use with extreme caution—alcohol can exaggerate this drug's hypoglycemic effect.

Tobacco Smoking: No interactions expected. I advise everyone to quit smoking.

▷ *Other Drugs*

The following drugs may *increase* the effects of repaglinide:

- cimetidine (Tagamet).
- erythromycins (see Drug Classes).
- itraconazole (Sporanox).
- ketoconazole (Nizoral).
- medicines that inhibit or compete for CYP 3A4 (a liver enzyme) will increase repaglinide because it is removed by that enzyme.
- mibefradil (Posicor) (removed from the U.S. market).
- nelfinavir (Viracept) and perhaps other protease inhibitors (see Drug Classes)—may increase blood levels.
- sildenafil (Viagra), since both drugs are removed by CYP3A4.
- Any medicine that interferes with cytochrome CYP3A4—will potentially increase repaglinide blood levels; in some cases, I expect that repaglinide dosing will need to be adjusted.

The following drugs may *decrease* the effects of repaglinide:

- carbamazepine (Tegretol), since it induces CYP3A4, which removes repaglinide from the body.
- corticosteroids (see Drug Classes).
- rifabutin (Mycobutin).
- rifampin (Rifadin, Rimactane).

▷ *Driving, Hazardous Activities:* This drug may cause dizziness, drowsiness, impaired vision and impaired hearing. Restrict activities as necessary.

Aviation Note: Diabetes *is a disqualification* for piloting. Consult a designated Aviation Medical Examiner.

Exposure to Sun: No restrictions.

Discontinuation: It is advisable not to interrupt or stop this drug without consulting your physician.

RIFABUTIN (RIF a byu tin)

Introduced: 1993   **Class:** Antimycobacterial agent (antitubercular)   **Prescription:** USA: Yes   **Controlled Drug:** USA: No; Canada: No   **Available as Generic:** USA: No; Canada: No

Brand Name: Mycobutin

Warning: Rifabutin prophylaxis must not be taken by people with active tuberculosis.

> **BENEFITS versus RISKS**
>
> | *Possible Benefits* | *Possible Risks* |
> |---|---|
> | PREVENTION OF DISSEMINATED MYCOBACTERIUM AVIUM-INTRACELLULARE COMPLEX IN PEOPLE WITH ADVANCED HIV INFECTION | NEUTROPENIA
 Low platelet counts |

▷ **Principal Uses**

As a Single Drug Product: Uses currently included in FDA-approved labeling: (1) Prevention of disseminated *Mycobacterium avium-intracellulare* complex in patients with advanced HIV infection; (2) combination treatment of *Mycobacterium avium-intracellulare* complex infection.

Other (unlabeled) generally accepted uses: (1) Some clinicians are using rifabutin in cases of resistant H. Pylori that can cause stomach ulcers.

How This Drug Works: Rifabutin inhibits DNA-dependent RNA polymerase (an enzyme critical to cells that are dividing) in *E. coli*. The exact mechanism of action of rifabutin in *Mycobacterium avium* or *Mycobacterium avium-intracellulare* complex is not known.

Available Dosage Forms and Strengths

Capsules (Mycobutin) — 150 mg

How to Store: Keep at room temperature, and avoid exposure to excessive humidity.

▷ **Recommended Dose Ranges** (Actual dose and schedule must be determined for each patient individually.)

Infants and Children: Safety and effectiveness of rifabutin in *Mycobacterium avium-intracellulare* complex prophylaxis has not been clearly established. Safety data comes from a trial of 22 children who were HIV positive.

Infants 1 year of age: 18.5 mg per kg of body mass per day.

Children 2–10 years: 8.6 mg per kg of body mass per day.

Adolescents up to 14 years: 4.0 mg per kg of body mass per day.

14 to 60 Years of Age: 300 mg once a day. Those prone to nausea and vomiting may take 150 mg two times a day with food.

Over 60 Years of Age: Same as 12 to 60 years of age.

Conditions Requiring Dosing Adjustments

Liver Function: At present, clear adjustments of dose in hepatic compromise are not defined, but the drug should be used with caution.

Kidney Function: Elimination of rifabutin may actually be increased in people with compromised kidneys, although the clinical effect is as yet unknown.

Author's Note: The information in this profile has been shortened to make room for more widely used medicines.

RIFAMPIN (ri FAM pin)

Other Name: Rifampicin

Introduced: 1967   **Class:** Antibiotic, rifamycins   **Prescription:** USA: Yes   **Controlled Drug:** USA: No; Canada: No   **Available as Generic:** Yes

Brand Names: Rifadin, Rifadin IV, Rifamate [CD], Rifater [CD], Rimactane, Rimactane/INH Dual Pack [CD], ❦Rofact

---

BENEFITS versus RISKS

Possible Benefits	*Possible Risks*
EFFECTIVE TREATMENT OF TUBERCULOSIS IN COMBINATION WITH OTHER DRUGS	DRUG-INDUCED KIDNEY OR LIVER DAMAGE
EFFECTIVE PREVENTION OF MENINGITIS	Blood cell or coagulation disorders
COMBINATION TREATMENT OF SOME STAPH INFECTIONS	Colitis (pseudomembranous)

▷ **Principal Uses**

As a Single Drug Product: Uses currently included in FDA-approved labeling: (1) Treats active tuberculosis—usually given concurrently with other antitubercular drugs to enhance its effectiveness; (2) also used to eliminate the meningitis germ (meningococcus) from the throats of healthy carriers so that it cannot be spread to others; (3) treats tuberculosis in coal workers with good outcomes when combined with other antitubercular drugs; (4) used to prevent tuberculosis in people exposed to patients with active disease.

Other (unlabeled) generally accepted uses: (1) Second-line agent in combination with doxycycline in treatment of brucellosis; (2) has a place in preventing *Haemophilus influenzae* infections in people exposed to patients with active disease; (3) combination therapy of lepromatous leprosy; (4) used with cotrimoxazole to eliminate methicillin-resistant Staphylococcus aureus (MRSA) from people who have the bacteria; (5) used with other drugs to treat Staph endocarditis.

As a Combination Drug Product [CD]: This drug is available in combination with isoniazid, another antitubercular drug that delays the development of drug-resistant strains of the tuberculosis germ.

How This Drug Works: This drug prevents the growth and multiplication of susceptible tuberculosis organisms by blocking specific enzyme systems that are involved in the formation of essential proteins.

Available Dosage Forms and Strengths

Capsules — 150 mg, 300 mg

▷ **Usual Adult Dosage Ranges**

For tuberculosis: 10 mg per kg of body mass per day, up to 600 mg once daily.

For meningococcus carriers: 600 mg once daily for 4 days. The total daily dose should not exceed 600 mg.

Note: Actual dose and schedule must be determined for each patient individually.

Conditions Requiring Dosing Adjustments

Liver Function: This drug can cause liver damage, and patients should be followed closely. In severe failure, the dose should be limited to 6 to 8 mg per kg of body mass twice a week.

Kidney Function: For patients with a creatinine clearance (see Glossary) of 10 to 50 ml/min, one researcher suggests that 50% to 100% of the usual dose should be given.

▷ **Dosing Instructions:** This drug is preferably taken with 8 ounces of water on an empty stomach (1 hour before or 2 hours after eating). However, it may be taken with food if necessary to reduce stomach irritation. The capsule may be opened and the contents mixed with applesauce or jelly to take it. If you forget a dose: Take the missed dose as soon as you remember it, unless it's nearly time for your next dose—if that is the case, skip the missed dose and take the next dose right on schedule. DO NOT double doses. Talk with your doctor if you find yourself missing doses.

Usual Duration of Use: Use on a regular schedule for several months usually determines effectiveness in promoting recovery from tuberculosis. Long-term use (possibly 1 to 2 years) requires ongoing physician supervision and periodic evaluation.

Typical Treatment Goals and Measurements (Outcomes and Markers)

Infections: The most commonly used measures of serious infections are white blood cell counts and differentials (the kind of blood cells that occur most often in your blood), and temperature. In tuberculosis, many clinicians start four medicines for the eight weeks it typically takes for sputum specimens containing this organism to grow to reveal their sensitivity patterns. While clinicians look for positive changes in 24–48 hours in typical infections, this kind of infection REQUIRES long-term treatment to kill it. NEVER stop an antibiotic because you start to feel better. The goals and time frame (see peak benefits above) should be discussed with you when the prescription is written.

▷ **This Drug Should Not Be Taken If**
  • you have had an allergic reaction to it previously.

▷ **Inform Your Physician Before Taking This Drug If**
  • you are pregnant.
  • you have a history of liver disease or impaired liver function.
  • you have active liver disease.
  • you consume alcohol daily.
  • you are taking an oral contraceptive—an alternate method of contraception is advised.
  • you are taking an anticoagulant.

Possible Side Effects (natural, expected and unavoidable drug actions)

Red, orange or brown discoloration of tears, sweat, saliva, sputum, urine or stool. Yellow coloring of the skin (not jaundice). **Note:** In the absence of illness symptoms, any discoloration is a harmless drug effect and does not mean toxicity. Possible fungal superinfections (see Glossary).

▷ **Possible Adverse Effects** (unusual, unexpected and infrequent reactions)

If any of the following develop, consult your physician promptly for guidance.

Mild Adverse Effects

Allergic reactions: skin rash, hives, itching, drug fever (see Glossary).

Headache, dizziness, blurred vision, impaired hearing, vague numbness and tingling—infrequent.

Joint and muscle pain—infrequent and often subsides after a few weeks.

Loss of appetite, heartburn, nausea, vomiting, abdominal cramps, diarrhea—infrequent.

Serious Adverse Effects
> Skin problems (Stevens-Johnson syndrome or toxic epidermal necrolysis)—
> case reports.
>
> Flu-like syndrome: fever, headache, dizziness, musculoskeletal pain, difficult
> breathing—case reports.
>
> Drug-induced liver damage, with or without jaundice—frequent.
>
> Kidney damage—infrequent.
>
> Drug-induced porphyria, pancreatitis, gallstones or pseudomembranous
> colitis—case reports.
>
> Excessively low blood platelet count: abnormal bleeding or bruising—rare.
>
> Blood-clotting problems (disseminated intravascular coagulopathy)—case
> report.
>
> Hemolytic anemia—case reports.
>
> Suppression of the adrenal gland—possible.
>
> Some case reports have been made regarding lung tumors (pulmonary
> malignancies). The cause-and-effect relationship is not yet defined.

▷ **Possible Effects on Sexual Function:** Altered timing and pattern of menstrua-
> tion—case reports.
>
> Decreased effectiveness of oral contraceptives.

▷ **Adverse Effects That May Mimic Natural Diseases or Disorders**
> Liver reactions may suggest viral hepatitis. Kidney reactions may suggest an
> infectious nephritis.

Possible Effects on Laboratory Tests
> Complete blood cell counts: decreased red cells, hemoglobin, white cells and
> platelets; increased eosinophils (allergic reaction).
>
> INR (protime): increased (when taken with warfarin).
>
> Liver function tests: increased liver enzymes (ALT/GPT, AST/GOT and alka-
> line phosphatase), increased bilirubin.

CAUTION
> 1. This drug may permanently discolor soft contact lenses.
> 2. This drug may reduce the effects of oral contraceptives—pregnancy
>   could occur. An alternate method of contraception is advised.
> 3. Resistance may develop rapidly if this drug is used alone to treat tuber-
>   culosis. Only use with other antitubercular drugs.
> 4. TAKE THE FULL course prescribed; this may be many months.

Precautions for Use
> *By Infants and Children:* Monitor closely for possible liver toxicity or deficiency
> of blood platelets.
>
> *By Those Over 60 Years of Age:* Natural changes in body composition and func-
> tion make you more susceptible to the adverse effects of this drug. Report
> promptly any indications of possible drug toxicity.

▷ **Advisability of Use During Pregnancy**
> *Pregnancy Category:* C. See Pregnancy Risk Categories at the back of this book.
> *Animal studies:* Cleft palate and spinal defects reported in rodent studies.
> *Human studies:* Adequate studies of pregnant women are not available.
> If possible, avoid use of drug during the first 3 months.

Advisability of Use If Breast-Feeding
> Presence of this drug in breast milk: Yes.
> Avoid drug or refrain from nursing.

Habit-Forming Potential: None.

Effects of Overdose: Nausea, vomiting, drowsiness, unconsciousness, severe liver damage, jaundice.

Possible Effects of Long-Term Use: Superinfections, fungal overgrowth of mouth or tongue.

Suggested Periodic Examinations While Taking This Drug (at physician's discretion)

Complete blood cell counts.

Liver and kidney function tests (frequent liver tests if used with pyrazinamide).

Hearing acuity tests if hearing loss is suspected.

▷ **While Taking This Drug, Observe the Following**

Foods: No restrictions.

Herbal Medicines or Minerals: Some patients use echinacea to attempt to boost their immune systems. Unfortunately, use of echinacea is not recommended in people with damaged immune systems. This herb may also actually weaken any immune system if it is used too often or for too long a time. DO NOT take mistletoe herb, oak bark or F.C. of marshmallow root, woody nightshade stem or licorice.

Beverages: No restrictions.

▷ *Alcohol:* It is best to avoid alcohol completely to reduce the risk of liver toxicity.

Tobacco Smoking: No interactions expected. I advise everyone to quit smoking.

▷ *Other Drugs*

Rifampin *taken concurrently* with
- halothane anesthesia may result in serious liver damage.

Rifampin may *decrease* the effects of
- amiodarone (Cordarone).
- amprenavir (Agenerase).
- antianxiety agents such as diazepam and perhaps other benzodiazepines (see Drug Classes).
- anticoagulants such as warfarin (Coumadin).
- anticonvulsant drugs such as phenytoin (Dilantin).
- barbiturates (see Drug Classes).
- BCG live-attenuated vaccine.
- beta blockers such as metoprolol or propranolol (see Drug Classes).
- birth control pills (oral contraceptives).
- buspirone (Buspar).
- some calcium channel blockers (see Drug Classes).
- carbamazepine (Tegretol)—may lead to carbamazepine toxicity.
- carvedilol (Coreg).
- chloramphenicol (Chloromycetin).
- clofibrate (Atromid-S).
- clozapine (Clozaril).
- cortisonelike drugs (see Drug Classes).
- cyclosporine (Sandimmune).
- dapsone.
- delavirdine (Rescriptor).
- digitalis preparations (Lanoxin, others).

- disopyramide (Norpace).
- donepezil (Aricept).
- doxycycline (various).
- enalapril (Vasotec).
- fluconazole (Diflucan).
- fosphenytoin (Cerebyx).
- some HMG-CoA reductase inhibitors (fluvastatin).
- indinavir (Crixivan) and nelfinavir (Viracept).
- itraconazole (Sporanox).
- leflunomide (Arava).
- losartan (Cozaar).
- ketoconazole (Nizoral).
- methadone (Dolophine).
- metoprolol (Lopressor).
- montelukast (Singulair).
- mexiletine (Mexitil).
- narcotics such as methadone (see Opioids in Drug Classes).
- nicardipine (Cardene).
- nifedipine (Adalat).
- olanzapine (Zyprexa).
- oral hypoglycemic agents (sulfonylureas such as tolbutamide: see Drug Classes).
- phenytoin (Dilantin).
- progestins.
- propafenone (Rythmol).
- quinidine (Quinaglute, others).
- repaglinide (Prandin).
- ritonavir (Norvir)—this combination may also lead to rifampin toxicity.
- rofecoxib (VIOXX).
- sildenafil (Viagra).
- sirolimus (Rapamune) or tacrolimus (Prograf).
- theophylline (Theo-Dur, others).
- tricyclic antidepressants (see Drug Classes).
- trimexate (Neutrexin).
- verapamil (Verelan).
- warfarin (Coumadin); increased INR testing is needed.
- zaleplon (Sonata).
- zidovudine (AZT); the therapeutic effect will be lessened by a decreased drug level.
- zolpidem (Ambien).

The following drug may **decrease** the effects of rifampin:

- para-aminosalicylic acid (PAS) and reduce its antitubercular effectiveness.

▷ *Driving, Hazardous Activities:* This drug may cause dizziness, drowsiness, impaired vision and impaired hearing. Restrict activities as necessary.

Aviation Note: The use of this drug *may be a disqualification* for piloting. Consult a designated Aviation Medical Examiner.

Exposure to Sun: No restrictions.

Discontinuation: It is advisable not to interrupt or stop this drug without consulting your physician. Intermittent use can increase risk of developing allergic reactions.

RISEDRONATE (RIH seh druh nate)

Introduced: 1999 **Class:** Third-generation bisphosphonate **Prescription:** USA: Yes **Controlled Drug:** USA: No **Available as Generic:** No **Brand Name:** Actonel

---

BENEFITS versus RISKS

Possible Benefits	*Possible Risks*
TREATMENT OF POST-MENOPAUSAL OSTEOPOROSIS	DIARRHEA
TREATS AND PREVENTS CORTICOSTEROID-CAUSED OSTEOPOROSIS	Irritation of the esophagus
SYMPTOM RELIEF IN PAGET'S DISEASE	Minor flu-like symptoms
MORE POTENT THAN PREVIOUSLY AVAILABLE BISPHOSPHONATES	

▷ **Principal Uses**

As a Single Drug Product: Uses currently included in FDA-approved labeling: (1) Treatment of postmenopausal osteoporosis; (2) treatment of Paget's disease; (3) prevention and treatment of corticosteroid-induced osteoporosis.

Other (unlabeled) generally accepted uses: None at present.

How This Drug Works: This medicine works at the brush border of the osteoclast cell. This prevents this cell from resorbing (gobbling up) bone while the osteoblast (bone-building cell) continues to work. This results in bone building and decreased fracture risk.

Available Dosage Forms and Strengths

Tablets—30 mg

Author's Note: Information in this profile will be broadened as more data are available.

RISPERIDONE (RIS peer i dohn)

Introduced: 1993 **Class:** Antipsychotic agent **Prescription:** USA: Yes **Controlled Drug:** USA: No; Canada: No **Available as Generic:** USA: No; Canada: No **Brand Name:** Risperdal

```
┌─────────────────────────────────────────────────────────────────────┐
│                        BENEFITS versus RISKS                          │
│        Possible Benefits                    Possible Risks            │
│  TREATMENT OF SCHIZOPHRENIA        Change in heart function           │
│    REFRACTORY TO OTHER             Involuntary movement disorder      │
│    AGENTS                          Neuroleptic malignant syndrome     │
│  DECREASED SIDE EFFECTS                                               │
│    COMPARED TO OTHER                                                  │
│    AVAILABLE DRUGS                                                    │
│  EFFECTIVE TREATMENT OF                                               │
│    CERTAIN PSYCHOTIC                                                  │
│    DISORDERS                                                         │
│  Medicines in this class are probably                                │
│    drugs of choice in older adults                                   │
│  May have a role in easing agitation                                 │
│    in dementia patients                                              │
└─────────────────────────────────────────────────────────────────────┘
```

▷ **Principal Uses**

As a Single Drug Product: Uses currently included in FDA-approved labeling: (1) Manages psychotic disorders such as chronic schizophrenia; (2) treats AIDS-related psychosis.

Other (unlabeled) generally accepted uses: (1) Treats acute schizophrenia; (2) treatment of aggression; (3) treatment of Tourette's syndrome; (4) can have a role in helping behavioral problems in people with mental retardation; (5) helps treatment-resistant obsessive-compulsive disorder and catatonia; (6) eases "sundown" agitation in dementia patients.

How This Drug Works: Balances two nerve transmitters (dopamine and serotonin), helping restore more normal thinking and mood.

Available Dosage Forms and Strengths

Oral solution — 1 mg/ml

Tablets — 0.25 mg, 0.5 mg, 1 mg, 2 mg, 3 mg, 4 mg

▷ **Recommended Dose Ranges** (Actual dose and schedule must be determined for each patient individually.)

Infants and Children: Safety and efficacy for those less than 18 years of age are not established.

18 to 60 Years of Age: Past starting dose was 1 mg taken twice daily. Newly approved dosing has shown doses up to 8 mg once daily to be effective. Doses in the twice-daily (BID) approach may be started as 1 mg twice daily and increased as needed and tolerated by 1 mg on the second and third day, for a total of 3 mg twice daily by the third day. If further dose changes are needed, they should be made at 1-week intervals. Doses greater than 8 mg per day are not recommended.

Over 60 Years of Age: Therapy is started with 0.5 mg twice daily. The dose is increased if needed and tolerated by 0.5 mg twice daily. Doses greater than 1.5 mg daily are achieved by small increases made at 1-week intervals. Careful attention must be paid to blood pressure and development of adverse effects.

Conditions Requiring Dosing Adjustments

Liver Function: The starting dose must be decreased and adjusted as for those over 60 years old. Additionally, there may be an increased amount of the active drug that results from each dose (increased free fraction), and as such a greater than expected effect may be seen.

Kidney Function: The starting dose must be decreased and adjusted as for those over 60 years old.

▷ **Dosing Instructions:** The tablet may be crushed, and the medication's effect is not changed by food. Water is the best liquid to take this medicine with. Cola or tea is NOT compatible with the liquid (solution) form. If you forget a dose: Take the missed dose as soon as you remember it, unless it's nearly time for your next dose—if that is the case, skip the missed dose and take the next dose right on schedule. DO NOT double doses. Talk with your doctor if you find yourself missing doses as there are a lot of timers and even beeper-based systems to help you.

Usual Duration of Use: Use on a regular schedule for 1 to 2 weeks usually determines effectiveness in helping control chronic schizophrenia. If long-term use is attempted, the lowest effective dose should be used. Periodic physician evaluation of response and dose is required.

Typical Treatment Goals and Measurements (Outcomes and Markers)

Psychosis: The general goal: to lessen the degree and severity of abnormal thinking, letting patients return to their daily lives. Specific measures of psychosis may involve testing or inventories and can be valuable in helping check benefits from this medicine.

Possible Advantages of This Drug

Treatment of schizophrenia resistant (refractory) to other therapy. Medicines in this class are probably drugs of choice in older adults.

▷ **This Drug Should Not Be Taken If**

- you had an allergic reaction to it previously.
- you had neuroleptic malignant syndrome (ask your doctor).

▷ **Inform Your Physician Before Taking This Drug If**

- you have a history of breast cancer.
- you have liver or kidney compromise.
- you are pregnant or plan to become pregnant or are breast-feeding your infant.
- you have had tardive dyskinesia in the past.
- you have a history of Parkinson's disease or seizures.
- you have a history of heart rhythm disturbances (especially QTc prolongation).
- you are unsure how much to take or how often to take it.

Possible Side Effects (natural, expected and unavoidable drug actions)

Increased prolactin levels may result in male and female breast tenderness and swelling.

Sleepiness.

Orthostatic hypotension (see Glossary)—rare.

Weight gain—infrequent.

▷ **Possible Adverse Effects** (unusual, unexpected and infrequent reactions)

If any of the following develop, consult your physician promptly for guidance.

Mild Adverse Effects

Allergic reactions: skin rash.

Difficulty in concentrating—rare.

Headache or increased dreaming—rare to infrequent.

Constipation, diarrhea or nausea—infrequent.

Palpitations—rare.

Increased urination—rare.

Serious Adverse Effects

Allergic reactions: anaphylactic reactions.

Abnormal heart function (prolonged QT interval)—rare.

Tardive dyskinesia (see Glossary) or neuroleptic malignant syndrome—case reports.

Parkinsonian tremor—case report.

Low sodium—rare.

Paresthesia—case reports.

Seizures—rare.

Lowered white blood cells or platelets—case reports.

Abnormal liver function—rare.

Pancreatitis—case reports.

▷ **Possible Effects on Sexual Function:** Diminished sexual desire; delayed or absent orgasm; erectile dysfunction including priapism; male or female breast tenderness or swelling; dry vagina or menstrual changes (hypermenorrhea)—rare. Ejaculation failure—case reports.

Possible Delayed Adverse Effects: Swelling and tenderness of male and female breast tissue.

Natural Diseases or Disorders That May Be Activated by This Drug: Some human cancers depend on prolactin for growth, and since risperidone increases prolactin, it should be used with *CAUTION* by people with previously diagnosed breast cancer.

Possible Effects on Laboratory Tests

Liver function tests: increased SGPT, SGOT and LDH.

Complete blood counts: decreased platelets, white blood cells and hemoglobin.

Prolactin: increased.

CAUTION

1. This drug should be used with great caution, if at all, by patients with cancer.
2. Call your doctor promptly if you have an increased tendency to infection or abnormal bleeding or bruising while taking this drug.
3. This drug should be used with great caution, if at all, by patients with a history of seizures.

Precautions for Use

By Infants and Children: Safety and effectiveness for those under 18 years of age are not established.

By Those Over 60 Years of Age: The starting dose of 0.5 mg twice daily is used for patients who are elderly or debilitated, and slower increases in dose as needed and tolerated are indicated. Great care should be taken in patient's with heart disease. You may be more likely to experience postural hypotension (see Glossary) and problems with motor skills. Those with prostate problems may have increased risk of urine retention.

▷ **Advisability of Use During Pregnancy**

Pregnancy Category: C. See Pregnancy Risk Categories at the back of this book.

Animal studies: Increased rat pup death during the first few days of lactation.

Human studies: Adequate studies of pregnant women are not available. One case report of lack of formation of the corpus callosum of the brain in a fetus exposed to this drug while in the uterus.

Ask your doctor for guidance.

Advisability of Use If Breast-Feeding

Presence of this drug in breast milk: Yes.

Avoid drug or refrain from nursing.

Habit-Forming Potential: None.

Effects of Overdose: Drowsiness, hypotension, tachycardia, low sodium and potassium, ECG changes (prolonged QT interval) and seizure.

Suggested Periodic Examinations While Taking This Drug (at physician's discretion)

Liver function tests.

Electrolytes (sodium and potassium).

ECG.

Prolactin levels.

▷ **While Taking This Drug, Observe the Following**

Foods: No restrictions.

Herbal Medicines or Minerals: Since risperidone and St. John's wort may act to increase serotonin, the combination is not advised. St. John's wort may also worsen sensitivity to the sun. Ma huang and yohimbe are also best avoided while taking this medicine. Kava kava and valerian may worsen drowsiness. Because part of the way that ginseng works is as an MAO inhibitor, DO NOT combine with risperidone.

Beverages: No restrictions.

▷ *Alcohol:* Patients should avoid alcohol while taking risperidone.

Tobacco Smoking: No interactions expected. I advise everyone to quit smoking.

Marijuana Smoking: Increased somnolence.

▷ *Other Drugs*

Risperidone may ***decrease*** the effects of

• levodopa (Sinemet, others).

Risperidone ***taken concurrently*** with

• bupropion (Zyban, Wellbutrin) can lead to increased blood levels and toxicity from "normal" doses of risperidone. Caution, careful patient monitoring and possible dose reductions are prudent if these medicines must be combined.

• carbamazepine (Tegretol) will decrease the drug level and perhaps the therapeutic effects of risperidone.

• other centrally acting medicines may result in increased central effects.

• clozapine (Clozaril) may decrease the therapeutic effects of risperidone.

• lithium (Lithobid, others) may lead to increased adverse effects.

• medicines that inhibit the liver enzyme Cytochrome P450 2D6 will increase risperidone levels and may lead to toxicity with "normal" doses. Medicines that increase cytochrome P450 2D6 will blunt the benefits of risperidone.

• methadone (various) may decrease methadone levels and lead to withdrawal symptoms.

• paroxetine (Paxil) and perhaps other SSRIs may lead to serotonin syndrome.

- phenytoin (Dilantin) or fosphenytoin (Cerebyx) may decrease risperidone blood levels and blunt risperidone therapeutic benefits.
- propafenone (Rythmol) may lead to propafenone toxicity.
- ritonavir (Norvir) and perhaps other protease inhibitors (see Drug Classes) may lead to toxicity.
- tramadol (Ultram) may increase seizure risk.
- venlafaxine (Effexor) may increase risperidone toxicity risk.
- zotepine (Nipolept) may increase seizure risk.

▷ *Driving, Hazardous Activities:* This drug may cause drowsiness and difficulty in concentrating. Restrict activities as necessary.

Aviation Note: The use of this drug *is a disqualification* for piloting. Consult a designated Aviation Medical Examiner.

Exposure to Sun: Use caution—this drug may cause photosensitivity.

Discontinuation: Consult your doctor before stopping this medication.

RIZATRIPTAN (rye zah TRIP tan)

Introduced: 1998 **Class:** Antimigraine, serotonin-1-receptor agonist **Prescription:** USA: Yes **Controlled Drug:** USA: No; Canada: No **Available as Generic:** USA: No; Canada: No

Brand Names: Maxalt, Maxalt-MLT

BENEFITS versus RISKS	
Possible Benefits	*Possible Risks*
RAPID AND EFFECTIVE RELIEF OR PREVENTION OF MIGRAINE	Fainting
	Small increases in blood pressure
GENERALLY WELL TOLERATED	Exacerbation of ischemic heart disease
Relieves photophobia (light sensitivity)	(should not be given to those patients)
Relieves phonophobia (sound sensitivity)	Not to be used in hemiplegic or basilar migraine
Relieves nausea and vomiting	Not to be used in significant cardiovascular disease
More potent than some of the other "triptans" currently available	

▷ **Principal Uses**

As a Single Drug Product: Uses currently included in FDA-approved labeling: Acute treatment of migraine with or without aura in adults.

Other (unlabeled) generally accepted uses: None at present.

How This Drug Works: Rizatriptan acts on blood vessels (by acting as a serotonin-1D agonist) to cause vasoconstriction (shrinking of the blood vessels). This relieves swelling, thought to be the cause of migraine. It is more potent dose-to-dose than sumatriptan (Imitrex).

Available Dosage Forms and Strengths

Tablets — 5 mg, 10 mg

Tablets, orally disintegrating (MLT) — 5 mg, 10 mg

Possible Advantages of This Drug: Offers a novel dosage form that is an orally disintegrating tablet. The convenience of this form makes it unobtrusive and easy to take. This medicine is more potent than sumatriptan (mg-to-mg) and may lead to better effects in stopping a migraine headache. Head-to-head trials are needed.

Author's Note: Information in this profile will be broadened as more data become available.

SALMETEROL (Sal ME Ter Ohl)

Introduced: 1994   **Class:** Bronchodilator   **Prescription:** USA: Yes
Controlled Drug: USA: No; Canada: Not available in Canada   **Available as Generic:** USA: No
Brand Names: ❧Advair [CD], Advair Diskus, Aeromax, Serevent

BENEFITS versus RISKS	
Possible Benefits	*Possible Risks*
LONG-ACTING RELIEF OF BRONCHIAL ASTHMA PREVENTION OF NOCTURNAL ASTHMA SYMPTOMS	Rapid heart rate (tachycardia)

▷ **Principal Uses**

As a Single Drug Product: Uses currently included in FDA-approved labeling: (1) Treatment and prevention of bronchospasm in asthma; (2) prevention of nocturnal asthma; (3) prevention of exercise-induced bronchospasm.

Other (unlabeled) generally accepted uses: May have a role in treating chronic obstructive pulmonary disease (COPD).

As a Combination Drug Product [CD]: This drug has been available in combination with fluticasone in Canada and now in this country. Fluticasone is a corticosteroid that fights inflammation and asthma in a different way than salmeterol (a long-acting beta-2 agonist). This profile will focus on the single medicine form.

How This Drug Works: Acts at specific sites (beta-2) in the lung and opens the airways (bronchodilation), decreasing airway reactivity and increasing movement of mucus. It also blocks release of chemicals from cells (mast) that worsen asthma.

Available Dosage Forms and Strengths

Advair Diskus form — 100/50, 250/50 and 500 mcg fluticasone and 50 mcg of salmeterol per use.

Inhaler — 13-g canister that gives 21 mcg of salmeterol per use.

Serevent Diskus — 50 mcg of salmeterol per use.

▷ **Recommended Dose Ranges** (Actual dose and schedule must be determined for each patient individually.)

Infants and Children: Safety and efficacy in those less than 12 years of age not established.

12 to 60 Years of Age: For prevention of asthma: Two inhalations (42 mcg) twice daily in the morning and evening. Doses are taken 12 hours apart.

Combination form: For asthma: *Fluticasone/salmeterol combination:* the starting dose is 100 mcg fluticasone and 50 mcg of salmeterol in people who are not presently taking an inhaled steroid (corticosteroid). If they are taking an inhaled corticosteroid such as budesonide and the steroid dose is less than or equal to 400 mcg a day, then the combination inhaler containing 100 mcg of fluticasone and 50 mcg of salmeterol is substituted and is taken twice a day. Other doses of budesonide or other corticosteroids require different combinations of fluticasone/salmeterol to get the best results.

For prevention of exercised-induced asthma: Two inhalations at least 30 to 60 minutes before exercise. Additional doses of salmeterol should not be taken for 12 hours.

Over 60 Years of Age: Same as 12 to 60 years of age.

Conditions Requiring Dosing Adjustments

Liver Function: Use with caution, as the drug may accumulate in liver failure.

Kidney Function: Salmeterol has not been studied in kidney failure patients.

▷ **Dosing Instructions:** Follow written instructions closely. This drug has not been studied with a spacer. Shake well before using. If you forget a dose: use the missed dose as soon as you remember it, unless it's nearly time for your next dose—if that is the case, skip the missed dose and use the next dose right on schedule. Talk with your doctor if you find yourself missing doses.

Usual Duration of Use: Use on a regular schedule for 4 to 6 weeks usually determines effectiveness in preventing asthma attacks. Long-term use (months to years) requires periodic physician evaluation of response and dose adjustment.

Typical Treatment Goals and Measurements (Outcomes and Markers)

Asthma: Signs and symptoms of asthma such as difficulty breathing (dyspnea), cough, light-headedness and wheezing should lessen. Forced expiratory volume at one second (FEV1) and/or peak expiratory flow rate (PEF) are checked by most pulmonologists as indicators of successful treatment. If the usual benefit is not realized, call your doctor.

Possible Advantages of This Drug

Longer-acting beta-2 agent than previously available. Combination form offers two mechanisms of action and may last 12 hours or longer in some patients.

▷ **This Drug Should Not Be Taken If**
- you had an allergic reaction to it previously.
- you currently have an irregular heart rhythm.
- you are taking, or have taken within the past 2 weeks, any monoamine oxidase (MAO) type A inhibitor.
- you have sudden onset asthma or status asthmaticus. (Fluticasone or fluticasone/salmeterol WON'T WORK.)

▷ **Inform Your Physician Before Taking This Drug If**
- your breathing does not improve after taking this drug.
- you have an overactive thyroid (hyperthyroidism).
- you have diabetes.
- you have a history of heart problems.
- you have abnormally high blood pressure.
- you are unsure how much to take or how often to take it.

Possible Side Effects (natural, expected and unavoidable drug actions)

Dryness or irritation of the mouth or throat, altered taste. Nervousness, tremor or palpitations.

▷ **Possible Adverse Effects** (unusual, unexpected and infrequent reactions)
　　If any of the following develop, consult your physician promptly for guidance.
　Mild Adverse Effects
　　Allergic reactions: skin rash and urticaria.
　　Rhinitis and laryngitis—possible.
　　Rapid heart rate (tachycardia)—case reports.
　　Headache, tremor, dizziness and nervousness—infrequent.
　Serious Adverse Effects
　　Allergic reactions: not defined.
　　Paradoxical bronchospasm—possible.
　　Respiratory arrest—case reports.

▷ **Possible Effects on Sexual Function:** Not defined.

Possible Delayed Adverse Effects: None defined at present.

▷ **Adverse Effects That May Mimic Natural Diseases or Disorders**
　　Rapid heart rate may mimic heart disease. Bronchospasm may mimic asthma.

Natural Diseases or Disorders That May Be Activated by This Drug
　　Latent coronary artery disease. Diabetes or high blood pressure.

Possible Effects on Laboratory Tests
　　Blood cholesterol profile: may be increased.
　　Blood glucose level: increased.

CAUTION
　1. Use of this drug by inhalation with beclomethasone aerosol (Beclovent, Vanceril) may increase the risk of fluorocarbon propellant (fluorocarbons being eliminated) toxicity. Use salmeterol aerosol 20 to 30 minutes **before** beclomethasone aerosol to reduce toxicity and enhance penetration of beclomethasone into the lungs.
　2. Serious heart rhythm problems or cardiac arrest can result from excessive and prolonged use.
　3. Call your doctor if asthma symptoms appear more often than usual, or if you begin to increase use of the immediate bronchodilator.
　4. *Guidelines for the Diagnosis and Management of Asthma* from the National Institutes of Health state that salmeterol should NOT be used for acute symptoms or asthma exacerbations.
　5. Combination form works primarily locally in the lung. Because of this, blood (plasma) levels don't predict the benefit (therapeutic effect). Additionally, Advair Diskus form should NOT be used to transfer people who have required systemic steroids due to possible adrenal insufficiency.

Precautions for Use
　By Infants and Children: Safety and effectiveness for those under 12 not established.
　By Those Over 60 Years of Age: Avoid increased use. If asthma is not controlled as it has been in the past, call your doctor.

▷ **Advisability of Use During Pregnancy**
　Pregnancy Category: C. See Pregnancy Risk Categories at the back of this book.
　Animal studies: Rabbit studies have revealed cleft palate, limb and paw flexures and delayed bone formation.

Human studies: Adequate studies of pregnant women are not available. Ask your doctor for guidance.

Advisability of Use If Breast-Feeding
Presence of this drug in breast milk: Yes, but extent not defined.
Avoid drug or refrain from nursing.

Habit-Forming Potential: None.

Effects of Overdose: Exaggeration of pharmacological effects: tachycardia and/or arrhythmia, muscle cramps, cardiac arrest and death.

Suggested Periodic Examinations While Taking This Drug (at physician's discretion)
Blood pressure checks.
Evaluations of heart (cardiac) status.

▷ **While Taking This Drug, Observe the Following**
Foods: No restrictions.
Herbal Medicines or Minerals: Using St. John's wort, ma huang, ephedrine-like compounds or kola while taking this medicine may result in unacceptable central nervous system stimulation. Fir or pine needle oil should NOT be used by asthmatics. Ephedra alone does carry a German Commission E monograph indication for asthma treatment. If you are allergic to plants in the Asteraceae family (aster, chrysanthemum, daisy or ragweed), you may also be allergic to echinacea, chamomile, feverfew and St. John's wort. Since part of the way ginseng works may be as an MAO inhibitor, do not combine ginseng with salmeterol.
Beverages: Avoid excessive caffeine as in coffee, tea, cola and chocolate.
▷ *Alcohol:* No interactions expected.
Tobacco Smoking: No interactions expected. Asthma may be worsened by irritation from smoking. I advise everyone to quit smoking.
▷ *Other Drugs*
Salmeterol ***taken concurrently*** with
• monoamine oxidase (MAO) type A inhibitors can cause extreme increases in blood pressure and heart stimulation.
The following drugs may **increase** the effects of salmeterol:
• methylxanthines such as caffeine or theophylline.
• tricyclic antidepressants.
▷ *Driving, Hazardous Activities:* This drug may cause nervousness or dizziness. Restrict activities as necessary.
Aviation Note: The use of this drug **is a disqualification** for piloting. Consult a designated Aviation Medical Examiner.
Exposure to Sun: No restrictions.
Heavy Exercise or Exertion: Use caution—this may stress the protective effects of this drug.

SELEGILINE (se LEDGE i leen)

Other Name: Deprenyl
Introduced: 1981   **Class:** Anti-Parkinsonism, monoamine oxidase (MAO) type B inhibitor   **Prescription:** USA: Yes   **Controlled Drug:** USA: No; Canada: No   **Available as Generic:** USA: Yes

Brand Names: ✽Apo-Selegiline, Carbex,✽Dom-Selegiline, Eldepryl, ✽Med-Selegiline, ✽Novo-Selegiline, ✽PMS-Selegiline

BENEFITS versus RISKS	
Possible Benefits	*Possible Risks*
EFFECTIVE INITIAL TREATMENT OF PARKINSON'S DISEASE when started at the onset of symptoms	ABNORMAL INVOLUNTARY MOVEMENTS
ADDITIVE RELIEF OF SYMPTOMS OF PARKINSON'S DISEASE when used concurrently with levodopa/carbidopa	HALLUCINATIONS
PERMITS REDUCTION IN SINEMET DOSE	INITIAL FALL IN BLOOD PRESSURE/ORTHOSTATIC HYPOTENSION
May have a role in Alzheimer's disease	

▷ **Principal Uses**

As a Single Drug Product: Uses currently included in FDA-approved labeling: (1) Used to start drug treatment of very early Parkinson's disease (soon after onset of symptoms), thus delaying the use of levodopa/carbidopa; (2) also used as an adjunct to levodopa/carbidopa treatment of Parkinson's disease if intolerable abnormal movements (dyskinesia) and/or increasing "on-off" episodes occur—addition of selegiline (a) permits reduction of the daily dose of levodopa with consequent lessening of dyskinesia and erratic drug response and (b) provides additional relief of Parkinsonian symptoms.

Other (unlabeled) generally accepted uses: (1) Some improvement achieved in Alzheimer's disease (some trials also used high-dose vitamin E) in patients treated with this drug; (2) narcolepsy; (3) may have a role in attention deficit hyperactivity disorder (ADHD) where methylphenidate is not tolerated; (4) may work as adjunctive treatment in some schizophrenia cases; (5) has some benefit in depression and bipolar disorder.

How This Drug Works: By inhibiting monoamine oxidase type B (the enzyme that inactivates dopamine in the brain) and by slowing the restorage of released dopamine at nerve terminals, this drug helps correct dopamine deficiency responsible for rigidity, tremor and sluggish movement characteristic of Parkinson's disease.

Available Dosage Forms and Strengths

Capsules —5 mg

Tablets —5 mg

Author's Note: The capsule form of this medicine may eventually replace the tablet form and is an astute attempt by the company to help avoid confusion with other white tablets or counterfeit copies of Eldepryl.

▷ **Usual Adult Dosage Ranges:** *Parkinsonism*: 5 mg once or twice daily. The usual maintenance dose is 5 mg after breakfast and 5 mg after lunch. Daily dose of 10 mg is adequate to achieve optimal benefit. Higher doses do not result in further improvement and are not advised. During gradual introduction of selegiline, dose of levodopa/carbidopa (Sinemet) may be cautiously decreased. Sinemet dose should be reduced by 10% to 20% when selegiline is started. **Note: Actual dose and schedule must be determined for each patient individually.**

Conditions Requiring Dosing Adjustments

Liver Function: This drug is extensively metabolized in the liver. Patients with liver compromise should be followed closely.

Kidney Function: No dosing changes thought to be needed. It can cause prostatic enlargement (hypertrophy). Used with urine outflow problems.

▷ **Dosing Instructions:** The tablet may be crushed and taken with food or milk to reduce stomach irritation. If you forget a dose: Take the missed dose as soon as you remember it, unless it's nearly time for your next dose—if that is the case, skip the missed dose and take the next dose right on schedule. DO NOT double doses. Taking this medicine with breakfast and/or dinner is usually best because taking it with dinner can disrupt your sleep. Talk with your doctor if you find yourself missing doses or have difficulty sleeping.

Usual Duration of Use: Use on a regular schedule for 4 to 6 weeks usually determines effectiveness in controlling the symptoms of Parkinson's disease and permitting reduction of levodopa/carbidopa dose. Long-term use (months to years) requires periodic physician evaluation and goal assessment.

Typical Treatment Goals and Measurements (Outcomes and Markers)

Parkinson's disease: The general goal is to minimize symptoms (tremor, sluggish movements, analysis of walking or gait, etc.) to the fullest extent possible. Additionally, many neurologists use Hahn-Yahr scores and the time it takes to maximum amount of finger tapping as indicators of the benefits of this drug.

Possible Advantages of This Drug

It may provide a more effective and uniform control of Parkinsonian symptoms and a significant reduction of some adverse effects associated with long-term levodopa therapy.

▷ **This Drug Should Not Be Taken If**
- you have had an allergic reaction to it previously.
- you have Huntington's disease, hereditary (essential) tremor or tardive dyskinesia (see Glossary).
- you are pregnant or breast-feeding.
- you take meperidine (Demerol).

▷ **Inform Your Physician Before Taking This Drug If**
- you have constitutionally low blood pressure.
- you have peptic ulcer disease.
- you are taking levodopa.
- you have a history of heart rhythm disorder.
- you are taking any antihypertensive drugs, antidepressants or antipsychotic drugs (see Drug Classes).

Possible Side Effects (natural, expected and unavoidable drug actions)

Weakness, orthostatic hypotension (see Glossary), dry mouth, insomnia—all rare.

▷ **Possible Adverse Effects** (unusual, unexpected and infrequent reactions)

If any of the following develop, consult your physician promptly for guidance.

Mild Adverse Effects
> Headache, dizziness, blurred vision, agitation—rare.
> Palpitations, fainting—rare.
> Altered taste—rare.
> Nausea and vomiting, stomach pain, anorexia—rare to frequent.

Serious Adverse Effects
> Dyskinesias: abnormal involuntary movements—infrequent.
> Confusion and hallucinations, depression, psychosis, vivid dreams—rare.
> Aggravation of peptic ulcer, gastrointestinal bleeding—rare.
> Growth of the prostate—rare.

▷ **Possible Effects on Sexual Function:** Transient decreases in penile sensation and anorgasmia have rarely been reported if doses exceed 10 mg per day. Increased libido may occur.

▷ **Adverse Effects That May Mimic Natural Diseases or Disorders**
> Effects on mental function and behavior may resemble psychotic disorders.

Natural Diseases or Disorders That May Be Activated by This Drug
> Peptic ulcer disease.

Possible Effects on Laboratory Tests
> None reported.

CAUTION
1. This drug can start dyskinesias and intensify existing dyskinesias. Watch carefully for tremors, twitching or abnormal, involuntary movements of any kind. Report these promptly.
2. This drug potentiates the effects of levodopa. When added to current levodopa treatment, adverse effects of levodopa may develop or be intensified. Levodopa dose must be reduced by 10% to 20% when treatment with selegiline begins.
3. Tell your doctor promptly if you become pregnant or plan pregnancy. The manufacturer does not recommend the use of this drug during pregnancy.
4. Some foods (tyramine containing—see Glossary) have lead to rare increases in blood pressure with selegiline doses greater than 10 mg. Talk to your doctor.

Precautions for Use
> *By Infants and Children:* This drug is not utilized by this age group.
> *By Those Over 60 Years of Age:* This drug is well tolerated by the elderly. Observe closely for any tendency to light-headedness or faintness, especially on arising from a lying or sitting position.

▷ **Advisability of Use During Pregnancy**
> *Pregnancy Category:* C. See Pregnancy Risk Categories at the back of this book.
> *Animal studies:* No birth defects due to this drug were found in rat studies.
> *Human studies:* Adequate studies of pregnant women are not available.
> The manufacturer advises that this drug should not be taken during pregnancy.

Advisability of Use If Breast-Feeding
> Presence of this drug in breast milk: Unknown.
> Avoid drug or refrain from nursing.

Habit-Forming Potential: None.

Effects of Overdose: Nausea, vomiting, palpitations, low blood pressure, agitation, severe involuntary movements, hallucinations.

Possible Effects of Long-Term Use: None reported.

Suggested Periodic Examinations While Taking This Drug (at physician's discretion)

Regular evaluation of drug response, heart function and blood pressure status.

▷ **While Taking This Drug, Observe the Following**

Foods: CAUTION should be used regarding foods containing tyramine (see Glossary for a list), although the reaction with this drug may not be as severe as that seen with other MAO inhibitors.

Herbal Medicines or Minerals: St. John's wort: *CAUTION* is advised because of possible serotonin syndrome. St. John's wort may also worsen sensitivity to the sun. Since part of the way ginseng works may be as an MAO inhibitor, do not combine ginseng with selegiline. Ma huang and yohimbe are also best avoided while taking this medicine. Calabar bean (chop nut, fabia, ordeal nut, others) is unsafe when taken by mouth (physostigmine is the active ingredient) and should never be taken by people with Parkinson's disease. Octacosanol (a cousin of vitamin E) can worsen movement problems and should also be avoided.

Beverages: No restrictions. May be taken with milk.

▷ *Alcohol:* Use *CAUTION* until the combined effects have been determined. Alcohol may exaggerate the blood-pressure-lowering and sedative effects of this drug. Aged wines, etc., containing tyramine may cause a reaction of varying severity.

Tobacco Smoking: No interactions expected. I advise everyone to quit smoking.

Marijuana Smoking: Additive drowsiness may occur.

▷ *Other Drugs*

Selegiline *taken concurrently* with

- albuterol (Ventolin, others) may result in increased adverse vascular effects.
- amphetamine (Dexedrine, others) can cause a severe increase in blood pressure.
- antidepressants (see Drug Classes) such as amitriptyline (Elavil) may cause neurotoxic reactions such as seizures.
- antihypertensive drugs (and Other Drugs that can lower blood pressure) require careful monitoring for excessive drops in pressure; dose adjustments may be necessary.
- benzodiazepines (see Drug Classes) may result in increased central nervous system depression.
- beta two type agonist medicines may increase risk of rapid heart rate, hypomania or agitation.
- birth control pills (oral contraceptives) may increase risk of selegiline toxicity.
- bupropion (Wellbutrin) may cause seizures.
- buspirone (Buspar) may result in increases in blood pressure.
- carbamazepine (Tegretol) may result in high fevers and seizures—still, some studies found benefits in resistant depression.
- citalopram (Celexa) may lead to toxicity—DO NOT COMBINE.
- cyclobenzaprine (Flexeril) may lead to toxicity—DO NOT COMBINE.

- dextromethorphan (various), a cough suppressant used in many nonprescription cough medicines, has been reported to cause toxicity with low blood pressure, spasms, high fevers and some deaths—these medicines should not be combined.
- ephedrine (various) can result in severe increases in temperature.
- fluoxetine (Prozac) may cause serotonin toxicity syndrome.
- fluvoxamine (Luvox) may result in extreme agitation, rigidity, excessive temperatures and coma—DO NOT combine these medicines.
- lithium (Lithobid) may increase risk of the serotonin toxicity syndrome.
- meperidine (Demerol) may cause a life-threatening reaction of unknown cause; avoid this combination.
- methyldopa (Aldomet) MAY LEAD TO HYPERTENSIVE CRISIS—DO NOT COMBINE.
- methylphenidate (Concerta, others) MAY LEAD TO HYPERTENSIVE CRISIS—DO NOT COMBINE.
- mirtazapine (Remeron) may lead to adverse seizures.
- morphine (MS Contin, various) may lead to excessive CNS and lowered blood pressure effects—DO NOT COMBINE.
- nefazodone (Serzone) may lead to serotonin syndrome—DO NOT COMBINE.
- oral hypoglycemic agents (see Oral Antidiabetic Drugs in Drug Classes) may cause very low blood sugars.
- paroxetine (Paxil) may result in central nervous system toxicity.
- phenothiazines (see Drug Classes) may result in increased occurrence of movement disorders.
- phentermine (Fastin) may lead to hypertensive crisis—DO NOT COMBINE.
- phenylpropanolamine (various) or phenylephrine (various) can cause severe increases in temperature and blood pressure—DO NOT combine.
- pseudoephedrine (various) can cause severe increases in temperature and blood pressure—DO NOT combine (this includes combination forms of pseudoephedrine such as loratadine/pseudoephedrine [Claritin-D]).
- sertraline (Zoloft) may result in central nervous system toxicity.
- sibutramine (Meridia) may lead to toxicity.
- sumatriptan (Imitrex) may lead to toxicity.
- tramadol (Ultram) may lead to seizures.
- tryptophan may cause a fatal serotonin syndrome.
- venlafaxine (Effexor) can result in central and autonomic nervous system toxicity.

The following drugs may *decrease* the effects of selegiline and diminish its effectiveness:
- chlorprothixene (Taractan).
- haloperidol (Haldol).
- metoclopramide (Reglan).
- phenothiazines (see Drug Classes).
- reserpine (Ser-Ap-Es, etc.), in high doses.
- thiothixene (Navane).

▷ *Driving, Hazardous Activities:* This drug may cause dizziness, drowsiness, impaired coordination or fainting. Restrict activities as necessary.

Aviation Note: The use of this drug *is a disqualification* for piloting. Consult a designated Aviation Medical Examiner.

Exposure to Sun: Use caution—photosensitivity has been reported.

Exposure to Heat: Use caution until the combined effects have been determined. Hot environments can cause lowering of blood pressure.

Discontinuation: **Do not stop this drug abruptly**. Sudden withdrawal can cause prompt increase in Parkinsonian symptoms and deterioration of control. Consult your physician regarding a schedule for gradual withdrawal and concurrent adjustment of Sinemet or other appropriate drugs.

SERTRALINE (SER tra leen)

Introduced: 1986   **Class:** Antidepressant   **Prescription:** USA: Yes
Controlled Drug: USA: No; Canada: No   Available as Generic: USA: No
Brand Name: Zoloft, ✺Apo-sertraline, ✺Gen-sertraline, ✺Novo-sertraline

---

BENEFITS versus RISKS

Possible Benefits	*Possible Risks*
EFFECTIVE TREATMENT OF DEPRESSION	Male sexual dysfunction
TREATS PANIC DISORDER	Seizures
TREATMENT OF OBSESSIVE-COMPULSIVE DISORDER	
TREATS POST-TRAUMATIC STRESS DISORDER (PTSD)	

▷ **Principal Uses**

As a Single Drug Product: Uses currently included in FDA-approved labeling: Treats (1) major depression; (2) obsessive-compulsive disorder; (3) panic disorder: (4) eases post-traumatic stress disorder.

Other (unlabeled) generally accepted uses: (1) May have a role in treating obesity—rat studies have shown a decrease in eating that depends on the dose that is taken, and studies in humans are being conducted; (2) may help some kinds of sexual problems (premature ejaculation); (3) helps clozapine-caused (induced) obsessive-compulsive disorder; (4) eases symptoms in premenstrual dysphoric syndrome (PMDS); (5) can ease the feeling of loss of breath in mild to severe obstructive lung disease.

How This Drug Works: This drug relieves depression by slowly restoring to normal levels a specific constituent of brain tissue (serotonin) that transmits nerve impulses.

Available Dosage Forms and Strengths

Tablets — 25 mg, 50 mg, 100 mg

▷ **Recommended Dose Ranges** (Actual dose and schedule must be determined for each patient individually.)

Infants and Children: In children 6 to 12 years old: 25 mg once daily has been approved to treat obsessive-compulsive disorder.

12 to 60 Years of Age: Depression: Initially 50 mg once daily, taken in the morning or evening. The dose is then slowly increased, as needed and tolerated, in increments of 50 mg at intervals of 1 week. The total daily dose should not exceed 200 mg.

Panic Disorder: Dosing is started at 25 mg a day (morning or evening). After seven days, the dose can be increased to 50 mg once daily. If needed and tolerated, the dose can then be increased (at 7 day intervals) to a 200 mg per day maximum.

PTSD: Similar to dosing for depression.

Over 60 Years of Age: Same as 12 to 60 years of age. Adjust dose as appropriate for impaired liver or kidney function.

Conditions Requiring Dosing Adjustments

Liver Function: Drug is a rare cause of liver damage. Patients with liver disease should be watched closely and lower doses used.

Kidney Function: The role of the kidneys is unknown.

▷ **Dosing Instructions:** The tablet may be crushed and is best taken with food to enhance absorption, but it may be taken at any time with or without food. The oral liquid form (concentrate) has 20 mg in each ml. Use the calibrated dropper to get the right dose. Just before you are going to take it, the dose can be mixed with 4 ounces of water, orange juice, ginger ale or other suitable liquid (talk to your pharmacist). It is ok if a haze appears once the concentrate has been added to the liquid. Taking this medicine regularly is important. If you forget a dose: Skip the missed dose and take the next dose right on schedule. DO NOT double doses. Talk with your doctor if you find yourself missing doses.

Usual Duration of Use: Use on a regular schedule for 4 to 8 weeks usually determines effectiveness in relieving depression and pattern of both favorable and unfavorable drug effects. Clinical studies suggest that people who respond during the first 8 weeks of treatment will benefit from another 8 weeks of sertraline therapy. Benefits of use in obsessive-compulsive disorder (OCD) have not been shown longer than 12 weeks in clinical trials. Since OCD tends to be ongoing, patients who benefit from this medicine should discuss the benefits and risks of continued sertraline. Long-term use requires periodic physician evaluation. The lowest effective dose should be used.

Typical Treatment Goals and Measurements (Outcomes and Markers)

Depression: The general goal: to lessen the degree and severity of depression, letting patients return to their daily lives. Specific measures of depression involve testing or inventories and can be valuable in helping check benefits from this medicine.

Panic disorder: Goals for panic tend to be more vague and subjective than hypertension or cholesterol. Frequently, the patient (in conjunction with physician assessment) will largely decide if panic has been modified to a successful extent. Additionally, decreased number of trips to the hospital or ER visits may be a useful measure. The ability of the patient to return to normal activities is a hallmark of successful treatment.

Possible Advantages of This Drug

Does not cause weight gain, a common side effect of tricyclic antidepressants. Less likely to cause dry mouth, constipation, urinary retention, orthostatic hypotension (see Glossary) and heart rhythm disturbances than tricyclic antidepressants. May have fewer drug interactions than other medicines in this same class.

▷ **This Drug Should Not Be Taken If**
- you have had an allergic reaction to it previously.
- you took a monoamine oxidase (MAO) type A inhibitor (see Drug Classes) in the last 14 days.

▷ **Inform Your Physician Before Taking This Drug If**
- you had any adverse effects from antidepressant drugs.
- you have impaired liver or kidney function.
- you have Parkinson's disease.
- you or a loved one does not understand or want to face the risk of possible suicide; careful follow-up by care givers and your physician is prudent.
- you have had a recent heart attack.
- you have a seizure disorder.
- you have a bleeding problem or take a diuretic.
- you are pregnant or plan pregnancy while taking this drug.

Possible Side Effects (natural, expected and unavoidable drug actions)
Decreased appetite, weight loss (average 1 to 2 lb).

▷ **Possible Adverse Effects** (unusual, unexpected and infrequent reactions)
If any of the following develop, consult your physician promptly for guidance.

Mild Adverse Effects
Allergic reactions: skin rash, itching—rare.
Headache, nervousness, insomnia, fatigue, tremor, dizziness, impaired concentration—rare.
Abnormal vision, numbness and tingling—rare.
Confusion—rare.
Alopecia—infrequent.
Night sweats—case report.
Chest pain and increased blood pressure—rare.
Paresthesias—rare.
Dry mouth, altered taste, nausea, vomiting, diarrhea, tongue ulceration—rare to frequent.

Serious Adverse Effects
Allergic reactions: dermatitis (various forms)—rare.
Drug-induced seizures—rare.
Hemorrhage into the anterior chamber of the eye or anemia—rare.
Hallucinations—case reports.
Increased blood cholesterol (hypercholesterolemia)—infrequent.
Low blood sugar—case reports.
Bronchospasm—infrequent.
QT interval changes—case reports.
Movement disorders (extrapyramidal reactions)—case reports.
Neuroleptic malignant syndrome—case reports with other SSRIs.
Low blood sodium—rare.
SIADH—case reports (may also occur with other selective serotonin reuptake inhibitors).

▷ **Possible Effects on Sexual Function:** Male sexual dysfunction: delayed ejaculation—may be frequent.
Female sexual dysfunction: inhibited orgasm—rare.
Swelling and tenderness of male (gynecomastia) and female breast tissue—case reports.
Infrequent dysmenorrhea, intermenstrual bleeding, atrophic vaginitis, painful erections (priapism)—possible, case reports.
May help some kinds of sexual disorders.

Natural Diseases or Disorders That May Be Activated by This Drug
  Latent epilepsy.

Possible Effects on Laboratory Tests
  Blood total cholesterol and triglyceride levels: increased—infrequent.
  Blood uric acid levels: decreased.
  Hemoglobin or hematocrit: decreased—rare.
  Liver function tests: increased liver enzymes (ALT/GPT, AST/GOT and alkaline phosphatase).
  Blood sodium: decreased (with rare SIADH).

CAUTION
  1. If any type of skin reaction develops (rash, hives, etc.), stop this drug and call your doctor promptly.
  2. If dryness of the mouth develops and persists for more than 2 weeks, consult your dentist for guidance.
  3. Ask your doctor or pharmacist before taking any other prescription or over-the-counter drug while taking sertraline.
  4. If you are advised to take any monoamine oxidase (MAO) type A inhibitor (see Drug Classes), allow an interval of 5 weeks after discontinuing this drug before starting the MAO inhibitor.
  5. It is advisable to withhold this drug if electroconvulsive therapy (ECT, "shock" treatment) is to be used to treat your depression.
  6. Movement reactions if they happen usually occur in the first month of treatment and close patient follow up is advisable.

Precautions for Use
  By Infants and Children: Safety and effectiveness for those under 12 years of age are not established.
  By Those Over 60 Years of Age: The lowest effective dose should be used for maintenance treatment and adjusted as needed for reduced kidney function.

▷ **Advisability of Use During Pregnancy**
  Pregnancy Category: C. See Pregnancy Risk Categories at the back of this book.
  Animal studies: Delayed bone development due to this drug found in rat and rabbit studies.
  Human studies: Adequate studies of pregnant women are not available.
  Use this drug only if clearly needed. Ask your physician for guidance.

Advisability of Use If Breast-Feeding
  Presence of this drug in breast milk: Yes, variable amounts.
  One small study found undetectable blood levels in infants who were breast-fed while their mothers were taking sertraline. Another found detectable levels. May be a drug of choice for mothers who breast-feed their infants. Discuss breast-feeding with your doctor.

Habit-Forming Potential: None.

Effects of Overdose: Agitation, restlessness, excitement, nausea, vomiting, seizures.

Possible Effects of Long-Term Use: None reported.

Suggested Periodic Examinations While Taking This Drug (at physician's discretion)
  None.

▷ **While Taking This Drug, Observe the Following**

Foods: May increase peak blood level.

Herbal Medicines or Minerals: Since sertraline and St. John's wort may act to increase serotonin, the combination is not advised. Because part of the way ginseng and ginkgo works may be as a MAO inhibitor, the combination is not advisable. Ma huang, yohimbe, Indian snakeroot and kava kava are also best avoided while taking this medicine.

Calcium now has excellent data (1,200–1,600 mg per day unless contraindicated) in helping prevent premenstrual dysphoric syndrome (PMDS). This may be an intelligent first-line therapy or valuable adjunctive use. Talk to your doctor to see if this makes sense for you.

Beverages: No restrictions. May be taken with milk.

▷ *Alcohol:* Avoid completely.

Tobacco Smoking: No interactions expected. I advise everyone to quit smoking.

▷ *Other Drugs*

Sertraline may **increase** the effects of

- astemizole (Hismanal—see medicines removed from the market), leading to torsade de pointes or other heart rhythm problems—DO NOT COMBINE.
- carbamazepine (Tegretol, others), leading to toxicity. Careful patient monitoring and more frequent carbamazepine levels are prudent.
- clozapine (Clozaril), leading to clozapine toxicity.
- dextromethorphan (in many cough "DM" suppressants).
- diazepam (Valium) and perhaps other benzodiazepines (see Drug Classes).
- diltiazem (Cardizem).
- dofetilide (Tikosyn), leading to toxicity. CAUTION and more frequent blood levels are prudent.
- fosphenytoin (Cerebyx) or phenytoin (Dilantin). Blood level checks are prudent if these medicines must be combined.
- lamotrigine (Lamictal).
- naratriptan (Amerge), sumatriptan (Imitrex) and rizatriptan (Maxalt), leading to loss of coordination and weakness.
- propafenone (Rythmol), leading to toxicity. Blood levels and clinical monitoring is prudent.
- sibutramine (Meridia), which may lead to toxicity (serotonin syndrome)—DO NOT COMBINE.
- theophylline (Theo-Dur, others) may lead to theophylline toxicity.
- tolbutamide (Orinase).
- warfarin (Coumadin) and related oral anticoagulants; more frequent INR (prothrombin time or protime) testing is needed. Ongoing warfarin doses should be based on INR results.

Sertraline *taken concurrently* with

- antidiabetic drugs (insulin, oral hypoglycemics: see Oral Antidiabetic Drugs in Drug Classes) may increase the risk of hypoglycemic reactions; monitor blood and urine sugar levels carefully.
- benzodiazepines removed by the CYP 3A4 family of liver enzymes (such as triazolam or alprazolam) may lead to benzodiazepine toxicity.
- bupropion (Wellbutrin, Zyban) may lead to sertraline toxicity. Caution and dosing in the lower end of the dose range are prudent.
- cimetidine (Tagamet, Tagamet HB 200) may lead to sertraline toxicity. Careful patient monitoring and lower sertraline doses are prudent.

- erythromycin (various) led to a serotonin syndrome in a 12-year-old boy; other macrolide antibiotics such as clarithromycin may also lead to this effect. Doses of sertraline should be lowered if these medicines must be combined.
- flecainide (Tambocor) may lead to flecainide toxicity.
- lithium (Lithobid, others) may lead to changes. Lithium blood levels are prudent.
- metoclopramide (Reglan) may lead to sertraline toxicity.
- monoamine oxidase (MAO) type A inhibitors may cause confusion, agitation, high fever, seizures and dangerous elevations of blood pressure—avoid the concurrent use of these drugs.
- quinidine (Quinaglute, others) may lead to quinidine toxicity—CAUTION is advised.
- ritonavir (Norvir) and perhaps other protease inhibitors (see Drug Classes) may lead to toxicity.
- terfenadine (Seldane) may lead to toxicity.
- tramadol (Ultram) may lead to seizures.
- zolpidem (Ambien) may lead to hallucinations—DO NOT COMBINE.

▷ *Driving, Hazardous Activities:* This drug may cause drowsiness, dizziness, impaired judgment and altered vision. Restrict activities as necessary.

Aviation Note: The use of this drug *is a disqualification* for piloting. Consult a designated Aviation Medical Examiner.

Exposure to Sun: Use caution—this drug may (rarely) cause photosensitivity (see Glossary).

Discontinuation: The slow elimination of this drug from the body makes it unlikely that any withdrawal effects will result from abrupt discontinuation. However, call your doctor if you plan to stop this drug for any reason.

SIBUTRAMINE (si BUTE rah meen)

Introduced: 1998 **Class:** Serotonin reuptake inhibitor, anorexiant, weight loss agent **Prescription:** USA: Yes **Controlled Drug:** USA: C-IV*; Canada: Yes **Available as Generic:** USA: No
Brand Name: Meridia

BENEFITS versus RISKS	
Possible Benefits	*Possible Risks*
EFFECTIVE WEIGHT LOSS	SIGNIFICANT INCREASES IN
ASSOCIATED DECREASES IN	BLOOD PRESSURE AND HEART
TRIGLYCERIDE AND HDL	RATE (DIASTOLIC)
LEVELS WITH WEIGHT LOSS	Increased premature (asymptomatic)
	heart contractions

▷ **Principal Uses**

As a Single Drug Product: Uses currently included in FDA-approved labeling: Used to manage obesity, including weight loss and maintaining weight loss in people on a reduced-calorie diet. Used in those with an initial body mass index (BMI: see Glossary) greater than or equal to 30 kg per square meter or 27 kg per square meter if there are other risk factors (such as diabetes, hyperlipidemia or hypertension).

Other (unlabeled) generally accepted uses: (1) May have a role in treating depression; (2) could help some cases of peripheral neuropathy.

How This Drug Works: This medicine helps treat obesity by decreasing the desire to eat by blocking reuptake of nerve transmitters (norepinephrine serotonin and dopamine) in brain synapses. People who took the drug in clinical studies were satisfied more quickly when they ate. Since metabolism is also increased, they used more of the food that they did eat than patients not receiving the medicine. Most of this effect comes from two active compounds (metabolites) that the body changes sibutramine into (M1 and M2).

Available Dosage Forms and Strengths

Capsules — 5 mg, 10 mg, 15 mg

▷ **Recommended Dosage Ranges** (Actual dose and schedule must be determined for each patient individually.) Dosing is started at 10 mg once a day in the morning. This dose may be decreased to 5 mg daily if not tolerated (using blood pressure and heart rate as guides). If weight loss does not reach goals after 4 weeks, the dose can be increased to 15 mg daily. The daily maximum is 15 mg.

Conditions Requiring Dosing Adjustments

Liver Function: This drug is changed in the liver; however, dose changes are not thought to be needed in mild to moderate liver failure. Drug should NOT be used in severe liver failure.

Kidney Function: No changes needed in mild to moderate kidney failure. Drug should NOT be used in severe kidney failure.

▷ **Dosing Instructions:** Capsule may be taken before or following food. It was usually taken in the morning in clinical trials. If the starting dose of 10 mg isn't tolerated (using heart rate and blood pressure as a guide), discuss this with your doctor. The dose is usually then lowered to 5 mg daily in those cases. If you forget a dose: Take the missed dose as soon as you remember it, unless it's nearly time for your next dose—if that is the case, skip the missed dose and take the next dose right on schedule. DO NOT double up on doses. Talk with your doctor if you find yourself missing doses.

Usual Duration of Use: This medicine has only been used up to a year in clinical studies. Longer-term use should be discussed with your doctor. One study found that 77% of those who took the medicine as part of a program not only lowered cholesterol but also helped achieve and maintain significant weight loss. Ongoing use requires periodic physician follow-up.

Typical Treatment Goals and Measurements (Outcomes and Markers)

Weight loss: The goal is to lower body weight or maintain weight loss. Body weight, percent body fat and laboratory tests such as triglycerides, VLDL, LDL and HDL can be checked to assess successful combination treatment. Be sure to talk to your doctor about the benefits of losing some weight and keeping it off versus crash or fad diets and weight yo-yoing.

Possible Advantages of This Drug

Use has not been associated with heart valve problems seen with dexfenfluramine (Redux). The STORM study (Sibutramine Trial in Obesity Reduction and Maintenance) showed that 67% of people who took sibutramine maintained their six-month weight loss for up to two years. In a more recent European study, 77% of people who took the medicine as part of an organized program lowered cholesterol and maintained significant weight loss.

▷ **This Drug Should Not Be Taken If**
- you had an allergic reaction to any form of it previously.
- you've had a stroke.
- you are anorexic.
- you have a history of abnormal heart rhythms.
- you have pulmonary hypertension.
- you have poorly controlled or uncontrolled high blood pressure.
- you have congestive heart failure or disease of the coronary arteries.
- other causes of obesity such as untreated low thyroid function (hypothyroidism) were not ruled out.
- you have glaucoma.
- you take, or have taken within the last 14 days, a monoamine oxidase (MAO) inhibitor (see Drug Classes).
- you have severe kidney or liver disease.

▷ **Inform Your Physician Before Taking This Drug If**
- you have heart (cardiovascular) disease or have had an unfavorable reaction to any serotonin reuptake inhibitor.
- you have narrow-angle glaucoma.
- you have a history of abnormal heart rhythms or high blood pressure.
- you have a history of kidney or liver compromise.
- you have a history of gallstones.
- you have a history of psychiatric disorders or drug abuse.
- you have taken other weight loss medicines (anorexiants) in the last year.
- you have a seizure disorder.
- you develop unexplained difficulty in breathing, fainting, chest pain or swelling of the ankles. These may be early symptoms of pulmonary hypertension.

Possible Side Effects (natural, expected and unavoidable drug actions)
Since some weight loss agents that cause increased levels of serotonin have been associated with development of a fatal lung problem (primary pulmonary hypertension, or PPH), it is prudent to talk about this with your doctor. It is unknown if sibutramine can cause this problem.

▷ **Possible Adverse Effects** (unusual, unexpected and infrequent reactions)
If any of the following develop, consult your physician promptly for guidance.

Mild Adverse Effects
Allergic reaction: skin rash.
Headache and anorexia—frequent.
Sleep disturbances—infrequent.
Dry mouth or constipation—frequent (but may ease over time).
Palpitations or tachycardia—rare.
Fast heart rate (tachycardia)—infrequent.
Increased liver enzymes—frequent (questionable cause).

Serious Adverse Effects
High blood pressure (increased up to 30% of the level present before starting the medicine) as well as some cases of increased diastolic pressure—infrequent.
Low blood platelets—case reports.

▷ **Possible Effects on Sexual Function:** Painful menstruation—infrequent.

Natural Diseases or Disorders That May Be Activated by This Drug

High blood pressure controlled by other medicines may return. Untreated high blood pressure may be worsened.

Possible Effects on Laboratory Tests

Drug testing: may cause false positive tests for amphetamines.

CAUTION

1. It is best to carry a card noting that you are taking this drug. A medicine alert bracelet is also a good idea.
2. This medicine may cause false positive urine drug tests for amphetamines.
3. Other conditions (organic causes) leading to obesity (such as low activity of the thyroid gland—hypothyroidism) should be ruled out prior to starting this medicine.
4. Safety and efficacy of use of sibutramine with other weight loss agents have NOT been established. Combination therapy is NOT recommended.
5. This medicine has NOT been found to cause lung problems (primary pulmonary hypertension or PPH); however, other drugs that increase serotonin were subsequently found to do this. If you develop unexplained difficulty in breathing, fainting, chest pain or swelling of the ankles, call your doctor. These may be early symptoms of pulmonary hypertension.
6. Because of the increased risk of increased blood pressure, periodic checks of blood pressure are prudent.
7. Nonprescription medicines such as pseudoephedrine, ephedrine or phenylpropanolamine can increase heart rate or blood pressure. Talk with your pharmacist or doctor BEFORE you combine any type of decongestant, cough, allergy or cold medicine.

Precautions for Use

By Infants and Children: Safety and effectiveness have not been established in those less than 16 years old.

By Those Over 60 Years of Age: The drug levels this medicine achieves and the places in the body where this medicine goes are no different for those over 60 than those under 60. *CAUTION* should be used (as with all medicines active in the central nervous system) in treating elderly patients with sibutramine. Since there is also a higher occurrence of high blood pressure and heart disease, caution and lower doses appear prudent.

▷ **Advisability of Use During Pregnancy**

Pregnancy Category: C. See Pregnancy Risk Categories at the back of this book.

Human studies: Adequate studies of pregnant women are not available.

NOT recommended for pregnant women.

Advisability of Use If Breast-Feeding

Presence of this drug in breast milk: unknown in humans.

Avoid drug or refrain from nursing.

Habit-Forming Potential: The possibility of physical dependence is low. Further study is needed to confirm an accurate probability of dependence risk. There was no evidence of addictive or drug-seeking behavior in premarketing studies.

Effects of Overdose: Few cases of overdose have been reported. Rapid heart rate was seen in one overdose.

Possible Effects of Long-Term Use: Weight loss (the desired effect). Increased blood pressure.

Suggested Periodic Examinations While Taking This Drug
Periodic weigh-ins.
Liver function tests.
Checks for early signs of primary pulmonary hypertension and hypertension in general are prudent.
Periodic blood pressure checks are prudent.

▷ **While Taking This Drug, Observe the Following**
Foods: Follow prescribed portion control and menu choices. Tryptophan (found in some health food stores) increases risk of serotonin syndrome.
Herbal Medicines or Minerals: Combining this medicine with St. John's wort IS NOT advised because of possible serotonin syndrome. Since part of the way ginseng works may be as an MAO inhibitor, do not combine ginseng with sibutramine. Ma huang, kola, ephedra and yohimbe are also best avoided while taking this medicine.
Nutritional Support: Dietary counseling and physician- or dietitian-directed menus and portion control are suggested.
Beverages: No restrictions except as described in your dietary guidelines.
▷ *Alcohol:* The manufacturer does not recommend use of excessive alcohol and sibutramine.
Tobacco Smoking: No interactions are described in current literature. I advise everyone to quit smoking.
▷ *Other Drugs*
Sibutramine *taken concurrently* with
- antimigraine agents (such as sumatriptan or Imitrex) and dihydroergotamine may rarely result in a serotonin syndrome—DO NOT combine.
- central nervous system active medicines (see Drug Classes of benzodiazepines, opioids [fentanyl, etc.], phenothiazines and others) may have additive effects—CAUTION is advised.
- dextromethorphan (various brands of cough medicine) may increase risk of serotonin syndrome—DO NOT COMBINE.
- fentanyl (Duragesic, others) increases risk of serotonin syndrome—DO NOT COMBINE.
- lithium (Lithobid, others) increases risk of serotonin syndrome—DO NOT COMBINE.
- meperidine (Demerol, others) increases risk of serotonin syndrome—DO NOT COMBINE.
- monoamine oxidase (MAO) inhibitors (see Drug Classes) may result in serious, even fatal reactions. Fourteen days should pass between stopping an MAO inhibitor and starting sibutramine.
- pentazocine (Talwin, others) increases risk of serotonin syndrome—DO NOT COMBINE.
- selective serotonin reuptake inhibitors (SSRIs: see Drug Classes) increases risk of serotonin syndrome—DO NOT COMBINE.
- tricyclic antidepressants (some, such as desipramine [Norpramin] and amitriptyline [Elavil]) increase serotonin syndrome risk.

- tryptophan (various) increases risk of serotonin syndrome—DO NOT COMBINE.

Sibutramine *taken concurrently* with the following may result in increased sibutramine levels:

- erythromycins (see Drug Classes).
- itraconazole (Sporanox).
- ketoconazole (Nizoral).
- mibefradil (Posicor) (recently removed from the U.S. market).
- nelfinavir (Viracept) and perhaps other protease inhibitors (see Drug Classes)—may increase blood levels.
- any medicine that interferes with cytochrome CYP3A4 or is removed from the body by those enzymes will potentially increase sibutramine blood levels. For example, if sildenafil (Viagra) and sibutramine are combined, I expect that doses of one or both drugs may need to be adjusted.

The following drugs may *decrease* the effects of sibutramine:

- rifabutin (Mycobutin).
- rifampin (Rifadin, Rimactane).

▷ *Driving, Hazardous Activities:* Use caution.

Aviation Note: The use of this drug *may be a disqualification* for piloting. Consult a designated Aviation Medical Examiner.

Exposure to Sun: No restrictions at present.

Occurrence of Unrelated Illness: Since weight loss may modify the need for medicines used to control blood pressure and lipids, the medicines used in these conditions may need to be adjusted.

Discontinuation: Ask your doctor for help if you are considering stopping this medicine.

SILDENAFIL CITRATE (sill DEN ah fill)

Introduced: 1998   **Class:** Anti-impotence   **Prescription:** USA: Yes
Controlled Drug: USA: No; Canada: No   **Available as Generic:** USA: No; Canada: No
Brand Name: Viagra

BENEFITS versus RISKS	
Possible Benefits	*Possible Risks*
SUCCESSFUL ACHIEVEMENT OF AN ERECTION	SERIOUS (HEART) DISEASE DRUG INTERACTIONS
SUFFICIENT ERECTION TO ACHIEVE INTERCOURSE	LIFE-THREATENING DRUG INTERACTIONS
May work in female orgasm problems (Italian data)	Drug-induced vision changes Headache

▷ **Principal Uses**

As a Single Drug Product: Uses currently included in FDA-approved labeling: (1) Treats difficulties getting or maintaining an erection (erectile dysfunction); (2) clinical trials that led to FDA approval for this medicine also showed better success rates for sexual intercourse for those using sildenafil versus placebo.

Other (unlabeled) generally accepted uses: Many anecdotal reports of improvement in sexuality (enhancement) and benefits in females have been made. A 12-week study of 33 women after menopause found that there was no significant change in sexual desire after 12 weeks of Viagra. Recent Italian data found benefits.

▷ **How This Drug Works:** Causes smooth muscle in the penis to relax, increasing blood flow into the penis, resulting in erection. Sildenafil causes release of nitric oxide (NO) in part of the penis called the corpus cavernosum. This then increases an enzyme called guanylate cyclase. This enzyme increases cyclic guanosine monophosphate (CGMP). The CGMP causes the smooth muscle in the penis to relax. Once the smooth muscle relaxes, blood flows into the penis, resulting in erection.

Available Dosage Forms and Strengths
Tablets — 25 mg, 50 mg, 100 mg

▷ **Recommended Dose Ranges** (Actual dose and schedule must be determined for each patient individually.)

Infants and Children: Not used in this age group.

18 to 65 Years of Age: Doses typically range from 25–100 mg used once daily. The dose that your doctor chooses is taken from half an hour up to four hours before sexual activity. This medicine has worked in more than 70% of patients who took the 50–100 mg daily dose. For people who are taking medicines that inhibit a liver enzyme called cytochrome P450 3A4 (such as itraconazole, ketoconazole or some macrolide antibiotics such as erythromycin), the 25 mg dose is used by clinicians who have patients who take one of those medicines at the same time as sildenafil. Further caution is required and it would be a benefit-to-risk decision if multiple 3A4 inhibitors are being taken and sildenafil is being considered. Additionally, some medicines used in combination therapy of HIV/AIDS may interact and caution and lower doses are prudent and use is a benefit to risk decision for your doctor. (See additional medicine combination comments in the drug interactions section below.)

Over 65 Years of Age: Because plasma levels of sildenafil may be increased in this age group, doses should be reduced to 25 mg once daily. If kidney function has decreased to less than 30 ml/min further in a patient in this age group, further benefit to risk decision should be given.

Conditions Requiring Dosing Adjustments
Liver Function: A starting dose of 25 mg is prudent in liver disease.
Kidney Function: Caution is advised, as one measure of drug levels is doubled in those with compromised kidneys.

▷ **Dosing Instructions:** The tablet may be crushed and taken without regard to eating (high-fat meals decreased absorption time and may make the medicine take longer to work). It can be taken an hour before sexual activity, and the manufacturer mentions an acceptable range of half an hour to four hours before sexual activity. If you forget a dose: This medicine is usually taken one hour before you want to have sexual intercourse. DO NOT take the medicine more than once a day.

Usual Duration of Use: Use is only recommended ONCE daily. If use is to be ongoing on a daily basis, this should be discussed with your doctor.

Typical Treatment Goals and Measurements (Outcomes and Markers)
Erectile dysfunction: The general goal is to help you attain an erection that will

help you have sex. Typical desired results are stiffness or tone of the penis and how often you have an erection in response to this medicine.

Possible Advantages of This Drug: Avoids direct injections into the penis. Avoids surgical placement of an implant. Excellent response rate.

▷ **This Drug Should Not Be Taken If**
- you have had an allergic reaction to it previously.
- you have a disease or condition that would result in serious health hazard if lowering of the blood pressure or sexual activity occurred.
- you are taking any nitrate (see Drug Classes). NEVER combine these medicines (see also "Other Drug" interactions).
- You have pre-existing cardiovascular disease and sexual activity is inadvisable.
- You have not fully discussed this medicine with your doctor and have obtained it from an alternative source.
- You have not told your doctor about all the medicines you are taking.

▷ **Inform Your Physician Before Taking This Drug If**
- you have liver or kidney disease.
- the drug was prescribed for you without a complete medical history or physical examination.
- you have a history of heart disease (such as congestive heart failure, past heart attack, unstable angina, arrhythmias or coronary ischemia).
- you have multiple myeloma, leukemia or sickle cell syndrome (may predispose you to painful and sustained erections called priapism).
- you are over 65 and a 50-mg dose has been prescribed.
- you have vision changes while taking this medicine.
- you have cataracts or impaired vision (such as retinitis pigmentosa).
- you have had structural damage to the penis (Peyronie's disease: see Glossary).
- you are taking a medicine that blocks or enhances the liver cytochrome system (CYP3A4 or 2C9) (Talk to your doctor or pharmacist about this).
- you are prone to heartburn or have other stomach conditions.
- you do not have any improvement in erections or sexual performance while taking this medicine.
- you are unsure how much to take or how often to take this medicine.

Possible Side Effects (natural, expected and unavoidable drug actions)
Changes in vision (blue tint) or dry eyes—up to 3% in clinical trials. Nasal congestion—possible.

▷ **Possible Adverse Effects** (unusual, unexpected and infrequent reactions)
If any of the following develop, consult your physician promptly for guidance.
Mild Adverse Effects
Allergic reactions: rash.
Headache—infrequent to frequent.
Flushing—infrequent to frequent.
Indigestion—infrequent.
Sensitivity to light or blurred vision—possible to infrequent (more likely with the 100 mg dose).
Inability to distinguish between blue and green—possible and may be dose-related.

Serious Adverse Effects

DEATH RESULTING FROM DRUG INTERACTIONS—possible.

Temporary vision loss—case reports.

Decrease in blood supplied to the heart muscle (myocardial ischemia)—rare.

Heart attack—case reports.

Arrhythmias—case reports from two patients who had previous heart attacks.

▷ **Possible Effects on Sexual Function:**

Abnormal ejaculation—case reports.

Sustained and painful erection (priapism)—case reports.

Possible Delayed Adverse Effects: None reported to date.

Natural Diseases or Disorders That May Be Activated by This Drug

Patient perception of any pre-existing retinal disease may be worsened if sildenafil haze or bluish vision-tinting happens. Some cardiovascular conditions may be worsened by this drug

Possible Effects on Laboratory Tests

None reported.

CAUTION

Author's Note: Early case reports of six deaths were reviewed by the FDA in May 1998. A total of 30 deaths were reviewed as of June 1998. Based on the review, Viagra itself was NOT found to be the cause of the deaths and NO CHANGES were made to the package insert. Subsequently, new and expanded safety information was added to required FDA labeling including drug interaction data. During this controversial and rapidly changing period, conflicting reports, possible interactions as absolute contraindications and unclear benefit-to-risk decisions were reported and evolved or failed to evolve. Talk to your doctor or pharmacist about the most current combinations of medicines which are thought to be inappropriate versus those requiring lower doses and those that should never be undertaken. Because a medicine has serious possible interactions does not mean that it is an undesirable medicine, only that some combinations are not prudent.

1. Because of the possibility of SERIOUS drug interactions, keep a card in your purse or wallet or get a medicine alert bracelet to wear that says you are taking sildenafil.

2. If this medicine does not help you get or maintain an erection, it is important that you follow up with your doctor.

3. Safety and efficacy of sildenafil combined with other treatments for erectile problems (dysfunction) have not been established and may not be recommended by your doctor.

4. Some people use illegal "poppers," which are actually ampules of alkyl nitrites, to enhance sexual activity. These should NEVER be combined with Viagra.

5. The American Academy of Ophthalmology recommended further studies of sildenafil's long-term effects on the eyes and also warned that those with conditions of the retina should take the drug in the lowest effective dose and with caution. Promptly report altered or impaired vision so that appropriate evaluation can be made.

6. The manufacturer notes that it is important to have a physical exam and

medical history taken to properly diagnose problems with erections (erectile dysfunction) and to identify (where possible) any underlying disease or condition that may actually be the cause of the problem (such as diabetes).

7. If your erection lasts more than 4 hours, go to the nearest emergency room. Such persistent erections may lead to damage of the penis that is not reversible.

Precautions for Use

By Infants and Children: Safety and effectiveness for those under 18 not established.

By Those Over 60 Years of Age: Because this medicine is more slowly removed from the body in this age group, drug levels may be higher. 25 mg is the recommended starting dose.

▷ **Advisability of Use During Pregnancy**

Pregnancy Category: B. See Pregnancy Risk Categories at the back of this book.

Animal studies: no evidence of embryotoxicity, fetotoxicity or teratogenicity in rats and rabbits.

Human studies: Adequate studies of pregnant women are not available.
NOT indicated for use in women, children or newborns.

Advisability of Use If Breast-Feeding

Presence of this drug in breast milk: Unknown.
Avoid drug or refrain from nursing.

Habit-Forming Potential: None.

Effects of Overdose: Adverse effects were similar to accepted dosing adverse effects, but increased in frequency with clinical trials of 800 mg doses. Supportive care is indicated with the caveat of extremely careful cardiac monitoring in those with existing heart disease.

Possible Effects of Long-Term Use: Not defined.

Suggested Periodic Examinations While Taking This Drug (at physician's discretion)

Follow-up on success in achieving an erection and having intercourse.
Complete eye examination at beginning of treatment and at any time that significant change in vision occurs. Ask your doctor for help.

▷ **While Taking This Drug, Observe the Following**

Foods: Grapefruit juice can be an inhibitor of CYP3A4. DO NOT combine. Water is the safest liquid to take this medicine with.

Herbal Medicines or Minerals: Using St. John's wort, ma huang or kola while taking this medicine may result in unacceptable heart stimulation. Since St. John's wort and sildenafil may increase sun sensitivity, the combination is NOT advised. There are no data regarding combining yohimbe (Pausinystala yohimbe) with sildenafil, and yohimbe can lead to serious heart complications. The combination is NOT advised. Numan has had some small cohort studies, but has also not been studied and cannot be recommended in combination with sildenafil.

Beverages: Grapefruit juice can be an inhibitor of the enzyme that removes sildenafil from the body (CYP3A4). DO NOT combine as toxicity may result. Drug may be taken with milk or water.

▷ *Alcohol:* Excess alcohol intake may blunt the benefits of this medicine.

Tobacco Smoking: No interactions expected. I advise everyone to quit smoking.

Marijuana Smoking: The active ingredient (cannabinoids) found in marijuana can act as an inhibitor of the principal enzyme (CYP3A4) that removes sildenafil from the body. COMBINATION IS NOT RECOMMENDED.

▷ *Other Drugs*

Sildenafil may increase the effects of
- nitrates (see Drug Classes)—NEVER COMBINE.

The following drugs may ***increase*** the effects of sildenafil:
- cimetidine (Tagamet).
- delavirdine (Rescriptor).
- diltiazem (Cardizem).
- erythromycins (erythromycin and clarithromycin: see Drug Classes).
- indinavir (Crixivan), nelfinavir (Viracept), saquinavir (Viracept) and perhaps other protease inhibitors (see Drug Classes).
- itraconazole (Sporanox).
- ketoconazole (Nizoral).
- metronidazole (Flagyl).
- mibefradil (Posicor) (removed from the U.S. market).
- nitroprusside (Nitropress).
- ritonavir (Norvir) can increase sildenafil blood levels by up to 1,000%. A maximum dose of 25 mg every 48 hours is suggested along with careful patient monitoring.
- sertraline (Zoloft).
- Any medicine that interferes with cytochrome (CYP3A4-major or 2C9-minor, such as sibutramine [Meridia], which uses CYP3A4) will potentially increase (or decrease) sildenafil blood levels. In some cases, I expect that sildenafil dosing will need to be adjusted, and in others, the combination should be avoided.

Sildenafil ***taken concurrently*** with
- amyl nitrite will result in serious decreases in blood pressure—DO NOT COMBINE.
- medicines that cause vision changes (see Table 4) may result in additive vision problems.
- oral hypoglycemic agents tolbutamide (Orinase an inhibitor of 2C9), and glipizide (Glucotrol)—one early case report of a serious interaction are representative of medicines which may lead to problems and in the case of glipizide had one reported problem. Talk to your doctor about the latest information on possible interactions of these medicines with sildenafil.

The following drugs may ***decrease*** the effects of sildenafil:
- carbamazepine (Tegretol).
- phenytoin (Dilantin).
- rifabutin (Mycobutin).
- rifampin (Rifadin, Rimactane).

▷ *Driving, Hazardous Activities:* No restrictions.

Aviation Note: The use of this drug ***may be a disqualification*** for piloting. Consult a designated Aviation Medical Examiner.

Exposure to Sun: May increase sensitivity of your eyes to sunlight. Talk to your doctor about sunglasses or other protective measures.

Discontinuation: Talk to your doctor about your results from taking this drug.

SIMVASTATIN (sim vah STA tin)

Introduced: 1986   **Class:** Anticholesterol   **Prescription:** USA: Yes
Controlled Drug: USA: No; Canada: No   **Available as Generic:** USA: No;
Canada: No
Brand Name: Zocor

BENEFITS versus RISKS

Possible Benefits	*Possible Risks*
EFFECTIVE REDUCTION OF TOTAL BLOOD CHOLESTEROL AND LDL CHOLESTEROL	Drug-induced liver problems (hepatitis)—rare
INCREASES HDL-C (GOOD CHOLESTEROL) IN PATIENTS WITH PRIMARY HYPER-CHOLESTEROLEMIA AND MIXED DYSLIPIDEMIA	Drug-induced muscle damage (myositis)—rare
	Decreased coenzyme Q10
TREATS ISOLATED HYPER-TRIGLYCERIDEMIA AND TYPE THREE HYPER-LIPOPROTEINEMIA	
REDUCES RISK FROM CORONARY DISEASE	
REDUCES DEATH FROM CORONARY REVASCULARIZATION	
REDUCES NONFATAL MYOCARDIAL INFARCTIONS	
REDUCES RISK OF STROKES	

▷ **Principal Uses**

As a Single Drug Product: Uses currently included in FDA-approved labeling:
(1) Used by patients with elevated cholesterol to reduce death from heart
disease and decrease the number of nonfatal heart attacks; (2) treats high
total blood cholesterol levels (in people with types IIa and IIb hypercholesterolemia)—used in conjunction with a cholesterol-lowering diet (it should
not be used until an adequate trial of nondrug methods for lowering cholesterol has proved to be ineffective); (3) stops progression and decreases
number of deaths of patients with coronary artery disease; (4) decreases
risk of strokes; (5) treats isolated hypertriglyceridemia and type three
hyperlipoproteinemia; (6) increases HDL-C in people with primary hypercholesterolemia and mixed dyslipidemia.

Other (unlabeled) generally accepted uses: (1) Used in combination with
estrogen (in one study of women averaging 57 years old) lowered LDL,
increased HDL and reduced undesirable blood-clotting factors and inflammation; (2) may help reduce lipid disorders that occur in kidney problems
(nephrotic syndrome); (3) combination therapy in preventing gallstones;
(4) may have a role after heart transplants to decrease death and lower
LDL-C levels.

How This Drug Works: Blocks the liver enzyme starting production of cholesterol. Reduces low-density lipoproteins (LDL), the fraction of cholesterol
thought to increase risk of coronary heart disease. May also increase high-
density lipoproteins (HDL), the cholesterol fraction that reduces the risk of
heart disease.

Available Dosage Forms and Strengths

Tablets — 5 mg, 10 mg, 20 mg, 40 mg, 80 mg

▷ **Recommended Dosage Ranges** (Actual dose and schedule must be determined
for each patient individually.)

Infants and Children: Under 2 years of age—do not use this drug.

2 to 20 years of age: dose not established.

20 to 60 Years of Age: Initially 20 mg daily, taken at bedtime. Dose is
increased as needed to reach desired goals (such as decreased LDL-C percent). The drug is then increased as needed and tolerated by increments of
5 to 10 mg at intervals of 4 weeks. The total daily dose should not exceed
80 mg. For patients who require more than a 45 percent decrease in bad
cholesterol (LDL), the starting dose is 40 mg per day.

Over 60 Years of Age: Initially 5 mg daily. Increase dose as needed and tolerated
by increments of 5 mg at intervals of 4 weeks. The total daily dose should
not exceed 40 mg.

Conditions Requiring Dosing Adjustments

Liver Function: This drug achieves a high concentration in the liver and is subsequently eliminated in the bile. It can be a rare cause of liver damage, and
patients should be followed closely.

Kidney Function: In severe kidney failure, the dose should be started at 5 mg
and the patient closely followed.

Heart Transplants: People who are getting immunosuppressive therapy should
be started on 5 mg of simvastatin. The maximum dose in these patients
should be 10 mg.

▷ *Dosing Instructions:* The tablet may be crushed and taken without regard to
eating, preferably at bedtime (the highest rates of cholesterol production
occur between midnight and 5 a.m.). If you forget a dose: Take the missed
dose as soon as you remember it, unless it's nearly time for your next
dose—if that is the case, skip the missed dose and take the next dose right
on schedule. DO NOT double doses. Talk with your doctor if you find yourself missing doses as there are many effective reminder systems available.

Usual Duration of Use: Use on a regular schedule for 4 to 6 weeks usually determines effectiveness in reducing blood levels of total and LDL cholesterol.
Long-term use (months to years) requires periodic physician evaluation of
response and dose adjustment. Consult your physician on a regular basis.

Typical Treatment Goals and Measurements (Outcomes and Markers)

Cholesterol: The National Institutes of Health has released ATP III as part of
the update to the National Cholesterol Education Program or NCEP. Key
points in these new guidelines include acknowledging diabetes as one of
the conditions that increases risk of heart disease, modifying risk factors
and recommending routine testing for all of the cholesterol fractions
(lipoprotein profile) versus total cholesterol alone. These new guidelines
also recommend a desirable total cholesterol of 200 mg/dl as before, but
change optimal LDL to 100 mg/dl, 130–159 mg/dl as borderline high,

160 mg/dl as high and cite 190 mg/dl as very high. One other noteworthy change is that "good cholesterol" or HDL has been made more important. The "too low" measure for HDL has been increased to 40 mg/dl. Take your medicine and reach these new targets! Electron beam computed tomography (EBCT) is an important tool to use in conjunction with these laboratory studies. Findings show that even patients who meet cholesterol goals (particularly females over 55) can still be at significant cardiovascular risk. EBCT then defines that risk by giving a calcium score and a "virtual tour" of the coronary arteries.

Possible Advantages of This Drug: Several studies indicate that HMG-CoA reductase inhibitors are more effective and better tolerated than other drugs currently available for reducing total and LDL cholesterol. Simvastatin increased HDL levels by 6.7% in one study.

▷ **This Drug Should Not Be Taken If**
- you have had an allergic reaction to it previously.
- you have active liver disease.
- your liver enzyme levels (serum transaminases) have increased without explanation.
- you are pregnant or breast-feeding your infant.

▷ **Inform Your Physician Before Taking This Drug If**
- you have previously taken any Other Drugs in this class: lovastatin (Mevacor) or pravastatin (Pravachol).
- you have a history of liver disease or impaired liver function.
- you are taking any of the medicines listed in the "Other Drugs" section of this profile.
- you are not using any method of birth control or you are planning pregnancy.
- you regularly consume substantial amounts of alcohol.
- you have cataracts or impaired vision.
- you have any type of chronic muscular disorder.
- you develop muscle pain, weakness or soreness that is unexplained while taking this medicine.
- you plan to have major surgery in the near future.

Possible Side Effects (natural, expected and unavoidable drug actions)
Development of abnormal liver function tests without associated symptoms. Decreased co-enzyme Q10 (co-Q10 or ubiquinone).

▷ **Possible Adverse Effects** (unusual, unexpected and infrequent reactions)
If any of the following develop, consult your physician promptly for guidance.
Mild Adverse Effects
Allergic reactions: rash.
Headache, dizziness or fatigue—infrequent.
Nausea, excessive gas, constipation, diarrhea—rare to infrequent.
Lowering of blood pressure—possible.
Serious Adverse Effects
Marked and persistent abnormal liver function tests with focal hepatitis—rare.
Acute myositis (muscle pain and tenderness)—infrequent.
Rhabdomyolysis—rare.

Potential for cataracts—based on animal data, not reported in humans.

Lowered blood platelets (thrombocytopenia)—rare.

Neuropathy—case report.

Depression—rare.

Protein in the urine—rare.

Lichen planus skin rash—rare.

▷ **Possible Effects on Sexual Function:** Impotence—case reports.

Possible Delayed Adverse Effects: Increased liver enzymes. Lowered levels of co-enzyme Q 10.

Natural Diseases or Disorders That May Be Activated by This Drug

Latent liver disease.

Possible Effects on Laboratory Tests

Blood alanine aminotransferase (ALT) enzyme level: increased (with higher doses of drug).

Blood total cholesterol, LDL cholesterol and triglyceride levels: decreased.

Blood HDL cholesterol level: increased.

Bone mineral density tests (DEXA, PDEXA and quantitative ultrasound) will remain the same or increase in many cases (beneficial effect).

CAUTION

1. If pregnancy occurs while taking this drug, stop the drug immediately and call your physician.
2. Report promptly any development of muscle pain or tenderness, especially if accompanied by fever or weakness (malaise).
3. Promptly report altered or impaired vision so that appropriate evaluation can be made.

Precautions for Use

By Infants and Children: Safety and effectiveness for those under 17 years of age are not established.

By Those Over 60 Years of Age: Inform your physician regarding any personal or family history of cataracts. Comply with all recommendations regarding periodic eye examinations. Report promptly any alterations in vision.

▷ **Advisability of Use During Pregnancy**

Pregnancy Category: X. See Pregnancy Risk Categories at the back of this book.

Animal studies: Mouse and rat studies reveal skeletal birth defects due to a closely related drug of this class.

Human studies: Adequate studies of pregnant women are not available.

This drug should be avoided during entire pregnancy.

Advisability of Use If Breast-Feeding

Presence of this drug in breast milk: Unknown, but expected since a similar drug from this class does go into breast milk.

Avoid drug or refrain from nursing.

Habit-Forming Potential: None.

Effects of Overdose: Increased indigestion, stomach distress, nausea, diarrhea.

Possible Effects of Long-Term Use: Abnormal liver function with focal hepatitis.

Suggested Periodic Examinations While Taking This Drug (at physician's discretion)

Blood cholesterol studies: total cholesterol, HDL and LDL fractions.

Liver function tests before treatment, 6 and 12 weeks after treatment is started, after dose increases and also every 6 months thereafter. In patients who have had an increase in liver enzymes, testing should continue frequently until the enzymes return to normal. IF THE ENZYMES INCREASE TO 3 TIMES THE UPPER LIMIT OF NORMAL, SIMVASTATIN SHOULD BE STOPPED.

Author's Note: A related medicine called cerivastatin (Baycol) was removed from the market because of liver changes. It is unknown at the time of this writing if the FDA will review similar medicines and ask for more frequent checks of liver function.

A complete eye examination at beginning of treatment and at any time that significant change in vision occurs is prudent. Ask your doctor for help.

EBCT can help define blood vessel damage (calcium score).

▷ **While Taking This Drug, Observe the Following**

Foods: Follow a standard low-cholesterol diet. Combination use of B vitamin supplements may help lower additional heart disease risk factors such as homocysteine.

Herbal Medicines or Minerals: No data exist from well-designed clinical studies about garlic and simvastatin combinations and can not presently be recommended. Additionally, garlic may inhibit blood-clotting (platelet) aggregation—something to consider if you are already taking a platelet inhibitor. The FDA has allowed one dietary supplement called Cholestin to continue to be sold. This preparation actually contains lovastatin. Since use of two HMG-CoA inhibitors may increase risk of rhabdomyolysis or myopathy, the combination is NOT advised. Because St. John's wort and this medicine can increase sun sensitivity, the combination is not advised.

Using plant stanol ester products (Benecol) with this medicine can help further lower total and LDL cholesterol. Soy products (milk, tofu, etc.) contain phytoestrogens that have led to an FDA-approved health claim for reducing risk of heart disease (if they have at least 6.25 g of soy protein per serving). Substituting soy for some of the meat in your diet can also help further lower cholesterol. Because this medicine can deplete co-enzyme Q10, supplementation may be needed.

Beverages: DO NOT take this medicine with grapefruit juice. Blood levels may be markedly increased, increasing risk of muscle damage. May be taken with milk or water.

▷ *Alcohol:* No interactions expected. Use sparingly.

Tobacco Smoking: No interactions expected. I advise everyone to quit smoking.

▷ *Other Drugs*

Simvastatin may ***increase*** the effects of

- digoxin (Lanoxin).
- warfarin (Coumadin); more frequent testing of INR (prothrombin time or protime) will be needed.

Simvastatin ***taken concurrently*** with

- amprenavir (Agenerase), indinavir (Crixivan), ritonavir (Norvir) and perhaps other protease inhibitors may increase simvastatin levels and the risk of muscle damage (myopathy).
- clarithromycin (Biaxin) and erythromycin (various) may increase risk of muscle damage. DOSE REDUCTION AND CAREFUL PATIENT MONITORING ARE REQUIRED IF THESE MEDICINES MUST BE COMBINED.
- clofibrate (Atromid-S) or other fibrates may result in increased risk of serious muscle toxicity. DOSE REDUCTION AND CAREFUL PATIENT

MONITORING ARE REQUIRED IF THESE MEDICINES MUST BE COMBINED.

- colesevelam (Welchol) results in better lowering of LDL-C.
- cyclosporine (Sandimmune) can result in kidney failure and myopathy.
- gemfibrozil (Lopid) may alter absorption and excretion of simvastatin and may also increase risk of muscle damage (rhabdomyolysis)—NOT RECOMMENDED.
- itraconazole (Sporanox) or ketoconazole (Nizoral) seriously increases risk of muscle damage—DO NOT COMBINE.
- medicines that change cytochrome P450 3A4 (inhibitors will increase simvastatin levels and inducers will blunt simvastatin therapeutic effects).
- nefazodone (Serzone) may increase risk of muscle damage. DOSE REDUCTION MAY BE PRUDENT AND CAREFUL PATIENT MONITORING IS REQUIRED IF THESE MEDICINES MUST BE COMBINED.
- niacin may cause an increased frequency of muscle problems (myopathy) when combined with a related medicine (lovastatin). DOSE REDUCTION AND CAREFUL PATIENT MONITORING ARE REQUIRED IF THESE MEDICINES MUST BE COMBINED.
- quinupristin/dalfopristin (Synercid) may increase the risk for myopathy by increasing simvastatin blood levels.
- verapamil (Verelan) may increase risk of muscle damage. DOSE REDUCTION AND CAREFUL PATIENT MONITORING ARE REQUIRED IF THESE MEDICINES MUST BE COMBINED.

The following drug may *decrease* the effects of simvastatin:

- cholestyramine (Questran) may reduce absorption of simvastatin; take simvastatin 1 hour before or 4 hours after cholestyramine.
- fosphenytoin (Cerebyx) or phenytoin (Dilantin) may increase the body chemicals (enzymes) that remove simvastatin and blunt simvastatin benefits. Careful patient monitoring and dose increases may be needed.

▷ *Driving, Hazardous Activities:* No restrictions.

Aviation Note: The use of this drug *may be a disqualification* for piloting. Consult a designated Aviation Medical Examiner.

Exposure to Sun: One case of skin reaction to the sun (photosensitivity/photodermatitis) has been reported.

Discontinuation: Do not stop this drug without your physician's knowledge and guidance. There may be a significant increase in blood cholesterol levels following discontinuation of this drug.

SPIRONOLACTONE (speer on oh LAK tohn)

Introduced: 1959   **Class:** Diuretic, aldosterone receptor antagonist   **Prescription:** USA: Yes   **Controlled Drug:** USA: No; Canada: No   **Available as Generic:** USA: Yes

Brand Names: Alatone, Aldactazide [CD], Aldactone, ✷Apo-Spirozide, ✷Novospiroton, ✷Novospirozine [CD], ✷Sincomen, Spironazide

BENEFITS versus RISKS	
Possible Benefits	*Possible Risks*
REDUCES RISK OF DEATH AND HOSPITALIZATION BY 30% WHEN USED AS PART OF COMBINATION THERAPY OF SEVERE HEART FAILURE	ABNORMALLY HIGH BLOOD POTASSIUM LEVEL with excessive use
EFFECTIVE PREVENTION OF POTASSIUM LOSS when used adjunctively with other diuretics	Enlargement of male breast tissue Masculinization effects in women: excessive hair growth, deepening of the voice
EFFECTIVE DIURETIC IN REFRACTORY CASES OF FLUID RETENTION when used adjunctively with other diuretics	Liver damage (case reports)

▷ **Principal Uses**

As a Single Drug Product: Uses currently included in FDA-approved labeling: (1) Manages congestive heart failure and disorders of the liver and kidney that are accompanied by excessive fluid retention (edema); (2) also used with other measures to treat high blood pressure where prevention of potassium loss is needed; (3) used to decrease fluid in patients who have failed glucocorticoid treatment and have nephrotic syndrome; (4) works to restore blood potassium to normal in drug caused (induced) low potassium (hypokalemia); (5) used in congestive heart failure (CHF) to reduce frequency of hospitalizations and death in patients with moderate to severe (NYHA class III when the principal study began and up to class IV) heart failure when used in combination with standard CHF treatment (usually a loop diuretic an ACE inhibitor [if tolerated] and in some cases digoxin).

Other (unlabeled) generally accepted uses: (1) May have an adjunctive role in treating acne; (2) can help treat lung problems (bronchopulmonary dysplasia) and slow the disease process; (3) can help precocious puberty in females; (4) eases fluid buildup in premenstrual syndrome; (5) may help women with excessive facial hair growth (hirsutism); (6) may protect against mountain sickness.

As a Combination Drug Product [CD]: This drug is available in combination with hydrochlorothiazide, a different kind of diuretic that promotes the loss of potassium from the body. Spironolactone is used in this combination to counteract the potassium-wasting effect of the thiazide diuretic.

How This Drug Works: By inhibiting the action of aldosterone (an adrenal gland hormone), this drug prevents the reabsorption of sodium and the excretion of potassium by the kidney. Thus the drug promotes the excretion of sodium (and water with it) and the retention of potassium. In heart failure, spironolactone works to protect the heart from too much aldosterone (a hormone that can lower the ability of the heart to pump).

Available Dosage Forms and Strengths

Tablets—25 mg, 50 mg, 100 mg

▷ **Usual Adult Dosage Ranges:** For *edema*: Initially 100 mg per day in one dose or divided into several doses. The dose is then adjusted according to individual response. The usual maintenance dose is 50 to 200 mg daily, divided into two to four doses. If response is not adequate after 5 days, a second fluid medicine (diuretic) is added.

For hypertension: two to four Aldactazide tablets in one dose or separated into several equal doses.

In moderate to severe heart failure: Many clinicians are recommending use of 25 mg per day in combination with an ACE inhibitor, a loop diuretic and possibly digoxin. **Note: Actual dosage and administration schedule must be determined for each patient individually.**

Conditions Requiring Dosing Adjustments

Liver Function: This drug can be a rare cause of liver damage and patients should be followed closely.

Kidney Function: For patients with mild kidney failure, the drug can be taken every 12 hours in the usual dose. In moderate kidney failure (GFR 10–50 ml/min), spironolactone can be taken every 12 to 24 hours in the usual dose. In severe kidney failure (GFR less than 10 ml/min or creatinine greater than 2.5 mg/dL), this drug should not be taken. Spironolactone is contraindicated in acute renal failure and severe chronic renal compromise.

▷ **Dosing Instructions:** The tablet may be crushed and taken with or following meals to promote absorption of the drug and reduce stomach irritation. If you forget a dose: Take the missed dose as soon as you remember it, unless it's nearly time for your next dose—if that is the case, skip the missed dose and take the next dose right on schedule. DO NOT double doses. Talk with your doctor if you find yourself missing doses.

Usual Duration of Use: Use on a regular schedule for 5 to 10 days usually determines effectiveness in clearing edema, and for 2 to 3 weeks to determine its effect on hypertension. Because patient response may vary in congestive heart failure (CHF) and the aldosterone antagonism data are new, discuss goals of CHF use individually. Long-term use (months to years) requires physician supervision and periodic evaluation.

Typical Treatment Goals and Measurements (Outcomes and Markers)

Congestive heart failure: The goal is to help remove excess fluid (edema) and hence decrease blood pressure while helping ease the amount of work the heart has to do. Additionally, when this medicine is combined with standard CHF treatment, death and adverse consequences of CHF as well as the number of times a given patient will generally have to be hospitalized are reduced. Clinical signs and symptoms such as ankle swelling, difficulty breathing and walking or exercise tolerance may also improve.

Blood pressure: The most recent treatment guidelines (JNC VI) actually define optimal blood pressure (BP) as less than 120/80 and high normal as 139/89. The American Diabetes Association has chosen a target of 130/80 as the blood pressure goal for people living with diabetes. Most clinicians try to achieve a BP that achieves the best balance of lower cardiovascular risk while avoiding the problem of too low a blood pressure. Additionally, it is important to make sure that loss or retention of body chemicals (electrolytes such as sodium, potassium and magnesium) is not excessive and adjustment is needed. The goal and time frame should be discussed with you when the prescription is written.

▷ **This Drug Should Not Be Taken If**
- you have had an allergic reaction to it previously.
- you have severely impaired liver or kidney function.
- your kidneys are not making any urine.
- your blood potassium is excessively high (hyperkalemia).
- your creatinine is greater than 2.5 mg/dL.

▷ **Inform Your Physician Before Taking This Drug If**
- you have a history of liver or kidney disease.
- you have diabetes.
- you take an anticoagulant, antihypertensives, a digitalis preparation, another diuretic, lithium, or a potassium preparation.
- your blood chemistry (electrolytes) are out of balance.
- you plan to have surgery under general anesthesia in the near future.
- you have a potassium-rich diet. Talk to your doctor and see Table 13.

Possible Side Effects (natural, expected, and unavoidable drug actions)
Abnormally high blood potassium levels—possible and may be frequent; abnormally low blood sodium levels or dehydration—infrequent.

▷ **Possible Adverse Effects** (unusual, unexpected, and infrequent reactions)
If any of the following develop, consult your physician promptly for guidance.

Mild Adverse Effects
Allergic Reactions: Skin rash, hives, itching, drug fever (see Glossary).
Headache, dizziness, unsteadiness, weakness, drowsiness, lethargy, confusion—infrequent.
Dry mouth, nausea, vomiting, diarrhea—infrequent.
Masculine pattern of hair growth and deepening of the voice in women—case reports.
Taste disturbances—possible.

Serious Adverse Effects
Allergic reactions: Abnormally low blood platelet count—rare.
Systemic lupus erythematosus like syndrome—case reports.
Symptomatic potassium excess: confusion, numbness and tingling in lips and extremities, fatigue, weakness, shortness of breath, slow heart rate, low blood pressure—possible.
Stomach ulceration with bleeding—case reports.
Disruption in the acid—base balance of body (hyperchloremic or hyperkalemic acidosis)—possible.
Liver toxicity (hepatitis)—case reports.
Porphyria or systemic-lupus-erythematosus-like syndrome—case reports.
Excessively low white blood cells (granulocytes) or platelets—case reports.
Thinning of the bones—case report.
This medicine is a tumorigen in chronic rat toxicity studies. Current labeling notes that unnecessary use of this medicine should be avoided.

▷ **Possible Effects on Sexual Function**
Decreased libido or impaired erection or impotence—possible.
Male breast enlargement and tenderness (gynecomastia) (increases with higher doses). Some gynecomastia reports were associated with impo-

tence. Female breast enlargement; altered timing and pattern of menstruation; postmenopausal bleeding.

Decreased vaginal secretion—case reports.

Possible Effects on Laboratory Tests

White blood cell count: possibly decreased.

Blood platelet count: possibly decreased.

Blood potassium level: increased.

Blood uric acid level: no effect in some; increased and decreased in others.

CAUTION

1. Do not take potassium supplements or increase intake of potassium-rich foods (see Table 13) while taking this drug.
2. Do not stop this drug abruptly unless abnormally high blood levels of potassium develop.
3. Ordinary doses of aspirin (600 mg) may reverse the diuretic effect of this drug. Discuss aspirin or NSAID use with your doctor.
4. Avoid excessive use of salt substitutes containing potassium; these are potential causes of potassium excess.
5. Spironolactone may interfere with laboratory checks of cortisol and digoxin levels.

Precautions for Use

By Infants and Children: Limit the continual use of this drug in children to 1 month.

Observe closely for indications of potassium accumulation.

By Those Over 60 Years of Age: The natural decline in kidney function may predispose to potassium retention in the body. Watch for indications of potassium excess: slow heart rate, irregular heart rhythms, low blood pressure, confusion, drowsiness. The excessive use of diuretics can cause harmful loss of body water (dehydration), increased viscosity of the blood, and an increased tendency of the blood to clot, predisposing to stroke, heart attack, or thrombophlebitis.

▷ **Advisability of Use During Pregnancy**

Pregnancy Category: D by one researcher. See Pregnancy Risk Categories at the back of this book.

Animal studies: This drug causes feminization of male rat fetuses.

Human studies: Adequate studies of pregnant women are not available.

This drug should not be used during pregnancy unless a very serious complication of pregnancy occurs for which this drug is significantly beneficial.

Advisability of Use If Breast-Feeding

Presence of this drug in breast milk: A metabolic end product (canrenone) is present.

Avoid drug or refrain from nursing.

Habit-Forming Potential: None.

Effects of Overdosage: Thirst, drowsiness, fatigue, weakness, nausea, vomiting, confusion, irregular heart rhythm, low blood pressure.

Possible Effects of Long-Term Use: Potassium accumulation to abnormally high blood levels. Male breast enlargement.

Suggested Periodic Examinations While Taking This Drug (at physician's discretion)

Measurements of blood sodium, potassium, magnesium and chloride levels. Kidney and liver function tests.

▷ **While Taking This Drug, Observe the Following**

Foods: Talk to your doctor about possible need to avoid high-potassium foods (see Table 13). Avoid excessive restriction of salt.

Herbal Medicines or Minerals: Hawthorn (Crataegus variety) and co-enzyme Q10 (co-Q10) can affect the way the heart works. BE CERTAIN to tell your doctor that you are taking or are considering taking these herbs if you are taking spironolactone or if a spironolactone prescription is being considered for you or a loved one. Issues remain regarding optimum doses, monitoring strategies and possible interactions for co-Q10. One objective review recognized co-Q10 as adjunctive therapy for congestive heart failure. Co-Q10 may also interact badly with aspirin. Soy products (milk, tofu, etc.) contain phytoestrogens that have led to an FDA-approved health claim for reducing risk of heart disease (if they have at least 6.25 g of soy protein per serving). It is important that potassium and magnesium levels be kept in the normal range while you are taking spironolactone.

Couch grass or nettle should NOT be taken by patients who have increased fluid (edema) caused by heart weakness. Ginseng may increase blood pressure, blunting some of the benefits of this medicine. Eleuthero root, hawthorn, saw palmetto, ma huang, goldenseal and licorice may also cause increased blood pressure. Couch grass may worsen edema due to heart or kidney problems. Indian snakeroot, calcium and garlic may help lower blood pressure.

Beverages: No restrictions. May be taken with milk.

▷ *Alcohol:* Use with caution. Alcohol may enhance the drowsiness and the blood-pressure-lowering effect of this drug.

Tobacco Smoking: No interactions expected, but I advise everyone to quit smoking.

▷ *Other Drugs*

Spironolactone may *increase* the effects of
- digoxin (Lanoxin). Cautious and increased checks of digoxin levels are prudent.

Spironolactone may *decrease* the effects of
- anticoagulants (Coumadin, etc.). Increased frequency of INR (prothrombin time or protime) testing is needed.

Spironolactone *taken concurrently* with
- arginine (various) may lead to excessive potassium levels.
- captopril (Capoten) or other ACE inhibitors (see Drug Classes) may cause further increases in blood potassium levels. More frequent laboratory tests are prudent.
- cortisone-like drugs (fludrocortisone, others) may lead to excessive potassium loss.
- cyclosporine (Sandimmune) may result in very elevated potassium levels.
- digitoxin (Crystodigin) may cause either increased or decreased digitoxin effects (unpredictable).
- lithium (Lithobid, others) may cause accumulation of lithium to toxic levels.

- norepinephrine (various) may blunt norepinephrine effects.
- potassium preparations may cause excessively high blood potassium levels.
- tacrolimus (Prograf) may lead to excessive potassium levels. USE IS NOT ADVISED.
- valsartan (Diovan) may lead to increased potassium levels. More frequent potassium checks are prudent.
- warfarin (Coumadin) may blunt effectiveness of warfarin. More frequent INR checks are prudent. Dose adjustments may be needed.

The following drugs may *decrease* the effects of spironolactone

- aspirin (higher doses) or other NSAIDs (see Drug Classes)—may reduce its diuretic effectiveness.

▷ *Driving, Hazardous Activities:* This drug may cause dizziness and drowsiness. Restrict activities as necessary.

Aviation Note: The use of this drug *may be a disqualification* for piloting. Consult a designated Aviation Medical Examiner.

Exposure to Sun: No restrictions.

Discontinuation: With high dosage or prolonged use, it is advisable to withdraw this drug gradually. Ask your physician for guidance.

STAVUDINE (STAV u dine)

Other Name: D4T

Introduced: 1994   **Class:** Antiretroviral, Anti-HIV, Anti AIDS   **Prescription:** USA: Yes   **Controlled Drug:** USA: No; Canada: No   **Available as Generic:** USA: No; Canada: No

Brand Name: Zerit

BENEFITS versus RISKS	
Possible Benefits	*Possible Risks*
INCREASED CD4 COUNTS IN ADULTS WITH ADVANCED HIV	PERIPHERAL NEUROPATHY Pancreatitis
LESS LIKELY THAN OTHER AGENTS TO DEVELOP RESISTANCE	
AVOIDS BONE MARROW TOXICITY OF ZIDOVUDINE	
EFFECTIVE COMBINATION THERAPY OF HIV	
PART OF A COMBINATION REGIMEN (HAART) REDUCING HIV TO UNDETECTABLE LEVELS	

▷ **Principal Uses**

As a Single Drug Product: Uses currently included in FDA-approved labeling: Treatment of HIV in adults and children as part of combination therapy (a study of stavudine plus didanosine plus nevirapine is an effective triple medicine combination).

Author's Note: Adherence—taking medicines for HIV exactly on time and in the right amount—is ABSOLUTELY critical to getting the best possi-

ble results or outcomes. **The new antiretroviral therapy guidelines from NIAID take into account how easily the medicine treating HIV can fit into a patient's life (twice daily dosing is a distinct advantage).** Other (unlabeled) generally accepted uses: None at present.

How This Drug Works: This drug inhibits HIV reproduction (replication) by (1) inhibiting an HIV enzyme (reverse transcriptase), which blocks the ability of the virus to make nuclear material, and (2) inhibiting an enzyme (DNA polymerase-gamma and-beta), which blocks the ability to make DNA in the mitochondria.

Available Dosage Forms and Strengths

Capsules — 15 mg, 20 mg, 30 mg, 40 mg
Powder — 1 mg/ml

▷ **Recommended Dose Ranges** (Actual dose and schedule must be determined for each patient individually.)

Infants and Children: Children weighing less than 30 kg are given 2 mg per kg per day separated into two equal doses 12 hours apart. Those weighing greater than 30 kg are given the adult dose.

18 to 60 Years of Age: Patients with a body mass of 60 kg (132 lb) or more should take 40 mg twice daily. Patients with a body mass of less than 60 kg should take 30 mg twice daily. For those who have had to stop because of peripheral neuropathy (after complete resolution of symptoms)—20 mg twice daily for patients with a body mass of 60 kg or more; 15 mg twice daily for those with a body mass less than 60 kg. Some suggestion has been made that doses greater than 1 mg per kg per day carry a greater risk of peripheral neuropathy. If peripheral neuropathy does happen, most clinicians will interrupt stavudine treatment. For patients in whom symptoms (tingling and numbness or pain in the hands or feet) resolve completely, stavudine can be restarted at 20 mg twice daily for people who weigh 60 kg or more or at 15 mg twice a day for those less than 60 mg. Some clinicians separate the total daily dose into three equal doses given three times a day.

Over 65 Years of Age: This drug has not been studied in those over 65.

Conditions Requiring Dosing Adjustments

Liver Function: If liver enzymes increase significantly, therapy may need to be stopped and then reintroduced with 20 mg daily for those weighing more than 60 kg and 15 mg daily if less than 60 kg.

Kidney Function: Patients with mild kidney compromise (creatinine clearance greater than 50 ml/min) take the usual weight-adjusted dose for adults. Mild to moderate kidney compromise (creatinine clearance 26 to 50 ml/min) should take one-half of the usual weight-adjusted dose every 12 hours. In severe kidney compromise (creatinine clearance 10 to 25 ml/min), one-half the usual weight-adjusted dose should be taken every 24 hours.

▷ **Dosing Instructions:** This drug may be taken without regard to food. Not missing doses (adherence) is critical, as missed doses will make resistance more likely. The oral solution should be mixed (reconstituted) with water by your pharmacist by adding 202 ml of purified water to the dry powder. SHAKE THE CONTAINER VIGOROUSLY BEFORE you give or take a dose. The reconstituted medicine should be refrigerated and expires 30 days after it is mixed. If you forget a dose: Take the missed dose as soon as you remember it, unless it's nearly time for your next dose—if that is the case, skip the missed dose and take the next dose right on schedule. DO NOT double doses. IT IS ABSOLUTELY CRITICAL to take HIV medicines exactly as prescribed. Talk with your doctor if you find yourself missing doses. There are beeper-based systems that can be a great help.

Usual Duration of Use: Use on a regular schedule for several months usually determines effectiveness in shutting down HIV replication and increasing CD4 counts. Long-term use (months to years) requires periodic physician evaluation of response (viral burden and CD4).

Typical Treatment Goals and Measurements (Outcomes and Markers)

HIV: Goals for HIV treatment presently are maximum suppression of viral replication, maximum lowering of the amount of virus in your body (viral load or burden), and maximum patient survival. Markers of successful therapy include undetectable viral load, increased CD4 cells, absence of indicator or opportunistic infections (OIs) and in the case of the HIV-positive patient, failure of the infection to progress to AIDS.

Possible Advantages of This Drug

More favorable side-effect profile than other nucleoside analogs. Favorable profile for combination therapy. Favorable twice-daily dosing.

▷ **This Drug Should Not Be Taken If**
  • you had an allergic reaction to it previously.

▷ **Inform Your Physician Before Taking This Drug If**
  • you have had peripheral neuropathy caused by Other Drugs before.
  • you have kidney or liver compromise.
  • you have had pancreatitis.
  • your bone marrow is depressed.
  • you have vitamin B_{12} deficiency or folic acid deficiency.
  • you are unsure how much to take or how often to take it.

Possible Side Effects (natural, expected and unavoidable drug actions)
Chills or fever—infrequent.
Peripheral neuropathy—infrequent to frequent.
Pancreatitis—infrequent.

▷ **Possible Adverse Effects** (unusual, unexpected and infrequent reactions)
If any of the following develop, consult your physician promptly for guidance.

Mild Adverse Effects
Allergic reactions: skin rash.
Nausea and vomiting or abdominal pain—infrequent.
Increased liver enzymes—frequent.
Lipodystrophy—possible

Author's Note: Current controversy as to possible lipid changes (lipodystrophy or LD) from protease inhibitors and/or nucleoside reverse transcriptase inhibitors involves presence of mild changes versus moderate to severe problems. The HOPS data found that risk of LD increases with increasing time on antiretrovirals and that LD increases with an increasing number of nondrug factors (age 40 or older, HIV infection 7 or more years, AIDS 2 or more years, hemophiliacs, nadir CD4 count less than 100 or less than 15 and time since nadir 3 or more years). Patients who did not have these risk factors DID NOT develop significant LD in the HOPS data.

Serious Adverse Effects
Allergic reactions: anaphylactic reactions—rare.
Anemia—case reports.
Low white blood cell or platelet counts—rare to infrequent in phase three data, not found in later data.
Lactic acidosis—case reports with nucleoside analogs.
Severe liver problems (hepatomegaly with statuses)—case reports with nucleoside analogs.

▷ **Possible Effects on Sexual Function:** Impotence—rare in phase three data. One case report of swelling of male breast tissue (gynecomastia).

Possible Delayed Adverse Effects: Peripheral neuropathy—up to 24%.

▷ **Adverse Effects That May Mimic Natural Diseases or Disorders**
Increased liver function tests may mimic hepatitis.

Possible Effects on Laboratory Tests
Liver function tests: increased.
Amylase: increased.
Complete blood counts: decreased platelets and white blood cells—possible.

CAUTION
1. Stavudine or undetectable viral burden **does not** remove risk of giving (transmission) HIV to others through sexual contact or blood contamination.
2. Promptly report the development of stomach pain and vomiting; this could indicate pancreatitis.
3. Report development of pain, numbness, tingling or burning in the hands or feet, as this may be peripheral neuropathy.

Precautions for Use
By Infants and Children: Watch carefully for adverse effects.
By Those Over 65 Years of Age: Age-related decline in kidney function may require dosing changes.

▷ **Advisability of Use During Pregnancy**
Pregnancy Category: C. See Pregnancy Risk Categories at the back of this book.
Animal studies: Clinical doses in rats have not revealed teratogenicity, but doses of 399 times those used in humans have resulted in skeletal problems. Increased early rat death has also occurred at 399 times the human dose.
Human studies: Adequate studies of pregnant women are not available.
Ask your doctor for guidance.

Advisability of Use If Breast-Feeding
Presence of this drug in breast milk: Yes.
Refrain from nursing if you are HIV positive or are taking this drug. HIV can be transmitted through breast milk.

Habit-Forming Potential: None.

Effects of Overdose: Adults treated with 12 to 24 times the recommended daily dose revealed no acute toxicity.

Possible Effects of Long-Term Use: Peripheral neuropathy and hepatic toxicity.

Suggested Periodic Examinations While Taking This Drug (at physician's discretion)
Liver function tests.

Amylase and complete blood counts.

CD4 or viral load measurement.

▷ **While Taking This Drug, Observe the Following**

Foods: No restrictions.

Herbal Medicines or Minerals: Some patients use echinacea to attempt to boost their immune systems. Unfortunately, use of echinacea is not recommended in people with damaged immune systems. This herb may also actually weaken any immune system if it is used too often or for too long a time.

Beverages: No restrictions.

▷ *Alcohol:* No interactions expected.

Tobacco Smoking: No interactions expected. I advise everyone to quit smoking.

▷ *Other Drugs*

Stavudine *taken concurrently* with

- Other Drugs such as metronidazole (Flagyl) that can cause peripheral neuropathy should be avoided if possible.

Stavudine may *increase* the effects of

- didanosine (Videx) at specific drug concentration ratios. Careful monitoring for liver toxicity should be undertaken.

Stavudine may *decrease* the effects of

- didanosine (Videx) at specific drug concentration ratios.
- zidovudine (AZT) at specific drug concentration ratios. The combination is NOT recommended

▷ *Driving, Hazardous Activities:* This drug may cause dizziness. Restrict activities as necessary.

Aviation Note: The use of this drug *may be a disqualification* for piloting. Consult a designated Aviation Medical Examiner.

Exposure to Sun: No restrictions.

Discontinuation: Do not stop this drug without your doctor's knowledge and guidance.

STRONTIUM-89 (STRON tee um)

Introduced: 1993   **Class:** Systemic radionuclide, pain syndrome modifier
Prescription: USA: Yes   **Controlled Drug:** USA: No;   Canada: No
Available as Generic: USA: No; Canada: No
Brand Name: Metastron

BENEFITS versus RISKS	
Possible Benefits	*Possible Risks*
EFFECTIVE RELIEF OF PRIMARY OR METASTATIC (SUCH AS FROM PROSTATE OR BREAST CANCER) CANCER OF THE BONE PAIN	BONE MARROW TOXICITY (decreased white blood cells and platelets) Transient increase in bone pain

▷ **Principal Uses**

As a Single Drug Product: Uses currently included in FDA-approved labeling: Used to treat metastatic bone cancer pain.

Other (unlabeled) generally accepted uses: None at present.

How This Drug Works: This radiopharmaceutical is selectively taken up by areas of bone cancer. Once it accumulates in cancerous areas, it emits radiation directly at the site of the cancer.

Available Dosage Forms and Strengths

Injection — 10.9 to 22.6 mg of strontium in a total of 1 ml of water

▷ **Recommended Dose Ranges** (Actual dose and schedule must be determined for each patient individually.)

Infants and Children: Safety and efficacy for those less than 18 years old are not established.

18 to 60 Years of Age: A dose of 1.5–2.2 megabecquerels/kg or 40–60 microcuries/kg of body weight is given intravenously over 1 to 2 minutes. The dose may be repeated at 90-day intervals, if needed and is based on original response and hematological status.

Over 60 Years of Age: Same as 18 to 60 years of age.

Conditions Requiring Dosing Adjustments

Liver Function: Dosing changes in liver compromise do not appear to be needed.

Kidney Function: This agent is primarily removed by the kidneys, but decreases in doses are not presently defined.

▷ **Dosing Instructions:** You may eat and drink as you normally would. During the first week after injection, strontium-89 will be present in the blood and the urine. A normal toilet should be used in preference to a urinal. If you forget a dose: CALL your doctor for instructions. This medicine must be taken on a regular basis.

Usual Duration of Use: Use of previously prescribed pain medicine will be expected for 7 to 21 days after the injection. A maximum of 42 days after injection has been needed to determine peak effectiveness in controlling bone cancer pain. The dose may be repeated (if blood tests are acceptable) 90 days after the prior dose was given. See your physician on a regular basis.

Typical Treatment Goals and Measurements (Outcomes and Markers)

Pain: Most clinicians treating pain use a device called an algometer to check your pain. This looks like a small ruler, but lets the clinician better understand your pain. The goals of treatment then relate to where the level of pain started (for example, a rating of seven on a zero to ten scale) and what the cause of the pain was. Pain medicines may also be used together (in combination) in order to get the best result or outcome. Relief of bone pain is a hallmark of successful treatment with this medicine. Decreasing use of primary pain medicine as well as rescue doses can be used to track response. Sleep patterns should also improve. If your pain control is not acceptable to YOU (remember, in hospitals and outpatient settings, etc. pain control is a patient right), call your doctor.

Possible Advantages of This Drug

Effective control of bone cancer pain without the risks or compromise of narcotics. This medicine may also allow lower doses of medicines such as morphine with excellent pain control—thereby reducing the risk of adverse effects from the opioid (such as morphine).

▷ **This Drug Should Not Be Taken If**

• you had an allergic reaction to it previously.
• you have cancer that does not involve the bone.

▷ **Inform Your Physician Before Taking This Drug If**
   • you have a history of low platelets or white blood cell counts.
   • you take other drugs that may lower white cells or platelets.
   • you have an increased calcium.
   • you do not understand how to appropriately dispose of your urine.

Possible Side Effects (natural, expected and unavoidable drug actions)
   May cause a calciumlike flushing when injected. May cause transient (up to 72 hours) increase in bone pain.

▷ **Possible Adverse Effects** (unusual, unexpected and infrequent reactions)
   If any of the following develop, consult your physician promptly for guidance.
   Mild Adverse Effects
   Allergic reactions: not defined.
   Chills and fever—possible.
   Serious Adverse Effects
   Allergic reactions: none defined.
   Bone marrow toxicity: 20–30% decrease in white cell or platelet counts—may be dose-related.
   Bacterial infection of blood (septicemia) following drug-induced decreases in white blood cells—possible.
   Animal data shows that this drug is a possible carcinogen.

▷ **Possible Effects on Sexual Function:** None reported.

Possible Delayed Adverse Effects: Lowering of white blood cells (recovery in up to 6 months) and blood platelets (lowest count 5 to 16 weeks after therapy).

Natural Diseases or Disorders That May Be Activated by This Drug
   Aplastic anemia.

Possible Effects on Laboratory Tests
   White blood cell counts: decreased.
   Platelet counts: decreased.

CAUTION
   1. Promptly report any signs of infection (lethargy, temperature, sore throat).
   2. It may take up to 21 days for this agent to work. Narcotics will need to be continued.
   3. Your blood and urine will contain radioactive strontium for 7 days after injection. Ask your doctor for help on appropriate disposal.
   4. This drug is a potential carcinogen.
   5. Promptly report any abnormal bleeding or bruising.

Precautions for Use
   By Infants and Children: Safety and effectiveness for those under 18 years of age are not established.
   By Those Over 60 Years of Age: Specific changes are not presently needed.

▷ **Advisability of Use During Pregnancy**
   Pregnancy Category: D. See Pregnancy Risk Categories at the back of this book.
   Animal studies: Adequate studies evaluating potential to cause birth defects have not been performed.
   Human studies: Adequate studies of pregnant women are not available.
   This drug may cause fetal harm. Ask your doctor for advice.

Advisability of Use If Breast-Feeding

Presence of this drug in breast milk: This drug acts like calcium and is expected to be present in breast milk.

Avoid drug or refrain from nursing.

Habit-Forming Potential: None.

Effects of Overdose: May result in acute radiation syndrome with initial nausea and vomiting followed by depressed white cells and platelets and tendency to infections. Careful dose calculations are indicated, as this drug emits beta-radiation.

Possible Effects of Long-Term Use: Not indicated for long-term use.

Suggested Periodic Examinations While Taking This Drug (at physician's discretion)

Complete blood counts should be tested once every other week during therapy.

▷ **While Taking This Drug, Observe the Following**

Foods: No restrictions.

Herbal Medicines or Minerals: Some patients use echinacea to attempt to boost their immune systems. Unfortunately, use of echinacea is not recommended in people with damaged immune systems. This herb may also actually weaken any immune system if it is used too often or for too long a time.

Beverages: No restrictions.

▷ *Alcohol:* No interactions expected.

Tobacco Smoking: No interactions expected. I advise everyone to quit smoking.

Marijuana Smoking: No interactions expected.

▷ *Other Drugs*

Strontium-89 *taken concurrently* with

• medications that lower white blood cells or platelets may result in severe decreases in white blood cells.

▷ *Driving, Hazardous Activities:* This drug may cause a transient increase in bone pain. Restrict activities as necessary.

Aviation Note: The use of this drug *may be a disqualification* for piloting. Consult a designated Aviation Medical Examiner.

Exposure to Sun: No restrictions.

Discontinuation: Dosing may be repeated if blood counts are acceptable.

SUCRALFATE (soo KRAL fayt)

Introduced: 1978   **Class:** Antiulcer, gastrointestinal drug   **Prescription:** USA: Yes   **Controlled Drug:** USA: No; Canada: No   **Available as Generic:** Yes

Brand Names: ✤Apo-Sucralfate, Carafate, ✤Dom-Sucralfate, ✤Novo-Sucralfate, ✤Sulcrate

BENEFITS versus RISKS	
Possible Benefits	*Possible Risks*
EFFECTIVE TREATMENT IN DUODENAL ULCER DISEASE	Constipation
	Skin rash, hives, itching
No serious adverse effects	Aluminum toxicity in kidney compromise

▷ **Principal Uses**

As a Single Drug Product: Uses currently included in FDA-approved labeling: Treats and prevents recurrence of duodenal ulcer disease in adults and children. Effective when used alone, but may be used with antacids for pain relief.

Other (unlabeled) generally accepted uses: (1) May be useful in treating stomach (gastric ulcers) if other therapy isn't tolerated; (2) can reduce the frequency of diarrhea caused by radiation therapy; (3) may have a role as a douche in promoting healing of vaginal ulcerations that are resistant to other measures; (4) can ease the pain and spasms associated with tonsillectomy.

How This Drug Works: Promotes ulcer healing by (1) forming a protective coating over the ulcer and ulcer margins, preventing further damage; (2) inhibiting the digestive action of pepsin; and (3) stimulating active healing (tissue repair).

Available Dosage Forms and Strengths

Tablets — 1 g

Suspension — 1 g/10 ml, 1 gram/5 ml in Canada

▷ **Usual Adult Dosage Ranges:** 1 g four times daily.

Note: Actual dose and schedule must be determined for each patient individually.

Conditions Requiring Dosing Adjustments

Liver Function: Sucralfate is not absorbed.

Kidney Function: Sucralfate is not absorbed, but some increased risk of aluminum absorption and toxicity is possible in dialysis and ongoing (chronic) kidney failure patients.

▷ **Dosing Instructions:** Take with water on an empty stomach at least 1 hour before or 2 hours after each meal and at bedtime. Swallow the tablets whole; do not alter or chew. Take the full course prescribed. If you forget a dose: Take the missed dose as soon as you remember it, unless it's nearly time for your next dose—if that is the case, skip the missed dose and take the next dose right on schedule. DO NOT double doses. Talk with your doctor if you find yourself missing doses.

Usual Duration of Use: Use on a regular schedule for 6 to 8 weeks is usually needed for peak effect in promoting the healing of ulcers. Use beyond 8 weeks must be determined by your physician. Current therapy also often involves treatment with an antibiotic to address *Helicobacter pylori*.

Typical Treatment Goals and Measurements (Outcomes and Markers)

Ulcers: The role of Helicobacter pylori in ulcers is no longer questioned and omeprazole (a proton pump inhibitor) is widely recognized as the standard for short-term treatment of stomach ulcers. When H. pylori is present, single-medicine therapy is not recommended. Additionally, an antibiotic is often used with other agents. The goal is to heal the ulcer area and prevent re-occurrence of the ulceration. Symptom relief (pain, etc.) as well as endoscopic examination help define success of treatment.

▷ **This Drug Should Not Be Taken If**

• you have had an allergic reaction to it previously.

▷ **Inform Your Physician Before Taking This Drug If**

• you have chronic constipation.

• you have chronic kidney failure.

• you are taking any other drugs at this time.

Possible Side Effects (natural, expected and unavoidable drug actions)
Constipation—infrequent.

▷ **Possible Adverse Effects** (unusual, unexpected and infrequent reactions)
If any of the following develop, consult your physician promptly for guidance.

Mild Adverse Effects
Allergic reactions: skin rash, hives, itching.
Dizziness, light-headedness, drowsiness—infrequent.
Dry mouth, indigestion, nausea, cramping, diarrhea—infrequent.

Serious Adverse Effects
Increased risk of aluminum toxicity (seizures, jerks and encephalopathy) with patients in end-stage kidney failure.
Bezoar (a clumping of food) formation in the esophagus or proximal stomach—possible.

▷ **Possible Effects on Sexual Function:** None reported.

Possible Effects on Laboratory Tests: None reported.

CAUTION
1. If antacids are needed to relieve ulcer pain, do not take them within half an hour before or 2 hours after the dose of sucralfate.
2. This drug may impair the absorption of *Other Drugs* if they are taken close together. Avoid taking any *Other Drugs* within 2 hours of taking sucralfate. This applies especially to cimetidine (Tagamet), phenytoin (Dilantin) and tetracyclines.
3. Even though a response is gained from this medicine, the presence of a response alone does not rule out a stomach cancer.
4. If this medicine is used in chronic kidney failure or dialysis patients, aluminum toxicity may occur.

Precautions for Use
By Infants and Children: This drug has been used to treat reflux esophagitis or long-standing (chronic) duodenal ulcers in those 3 months to 13 years. In esophagitis, 500 mg was used four times daily in those less than 6 years old. Adult dose and interval was used for those 6 or older. Duodenal ulcer treatment used adult doses.
By Those Over 60 Years of Age: Specific changes not presently needed.

▷ **Advisability of Use During Pregnancy**
Pregnancy Category: B. See Pregnancy Risk Categories at the back of this book.
Animal studies: No birth defects reported in mouse, rat and rabbit studies.
Human studies: Adequate studies of pregnant women are not available.
This drug should be used only if clearly needed. Ask your physician for guidance.

Advisability of Use If Breast-Feeding
Presence of this drug in breast milk: Unknown.
Watch nursing infant closely, and stop drug or nursing if adverse effects develop.

Habit-Forming Potential: None.

Effects of Overdose: Nausea, stomach cramping, possible diarrhea.

Possible Effects of Long-Term Use: Deficiencies of vitamins A, D, E and K due to impaired absorption from the intestine.

Suggested Periodic Examinations While Taking This Drug (at physician's discretion)

Follow-up on resolution of ulcer symptoms.

▷ **While Taking This Drug, Observe the Following**

Foods: Protein-rich foods increase stomach acid secretion. Garlic, onions, citrus fruits and tomatoes may also increase acid secretion. Follow diet prescribed by your physician.

Herbal Medicines or Minerals: Kola and ma huang may increase stomach acid, blunting the benefits of this medicine. Black cohosh root, ginkgo and squill are contraindicated in gastrointestinal disturbances. Licorice root has a Commission E monograph indication for gastrointestinal ulcers, but use with sucralfate has not been studied. Talk to your doctor BEFORE adding any herbals to these medicines.

Beverages: Caffeine may increase stomach acid. Talk to your doctor about restricting consumption. This drug is preferably taken with water.

▷ *Alcohol:* No interactions with drug expected, but alcohol is best avoided because of its irritant effect on the stomach.

Tobacco Smoking: Nicotine can delay ulcer healing and reduce the effectiveness of this drug. Avoid all forms of tobacco.

▷ *Other Drugs*

Sucralfate may ***decrease*** the effects of

- anagrelide (Agrylin).
- cimetidine (Tagamet).
- ciprofloxacin (Cipro), enoxacin (Penetrex), fleroxacin (Megalone), gatifloxacin (Tequin), grepafloxacin (Raxar), levofloxacin (Levaquin), lomefloxacin (Maxaquin), moxifloxacin (Avelox), norfloxacin (Noroxin), ofloxacin (Floxin), sparfloxacin (Zagam) or other quinolone antibiotics. Give these medicines 4 hours before or 8 hours after sucralfate.
- digoxin (Lanoxin).
- ketoconazole (Nizoral).
- lansoprazole (Prevacid)—separate doses by half an hour.
- levothyroxine (various)—blood levels are prudent.
- phenytoin (Dilantin, etc.).
- quinidine (Quinaglute).
- tetracycline (Achromycin, Tetracyn, etc.).
- warfarin (Coumadin, etc.) and reduce its anticoagulant effect; increased frequency of INR testing (prothrombin time or protime) is needed.

▷ *Driving, Hazardous Activities:* This drug may cause dizziness or drowsiness. Restrict activities as necessary.

Aviation Note: The use of this drug ***may be a disqualification*** for piloting. Consult a designated Aviation Medical Examiner.

Exposure to Sun: No restrictions.

SULFAMETHOXAZOLE (sul fa meth OX a zohl)

Please see the sulfonamide antibiotic family profile.

SULFASALAZINE (sul fa SAL a zeen)

Introduced: 1949 **Class:** Bowel anti-inflammatory, sulfonamides **Prescription:** USA: Yes **Controlled Drug:** USA: No; Canada: No **Available as Generic:** USA: Yes; Canada: No

Brand Names: Azaline, Azulfidine, Azulfidine EN-Tabs, ❦PMS Sulfasalazine, ❦PMS Sulfasalazine E.C., ❦Salazopyrin, ❦Salazopyrin EN, ❦SAS-Enema, ❦SAS Enteric-500, SAS-500

BENEFITS versus RISKS	
Possible Benefits	*Possible Risks*
EFFECTIVE SUPPRESSION OF INFLAMMATORY BOWEL DISEASE	Allergic reactions: mild to severe skin reactions
SYMPTOMATIC RELIEF OF REGIONAL ENTERITIS AND ULCERATIVE COLITIS	Blood cell disorders: aplastic anemia, hemolytic anemia, abnormally low white cell or platelet counts
HELPFUL IN REFRACTORY RHEUMATOID ARTHRITIS	Drug-induced liver damage
	Drug-induced kidney damage
	Seizures

▷ **Principal Uses**

As a Single Drug Product: Uses currently included in FDA-approved labeling: (1) Treats inflammatory disease of the lower intestinal tract and then helps retain remissions: regional enteritis (Crohn's disease) and ulcerative colitis—it is usually taken by mouth, but may also be used in retention enemas; (2) helps rheumatoid arthritis.

Other (unlabeled) generally accepted uses: (1) Short-term use in therapy of ankylosing spondylitis; (2) treatment of mild to moderate psoriasis; (3) may have a role in juvenile arthritis.

How This Drug Works: Suppresses the formation of prostaglandins and related tissue substances that cause inflammation, diarrhea, and tissue destruction.

Available Dosage Forms and Strengths

Oral suspension — 250 mg/5 ml

Tablets — 500 mg

Tablets, enteric coated — 500 mg

▷ **Usual Adult Dosage Ranges:** *Ulcerative colitis*: Some clinicians start with 3 to 4 g per day of this medicine, separated into equal doses given every 6 to 8 hours until symptoms are adequately controlled. For maintenance, 500 mg every 6 hours. Some clinicians use a starting dose of 1–2 g a day in order to minimize stomach and intestinal adverse effects. Some patients tolerate up to 6 g a day, but doses of 4 g a day or greater bring increased risk of adverse effects. If diarrhea occurs, the dose is often decreased to the earlier dose that worked and did not cause diarrhea. Some patients do not remove this medicine well (slow acetylators) and are given 2.5 to 3 g a day.

Rheumatoid arthritis (when salicylates or NSAIDs have not worked): 2 to 3 g daily is taken in equally divided doses. If the delayed-release form (Azulfidine EN-Tabs) is used, 500 mg is taken for 1 week in the evening, then 500 mg twice daily for a week, then 500 mg in the morning and 1 g in the evening for a week and continuing with 1 g twice a day.

Note: Actual dose and schedule must be individually determined.

Conditions Requiring Dosing Adjustments

Liver Function: This drug can be a cause of liver damage, and patients should be followed closely.

Kidney Function: Empiric decreases in doses should be considered. This drug should be used with **CAUTION** in kidney compromise.

▷ **Dosing Instructions:** This drug is preferably taken with 8 ounces of water on an empty stomach, 1 hour before or 2 hours after eating. However, it may be taken with or following food to reduce stomach irritation. Intervals between doses (day and night) should be no longer than 8 hours. The regular tablet may be crushed; the enteric-coated tablet should be swallowed whole without alteration. If you forget a dose: Take the missed dose as soon as you remember it, unless it's nearly time for your next dose—if that is the case, skip the missed dose and take the next dose right on schedule. DO NOT double doses. Talk with your doctor if you find yourself missing doses. There are many effective medicine reminder systems to help you.

Usual Duration of Use: Use on a regular schedule for 1 to 3 weeks usually determines effectiveness in controlling the symptoms of regional enteritis or ulcerative colitis. Benefits in rheumatoid arthritis may be seen in 4 to 12 weeks. Long-term use (months to years) requires physician supervision.

Typical Treatment Goals and Measurements (Outcomes and Markers)

Inflammatory bowel disease: The goal is to cause (induce) a remission and maintain it. Symptoms that will resolve include rectal bleeding and diarrhea. More involved exams will reveal an absence of bowel ulceration and easing of friability or granularity of the bowel itself.

▷ **This Drug Should Not Be Taken If**
- you are allergic to any sulfonamide drug (see Drug Classes) or aspirin (or other salicylates).
- you are in the final month of pregnancy (near term).
- it has been prescribed for an infant less than 2 years old.
- you have a urinary or intestinal obstruction or porphyria.
- you are breast-feeding.

▷ **Inform Your Physician Before Taking This Drug If**
- you are allergic to any sulfonamide: acetazolamide, thiazide diuretics or sulfonylurea antidiabetics (see Drug Classes).
- you are allergic by nature: history of hay fever, asthma, hives, eczema.
- you have asthma.
- you have impaired liver or kidney function.
- you have a glucose-6-phosphate dehydrogenase (G6PD) deficiency or are known to be a slow acetylator.
- you have a personal or family history of porphyria.
- you have had a drug-induced blood cell or bone marrow disorder.
- you currently take any oral anticoagulant, antidiabetic drug or phenytoin.
- you plan to have surgery under pentothal anesthesia soon.

Possible Side Effects (natural, expected and unavoidable drug actions)

Brownish coloration of the urine—of no significance. Skin pigmentation. Superinfections, bacterial or fungal (see Glossary).

▷ **Possible Adverse Effects** (unusual, unexpected and infrequent reactions)
If any of the following develop, consult your physician promptly for guidance.

Mild Adverse Effects

Allergic reactions: skin rashes, hives, itching.

Headache—frequent.

Dizziness—infrequent.

Discoloration (yellow stains) on contact lenses—possible.

Ringing in the ears—case reports.

Loss of appetite, irritation of mouth or tongue, nausea, vomiting, diarrhea—infrequent to frequent.

Taste disorders—rare.

Serious Adverse Effects

Allergic reactions: drug fever (see Glossary), swollen glands, painful joints, anaphylaxis (see Glossary).

Allergic pneumonitis, allergic liver damage (hepatitis).

Severe skin reactions (Stevens-Johnson syndrome or toxic epidermal necrolysis).

Idiosyncratic reactions: hemolytic anemia (see Glossary).

Bone marrow depression (see Glossary): fever, sore throat, abnormal bleeding/bruising—rare to infrequent.

Pancreatitis, myopathy or drug-induced lupus erythematosus—case reports.

Hearing loss—case reports.

Folic acid deficiency—possible.

Kidney damage—case reports.

Peripheral neuropathy (see Glossary)—case reports.

Inflammation of tissue around the heart (pericarditis)—case reports.

▷ **Possible Effects on Sexual Function:** Decreased production of sperm, reversible infertility—case reports.

▷ **Adverse Effects That May Mimic Natural Diseases or Disorders**

Liver reactions may suggest viral hepatitis. Lung reactions may suggest an infectious pneumonia.

Natural Diseases or Disorders That May Be Activated by This Drug

Goiter, acute intermittent porphyria.

Possible Effects on Laboratory Tests

Complete blood cell counts: decreased red cells, hemoglobin, white cells and platelets; increased eosinophils (allergic reaction).

Liver function tests: increased enzymes (ALT/GPT, AST/GOT, alkaline phosphatase) or bilirubin.

Sperm count: decreased; abnormal sperm common; effects reversible on discontinuation of drug.

CAUTION

1. A large intake of water (up to 2 quarts daily) is necessary to ensure an adequate volume of urine.

2. Shake liquid dose forms well before measuring each dose.

Precautions for Use

By Infants and Children: Safety and effectiveness for those under 2 years of age are not established.

By Those Over 60 Years of Age: Observe for the development of reduced urine volume, fever, sore throat, abnormal bleeding or bruising or skin irritation with itching, particularly in the anal or genital regions.

▷ **Advisability of Use During Pregnancy**

Pregnancy Category: B; however, this drug should not be used near the time of the birth of the baby. See Pregnancy Risk Categories at the back of this book.

Animal studies: Cleft palate and skeletal birth defects due to sulfonamides reported in mice and rats.

Human studies: No increase in birth defects reported in 4,584 exposures to various sulfonamides during pregnancy.

Avoid use of drug during the final month of pregnancy because of possible adverse effects on the newborn infant.

Advisability of Use If Breast-Feeding

Presence of this drug in breast milk: Yes.

Avoid drug or refrain from nursing.

Habit-Forming Potential: None.

Effects of Overdose: Headache, dizziness, nausea, vomiting, abdominal cramping, toxic fever, coma, jaundice, kidney failure.

Possible Effects of Long-Term Use: Development of goiter, with or without hypothyroidism. An orange-yellow discoloration of the skin has been reported. This is not jaundice.

Suggested Periodic Examinations While Taking This Drug (at physician's discretion)

Complete blood cell counts, weekly for the first 8 weeks.

Urine analysis weekly.

Liver and kidney function tests.

▷ **While Taking This Drug, Observe the Following**

Foods: Follow prescribed diet. See iron salt interaction below.

Herbal Medicines or Minerals: Since St. John's wort and sulfasalazine may increase sun sensitivity, the combination is NOT advised. Flaxseed, peppermint oil and psyllium husk have Commission E monograph indications for irritable bowel syndrome. This is NOT the same as ulcerative colitis, and those products have not been studied in ulcerative colitis. Aloe, buckhorn berry or bark, cascara sagrada bark, rhubarb root and senna should not be taken by people living with ulcerative colitis.

Beverages: No restrictions. May be taken with milk.

▷ *Alcohol:* Use caution. Sulfonamide drugs can increase the intoxicating effects of alcohol.

Tobacco Smoking: No interactions expected. I advise everyone to quit smoking.

▷ *Other Drugs*

Sulfasalazine may *increase* the effects of

- anticoagulants (Coumadin, etc.) and increase bleeding risk; more frequent INR (prothrombin time) testing is needed.
- sulfonylureas or other oral hypoglycemic agents (see Sulfonylureas and Oral Antidiabetic Drugs in Drug Classes) and increase the risk of hypoglycemia.

Sulfasalazine may *decrease* the effects of

- digoxin (Lanoxin).
- live typhoid vaccine (Vivotif).

Sulfasalazine *taken concurrently* with
- ampicillin and perhaps other penicillins may lower therapeutic benefits from sulfasalazine.
- some barbiturates (see Drug Classes) may result in decreased sulfasalazine therapeutic benefits.
- calcium supplements (calcium gluconate) may result in decreased therapeutic benefits from sulfasalazine.
- folic acid (various) may decrease folate absorption.
- iron salts or calcium may decrease sulfasalazine's benefits.
- varicella vaccine (Varivax) may result in Reye's syndrome; avoid taking this medicine for 6 weeks following varicella vaccine.

▷ *Driving, Hazardous Activities:* This drug may cause dizziness. Restrict activities as necessary.

Aviation Note: The use of this drug *may be a disqualification* for piloting. Consult a designated Aviation Medical Examiner.

Exposure to Sun: Use caution—some sulfonamide drugs can cause photosensitivity (see Glossary).

SULFONAMIDE ANTIBIOTIC FAMILY

Sulfamethoxazole (sul fa meth OX a zohl) **Sulfisoxazole** (sul fi SOX a zohl)

Introduced: 1961, 1949, respectively   **Class:** Anti-infective, sulfonamides
Prescription: USA: Yes   **Controlled Drug:** USA: No; Canada: No
Available as Generic: Yes

Brand Names: Sulfamethoxazole: ✤Apo-Sulfamethoxazole, ✤Apo-Sulfatrim [CD], ✤Apo-Sulfatrim DS [CD], Azo Gantanol [CD], Bactrim [CD], Bactrim DS [CD], Bethaprim [CD], Comoxol [CD], Cotrim [CD], Gantanol, ✤Novo-Trimel [CD], ✤Novo-Trimel DS [CD], ✤Nu-Cotrimox, ✤Protrin [CD], ✤Protrin DF [CD], ✤Roubac [CD], Septra [CD], Septra DS [CD], Sulfatrim [CD], ✤Uro Gantanol [CD], Uroplus DS [CD], Uroplus SS [CD], Vagitrol, Sulfisoxazole: Azo Gantrisin [CD], Azo-Sulfisoxazole, Eryzole [CD], Gantrisin, Gulfasin, Lipo Gantrisin, ✤Novosoxazole, Pediazole [CD], SK-Soxazole, Sulfalar, Vagila

---

BENEFITS versus RISKS

Possible Benefits	*Possible Risks*
EFFECTIVE ANTIMICROBIAL ACTION AGAINST SUSCEPTIBLE BACTERIA AND PROTOZOA	Allergic reactions: mild to severe skin reactions, anaphylaxis, myocarditis
Effective adjunctive prevention and treatment of *Pneumocystis carinii* pneumonia (AIDS-related-sulfamethoxazole)	Blood cell disorders: aplastic anemia, hemolytic anemia, abnormally low white cell or platelet counts
	Drug-induced liver or kidney damage

▷ **Principal Uses**

As a Single Drug Product: Uses currently included in FDA-approved labeling: (1) Sulfamethoxazole is used to treat some bacterial or protozoan infections: chancroid, cystitis and other infections of the urinary tract. **Sulfamethoxazole should not be used to treat group A streptococcal infections.**

(2) Sulfisoxazole is used in treating ear infections (otitis media), chloroquine-resistant malaria and toxoplasmosis.

Other (unlabeled) generally accepted uses: (1) Treats *Chlamydia* infections; (2) combination therapy of resistant *Mycobacterium kansasii* infections; (3) sulfisoxazole may work in long-term prevention of ear infections; (4) some patients with rheumatoid arthritis have shown benefit from sulfamethoxazole.

As a Combination Drug Product [CD]: These medicines are available in combination with phenazopyridine, an analgesic to ease discomfort associated with acute urethral infections. Sulfamethoxazole is also available in combination with another antibacterial drug, trimethoprim; in some countries this combination is given the generic name cotrimoxazole. This combination is quite effective in the treatment of certain types of middle ear infection, bronchitis, pneumonia and certain infections of the intestinal tract and urinary tract. It is now used as primary prevention and treatment for Pneumocystis carinii pneumonia associated with AIDS.

Author's Note: This medicine in the combination form has assumed a major role in helping prevent a prevalent opportunistic infection in HIV-positive people (PCP pneumonia).

How These Drugs Work: Prevent the growth and multiplication of susceptible bacteria or protozoa by interfering with their formation of folic acid, an essential nutrient.

Available Dosage Forms and Strengths

Sulfamethoxazole:
        Oral suspension — 500 mg/5 ml
                Tablets — 500 mg, 1 g
Sulfisoxazole:
    Emulsion, prolonged action — 1 g/5 ml
                Eyedrops — 4%
            Eye ointment — 4%
                Injection — 400 mg/ml
    Pediatric suspension — 500 mg/5 ml
                Syrup — 500 mg/5 ml
                Tablets — 500 mg

▷ **Recommended Dosage Ranges** (Actual dose and schedule must be determined for each patient individually.)

Infants and Children:

Sulfamethoxazole: Children over 2 months—50 to 60 mg per kg of body mass to start and then 25 to 30 mg per kg of body mass every 12 hours, up to a maximum of 75 mg per kg of body mass daily.

Sulfisoxazole: Children over 2 months—50 mg per kg of body mass to start and then 100 mg per kg of body mass per day, divided into equal doses given two to four times daily.

Recommended Dosage Range:

Sulfamethoxazole: Initially 2 g and then 1 g every 8 to 12 hours, depending upon the severity of the infection. The total daily dose should not exceed 3 g.

Sulfisoxazole: Initially 2 to 4 g (may not be required in urinary tract infections) and then 750 to 1,500 mg (1.5 g) every 4 hours or 1 to 2 g every 6 hours, depending upon the severity of the infection. The total daily dose should not exceed 8 g.

Conditions Requiring Dosing Adjustments

Liver Function: Patients with compromised livers should be followed closely, but specific guidelines for decreasing doses are not defined. Sulfisoxazole may cause liver damage.

Kidney Function: Doses should be decreased for patients with compromised kidneys. For patients with mild to moderate kidney failure, sulfisoxazole can be taken every 6 hours in the usual dose. In moderate to severe kidney failure, it can be taken every 12 to 24 hours in the usual dose. In severe kidney failure, it can be taken once a day. It should be used with *CAUTION* in renal compromise. Increased elimination of this drug may be seen in patients with alkaline urine. For sulfamethoxazole: Specific dosing changes have not been made for the single agent. For cotrimoxazole, it has been recommended that the dosing interval be increased for patients with impaired kidneys.

▷ **Dosing Instructions:** The tablet may be crushed and is preferably taken on an empty stomach, 1 hour before or 2 hours after eating. However, both drugs may be taken with or following food to reduce stomach irritation. Be certain to drink liberal amounts of water while taking this medicine if you are not restricted from doing so. If you forget a dose: Take the missed dose as soon as you remember it, unless it's nearly time for your next dose—if that is the case, skip the missed dose and take the next dose right on schedule. DO NOT double doses. Talk with your doctor if you find yourself missing doses as compliance ensures treatment or best possible prevention of infection.

Usual Duration of Use: Use on a regular schedule for 4 to 7 days usually determines effectiveness in controlling responsive infections. Treatment should be continued until the patient is free of symptoms for 48 hours. Limit treatment to no more than 14 days if possible. Preventive use of trimethoprim/sulfamethoxazole will be ongoing.

Typical Treatment Goals and Measurements (Outcomes and Markers)

Infections: The most commonly used measures of serious infections are white blood cell counts and differentials (the kind of blood cells that occur most often in your blood), and temperature. Many clinicians look for positive changes in 24–48 hours. NEVER stop an antibiotic because you start to feel better. For treating infections, the full course is REQUIRED to kill the bacteria. Prophylaxis (for example of PCP) often requires ongoing use. The goals and time frame (see peak benefits above) should be discussed with you when the prescription is written.

Currently a Drug of Choice

Sulfamethoxazole (when combined with trimethoprim) is the drug of choice for preventing pneumonia (due to *Pneumocystis carinii*) in HIV-positive patients or those with AIDS.

▷ **These Drugs Should Not Be Taken If**

- you are allergic to any sulfonamide drug (see Drug Classes).
- you are in the final month of pregnancy.
- you are breast-feeding your infant.
- it has been prescribed for an infant less than 2 months old (unless congenital toxoplasmosis is being treated—sulfisoxazole).

▷ **Inform Your Physician Before Taking These Drugs If**
- you are allergic to any sulfonamide derivative: acetazolamide, thiazide diuretics, sulfonylurea antidiabetics (see Drug Classes).
- you are allergic by nature: history of hay fever, asthma, hives, eczema.
- you have impaired liver or kidney function.
- you have a personal or family history of porphyria.
- you have had a drug-induced blood cell or bone marrow disorder.
- you have a glucose-6-phosphate dehydrogenase (G6PD) deficiency in your red blood cells (ask your doctor).
- you currently take any oral anticoagulant, antidiabetic drug or phenytoin.
- you plan to have surgery under pentothal anesthesia while taking this drug.

Possible Side Effects (natural, expected and unavoidable drug actions)
Brownish coloration of the urine—of no significance. Superinfections, bacterial or fungal (see Glossary).

▷ **Possible Adverse Effects** (unusual, unexpected and infrequent reactions)
If any of the following develop, consult your physician promptly for guidance.

Mild Adverse Effects
Allergic reactions: skin rashes, hives, itching, localized swellings, reddened eyes, temporary myopia.
Myopia—infrequent.
Headache, dizziness, unsteadiness, ringing in the ears—possible.
Loss of appetite, irritation of mouth or tongue, nausea, vomiting, abdominal pain, diarrhea—infrequent.

Serious Adverse Effects
Allergic reactions: drug fever (see Glossary), swollen glands, painful joints, anaphylaxis (see Glossary).
Allergic reaction in the heart muscle (myocarditis), allergic pneumonitis, allergic hepatitis.
Severe skin reactions—rare.
Idiosyncratic reactions: hemolytic anemia (see Glossary)—possible.
Bone marrow depression (see Glossary): fatigue, weakness, fever, sore throat, abnormal bleeding or bruising—case reports.
Liver damage—rare.
Pancreatitis—case reports.
Kidney damage: bloody or cloudy urine, reduced urine volume—possible.
Psychotic reactions, hallucinations, seizures, hearing changes (loss or vestibular symptoms), peripheral neuropathy (see Glossary)—case reports.
Severe hypoglycemia—case report (sulfamethoxazole).
Methemoglobinemia—rare.
Drug-induced lupus erythematosus or blood-clotting problems (hypoprothrombinemia)—rare.
Drug-induced disulfiramlike reaction (sulfisoxazole)—possible.

▷ **Possible Effects on Sexual Function:** None reported.
▷ **Adverse Effects That May Mimic Natural Diseases or Disorders**
Liver reactions may suggest viral hepatitis. Lung reactions may suggest an infectious pneumonia.

Natural Diseases or Disorders That May Be Activated by These Drugs
Goiter, acute intermittent porphyria, polyarteritis nodosa, systemic lupus erythematosus (questionable).

Possible Effects on Laboratory Tests

Complete blood cell counts: decreased red cells, hemoglobin, white cells and platelets; increased eosinophils (allergic reaction).

INR (prothrombin time): increased (when taken concurrently with warfarin).

Liver function tests: increased enzymes (ALT/GPT, AST/GOT, alkaline phosphatase) or bilirubin.

CAUTION

1. A large intake of water (up to 2 quarts daily) is necessary to ensure an adequate volume of urine.
2. Shake liquid dose forms well before measuring each dose.

Precautions for Use

By Infants and Children: These drugs should not be used in infants under 2 months of age.

By Those Over 60 Years of Age: Small doses taken at longer intervals often achieve adequate blood and tissue drug levels. Observe for the development of reduced urine volume, fever, sore throat, abnormal bleeding or bruising, or skin irritation with itching, particularly in the anal or genital regions.

▷ **Advisability of Use During Pregnancy**

Pregnancy Category: C; however, these drugs **SHOULD NOT BE TAKEN** (are contraindicated) near the time of the birth of the baby. See Pregnancy Risk Categories at the back of this book.

Animal studies: Cleft palate and skeletal birth defects reported in mice and rats.

Human studies: No increase in birth defects reported in 4,584 exposures to various sulfonamides during pregnancy.

Avoid use of drug during the final 3 months of pregnancy because of Possible Adverse Effects on the newborn infant.

Advisability of Use If Breast-Feeding

Presence of these drugs in breast milk: Yes.

Avoid drug or refrain from nursing.

Habit-Forming Potential: None.

Effects of Overdose: Headache, dizziness, nausea, vomiting, abdominal cramping, toxic fever, coma, jaundice, kidney failure.

Possible Effects of Long-Term Use

Superinfections, bacterial or fungal. Development of goiter, with or without hypothyroidism. Excessive loss of vitamin C via urine.

Suggested Periodic Examinations While Taking These Drugs (at physician's discretion)

Complete blood cell counts, weekly for the first 8 weeks.

Urine analysis weekly.

Liver and kidney function tests.

▷ **While Taking These Drugs, Observe the Following**

Foods: No restrictions.

Herbal Medicines or Minerals: Since St. John's wort and these medicines may increase sun sensitivity, the combination is NOT advised. Some patients use echinacea to attempt to boost their immune systems. Unfortunately, use of echinacea is not recommended in people with damaged immune systems. This herb may also actually weaken any immune system if it is used too often or for too long a time. DO NOT take mistletoe herb, oak bark or F.C.

of marshmallow root and licorice extracts. Pure cranberry juice may help keep harmful bacteria from attaching to the bladder wall and may be useful in helping to prevent urinary tract infections.

Beverages: No restrictions. May be taken with milk. Note recommendations for increased fluid intake.

▷ *Alcohol:* Use caution. Sulfonamide drugs can increase the intoxicating effects of alcohol and may also lead to a disulfiram (see Glossary) reaction.

Tobacco Smoking: No interactions expected. I advise everyone to quit smoking.

▷ *Other Drugs*

These medicines may ***increase*** the effects of
- amantadine (Symmetrel) and cause abnormal heart rhythms and CNS stimulation (confusion, disorientation).
- anticoagulants (Coumadin, etc.) and increase the risk of bleeding; more frequent INR testing (prothrombin time or protime) is needed. Ongoing warfarin doses should be decided based on laboratory results.
- metformin (Glucophage) and lead to increased risk of lowered blood sugar or lactic acidosis.
- methotrexate (Mexate) and cause severe blood toxicity.
- sulfonylureas (see Drug Classes) or other oral hypoglycemic agents and increase the risk of excessively low blood sugar (hypoglycemia).
- zidovudine (AZT) and lamivudine and result in zidovudine or lamivudine toxicity in the single product or in their combination forms.

These medicines may ***decrease*** the effects of
- birth control pills (oral contraceptives).
- cyclosporine (Sandimmune) and reduce its immunosuppressive effect.
- live typhoid vaccine (Vivotif).
- penicillins (see Drug Classes).

These medicines ***taken concurrently*** with
- metronidazole (Flagyl) may lead to a disulfiram reaction.

▷ *Driving, Hazardous Activities:* These drugs may cause dizziness. Restrict activities as necessary.

Aviation Note: The use of these drugs ***may be a disqualification*** for piloting. Consult a designated Aviation Medical Examiner.

Exposure to Sun: Use caution. Some sulfonamide drugs can cause photosensitivity (see Glossary).

SULINDAC (sul IN dak)

Please see the acetic acid (nonsteroidal anti-inflammatory drug) family profile.

SUMATRIPTAN (soo ma TRIP tan)

Introduced: 1993   **Class:** Antimigraine drug, serotonin-1-receptor agonist
Prescription: USA: Yes   **Controlled Drug:** USA: No; Canada: No   **Available as Generic:** USA: No; Canada: No
Brand Names: Imitrex, Imitrex Nasal Spray

BENEFITS versus RISKS	
Possible Benefits	**Possible Risks**
RAPID AND EFFECTIVE RELIEF OR PREVENTION OF MIGRAINE	Fainting
GENERALLY WELL TOLERATED	Myocardial infarction (probably secondary to coronary vasospasm)
NASAL SPRAY FORM	Serious atrial and ventricular arrhythmias
Relieves photophobia (light sensitivity)	Exacerbation of ischemic heart disease (should not be given to those patients)
Relieves phonophobia (sound sensitivity)	Not to be used in hemiplegic or basilar migraine
Relieves nausea and vomiting	Not to be used in significant cardiovascular disease
	Not compatible with patients with seizure disorders

▷ **Principal Uses**

As a Single Drug Product: Uses currently included in FDA-approved labeling: (1) Acute treatment of migraine with or without aura in adults; (2) treatment of cluster headache in adults.

Other (unlabeled) generally accepted uses: Treatment of posttraumatic headaches.

How This Drug Works: Sumatriptan acts on blood vessels to cause vasoconstriction (shrinking of the blood vessels). This relieves swelling, thought to be the cause of migraine. The drug binds to receptor arteries such as the basilar artery and in vasculature (blood vessels) associated with the dura mater (part of the lining of the brain).

Available Dosage Forms and Strengths

Nasal spray—5 mg/100 mcl, 20 mg/100 mcl

Sumatriptan succinate (Imitrex) injection SELFdose system kit—2 syringes with 6 mg in 0.5 ml of liquid in each 1-ml size syringe, a dosing device and instructions.

Unit-of-use syringes—6 mg in 0.5 ml of liquid in a 1-ml syringe in a carton of two syringes.

6 mg single-dose vials—0.5 ml of liquid in a 2-ml vial.

All the liquid should be a colorless to pale yellow clear solution. Particles or precipitates should NEVER appear.

Tablets—25 mg, 50 mg, 100 mg

How to Store

Keep out of reach of children. Store at room temperature in a room where the temperature will not exceed 86 degrees F (30 degrees C). Keep away from heat and light.

▷ **Recommended Dosage Ranges** (Actual dose and schedule must be determined for each patient individually.)

Infants and Children: The safety and effectiveness in pediatrics have not been determined.

18 to 60 Years of Age:

Subcutaneous: Maximum adult dose is 6 mg. The dose should be taken as soon as possible after the symptoms of acute migraine are recognized. Controlled clinical trials have failed to demonstrate a benefit of repeated injections if the initial injection is unsuccessful. If symptoms return, a second 6-mg injection may be taken 12 hours after the first injection. If side effects occur, use the lowest dose in the approved dose range that is effective for you. Daily maximum is 12 mg.

Oral: 25 mg taken with water or other acceptable liquids as soon as possible after a headache starts. The dose chosen must balance possible benefit of the higher dose with increased risk of adverse effects of higher doses. Take the dose your doctor prescribes as soon as headache pain starts. If the headache returns or if there is a partial response, single tablets can be taken at least two hours after the first dose (up to 100 mg a day). Maximum daily oral dose is 100 mg. There is evidence that any dose more than 100-mg provides more relief. If symptoms come back, subsequent doses can be taken (talk this over with your doctor first) separated by two hours after the last dose and taken up to a total of 300 mg in 100-mg increments in 24 hours.

Nasal: 5 to 20 mg as a one-time dose. Newly labeled dosing notes that more patients taking the 20 mg dose had headache relief. The dose chosen must balance possible benefit of the higher dose with increased risk of adverse effects of higher doses. Take the dose prescribed as soon as headache pain starts. For example, 10 mg may be taken by 5 mg in each nostril. A 20-mg dose can be taken as 10 mg in each nostril. Data exists that shows that single doses more than 20 mg do not give additional benefit. If symptoms return, the dose can be taken once again (two hours after the first dose was taken), but the daily maximum of 40 mg must not be exceeded. Safety in treating more than 4 headaches in 30 days is unknown with any dosage form.

Over 65 Years of Age: Safety and effectiveness have not been evaluated in this age group. Since declines in renal and hepatic function and coronary artery disease are more common in those over 65, the possibility of an increase in side effects would be expected.

Conditions Requiring Dosing Adjustments

Liver Function: Oral tablets will give unpredictable variations in blood levels if used in liver disease. Maximum dose is 50 mg.

Kidney Function: No changes in dose thought to be needed in kidney disease.

Dosing Instructions: The injection form must be given subcutaneously, not intravenously. Intravenous injection must be avoided because of potential to cause coronary vasospasm (constriction of the blood vessels that supply the heart). This medicine should be colorless to pale yellow and clear. Particles should never be present. There is extensive information on self-injection available from your doctor or pharmacist. The first dose is usually given in the doctor's office. The tablet form may take more than an hour to work. The tablet form may be taken with food. Follow directions for the nasal form closely. If you forget a dose: This medicine is used when you get a migraine headache, NOT on an ongoing basis.

Usual Duration of Use: The maximum dose is two 6-mg doses (injections) in 24 hours. This medication relieves existing migraines and will not change the frequency or number of attacks. Recurring use of this medicine will be needed. If your migraines increase in frequency or severity, consult your doctor. If this medicine is not effective in helping your migraine, call your doctor.

Typical Treatment Goals and Measurements (Outcomes and Markers)

Migraine pain: Most clinicians treating pain use a device called an algometer to check your pain. This looks like a small ruler, but lets the clinician better understand your pain. The goals of treatment then relate to where the level of pain started (for example, a rating of seven on a zero to ten scale) and what the cause of the pain was. Pain medicines may also be used together (in combination) in order to get the best result or outcome. Specific results to migraine relate to stopping (aborting) an attack or easing the severity of an attack. Once again, the role of prophylactic medicines is clear in helping some patients avoid attacks altogether. A migraine diary can help you identify trigger foods as well as medication response.

▷ **This Drug Should Not Be Taken If**
- you had an allergic reaction to it previously.
- you are unfamiliar with the subcutaneous route. Particular care must be taken to avoid intravenous use because this may lead to coronary vasospasm (constriction of the blood vessels that supply the heart).
- you have ischemic heart disease with symptoms such as angina pectoris or silent ischemia, or history of MI (myocardial infarction).
- you have a seizure disorder.
- you have Prinzmetal's angina (a specific kind of chest pain).
- you have uncontrolled hypertension (high blood pressure).
- you have basilar or hemiplegic migraine.
- you have taken an MAO inhibitor within the last 2 weeks.
- you have (within 24 hours) taken an ergotamine preparation.

▷ **Inform Your Physician Before Taking This Drug If**
- you are pregnant or plan to become pregnant.
- you are breast-feeding your infant.
- you have high blood pressure.
- you have chest pain, heart disease or irregular heartbeats.
- you have taken or have prescriptions for other migraine medications.
- you have allergies or trouble taking other medications, whether prescription or over the counter.
- you have liver or kidney disease.
- you are uncertain of how much to take or when to take this medicine.
- you do not understand the subcutaneous injection technique.
- you have Raynaud's phenomenon.

Possible Side Effects (natural, expected and unavoidable drug actions)

Excessive thirst and frequent urination. Transient rises in blood pressure. Vision changes—rare. Taste changes—frequent.

▷ **Possible Adverse Effects** (unusual, unexpected and infrequent reactions)

If any of the following develop, consult your physician promptly for guidance.

Mild Adverse Effects

Allergic reactions: red, itching skin; skin rash and tenderness.

Atypical sensations such as tingling (rare with injection, infrequent with tablet form).

Confusion and other mental changes or dizziness—rare.

Flushing—rare.

Tightness in the chest or jaw—infrequent.

Gastroesophageal reflux and diarrhea—case report.

Pain at the injection site; joint pain, weakness and stiffness—rare.

Serious Adverse Effects

Allergic reactions: anaphylactic reactions.

Syncope (fainting), CVA, dysphasia, seizure—rare.

Serious changes in heart rate and rhythm—rare.

Raynaud's phenomenon, dyspnea (difficulty breathing)—rare.

Kidney stones (renal calculi)—rare.

Prinzmetal's angina—rare.

Heart attack (myocardial infarction)—rare.

▷ **Possible Effects on Sexual Function:** Dysmenorrhea, erection problems—case reports.

Possible Delayed Adverse Effects: None identified.

▷ **Adverse Effects That May Mimic Natural Diseases or Disorders**

Changes in heart rate and rhythm may mimic a number of cardiac conditions. Drug-induced acute renal failure (ARF) may mimic non-drug-induced ARF. Drug-induced hypertension may mimic hypertension from other causes. Urological symptoms may mimic benign prostatic hypertrophy. Sumatriptan can mimic Raynaud's phenomenon.

Natural Diseases or Disorders That May Be Activated by This Drug

Hypertension.

Possible Effects on Laboratory Tests

Liver function tests: rare increases in SGOT and SGPT.

CAUTION

1. Do not use sumatriptan if you are pregnant.
2. Call your doctor if you have any pain or tightness in the chest or throat when you use this medicine.
3. Do not use sumatriptan if you have used an ergotamine preparation within the last 24 hours.
4. This medication is **not** to be used intravenously.
5. **If** you are diagnosed as having ischemic heart disease after sumatriptan has been prescribed for you, do not use the medicine again.

Precautions for Use

By Infants and Children: Safety and effectiveness for those under 18 years of age are not established.

By Those Over 65 Years of Age: Not established.

▷ **Advisability of Use During Pregnancy**

Pregnancy Category: C. See Pregnancy Risk Categories at the back of this book.

Animal studies: Sumatriptan has been lethal to rabbit embryos when given in doses that were threefold higher than those produced by a 6-mg dose. Term fetuses from rabbits treated with sumatriptan exhibited an increase in cervicothoracic vascular defects and minor skeletal abnormalities.

Human studies: Adequate studies of pregnant women are not available.

Ask your physician for guidance.

Advisability of Use If Breast-Feeding

Presence of this drug in breast milk: Yes.

Use of this medication by nursing mothers is a benefit-to-risk decision to be made by a physician.

Habit-Forming Potential: Not clearly defined.

Effects of Overdose: Patients have received doses of 8 to 12 mg without adverse effects. Healthy volunteers have taken up to 16 mg subcutaneously without serious adverse events. Coronary vasospasm has resulted from intravenous doses. Animal data presents convulsions, tremor, flushing, decreased breathing and activity, cyanosis, ataxia and paralysis.

Possible Effects of Long-Term Use: Not defined.

Suggested Periodic Examinations While Taking This Drug (at physician's discretion)

Liver function tests.

Electrocardiogram.

▷ **While Taking This Drug, Observe the Following**

Foods: No restrictions; however, some foods or additives such as monosodium glutamate or chocolate may be a risk factor for migraines. Skipping meals can also be a risk factor for migraines. Keeping a migraine diary can help identify triggers.

Herbal Medicines or Minerals: Using St. John's wort, ma huang or kola while taking this medicine may trigger a migraine. Trigger compounds must be individually identified. Since part of how ginseng works (mechanism of action) may involve an MAO inhibitor, combination with sumatriptan is NOT recommended. Using ma huang or ephedrine-like compounds (ephedra) may result in additive and undesirable vasoconstriction. If you are allergic to plants in the Asteraceae family (aster, chrysanthemum, daisy or ragweed), you may also be allergic to echinacea, chamomile, feverfew and St. John's wort. St. John's wort can cause changes in the liver enzymes that help remove this medicine—talk to your doctor before combining any herbal medicine or mineral with ergotamine.

Beverages: An individual trigger beverage list should be identified.

▷ *Alcohol:* May cause additive sedation. Alcohol may also be a precipitating factor for migraine.

Tobacco Smoking: No interactions expected. I advise everyone to quit smoking.

Marijuana Smoking: May cause additive dizziness, drowsiness and lethargy; may cause additive increases in blood pressure.

▷ *Other Drugs*

Sumatriptan *taken concurrently* with

- citalopram (Celexa) may lead to loss of coordination and excessive reflex response—DO NOT COMBINE.
- ergotamine-containing preparations (see Drug Classes) may result in additive vasospasm (prolonged constriction of the blood vessels)—these medicines SHOULD NOT be taken within 24 hours of any sumatriptan dose. There is a case report of heart attack after sumatriptan was combined with methysergide.
- fluoxetine (Prozac) may result in coordination problems.
- fluvoxamine (Luvox) and other SSRIs may result in coordination problems.
- monoamine oxidase (MAO) inhibitors (see Drug Classes) may result in toxic levels of sumatriptan—MAO inhibitors and sumatriptan should

never be combined. It is important that 14 days go by after your last dose of an MAO inhibitor before you take any form of sumatriptan.

- naratriptan (Amerge) or other 5HT1 agonists may lead to prolonged spasm of the blood vessels—DO NOT COMBINE.
- paroxetine (Paxil) may result in coordination problems.
- sertraline (Zoloft) may result in coordination problems.
- sibutramine (Meridia) may increase risk of serotonin syndrome—DO NOT COMBINE.
- venlafaxine (Effexor) may result in coordination problems.

▷ *Driving, Hazardous Activities:* This drug may cause dizziness and drowsiness. Restrict activities as necessary.

Aviation Note: The use of this drug ***may be a disqualification*** for piloting. Consult a designated Aviation Medical Examiner.

Exposure to Sun: No restrictions.

Exposure to Cold: Use **CAUTION** until tolerance is determined. Cold may enhance sumatriptan vasoconstriction.

Heavy Exercise or Exertion: Strenuous exercise can be a risk factor for migraines in some patients.

Special Storage Instructions: Keep this medicine out of reach of children. Store at room temperature in a room where the temperature will not exceed 86 degrees F (30 degrees C). Keep away from heat and light.

Observe the Following Expiration Times: There is an expiration date printed on the treatment package. Throw the medication away if it has expired. The autoinjector may be used again.

SYNTHETIC CONJUGATED ESTROGENS, A (CHEMICALLY DERIVED FROM PLANTS [YAMS AND SOY])

Other Names: Sodium estrone sulfate, sodium equilin sulfate, sodium 17 alpha-dihydroequilin sulfate, sodium 17 alpha estradiol sulfate, sodium 17 beta dihydroequilin sulfate, sodium 17 beta estradiol sulfate, sodium equilin sulfate (higher molecular weight), sodium 17 alpha dihydroequilin sulfate, and sodium 17 beta dihydroequilin sulfate (higher molecular weight). All of these compounds are present in Cenestin.

Author's Note: Since this medicine contains compounds that work like the estrogen that the body makes before menopause (estrogenic substances) and because the compounds were derived from plants (versus horse urine for many other estrogen replacement medicines), the FDA approved Cenestin as an entirely new class. Many of the warnings, etc., in this profile are those for estrogens in general. Reports from prescribing of this medicine (Phase Four) will determine further uses (indications) for this medicine as well as the full scope of specific possible side effects and benefits. Alternative synthetic conjugated estrogen combinations such as Cenestin are further detailed below in the synthetic conjugated estrogen alternative profile. Controversy has erupted based on results from the HERS (Heart and estrogen/progestin Replacement Study) trial regarding benefits of

estrogen/progestin combination in preventing a second heart attack (secondary prevention). Controversy results from higher use of statins (HMG-CoA reductase inhibitors—see Drug Classes) in the control group and high use of beta blockers and aspirin in both study and control groups. Additional studies include the Women's Health Initiative (WHI) and the WISDOM research. Newer data from the two-year Women's Health, Osteoporosis, Progestin, Estrogen study (HOPE) points to the use of 1.5 mg of progestin with 0.45 or 0.3 mg of estrogen being equal in benefits to higher doses. An important new direction in research may be use of lower doses of estrogens combined with lower doses of progestins to define cardiovascular, bone health and other benefits while avoiding or lowering risks.

Introduced: 1999   **Class:** Female sex hormones   **Prescription:** USA: Yes
Controlled Drug: USA: No; Canada: No   **Available as Generic:** USA: No; Canada: No
Brand Names: Cenestin, ✤C.E.S.

<table>
<tr><th colspan="2">BENEFITS versus RISKS</th></tr>
<tr><th>*Possible Benefits*</th><th>*Possible Risks*</th></tr>
<tr><td>RELIEF OF MENOPAUSAL HOT FLASHES AND NIGHT SWEATS</td><td>INCREASED RISK OF CANCER OF THE UTERUS (endometrium—possible and expected to be more probable with longer use)</td></tr>
<tr><td>Possible prevention or relief of atrophic vaginitis or atrophy of the vulva and urethra</td><td>INCREASED RISK OF BREAST CANCER (possible and expected to be more probable with longer use)</td></tr>
<tr><td>Works to help prevent postmenopausal osteoporosis</td><td>Increased frequency of gallstones</td></tr>
<tr><td>Works in older women to increase bone mineral density</td><td>Fluid retention</td></tr>
<tr><td>May have a mental tonic effect</td><td>Postmenopausal spotting</td></tr>
<tr><td>May help improve memory</td><td>Increased blood pressure</td></tr>
<tr><td></td><td>Deep vein thrombophlebitis and thromboembolism (but less likely with conjugated estrogens than other estrogens)</td></tr>
<tr><td></td><td>Doses of 5 mg per day may increase risk of nonfatal heart attack (because of increased clotting risk change above)</td></tr>
</table>

▷ **Principal Uses**

As a Single Drug Product: Uses currently included in FDA-approved labeling: "Replacement" therapy in moderate to severe menopausal symptoms (vasomotor symptoms).

Other (unlabeled) generally accepted uses: (1) a study of 46 women (at Yale) after menopause found that estrogen (not this specific product) increased activity in the brain in a region associated with memory.

How This Drug Works: When used to correct hormonal deficiency states, estrogens restore normal cellular activity by increasing nuclear material and protein synthesis. Frequency and intensity of menopausal symptoms are reduced when normal levels of estrogen are restored.

Available Dosage Forms and Strengths

    Tablets—0.625 mg, 0.9 mg, 1.25 mg

▷ **Usual Adult Dosage Ranges:** *For moderate to severe symptoms associated with menopause*: Dosing is started at 0.625 mg a day. The dose may be increased to a maximum of 1.25 mg daily if needed and tolerated. The lowest effective dose should be used and attempts to stop and taper medicine made at three- to six-month intervals. **Note: Actual dose and schedule must be determined for each patient individually.**

Conditions Requiring Dosing Adjustments

    Liver Function: Since this medicine is metabolized in the liver, blood levels should be checked and the dose adjusted as needed in liver compromise. Estrogens should not be used in acute or severe liver compromise. This drug can be lithogenic (capable of causing stones) in bile.

    Kidney Function: No expected dosing changes in kidney compromise.

▷ **Dosing Instructions:** The effect of food on this medicine is not known. At present, it is best to take this medicine on an empty stomach. If you forget a dose: Take the missed dose as soon as you remember it, unless it's nearly time for your next dose—if that is the case, skip the missed dose and take the next dose right on schedule. DO NOT double doses. Talk with your doctor if you find yourself missing doses.

Usual Duration of Use: Regular use for 10 to 20 days needed to see effectiveness in easing menopausal symptoms. Long-term use requires periodic evaluation by your doctor. Attempts to stop or lower the dose (taper) this medicine should be made at 3- to 6-month intervals.

Typical Treatment Goals and Measurements (Outcomes and Markers)

    Menopause: Most clinicians treating menopause seek goals of reduction or cessation of hot flashes, greater sense of well-being and avoidance of rapid bone loss (which can also be measured by some lab tests and DEXA testing). Longer term use of estrogen is associated with increased risk of cancer, so trends may develop toward shorter term therapy than in the past.

Possible Advantages of This Drug

    THIS DRUG IS NOT derived from horse urine and avoids the possible allergic potential of products that are. Effective with once-a-day dose.

▷ **This Drug Should Not Be Taken If**
- you have had an allergic reaction to it previously.
- you have a history of thrombophlebitis, embolism, heart attack or stroke.
- you have seriously impaired liver function or recent onset of liver disease.
- you have abnormal and unexplained vaginal bleeding.
- you are pregnant.
- you have or are suspected to have breast cancer (may eventually be used to treat some kinds of breast cancer).
- you have known or suspected estrogen-dependent cancer (your doctor will determine this).

▷ **Inform Your Physician Before Taking This Drug If**
- you have had an unfavorable reaction to estrogen therapy previously.
- you have a history of breast or reproductive organ cancer.
- you have fibrocystic breast changes, fibroid tumors of the uterus, endometriosis, migraine headaches, epilepsy, asthma, heart disease, high blood pressure, gallbladder disease, diabetes or porphyria.

- you have retention of fluid.
- you have elevated calcium and kidney disease.
- you smoke tobacco on a regular basis.
- you have a history of blood-clotting disorders.
- you plan to have surgery in the near future.

Possible Side Effects (natural, expected and unavoidable drug actions)

Fluid retention, weight gain, "breakthrough" bleeding (spotting), altered menstrual pattern, resumption of menstrual flow ("periods") after natural cessation (postmenopausal bleeding).

▷ **Possible Adverse Effects** (unusual, unexpected and infrequent reactions)

If any of the following develop, consult your physician promptly for guidance.

Mild Adverse Effects

Allergic reactions: skin rash—reported with other estrogens.

Headache, nervous tension, depression, accentuation of migraine headaches—infrequent.

Vision change (steepening of the curve of the cornea)—possible.

Nausea, vomiting, bloating, diarrhea—infrequent to frequent.

Tannish pigmentation of the face—possible.

Serious Adverse Effects

Allergic reactions: anaphylaxis—case reports with other estrogens.

Idiosyncratic reaction: not reported with this product.

Can produce or worsen high blood pressure—more likely with higher doses.

Gallbladder disease—two-to fourfold increased risk.

Intolerance to sugar—possible.

Thrombophlebitis (inflammation of a vein with formation of blood clot): pain or tenderness in thigh or leg, with or without swelling of foot or leg— low dose has minimal increased risk; higher doses may carry more risk.

Pulmonary embolism (movement of blood clot to lung): sudden shortness of breath, pain in chest, coughing, bloody sputum—possible.

Systemic lupus erythematosus or worsening of porphyria—rare.

Stroke (blood clot in brain): headaches, blackout, sudden weakness or paralysis of any part of the body, severe dizziness, altered vision, slurred speech, inability to speak—case reports with other estrogens.

Endometrial cancer—increased risk (how long increased risk continues if the drug is stopped is not clear). There is no evidence that natural estrogens are more or less likely than other estrogens to increase risk. Longer periods of use are associated with increased risk.

Nonfatal heart attack (blood clot in coronary artery): sudden pain in chest, neck, jaw or arm; weakness; sweating; nausea. Has been associated with women taking higher doses and with men using estrogen to treat prostate cancer; however, this is not clearly decided as yet with this product. Estrogen in lower doses appears to decrease overall risk of heart attack.

Breast cancer—increased risk possible although only a slight increase in risk. One study that followed 46,355 women after menopause found that use of estrogen with or without a progestin was associated with a slightly increased breast cancer risk. Risk appeared to increase by combination with a progestin (in contrast to earlier findings) and increased as the length of time the estrogen was taken grew.

Benign liver adenomas or blood clots in the liver—reported with oral contraceptives.

▷ **Possible Effects on Sexual Function:** Swelling and tenderness of breasts, milk production. Increased vaginal secretions.

Possible Delayed Adverse Effects: Estrogens taken during pregnancy may predispose a female child to the later development of cancer of the vagina or cervix following puberty.

▷ **Adverse Effects That May Mimic Natural Diseases or Disorders**

Blood clots may mimic clots forming for other reasons.

Natural Diseases or Disorders That May Be Activated by This Drug

Latent hypertension, diabetes mellitus, acute intermittent porphyria.

Possible Effects on Laboratory Tests

Serum folate: may be decreased (the effect of possible lowering of folate by Cenestin on red blood cells is not yet defined).

Glucose tolerance test (GTT): decreased tolerance.

Liver function tests: increased with other estrogens if a rare liver clot forms.

CAUTION

1. Yearly mammography is needed for ALL women who take this medicine who are more than 50 years old.
2. Bone mineral density tests (DEXA or PDEXA) are prudent to see whether this medicine is helping bone mass.
3. While this product is derived from plants (yam and soy), it was approved by the FDA as an estrogen and as such may carry the benefits and risks of existing estrogens. Many consumers think that because something is derived from a natural source, it is somehow safer. This tablet is a blend of nine estrogenic compounds derived from soy and yams and may or may not carry similar risks and benefits of existing estrogens. Ongoing use will define how possible side effects or benefits of prior estrogens apply to Cenestin. Any unusual vaginal bleeding should be immediately reported your doctor.
4. Repeated data found that estrogen replacement therapy was associated with a small increase in breast cancer risk. One study found that combining estrogen with progestin increased risk of breast cancer. Risk was also found to increase the longer hormone replacement therapy (HRT) is taken. This area is now controversial, and is a benefit-to-risk decision. From some studies, it appeared that taking HRT for two to three years for menopausal symptoms wasn't likely to increase breast cancer risk.

Precautions for Use

By Those Over 60 Years of Age: Will help women who are at increased risk for osteoporosis. In this age group, it may be advisable to attempt relief of hot flashes with nonestrogenic medicines. During use, report promptly any indications of impaired circulation: speech disturbances, altered vision, sudden hearing loss, vertigo, sudden weakness or paralysis, angina, leg pains.

▷ **Advisability of Use During Pregnancy**

Pregnancy Category: X. See Pregnancy Risk Categories at the back of this book.

Animal studies: Genital defects reported in mice and guinea pigs; cleft palate reported in rodents from other estrogens.

Human studies: Information from studies of pregnant women indicates that estrogens can masculinize the female fetus. In addition, limb defects and heart malformations have been reported. It is now known that estrogens taken during pregnancy can predispose the female child to the development of cancer of the vagina or cervix following puberty.

Avoid estrogens completely during entire pregnancy.

Advisability of Use If Breast-Feeding

Presence of this drug in breast milk: Yes, in minute amounts.

Estrogens in large doses can suppress milk formation. Breast-feeding is considered to be safe during the use of estrogens. Malnourished mothers may have unacceptable decreases in protein and nitrogen in their breast milk if this drug is used while breast-feeding. Estrogens should NOT be used to try to stop breast milk formation after giving birth, as this may increase risk of blood clots.

Habit-Forming Potential: There has been some suggestion of estrogens having potential for psychological dependence and tolerance because of their mood-elevating properties, but clinical reports have not been presented.

Effects of Overdose: Nausea, vomiting, fluid retention, abnormal vaginal bleeding, breast enlargement and discomfort.

Possible Effects of Long-Term Use: High blood pressure, gallbladder disease with gallstone formation. Increased growth of benign fibroid tumors of the uterus reported with other estrogens. Several reports suggest possible association between the long-term use (10+ years) of estrogens and the development of cancer of the lining of the uterus. Further studies are needed to establish a definite cause-and-effect relationship (see Glossary). Prudence dictates that women who have a uterus should use estrogens only when symptoms justify it and with proper supervision.

Suggested Periodic Examinations While Taking This Drug (at physician's discretion)

Yearly mammography for ALL women who take this medicine and are more than 50 years old.

Regular (every 6 months) evaluation of the breasts and pelvic organs, including Pap smears.

Liver function tests as indicated.

▷ **While Taking This Drug, Observe the Following**

Foods: Avoid excessive use of salt if fluid retention occurs. Combined use of calcium and vitamin D can be a further step to help avoid osteoporosis.

Herbal Medicines or Minerals: Black cohosh appears to work by (1) suppressing luteinizing hormone; (2) binding to estrogen receptors in the pituitary and inhibiting luteinizing hormone release and (3) binding to estrogen receptors in the pituitary. The net effect is that this herb eases symptoms of menopause, but little is known about long-term use or heart and bone protective effects. This herb may interfere with the benefits of estrogen replacement therapy. Talk to your doctor before starting black cohosh if you are currently taking any form of estrogen. Use of St. John's wort, echinacea or ginkgo completely stopped or lowered the ability of sperm to penetrate eggs in one study. DO NOT use these herbs if you are using a conjugated estrogen product to augment mucous quality and help infertility. St. John's wort may also increase sun sensitivity.

Beverages: No restrictions. May be taken with milk.

▷ *Alcohol:* No interactions expected.

Tobacco Smoking: Some studies show that heavy smoking (15 or more cigarettes daily) in association with use of estrogen-containing oral contraceptives significantly increases risk of heart attack (coronary thrombosis). I advise everyone to stop smoking.

▷ *Other Drugs*

Estrogens *taken concurrently* with

- alendronate (Fosamax) have not been specifically studied but had beneficial effects in one part of a larger study using a different medicine. The combination of a different kind of estrogen used with alendronate is now approved in Canada.
- oral antidiabetic drugs (see Drug Classes) or oral blood-sugar-lowering medicines may cause loss of glucose control and high blood sugars.
- progestins (various) may increase risk of breast cancer versus estrogen use by itself.
- thyroid hormones may increase the bound (inactive) drug and require an increase in thyroid dose.
- tricyclic antidepressants (Elavil, Sinequan, etc.) may enhance their adverse effects and reduce their antidepressant effectiveness.
- vitamin C (ascorbic acid, various brands) in higher doses may result in increased estrogen effects—a lower dose of estrogens may be indicated if higher-dose vitamin C will be taken on an ongoing basis.
- warfarin (Coumadin) may cause alterations of prothrombin activity; increased doses may be needed, and more frequent INR testing is indicated.

The following drugs may decrease the effects of estrogens:

- carbamazepine (Tegretol).
- phenobarbital (various).
- phenytoin (Dilantin) or fosphenytoin (Cerebyx).
- primidone (Mysoline).
- rifampin (Rifadin, Rimactane).

Author's Note: The possible drug interactions above are those detailed for existing estrogens in the estrogen profile earlier in this book.

▷ *Driving, Hazardous Activities:* Usually no restrictions. Talk to your doctor for assessment of individual risk and for guidance regarding specific restrictions.

Aviation Note: Usually no restrictions, but watch for the rare occurrence of disturbed vision (curvature changes) and restrict activities accordingly. Consult a designated Aviation Medical Examiner.

Exposure to Sun: Caution—existing estrogens may cause photosensitivity (see Glossary).

Discontinuation: It's best to stop estrogens periodically to see if they are still needed (every three to six months). The dose is reduced gradually to prevent acute withdrawal hot flashes. Avoid continual, uninterrupted use of large doses. Stop altogether when a definite need for replacement therapy has ended. Ask your doctor for help.

TACRINE (TA kreen)

Please see the anti-Alzheimer's drug family profile.

TAMOXIFEN (ta MOX i fen)

Introduced: 1973   **Class:** Anticancer, chemotherapy, selective estrogen receptor modulator (SERM)   **Prescription:** USA: Yes   **Controlled Drug:** USA: No; Canada: No   **Available as Generic:** Yes

Brand Names: ✤Alpha-Tamoxifen, ✤Apo-Tamox, ✤Dom-Tamoxifen, Nolvadex, ✤Nolvadex-D, ✤Novo-Tamoxifen, ✤PMS-Tamoxifen, ✤Tamofen, ✤Tamone

---

BENEFITS versus RISKS

Possible Benefits	*Possible Risks*
DECREASED RISK OF BREAST CANCER	UTERINE CANCER
PREVENTION OF BREAST CANCER IN HIGH RISK FEMALES	Severe increase in tumor or bone pain, transient thrombophlebitis, pulmonary embolism
EFFECTIVE ADJUNCTIVE TREATMENT IN ADVANCED BREAST CANCER	Abnormally high blood calcium levels
MAY INCREASE THE CHANCES OF BREAST CONSERVATION	Eye changes:corneal opacities, retinal injury
ADDITION OF TAMOXIFEN TO LUMPECTOMY AND RADIATION TREATMENT REDUCES OCCURRENCE OF INVASIVE BREAST CANCER IN WOMEN WITH DUCTAL CARCINOMA IN SITU	

▷ **Principal Uses**

As a Single Drug Product: Uses currently included in FDA-approved labeling: (1) An alternative to estrogens and androgens (male sex hormones) to treat advanced breast cancer in postmenopausal women; (2) treats advanced breast cancer in women that has spread (metastasized) from a prior site; (3) used to delay or prevent the recurrence of breast cancer in high risk females (47% reduced occurrence of a second breast cancer with 5 years of treatment).

Other (unlabeled) generally accepted uses: (1) May have a role in treating cancer of the liver or lung; (2) used to stimulate ovulation in premenopausal women with infertility; (3) used to treat rare desmoid tumors; (4) helps prevent osteoporosis in women in whom the drug is being used to prevent the recurrence of cancer; (5) can help retroperitoneal fibrosis; (6) could have a role in treating tenderness and swelling of male breast tissue (gynecomastia) of unknown cause (idiopathic); (7) in a study of 1,804 women, addition of tamoxifen to radiation therapy and lumpectomy in women with ductal carcinoma in situ led to a 43% decrease in invasive breast cancer in the same breast or in the opposite breast versus a dummy pill or placebo.

Author's Note: Tamoxifen reduced breast cancer rates by almost half in a very large (13,388 patients) cancer prevention study performed by the National Cancer Institute over a period of 6 years. The FDA has

launched a new oncology tools website. Visit this at www.fda.gov/cder/cancer. There is a listing of cancer medicine trials on the World Wide Web at http://cancertrials.nci.nih.gov. The STAR (Study of Tamoxifen and Raloxifene) trial is underway. This is a National Cancer Institute study evaluating 20,000 women who are at risk for breast cancer. They will be given either 20 mg per day of tamoxifen or 60 mg of raloxifene each day for five years. For more information, you can reach the National Cancer Institute at 1-800-422-6237.

How This Drug Works: It is thought that by blocking the uptake of estradiol (estrogen), this drug removes or reduces a stimulus to breast cancer cells. It acts as a selective estrogen receptor modulator, or SERM.

Available Dosage Forms and Strengths
Tablets — 10 mg, 20 mg
Tablets (Canada) — 15.2 mg, 30.4 mg

▷ **Usual Adult Dosage Ranges:** *Breast cancer:* A loading dose of 40 mg four times a day for one day then 20 mg daily is used. The range of ongoing doses is from 20 to 40 mg. Doses more than 20 mg are given in equal doses twice a day. Dosing is continued for 5 years. *Prevention of breast cancer:* At this time, both age and risk factors are used to determine the BENEFITS versus RISKS of giving the medicine. Health care professionals may obtain a *Gail Model Risk Assessment Tool by calling 1-800-544-2007. For reduction of breast cancer in high-risk women:* 20 mg daily for five years is given. The STAR trial is expected to provide further information.

Note: Actual dose and schedule must be determined for each patient individually.

Conditions Requiring Dosing Adjustments
Liver Function: Dose decreases are not defined in liver disease.
Kidney Function: Dose decreases are not thought to be needed in mild to moderate kidney disease. No studies are available in severe disease.

▷ **Dosing Instructions:** The tablet may be crushed and taken either on an empty stomach or with food. If you forget a dose: Take the missed dose as soon as you remember it, unless it's nearly time for your next dose—if that is the case, skip the missed dose and take the next dose right on schedule. DO NOT double up on doses. Talk with your doctor if you find yourself missing doses—there are effective beeper-based systems to help you remember your medicine.

Usual Duration of Use: Use on a regular schedule for 4 to 10 weeks usually determines effectiveness in controlling growth and spread of advanced breast cancer. In the presence of bone involvement, treatment for several months may be required to evaluate effectiveness. Ongoing use for prevention of breast cancer still requires careful examinations and long-term use. Ongoing use (months to years) requires physician supervision and periodic evaluation.

Typical Treatment Goals and Measurements (Outcomes and Markers)
Breast cancer: Treatment of existing cancer seeks to attain a complete remission. The minimum goal is to shrink (regress) the size of the tumor and decrease the probability of spread. Checks of coagulation (such as clotting factor assay) can help define how activated the coagulation system has

become. In breast cancer prophylaxis, the goal is to prevent breast cancer in females who carry significant risk factors for breast cancer.

▷ **This Drug Should Not Be Taken If**
- you had a serious allergic or adverse reaction to it before.
- you have active phlebitis.
- you have a significant deficiency of white blood cells or blood platelets.
- you are pregnant.

▷ **Inform Your Physician Before Taking This Drug If**
- you have a history of thrombophlebitis or pulmonary embolism
- you take birth control pills.
- you have a history of abnormally high blood calcium levels.
- you have a history of any type of blood cell or bone marrow disorder.
- you have cataracts or other visual impairment.
- you have impaired liver function.
- you have high cholesterol.
- you plan to have surgery in the near future.

Possible Side Effects (natural, expected and unavoidable drug actions)
Hot flashes—frequent.
Fluid retention, weight gain.

▷ **Possible Adverse Effects** (unusual, unexpected and infrequent reactions)
If any of the following develop, consult your physician promptly for guidance.
Mild Adverse Effects
Allergic reactions: skin rash.
Visual impairment—infrequent.
Increased calcium—infrequent.
Headache, dizziness, drowsiness, depression, fatigue, confusion—infrequent.
Nausea, vomiting—frequent.
Itching in genital area, loss of hair—infrequent.
Serious Adverse Effects
Initial "flare" of severe pain in tumor or involved bone—possible.
Development of thrombophlebitis, risk of pulmonary embolism—increased risk.
Eye changes: corneal opacities, retinal injury—case reports.
Delusions—rare.
Increased uterine cancer risk (increased karyopyknotic index of vaginal epithelium)—possible, but many researchers now believe that the benefits far outweigh the risks.
Development of abnormally high blood calcium levels—possible.
Transient decreases in white blood cells and blood platelets—frequent.
Neutropenia or decrease in all blood cells (pancytopenia)—case reports.
Liver toxicity—rare.

▷ **Possible Effects on Sexual Function:** Premenopausal—altered timing and pattern of menstruation. Postmenopausal—vaginal bleeding, decreased libido.
Abnormal and painful erections (priapism)—case reports.
This drug may be effective in treating the following conditions:
- male infertility due to abnormally low sperm counts.
- male breast enlargement and tenderness.
- chronic female breast pain (mastodynia).

Possible Effects on Laboratory Tests

Complete blood cell counts: decreased red cells, hemoglobin, white cells and platelets.

Blood calcium level: increased.

Blood thyroid hormone levels: T3, T4 and free T4 increased.

Liver function tests: increased liver enzyme (AST/GOT), increased bilirubin (one case report).

Sperm count: increased or decreased.

CAUTION

1. If this drug is used prior to your menopause, it may induce ovulation and predispose to pregnancy. Since this drug should not be used during pregnancy, some method of contraception (other than oral contraceptives) is advised.

2. Do not take any form of estrogen while taking this drug; estrogens can inhibit tamoxifen's effectiveness.

3. Tamoxifen has been shown to cause an increased risk of uterine cancer. Women who have received or are receiving this drug should have regular gynecological examinations. Report menstrual irregularity, abnormal vaginal bleeding or vaginal discharge, pelvic pain or pressure promptly to your doctor.

4. High risk females in the BCPT were defined as a five-year predicted risk greater than 1.67%. The model used (Gail Model) can be obtained by your health care professional from Zeneca by calling 1-800-345-4334 or by calling 1-800-544-2007. Even though this medicine is taken, all risk of breast cancer is NOT removed, and the usual detection and screening measures should be continued.

▷ **Advisability of Use During Pregnancy**

Pregnancy Category: D. See Pregnancy Risk Categories at the back of this book.

Animal studies: No birth defects due to this drug reported.

Human studies: Adequate studies of pregnant women are not available.

This drug can have estrogenic effects. It should not be used during pregnancy.

Advisability of Use If Breast-Feeding

Presence of this drug in breast milk: Unknown.

Avoid drug or refrain from nursing.

Habit-Forming Potential: None.

Effects of Overdose: Severe extension of the pharmacological effects.

Possible Effects of Long-Term Use: Development of abnormally high blood calcium levels.

Suggested Periodic Examinations While Taking This Drug (at physician's discretion)

Complete blood cell counts.

Measurements of blood calcium levels.

Complete eye examinations if impaired vision occurs.

Women who have been given or are now receiving tamoxifen must have regular gynecological examinations.

▷ **While Taking This Drug, Observe the Following**

Foods: No restrictions.

Herbal Medicines or Minerals: Some patients use echinacea to attempt to boost their immune systems. Unfortunately, use of echinacea is not recommended in people with damaged immune systems. This herb may also actually weaken any immune system if it is used too often or for too long a time. Black cohosh estrogenic effects may have an undesirable effect on tamoxifen and combination in not advisable. Very early research from the University of Illinois at Chicago (www.uic.edu/depts/paff/opa/releases/2001/tamoxandsoy release.html) in rats shows that a soy rich diet may enhance the effects of tamoxifen. Talk to your doctor to find out about further research on soy and this March 2001 study.

Beverages: No restrictions. May be taken with milk.

▷ *Alcohol:* No interactions expected.

Tobacco Smoking: No interactions expected. I advise everyone to quit smoking.

Marijuana Smoking: Animal studies show an increased suppression of the immune system; significance in humans is not known.

▷ *Other Drugs*

The following drugs may *decrease* the effects of tamoxifen:
- estrogens.
- oral contraceptives (those that contain estrogens).

Tamoxifen *taken concurrently* with
- allopurinol (Zyloprim) may worsen allopurinol toxicity to the liver.
- clopidogrel (Plavix) may result in higher than expected tamoxifen levels; no reports of adverse effects from this reaction have been made, but caution is advised.
- cyclophosphamide (Cytoxan) may increase blood clot (thromboembolism) risk.
- cyclosporine (Sandimmune) may increase cyclosporine levels and cause toxicity.
- medicines that inhibit CYP2C9 (such as fluconazole, fluvastatin and zafirlukast) may lead to increased tamoxifen levels—talk to your doctor about this.
- methotrexate (Mexate, Rheumatrex) may increase blood clot (thromboembolism) risk.
- mitomycin will cause increased risk of hemolytic uremic syndrome.
- pneumococcal and perhaps other vaccines will blunt the vaccine's immune response (benefit).
- ritonavir (Norvir) and perhaps other protease inhibitors (see Drug Classes) may lead to toxicity.
- warfarin (Coumadin) presents an increased risk of bleeding; increased frequency of INR (prothrombin time or protime) testing is needed.

▷ *Driving, Hazardous Activities:* This drug may cause dizziness or drowsiness. Restrict activities as necessary.

Aviation Note: The use of this drug *may be a disqualification* for piloting. Consult a designated Aviation Medical Examiner.

Exposure to Sun: No restrictions.

TAMSULOSIN (TAM su low sin)

Introduced: 1997 **Class:** Antiprostatism, alpha 1 (A) blocker **Prescription:** USA: Yes **Controlled Drug:** USA: No **Available as Generic:** No **Brand Name:** Flomax

---

BENEFITS versus RISKS

Possible Benefits	*Possible Risks*
MODEST IMPROVEMENT IN BENIGN PROSTATIC HYPERPLASIA ONCE-DAILY DOSING More selective for the genitourinary tract than other therapies	Headache Runny nose

---

▷ **Principal Uses**

 As a Single Drug Product: Uses currently included in FDA-approved labeling: Treats symptomatic benign prostatic hyperplasia (BPH).

 Other (unlabeled) generally accepted uses: None at present.

How This Drug Works: Relaxes smooth muscle around the bladder neck and prostate (by binding to a very specific alpha 1A receptor), allowing opening of the urethra and increased urine flow.

Available Dosage Forms and Strengths

 Capsules — 0.4 mg

▷ **Usual Adult Dosage Ranges:** Started with 0.4 mg once daily. If response is not acceptable after 2 to 4 weeks, the dose can be increased to 0.8 mg once a day. **Note: Actual dose and schedule must be determined for each patient individually.**

Conditions Requiring Dosing Adjustments

 Liver Function: No dose changes needed in moderate liver disease.

 Kidney Function: Dose changes not needed in those with creatinine clearance (see Glossary) as low as 10 ml/min. Not studied in more compromised kidney failure patients.

Dosing Instructions: Best if not taken with food since this decreases absorption. Take this medicine half an hour before the same meal every day. If you forget a dose: Take the missed dose as soon as you remember it, unless it is nearly time for your next dose—if that is the case, omit the missed dose and take the next scheduled dose right on schedule. DO NOT double doses. Do NOT chew, crush or break the capsules. If you forget this medicine for several days, treatment should be resumed with the 0.4 mg dose and dose increased as previously required and scheduled.

Usual Duration of Use: Benefits may be seen very quickly with the first dose and with symptoms resolving within the first week of regular treatment. Use on a regular schedule for 14 weeks may be needed to see this drug's peak benefit.

Typical Treatment Goals and Measurements (Outcomes and Markers)

 BPH: Urologists use improvement in urinary flow as well as subjective measures such as relief of difficulty urinating and lowered feeling of urgency. There is a score set called the American Urological Association (AUA) symptom scores as well as the Boyarsky symptom scores. Digital rectal examination for prostate cancer should be done periodically.

Possible Advantages of This Drug: May give you symptomatic relief of benign prostatic hyperplasia (BPH) without surgery. Goes to work quickly (faster onset) than previously available medicines. No clinically significant drug interactions.

▷ **This Drug Should Not Be Taken If**
- you had an allergic reaction to it previously or if you are a woman or child.

▷ **Inform Your Physician Before Taking This Drug If**
- you have impaired liver function or liver disease.
- you have not had prostate cancer ruled out and this is a new prescription.
- you have kidney problems of any nature.

Possible Side Effects (natural, expected and unavoidable drug actions)
Excessive lowering of blood pressure on standing (orthostatic hypotension).

▷ **Possible Adverse Effects** (unusual, unexpected and infrequent reactions)
If any of the following develop, consult your physician promptly for guidance.

Mild Adverse Effects
Allergic reactions: skin rash, hives—rare.
Amblyopia—rare.
Runny nose—may be frequent.
Headache or dizziness—may be frequent.
Back pain (up to 8% in one trial).
Nausea or diarrhea—infrequent.
Slight decreases in red blood cell counts or hemoglobin—possible.
Increased liver function tests—rare.

Serious Adverse Effects
Allergic reactions: hypersensitivity reactions—case reports.

Possible Effects on Sexual Function: Abnormal ejaculation (up to 18%) and rare cases of decreases libido have been reported.

Possible Delayed Adverse Effects: Not reported.

Possible Effects on Laboratory Tests
Slight decreases in hemoglobin and red blood cells.

CAUTION
1. A digital rectal exam and other prostate cancer exams are prudent before this medicine is started. PSA will be falsely decreased by this medicine.

Precautions for Use
By Infants and Children: Safety and effectiveness for infants and children are not established.
By Those Over 60 Years of Age: No specific precautions other than changes related to decreased liver function.

▷ **Advisability of Use During Pregnancy**
Pregnancy Category: B. See Pregnancy Risk Categories at the back of this book.
Human studies: Contraindicated in women.

Advisability of Use If Breast-Feeding
Unknown, but tamsulosin is NOT indicated for women.

Habit-Forming Potential: None.

Effects of Overdose: Extension effects of the pharmacological and adverse effects.

Possible Effects of Long-Term Use: Adverse effects of long-term use are similar to short-term use effects.

Suggested Periodic Examinations While Taking This Drug (at physician's discretion)

Patients should be monitored for signs and symptoms of orthostatic hypotension.

Patients should be monitored for improvement in symptoms of BPH.

While Taking This Drug, Observe the Following

Foods: This medicine is best taken on an empty stomach.

Herbal Medicines or Minerals: Saw palmetto works by anti-androgenic and anti-inflammatory actions. The combination of this herb and tamsulosin has not been studied, but both drugs appear to work by different mechanisms. Talk to your doctor before combining.

Beverages: No restrictions.

Alcohol: No restrictions.

Tobacco Smoking: No interactions expected. I advise everyone to quit smoking.

Marijuana Smoking: No interactions expected.

Other Drugs

Tamsulosin *taken concurrently* with

- beta blockers (see Drug Classes) may increase extent of first dose orthostatic hypotension. Caution is advised.
- cimetidine (Tagamet) may increase tamsulosin blood levels and extent of first dose orthostatic hypotension as well as dizziness. Caution is advised.
- medicines that change liver enzymes in the cytochrome P450 class. The specific enzymes involved in removing tamsulosin have not been fully characterized, but combining medicines that change that liver enzyme system may have an effect on tamsulosin levels. Caution is advised.
- warfarin (Coumadin) may change the effects of tamsulosin or warfarin. More frequent checks of INR and careful patient check for unexpected adverse effects are prudent.

▷ *Driving, Hazardous Activities:* No restrictions.

Aviation Note: No restrictions.

Exposure to Sun: No restrictions.

Special Storage Instructions: Keep at room temperature. Avoid exposure to extreme humidity.

TERAZOSIN (ter AY zoh sin)

Introduced: 1987   **Class:** Antihypertensive   **Prescription:** USA: Yes
Controlled Drug: USA: No   **Available as Generic:** Yes
Brand Names: ✿Apo-Terazosin, Hytrin, Novo-Terazosin

BENEFITS versus RISKS	
Possible Benefits	*Possible Risks*
EFFECTIVE TREATMENT OF MILD TO MODERATE HYPERTENSION	"First-dose" drop in blood pressure with fainting
LOWERED LOW-DENSITY LIPOPROTEINS AND TOTAL CHOLESTEROL	Fluid retention
LOWERED TRIGLYCERIDE LEVELS	
TREATS BENIGN PROSTATIC HYPERPLASIA	

Author's Note: Data from the ALLHAT trial found that alpha blockers such as this medicine are not drugs of first choice in high blood pressure. Information in this profile has been shortened for more widely used medicines.

TERBUTALINE (ter BYU ta leen)

Introduced: 1974 **Class:** Antiasthmatic, bronchodilator **Prescription:** USA: Yes **Controlled Drug:** USA: No; Canada: No **Available as Generic:** No
Brand Names: Brethaire, Brethine, Bricanyl, ✤Bricanyl Spacer, ✤Med-Broncodil

BENEFITS versus RISKS	
Possible Benefits	*Possible Risks*
VERY EFFECTIVE RELIEF OF BRONCHOSPASM	Increased blood pressure Fine hand tremor Irregular heart rhythm (with excessive use)

▷ **Principal Uses**

As a Single Drug Product: Uses currently included in FDA-approved labeling: Relieves acute bronchial asthma and reduces frequency and severity of chronic, recurrent asthmatic attacks.

Other (unlabeled) generally accepted uses: (1) May have a role in helping ease fetal distress in some patients; (2) used to help stop premature labor and continue pregnancies to more than 36 weeks; (3) an alternative to intravenous isoproterenol in therapy of status asthmaticus; (4) relieves reversible bronchospasm associated with chronic bronchitis and emphysema; (5) eases extended and painful erections (priapism).

How This Drug Works: Stimulates sympathetic nerve terminals dilating constricted bronchial tubes, improving the ability to breathe.

Available Dosage Forms and Strengths

Aerosol (per actuation) — 0.2 mg
Aerosol (Canada) (per actuation) — 0.25 mg
Injection — 1 mg/ml
Tablets — 2.5 mg, 5 mg

▷ **Usual Adult Dosage Ranges:** *Aerosol:* 0.4 mg taken in two separate inhalations 1 minute apart; repeat every 4 to 6 hours as needed.

Tablets: 2.5 to 5 mg taken every 6 hours. The total daily dose should not exceed 15 mg.

Use of the injectable has been undertaken with a MiniMed 404SP pump to give continuous under the skin (subcutaneous) doses of 50–100 micrograms per hour. This treatment has been started in hospitals and then continued in a nursing home or a home IV service until the pregnancy has continued for 37 weeks.

Note: Actual dose and schedule must be determined for each patient individually.

Conditions Requiring Dosing Adjustments

Liver Function: Extensively metabolized in the liver, but dosing guidelines in liver disease are not available.

Kidney Function: For patients with moderate to severe kidney failure, 50% of the usual dose can be taken at the usual time. In severe failure, the drug should not be used.

▷ **Dosing Instructions:** Tablets may be crushed and taken on an empty stomach or with food or milk. For aerosol, follow the written instructions carefully. Do not overuse. If you forget a dose: Use the inhaler as soon as you remember it, unless it's nearly time for your next dose—if that is the case, skip the missed dose and take the next dose right on schedule. Use the remaining doses for the day at evenly spaced dosing intervals, and then return to your usual schedule. Talk with your doctor if you find yourself missing doses. If you think your inhaler container (canister) is empty, get a bowl of cold water and place the canister in it—if the canister floats, there is no medicine left in it.

Usual Duration of Use: Individualized. Do not use beyond the time necessary to stop (terminate) episodes of asthma. Unlabeled use as a tocolytic in preterm labor often continues until 37 weeks of pregnancy.

Typical Treatment Goals and Measurements (Outcomes and Markers)

Asthma: Signs and symptoms of asthma such as difficulty breathing (dyspnea), cough, light-headedness and wheezing should lessen. Forced expiratory volume at one second (FEV1) and/or peak expiratory flow rate (PEF) are checked by most pulmonologists as indicators of successful treatment. If the usual benefit is not realized, after the time to peak effect (see above) was expected, call your doctor.

Possible Advantages of This Drug: Rapid onset of action. Long duration of action. Highly effective relief of asthma.

▷ **This Drug Should Not Be Taken If**
- you had an allergic reaction to any form of it previously.
- you currently have an irregular heart rhythm.
- you took a monoamine oxidase (MAO) type A inhibitor (see Drug Classes) in the last 14 days.

▷ **Inform Your Physician Before Taking This Drug If**
- you are overly sensitive to other drugs that stimulate the sympathetic nervous system.
- you are currently using epinephrine (Adrenalin, Primatene Mist, etc.) to relieve asthmatic breathing.
- you have a seizure disorder.
- you have liver or kidney failure.
- you have any type of heart or circulatory disorder, especially high blood pressure or coronary heart disease.
- you have diabetes or an overactive thyroid gland (hyperthyroidism).
- you are taking any form of digitalis or any stimulant drug.

Possible Side Effects (natural, expected and unavoidable drug actions)

Aerosol—dryness or irritation of mouth or throat, altered taste. Tablet—nervousness, tremor, palpitation.

▷ **Possible Adverse Effects** (unusual, unexpected and infrequent reactions)

If any of the following develop, consult your physician promptly for guidance.

Mild Adverse Effects

Allergic reactions: skin rashes.

Headache, dizziness, drowsiness, restlessness, insomnia—infrequent.

Rapid, pounding heartbeat; increased sweating; muscle cramps in arms and legs—infrequent to frequent.

Nausea, heartburn, vomiting—rare with oral form, frequent with IV.

Increased blood sugar—frequent (40% abnormal one-hour glucose).

Serious Adverse Effects

Rapid or irregular heart rhythm, intensification of angina, increased blood pressure—infrequent.

Chest pain with heartbeat changes (ST depression)—reported when oral and intravenous therapy is combined in preterm labor.

Lowered blood calcium or potassium (especially with intravenous use)—possible.

Liver toxicity—case reports.

Severe lowering of blood pressure (hypotension)—case reports.

Increased blood sugar—infrequent.

Ketoacidosis—case reports.

Fluid around the lungs (pulmonary edema)—case reports.

▷ **Possible Effects on Sexual Function:** None reported.

Natural Diseases or Disorders That May Be Activated by This Drug

Latent coronary artery disease, diabetes or high blood pressure.

Possible Effects on Laboratory Tests

Blood total cholesterol and LDL cholesterol levels: no effect.

Blood HDL cholesterol level: increased.

Blood triglyceride levels: no effect.

Blood thyroid hormone levels: T3 increased; T4 decreased; free T4 no effect.

Glucose tolerance test: abnormal test.

Liver function tests: may be elevated.

CAUTION

1. Combination of this drug by aerosol with beclomethasone aerosol (Beclovent, Vanceril) may increase risk of fluorocarbon propellant (being phased out) toxicity. Best to use this aerosol 20 to 30 minutes before beclomethasone aerosol. This reduces toxicity risk and will help beclomethasone get into the lungs.

2. **Avoid excessive use of aerosol inhalation.** Excessive or prolonged inhalation use can reduce effectiveness and cause serious heart rhythm disturbances, including cardiac arrest.

3. Do not use this drug with epinephrine. These two drugs may be used alternately, allowing 4 hours between doses.

4. If you do not respond to your usually effective dose, ask your doctor for help. Do not increase the size or frequency of the dose without your physician's approval.

Precautions for Use

By Infants and Children: Manufacturer DOES NOT recommend use in those under 12 years of age.

By Those Over 60 Years of Age: Avoid excessive and continual use. If acute asthma is not relieved promptly, other drugs will be needed. Watch for nervousness, palpitations, irregular heart rhythm and muscle tremors. Use with extreme caution if you have hardening of the arteries, heart disease or high blood pressure.

▷ **Advisability of Use During Pregnancy**

    Pregnancy Category: B. See Pregnancy Risk Categories at the back of this book.

    Animal studies: No significant birth defects reported in mouse and rat studies.

    Human studies: Adequate studies of pregnant women are not available.

       Use only if clearly needed. Ask your physician for guidance.

Advisability of Use If Breast-Feeding

    Presence of this drug in breast milk: Yes.

    Monitor nursing infant closely, and discontinue drug or nursing if adverse effects develop.

Habit-Forming Potential: None.

Effects of Overdose: Nervousness, palpitation, rapid heart rate, sweating, headache, tremor, vomiting, chest pain.

Possible Effects of Long-Term Use: Loss of effectiveness. See "CAUTION" above.

Suggested Periodic Examinations While Taking This Drug (at physician's discretion)

    Blood pressure measurements.

    Evaluation of heart status.

▷ **While Taking This Drug, Observe the Following**

    Foods: No restrictions.

    Herbal Medicines or Minerals: Using St. John's wort, ma huang, ephedrine-like compounds or kola while taking this medicine may result in unacceptable central nervous system stimulation. Fir or pine needle oil should NOT be used by asthmatics. Ephedra alone does carry a German Commission E monograph indication for asthma treatment. If you are allergic to plants in the Asteraceae family (aster, chrysanthemum, daisy or ragweed), you may also be allergic to echinacea, chamomile, feverfew and St. John's wort. Since part of the way ginseng works may be as an MAO inhibitor, do not combine ginseng with terbutaline.

    Beverages: Avoid excessive use of caffeine-containing beverages: coffee, tea, cola, chocolate.

▷   *Alcohol:* No interactions expected.

    Tobacco Smoking: No interactions expected. I advise everyone to quit smoking.

▷   *Other Drugs*

       Terbutaline ***taken concurrently*** with

- monoamine oxidase (MAO) type A inhibitors may cause excessive increase in blood pressure and undesirable heart stimulation (see Drug Classes).
- succinylcholine (Anectine) may lead to increased neuromuscular blockade which may require neostigmine.
- theophylline (Theo-Dur, others) may cause decreased theophylline effectiveness.

       The following drugs may ***decrease*** the effects of terbutaline:

- beta blockers (see Drug Classes)—may impair terbutaline's effectiveness.

▷   *Driving, Hazardous Activities:* Usually no restrictions. Use caution if excessive nervousness or dizziness occurs.

    Aviation Note: The use of this drug ***is a disqualification*** for piloting. Consult a designated Aviation Medical Examiner.

    Exposure to Sun: No restrictions.

    Heavy Exercise or Exertion: Use caution—excessive exercise can induce asthma in some patients.

TESTOSTOSTERONE (Tes TOS tur own)

Other Names: Chlorotrianisene, conjugated estrogens, esterified estrogens, estradiol, estriol, estrone, estropipate, quinestrol

Introduced: 2000 (Gel)   **Class:** Male sex hormone   **Prescription:** USA: Yes   **Controlled Drug:** USA: No; Canada: No   **Available as Generic:** USA: No; Canada: No

Brand Names: AndroGel 1%, Andriol, Androderm, Testoderm
Author's Note: Information in this profile will be broadened once more data and outcomes are available.

TETRACYCLINE ANTIBIOTIC FAMILY (te trah SI kleen)

Other Names: Doxycycline, tetracycline

Introduced: 1953, 1967   **Class:** Antibiotic, tetracyclines   **Prescription:** USA: Yes   **Controlled Drug:** USA: No; Canada: No   **Available as Generic:** Yes

Brand Names: Doxycycline: ✿Apo-Doxy, ✿Apo-Doxy-Tabs, Atridox (gum line delivery form), ✿Doryx, Doryx, Doxy Caps, Doxychel, ✿Doxycin, Doxy-Lemmon, Doxy 100, Doxy Tabs, Doxy 200, Monodox, ✿Novo-Doxylin, Periostat, Vibramycin, Vibra-Tabs, ✿Vibra-Tabs C-Pak, Tetracycline: Achromycin, Achromycin Ophthalmic, Achromycin V, ✿Acrocidin, Actisite, ✿Apo-Tetra, Aureomycin, Bristacycline, Contimycin, Cyclinex, Cyclopar, Lemtrex, ✿Medicycline, Mysteclin-F [CD], ✿Neo-Tetrine, ✿Nor-Tet, ✿Novo-Tetra, ✿Nu-Tetra, Panmycin, Retet, Robitet, SK-Tetracycline, Sumycin, Teline, Tetra-C, Tetracap, Tetra-Con, Tetracyn, Tetralan, Tetram, Tetrex-F, Tropicycline

BENEFITS versus RISKS	
Possible Benefits	*Possible Risks*
EFFECTIVE TREATMENT OF INFECTIONS DUE TO SUSCEPTIBLE BACTERIA AND PROTOZOA	ALLERGIC REACTIONS, MILD TO SEVERE: ANAPHYLAXIS, DRUG-INDUCED HEPATITIS
	Drug-induced colitis
	Superinfections (bacterial or fungal)
	Blood cell disorders: hemolytic anemia, abnormally low white cell and platelet counts
	Kidney toxicity

▷ **Principal Uses**

As a Single Drug Product: Uses currently included in FDA-approved labeling: (1) Treats a broad range of infections caused by susceptible bacteria and protozoa (short-term use); (2) treats severe, resistant pustular acne (long-term use) (tetracycline); (3) used in a sustained-release form (Actisite) to treat gum disease (periodontitis) in adults (tetracycline) and a new doxycycline form (Periostat) is used to treat periodontitis; (4) doxycycline treats syphilis in penicillin-allergic people; (5) helpful in acne; (6) helps prevent malaria in travelers; (7) tetracycline is the drug of choice for cholera; (8) doxycycline is of use in anthrax, brucellosis, cholera, and plague.

Other (unlabeled) generally accepted uses: (1) Combination antibiotic treatment of duodenal ulcers caused by Helicobacter pylori; (2) used in vaginal and vulval cysts (Gartner's) and in vaginal hydrocele; (3) topical tetracycline is useful in chronic eye problems (blepharitis); (4) treats cancer (malignant) fluid (pericardial effusion) buildup around the heart; (5) has a role in acne rosacea in decreasing the number of papules or nodules; (7) doxycycline: a) treats early Lyme disease used to treat stage one Lyme disease (new data found that 87% of people who took doxycycline within 72 hours of a tick bite DID NOT develop Lyme disease; (b) treats sexual assault victims; (c) treats prostatitis; (d) can help in some cases of PMS; (e) may treat some cases of male infertility of unexplained origin; (f) helps treat rheumatoid arthritis.

As a Combination Drug Product [CD]: Tetracycline is available combined with amphotericin B, an antifungal antibiotic that is provided to reduce the risk of developing an overgrowth of yeast organisms (superinfection) of the gastrointestinal tract.

How These Drugs Work: Prevent growth and multiplication of susceptible organisms by interfering with formation of essential proteins. Periostat seems to work by its anticolligenase and anti-inflammatory properties.

Available Dosage Forms and Strengths
   Doxycycline:
               Capsules — 50 mg, 100 mg
          Capsules, coated pellets — 100 mg
        Capsule, delayed release — 100 mg
            Injection (per vial) — 100 mg, 200 mg
            Oral suspension — 25 mg/5 ml
                   Syrup — 50 mg/5 ml
               Tablets — 50 mg, 100 mg
   Tetracycline:
               Capsules — 100 mg, 250 mg, 500 mg
               Ointment — 3%
        Ointment, ophthalmic — 10 mg/g
   Periodontal fiber (per fiber) — 12.7 mg
            Solution, topical — 2.2 mg/ml
        Suspension, ophthalmic — 10 mg/ml
            Suspension, oral — 125 mg/5 ml
               Tablets — 250 mg, 500 mg

▷ **Usual Adult Dosage Ranges:**
   Doxycycline: 100 mg every 12 hours the first day and then 100 mg once daily. Some severe infections may require ongoing therapy of 100 mg every 12 hours. Total daily dose should not exceed 300 mg.
   Tetracycline: 250 to 500 mg every 6 hours, or 500 to 1,000 mg every 12 hours. The total daily dose should not exceed 4,000 mg (4 g). **Note: Actual dose and schedule must be determined for each patient individually.**

Typical Treatment Goals and Measurements (Outcomes and Markers)
   Infections: The most commonly used measures of serious infections are white blood cell counts and differentials (the kind of blood cells that occur

most often in your blood), and temperature. Many clinicians look for positive changes in 24–48 hours. NEVER stop an antibiotic because you start to feel better. For many infections, a full 14 days is REQUIRED to kill the bacteria. The goals and time frame (see peak benefits above) should be discussed with you when the prescription is written.

Conditions Requiring Dosing Adjustments

Liver Function: Doxycycline: Patients with both liver and kidney compromise should have the dose decreased. Drug can cause liver problems, and a benefit-to-risk decision should be made for people with liver disease.

Tetracycline: Is a possible cause of hepatoxicity. A benefit-to-risk decision should be made for patients with compromised livers to use this drug. Daily maximum in liver disease is 1 g.

Kidney Function: Patients with mild to moderate kidney failure can take the usual dose every 8 to 12 hours. Patients with moderate to severe kidney failure take the usual dose every 12 to 24 hours. In severe kidney failure (creatinine clearance less than 10 ml/min), tetracycline should be avoided.

Malnutrition: Doxycycline: Lower than expected levels may occur in patients with malnutrition. If clinical progress is not as expected, the dose may need to be increased.

▷ **Dosing Instructions:** The tablet may be crushed and the capsule opened and preferably taken on an empty stomach, 1 hour before or 2 hours after eating. However, to reduce stomach irritation, it may be taken with crackers that contain insignificant amounts of iron, calcium, magnesium or zinc. Avoid all dairy products for 2 hours before and after taking this drug. (Unlike other tetracyclines, doxycycline absorption is not significantly changed by food or milk.) Take at the same time each day, with a full glass of water. Take the full course prescribed. If you forget a dose: Take the missed dose as soon as you remember it, unless it's nearly time for your next dose—if that is the case, skip the missed dose and take the next dose right on schedule. DO NOT double up on doses. Taking your medicine exactly as prescribed will get the best results. Talk with your doctor if you find yourself missing doses.

Usual Duration of Use: The time required to control the acute infection and be free of fever and symptoms for 48 hours. This varies with the nature of the infection. Long-term use (months to years, as for treatment of acne) requires supervision and periodic evaluation. Treatment of stage one Lyme disease requires 3 to 4 weeks in adults even though one doxycycline dose may prevent a high percentage of Lyme infections.

▷ **These Drugs Should Not Be Taken If**
  • you are allergic to any tetracycline (see Drug Classes).
  • you are pregnant or breast-feeding.
  • you have severe liver disease.

▷ **Inform Your Physician Before Taking This Drug If**
  • it is prescribed for a child under 8 years of age.
  • you have a history of liver or kidney disease.
  • you have systemic lupus erythematosus.
  • you are taking any penicillin drug.
  • you are taking any anticoagulant drug.
  • you will have surgery with general anesthesia.

Possible Side Effects (natural, expected and unavoidable drug actions)
> Superinfections (see Glossary), often due to yeast organisms—these can occur in the mouth, intestinal tract, rectum and/or vagina, resulting in rectal and vaginal itching. Tooth discoloration (when used in children less than 8 years old). Metallic taste.

▷ **Possible Adverse Effects** (unusual, unexpected and infrequent reactions)
> **If any of the following develop, consult your physician promptly for guidance.**

Mild Adverse Effects
> Allergic reactions: skin rash, hives, itching of hands and feet, swelling of face or extremities.
> Loss of appetite, stomach irritation, taste disorders, nausea, vomiting, diarrhea—infrequent.
> Warts—very rare and of questionable causality (tetracycline).
> Irritation of mouth or tongue, "black tongue," sore throat, abdominal cramping or pain—infrequent.

Serious Adverse Effects
> Allergic reactions: anaphylactic reaction (see Glossary), asthma, fever, swollen joints and lymph glands.
> Serious skin problems (Stevens-Johnson syndrome, Jarisch-Herxheimer reaction)—case reports.
> Drug-induced hepatitis with jaundice—case reports.
> Permanent discoloration and/or malformation of teeth if taken by children under 8, including unborn child and infant.
> Drug-induced colitis, myasthenia gravis or pancreatitis—case reports.
> Worsening of existing systemic lupus erythematosus—case reports.
> Rare blood cell disorders: hemolytic anemia (see Glossary); abnormally low white blood cell count, causing fever and infections; abnormally low blood platelet count—case reports.
> Impairment of blood clotting—case reports.
> Increased intracranial pressure (pseudotumor cerebri) or kidney problems—rare (tetracycline).
> Drug-induced porphyria, esophageal ulcers or low blood potassium—case reports (tetracycline).

▷ **Possible Effects on Sexual Function:** Decreased effectiveness of oral contraceptives taken concurrently (several case reports of pregnancy). Decreased male fertility—case reports (tetracycline).

▷ **Adverse Effects That May Mimic Natural Diseases or Disorders**
> Drug-induced hepatitis may suggest viral hepatitis.

Natural Diseases or Disorders That May Be Activated by This Drug
> Systemic lupus erythematosus.

Possible Effects on Laboratory Tests
> Complete blood cell counts: decreased red cells, hemoglobin, white cells and platelets; increased eosinophils (allergic reaction).
> Blood lupus erythematosus (LE) cells: positive.
> Blood amylase level: increased (toxic effect in pregnant women).
> Liver function tests: increased enzymes (ALT/GPT, AST/GOT, alkaline phosphatase) or bilirubin.

Kidney function tests: increased blood creatinine and urea nitrogen (BUN) levels (kidney damage).

Urine sugar tests: false-positive results with Benedict's solution and Clinitest.

CAUTION

1. Antacids, dairy products and preparations containing aluminum, bismuth, calcium, iron, magnesium or zinc can prevent adequate absorption and reduce effectiveness significantly.
2. Troublesome and persistent diarrhea can occur. If diarrhea persists for more than 24 hours, call your doctor.
3. If general anesthesia is required while taking this drug, the choice of anesthetic agent must be selected carefully to prevent kidney damage.

Precautions for Use

By Infants and Children: If possible, tetracyclines should not be given to children under 8 years of age because of the risk of permanent discoloration and deformity of the teeth. Rarely, infants may develop increased intracranial pressure within the first 4 days of receiving this drug. Tetracyclines may inhibit normal bone growth and development.

By Those Over 60 Years of Age: Dose must be carefully individualized based on kidney function. Natural skin changes may predispose to severe and prolonged itching reactions in the genital and anal regions.

▷ **Advisability of Use During Pregnancy**

Pregnancy Category: D. See Pregnancy Risk Categories at the back of this book.

Animal studies: Tetracycline causes limb defects in rats, rabbits and chickens.

Human studies: Information from studies of pregnant women indicates that this drug can cause impaired development and discoloration of teeth and other developmental defects.

It is advisable to avoid these drugs completely during entire pregnancy.

Advisability of Use If Breast-Feeding

Presence of these drugs in breast milk: Yes.

Avoid drug or refrain from nursing.

Habit-Forming Potential: None.

Effects of Overdose: Stomach burning, nausea, vomiting, diarrhea.

Possible Effects of Long-Term Use: Superinfections; impairment of bone marrow, liver or kidney function—rare.

Suggested Periodic Examinations While Taking This Drug (at physician's discretion)

Complete blood cell counts.

Liver and kidney function tests.

During extended use, sputum and stool examinations may detect early superinfection due to yeast organisms.

▷ **While Taking This Drug, Observe the Following**

Foods: Avoid cheeses, yogurt, ice cream, iron-fortified cereals and supplements and meats for 2 hours before and after taking this drug.

Herbal Medicines or Minerals: Some patients use echinacea to attempt to boost their immune systems. Use of echinacea is not recommended in people with damaged immune systems. This herb may also actually weaken any immune system if it is used too often or for too long a time. No data exist for combination use with tetracyclines. Mistletoe has been used in similar fashion and there are also NO DATA for combining it with tetracyclines. Calcium, zinc and iron can combine with these drugs and reduce absorption significantly. St. John's wort and this medicine can intensify reactions to the sun—extreme caution is advised.

Beverages: Avoid all forms of milk for 2 hours before and after taking.

▷   *Alcohol:* Reduces doxycycline blood levels. Alcohol should be avoided with doxycycline and perhaps another tetracycline substituted, particularly for those who have drinking problems. Alcohol is also best avoided if you have active liver disease.

Tobacco Smoking: No interactions expected. I advise everyone to quit smoking.

▷   *Other Drugs*

Tetracyclines may ***increase*** the effects of
- cyclosporine (Sandimmune, Neoral).
- digoxin (Lanoxin) and cause digitalis toxicity.
- lithium (Eskalith, Lithane, etc.) and increase the risk of lithium toxicity.
- oral anticoagulants such as warfarin (Coumadin) and make it necessary to reduce their dose; increased INR (prothrombin time or protime) testing is needed.

Tetracyclines may ***decrease*** the effects of
- birth control pills (oral contraceptives) and impair their effectiveness in preventing pregnancy.
- penicillins (see Drug Classes) and impair their effectiveness in treating infections.

Tetracyclines ***taken concurrently*** with
- furosemide (Lasix) increases blood urea nitrogen (BUN).
- isotretinoin (Accutane) may worsen tetracycline-caused increased intracranial pressure and cause additive toxicity.
- methoxyflurane anesthesia may impair kidney function.
- theophylline (Theo-Dur) may result in variable changes in drug levels; more frequent theophylline blood levels are needed if these medicines are to be combined.
- warfarin (Coumadin) poses an increased risk of bleeding; INR (prothrombin time or protime) testing should be checked more frequently and doses adjusted if needed.

The following drugs may ***decrease*** the effects of tetracyclines:
- antacids (aluminum or magnesium preparations, sodium bicarbonate, etc.)—may reduce drug absorption.
- bismuth subsalicylate (Pepto-Bismol, others).
- calcium supplements (various brands).
- carbamazepine (Tegretol).
- cholestyramine (Questran) and other cholesterol-lowering resins.
- colestipol (Colestid) and perhaps colesevelam (Welchol).
- iron, zinc, magnesium and mineral preparations—may reduce drug absorption.
- phenobarbital.
- phenytoin (Dilantin) or fosphenytoin (Cerebyx).
- quinapril (Accupril).
- rifampin (Rifadin, others).

- sucralfate (Carafate).
- zinc salts.

▷ *Driving, Hazardous Activities:* Usually no restrictions. However, this drug may cause nausea or diarrhea. Restrict activities as necessary.

Aviation Note: The use of these drugs ***may be a disqualification*** for piloting. Consult a designated Aviation Medical Examiner.

Exposure to Sun: Use caution—some tetracyclines can cause photosensitivity (see Glossary).

THEOPHYLLINE (thee OFF i lin)

Introduced: 1900   **Class:** Antiasthmatic, bronchodilator, xanthines   **Prescription:** USA: Yes   **Controlled Drug:** USA: No; Canada: No   **Available as Generic:** Yes

Brand Names: Accurbron, ✸Acet-Am, A.E.A., Aerolate, Aminodrox-Forte, ✸Apo-Oxtriphylline, ✸Aquaphyllim, ✸Asbron [CD], Asmalix, Azpan, Brocomar [CD], Bronchial Gelatin Capsule, Broncomar [CD], Bronkaid Tablets [CD], Bronkodyl, Bronkolixir [CD], Bronkotabs, Bronkotabs [CD], Constant-T, Duraphyl, Elixicon, Elixomin, Elixophyllin, For-Az-Ma [CD], Isuprel Compound [CD], Labid, Lanophyllin, Lixolin, Lodrane, Lodrane CR, Marax [CD], Marax DF [CD], Mudrane GG Elixir [CD], Phedral [CD], Phyllocontin, Physpan, ✸PMS Theophylline, Primatene, ✸Pulmophylline, Quadrinal [CD], Quibron [CD], Quibron Plus [CD], Quibron-T Dividose, Quibron-300 [CD], Quibron-T/SR, Respbid, Slo-Bid, Slo-Bid Gyrocaps, Slo-Phyllin, Slo-Phyllin GG [CD], Slo-Phyllin Gyrocaps, Somophyllin, Somophyllin-12, Sustaire, Tedral [CD], Tedral SA [CD], T.E.H. [CD], T.E.P., Thalfed, Theobid Duracaps, ✸Theo-Bronc, Theochron, Theoclear, Theoclear L.A., Theocord, Theo-Dur, Theo-Dur Sprinkle, Theolair, Theolair-SR, Theolate [CD], Theolixir, Theomar [CD], Theomax DF, Theon, Theophyl-SR, Theospan-SR, Theo-SR, Theo-Time, Theo-24, Theovent, Theox, Theozine, Therex [CD], Uni-Dur, ✸Uniphyl, Vitaphen [CD]

BENEFITS versus RISKS	
Possible Benefits	*Possible Risks*
EFFECTIVE PREVENTION AND RELIEF OF ACUTE BRONCHIAL ASTHMA	NARROW TREATMENT RANGE FREQUENT STOMACH DISTRESS Gastrointestinal bleeding
MODERATELY EFFECTIVE CONTROL OF CHRONIC, RECURRENT BRONCHIAL ASTHMA	Central nervous system toxicity, seizures Heart rhythm disturbances
Moderately effective symptomatic relief in chronic bronchitis and emphysema	

▷ **Principal Uses**

As a Single Drug Product: Uses currently included in FDA-approved labeling: (1) Used to relieve shortness of breath and wheezing of acute bronchial asthma and to prevent the recurrence of asthmatic episodes; (2) useful in relieving asthmalike symptoms associated with some types of chronic bronchitis, chronic obstructive pulmonary disease and emphysema.

Other (unlabeled) generally accepted uses: (1) May have a role in combination therapy of cystic fibrosis; (2) can help decrease excessive production of red blood cells in kidney transplant patients; (3) may have a role in helping decrease the risk of sudden infant death syndrome (SIDS); (4) may have a supportive role with steroids and other agents in helping prevent rejection of transplanted kidneys; (5) can help ease essential tremor; (6) decreases risk of breathing cessation in neonatal apnea; (7) helps in treating SIDS children; (8) may have a role in treating sleep apnea; (9) one small study found it effective in stopping ACE inhibitor (see Drug Classes) cough.

As a Combination Drug Product [CD]: Available combined with several other drugs that manage bronchial asthma and related conditions. Ephedrine is added to enhance opening of the bronchi (bronchodilation); guaifenesin is added to thin mucus in the bronchial tubes (an expectorant effect); and mild sedatives such as phenobarbital are added to allay anxiety often seen in acute attacks of asthma.

How This Drug Works: By inhibiting the enzyme phosphodiesterase, this drug produces an increase in the tissue chemical cyclic AMP. This causes relaxation of the muscles in the bronchial tubes and blood vessels of the lung, resulting in relief of bronchospasm, expanded lung capacity and improved lung circulation.

Available Dosage Forms and Strengths
Capsules — 100 mg, 200 mg, 250 mg, 260 mg
Capsules, prolonged action — 50 mg, 60 mg, 65 mg, 75 mg, 100 mg, 125 mg, 130 mg, 200 mg, 250 mg, 260 mg, 300 mg
Elixir — 27 mg/5 ml, 50 mg/5 ml
Oral solution — 27 mg/5 ml, 53.3 mg/5 ml
Oral suspension — 100 mg/5 ml
Syrup — 27 mg/5 ml, 50 mg/5 ml
Tablets — 100 mg, 125 mg, 200 mg, 250 mg, 300 mg
Tablets, prolonged action — 50 mg, 60 mg, 65 mg, 75 mg, 100 mg, 125 mg, 130 mg, 200 mg, 225 mg, 250 mg, 260 mg, 300 mg, 350 mg, 400 mg, 450 mg, 500 mg, 600 mg

▷ **Recommended Dosage Ranges** (Actual dose and schedule must be determined for each patient individually.)

Infants and Children: Sudden asthma attack (not currently taking theophylline)—loading dose of 5 mg per kg of body mass. For acute attack (while currently taking theophylline)—a single dose of 2.5 mg per kg of body mass, if no signs of theophylline toxicity. Check blood levels of theophylline.

For ongoing use during acute attack—dose is based on age: Up to 6 months of age—0.07 for each week of age + 1.7 = the mg per kg of body mass, given every 8 hours. 6 months to 1 year of age—0.05 for each week of age + 1.25 = the mg per kg of body mass, given every 6 hours. 1 to 9 years of age—5 mg per kg of body mass, every 6 hours. 9 to 12 years of age—4 mg per kg of body mass, every 6 hours. 12 to 16 years of age—3 mg per kg of body mass, every 6 hours.

For ongoing use to prevent asthma—dose is based on age: Once slow dosing increase is accomplished, daily doses are adjusted to reach blood levels of 10 to 15 mcg/ml.

16 to 60 Years of Age:

For acute attack of asthma (not currently taking theophylline): Loading dose of 5 mg per kg of body mass. For acute attack while currently taking theophylline—a single dose of 2.5 mg per kg of body mass, if no indications of theophylline toxicity. Monitor blood levels of theophylline.

For maintenance during acute attack: For nonsmokers: 3 mg per kg of body mass, every 8 hours; for smokers: 4 mg per kg of body mass, every 6 hours.

For chronic treatment to prevent recurrence of asthma: Initially 6 to 8 mg per kg of body mass, in three or four divided doses at 6- to 8-hour intervals, up to a maximum of 400 mg daily. Increase dose as needed and tolerated by increments of 25% every 2 to 3 days. The total daily dose should not exceed 13 mg per kg of body mass or 900 mg, whichever is less. Prolonged-action formulations may allow twice-daily dosing with good results.

For once daily dosing: The Slo-bid Gyrocaps and the Theo-Dur forms may work in adult non-smokers when they are given once a day. The strategy here is usually to establish a therapeutic blood level using the twice daily approach, and then using that effective dose. The once a day dose is then twice the two times a day dose. This new once daily dose is started 12 hours after the last twice a day dose. Blood levels should be checked as the peak and trough levels may be higher or lower than with the twice a day approach. If problems consistent with toxicity happen, the patient should be returned to the twice a day dosing strategy.

Over 60 Years of Age: Theophylline is removed some 30% more slowly than in younger patients. Decreased doses and more frequent blood levels are prudent.

Conditions Requiring Dosing Adjustments

Liver Function: The dose must be lowered and blood levels obtained frequently. Doses may need to be decreased by 50% in some cases.

Kidney Function: Lower doses and more frequent blood levels are indicated.

▷ **Dosing Instructions:** May be taken with or following food to reduce stomach irritation. The regular capsules may be opened, and the regular tablets may be crushed. The prolonged-action forms should be swallowed whole and not altered. Shake the oral suspension well before measuring each dose. Do not refrigerate liquid dose forms. Blood levels are critical for this medicine. If theophylline has been taken previously, a blood level is often checked and then clinicians use 1 mg/kg for each 2 mcg/ml increase in blood level that is wanted. If you forget a dose: Take the missed dose as soon as you remember it, unless it's nearly time for your next dose—if that is the case, skip the missed dose and take the next dose right on schedule. JUST THE RIGHT BLOOD LEVEL is very important for this medicine. DO NOT double up doses. Talk with your doctor if you find yourself forgetting this drug. Timers and beeper-based reminder services can be very helpful.

Usual Duration of Use: Use on a regular schedule for 48 to 72 hours usually determines effectiveness in controlling the breathing impairment associated with bronchial asthma and chronic lung disease. Long-term use requires supervision and periodic physician evaluation.

Typical Treatment Goals and Measurements (Outcomes and Markers)

Asthma: Signs and symptoms of asthma such as difficulty breathing (dyspnea), cough, light-headedness and wheezing should lessen. Exercise ability should increase. Forced expiratory volume at one second (FEV1) and/or peak expiratory flow rate (PEF) are checked by most pulmonologists as indicators of successful treatment. If the usual benefit is not realized, or if symptoms improve and then worsen, call your doctor.

▷ **This Drug Should Not Be Taken If**

- you have had an allergic reaction to it or to aminophylline, dyphylline or oxtriphylline.
- you have active peptic ulcer disease.
- you have an uncontrolled seizure disorder.
- you had a blood level drawn and it is in the "toxic" range.

▷ **Inform Your Physician Before Taking This Drug If**

- you have had an unfavorable reaction to any xanthine (see Drug Classes).
- you have a seizure disorder of any kind.
- you have a history of peptic ulcer disease.
- you have a history of underactive thyroid (hypothyroidism).
- you have impaired liver or kidney function.
- you take any of the drugs listed in the "Other Drugs" section below.
- you have hypertension, heart disease or any type of heart rhythm disorder.

Possible Side Effects (natural, expected and unavoidable drug actions)

Nervousness, insomnia, rapid heart rate, increased urine volume.

▷ **Possible Adverse Effects** (unusual, unexpected and infrequent reactions)

If any of the following develop, consult your physician promptly for guidance.

Mild Adverse Effects

Allergic reactions: skin rash, hives.

Headache, dizziness, irritability, tremor, fatigue, weakness—infrequent.

Loss of appetite, nausea, vomiting (may be an early warning of toxicity), abdominal pain, diarrhea, excessive thirst—infrequent.

Stuttering—case report.

Flushing of face—case reports.

Serious Adverse Effects

Allergic reactions: severe skin rash (Stevens-Johnson syndrome)—case reports.

Idiosyncratic reactions: marked anxiety, confusion, behavioral disturbances.

Central nervous system toxicity: muscle twitching, seizures—dose-related.

Heart rhythm abnormalities, rapid breathing, low blood pressure—variable and dose-related.

Gastrointestinal bleeding—rare.

Defects in clotting (coagulation)—case reports.

Drug-induced abnormal urine production (SIADH) or porphyria—case reports.

Worsening of ulcers—possible.

Liver toxicity—case reports.

▷ **Possible Effects on Sexual Function:** None reported.

Natural Diseases or Disorders That May Be Activated by This Drug

Latent peptic ulcer disease.

Possible Effects on Laboratory Tests

Blood uric acid level: increased.

Fecal occult blood test: positive (large doses may cause stomach bleeding).

Triglycerides: may be increased with prolonged use.

CAUTION

1. This drug should not be taken at the same time as other antiasthmatic drugs unless your doctor prescribes the combination. Serious overdose could result.
2. If you develop severe weakness or confusion, irregular heart beats, shakes (tremors) or muscle twitching while taking this medicine—CALL YOUR DOCTOR immediately.
3. influenza vaccines may delay the elimination of this drug and cause accumulation to toxic levels.

Precautions for Use

By Infants and Children: Do not exceed recommended doses. Watch for toxicity: irritability, agitation, tremors, lethargy, fever, vomiting, rapid heart rate and breathing, seizures. Blood level tests are needed during long-term use.

By Those Over 60 Years of Age: Small starting doses are indicated. You may be at increased risk for stomach irritation, nausea, vomiting or diarrhea. When used concurrently with coffee (caffeine) or nasal decongestants, this drug may cause excessive stimulation and a hyperactivity syndrome.

▷ Advisability of Use During Pregnancy

Pregnancy Category: C. See Pregnancy Risk Categories at the back of this book.

Animal studies: Significant birth defects due to this drug reported in mice.

Human studies: Adequate studies of pregnant women are not available. No increase in birth defects reported in 394 exposures to this drug.

Avoid this drug during the first 3 months. Use it otherwise only if clearly needed. Ask your physician for guidance.

Advisability of Use If Breast-Feeding

Presence of this drug in breast milk: Yes.

Avoid drug or refrain from nursing.

Habit-Forming Potential: None.

Effects of Overdose: Nausea, vomiting, restlessness, irritability, confusion, delirium, seizures, high fever, weak pulse, coma.

Possible Effects of Long-Term Use: Gastrointestinal irritation.

Suggested Periodic Examinations While Taking This Drug (at physician's discretion)

Periodic testing of blood theophylline levels (see "Therapeutic Drug Monitoring," chapter 2). Time to sample blood for theophylline level: 2 hours after regular (standard) dose forms; 5 hours after sustained-release dose forms. Recommended therapeutic range: 10 to 20 mcg/ml.

▷ While Taking This Drug, Observe the Following

Foods: No restrictions.

Herbal Medicines or Minerals: Using St. John's wort, ma huang, ephedrine-like compounds or kola while taking this medicine may result in increased sensation of jitteriness or nervousness (central nervous system stimulation). There is one case report of decreased removal (clearance) of theophylline from the body if it is combined with St. John's wort. Caution and more frequent testing of blood levels are prudent. Fir or pine needle oil should NOT be used by asthmatics. Ephedra alone does carry a German Commission E monograph indication for asthma treatment. If you are allergic to plants in the Asteraceae family (aster, chrysanthemum, daisy or ragweed), you may also be allergic to echinacea, chamomile, feverfew and St. John's wort. Ipriflavone can increase theophylline levels—requiring theophylline dosage adjustments. Talk to your doctor BEFORE adding any herbal medicine to theophylline.

Beverages: Avoid excessive use of caffeine-containing beverages: coffee, tea, cola or chocolate; this combination could cause nervousness and insomnia.

▷ *Alcohol:* Large doses may decrease removal by up to 30%. May have additive effect on stomach irritation.

Tobacco Smoking: May hasten the elimination of this drug and reduce its effectiveness. I advise everyone to quit smoking.

Marijuana Smoking: May hasten the elimination of this drug and reduce its effectiveness. Higher doses may be necessary to maintain a therapeutic blood level.

▷ *Other Drugs*

Theophylline may *decrease* the effects of
- adenosine (Adenocard).
- benzodiazepines (See Drug Classes).
- lithium (Lithane, Lithobid, etc.).
- zafirlukast (Accolate).

Theophylline *taken concurrently* with
- halothane (anesthesia) may cause heart rhythm abnormalities.
- phenytoin (Dilantin) may cause decreased effects of both drugs. Monitor blood levels and adjust doses as appropriate.
- tacrolimus (Prograf) may cause increased levels of tacrolimus—more frequent tacrolimus blood levels are prudent.

The following drugs may *increase* the effects of theophylline:
- allopurinol (Lopurin, Zyloprim).
- amiodarone (Cordarone).
- birth control pills (oral contraceptives—estrogens).
- cimetidine (Tagamet).
- ciprofloxacin (Cipro).
- clarithromycin (Biaxin).
- diltiazem (Cardizem).
- disulfiram (Antabuse).
- doxycycline and other tetracyclines.
- enoxacin (Penetrex).
- ephedrine (various).
- erythromycin (E-Mycin, Erythrocin, etc.).
- famotidine (Pepcid).
- flu vaccine (influenza vaccine).
- fluvoxamine (Luvox).
- furosemide (Lasix).
- grepafloxacin (Raxar).
- imipenem/cilastatin (Primaxin).
- interferon alfa.
- ipriflavone (various).
- isoniazid (INH).

- methotrexate (Mexate).
- mexiletine (Mexitil).
- nicotine (Nicorette, Pro-Step, others).
- norfloxacin (Noroxin).
- ofloxacin (Floxin).
- pentoxifylline (Trental).
- perfloxacin (Perflacine-France).
- propafenone (Rythmol).
- ranitidine (Zantac).
- sertraline (Zoloft).
- tacrine (Cognex).
- thiabendazole.
- ticlopidine (Ticlid).
- troleandomycin (TAO).
- trovafloxacin (Trovan).
- verapamil (Calan, Verelan).
- viloxazine.
- zafirlukast (Accolate).
- zileuton (Zyflo)-may require 50% dose decreases.

The following drugs may *decrease* the effects of theophylline:
- barbiturates (phenobarbital, etc.).
- beta blockers (see Drug Classes).
- carbamazepine (Tegretol).
- isoproterenol.
- fosphenytoin (Cerebyx) or phenytoin (Dilantin).
- lansoprazole (Prevacid).
- primidone (Mysoline).
- rifampin (Rifadin, Rimactane, etc.).
- ritonavir (Norvir) and perhaps other protease inhibitors (see Drug Classes).
- sulfinpyrazone (Anturane).

▷ *Driving, Hazardous Activities:* This drug may cause dizziness. Restrict activities as necessary.

Aviation Note: The use of this drug *may be a disqualification* for piloting. Consult a designated Aviation Medical Examiner.

Exposure to Sun: No restrictions.

Occurrence of Unrelated Illness: Sudden viral respiratory infections or fever may slow drug removal. Watch for signs of toxicity, as dosing must be changed if this occurs. More frequent blood levels are needed. Seizure disorders may be worsened by this medicine. Use with extreme caution by seizure patients. Theophylline used with extreme caution in active peptic ulcer disease or heart arrhythmias (cardiac, not including slow or bradyarrhythmias).

Discontinuation: Avoid prolonged or unnecessary use of this drug. When your asthma resolves, withdraw this drug gradually over several days.

THIAZIDE DIURETICS FAMILY

Bendroflumethiazide   (ben droh FLOO meh THI a zide)   **Chlorothiazide** (klor oh THI a zide)   **Chlorthalidone**   (KLOR thal i dohn)   **Hydro-**

chlorothiazide (hi droh klor oh THI a zide)   **Hydroflumethiazide** (hi droh flu meh THI a zide) Methyclothiazide (METH i klo THI a zide)   **Metolazone** (me TOHL a zohn)   **Trichlormethiazide** (tri klor me THI a zide)

Introduced 1960, 1957, 1960, 1959, 1961, 1959, 1974, 1962, respectively   **Class** Antihypertensive, diuretic, thiazides   **Prescription** USA: Yes   **Controlled Drug:** USA: No; Canada: No   **Available as Generic** USA: Yes, hydrochlorothiazide and combination with triamterene and with bisoprolol also; Canada: Yes

Brand Names: Bendroflumethiazide: Naturetin, Chlorothiazide: Aldochlor [CD], Diachlor, Diupres [CD], Diurigen, Diuril, SK-Chlorothiazide, ✤Supres [CD], Chlorthalidone: ✤Apo-Chlorthalidone, Combipres [CD], Demi-Regroton [CD], Hygroton, ✤Hygroton-Resperpine [CD], Hylidone, ✤Novothalidone, Regroton [CD], Tenoretic, Thalitone, ✤Uridon, Hydrochlorothiazide: Atacand HCT [CD], Aldactazide [CD], Aldoril D30/D50 [CD], Aldoril-15/25 [CD], ✤Apo-Amilzide, ✤Apo-Hydro, ✤Apo-Methazide [CD], ✤Apo-Triazide [CD], Apresazide [CD], Apresoline-Esidrix [CD], Capozide [CD], ✤Co-Betaloc [CD], Diaqua, ✤Diuchlor H, Dyazide [CD], Esidrex, Ezide, H-H-R, H.H.R., HydroDiuril, Hydromal, Hydro-Par, Hydropres [CD], Hydroserpine [CD], Hydroserpine Plus [CD], Hydro-T, Hydro-Z-50, Hyzaar [CD], Inderide [CD], Inderide LA [CD], ✤Ismelin-Esidrex [CD], Lopressor HCT [CD], Maxzide [CD], Maxzide-25 [CD], M Dopazide [CD], Microzide, Mictrin, ✤Moduret [CD], Moduretic [CD], ✤Natrimax, ✤Neo-Codema, Normozide [CD], ✤Novo-Doparil [CD], ✤Novo-Hydrazide, ✤Novo-Spirozine [CD], ✤Novo-Triamzide [CD], Oretic, Oreticyl [CD], ✤PMS Dopazide [CD], Prinzide [CD], Ser-Ap-Es [CD], Serpasil-Esidrex [CD], SK-Hydrochlorothiazide, Thiuretic, Timolide [CD], Trandate HCT [CD], Unipres [CD], Uniretic [CD] ✤Urozide, Vaseretic [CD], ✤Viskazide [CD], Zestoretic [CD], Ziac [CD], Zide, Hydroflumethiazide: Diucardin, Saluron, Methyclothiazide: Aquatensen, ✤Duretic, Enduron, Metolazone: Diulo, Microx, Mykrox, Zaroxolyn, Trichlormethiazide: Diurese, Marazide II, Metahydrin, Naqua, Naquival [CD]

BENEFITS versus RISKS	
Possible Benefits	*Possible Risks*
EFFECTIVE, WELL-TOLERATED DIURETICS	Loss of body potassium and magnesium (especially with higher
POSSIBLY EFFECTIVE IN MILD HYPERTENSION	doses)
ENHANCES EFFECTIVENESS OF OTHER ANTIHYPERTENSIVES	Cardiac arrhythmias caused by decreased electrolytes (studied in chlorthalidone and
Beneficial in treatment of diabetes insipidus	hydrochlorothiazide)
	Increased blood sugar, uric acid or calcium
	Rare blood cell disorders
	Rare liver toxicity (chlorothiazide or hydrochlorothiazide)

▷ **Principal Uses**

As a Single Drug Product: Uses currently included in FDA-approved labeling: (1) Increases the volume of urine (diuresis) to correct fluid retention (edema) seen in congestive heart failure, corticosteroid or estrogen use, and certain types of liver and kidney disease; (2) starting therapy for high blood pressure (hypertension).

Author's Note: One large study showed that hydrochlorothiazide achieves benefits (outcomes) in decreasing left ventricular size equal to more expensive agents, such as ACE inhibitors. A review of ten studies found that diuretics versus beta blockers should be the first-line medicines for treating high blood pressure in the elderly.

Other (unlabeled) generally accepted uses: (1) Prevention of kidney stones that contain calcium; (2) may help decrease the frequency of hip fractures in the elderly; (3) methyclothiazide has been used to help maintain blood calcium levels in Paget's disease; (4) may have a role in helping prevent osteoporosis (by correcting abnormally high elimination of calcium in the urine or hypercalciuria); (5) used in diabetes insipidus (nephrogenic) in decreasing the urine volume.

As Combination Drug Products [CD]: Used to treat blood pressure that has not responded to single-drug therapy by combining beta blockers or angiotensin II receptor blockers with this diuretic.

How These Drugs Work: By increasing removal of salt and water in the urine, these drugs reduce fluid volume and body sodium. They also relax walls of smaller arteries. The combined effect of these two actions (reduced blood volume in expanded space) lowers blood pressure.

Available Dosage Forms and Strengths

Bendroflumethiazide:

Tablets — 5 mg, 10 mg

Chlorothiazide:

Injection — 500 mg/20 ml
Oral suspension — 250 mg/5 ml
Tablets — 250 mg, 500 mg

Chlorthalidone:

Tablets — 25 mg, 50 mg, 100 mg

Hydrochlorothiazide:

Solution — 50 mg/5 ml
Solution, intensol — 100 mg/ml
Tablets — 12.5 mg, 25 mg, 50 mg, 100 mg

Hydrochlorothiazide combinations:

Bisoprolol and hydrochlorothiazide — 2.5 mg/6.25 mg, 5 mg/6.25 mg, 10 mg/6.25 mg
Candesartan and hydrochlorothiazide — 16 mg/12.5 mg, 32 mg/12.5 mg
Losartan and hydrochlorothiazide — 50 mg/12.5 mg, 100 mg/12.5 mg

Methyclothiazide:

Tablets — 2.5 mg, 5 mg

Metolazone:

Tablets — 0.5 mg, 2.5 mg, 5 mg, 10 mg

Trichlormethiazide:

Tablets — 2 mg, 4 mg

▷ **Usual Adult Dosage Ranges:** *Bendroflumethiazide:* As antihypertensive—12.5 to 5 mg daily, in a single dose.

Chlorothiazide: As antihypertensive—500 to 1,000 mg per day to start, and 500 to 2,000 mg daily as a maintenance dose. As a diuretic—500 to 2,000 mg per day, using the smallest effective dose. Daily maximum is 2,000 mg.

Chlorthalidone: As antihypertensive—15 to 30 mg daily, and then up to 50 mg daily if needed. As a diuretic—30 to 60 mg daily and then the smallest effective dose is used (maintenance dose). Some patients have required 120 mg daily.

Hydrochlorothiazide: As antihypertensive—12.5 to 100 mg daily initially; 12.5 to 200 mg daily for maintenance. As diuretic—variable; 12.5 to 200 mg daily. Many patients require 100–200 mg; the smallest effective dose should be determined (see "CAUTION" below). The total daily dose should not exceed 200 mg. Microzide is a new once-daily formulation (12.5 mg) of this medicine. Combination forma are started using the lowest dose combination form and then are increased as needed and tolerated.

Author's Note: Many patients with mild to moderate high blood pressure get acceptable blood-pressure-lowering results from 12.5 mg of hydrochlorothiazide. If results are obtained with this dose, it can minimize loss of potassium and magnesium as well!

Methyclothiazide: As antihypertensive or diuretic—2.5 to 5 mg daily. Maximum daily diuretic dose is 10 mg. Pediatric dose—0.05 to 0.2 mg per kg of body mass daily.

Trichlormethiazide: As antihypertensive or diuretic—therapy may be started with 1 to 4 mg twice daily. Usual maintenance dose is 1 to 4 mg once daily.

Note: Actual dose and schedule must be determined for each patient individually.

Conditions Requiring Dosing Adjustments

Liver Function: Electrolyte balance is critical in liver failure. These drugs may precipitate encephalopathy. Hydrochlorothiazide and chlorothiazide are also a rare cause of cholestatic jaundice and should be used with caution in liver failure.

Kidney Function: These drugs can be used with caution by patients with mild kidney failure and are not effective for patients with moderate failure. They should not be used in severe kidney failure; they can be a rare cause of kidney damage.

▷ **Dosing Instructions:** The tablets may be crushed and taken with or following meals to reduce stomach irritation. They are best taken in the morning to avoid nighttime urination. If you forget a dose: Take the missed dose as soon as you remember it, unless it's nearly time for your next dose—if that is the case, skip the missed dose and take the next dose right on schedule. DO NOT double up on doses. Talk with your doctor if you find yourself missing doses because the best results come from keeping your blood pressure under tight control.

Usual Duration of Use: Regular use for 2 to 3 weeks determines benefits in lowering high blood pressure. Long-term use requires follow-up with your doctor. If goals for blood pressure are not met, dose increases, combination treatment or changing medicines is appropriate. Take control of blood pressure for life.

Typical Treatment Goals and Measurements (Outcomes and Markers)

Blood pressure: The most recent treatment guidelines (JNC VI) actually define optimal blood pressure (BP) as less than 120/80 and high normal as 139/89. The American Diabetes Association has chosen a target of 130/80 as the blood pressure goal for people living with diabetes. Most clinicians try to achieve a BP that achieves the best balance of lower cardiovascular risk while avoiding the problem of too low a blood pressure. Additionally, it is important to make sure that loss of body chemicals (electrolytes such as potassium and magnesium) is not excessive and is replaced if needed. The goal and time frame (see peak benefits above) should be discussed with you when the prescription is written.

Possible Advantages of These Drugs

Hydrochlorothiazide was studied in more than 1,100 Veterans Administration patients with mild to moderate high blood pressure. It was found to have met blood pressure reduction goals while offering decreased left ventricular mass. These outcomes or results were accomplished using low-dose therapy, avoiding many of the undesirable changes in blood chemistry that can be seen with higher doses. This was also accomplished at a fraction of the cost of ACE inhibitors or calcium channel blockers. Diuretics such as these are drugs of first choice for African Americans with high blood pressure versus prior preference given to calcium channel blockers.

▷ **These Drugs Should Not Be Taken If**
- you had an allergic reaction to any form of it previously.
- your kidneys are not making urine.

▷ **Inform Your Physician Before Taking These Drugs If**
- you are allergic to any form of "sulfa" drug.
- you are pregnant or planning pregnancy.
- you have a history of kidney or liver disease.
- you have a history of pancreatitis or lupus erythematosus.
- you have developed swelling (angioedema) of the tongue, face or throat (medicine should be stopped).
- you have asthma or allergies to other medicines.
- you have had testing of electrolytes ordered by another physician, which your doctor has not seen.
- you develop muscle cramps, weakness or abnormal heartbeats while taking one of these medicines.
- you have diabetes, gout or lupus erythematosus.
- you are allergic to the dye tartrazine, as some of these medicines contain it.
- you take any form of cortisone, digitalis, oral antidiabetic drug or insulin.
- you will have surgery with general anesthesia.

Possible Side Effects (natural, expected and unavoidable drug actions)

Light-headedness on arising from sitting or lying position (see Orthostatic Hypotension in Glossary). Increased blood sugar or uric acid level; decreased blood potassium, zinc or magnesium level. Decreased blood magnesium, combined with loss of potassium, may lead to increased risk of sudden cardiac death (high doses for extended periods).

▷ **Possible Adverse Effects** (unusual, unexpected and infrequent reactions)
If any of the following develop, consult your physician promptly for guidance.

Mild Adverse Effects

Allergic reactions: skin rashes, hives, drug fever (see Glossary).

Muscle aches—case report.

Headache, dizziness, blurred or yellow vision—infrequent.

Reduced appetite, indigestion, nausea, vomiting, diarrhea—infrequent.

Serious Adverse Effects

Allergic reactions: hepatitis with jaundice (see Glossary), anaphylactic reaction (see Glossary), severe skin reactions.

Inflammation of the pancreas—case reports.

Bone marrow depression (see Glossary): fever, sore throat, abnormal bleeding/bruising—case reports.

Data from studies of hydrochlorothiazide and chlorthalidone suggest that potassium and magnesium loss associated with higher-dose therapy increases the risk of sudden cardiac death.

Acute gout in some patients (because these medicines decrease uric acid removal).

Loss of blood glucose control—possible.

Short-term (less than 1 year) increase in serum lipids (returns to pretreatment levels in about 1 year).

▷ **Possible Effects on Sexual Function:** Decreased libido (hydrochlorothiazide, chlorthalidone); impotence (bendroflumethiazide, chlorothiazide, hydrochlorothiazide)—case reports.

▷ **Adverse Effects That May Mimic Natural Diseases or Disorders**

Liver reaction may suggest viral hepatitis.

Natural Diseases or Disorders That May Be Activated by These Drugs

Diabetes, gout, systemic lupus erythematosus. Those with asthma or drug allergies are more likely to have allergic reactions.

Possible Effects on Laboratory Tests

Complete blood counts: decreased red cells, hemoglobin, white cells and platelets.

Blood amylase level: increased (possible pancreatitis).

Blood calcium or uric acid level: increased.

Blood sodium and chloride levels: decreased.

Blood cholesterol and triglyceride levels: increased, short term.

Blood glucose level: increased.

Glucose tolerance test (GTT): decreased.

Blood lithium level: increased.

Blood potassium and magnesium level: decreased.

Blood urea nitrogen (BUN) level: increased with long-term use.

Liver function tests (hydrochlorothiazide and chlorothiazide): increased liver enzymes (ALT/GPT, AST/GOT and alkaline phosphatase), increased bilirubin.

CAUTION

1. One study found a strong association between higher doses of hydrochlorothiazide and chlorthalidone and combination drugs con-

taining these diuretics and electrolyte loss and sudden cardiac death. This appeared to be a result of magnesium and potassium loss and may be circumvented by close following of those electrolytes.

2. Take these exactly as prescribed. Excessive loss of sodium and potassium can lead to loss of appetite, nausea, fatigue, weakness, confusion and tingling in the extremities.

3. If you take digitalis (digitoxin, digoxin), adequate potassium is critical. Periodic testing and high-potassium foods may be needed to prevent potassium deficiency—a potential cause of digitalis toxicity (see Table 13, "High Potassium Foods," Section Six).

Precautions for Use

By Infants and Children: Overdose could cause serious dehydration. Significant potassium loss can occur within the first 2 weeks of drug use.

By Those Over 60 Years of Age: Starting doses may be as low as 12.5 mg. Increased risk of impaired thinking, orthostatic hypotension, potassium loss and blood sugar increase. Overdose or extended use can cause excessive loss of body water, thickening (increased viscosity) of blood and increased tendency for the blood to clot—predisposing to stroke, heart attack or thrombophlebitis (vein inflammation with blood clot).

▷ ### Advisability of Use During Pregnancy

Pregnancy Category: Metolazone: B by manufacturer, D by other researchers. All other thiazides in this class are D. See Pregnancy Risk Categories at the back of this book. Some combination forms are C during the first trimester and D during the second and third trimesters.

Animal studies: No birth defects found in rat studies.

Human studies: Reports are conflicting and inconclusive.

Use of thiazides can cause maternal complications that may cause adverse fetal effects, including death. They should not be used in pregnancy unless a very serious complication occurs for which these drugs work. Ask your doctor for guidance.

Advisability of Use If Breast-Feeding

Presence of these drugs in breast milk: Yes.

Avoid drugs or refrain from nursing.

Habit-Forming Potential: None.

Effects of Overdose: Dry mouth, thirst, lethargy, weakness, muscle cramping, nausea, vomiting, drowsiness progressing to stupor or coma.

Possible Effects of Long-Term Use: Impaired balance of water, salt, magnesium and potassium in blood and body tissues. Impaired tolerance of glucose. Pathological changes in parathyroid glands with increased blood calcium levels and decreased blood phosphate levels.

Suggested Periodic Examinations While Taking These Drugs (at physician's discretion)

Complete blood cell counts.

Measurements of blood levels of sodium, potassium, chloride, magnesium, sugar and uric acid.

Kidney and liver function tests.

Repeat bone mineral density test if this drug is used to decrease calcium loss.

▷ **While Taking These Drugs, Observe the Following**

Foods: Ask your doctor if you need to eat foods rich in potassium. See Table 13, "High-Potassium Foods," Section Six, if needed. Follow your physician's advice regarding the use of salt.

Herbal Medicines or Minerals: Ginseng and ginkgo may increase blood pressure, blunting the benefits of this medicine. Hawthorn, saw palmetto, ma huang and licorice may also cause increased blood pressure. Licorice can also cause potassium loss and is especially NOT to be combined with a thiazide. Indian snakeroot has a German Commission E monograph indication for hypertension, but has not been studied with thiazides. Eleuthero root and ephedra should be avoided by people living with hypertension. Calcium and garlic may lower blood pressure. Use caution and work with your doctor to make sure blood pressure is not lowered too much. Calcium may also accumulate to a greater degree than expected since thiazides decrease removal of calcium in the urine. Because St. John's wort and some of these medicines may increase sun sensitivity, the combination is NOT advised. Talk to your doctor BEFORE combining any herbal medicine with this medicine. Diuretics are well known for depleting magnesium, zinc and potassium. These minerals should be routinely checked and supplemented if the medicines have lowered blood mineral levels.

Beverages: No restrictions. This drug may be taken with milk.

▷ *Alcohol:* Use with caution—alcohol may exaggerate the blood-pressure-lowering effects of these drugs and cause orthostatic hypotension.

Tobacco Smoking: No interactions expected. I advise everyone to quit smoking.

▷ *Other Drugs*

These drugs may ***increase*** the effects of
- other antihypertensive drugs; dose adjustments may be necessary to prevent excessive lowering of blood pressure.
- fluconazole (Diflucan).
- lithium (Lithobid, others) and cause lithium toxicity.

These drugs may ***decrease*** the effects of
- oral anticoagulants such as warfarin (Coumadin); increased frequency of INR (prothrombin time) testing is needed.
- oral antidiabetic drugs (sulfonylureas—see Drug Classes and others); dose adjustments may be needed for better blood sugar control.

These drugs ***taken concurrently*** with
- allopurinol (Zyloprim) may decrease kidney function.
- amphotericin B (Abelcet, Fungizone) may result in additive potassium loss; increased frequency of laboratory testing is needed.
- calcium may result in the milk-alkali syndrome with increased calcium, alkalosis and kidney failure.
- carbamazepine (Tegretol) may result in low sodium levels and symptomatic hyponatremia.
- cortisone or other corticosteroid medicines may result in excessive potassium loss with resultant heart rhythm changes and lethargy.
- cyclophosphamide (Cytoxan) may increase immunosuppression.
- digitalis preparations (digitoxin, digoxin) require careful monitoring and dose changes to prevent low potassium levels and serious disturbances of heart rhythm.

- methotrexate (Mexate) may increase immunosuppression.
- nonsteroidal anti-inflammatory drugs (see Drug Classes), such as sulindac (Clinoril) and naproxen (Naprosyn, Aleve, Anaprox, others), may result in decreased thiazide effectiveness.
- probenecid (various) may result in increased thiazide blood levels. Checks of thiazide response are prudent.

The following drugs may *decrease* the effects of these thiazides:

- cholestyramine (Cuemid, Questran)—may interfere with their absorption.
- colestipol (Colestid)-may interfere with their absorption.

Take cholestyramine and colestipol 1 hour before any oral diuretic.

▷ *Driving, Hazardous Activities:* Use caution until the possible occurrence of orthostatic hypotension, dizziness or impaired vision has been determined.

Aviation Note: The use of these drugs *may be a disqualification* for piloting. Consult a designated Aviation Medical Examiner.

Exposure to Sun: These drugs can cause photosensitivity (see Glossary). Use caution until sensitivity has been determined.

Exposure to Heat: Caution-excessive perspiring could cause additional loss of salt and water from the body.

Heavy Exercise or Exertion: Avoid exertion that produces light-headedness, excessive fatigue or muscle cramping. Isometric exercises can raise blood pressure significantly. Ask your doctor for help regarding participation in this form of exercise.

Occurrence of Unrelated Illness: Vomiting or diarrhea can produce a serious imbalance of important body chemistry. Ask your doctor for help.

Discontinuation: These drugs should not be stopped abruptly following long-term use; sudden discontinuation can cause serious thiazide-withdrawal fluid retention (edema). The dose should be reduced gradually. It may be advisable to discontinue this drug 5 to 7 days before major surgery. Ask your physician, surgeon and/or anesthesiologist for guidance.

THIAZOLIDINEDIONE FAMILY (THIGH ah zoh li dean die ohn)

Rosiglitazone (ROSS ih glit a zoan) **Pioglitazone** (PEE oh glit a zoan)

Introduced: 1999, 1999 **Class:** Antidiabetic, thiazolidinedione **Prescription:** USA: Yes **Controlled Drug:** USA: No; Canada: No **Available as Generic:** No

Brand Name: Rosiglitazone: Avandia, Pioglitazone: Actos

BENEFITS versus RISKS	
Possible Benefits	*Possible Risks*
COMBINATION USE OF ROSIGLITAZONE OR PIOGLITAZONE WITH METFORMIN MAY SLOW DIABETES PROGRESSION AS WELL AS HELP AVOID LONG-TERM COMPLICATIONS OF DIABETES ITSELF DECREASED INSULIN RESISTANCE EFFECTIVE CONTROL OF BLOOD SUGAR (GLUCOSE) POSSIBLE AVOIDANCE OF LONG-TERM EFFECTS (BLOOD VESSEL, NERVE, KIDNEY, HIGH BLOOD PRESSURE and HEART ADVERSE EFFECTS) FROM DIABETES FAVORABLE SIDE EFFECT PROFILE VERSUS TROGLITAZONE ROSIGLITAZONE AVOIDS CYP3A4 ELIMINATION OF PIOGLITAZONE (uses CYP2C8 and has fewer potential drug-drug interactions) May have a role in some kinds of infertility where insulin resistance may be part of the problem (such as polycystic ovary syndrome or PCOS)	Hypoglycemia Edema Worsening of existing heart failure Case reports of rosiglitazone and heart failure

▷ **Principal Uses**

As a Single Drug Product: Uses currently included in FDA-approved labeling: (1) Helps control Type 2 diabetes mellitus (adult, maturity-onset); (2) helps people who have not responded to diet alone or to a maximum dose of metformin (Glucophage); (3) pioglitazone can be used in combination with metformin, a sulfonylurea or insulin.

Other (unlabeled) generally accepted uses: (1) may help improve resistance to insulin and may help some patients with syndromes such as Werner syndrome or PCOS where insulin resistance is part of the problem; (2) rosiglitazone may be effective if used with a sulfonylurea.

How These Drugs Work: Work to make insulin more effective (decrease cellular resistance as a peroxisome proliferator activated receptor gamma activator-PPAR gamma). This increases the number of GLUT-4 transporters. Probably also work to decrease local and systemic lipid availability.

Available Dosage Forms and Strengths

Rosiglitazone:
Tablets — 1 mg (Canada), 2 mg, 4 mg, 8 mg
Pioglitazone:
Tablets — 15 mg, 30 mg and 45 mg

▷ **Usual Adult Dosage Ranges**

Rosiglitazone: Used alone (monotherapy): Initially 4 mg once daily or separated into two 2 mg given twice daily. The dose may be increased, if needed and tolerated, after 12 weeks to 4 mg twice daily or 8 mg once daily.

Combined with metformin: Same as monotherapy.

Pioglitazone: Used alone in Type 2 diabetes, the starting dose is 15 or 30 mg once a day. If the response is not at target, the dose may be slowly increased to 45 mg once a day.

Combined with insulin: The starting dose is 15 or 30 mg once a day. Once pioglitazone is started, if low blood sugar (hypoglycemia) happens or if plasma sugar (glucose) is 100 mg/deciliter or less, the dose of insulin should be lowered by 10 to 25%. If combined with metformin, the prior metformin dose can be continued as hypoglycemia is unlikely.

Combined with a sulfonylurea: 15 or 30 mg once daily is used. The sulfonylurea dose will have to be decreased if hypoglycemia occurs.

Note: Actual dose and schedule must be determined for each patient individually.

Conditions Requiring Dosing Adjustments

Liver Function:

Rosiglitazone: should NOT be started if there is active liver disease or if ALT is more than 2.5 times the upper normal limit. In mild to moderate liver disease, rosiglitazone blood levels and the time rosiglitazone stays in the body increase. Decreases in dose or increases in dosing interval are required.

Pioglitazone: Should NOT be used in people with increased liver enzymes (transaminases such as an alanine aminotransferase more than 2.5 times the upper normal) or in patients with clinical signs/symptoms/evidence of active liver disease.

Kidney Function:

Rosiglitazone or pioglitazone: Dosing changes are probably not needed in kidney compromise.

▷ **Dosing Instructions:** May be taken with or without food. Skipping meals while taking these medicines is NOT advised, as the medicine will still continue to increase insulin sensitivity even if the sugar (glucose) from a meal is not there—making hypoglycemia more likely. The tablets may be crushed to make it easier to take. If you are taking these medicines with the maximum dose of metformin, lower ongoing doses of rosiglitazone or pioglitazone may be effective for you. If you are taking these medicines with a sulfonylurea and low blood sugar occurs, the sulfonylurea dose will have to be decreased. If you forget a dose: Take the missed dose as soon as you remember it, unless it's nearly time for your next dose—if that is the case, skip the missed dose and take the next dose right on schedule. DO NOT double doses. Talk with your doctor if you find yourself missing doses. Taking these medicines the right way and keeping blood sugar in tight control gets the best long-term results.

Usual Duration of Use: Use on a regular schedule for 12 weeks usually determines peak effectiveness in controlling diabetes for rosiglitazone. Benefits for both medicines as checked by hemoglobin A1C (glycosylated hemoglobin) or insulin resistance may require longer therapy. Failure to respond after the 12-week period requires a dose increase for rosiglitazone and failure to respond after an acceptable period for pioglitazone also requires a dose increase. Effective use can only be determined by periodic measurement of the blood sugar. See your doctor on a regular basis.

Typical Treatment Goals and Measurements (Outcomes and Markers)

Blood sugar: The general goal for blood sugar is to return it to the usual "normal" range (generally 80–120 mg/dl), while avoiding risks of excessively low blood sugar. One study (the United Kingdom Prospective Diabetes Study or UKPDS) used a fasting plasma sugar (glucose) of less than 108 mg/dl. The Diabetes Control and Complications Trial (DCCT) attempted to achieve near normal glycosylated hemoglobin and found reduced undesirable small blood vessel (microvascular) changes. Using glycosylated hemoglobin as a marker or resolution of insulin resistance will require a longer time period to response than blood sugar. Work with your doctor to get the best individualized results.

Fructosamine and glycosylated hemoglobin: Fructosamine levels (a measure of the past 2 to 3 weeks of blood sugar control) should be less than or equal to 310 micromoles per liter. Glycosylated hemoglobin or hemoglobin A1C (a measure of the past 2–3 months of blood sugar control) should be less than or equal to 7.0%.

Possible Advantages of These Drugs

Offer a novel mechanism of action. Appear to avoid the liver damage potential of troglitazone. Rosiglitazone does not use the CYP3A4 enzyme (a more widely used enzyme) for removal from the body (uses CYP 2C8) and therefore has fewer potential drug-drug interactions than pioglitazone (which uses both). Pioglitazone may have a more favorable effect on good and bad cholesterol.

▷ **These Drugs Should Not Be Taken If**
- you have had an allergic reaction to them previously.
- you have active liver disease or if ALT (ask your doctor) is more than 2.5 times the upper normal limit.
- you have Type 1 diabetes (monotherapy) or are in ketoacidosis.

▷ **Inform Your Physician Before Taking This Drug If**
- you are over 60 years old.
- your diabetes has been unstable or "brittle" in the past.
- you are pregnant or have been unable to ovulate (both drugs may cause ovulation to restart in premenopausal women with insulin resistance who previously did not ovulate. Adequate contraception will be needed.
- you do not know how to recognize or treat hypoglycemia (see Glossary).
- you have an infection and a fever.
- you have a deficiency of red blood cells (anemia)—ask your doctor.
- you have liver or kidney damage.
- you have or develop an accumulation of fluid in your body (edema).
- you have heart failure in New York Class three or four (both drugs increase plasma volume).
- you are nursing your child.

Possible Side Effects (natural, expected and unavoidable drug actions)

If drug dose is excessive or food intake is delayed or inadequate, abnormally low blood sugar (hypoglycemia) may occur.

▷ **Possible Adverse Effects** (unusual, unexpected and infrequent reactions)
   If any of the following develop, consult your physician promptly for guidance.
   Mild Adverse Effects
   Allergic reactions: not reported—rare.
   Headache—infrequent.
   Hypoglycemia—possible.
   Weight gain—possible.
   Muscle aches—infrequent (pioglitazone).
   Fluid retention (edema)—infrequent.
   Increased liver enzymes—very rare (happened within the first two weeks of treatment).
   Diarrhea—rare.
   Serious Adverse Effects
   Allergic reactions: not reported.
   Idiosyncratic reactions: not reported.
   Worsening of congestive heart failure—possible (due to infrequent increased body fluid)—rosiglitazone plus insulin may worsen it further.
   Retinopathy aggravation—case report (pioglitazone).
   Hypoglycemia—possible.
   Anemia—possible—usually mild.
   Liver toxicity—very rare.

▷ **Possible Effects on Sexual Function:** If insulin resistance has been a cause of infertility, these drugs may enable you to become fertile.

▷ **Adverse Effects That May Mimic Natural Diseases or Disorders**
   Fluid accumulation may mimic edema from congestive heart failure.

Natural Diseases or Disorders That May Be Activated by This Drug
   Increased fluid in the body (plasma volume expansion) may worsen congestive heart failure.

Possible Effects on Laboratory Tests
   Complete blood cell count: decreased red cells, hemoglobin and hematocrit—mild.
   Blood glucose, fructosamine or glycosylated hemoglobin level: decreased.
   Liver function tests (ALT): possibly increased.
   LDL: increased by up to 19% for rosiglitazone (inconsistent change for pioglitazone).
   Total cholesterol: increased.
   HDL: increased (beneficial effect) by up to 14% for rosiglitazone and 19% for pioglitazone.

CAUTION
   1. These drugs must be regarded as only one part of the total program for the management of your diabetes. It is not a substitute for a properly prescribed diet, insulin and regular exercise.
   2. A similar medicine caused serious liver reactions. While these medicines HAVE NOT caused such reactions, liver enzyme testing is required.
   3. These drugs may cause you to ovulate if insulin resistance has been the cause of a failure to ovulate.

Precautions for Use

By Infants and Children: Safety and efficacy have not been established in this age group.

By Those Over 65 Years of Age: Any medicine with the potential to lower blood sugar should be used with caution in this age group and monitored closely to prevent hypoglycemic reactions. Repeated episodes of hypoglycemia in the elderly can cause brain damage. Clinical trials did not reveal differences in safety or effectiveness in those over 65 for either medicine.

▷ **Advisability of Use During Pregnancy**

Pregnancy Category: C (both medicines). See Pregnancy Risk Categories at the back of this book.

Animal studies: Rosiglitazone in treated rats and rabbits (during mid-late gestation) showed growth retardation and was associated with fetal death. Pioglitazone in treated rats and rabbits showed delayed parturition and embryotoxicity at high doses.

Human studies: Adequate studies of pregnant women are not available for either medicine.

Because uncontrolled blood sugar levels during pregnancy are associated with a higher incidence of birth defects, many experts recommend that insulin (instead of an oral agent) be used as necessary to control diabetes during the entire pregnancy.

Advisability of Use If Breast-Feeding

Presence of this drug in breast milk: Yes for rosiglitazone, unknown for pioglitazone.

Avoid drug or refrain from nursing.

Habit-Forming Potential: None.

Effects of Overdose: Limited experience is available for both medicines. Single doses of rosiglitazone of 20 mg by mouth were well tolerated. One pioglitazone patient took 180 mg for seven days without any reported ill effects. If an overdose occurs of either drug, supportive treatment consistent with the patient's signs and symptoms should be provided.

Possible Effects of Long-Term Use: Normalization of fructosamine, hemoglobin A1C, decreased LDL, increased HDL. Pioglitazone may have a more favorable effect on good and bad cholesterol.

Suggested Periodic Examinations While Taking This Drug (at physician's discretion)

Complete blood cell counts.

Liver function (serum transaminases) must be tested at the beginning of treatment, every two months for the first year and then periodically thereafter.

Follow-up tests (such as finger stick testing) of blood sugar.

Fructosamine (now available as a finger stick self-test).

Glycosylated hemoglobin.

HDL and LDL.

▷ **While Taking This Drug, Observe the Following**

Foods: Follow the diabetic diet prescribed by your physician. Vitamin C in high doses may worsen blood sugar control.

Herbal Medicines or Minerals: Using chromium may change the way your body is able to use sugar. Some health food stores advocate vanadium as mimicking the actions of insulin, but possible toxicity and need for rigorous studies presently preclude recommending it. DHEA may change sensitivity to insulin or insulin resistance. Hawthorn, ginger, garlic, ginseng and licorice, nettle and yohimbe may change blood sugar. Since this may require adjustment of hypoglycemic medicine dosing, talk to your doctor BEFORE combing any of these herbal medicines with these medicines. Echinacea pupurea (injectable) and blonde psyllium seed or husk should NOT be taken by people living with diabetes. Talk to your doctor BEFORE combining any herbal medicine with these drugs.

Beverages: As directed in the diabetic diet. May be taken with milk.

▷ *Alcohol:* Single doses did not increase risk of sudden lowering of blood sugar (hypoglycemia). Use with caution. Repeated or large doses of alcohol can lower blood sugar, and chronic high doses can impact liver function.

Tobacco Smoking: No interaction expected. I advise everyone to quit smoking.

▷ *Other Drugs*

The following drugs may *decrease* the effects of rosiglitazone:
- beta blocker (see drug classes).
- cholestyramine (Questran).
- corticosteroids (see Drug Classes).
- thiazide diuretics (see Drug Classes).

These medicines *taken concurrently* with
- birth control pills (oral contraceptives) lead to loss of control with one medicine in this same class. Pills containing ethinyl estradiol of norethindrone may not work.
- medicines metabolized by CYP 2C8 or decreasing this enzyme may increase blood levels of rosiglitazone.
- medicines that increase levels of CYP 2C8 may decrease the effects of rosiglitazone.
- medicines metabolized by CYP 3A4 or inhibiting this enzyme (such as many macrolide antibiotics, azole antifungals, protease inhibitors and zafirlukast or zileuton) may increase blood levels of pioglitazone.
- medicines that increase levels of CYP 3A4 (such as carbamazepine, fosphenytoin, phenytoin, rifampin or dexamethasone) may decrease the effects of pioglitazone.
- protease inhibitors (PIs—see Drug Classes) may result in loss of glucose control because PIs as a class can cause glucose intolerance.
- sulfonylureas (see Drug Classes) can work to effectively lower blood sugar, but may also lower blood sugar too much. Combination use requires blood sugar checks and adjustments of sulfonylurea dosing if the blood sugar goes too low. This is also true of other medicines that lower blood sugar.

▷ *Driving, Hazardous Activities:* Regulate your dose schedule, eating schedule and physical activities very carefully to prevent hypoglycemia. Be able to recognize the early symptoms of hypoglycemia so that you can avoid hazardous activities and take corrective measures.

Aviation Note: Diabetes *is a disqualification* for piloting. Consult a designated Aviation Medical Examiner.

Exposure to Sun: Not defined.

Occurrence of Unrelated Illness: Acute infections, illnesses causing vomiting or diarrhea, serious injuries and surgical procedures can interfere with diabetic control and may require insulin. If any of these conditions occur, call your doctor promptly.

Discontinuation: Talk with your doctor before changing the dosing schedule of this medicine or considering stopping these medicines.

THIORIDAZINE (thi oh RID a zeen)

Introduced: 1959   **Class:** Antipsychotic; tranquilizer, major; phenothiazines
Prescription: USA: Yes   **Controlled Drug:** USA: No; Canada: No   **Available as Generic:** USA: Yes; Canada: Yes
Brand Names: ❧Apo-Thioridazine, Mellaril, Mellaril-S, Millazine, ❧Novoridazine, ❧PMS-Thioridazine, SK-Thioridazine

BENEFITS versus RISKS	
Possible Benefits	*Possible Risks*
EFFECTIVE CONTROL OF ACUTE MENTAL DISORDERS	TARDIVE DYSKINESIA (SERIOUS TOXIC BRAIN EFFECT) with long-term use
Relief of anxiety, agitation and tension	NEUROLEPTIC MALIGNANT SYNDROME
Behavior problems that are resistant to other medicines	MAY PROLONG HEART BEAT INTERVALS AND LEAD TO FATAL HEART RHYTHM PROBLEMS
	Liver damage with jaundice (infrequent)
	Blood cell disorder: abnormally low white blood cell count

▷ **Principal Uses**

As a Single Drug Product: Uses currently included in FDA-approved labeling: (1) Helps manage symptoms of psychotic disorders, moderate to marked depression with significant anxiety and nervous tension, and agitation, anxiety, depression and exaggerated fears in the elderly; (2) used in severe behavioral problems in children characterized by hyperexcitability, short attention span and rapid swings in mood (temper tantrums); (3) eases agitation in Alzheimer's disease.

Other (unlabeled) generally accepted uses: (1) May have a role in treating alcohol withdrawal in patients who cannot tolerate benzodiazepines; (2) can be used to treat unexplained infertility; (3) may help control premature ejaculation and nocturnal emissions in men; (4) can help borderline personality disorder; (5) of use in some chronic pain syndromes; (6) may be of use in hypersexuality.

Author's Note: Information in this profile has been shortened to make room for more widely used medicines.

THIOTHIXENE (thi oh THIX een)

Introduced: 1967   **Class:** Tranquilizer, major; thioxanthenes   **Prescription:** USA: Yes   **Controlled Drug:** USA: No; Canada: No   **Available as Generic:** USA: Yes; Canada: No
Brand Name: Navane

+---+
| **BENEFITS versus RISKS** |
| *Possible Benefits*   *Possible Risks* |
| EFFECTIVE CONTROL OF ACUTE   SERIOUS TOXIC EFFECTS ON |
| MENTAL DISORDERS   BRAIN with long-term use |
| MAY BE EFFECTIVE WHEN   Liver damage with jaundice |
| OTHER ANTIPSYCHOTIC   Blood cell disorder: abnormally low |
| MEDICINES HAVE FAILED   white blood cell count |
+---+

▷ **Principal Uses**

As a Single Drug Product: Uses currently included in FDA-approved labeling: (1) Relieves psychotic thinking and behavior associated with acute psychoses, episodes of mania and paranoia and acute schizophrenia; (2) effective in delusions.

Other (unlabeled) generally accepted uses: Can be of use in significant borderline personality disorder.

How This Drug Works: By inhibiting dopamine, this drug corrects an imbalance of nerve impulse transmissions (at both D1 and D2 receptors) that is thought to be responsible for certain mental disorders.

Available Dosage Forms and Strengths

Capsules — 1 mg, 2 mg, 5 mg, 10 mg, 20 mg

Concentrate — 5 mg/ml

Injections — 2 mg/ml, 5 mg/ml

▷ **Usual Adult Dosage Ranges:** Initially 2 to 5 mg two or three times daily. Dose may be increased by 2 mg at 3- to 4-day intervals as needed and tolerated. Usual dose range is 20 to 30 mg daily. The total daily dose should not exceed 60 mg. **Note: Actual dose and schedule must be determined for each patient individually.**

Conditions Requiring Dosing Adjustments

Liver Function: This drug should be used with caution in liver compromise.

Kidney Function: Patients with compromised kidneys should be closely followed.

▷ **Dosing Instructions:** The capsules may be opened and taken with or following meals to reduce stomach irritation. The liquid concentrate must be diluted just before dosing by adding it to 8 ounces of water, milk, fruit juice or carbonated beverage. If you forget a dose: Take the missed dose as soon as you remember it, unless it's nearly time for your next dose—if that is the case, skip the missed dose and take the next dose right on schedule. DO NOT double up on doses. Talk with your doctor if you find yourself missing doses.

Usual Duration of Use: Use on a regular schedule for several weeks usually determines control of psychotic disorders. If not beneficial within 6 weeks, it should be stopped. Long-term use (months to years) requires periodic physician evaluation of response, appropriate dose adjustment and consideration of continued need.

Typical Treatment Goals and Measurements (Outcomes and Markers)

Schizophrenia: The general goal: to ease the severity of symptoms in order to let the patient resume his or her usual activities. There should be lessened time spent with prior intrusions of abnormal thinking into more normal life. Some psychiatrists or psychologists use specific question sets (brief psychiatric ratings scale, clinical global impressions scale) and/or positive effects on psychotic symptoms (such as clearer thinking, easing of delusions or hallucinations) as measures of success.

▷ **This Drug Should Not Be Taken If**
- you have had an allergic reaction to it previously.
- you have active liver disease.
- you have cancer of the breast.
- you have a current blood cell or bone marrow disorder.

▷ **Inform Your Physician Before Taking This Drug If**
- you are allergic or abnormally sensitive to other thioxanthene drugs or any phenothiazine drug (see Drug Classes).
- you have impaired liver or kidney function.
- you have any type of seizure disorder.
- you have diabetes, glaucoma or heart disease.
- you have a history of lupus erythematosus or low white blood cells or other blood dyscrasias.
- you have Parkinson's disease.
- you have had neuroleptic malignant syndrome.
- you are taking any drug with sedative effects.
- you drink alcohol daily.
- you plan to have surgery under general or spinal anesthesia in the near future.

Possible Side Effects (natural, expected and unavoidable drug actions)
Mild drowsiness (usually during the first 2 weeks), orthostatic hypotension (see Glossary), blurred vision, dry mouth, nasal congestion, constipation, impaired urination—possible.

▷ **Possible Adverse Effects** (unusual, unexpected and infrequent reactions)
If any of the following develop, consult your physician promptly for guidance.
Mild Adverse Effects
Allergic reactions: skin rash, hives, itching.
Lowering of body temperature, especially in the elderly (see Hypothermia in Glossary).
Fluid retention, weight gain—possible.
Dizziness, weakness, agitation, insomnia, impaired vision—infrequent to frequent.
Nausea, vomiting—infrequent.
Serious Adverse Effects
Allergic reactions: rare hepatitis with jaundice (see Glossary), anaphylactic reaction (see Glossary).
Idiosyncratic reactions: paradoxical worsening of psychotic symptoms.
Development of the neuroleptic malignant syndrome (see Glossary).
Abnormal production of urine and loss of blood sodium (SIADH)—case reports.
Depression, disorientation, seizures—case reports.
Pigmented spots (lenticular)—case report.
Abnormal fixed eye positioning (oculogyric crisis)—frequent extrapyramidal effect.

Rapid heart rate, heart rhythm disorders—possible.

Systemic lupus erythematosus or blood cell disorders: reduced white blood count—case reports.

Nervous system reactions: Parkinson-like disorders (see Glossary), severe restlessness, muscle spasms involving the face and neck, tardive dyskinesia (see Glossary)—infrequent.

Vitamin E may help reduce risk of movement disorders. Talk to your doctor.

Severe reduction in blood pressure—rare.

Possible Effects on Sexual Function: Altered timing and pattern of menstruation.

Impotence, priapism and retrograde ejaculation—rare.

Male breast enlargement and tenderness (gynecomastia)—case reports.

Female breast enlargement with milk production—rare.

▷ **Adverse Effects That May Mimic Natural Diseases or Disorders**

Nervous system reactions may suggest true Parkinson's disease or Reye's syndrome (see Glossary). Liver reactions may suggest viral hepatitis.

Natural Diseases or Disorders That May Be Activated by This Drug

Latent epilepsy, glaucoma, prostatism (see Glossary).

Possible Effects on Laboratory Tests

Complete blood cell counts: decreased red cells, hemoglobin, white cells and platelets; increased eosinophils.

Blood glucose level: increased and decreased (fluctuations).

Liver function tests: increased enzymes (ALT/GPT, AST/GOT, alkaline phosphatase) or bilirubin.

Urine pregnancy tests: false-positive result with some tests.

CAUTION

1. Many over-the-counter medications (see Glossary) for allergies, colds and coughs contain drugs that can interact unfavorably with this drug. Ask your doctor or pharmacist for help **before** using any such medications.

2. Antacids that contain aluminum and/or magnesium may limit drug absorption and effectiveness.

3. Call your doctor if your vision changes while taking this drug.

Precautions for Use

By Infants and Children: Use of this drug is not recommended for children under 12 years of age. Do not use this drug in the presence of symptoms suggestive of Reye's syndrome (see Glossary). Children with acute infectious diseases (flu-like infections, chicken pox, measles, etc.) are more prone to develop muscular spasms of the face, back and extremities when this drug is given.

By Those Over 60 Years of Age: Small starting doses are advisable. Increased risk of drowsiness, lethargy, constipation, lowering of body temperature (hypothermia) and orthostatic hypotension (see Glossary). This drug can worsen existing prostatism (see Glossary). You may also be more susceptible to the development of Parkinson-like reactions and/or tardive dyskinesia (see discussion of these terms in Glossary). These reactions must be recognized early since they may become unresponsive to treatment and irreversible.

▷ **Advisability of Use During Pregnancy**

    Pregnancy Category: C. See Pregnancy Risk Categories at the back of this book.

    Animal studies: No birth defects reported in rats, rabbits or monkeys.

    Human studies: Adequate studies of pregnant women are not available.

      Avoid drug during the first 3 months if possible. Avoid during the final month (possible effects on the newborn).

Advisability of Use If Breast-Feeding

    Presence of this drug in breast milk: Expected in small amounts, but no data are available.

    Avoid drug or refrain from nursing.

Habit-Forming Potential: None.

Effects of Overdose: Marked drowsiness, weakness, tremor, agitation, unsteadiness, deep sleep, coma, convulsions.

Possible Effects of Long-Term Use: Opacities in the cornea or lens of the eye, pigmentation of the retina. Tardive dyskinesia (see Glossary).

Suggested Periodic Examinations While Taking This Drug (at physician's discretion)

    Complete blood cell counts, especially between the 4th and 10th weeks of treatment.

    Liver function tests.

    Electrocardiograms.

    Complete eye examinations—eye structures and vision.

    Careful inspection of the tongue for early evidence of fine, involuntary, wave-like movements that could indicate the beginning of tardive dyskinesia.

▷ **While Taking This Drug, Observe the Following**

    Foods: No restrictions. Vitamin E may help reduce risk of movement disorders. Talk to your doctor.

    Herbal Medicines or Minerals: Since phenothiazines and St. John's wort may act to worsen sensitivity to the sun, caution is advised. Kava and valerian may worsen drowsiness. Since part of the way that ginseng works is as an MAO inhibitor, combination with this medicine is not advisable.

    Beverages: No restrictions. May be taken with milk.

▷   *Alcohol:* Avoid completely. Alcohol can increase the sedative action of thiothixene and accentuate its depressant effects on brain function and blood pressure. Thiothixene can increase the intoxicating effects of alcohol.

    Tobacco Smoking: No interactions expected. I advise everyone to quit smoking.

    Marijuana Smoking: Moderate increase in drowsiness; accentuation of orthostatic hypotension; increased risk of precipitating latent psychoses, confusing the interpretation of mental status and drug responses.

▷   *Other Drugs*

    Thiothixene may ***increase*** the effects of

    • all atropinelike drugs and cause nervous system toxicity.

    • all sedative drugs, especially barbiturates and narcotic analgesics and cause excessive sedation.

    Thiothixene may ***decrease*** the effects of

    • guanethidine (Ismelin, Esimil) and reduce its effectiveness in lowering blood pressure.

Thiothixene taken concurrently with
- ketorolac (Toradol) may result in hallucinations.
- lithium (Lithobid, others) may result in exaggerated neurotoxicity (rigidity and tremor).
- monoamine oxidase (MAO) inhibitors (see Drug Classes) may result in worsening of the depressive effects of thiothixene on the central nervous system and breathing.
- tramadol (Ultram) may increase seizure risk.
- zotepine (Nipolept) may increase seizure risk.

The following drugs may **decrease** the effects of thiothixene:
- antacids containing aluminum and/or magnesium.
- barbiturates (see Drug Classes).
- benztropine (Cogentin).
- trihexyphenidyl (Artane).

▷ *Driving, Hazardous Activities:* This drug can impair mental alertness, judgment and physical coordination. Avoid hazardous activities.

Aviation Note: The use of this drug *is a disqualification* for piloting. Consult a designated Aviation Medical Examiner.

Exposure to Sun: This drug can cause photosensitivity (see Glossary). Use caution until sensitivity has been determined.

Exposure to Heat: Use caution and avoid excessive heat as much as possible. This drug may impair the regulation of body temperature and increase the risk of heatstroke.

Exposure to Cold: Use caution and dress warmly. This drug can increase the risk of hypothermia in the elderly.

Discontinuation: After a period of long-term use, do not stop this drug suddenly. Gradual withdrawal over 2 to 3 weeks under physician supervision is recommended. Do not discontinue this drug without your physician's knowledge and approval. The relapse rate of schizophrenia after discontinuation is 50 to 60%.

TICLOPIDINE (ti KLOH pi deen)

Introduced: 1985   **Class:** Antiplatelet
Author's Note: Because of more widespread use of clopidogrel, this profile has been shortened.

TIMOLOL (TI moh lohl)

Introduced: 1972   **Class:** Anti-anginal, antiglaucoma, antihypertensive, beta blocker   **Prescription:** USA: Yes   **Controlled Drug:** USA: No; Canada: No   **Available as Generic:** USA: Yes; Canada: No

Brand Names: ♣Apo-Timolol, ♣Apo-Timop, Betimol, Blocadren, Cosopt [CD], ♣Dom-Timolol, ♣Novo-Timolol, ♣Timolide [CD], Timoptic, Timoptic Ouches, Timoptic-XE

```
                       BENEFITS versus RISKS
      Possible Benefits                    Possible Risks
EFFECTIVE, WELL-TOLERATED         CONGESTIVE HEART FAILURE IN
  ANTI-ANGINAL DRUG                 ADVANCED HEART DISEASE
EFFECTIVE ANTIGLAUCOMA            Worsening of angina in coronary heart
  DRUG                              disease (if drug is abruptly
ANTIHYPERTENSIVE DRUG in           withdrawn)
  mild to moderate hypertension   Masking of low blood sugar
EFFECTIVE PREVENTION OF            (hypoglycemia) in drug-treated
  MIGRAINE HEADACHES               diabetes
EFFECTIVE ADJUNCTIVE             Provocation of asthma
  PREVENTION (SECONDARY
  PREVENTION) OF RECURRENT
  HEART ATTACK
May have a role in combination
  glaucoma therapy with latanoprost
```

▷ **Principal Uses**

As a Single Drug Product: Uses currently included in FDA-approved labeling: (1) Treats classical effort-induced angina, certain types of heart rhythm disturbance and high blood pressure; (2) lowers increased internal eye pressure in chronic open-angle glaucoma; (3) beneficial when taken within 24 hours and for 28 days thereafter in decreasing the size of the heart damage, decreasing arrhythmias and preventing repeat heart attacks (myocardial infarction); (4) reduces frequency and severity of migraines.

Other (unlabeled) generally accepted uses: (1) Has been used by people who are afraid to fly on airplanes (air travel phobia); (2) may help decrease incidence of abnormal heart rhythms in the atria of the heart (atrial fibrillation and flutter); (3) helps prevent abnormally increased intraocular pressure after cataract surgery; (4) used in patients with detached (not torn) retinas.

As a Combination Drug Product [CD]: Available combined with hydrochlorothiazide to treat high blood pressure. Combination product includes two drugs with different mechanisms of action. This provides better effectiveness and convenience for long-term use.

How This Drug Works: Blocks certain actions of the sympathetic nervous system:
- reducing heart rate and contraction force, lowering blood ejection pressure and reducing oxygen needs of the heart, increasing blood flow to the heart (myocardial perfusion).
- reducing degree of blood vessel wall contraction, lowering blood pressure.
- prolonging conduction time of nerve impulses through the heart, of benefit in managing certain heart rhythm disorders.
- slowing formation of fluid (aqueous humor) in the anterior eye chamber, improving its drainage from the eye, lowering the internal eye pressure.

Available Dosage Forms and Strengths

Eye solutions — 0.25%, 0.5%
Timoptic-XE — 2.5 mg/ml and 5 mg/ml
Tablets — 5 mg, 10 mg, 20 mg

▷ **Usual Adult Dosage Ranges:** *Anti-anginal and antihypertensive:* Initially 10 mg two times daily; increase dose gradually every 7 days as needed and tolerated. Usual maintenance dose is 10 to 20 mg once a day or divided into two equal doses and taken twice daily. The total daily dose should not exceed 60 mg.

 Migraine headache prevention: Initially 10 mg two times daily; increase dose as needed to 10 mg in the morning and 20 mg at night.

 Preventing repeat heart attack: 10 mg twice daily.

 Anti-glaucoma: one drop in affected eye twice daily.

 Author's Note: Timoptic-XE form is a clear gel and is used once daily.

 Note: Actual dose and schedule must be determined for each patient individually.

Conditions Requiring Dosing Adjustments

 Liver Function: Prudent to decrease systemic (nonophthalmic) doses in people with liver diseases.

 Kidney Function: Patients with kidney compromise should be followed closely and the dose decreased if the medication appears to be accumulating.

▷ **Dosing Instructions:** Preferably taken 1 hour before eating to maximize absorption. The tablet may be crushed. Do not stop this drug abruptly. Eyedrops or gel must be used on an ongoing basis. Wash your hands before using the eye drops and do not touch the dropper end. If you forget a dose: Take the missed dose as soon as you remember it, unless it's 4 hours or less until your next dose—if that is the case, skip the missed dose and take the next dose right on schedule. DO NOT double up on doses. Talk with your doctor if you find yourself missing doses—there are beeper-based systems to help you remember your medicines.

Usual Duration of Use: Use on a regular schedule for 10 to 14 days usually determines effectiveness in preventing angina, controlling heart rhythm disorders and lowering blood pressure. Peak benefit may require continual use for 6 to 8 weeks. The long-term use of pill forms will be determined by the course of your symptoms and response to an overall treatment program (weight reduction, salt restriction, smoking cessation, etc.). Ophthalmic forms start to work in 15 to 20 minutes, but require ongoing doses to keep eye pressure low. Follow-up with your doctor is mandatory.

Typical Treatment Goals and Measurements (Outcomes and Markers)

 Blood pressure: The most recent treatment guidelines (JNC VI) actually define optimal blood pressure (BP) as less than 120/80 and high normal as 139/89. The American Diabetes Association has chosen a target of 130/80 as the blood pressure goal for people living with diabetes. Most clinicians try to achieve a BP that achieves the best balance of lower cardiovascular risk while avoiding the problem of too low a blood pressure. The goal and time frame to reach it (see peak benefits above) should be discussed with you when the prescription is written.

 Glaucoma: Ophthalmologists measure intraocular pressure (IOP), and then to check IOP lowering once this medicine is started. The chamber angle can be checked prior to treatment.

Possible Advantages of This Drug: XE form actually forms a clear gel from the initial application of a solution. Once-daily dosing is expected to help people remember to take their medicine (adherence benefit).

▷ **This Drug Should Not Be Taken If**
- you have bronchial asthma or severe obstructive lung disease.
- you have had an allergic reaction to it previously.
- you have Prinzmetal's variant angina (coronary artery spasm).
- you have congestive heart failure.
- you have an abnormally slow heart rate or a serious form of heart block.
- you took a monoamine oxidase (MAO) type A (see Drug Classes) in the last 14 days.

▷ **Inform Your Physician Before Taking This Drug If**
- you had an adverse reaction to a beta blocker (see Drug Classes).
- you have a history of serious heart disease or impaired circulation.
- you have a history of hay fever (allergic rhinitis), asthma, chronic bronchitis or emphysema.
- you have a history of overactive thyroid function (hyperthyroidism).
- you have a history of low blood sugar (hypoglycemia).
- you have impaired liver or kidney function.
- you have Raynaud's phenomenon.
- you have diabetes or myasthenia gravis.
- you currently take digitalis, quinidine or reserpine or any calcium-channel-blocker drug (see Drug Classes).
- you plan to have surgery under general anesthesia in the near future.

Possible Side Effects (natural, expected and unavoidable drug actions)
Lethargy and fatigability, cold extremities, slow heart rate, light-headedness in upright position (see Orthostatic Hypotension in Glossary).

▷ **Possible Adverse Effects** (unusual, unexpected and infrequent reactions)
If any of the following develop, consult your physician promptly for guidance.

Mild Adverse Effects
Allergic reactions: skin rash, itching.
Loss of hair involving the scalp, eyebrows and/or eyelashes. This effect can occur with use of the oral tablets or the eyedrops (used to treat glaucoma). Regrowth occurs with discontinuation of this drug.
Headache, dizziness, visual disturbances, vivid dreams—infrequent.
Indigestion, nausea, vomiting, diarrhea—infrequent.
Numbness and tingling in extremities, joint pain—case reports.

Serious Adverse Effects
Allergic reactions: laryngospasm, severe dermatitis.
Idiosyncratic reactions: acute behavioral disturbances—depression, hallucinations.
Chest pain, shortness of breath, precipitation of congestive heart failure—case reports.
Induction of bronchial asthma (in asthmatic individuals)—possible.
May mask warning signs of impending low blood sugar (hypoglycemia) in drug-treated diabetes.
Drug-induced myasthenia gravis—case reports.
Periodic cramping of the leg (intermittent claudication)—possible.
Stopping of breathing (respiratory arrest)—case report.
Author's Note: Some of the eyedrops or eye gel form can get into your body. While the listed possible reactions are mainly for the forms

taken by mouth (oral), they may possibly (although much less likely) happen with the eye forms.

▷ **Possible Effects on Sexual Function:** Decreased libido, impaired erection, impotence—case reports. **Note: All of these effects can occur with the use of timolol eyedrops at recommended dose, albeit less often.**

▷ **Adverse Effects That May Mimic Natural Diseases or Disorders**

Reduced blood flow to extremities may resemble Raynaud's phenomenon (see Glossary).

Natural Diseases or Disorders That May Be Activated by This Drug

Prinzmetal's variant angina, Raynaud's phenomenon, intermittent claudication, myasthenia gravis (questionable).

Possible Effects on Laboratory Tests

None reported.

CAUTION

1. ***Do not stop this drug suddenly*** without the knowledge and guidance of your doctor. Carry a note stating that you take this drug.
2. Ask your doctor or pharmacist before using nasal decongestants usually present in over-the-counter cold preparations and nose drops. These can cause sudden increases in blood pressure when taken concurrently with beta-blocker drugs.
3. Report development of tendency to emotional depression.

Precautions for Use

By Infants and Children: Safety and effectiveness for those under 12 years of age are not established. However, if this drug is used, watch for low blood sugar (hypoglycemia) during periods of reduced food intake.

By Those Over 60 Years of Age: High blood pressure should be reduced without creating risks associated with excessively low blood pressure. Small starting doses and frequent blood pressure checks are needed. Sudden, rapid and excessive lowering of blood pressure can predispose to stroke or heart attack. Watch for dizziness, unsteadiness, falling, confusion, hallucinations, depression or urinary frequency.

▷ **Advisability of Use During Pregnancy**

Pregnancy Category: C. See Pregnancy Risk Categories at the back of this book.

Animal studies: No significant increase in birth defects due to this drug.

Human studies: Adequate studies of pregnant women are not available.

Avoid use during the first 3 months if possible. Use only if clearly needed. Ask your physician for guidance.

Advisability of Use If Breast-Feeding

Presence of this drug in breast milk: Yes.

Monitor nursing infant closely, and discontinue drug or nursing if adverse effects develop.

Habit-Forming Potential: None.

Effects of Overdose: Weakness, slow pulse, low blood pressure, fainting, cold and sweaty skin, congestive heart failure, possible coma and convulsions.

Possible Effects of Long-Term Use: Reduced heart reserve and eventual heart failure in susceptible people with advanced heart disease.

Suggested Periodic Examinations While Taking This Drug (at physician's discretion)

Complete blood cell counts (because of adverse effects of other drugs of this class).

Measurements of blood pressure.

Evaluation of heart function.

Lowering of eye (intraocular) pressure with ophthalmic forms.

▷ **While Taking This Drug, Observe the Following**

Foods: No restrictions. Avoid excessive salt intake.

Herbal Medicines or Minerals: Ginseng may increase blood pressure, blunting the benefits of this medicine. Hawthorn, saw palmetto, ma huang, goldenseal, yohimbe and licorice may also cause increased blood pressure. Calcium and garlic may help lower blood pressure. Use caution and work with your doctor to make sure blood pressure is not lowered too much. Indian snakeroot has a German Commission E monograph indication for hypertension—talk to your doctor. Eleuthero root and ephedra should be avoided by people living with hypertension. Scopolia root has glaucoma as a possible side effect. DO NOT COMBINE. Henbane and belladonna should also be avoided. Talk to your doctor BEFORE combining any herbals with this drug.

Beverages: No restrictions. May be taken with milk.

▷ *Alcohol:* Use with caution. Alcohol may exaggerate this drug's ability to lower blood pressure and may increase its mild sedative effect.

Tobacco Smoking: Nicotine may reduce this drug's effectiveness. I advise everyone to quit smoking.

▷ *Other Drugs*

Timolol may ***increase*** the effects of

- amiodarone (Cordarone) and cause cardiac arrest and bradycardia.
- other antihypertensive drugs and cause excessive lowering of blood pressure; dose adjustments may be necessary (for example, alpha-1 blockers or dihydropyridine calcium channel blockers).
- ergot derivatives, increasing risk of decreased blood flow to arms and legs (peripheral ischemia).
- lidocaine (Xylocaine, etc.).
- reserpine (Ser-Ap-Es, etc.) and cause sedation, depression, slowing of the heart rate and lowering of blood pressure.
- verapamil (Calan, Isoptin) and cause excessive depression of heart function; monitor this combination closely.

Timolol may decrease the effects of

- theophyllines (Aminophyllin, Theo-Dur, etc.) and reduce their antiasthmatic effectiveness.

Timolol taken concurrently with

- clonidine (Catapres) requires close monitoring for rebound high blood pressure if clonidine is withdrawn while timolol is still being taken.
- epinephrine (Adrenalin, etc.) may cause marked rise in blood pressure and slowing of the heart rate.
- insulin may hide the symptoms of hypoglycemia (see Glossary).
- methyldopa may have paradoxical increases in blood pressure.
- oral hypoglycemic agents (see Oral Antidiabetic Drugs in Drug Classes)

such as acetohexamide (Dymelor) and glipizide (Glucotrol) may result in prolonged low blood sugar.

- quinidine (Quinaglute, others) may lead to excessive slowing of the heart.
- venlafaxine (Effexor) may result in increased risk of timolol toxicity.

The following drugs may increase the effects of timolol:

- chlorpromazine (Thorazine, etc.).
- cimetidine (Tagamet).
- fluoxetine (Prozac).
- fluvoxamine (Luvox).
- methimazole (Tapazole).
- propylthiouracil (Propacil).
- ritonavir (Norvir) and perhaps other protease inhibitors (see Drug Classes).
- zileuton (Zyflo).

The following drugs may decrease the effects of timolol:

- antacids (when taken at the same time).
- barbiturates (phenobarbital, etc.).
- indomethacin (Indocin) and possibly other "aspirin substitutes," or NSAIDs—may impair timolol's antihypertensive effect.
- rifabutin (Mycobutin).
- rifampin (Rifadin, Rimactane).

▷ *Driving, Hazardous Activities:* Use caution until the full extent of dizziness, lethargy and blood pressure change has been determined.

Aviation Note: The use of this drug **may be a disqualification** for piloting. Consult a designated Aviation Medical Examiner.

Exposure to Sun: No restrictions.

Exposure to Heat: Caution is advised. Hot environments can exaggerate the effects of this drug.

Exposure to Cold: Caution is advised. Cold environments can worsen circulatory deficiency in the extremities that may occur with this drug. The elderly should be careful to prevent hypothermia (see Glossary).

Heavy Exercise or Exertion: It is advisable to avoid exertion that produces lightheadedness, excessive fatigue or muscle cramping. The use of this drug may intensify the hypertensive response to isometric exercise.

Occurrence of Unrelated Illness: Fever can lower blood pressure and require adjustment of dose. Nausea or vomiting may interrupt the dosing schedule. Ask your doctor for help.

Discontinuation: It is advisable to avoid sudden discontinuation of this drug in all situations; this is especially true in the presence of coronary artery disease. If possible, gradual reduction of dose over a period of 2 to 3 weeks is recommended. Ask your physician for specific guidance.

TOLBUTAMIDE (tohl BYU ta mide)

Introduced: 1956   **Class:** Antidiabetic, sulfonylureas   **Prescription:** USA: Yes   **Controlled Drug:** USA: No; Canada: No   **Available as Generic:** Yes
Brand Names: ✣Apo-Tolbutamide, ✣Mobenol, ✣Novo-butamide, Oramide, Orinase, Orinase Diagnostic, SK-Tolbutamide

Warning: The brand names Orinase, Ornade and Ornex sound similar; this can lead to serious medication errors. Orinase is tolbutamide, used to treat diabetes. Ornade is chlorpheniramine and phenylpropanolamine, used to treat nasal and sinus congestion. Ornex is acetaminophen and phenyl-propanolamine, used to treat head colds and sinus pain. Make sure you get the correct drug.

Author's Note: The information in this profile has been shortened to make room for more widely used medicines.

TOLCAPONE (TOHL ka poan)

Introduced: 1998   **Class:** COMT inhibitor, anti-Parkinsonism   **Prescription:** USA: Yes   **Controlled Drug:** USA: No   **Available as Generic:** No
Brand Name: Tasmar
Author's Note: The information in this profile will be broadened in subsequent editions once concerns about possible liver toxicity are resolved.

TOLMETIN (TOHL met in)

Please see the acetic acid (nonsteroidal anti-inflammatory drug) family profile.

TOLTERODINE (tol TER oh dyne)

Introduced: 1998   **Class:** Muscarinic receptor antagonist, overactive bladder treatment   **Prescription:** USA: Yes   **Controlled Drug:** USA: No
Available as Generic: No
Brand Name: Detrol, Detrol LA

BENEFITS versus RISKS	
Possible Benefits	*Possible Risks*
EFFECTIVE TREATMENT OF OVERACTIVE BLADDER	CONSTIPATION
CONTROLS URGE TO URINATE	Dry mouth
LOWERS FREQUENCY OF URINATION	Blurred vision
DECREASES UNEXPECTED URGENT DESIRE TO URINATE (URGE INCONTINENCE)	
NEW ONCE DAILY FORM OFFERS INCREASED CONTROL AND ADHERENCE	

▷ **Principal Uses**
As a Single Drug Product: Uses currently included in FDA-approved labeling: (1) Treats symptoms of overactive bladders; (2) used to decrease excessive

urination (urinary frequency); (3) eases unexpected urgent desire to urinate followed by inability to control the bladder (urge incontinence).
Other (unlabeled) generally accepted uses: None at present.

How This Drug Works: Acts as an anticholinergic agent (competitive muscarinic receptor antagonist) with some selective action on the bladder.
This effect increases volume of residual urine and decreases maximum
detrusor pressure. This makes it more difficult to urinate, easing overactive bladder symptoms and helping urge incontinence.

Available Dosage Forms and Strengths
Capsules, extended release — 2 mg, 4 mg
Tablets — 1 mg, 2 mg

▷ **Usual Adult Dosage Ranges:** Started with 2 mg twice a day. The dose may be
lowered to 1 mg twice a day if the higher dose is not tolerated (people taking drugs inhibiting liver enzymes CYP3A4 and CYP2D6 should also be
given 1 mg twice daily). Detrol LA form is dosed at 4 mg once daily. As with
the immediate-release form, the dose is decreased (to 2 mg once daily) for
those taking drugs inhibiting CYP 3A4 or 2D6 or with lowered kidney or
liver function. **Note: Actual dose and schedule must be determined for
each patient individually.**

Conditions Requiring Dosing Adjustments
Liver Function: Dose should be decreased to 1 mg twice a day of the immediate-release form or 2 mg once daily of Detrol LA in liver disease. (As this
drug undergoes cytochrome P-450 2D6 and CYP3A4 metabolism.)
Kidney Function: Used with caution. The drug was not studied in kidney disease, but dose should be decreased to 1 mg of the immediate-release form
twice daily or to 2 mg once daily of Detrol LA.

▷ **Dosing Instructions:** The tablet may be crushed and taken without regard to food
(food does increase bioavailability—53% on average, but this is not thought
to be clinically significant). If you forget a dose: Take the missed dose as soon
as you remember it, unless it's nearly time for your next dose—if that is the
case, skip the missed dose and take the next dose right on schedule. DO NOT
double up on doses. Talk with your doctor if you find yourself missing doses.

Usual Duration of Use: Initial response to this medicine happens in about an
hour. The clinical trials leading to FDA approval showed some benefits of
use on a regular schedule in one trial at 4 weeks and peak and consistent
benefits at 12 weeks. It is important to follow up with your doctor regarding side effects (dose may need to be decreased) and therapeutic benefits.

Typical Treatment Goals and Measurements (Outcomes and Markers)
Bladder activity: Most urologists use patient reports of lowered desire or frequency of urination as a hallmark of successful therapy. A general sense of
decreased need to urinate immediately (urgency) is also useful. Some
physicians will use a bladder diary to help define, in absolute terms, the
beneficial effects of this medicine.

Possible Advantages of This Drug
May be more selective for the bladder than other medicines.

▷ **This Drug Should Not Be Taken If**
- you are allergic to tolterodine.
- you retain urine abnormally (retention of urine).

- you have a problem with retaining food or fluid in the stomach (gastric retention).
- you have narrow-angle glaucoma that is not controlled.

▷ **Inform Your Physician Before Taking This Drug If**
- you have liver or kidney disease.
- you have a history of ulcerative colitis.
- you have narrow-angle glaucoma controlled by medicines.
- your job requires visual acuity.
- you have heart or blood vessel disease.
- you have had a bowel obstruction or ulcerative colitis.
- you are breast-feeding your child.
- you are prone to constipation.
- you will have surgery under general anesthesia soon.

Possible Side Effects (natural, expected and unavoidable drug actions)
Dry mouth, nasal congestion, constipation—may be frequent.

▷ **Possible Adverse Effects** (unusual, unexpected and infrequent reactions)
If any of the following develop, consult your physician promptly for guidance.
Mild Adverse Effects
Allergic reactions: skin rash.
Dizziness—infrequent.
Blurred vision and increased light sensitivity—rare to infrequent.
Decreased salivation—infrequent.
Dryness of hands or feet—infrequent.
Serious Adverse Effects
Passing out (syncope)—case reports in clinical trials.
Cerebrovascular disorder—case reports . . . possibly related to the drug in clinical trials.
Urinary retention—case reports.

▷ **Possible Effects on Sexual Function:** None defined.

Natural Diseases or Disorders That May Be Activated by This Drug
Tendency to constipation may be worsened.
Narrow-angle glaucoma may be worsened.

Possible Effects on Laboratory Tests None defined.

CAUTION
1. Some people (about 7% of the population) are poor metabolizers of this drug. This means that the medicine may accumulate and more of an effect from a "normal dose" will be seen in those people. Once this pattern is identified, doses will need to be decreased to avoid getting too much of the medicine from a "normal" dose.
2. Talk to your doctor or dentist about sugarless candy or other measures to take if dry mouth becomes a problem.
3. **If** you are prone to constipation, it may be prudent to start a medicine to address possible constipation if this medicine is started.

Precautions for Use
By Infants and Children: Safety and effectiveness not established in pediatrics.
By Those Over 60 Years of Age: No dosage change is recommended by the man-

ufacturer. Mean blood concentrations of the drug and its metabolite were increased by 20–50%, but no overall safety differences were seen between older and younger patients who were studied.

▷ **Advisability of Use During Pregnancy**
Pregnancy Category: C. See Pregnancy Risk Categories at the back of this book.
Animal studies: No birth defects found in mice studies.
Human studies: Adequate studies of pregnant women are not available.
Use this drug only if clearly needed. Ask your doctor for help.

Advisability of Use If Breast-Feeding
Presence of this drug in breast milk: Yes in mice, unknown in humans.
Stop the medicine or discontinue nursing.

Habit-Forming Potential: None.

Effects of Overdose: Severe central anticholinergic effects.

Possible Effects of Long-Term Use: None reported.

Suggested Periodic Examinations While Taking This Drug (at physician's discretion)
Follow-up on decreased urination versus adverse effects.

▷ **While Taking This Drug, Observe the Following**
Foods: No restrictions.
Herbal Medicines or Minerals: Since St. John's wort and tolterodine may increase sun sensitivity, the combination is NOT advised. Caffeine-containing beverages as well as kola, ephedra and ma huang may increase blood pressure, eventually leading to possible increased fluid removal and increased need to urinate. Caution is advised.
Beverages: Grapefruit juice is not advisable. May be taken with water or milk. See caffeine note above (coffee and some teas). Some teas also contain substances that act as mild diuretics.
▷ *Alcohol:* Alcohol can increase loss of water from the body. This can work against the action of this medicine.
Tobacco Smoking: Nicotine may work counter to this medicine. Avoid all forms of tobacco.
▷ *Other Drugs*
Tolterodine *taken concurrently* with
• other medicines that inhibit CYP 3A4 or 2D6 (such as macrolide antibiotics, itraconazole, ketoconazole and others) may lead to excessive blood levels and toxicity risk.
• fluoxetine (Prozac) may lead to tolterodine toxicity.
• warfarin (Coumadin) may lead to increased bleeding risk. More frequent INRs are prudent.
▷ *Driving, Hazardous Activities:* This drug may cause blurred vision. Restrict activities as necessary.
Aviation Note: The use of this drug **may be a disqualification** for piloting. Consult a designated Aviation Medical Examiner.
Exposure to Sun: May increase sensitivity of your eyes to the sun.
Heavy Exercise or Exertion: Excessive exertion is cooled by sweating. This medicine may lead to drying of skin and decreased perspiration.
Discontinuation: Ask your physician for guidance.

TRAMADOL (TRAM ah doll)

Introduced: 1996   **Class:** Analgesic   **Prescription:** USA: Yes   **Con-trolled Drug:** USA: Yes; Canada: No   **Available as Generic:** USA: No; Canada: No
Brand Name: Ultram

BENEFITS versus RISKS

Possible Benefits	*Possible Risks*
EFFECTIVE TREATMENT OF PAIN	DROWSINESS
MINIMAL SIDE EFFECTS VERSUS	May decrease the seizure threshold
MORPHINE-LIKE AGENTS	Constipation
(OPIOIDS)	

▷ **Principal Uses**

As a Single Drug Product: Uses currently included in FDA-approved labeling: Used to provide symptomatic relief in all types of pain.

Other (unlabeled) generally accepted uses: (1) May have a role in pain where depression is also a therapeutic problem; (2) might have a role as an adjunct to anesthesia; (3) eases fibromyalgia pain.

How This Drug Works: Increases the availability of serotonin and norepineph-rine in certain brain centers and also works at opioid (see Glossary) centers, thereby relieving pain.

Available Dosage Forms and Strengths

Tablets — 50 mg

▷ **Usual Adult Dosage Ranges:** 50 to 100 mg every 4 to 6 hours. Most patients respond to 150 to 300 mg daily. The total daily dose should not exceed 400 mg. German data found clinicians using 0.7 mg per kg per dose and 5.6 mg per kg of body mass per day as a maximum for those over 18 years of age. **Note: Actual dose and schedule must be determined for each patient individually.**

Conditions Requiring Dosing Adjustments

Liver Function: Patients with cirrhosis should be closely watched for adverse effects and may take only 50 mg every 12 hours.

Kidney Function: For patients with creatinine clearances less than 30 ml/min, usual dose is taken every 12 hours, and the daily maximum is 200 mg.

▷ **Dosing Instructions:** May be taken without regard to meals. The tablet may be crushed. If excessive drowsiness or dizziness occurs, call your doctor. If you forget a dose: Take the missed dose as soon as you remember it, unless it's nearly time for your next dose—if that is the case, skip the missed dose and take the next dose right on schedule. DO NOT double doses. Talk with your doctor if you find yourself missing doses.

Usual Duration of Use: Peak effect usually happens in half an hour. Use on a regular schedule depends on the condition treated. Many chronic pain syndromes are treated with combinations of medicines. Long-term use requires supervision by your doctor.

Typical Treatment Goals and Measurements (Outcomes and Markers)

Pain: Most clinicians treating pain use a device called an algometer to check your pain. This looks like a small ruler, but lets the clinician better understand your pain. The goals of treatment then relate to where the level of pain started (for example, a rating of seven on a zero to ten scale) and what the cause of the pain was. Pain medicines may also be used together (in combination) in order to get the best result or outcome. If your pain control is not acceptable to YOU (remember, in hospitals and outpatient settings, etc. pain control is a patient right and the fifth vital sign), call your doctor. It is not unusual to have an immediate-release rescue dose available and then some percentage of previous day use added back to an extended-release form. Pain can be dynamic and adjustments are often required.

Possible Advantages of This Drug: Possible Advantages of This Drug: Avoids opioid side effects.

▷ **This Drug Should Not Be Taken If**
- you have had an allergic reaction to it previously.
- you are allergic to codeine or similar compounds.
- you are intoxicated by morphinelike drugs or alcohol.
- you are taking, or have taken within the last 14 days, a monoamine oxidase (MAO) inhibitor.

▷ **Inform Your Physician Before Taking This Drug If**
- you have a history of seizures or take medicines that may make seizures more likely.
- you have a history of alcoholism, epilepsy, narcotic addiction or thyroid gland problems.
- you are prone to constipation.
- you have impaired liver or kidney function.
- you are pregnant or breast-feeding your infant.
- you plan to have surgery under general anesthesia in the near future.

Possible Side Effects (natural, expected and unavoidable drug actions)
Drowsiness, light-headedness, blurred vision, dry mouth, constipation-infrequent to frequent.

▷ **Possible Adverse Effects** (unusual, unexpected and infrequent reactions)
If any of the following develop, consult your physician promptly for guidance.

Mild Adverse Effects
Allergic reactions: skin rash.
Rapid heart rate, palpitations—case reports.
Nausea, vomiting, diarrhea—infrequent to frequent.
Sweating—frequent.
Urinary retention—possible.

Serious Adverse Effects
Allergic reactions: anaphylaxis—case reports.
Behavioral effects: confusion, hallucinations—case reports.
Seizures—increased risk, especially in those with seizure disorders.
Lowered blood pressure—possible and dose-related.

▷ **Possible Effects on Sexual Function:** Decreased male or female libido—possible.

Possible Effects on Laboratory Tests
Liver enzymes: increased.

CAUTION
1. If you experience a significant degree of mouth dryness while using this drug, consult your dentist regarding the risk of gum erosion or

tooth decay. Ask for guidance in ways to keep the mouth comfortably moist.

2. If you have breathing problems (such as chronic obstructive pulmonary disease [COPD]), you may be at greater risk for respiratory depression.

3. DO NOT take this medicine if you are allergic to codeine (more likely to have a serious reaction).

Precautions for Use

By Infants and Children: Safety and effectiveness for use by those under 18 years of age have not been established.

By Those Over 60 Years of Age: Lower starting doses and adjustment to calculated creatinine clearance are prudent. During the first 2 weeks of treatment, observe for confusion or disorientation. Be aware of possible unsteadiness and incoordination that may predispose to falling. This drug may enhance prostatism (see Glossary).

▷ **Advisability of Use During Pregnancy**

Pregnancy Category: C. See Pregnancy Risk Categories at the back of this book.

Animal studies: Fetal deaths and birth defects reported at doses 3 to 15 times the human dose.

Human studies: Adequate studies of pregnant women are not available.

Avoid this drug completely during the first 3 months. Ask your physician for guidance.

Advisability of Use If Breast-Feeding

Presence of this drug in breast milk: Yes.

Avoid drug or refrain from nursing.

Habit-Forming Potential: May cause psychological or physical dependence.

Effects of Overdose: Marked drowsiness, weakness, confusion, tremors, stupor, coma, possible seizures.

Possible Effects of Long-Term Use: May increase likelihood of dependence.

Suggested Periodic Examinations While Taking This Drug (at physician's discretion)

Heart rate and blood pressure.

Bowel and bladder status.

Evaluation for tremor or hallucination.

Liver function tests.

▷ **While Taking This Drug, Observe the Following**

Foods: No restrictions.

Herbal Medicines or Minerals: Kava kava and valerian may worsen drowsiness. Since ginseng may act as an MAO inhibitor, DO NOT combine. St. John's wort can change (inducing or increasing) P450 enzymes, blunting the effects of this medicine. Talk to your doctor BEFORE you combine any herbal medicines with tramadol.

Beverages: No restrictions. May be taken with milk.

▷ *Alcohol:* Avoid completely. This drug can markedly increase the intoxicating effects of alcohol and accentuate its depressant action on brain functions.

Tobacco Smoking: No interactions expected. I advise everyone to quit smoking.

▷ *Other Drugs*

Tramadol may ***increase*** the effects of

- antihypertensive drugs and cause excessive lowering of blood pressure; dose adjustments may be necessary.

- drugs with sedative effects and cause excessive sedation (see Antihistamines, Opioids, Antianxiety Drugs, etc., in Drug Classes).
- tricyclic antidepressants (see Drug Classes), leading to seizures.
- warfarin (Coumadin), requiring dose adjustment; more frequent INR (pro-time) tests are prudent.

Tramadol **taken concurrently** with

- carbamazepine (Tegretol) may lower tramadol benefits.
- clonidine will lessen clonidine's therapeutic effect.
- clozapine (Clozaril) may increase seizure risk.
- cyclobenzaprine (Flexeril) increases seizure risk.
- digoxin (Lanoxin) may lead to digoxin toxicity—DO NOT COMBINE.
- fluoxetine (Prozac) may result in an increased seizure risk.
- fluvoxamine (Luvox) may result in an increased seizure risk.
- monoamine oxidase (MAO) inhibitors (see Drug Classes) may result in serious side effects (seizures, cardiovascular collapse)—DO NOT COMBINE.
- other drugs that cause central nervous system depression (see Benzodiazepines, Opioids and Tranquilizers in Drug Classes) may have additive effects.
- other drugs that increase seizure risks may have additive effects.
- some phenothiazines (see Drug Classes) may result in excessively lowered blood pressure.
- quinidine (Quinaglute, others) may change tramadol levels.
- ritonavir (Norvir) and perhaps other protease inhibitors (see Drug Classes) may lead to toxicity.
- sertraline (Zoloft) increases seizure risk.
- venlafaxine (Effexor) increases seizure risk.

▷ *Driving, Hazardous Activities:* This drug may cause dizziness or drowsiness. Restrict activities as necessary.

Aviation Note: The use of this drug *is a disqualification* for piloting. Consult a designated Aviation Medical Examiner.

Exposure to Sun: No restrictions.

Discontinuation: It is advisable to discontinue this drug gradually. Ask your physician for guidance in dose reduction over an appropriate period of time.

TRAVOPROST (TRAV oh prost)

Introduced: 2001   **Class:** Prostaglandin analogue, antiglaucoma   **Prescription:** USA: Yes   **Controlled Drug:** USA: No; Canada: No   **Available as Generic:** No
Brand Name: Travatan

BENEFITS versus RISKS	
Possible Benefits	*Possible Risks*
EFFECTIVE REDUCTION OF INTERNAL EYE PRESSURE FOR CONTROL OF ACUTE AND CHRONIC GLAUCOMA CONTROL OF OCULAR HYPERTENSION	Mild side effects with systemic absorption

▷ **Principal Uses**

    As a Single Drug Product: Uses currently included in FDA-approved labeling: (1) Used to manage glaucoma in patients who are intolerant of or who are not adequately controlled by other intraocular pressure lowering medicines; (2) lowers increased pressure in the eye (intraocular pressure).

    Other (unlabeled) generally accepted uses: (1) None as yet.

Possible Advantages of This Drug: Appears to have greater effectiveness in patients of African descent than other previously available agents.

Author's Note: Information in this profile will be broadened as clinical efficacy warrants.

TRAZODONE (TRAZ oh dohn)

Introduced: 1967   **Class:** Antidepressants   **Prescription:** USA: Yes **Controlled Drug:** USA: No; Canada: No   **Available as Generic:** USA: Yes; Canada: Yes

Brand Names: Desyrel, ✤Alti-Trazodone, ✤Apo-Trazodone, ✤Desyrel Dividose, ✤Novo-Trazodone, ✤PMS-Trazodone, Trialodine

BENEFITS versus RISKS	
Possible Benefits	*Possible Risks*
EFFECTIVE TREATMENT IN ALL TYPES OF DEPRESSIVE ILLNESS	Adverse behavioral effects
	Potential for causing heart rhythm disorders in people with heart disease

▷ **Principal Uses**

    As a Single Drug Product: Uses currently included in FDA-approved labeling: Used to provide symptomatic relief in all types of depression.

    Other (unlabeled) generally accepted uses: (1) May have a role in reducing the symptoms of agoraphobia; (2) may help drug-induced (such as MAO inhibitors) insomnia; (3) can have a role in combination therapy of some pain syndromes; (4) may be of help in essential tremor; (5) can ease bouts of repetitive screaming.

How This Drug Works: Increases availability of serotonin in certain brain centers and thereby relieves the symptoms of emotional depression.

Available Dosage Forms and Strengths

    Tablets — 50 mg, 100 mg, 150 mg, 300 mg

▷ **Usual Adult Dosage Ranges:** Initially 50 mg three times daily. The dose may be increased by 50 mg a day at intervals of 3 or 4 days, as needed and tolerated. In order to minimize excessive sleepiness, slower increases of 25–50 mg every two weeks may help. The total daily dose should not exceed 400 mg in people not in the hospital and a maximum dose of 600 mg a day for those who are hospitalized. The lowest effective dose should be used. **Note: Actual dose and schedule must be determined for each patient individually.**

Conditions Requiring Dosing Adjustments

    Liver Function: Blood levels should be obtained to guide dosing. May be a rare cause of liver damage, and patients should be followed closely.

Kidney Function: Metabolites are removed by the kidneys, but dose adjustment in renal compromise is not defined.

▷ **Dosing Instructions:** This drug is best taken with food to improve absorption. The tablet may be crushed. If excessive drowsiness or dizziness occurs, it is advisable to take a larger portion of the daily dose at bedtime and divide the remaining amount into two or three smaller doses to be taken during the day. If you forget a dose: Take the missed dose as soon as you remember it, unless it's nearly time for your next dose—if that is the case, skip the missed dose and take the next dose right on schedule. DO NOT double dose. Talk with your doctor if you find yourself missing doses.

Usual Duration of Use: Some relief in symptoms can be seen in as little as a week. Use on a regular schedule for 2 to 4 weeks usually determines maximum effectiveness in relieving the symptoms of depression. Long-term use (weeks to months) requires supervision and periodic evaluation by your physician.

Typical Treatment Goals and Measurements (Outcomes and Markers)
Depression: The general goal: to at least help lessen the degree and severity of depression, letting patients return to their daily lives. Some psychologists or psychiatrists use specific measures of depression (such as the Hamilton Depression scale) that involve testing or inventories. These can be valuable in helping check benefits from this medicine.

Possible Advantages of This Drug: Appears to have a better heart (cardiac) side effect profile than other antidepressants.

▷ **This Drug Should Not Be Taken If**
 • you have had an allergic reaction to it previously.
 • you are recovering from a recent heart attack (myocardial infarction).
 • you have carcinoid syndrome.
 • you are taking, or have taken within the past 14 days, any monoamine oxidase (MAO) type A inhibitor (see Drug Classes).

▷ **Inform Your Physician Before Taking This Drug If**
 • you have a history of alcoholism, epilepsy or heart disease (especially heart rhythm disorders).
 • you have impaired liver or kidney function.
 • you have a sustained erection (may be priapism).
 • you are pregnant or breast-feeding your infant.
 • you are taking any antihypertensive drugs.
 • you are going to have electroshock therapy (ECT).
 • you will have surgery with general anesthesia.

Possible Side Effects (natural, expected and unavoidable drug actions)
Drowsiness, light-headedness, blurred vision, weight gain, dry mouth, constipation.

▷ **Possible Adverse Effects** (unusual, unexpected and infrequent reactions)
If any of the following develop, consult your physician promptly for guidance.
Mild Adverse Effects
Allergic reactions: skin rash.
Headache, dizziness, fatigue, impaired concentration, nervousness, tremors—infrequent.
Rapid heart rate, palpitations—rare.

Peculiar taste, stomach discomfort, nausea, vomiting, diarrhea—infrequent.

Urinary retention—possible.

Cavities (dental caries)—case reports.

Muscular aches and pains—infrequent.

Serious Adverse Effects

Allergic reactions: serious skin rashes (erythema multiforme).

Behavioral effects: confusion, anger, hostility, delusions, hallucinations, nightmares—case reports.

Irregular heart rhythms, heart attack—case reports.

Low blood pressure, fainting (syncope)—case reports.

Erythema multiforme—case reports.

Abnormal white blood cell counts or hemolytic anemia—case reports.

Seizures—rare.

Liver toxicity—possible.

▷ **Possible Effects on Sexual Function:** Decreased male libido; increased female libido. Inhibited ejaculation, impotence, priapism (see Glossary) or altered timing and pattern of menstruation—case reports.

Possible Effects on Laboratory Tests: Liver enzymes: increased.

CAUTION

1. If you have significant mouth dryness while using this drug, ask your dentist about risk of gum erosion or tooth decay. Ask for help in ways to keep the mouth comfortably moist.

2. It is advisable to withhold this drug if electroconvulsive therapy (ECT) is to be used to treat your depression.

Precautions for Use

By Infants and Children: Safety and effectiveness for use by those under 18 years of age have not been established.

By Those Over 60 Years of Age: During the first 2 weeks of treatment, observe for the development of restlessness, agitation, excitement, forgetfulness, confusion or disorientation. Be aware of possible unsteadiness and incoordination that may predispose to falling. This drug may enhance prostatism (see Glossary).

▷ **Advisability of Use During Pregnancy**

Pregnancy Category: C. See Pregnancy Risk Categories at the back of this book.

Animal studies: Fetal deaths and birth defects reported.

Human studies: Adequate studies of pregnant women are not available.

Avoid this drug completely during the first 3 months. Ask your physician for guidance.

Advisability of Use If Breast-Feeding

Presence of this drug in breast milk: Yes.

Avoid drug or refrain from nursing.

Habit-Forming Potential: None.

Effects of Overdose: Marked drowsiness, confusion, tremors, low blood pressure, rapid heart rate, stupor, coma or seizures.

Possible Effects of Long-Term Use: None reported.

Suggested Periodic Examinations While Taking This Drug (at physician's discretion)

Complete blood cell counts. (This drug may cause slight reductions in white blood cell counts. This should be monitored closely if infection, sore throat or fever develops.)

Serial blood pressure readings and electrocardiograms.

▷ **While Taking This Drug, Observe the Following**

Foods: No restrictions.

Herbal Medicines or Minerals: Caution is advised with St. John's wort because of possible serotonin syndrome. Since part of the way ginseng works may be as an MAO inhibitor, do not combine ginseng with trazodone. Ma huang, Indian snakeroot and yohimbe are also best avoided while taking this medicine. Talk to your doctor BEFORE combining any herbal with this drug.

Beverages: No restrictions. May be taken with milk.

▷ *Alcohol:* Avoid completely. This drug can markedly increase the intoxicating effects of alcohol and accentuate its depressant action on brain functions.

Tobacco Smoking: No interactions expected. I advise everyone to quit smoking.

▷ *Other Drugs*

Trazodone may *increase* the effects of

- antihypertensive drugs and cause excessive lowering of blood pressure; dose adjustments may be necessary.
- drugs with sedative effects and cause excessive sedation.
- phenytoin (Dilantin) or fosphenytoin (Cerebyx) by raising its blood level; observe for phenytoin or fosphenytoin toxicity.
- tramadol (Ultram).

Trazodone *taken concurrently* with

- clonidine (Catapres) will lessen the therapeutic effect of clonidine.
- fluoxetine (Prozac) may result in an increased trazodone level and toxicity.
- monoamine oxidase (MAO) inhibitors (see Drug Classes) may result in undesirable side effects in some patients and beneficial therapeutic effects in others.
- other drugs that cause central nervous system depression (see Benzodiazepines, Opioids and Tranquilizers in Drug Classes) may have additive effects.
- paroxetine (Paxil) may result in toxicity (serotonin syndrome).
- some phenothiazines (see Drug Classes) may result in excessively lowered blood pressure.
- ritonavir (Norvir) and perhaps other protease inhibitors (see Drug Classes) may lead to toxicity.
- tramadol (Ultram) may increase seizure risk.
- warfarin (Coumadin) may result in decreased therapeutic benefits of warfarin; INR (prothrombin time or protime) should be checked more often if warfarin and trazodone are combined.

▷ *Driving, Hazardous Activities:* This drug may cause dizziness or drowsiness. Restrict activities as necessary.

Aviation Note: The use of this drug *is a disqualification* for piloting. Consult a designated Aviation Medical Examiner.

Exposure to Sun: No restrictions.

Discontinuation: It is advisable to discontinue this drug gradually. Ask your physician for guidance in dose reduction over an appropriate period of time.

TRIAMCINOLONE (tri am SIN oh lohn)

Introduced: 1985   **Class:** Antiasthmatic, cortisonelike drugs   **Prescription:** USA: Yes   **Controlled Drug:** USA: No; Canada: No   **Available as Generic:** Yes

Brand Name: Amcort, Aristocort, Aristocort R, Aristoform D, ✤Aristospan, Articulose LA, ✤Aureocort, Azmacort, Cenocort, Cenocort Forte, Flutex, ✤Kenacomb, Kenacort, Kenaject, Kenalog, Kenalog H, Kenalog IN, Kenalone, Mycogen II, Mycolog [CD], Mycomar, Mytrex [CD], Mytriacet II [CD], Nasacort, Nasacort AQ, SK-Triamcinolone, TAC-D, TAC–40, Triacet, ✤Triaderm Mild, ✤Triaderm Regular, Triam-A, Triam-Forte, Triamolone 40, Triderm, Tri-Kort, Trilog, Tristoject, ✤Viaderm-K.C.

BENEFITS versus RISKS

Possible Benefits	*Possible Risks*
EFFECTIVE CONTROL OF SEVERE, CHRONIC BRONCHIAL ASTHMA	Yeast infections of mouth and throat
EFFECTIVE SUPPRESSION OF A VARIETY OF INFLAMMATORY DISORDERS	Suppression of normal cortisone production
POSSIBLE REDUCTION IN SYSTEMIC STEROID USE	Euphoria and psychotic episodes
EFFECTIVE TREATMENT OF SEASONAL OR PERENNIAL ALLERGIC RHINITIS IN ADULTS AND CHILDREN	Cushing's syndrome ("moon face," obesity and "buffalo hump") Muscle wasting (with long-term use) Osteoporosis (with long-term use)

▷ **Principal Uses**

As a Single Drug Product: Uses currently included in FDA-approved labeling: (1) Inhaler form is used to treat chronic bronchial asthma in people who require cortisonelike drugs for asthma control—this is better than cortisone taken by mouth (swallowed) or injection because it works more locally on the respiratory tract, not requiring systemic distribution; this helps prevent some serious adverse effects that usually result from the long-term use of cortisone taken for systemic effects; (2) tablet form can be used in a variety of inflammatory disorders; (3) tablet form is used to ease drug reactions; (4) used as part of combination treatment of acute lymphocytic leukemia in children; (5) used in autoimmune hemolytic anemia; (6) nasal inhaler form helps adults and children with symptoms of seasonal or perennial allergic rhinitis; (7) combined with antibiotics in some countries for use as a wound dressing.

Other (unlabeled) generally accepted uses: (1) May have a role in postherpetic nerve pain (neuralgia); (2) corticosteroids may be of use with Pneumocystis carinii pneumonia in extreme cases where conventional therapy has not worked; (3) may help Guillain-Barré syndrome; (4) can help myasthenia gravis; (5) short-term therapy of psoriasis; (6) injection form relieves pseudogout.

As a Combination Drug Product [CD]: Available combined with antibiotics in some countries as a wound dressing.

How This Drug Works: By increasing the amount of cyclic AMP in appropriate tissues, this drug may thereby increase the concentration of epinephrine, which is an effective bronchodilator and antiasthmatic. Additional benefit is due to the drug's ability to reduce local allergic reaction and inflammation in the lining tissues of the respiratory tract.

Available Dosage Forms and Strengths

Inhalation aerosol (per metered spray) — 0.1 mg

Nasal inhaler — 55 mcg per actuation

Nasal spray — 55 mcg or 100 mcg per metered dose (100 mcg is Canada only)

Tablets — 1 mg, 2 mg, 4 mg, 8 mg

Topical cream — 0.025%, 0.1%, 0.25%

Topical ointment — 0.1%, 0.5%

Topical ointment — 0.25%, 0.5%

▷ **Recommended Dosage Ranges** (Actual dose and schedule must be determined for each patient individually.)

Infants and Children:

Up to 6 years of age: dose not established.

6 to 12 years of age: 0.1 to 0.2 mg (one or two metered sprays) three or four times a day. Adjust dose as needed and tolerated. Limit total daily dose to 1.2 mg (12 metered sprays).

12 to 60 Years of Age:

Inhalation: Initially 0.2 mg (two metered sprays) three or four times a day. For severe asthma—1.2 to 1.6 mg (12 to 16 metered sprays) per day, in divided doses. Adjust dose as needed and tolerated. It is usually used as two inhalations three to four times a day. Results are better when used in this fashion versus on an as-needed basis. Limit total daily dose to 1.6 mg (16 metered sprays). Nasacort AQ and Nasacort may prove effective with a starting dose of 220 mcg per day.

Tablets: 4 to 48 mg daily for inflammatory conditions.

Topical cream: 0.025% is usually applied to the affected area two to four times a day.

Over 60 Years of Age: Same as 12 to 60 years of age.

Conditions Requiring Dosing Adjustments

Liver Function: This drug is metabolized in the liver. Dosing changes in liver compromise are not defined.

Kidney Function: Dosing adjustments do not appear warranted for patients with compromised kidneys.

▷ **Dosing Instructions:** Inhalation form: May be used as needed without regard to eating. Shake the container well before using. Carefully follow the printed patient instructions provided with the unit. Rinse the mouth and throat (gargle) with water thoroughly after each inhalation; do not swallow the rinse water. The Nasacort AQ form is water-based for treatment of allergic rhinitis and does not contain chlorofluorocarbon propellants.

Oral tablets: May cause stomach upset and can be taken with meals or snacks.

If you forget a dose: Take, use or apply the missed dose as soon as you remember it, unless it's nearly time for your next dose—if that is the case, skip the missed dose and take the next dose right on schedule. DO NOT double up on doses. Talk with your doctor if you find yourself missing doses.

Usual Duration of Use: Use on a regular schedule for 1 to 2 weeks usually determines effectiveness in controlling severe, chronic asthma. Long-term use requires the supervision and guidance of a physician.

Typical Treatment Goals and Measurements (Outcomes and Markers)

Asthma: Frequency and severity of asthma attacks should ease. Some clinicians also use decreased frequency of rescue inhaler use as a further clinical indicator. It is critical that this medicine is used regularly to get the best results. Lung (pulmonary function) testing (FEV1 and others) and improvement in those tests also helps define results in asthma. Lastly, clinical signs and symptoms such as wheezing, tightness in the chest and exercise tolerance should all move in favorable directions.

An additional goal of therapy is to use the lowest effective dose. Some people keep their improvements when doses are lowered, while others relapse. Those with a less than two-fold improvement in airway response and people who stay in the moderate to severe asthma range despite appropriate dosing may be more likely to relapse if dosing decrease attempts are made. If the usual benefit of ongoing use is not realized, call your doctor.

Inflammation: The general goal is to relieve the swelling and the inflammatory response. Topical use in skin conditions gives a local effect to benefit discomfort, itching and swelling.

Allergic rhinitis: Symptoms such as itchy, runny nose, sore throat and postnasal drip should all ease once this medicine begins to work. Because there may be some seasonality to the pollen or molds that can cause rhinitis, talk to your doctor about exactly how he or she wants you to use this medicine.

▷ **This Drug Should Not Be Taken If**
- you have had an allergic reaction to it previously.
- you are having severe acute asthma or status asthmaticus that requires immediate relief.
- you have a form of nonallergic bronchitis with asthmatic features.
- you have a systemic fungal infection.
- the dental paste form has been prescribed and you have a bacterial, viral or fungal mouth infection.

▷ **Inform Your Physician Before Taking This Drug If**
- you are now taking, or have recently taken, any cortisone-related drug (including ACTH by injection) for any reason (see Drug Classes).
- you have a history of tuberculosis of the lungs.
- you have chronic bronchitis or bronchiectasis.
- you have diabetes, glaucoma, myasthenia gravis or peptic ulcer disease.
- you have had unexpected surgery (may delay wound healing).
- you have an underactive thyroid (hypothyroidism).
- you think you may have an active infection of any kind, especially a respiratory infection.
- you are taking any of the following drugs: warfarin, oral antidiabetic drugs, insulin or digoxin.

Possible Side Effects (natural, expected and unavoidable drug actions)

Yeast infections (thrush) of the mouth and throat. Irritation of mouth, tongue or throat. May cause euphoria, manic-depressive illness or paranoid states with long-term oral use. Can cause a syndrome (Cushing's) characterized by "moon face," obesity and poorly controlled high blood pressure.

▷ **Possible Adverse Effects** (unusual, unexpected and infrequent reactions)

If any of the following develop, consult your physician promptly for guidance.

Mild Adverse Effects

Allergic reactions: skin rash.

Easy bruising (ecchymosis)—infrequent.

Swelling of face, hoarseness, voice change, cough—possible to infrequent.

Serious Adverse Effects

Allergic reactions—rare.

Bronchospasm, asthmatic wheezing—rare.

Can be a cause of high blood pressure with long-term use.

Edema or swelling, especially with kidney or heart vessel disease—infrequent.

Decrease of circulating T lymphocytes—possible.

Drug-induced seizures, ulcer development, pancreatitis or osteoporosis—possible to infrequent.

Increased intracranial pressure (pseudotumor cerebri)—rare.

Osteonecrosis, avascular necrosis or aseptic necrosis of bone—possible.

Electrolyte disturbances (decreased blood potassium)—infrequent.

Excessive thyroid activity (hyperthyroidism).

Cataract formation or muscle wasting has occurred with long-term use.

Decreased growth in children, especially with high-dose and long-term therapy—possible.

Elevated blood sugar—possible.

Toxic megacolon—rare.

Toxic psychosis has occurred with other steroids.

Author's Note: The inhalation, nasal and topical cream forms avoid many of the systemic side effects of oral systemic use.

▷ **Possible Effects on Sexual Function:** None reported.

Natural Diseases or Disorders That May Be Activated by This Drug

Latent amebiasis, congestive heart failure, diabetes, glaucoma, hypertension, myasthenia gravis, peptic ulcer.

Cortisone-related drugs (used by inhalation) that produce systemic effects can impair immunity and lead to reactivation of "healed" or quiescent tuberculosis of the lungs. Individuals with a history of tuberculosis should be observed closely during use of cortisonelike drugs by inhalation.

Possible Effects on Laboratory Tests

Blood calcium levels: decreased.

Blood total cholesterol levels: increased.

Blood glucose or sodium levels: increased.

Blood potassium levels: decreased.

CAUTION

1. This drug is NOT for the immediate relief of acute asthma.
2. If you were using any cortisone-related drugs for asthma *before* switching to this inhaler, you may need to restart the former cortisone-related drug if you are injured, get an infection or require surgery. Tell your doctor about prior use of cortisone-related drugs.
3. If you experience a return of severe asthma while using this drug, call your doctor immediately. Additional treatment with cortisone-related drugs by mouth or injection may be required.

4. Carry a card noting (if applicable) that you have used cortisone-related drugs within the past year. During periods of stress, resumption of cortisone treatment may be required.
5. Approximately 5 to 10 minutes should separate the inhalation of bronchodilators such as albuterol, epinephrine, pirbuterol, etc. (which should be used first) and the inhalation of this drug. This sequence will permit greater penetration of triamcinolone into the bronchial tubes. This will also reduce the possibility of adverse effects from the propellants used in the two inhalers.
6. If you develop hip pain or back pain while taking this medicine—especially if therapy is long-term—call your doctor.

Precautions for Use
By Infants and Children: Safety and effectiveness for use of the oral inhaler by those under 6 years of age have not been established. To ensure adequate penetration of the drug and obtain maximal benefit, the use of a spacer device is recommended for inhalation therapy in children.
By Those Over 60 Years of Age: Individuals with chronic bronchitis or bronchiectasis should be observed closely for the development of lung infections.

▷ **Advisability of Use During Pregnancy**
Pregnancy Category: C. See Pregnancy Risk Categories at the back of this book.
Animal studies: Rat and rabbit studies reveal significant toxic effects on the embryo and fetus and multiple birth defects due to this drug.
Human studies: Adequate studies of pregnant women are not available.
Limit use to very serious illness for which no satisfactory treatment alternatives are available.

Advisability of Use If Breast-Feeding
Presence of this drug in breast milk: expected to be safe.
Ask your doctor for guidance.

Habit-Forming Potential: With recommended dose, a state of functional dependence (see Glossary) is not likely to develop.

Effects of Overdose: Indications of cortisone excess (due to systemic absorption)—fluid retention, flushing of the face, stomach irritation, nervousness.

Possible Effects of Long-Term Use: Significant suppression of normal cortisone production.

Suggested Periodic Examinations While Taking This Drug (at physician's discretion)
Inspection of mouth and throat for evidence of yeast infection.
Assessment of the status of adrenal gland function (cortisone production).
X-ray of the lungs of people with a prior tuberculosis history.
Bone mineral density tests to assess osteoporosis.

▷ **While Taking This Drug, Observe the Following**
Foods: No specific restrictions beyond those advised by your physician.
Herbal Medicines or Minerals: Increased calcium and vitamin D are prudent. During long-term use, take a vitamin D and vitamin C supplement. During wound repair, take a zinc supplement. Potassium loss may need to be replaced. Ask your doctor if glucosamine makes sense for you if you are taking the oral form.

Fir or pine needle oil should NOT be used by asthmatics. Ephedra alone does carry a German Commission E monograph indication for asthma treatment. If you are allergic to plants in the Asteraceae family (aster, chrysanthemum, daisy or ragweed), you may also be allergic to echinacea, chamomile, feverfew and St. John's wort.

Beverages: No specific restrictions.

▷ *Alcohol:* No interactions expected.

Tobacco Smoking: No interactions expected. I advise everyone to quit smoking.

▷ *Other Drugs*

The following drugs may ***increase*** the effects of triamcinolone:

- inhalant bronchodilators—albuterol, bitolterol, epinephrine, pirbuterol, etc.
- oral bronchodilators—aminophylline, ephedrine, terbutaline, theophylline, etc.

The following drugs may ***decrease*** the effects of triamcinolone:

- carbamazepine (Tegretol)—increases triamcinolone metabolism and may result in decreased effectiveness.
- phenobarbital (various).
- phenytoin (Dilantin) or fosphenytoin (Cerebyx)—increases triamcinolone metabolism and may result in decreased effectiveness.
- primidone (Mysoline)—increases steroid metabolism and may result in decreased triamcinolone metabolism.
- rifampin (Rifadin).

Triamcinolone ***taken concurrently*** with

- amphotericin B (Abelcet) may lead to additive potassium loss.
- aspirin may result in increased removal of aspirin from the body and may also lead to increased stomach irritation or ulceration. This effect may be immediate or delayed. Patients should be checked for loss of aspirin benefits and stomach upset of GI bleeding.
- cyclosporine (Sandimmune) may result in changes in the blood levels of both medicines.
- human growth hormone (HGH) may blunt HGH benefits.
- insulin (various forms) may lead to loss of glucose control.
- neuromuscular blocking agents (such as pancuronium—Pavulon or vercuronium—Norcuron) may prolong muscle weakness.
- oral hypoglycemic agents (see Oral Antidiabetic Drugs in Drug Classes) may result in loss of glucose control.
- thiazide diuretics (see Drug Classes) can result in loss of glucose control.
- vaccines (flu, rabies, rotavirus, others) may result in a less than optimal vaccine response.
- warfarin (Coumadin) can result in variation in the degree of anticoagulation; increased INR (prothrombin time or protime) testing is indicated.

▷ *Driving, Hazardous Activities:* No restrictions.

Aviation Note: The use of this drug and the disorder for which this drug is prescribed ***may be disqualifications*** for piloting. Consult a designated Aviation Medical Examiner.

Exposure to Sun: No restrictions.

Occurrence of Unrelated Illness: Acute infections, serious injuries and surgical procedures can create an urgent need for the administration of additional supportive cortisone-related drugs given by mouth and/or injection. Notify your physician immediately in the event of new illness or injury of any kind.

Special Storage Instructions: Store at room temperature. Avoid exposure to temperatures above 120 degrees F (49 degrees C). Do not store or use this inhaler near heat or open flame.

Discontinuation: If the regular use of this drug has made it possible to reduce or stop doses of cortisonelike drugs by mouth, do not discontinue this drug abruptly. Call your doctor if you must stop this drug for any reason. Restarting cortisone preparations may be required.

TRIAMTERENE (tri AM ter een)

Introduced: 1964   **Class:** Diuretic   **Prescription:** USA: Yes   **Controlled Drug:** USA: No; Canada: No   **Available as Generic:** Yes
Brand Names: ✿Apo-Triazide [CD], Dyazide [CD], Dyrenium, Maxzide [CD], Maxzide-25 [CD], ✿Novo-Triamzide [CD], ✿Nu-Triazide

BENEFITS versus RISKS	
Possible Benefits	*Possible Risks*
EFFECTIVE PREVENTION OF POTASSIUM LOSS when used adjunctively with other diuretics	ABNORMALLY HIGH BLOOD POTASSIUM LEVEL with excessive use
EFFECTIVE DIURETIC IN REFRACTORY CASES OF FLUID RETENTION when used adjunctively with other diuretics	Possible blood cell disorders: megaloblastic anemia, abnormally low white blood cell and platelet counts
	Possible kidney stone formation

Principal Uses

As a Single Drug Product: Uses currently included in FDA-approved labeling: (1) Used in combination with other drugs to treat high blood pressure (primarily used in situations where it is advisable to prevent loss of potassium from the body); (2) used as combination therapy of congestive heart failure or liver and kidney disorders accompanied by excessive fluid retention (edema).

Other (unlabeled) generally accepted uses: None.

As a Combination Drug Product [CD]: Available in combination with hydrochlorothiazide, a different kind of diuretic that promotes potassium loss from the body. Triamterene is used to counteract the potassium-wasting effect of the thiazide diuretic.

How This Drug Works: By inhibiting the enzyme system that starts the sodium-potassium exchange process, this drug prevents reabsorption of sodium and excretion of potassium by the kidney. This leads to excretion of sodium (and water with it) and potassium retention.

Available Dosage Forms and Strengths

Capsules — 50 mg, 100 mg
Capsules — triamterene 37.5 mg and hydrochlorothiazide 25 mg and also 75 mg/50 mg of each.

▷ **Usual Adult Dosage Ranges:** Initially 50 to 100 mg twice daily. The dose is then adjusted according to individual response. The usual ongoing dose is 100 to 200 mg daily, divided into two doses. The total daily dose should not exceed 300 mg.

Dyazide combination—one or two capsules daily for high blood pressure.

Note: Actual dose and schedule must be determined for each patient individually.

Conditions Requiring Dosing Adjustments

Liver Function: Dose should be reduced and used with extreme caution in liver disease.

Kidney Function: Patients with mild to moderate kidney failure may take the usual dose every 12 hours. In severe or progressive kidney failure, this medication should not be used.

▷ **Dosing Instructions:** May be taken with or following meals to promote absorption of the drug and reduce stomach irritation. The capsule may be opened. Intermittent or alternate-day use is recommended to minimize the risk of sodium and potassium imbalance. If you forget a dose: Take the missed dose as soon as you remember it, unless it's nearly time for your next dose—if that is the case, skip the missed dose and take the next dose right on schedule. DO NOT double doses. Talk with your doctor if you find yourself missing doses as the best control of blood pressure comes from taking your medicine exactly as prescribed.

Usual Duration of Use: Use on a regular schedule for 3 to 5 days usually determines effectiveness in clearing edema and for 2 to 3 weeks to determine its effect on hypertension. Long-term use (months to years) requires physician supervision and periodic evaluation. Take control of your blood pressure by taking those medicines!

Typical Treatment Goals and Measurements (Outcomes and Markers)

Blood Pressure: The most recent treatment guidelines (JNC VI) actually define optimal blood pressure (BP) as less than 120/80 and high normal as 139/89. The American Diabetes Association has chosen a target of 130/80 as the blood pressure goal for people living with diabetes. Most clinicians try to achieve a BP that achieves the best balance of lower cardiovascular risk while avoiding the problem of too low a blood pressure. The goal and time frame (see peak benefits above) should be discussed with you when the prescription is written.

▷ **This Drug Should Not Be Taken If**
- you have had an allergic reaction to it previously.
- you have severely impaired liver or kidney function.
- your kidney disease is progressive or you have a creatinine clearance greater than 2.5 mg/dl (ask your doctor).
- your blood potassium level is significantly elevated (ask your doctor).

▷ **Inform Your Physician Before Taking This Drug If**
- you have a history of liver or kidney disease.
- you have diabetes or gout.
- you are taking any of the following: antihypertensives, a digitalis preparation, another diuretic, lithium or a potassium preparation.
- you have a history of glucose-6-phosphate dehydrogenase (G6PD) deficiency (ask your doctor).
- you have a history of blood cell disorders.
- you will have surgery with general anesthesia.

Possible Side Effects (natural, expected and unavoidable drug actions)

With excessive use: abnormally high blood potassium levels, abnormally low blood sodium levels, dehydration. Blue coloration of the urine (of no significance).

▷ **Possible Adverse Effects** (unusual, unexpected and infrequent reactions)

If any of the following develop, consult your physician promptly for guidance.

Mild Adverse Effects

Allergic reactions: skin rash, itching.

Headache, dizziness, unsteadiness, weakness, drowsiness, lethargy—infrequent.

Dry mouth, nausea, vomiting, diarrhea—infrequent.

Serious Adverse Effects

Allergic reaction: anaphylactic reaction (see Glossary).

Symptomatic potassium excess: confusion, numbness and tingling in lips and extremities, fatigue, weakness, shortness of breath, slow heart rate, low blood pressure—possible.

Blood cell disorders: megaloblastic anemia, abnormally low white blood cell count or abnormally low blood platelet count—case reports.

Hemolytic anemia—in those with deficiency of G6PD in red cells.

Abnormal urine production (SIADH)—case reports.

Formation of kidney stones and kidney toxicity—rare.

Liver toxicity—rare.

▷ **Possible Effects on Sexual Function:** None reported.

Possible Effects on Laboratory Tests

Complete blood cell counts: decreased red cells, hemoglobin, white cells and platelets; increased eosinophils (allergic reaction).

Blood glucose level: increased in diabetics.

Blood lithium, potassium or uric acid level: increased.

Kidney function tests: increased blood creatinine and urea nitrogen (BUN) levels (kidney damage).

CAUTION

1. Do not take potassium supplements or increase your intake of potassium-rich foods while taking this drug.
2. Patients who take quinidine (Quinaglute, others) may have falsely increased laboratory test results if fluorescent measurement techniques are used.
3. Do not stop this drug abruptly unless abnormally high blood levels of potassium develop.
4. Avoid liberal use of salt substitutes with potassium in them (potential causes of potassium excess).

Precautions for Use

By Infants and Children: This drug is not recommended for use in children.

By Those Over 60 Years of Age: Natural decline in kidney function may predispose to potassium retention. Watch for potassium excess: slow heart rate, irregular heart rhythms, low blood pressure, confusion, drowsiness. Excessive use of diuretics can cause harmful loss of body water (dehydration), increased viscosity of the blood and an increased tendency of the blood to clot, predisposing to stroke, heart attack or thrombophlebitis.

▷ **Advisability of Use During Pregnancy**
   Pregnancy Category: B by one manufacturer, D by the FDA. See Pregnancy Risk
      Categories at the back of this book.
   Animal studies: No birth defects due to this drug were reported.
   Human studies: Adequate studies of pregnant women are not available.
      This drug should not be used during pregnancy unless a very serious com-
      plication of pregnancy occurs for which this drug is significantly benefi-
      cial.

Advisability of Use If Breast-Feeding
   Presence of this drug in breast milk: Yes.
   Avoid drug or refrain from nursing.

Habit-Forming Potential: None.

Effects of Overdose: Thirst, drowsiness, fatigue, nausea, vomiting, confusion,
   irregular heart rhythm, low blood pressure.

Possible Effects of Long-Term Use: Potassium accumulation to abnormally
   high blood levels.

Suggested Periodic Examinations While Taking This Drug (at physician's dis-
   cretion)
   Complete blood cell counts.
   Measurements of blood sodium, potassium and chloride levels.
   Kidney function tests.

▷ **While Taking This Drug, Observe the Following**
   Foods: Diets high in high-potassium foods (see Table 13, Section Six) may
      cause problems. Avoid excessive restriction of salt.
   Herbal Medicines or Minerals: Ginseng may increase blood pressure, blunting
      the benefits of these medicines. Hawthorn, saw palmetto, ma huang, gold-
      enseal, yohimbe and licorice may also increase blood pressure. Calcium
      and garlic may help lower blood pressure. Use caution and work with your
      doctor to make sure blood pressure is not lowered too much. Indian snake-
      root has a German Commission E monograph indication for hyperten-
      sion—talk to your doctor. Eleuthero root and ephedra should be avoided
      by people living with hypertension. CAUTION: St. John's wort may also
      lead to photosensitivity.
   Beverages: No restrictions. May be taken with milk.
▷ *Alcohol:* Use with caution. Alcohol may enhance drowsiness and the blood-
      pressure-lowering effect of this drug.
   Tobacco Smoking: No interactions expected. I advise everyone to quit smoking.
▷ *Other Drugs*
   Triamterene may *increase* the effects of
   • amantadine (Symmetrel).
   • digoxin (Lanoxin).
   • metformin (Glucophage).
   • methotrexate (Mexate), leading to bone marrow toxicity.
   • valsartan (Diovan), leading to potassium toxicity.
   Triamterene *taken concurrently with*
   • captopril (Capoten) or other ACE inhibitors may cause excessively high
      blood potassium levels.
   • cyclosporine (Sandimmune) SHOULD NOT BE COMBINED.
   • dofetilide (Tikosyn) may lead to excessive dofetilide levels. Careful patient

> monitoring and more frequent dofetilide levels are indicated if these medicines are combined.
- folic acid may reduce folic acid benefits.
- histamine (H2) blockers (see Drug Classes) may decrease triamterene absorption and its therapeutic effects.
- indomethacin (Indocin) may increase the risk of kidney damage.
- lithium may cause accumulation of lithium to toxic levels.
- NSAIDs (see Drug Classes) may blunt the blood-pressure-lowering effect of triamterene.
- potassium preparations may cause excessively high blood pressure.
- tacrolimus (Prograf) may lead to excessively high blood potassium levels. Combination should be avoided.

▷ *Driving, Hazardous Activities:* This drug may cause dizziness and drowsiness. Restrict activities as necessary.

Aviation Note: The use of this drug **may be a disqualification** for piloting. Consult a designated Aviation Medical Examiner.

Exposure to Sun: Use caution—this drug may cause photosensitivity (see Glossary).

Discontinuation: With high-dose or prolonged use, it is best to slowly withdraw this drug. Stopping it suddenly may cause rebound potassium removal and potassium deficiency. Ask your doctor for help.

TRICHLORMETHIAZIDE (tri KLOR meth i a zide)

Please see the thiazide diuretic family profile.

TRIFLUOPERAZINE (tri flu oh PER a zeen)

Introduced: 1958 **Class:** Tranquilizer, major; phenothiazines **Prescription:** USA: Yes **Controlled Drug:** USA: No; Canada: No **Available as Generic:** USA: Yes; Canada: No

Brand Names: ❧Apo-Trifluoperazine, ❧Novo-Flurazine, ❧Solazine, Stelabid [CD], Stelazine, Suprazine, ❧Terfluzine

---

BENEFITS versus RISKS

Possible Benefits	*Possible Risks*
EFFECTIVE CONTROL OF ACUTE MENTAL DISORDERS: beneficial effects on thinking, mood and behavior	SERIOUS TOXIC EFFECTS ON BRAIN with long-term use
	Liver damage with jaundice—infrequent
	Rare blood cell disorders: abnormally low red and white blood cell and platelet counts

---

▷ **Principal Uses**

As a Single Drug Product: Uses currently included in FDA-approved labeling: (1) Treats psychotic thinking and behavior seen in acute psychoses of unknown nature, mania, paranoid states and acute schizophrenia—very effective in withdrawn and apathetic people and those with agitation, delusions and hallucinations; (2) approved for treatment of anxiety disorders. Other (unlabeled) generally accepted uses: May have a role in combination therapy of some kinds of chronic pain.

How This Drug Works: By inhibiting the action of dopamine, this drug corrects an imbalance of nerve transmissions thought to be responsible for certain mental disorders.

Available Dosage Forms and Strengths
Concentrate — 10 mg/ml
Injection — 2 mg/ml
Tablets — 1 mg, 2 mg, 5 mg, 10 mg

▷ **Usual Adult Dosage Ranges**
For nonpsychotic anxiety: Initially 1 or 2 mg twice daily. The dose may be increased by 1 or 2 mg at 3- to 4-day intervals to a maximum dose of 4 mg for patients who are not in the hospital.
For psychosis: 2 to 5 mg twice a day. The dose is then increased every 3 or 4 days as needed and tolerated. Usual dose range is 15 to 20 mg daily. The total daily dose should not exceed 40 mg. Some rare cases have required 100 mg per day.
Note: Actual dose and schedule must be determined for each patient individually.

Conditions Requiring Dosing Adjustments
Liver Function: This drug should be used with caution in liver compromise.
Kidney Function: Patients with compromised kidneys should be closely followed.

▷ **Dosing Instructions:** The tablets may be crushed and taken with or following meals to reduce stomach irritation. If you forget a dose: Take the missed dose as soon as you remember it, unless it's nearly time for your next dose—if that is the case, skip the missed dose and take the next dose right on schedule. DO NOT double doses. Talk with your doctor if you find yourself missing doses. The best results are obtained when this medicine is taken on a regular basis.

Usual Duration of Use: Use on a regular schedule for several weeks usually determines effectiveness in psychotic disorders. If not significantly beneficial within 6 weeks, it should be stopped. Long-term use requires periodic physician evaluation.

Typical Treatment Goals and Measurements (Outcomes and Markers)
Schizophrenia: The general goal: to ease the severity of symptoms in order to let the patient resume his or her usual activities. There should be lessened time spent with prior intrusions of abnormal thinking into more normal life. Some clinicians use specific inventories or question sets to help determine benefits.

▷ **This Drug Should Not Be Taken If**
• you are allergic to any form of trifluoperazine.
• you have active liver disease.
• you have a current blood cell or bone marrow disorder.

▷ **Inform Your Physician Before Taking This Drug If**
• you are allergic or abnormally sensitive to any phenothiazine drug (see Drug Classes).
• you have impaired liver or kidney function.

- you have a history of anginal pain (this drug may worsen it).
- you have any type of seizure disorder.
- you have diabetes, glaucoma, retinopathy or heart disease.
- you have cancer of the breast.
- you have a history of lupus erythematosus.
- you are taking any drug with sedative effects.
- you have had neuroleptic malignant syndrome (ask your doctor).
- you will have surgery with general or spinal anesthesia

Author's Note: Information in this profile has been shortened to make room for more widely used medicines.

TRIMETHOPRIM (tri METH oh prim)

Introduced: 1966   **Class:** Anti-infective   **Prescription:** USA: Yes
Controlled Drug: USA: No; Canada: No   **Available as Generic:** USA: Yes;
Canada: No

Brand Names: Alti-Trimethoprim, ✤Apo-Sulfatrim [CD], ✤Apo-Sulfatrim DS
[CD], Bactrim [CD], Bactrim DS [CD], Bethaprim [CD], Comoxol [CD],
✤Coptin [CD], Cotrim [CD], ✤Novo-Trimel [CD], ✤Novo-Trimel DS [CD],
✤Nu-Cotrimox, Polytrim, Proloprim, ✤Protrin [CD], ✤Protrin DF [CD],
✤Roubac [CD], Septra [CD], Septra DS [CD], SMZ-TMP [CD], Sulfatrim
D/S, Trimpex, Uroplus DS [CD], Uroplus SS [CD]

BENEFITS versus RISKS	
Possible Benefits	*Possible Risks*
EFFECTIVE TREATMENT OF INFECTIONS DUE TO SUSCEPTIBLE MICROORGANISMS	Blood cell disorders: megaloblastic anemia, methemoglobinemia, abnormally low white cells or platelets
Effective adjunctive prevention and treatment of *Pneumocystis carinii* pneumonia (AIDS related)	May increase homocysteine with ongoing use

▷ **Principal Uses**

As a Single Drug Product: Uses currently included in FDA-approved labeling:
(1) Treats or prevents certain infections of the urinary tract not complicated by the presence of kidney stones or obstructions to the normal flow
of urine; (2) treats eye infections caused by sensitive organisms.

Other (unlabeled) generally accepted uses: (1) Used in combination with
dapsone to treat *Pneumocystis carinii* pneumonia in AIDS patients; (2)
may have a role in combination therapy of resistant acne; (3) prevention
(prophylaxis) of urinary tract infections; (4) some clinicians are using
trimethoprim/sulfamethoxazole (Bactrim or Septra) in combination with
permethrin (Nix) to treat head lice.

As a Combination Drug Product [CD]: Available combined with sulfamethoxazole (cotrimoxazole is used in some countries to identify this combination). Treats certain urinary tract infections, middle ear infections, chronic
bronchitis, acute enteritis and certain types of pneumonia. It is now used
as primary prevention and treatment of Pneumocystis carinii pneumonia
associated with AIDS.

How This Drug Works: Prevents growth and multiplication of susceptible organisms by inactivating enzyme systems needed for formation of essential nuclear elements and cell proteins.

Available Dosage Forms and Strengths

Ophthalmic — 1 mg/ml

Oral suspension, combination (per 5 ml) — 40 mg trimethoprim/200 mg sulfamethoxazole

Tablets — 100 mg, 200 mg

Tablets, combination — 80 mg trimethoprim/400 mg sulfamethoxazole 160 mg trimethoprim/800 mg sulfamethoxazole

▷ **Usual Adult Dosage Ranges:** *Orally for infections:* 100 mg every 12 hours for 10 days. For certain pneumonias, the same dose is taken every 6 hours. The total daily dose should not exceed 640 mg.

Ophthalmic: One drop in the affected eye every 3 hours (up to six doses a day) for 7 to 10 days.

Note: Actual dose and schedule must be determined for each patient individually.

Conditions Requiring Dosing Adjustments

Liver Function: Used with caution by patients with both liver and kidney disease.

Kidney Function: Patients with mild kidney compromise can take the usual dose every 12 hours. Patients with stable moderate to more compromised kidney failure (creatinine clearances of 15 to 50 ml/min) can take the usual dose every 18 hours. Should NOT be used in severe or worsening kidney failure.

▷ **Dosing Instructions:** The tablet may be crushed and may be taken with or following food if necessary to reduce stomach irritation. If you forget a dose: Take the missed dose as soon as you remember it, unless it's nearly time for your next dose—if that is the case, skip the missed dose and take the next dose right on schedule. DO NOT double up on doses. Talk with your doctor if you find yourself missing doses as compliance ensures the best treatment results or best possible prevention of infection.

Usual Duration of Use: Use on a regular schedule for 7 to 14 days usually determines effectiveness in controlling responsive infections. The actual duration of use will depend upon the nature of the infection. Prevention of (prophylaxis) of PCP in HIV positive patients with the combination form will be ongoing.

Typical Treatment Goals and Measurements (Outcomes and Markers)

Infections: The most commonly used measures of serious infections are white blood cell counts and differentials (the kind of blood cells that occur most often in your blood), and temperature. Many clinicians look for positive changes in 24–48 hours. NEVER stop an antibiotic because you start to feel better. For treating infections, the full course is REQUIRED to kill the bacteria. Prophylaxis (for example of PCP) often requires ongoing use. The goals and time frame (see peak benefits above) should be discussed with you when the prescription is written.

Currently a Drug of Choice

When combined with sulfamethoxazole, for preventing pneumonia (due to Pneumocystis carinii) in patients with AIDS.

▷ **This Drug Should Not Be Taken If**
- you have had an allergic reaction to it previously.
- you have an anemia due to folic acid deficiency (megaloblastic anemia).

▷ **Inform Your Physician Before Taking This Drug If**
- you have a history of folic acid deficiency.
- you have impaired liver or kidney function.
- you are pregnant or breast-feeding.
- you have a history of cardiovascular disease. This medicine may increase homocysteine levels.

Possible Side Effects (natural, expected and unavoidable drug actions)
None with short-term use.

▷ **Possible Adverse Effects** (unusual, unexpected and infrequent reactions)
If any of the following develop, consult your physician promptly for guidance.
Mild Adverse Effects
Allergic reactions: skin rash, itching, drug fever (see Glossary).
Headache, abnormal taste, sore mouth or tongue, nausea, vomiting, cramping, diarrhea—infrequent.
Serious Adverse Effects
Allergic reactions: severe dermatitis with peeling of skin (toxic epidermal necrolysis).
Blood cell disorders: megaloblastic anemia, methemoglobinemia, abnormally low white blood cell and platelet counts—rare.
Worsening of hyperkalemia (increased blood potassium)—possible.
Kidney or liver toxicity—rare.
Aseptic meningitis (of questionable causal relationship)—case reports.

▷ **Possible Effects on Sexual Function:** None reported.

Possible Effects on Laboratory Tests
Complete blood cell counts: decreased red cells, hemoglobin, white cells and platelets.
INR (prothrombin time): increased (when taken concurrently with warfarin).

CAUTION
1. Resistance may develop. If you do not show significant improvement within 2 days, call your physician.
2. Comply with your physician's request for periodic blood counts during long-term therapy.
3. This medicine may increase homocysteine levels. Talk to your doctor about checking levels if you will be taking this medicine on an ongoing basis. Taking a multivitamin appears prudent.

Precautions for Use
By Infants and Children: Safety and effectiveness for those under 2 months of age are not established.
By Those Over 60 Years of Age: The natural decline in liver and kidney function may require smaller doses. If you develop itching reactions in the genital or anal areas, report this promptly.

▷ **Advisability of Use During Pregnancy**
Pregnancy Category: C. See Pregnancy Risk Categories at the back of this book.
Animal studies: Birth defects due to this drug reported in rat and rabbit studies.

Human studies: Adequate studies of pregnant women are not available.
Avoid use of drug during the first 3 months and during the final 2 weeks of pregnancy. Use this drug otherwise only if clearly needed. Ask your physician for guidance.

Advisability of Use If Breast-Feeding
Presence of this drug in breast milk: Yes.
Avoid drug or refrain from nursing.

Habit-Forming Potential: None.

Effects of Overdose: Headache, dizziness, confusion, depression, nausea, vomiting, bone marrow depression, possible liver toxicity with jaundice.

Possible Effects of Long-Term Use: Impaired production of red and white blood cells and blood platelets.

Suggested Periodic Examinations While Taking This Drug (at physician's discretion)
Complete blood cell counts.

▷ **While Taking This Drug, Observe the Following**
Foods: Since this medicine may increase homocysteine levels, a multivitamin appears prudent.
Herbal Medicines or Minerals: Some patients use echinacea to attempt to boost their immune systems. Unfortunately, echinacea is not recommended in people with damaged immune systems. This herb may also actually weaken any immune system if it is used too often or for too long a time. DO NOT take mistletoe herb, oak bark or F.C. of marshmallow root and licorice extracts. Pure cranberry juice may help keep harmful bacteria from attaching to the bladder wall and may be useful in combination with antibiotics in helping to prevent urinary tract infections. TALK to your doctor BEFORE adding any herbal medicine.
Beverages: No restrictions. May be taken with milk.
▷ *Alcohol:* No interactions expected.
Tobacco Smoking: No interactions expected, but I advise everyone to quit smoking.
▷ *Other Drugs*
Trimethoprim may ***increase*** the effects of
- ACE inhibitors (see Drug Classes), resulting in dangerously increased potassium levels.
- amantadine (Symmetrel) and also result in increased levels of trimethoprim, resulting in toxicity.
- cyclosporine (Sandimmune) and result in increased kidney toxicity.
- dapsone and result in dapsone or trimethoprim toxicity.
- digoxin (Lanoxin), leading to toxicity.
- dofetilide (Tikosyn) may lead to heart toxicity. Avoid this combination.
- lamivudine (Epivir) and adjustments in lamivudine doses may be required.
- metformin (Glucophage) and other cationic drugs.
- methotrexate (Mexate), leading to toxicity.
- phenytoin (Dilantin) or fosphenytoin (Cerebyx) and cause phenytoin or fosphenytoin toxicity.
- procainamide (Procan SR) and result in procainamide toxicity.
- zidovudine (AZT), leading to increased toxicity risk.

The following drugs may *decrease* the effects of trimethoprim:
- cholestyramine (Questran) and perhaps other cholesterol-lowering medicines (see Drug Classes) of the same class—these will bind trimethoprim and blunt its beneficial effects by inhibiting absorption.
- rifampin (Rifadin, Rimactane).
- ritonavir (Norvir).

▷ *Driving, Hazardous Activities:* No restrictions.
Aviation Note: The use of this drug is *probably not a disqualification* for piloting. Consult a designated Aviation Medical Examiner.
Exposure to Sun: No restrictions.

TROGLITAZONE (troh GLIT a zoan)

Introduced: 1997   **Class:** Antidiabetic, thiazolidinedione
Author's Note: This medicine was voluntary removed from the market in March 2000. Please see the thiazolidinedione family profile for information on the to remaining "glitazones."

VALPROIC ACID (val PROH ik A sid)

Introduced: 1967   **Class:** Anticonvulsant   **Prescription:** USA: Yes
Controlled Drug: USA: No; Canada: No   **Available as Generic:** USA: Yes; Canada: Yes
Brand Names: ✿Alti-Valproic, ✿Apo-Divalproic, ✿Apo-Valproic, Atemperator, Depa, Depakene, Depakote (divalproex sodium), Deproic, ✿Epival, Myproic, ✿Novo-Divalproex, ✿Novo-valproic, ✿Nu-Valproic, Rhoproic, Valproic

BENEFITS versus RISKS	
Possible Benefits	*Possible Risks*
EFFECTIVE CONTROL OF MULTIPLE SEIZURE TYPES: ABSENCE SEIZURES, TONIC-CLONIC SEIZURES, MYOCLONIC SEIZURES, PSYCHOMOTOR SEIZURES, WHEN USED ADJUNCTIVELY WITH OTHER ANTISEIZURE DRUGS	LIVER TOXICITY, INFREQUENT BUT MAY BE SEVERE
	Reduction of blood platelets and impaired platelet function with risk of bleeding
HELPS CONTROL REFRACTORY MIGRAINES	Possible pancreatitis or liver toxicity
DIVALPROEX SODIUM HELPS MANIA	

▷ **Principal Uses**
As a Single Drug Product: Uses currently included in FDA-approved labeling: (1) Used to manage the following types of epilepsy: simple and complex absence seizures (petit mal); tonic-clonic seizures (grand mal); myoclonic seizures; complex partial seizures (psychomotor, temporal lobe epilepsy)—sometimes used adjunctively with other anticonvulsants as needed; (2) used for people

who do not respond to medicine once they have a migraine or have more than two migraines a month; (3) divalproex sodium (Depakote) is approved for use in treating mania; (4) eases mania in AIDS; (5) helps kleptomania.

Other (unlabeled) generally accepted uses: (1) Can help relieve the symptoms of trigeminal neuralgia; (2) can have a role in intractable hiccups; (3) some use in patients with epilepsy and hepatic porphyria; (4) may be of help for writer's cramp.

How This Drug Works: It is thought that by increasing the availability of the nerve impulse transmitter gamma-aminobutyric acid (GABA), this drug suppresses the spread of abnormal electrical discharges that cause seizures.

Available Dosage Forms and Strengths

Capsules — 250 mg

Capsules, sprinkle — 125 mg

Syrup — 250 mg/5 ml

Tablets, enteric coated — 125 mg, 250 mg, 500 mg

▷ **Usual Adult Dosage Ranges:** Starting dose is 10–15 mg per kg of body mass per day. The dose is increased cautiously by 5 to 10 mg per kg of body mass daily, every 7 days as needed and tolerated. The usual daily dose is from 1,000 mg to 1,600 mg in divided doses. The total daily dose should not exceed 60 mg per kg of body mass. Blood levels are used to guide ongoing dosing.

For migraines: Starting dose is 250 mg, which is then slowly increased, as needed and tolerated, to 500 to 1000 mg daily in divided doses. For the extended release tablet: 500 mg once a day to start for seven days, then increased to 1,000 mg a day as needed and tolerated.

Note: Actual dose and schedule must be determined for each patient individually.

Typical Treatment Goals and Measurements (Outcomes and Markers)

Seizures: The general goal for this medicine is effective seizure control. Neurologists tend to define effective on a case-by-case basis depending on the seizure type and patient factors. If seizure control is not effective, it's not unusual to use combination treatment. For this medicine, a balance must be struck between too little medicine and too much medicine. Blood levels are used to make sure that the amount of medicine is in just the right range.

Conditions Requiring Dosing Adjustments

Liver Function: This medicine SHOULD NOT be taken by patients with significant liver compromise or liver disease.

Kidney Function: No dosing changes thought to be needed in kidney disease.

▷ **Dosing Instructions:** Preferably taken 1 hour before meals, although it may be taken with or following food if necessary to prevent stomach irritation. The regular capsule should not be opened, and the tablet should not be crushed. The sprinkle capsule may be opened and the contents sprinkled on soft food. Do not give the syrup in carbonated beverages. Dilute in water or milk. If you forget a dose: Take the missed dose as soon as you remember it, unless it's nearly time for your next dose—if that is the case, skip the missed dose and take the next dose right on schedule. DO NOT double dose. Talk with your doctor if you find yourself missing doses. The best seizure control comes from keeping this medicine in just the right range. This most often results from taking just the right dose at just the right time.

Usual Duration of Use: Use on a regular schedule for 2 weeks usually determines effectiveness in reducing the frequency and severity of seizures. Long-term use (months to years) requires physician supervision and periodic evaluation. Use in seizure cases will be ongoing as will use in migraine prevention.

▷ **This Drug Should Not Be Taken If**
  • you have had an allergic reaction to it previously.
  • you have active liver disease.
  • you are pregnant.
  • you have an active bleeding disorder.

▷ **Inform Your Physician Before Taking This Drug If**
  • you have a history of liver disease, impaired liver function or pancreatitis.
  • you have a history of any type of bleeding disorder.
  • you are pregnant or planning pregnancy.
  • you have myasthenia gravis.
  • you are taking anticoagulants, other anticonvulsants or antidepressants—either the tricyclic type or monoamine oxidase (MAO) type A inhibitors (see Drug Classes).
  • you will have surgery or dental extraction.

Possible Side Effects (natural, expected and unavoidable drug actions)
  Drowsiness and lethargy.

▷ **Possible Adverse Effects** (unusual, unexpected and infrequent reactions)
  If any of the following develop, consult your physician promptly for guidance.
  Mild Adverse Effects
  Allergic reactions: skin rash—rare.
  Headache, dizziness, confusion, unsteadiness, tremor—dose-related.
  Slurred speech—infrequent.
  Nausea, indigestion, stomach cramps, diarrhea—infrequent.
  Weight gain—case reports.
  Bedwetting at night—case reports.
  Zinc, carnitine and selenium lowering—possible.
  Temporary loss of scalp hair—case reports.
  Serious Adverse Effects
  Idiosyncratic reactions: bizarre behavior, psychosis, hallucinations.
  Drug-induced hepatitis with jaundice (see Glossary).
  Children less than 2 years old have considerably increased risk of fatal hepatotoxicity.
  Blood ammonia level or blood glucose—increased.
  Drug-induced pancreatitis, porphyria, lowered thyroid gland function (hypothyroidism)—case reports.
  Selenium, zinc and carnitine levels—decreased.
  Reduced formation of blood platelets, impaired platelet function and anemia—case reports.
  Clotting (coagulation) defects—case reports (one case of lung bleeding).
  Worsening of demylinating disease—case report.
  Increased pressure in the head (pseudotumor cerebri)—case reports.
  Can cause a Reye's-like syndrome.

▷ **Possible Effects on Sexual Function:** Altered timing and pattern of menstruation. Female breast enlargement with milk production. Decreased libido—

case reports. Decreased effectiveness of oral contraceptives taken concurrently—CAUTION.

▷ **Adverse Effects That May Mimic Natural Diseases or Disorders**

Liver reactions may suggest viral hepatitis.

Possible Effects on Laboratory Tests

Complete blood cell counts: decreased white cells and platelets.

Bleeding time or INR (prothrombin time): increased.

Blood amylase level: increased (possible pancreatitis).

Liver function tests: increased enzymes (ALT/GPT, AST/GOT, alkaline phosphatase) or bilirubin.

CAUTION

1. The capsules and tablets should be swallowed whole to avoid irritation of the mouth and throat.
2. Carnitine, selenium and zinc supplementation may be needed. Talk to your doctor.
3. This drug can impair normal blood-clotting mechanisms. In the event of injury, dental extraction or need for surgery, inform your physician or dentist that you are taking this drug.
4. Because this drug can impair the normal function of blood platelets, it is best to avoid aspirin (which has the same effect).
5. Over-the-counter drug products that contain antihistamines (allergy and cold remedies, sleep aids) can enhance sedation.

Precautions for Use

By Infants and Children: The concurrent use of aspirin with this drug can cause abnormal bleeding or bruising. Children with mental retardation, organic brain disease or severe seizure disorders may be at increased risk for severe liver toxicity while taking this drug. Observe closely for the development of fever that could indicate the onset of a drug-induced Reye's syndrome (see Glossary). Avoid concurrent use of clonazepam (Klonopin); the combined use could result in continuous petit mal episodes.

By Those Over 60 Years of Age: Start treatment with small doses and increase dose cautiously. Observe closely for excessive sedation, confusion or unsteadiness that could predispose to falling and injury.

▷ **Advisability of Use During Pregnancy**

Pregnancy Category: D. See Pregnancy Risk Categories at the back of this book.

Animal studies: Palate and skeletal birth defects reported in mouse, rat and rabbit studies.

Human studies: Adequate studies of pregnant women are not available. There have been several reports of birth defects attributed to the use of this drug during early pregnancy.

Talk to your doctor about the advantages and disadvantages of using this drug. If it is used, it is advisable to keep the dose as low as possible.

Advisability of Use If Breast-Feeding

Presence of this drug in breast milk: Yes.

Discontinue drug or stop nursing.

Habit-Forming Potential: None.

Effects of Overdose: Increased drowsiness, weakness, unsteadiness, confusion, stupor progressing to coma.

Possible Effects of Long-Term Use: None reported.

Suggested Periodic Examinations While Taking This Drug (at physician's discretion)

Complete blood cell counts and baseline liver function tests should be done before treatment is started. During treatment, blood counts should be repeated every month and liver function tests repeated every 2 months. Amylase or other measures of possible pancreatitis are prudent.

▷ **While Taking This Drug, Observe the Following**

Foods: No restrictions.

Herbal Medicines or Minerals: Using kola or ma huang may result in unacceptable central nervous system stimulation. Valerian and kava kava may interact to increase drowsiness. St. John's wort may also cause increased sun sensitivity—caution is advised. Replacement of zinc and selenium is prudent. Carnitine replacement (intravenous) is needed in valproic acid–caused (induced) liver toxicity and overdose. Carnitine replacement may also be needed in infants and young children taking multiple seizure medicines as well as epileptic patients on a ketogenic diet who have low carnitine (hypocarnitinemia).

Beverages: Do not administer the syrup in carbonated beverages; this could liberate the valproic acid and irritate the mouth and throat. This drug may be taken with milk.

▷ *Alcohol:* Alcohol can increase the sedative effect of this drug. Also, this drug can increase the depressant effects of alcohol on brain function.

Tobacco Smoking: No interactions expected. I advise everyone to quit smoking.

▷ *Other Drugs*

Valproic acid may ***increase*** the effects of
- anticoagulants (Coumadin, etc.) and increase the risk of bleeding; increased frequency of INR (prothrombin time or protime) testing is needed.
- antidepressants (both monoamine oxidase [MAO] type A inhibitors and tricyclics) and cause toxicity.
- benzodiazepines (such as alprazolam).
- nimodipine (Nimotop) and cause nimodipine toxicity.
- phenobarbital and cause barbiturate intoxication.
- phenytoin (Dilantin) or fosphenytoin (Cerebyx) and cause phenytoin or fosphenytoin toxicity.
- zidovudine (AZT) and may lead to zidovudine toxicity.

Valproic acid ***taken concurrently*** with
- acyclovir (Zovirax) may lower valproic acid levels.
- antacids (Maalox) will decrease absorption and lower therapeutic benefits of valproic acid.
- antiplatelet drugs—aspirin, dipyridamole (Persantine), sulfinpyrazone (Anturane)—may enhance the inhibition of platelet function and increase the risk of bleeding.
- aspirin can lead to valproic acid toxicity.
- carbamazepine (Tegretol) may have a variable effect on blood levels; more frequent blood level testing is advised.
- cholestyramine (various) may blunt valproic acid benefits.
- clonazepam (Klonopin) may result in repeated episodes of absence seizures (absence status).

- cyclosporine (Sandimmune) may increase risk of liver toxicity.
- erythromycin (Ery-Tab, others) may increase the level of valproic acid and result in toxicity; the newer macrolides (azithromycin or clarithromycin) may also cause problems.
- felbamate (Felbatol) can lead to increased valproic acid levels.
- fluoxetine (Luvox) can lead to increased valproic acid levels. Blood levels and dosing adjusted to levels is prudent.
- isoniazid (INH) can cause valproic acid or isoniazid toxicity.
- rifampin (Rifater) may lead to valproic acid toxicity.
- ritonavir (Norvir) can lead to loss of valproic acid benefits.

▷ *Driving, Hazardous Activities:* This drug may cause drowsiness, dizziness or confusion. Restrict activities as necessary.

Aviation Note: The use of this drug *is a disqualification* for piloting. Consult a designated Aviation Medical Examiner.

Exposure to Sun: Caution: This drug has caused photosensitivity.

Discontinuation: Do not stop this drug suddenly. Abrupt withdrawal can cause repetitive seizures that are difficult to control.

VANCOMYCIN (van koh MI sin)

Introduced: 1974   **Class:** Anti-infective, glycopeptide antibiotic   **Prescription:** USA: Yes   **Controlled Drug:** USA: No; Canada: No   **Available as Generic:** USA: Yes; Canada: Yes

Brand Names: ✤PMS-Vancomycin, Vancocin, Vancoled, Vancor

Author's Note: Vancomycin is used to treat a variety of serious infections. It is given intravenously to treat some infections and orally to treat others. In the past, the information provided in this profile was limited to the use of vancomycin taken by mouth. Since resistant organisms have increased use of this medicine by vein (intravenously), this profile has been expanded to help patients understand vancomycin's broadened role in infectious disease.

BENEFITS versus RISKS	
Possible Benefits	*Possible Risks*
TREATS SERIOUS INFECTIONS CAUSED BY RESISTANT GRAM-POSITIVE ORGANISMS SUCH AS STAPH AND STREP	KIDNEY TOXICITY (with combined aminoglycoside use)
	Ringing in ears (tinnitus)
	Loss of hearing
TREATS ANTIBIOTIC-ASSOCIATED PSEUDOMEMBRANOUS COLITIS (oral form)	

▷ **Principal Uses**

As a Single Drug Product: Uses currently included in FDA-approved labeling: (1) Oral form is used in antibiotic-associated pseudomembranous colitis caused by *Clostridium difficile;* (2) the oral form is also used in enterocolitis caused by staphylococcal organisms; (3) the intravenous form is used to treat a variety of serious infections, such those in heart valves, bones (osteomyelitis), endocarditis and meningitis, including those caused by methicillin-resistant *Staphylococcus aureus* (MRSA) and other susceptible bacteria.

Other (unlabeled) generally accepted uses: (1) May have a role preventing central venous catheter infections (combined with heparin flush) in immunosuppressed pediatric patients.

How This Drug Works: By inhibiting the formation of bacterial cell walls and the production of RNA, this drug destroys susceptible strains of infecting bacteria.

Available Dosage Forms and Strengths

Capsules — 125 mg, 250 mg

Intravenous — 500 mg/15 ml, 1 g/15 ml

Oral solution — 250 mg/5 ml teaspoonful and 500 mg/5 ml

▷ **Recommended Dosage Ranges** (Actual dose and schedule must be determined for each patient individually.)

Infants and Children: 10 mg per kg of body mass every 6 hours, for 5 to 10 days. The total daily dose should not exceed 2,000 mg (2 g). Repeat course as necessary.

12 to 60 Years of Age: Intravenous: Many clinicians use a 15-mg-per-kg-of-body-mass loading dose and then calculate ongoing doses based on individual patient height, weight, kidney function and suspected bacteria (bacterial pathogen). Calculations are made in order to attain a peak blood level of 30–40 mcg/ml and a lowest blood level (trough) of 5–10 mcg/ml.

Oral dosing for pseudomembranous colitis caused by *Clostridium difficile:* 125 mg by mouth every 6 hours for 10 days.

Over 60 Years of Age: Intravenous dosing: The loading dose is the same as for younger patients. Ongoing doses may be much smaller and may need to be taken much less often than in younger patients (such as once a day or once every 2 days) because of the age-related declines in kidney function.

Oral dosing: Same as 12 to 60 years of age (vancomycin in pseudomembranous colitis is not absorbed).

Conditions Requiring Dosing Adjustments

Liver Function: The liver is not involved in the elimination of vancomycin.

Kidney Function: Oral vancomycin is minimally absorbed. Intravenous vancomycin MUST be taken in decreased dose or increased interval in kidney failure. This drug is also a potential cause of kidney failure and should only be taken if other alternatives are not available. Daily measures of kidney function and more frequent blood levels are indicated if this medicine is used by patients with compromised kidneys.

▷ **Dosing Instructions:** Oral form may be taken with or following food to reduce stomach irritation. Because of this drug's unpleasant taste, it is preferable to swallow the capsule whole without alteration. Use a measuring device to ensure accuracy of dose when taking the oral solution. Observe the expiration date. If you forget a dose: For oral dosing: Take the missed dose as soon as you remember it, unless it's nearly time for your next dose—if that is the case, skip the missed dose and take the next dose right on schedule. Take any remaining doses for the day at evenly spaced intervals, then return to your usual dosing schedule. For intravenous home therapy: If you miss a dose, call the home IV service or your doctor for instructions. Talk with your doctor if you find yourself missing doses because the best results come from taking this medicine right on time and keeping the blood levels or intestinal levels high enough to kill the infecting organism.

Usual Duration of Use

Oral use: Use on a regular schedule for 48 to 72 hours usually determines effectiveness in controlling infection in the colon. If response is prompt, treatment may be limited to 10 days. If symptoms warrant, oral treatment for C. difficile diarrhea may have to be continued for 14 to 21 days. Consult your physician on a regular basis.

Intravenous use: The length of treatment depends on the severity and site of the infection (for example, bone infections such as osteomyelitis may take 6 weeks to cure).

Typical Treatment Goals and Measurements (Outcomes and Markers)

Infections: The most commonly used measures of serious infections are white blood cell counts and differentials (the kind of blood cells that occur most often in your blood), and temperature. Many clinicians look for positive changes in 24–48 hours. NEVER stop an antibiotic because you start to feel better. For many infections, a full 14 days is REQUIRED to kill the bacteria. The goals and time frame (see peak benefits above) should be discussed with you when the prescription is written.

Currently a "Drug of Choice"

For treating metronidazole-treatment failures in antibiotic-associated pseudomembranous colitis caused by *Clostridium difficile* and in cases of methicillin-resistant *Staphylococcus aureus* (MRSA).

▷ **This Drug Should Not Be Taken If**

- you have had an allergic reaction to it previously.

▷ **Inform Your Physician Before Taking This Drug If**

- you have a history of Crohn's disease or ulcerative colitis.
- you have impaired kidney function.
- you are pregnant.
- you have any degree of hearing loss.
- you are taking cholestyramine (Questran) or colestipol (Colestid).

Possible Side Effects (natural, expected and unavoidable drug actions)

Bitter, unpleasant taste for the oral form. Kidney damage with long-term, high-dose use of the intravenous form. Red-man syndrome (lowering of blood pressure, sudden rash of neck, chest, face and extremities) and even cardiac arrest have occurred with too rapid vancomycin infusions. Doses should be given over one hour.

▷ **Possible Adverse Effects** (unusual, unexpected and infrequent reactions)

If any of the following develop, consult your physician promptly for guidance.

Mild Adverse Effects

Allergic reactions: skin rash (with large doses or prolonged use).

Nausea, vomiting—infrequent with oral form and rare with intravenous form.

Chills—infrequent.

Serious Adverse Effects

Allergic reactions: anaphylaxis.

Serious skin rashes (exfoliative dermatitis or Stevens-Johnson syndrome).

Ringing or buzzing in ears, sensation of ear fullness, loss of hearing—toxicity sign.

Lowering of white blood cells—reversible and seen with the intravenous form.

Lowering of white blood cells (granulocytes) and platelets—case reports and reversible with granulocyte colony stimulating factor (GCSF).

Cardiac arrest—rare.

Hearing loss—may be reversible and more likely with high-dose or long-term use.

Kidney toxicity—may be dose-dependent and more likely with higher doses and long-term use.

Pseudomembranous colitis—possible with the IV form.

Thrombophlebitis—infrequent with the intravenous form.

▷ **Possible Effects on Sexual Function:** None reported.

Natural Diseases or Disorders That May Be Activated by This Drug
Latent hearing loss, kidney failure.

Possible Effects on Laboratory Tests
Serum creatinine: increased (a sign of kidney toxicity).

CAUTION
1. Report promptly the development of fullness, ringing or buzzing in either ear. This may indicate the onset of nerve damage that could lead to hearing loss.
2. Do not take any medication to stop your diarrhea without calling your doctor. The bacterial toxin that causes colitis is eliminated by diarrhea; stopping the elimination could intensify and prolong your illness.
3. Blood levels MUST be used to guide intravenous dosing. Keep all appointments for laboratory work.

Precautions for Use
By Infants and Children: Some cases may require doses up to 50 mg per kg of body mass daily.
By Those Over 60 Years of Age: You may be more susceptible to drug-induced hearing loss. Use the minimum course of treatment required to cure your colitis or other infection.

▷ **Advisability of Use During Pregnancy**
Pregnancy Category: C. See Pregnancy Risk Categories at the back of this book.
Animal studies: Rat and rabbit studies reveal no drug-induced birth defects.
Human studies: Adequate studies of pregnant women are not available.
Use this drug only if clearly needed. Ask your doctor for help.

Advisability of Use If Breast-Feeding
Presence of this drug in breast milk: Yes.
Avoid drug or refrain from nursing.

Habit-Forming Potential: None.

Effects of Overdose: Possible nausea, vomiting, ringing in ears.

Possible Effects of Long-Term Use: Hearing loss.

Suggested Periodic Examinations While Taking This Drug (at physician's discretion)
Hearing tests.
Measures of kidney function and blood vancomycin levels with intravenous use.

▷ **While Taking This Drug, Observe the Following**
Foods: No restrictions.
Herbal Medicines or Minerals: Some patients use echinacea to attempt to boost their immune systems. Unfortunately, use of echinacea is not recommended in people with damaged immune systems. This herb may also actually weaken any immune system if it is used too often or for too long a time.
Beverages: No restrictions. May be taken with milk.

▷ *Alcohol:* No interactions expected. Use sparingly; alcohol may aggravate colitis.
Tobacco Smoking: No interactions expected. I advise everyone to quit smoking.

▷ *Other Drugs*

The following drugs may *decrease* the effects of vancomycin:
- cholestyramine (Questran).
- colestipol (Colestid).

Vancomycin *taken concurrently* with
- aminoglycoside antibiotics (see Drug Classes), such as gentamicin or tobramycin, may cause additive toxicity risk to the ears and kidneys.
- cyclosporine (Sandimmune) may result in increased toxicity risk.
- metformin (Glucophage) or other cationic drugs poses an increased risk of lactic acidosis.
- other medicines that cause kidney toxicity may pose an additive toxicity risk.
- rapacuronium (Raplon) can lead to extended neuromuscular blockade requiring neostigmine use.
- succinylcholine (Anectine) can lead to extended neuromuscular blockade requiring neostigmine use.
- warfarin (Coumadin) may cause increased bleeding risk; increased INR (prothrombin time or protime) testing is needed.

▷ *Driving, Hazardous Activities:* Usually no restrictions.
Aviation Note: The use of this drug is *probably not a disqualification* for piloting. Consult a designated Aviation Medical Examiner.
Exposure to Sun: No restrictions.
Special Storage Instructions: Refrigerate the oral solution. A home IV service will explain storage of the intravenous form.
Observe the Following Expiration Times: Provided on your prescription label by your pharmacist.
Discontinuation: To be determined by your physician.

VARICELLA VIRUS VACCINE (VAIR a sell ah)

Introduced: 1995 **Class:** Vaccine **Prescription:** USA: Yes **Controlled Drug:** USA: No; Canada: No **Available as Generic:** USA: No; Canada: No
Brand Name: Varivax

BENEFITS versus RISKS	
Possible Benefits	*Possible Risks*
PREVENTION OF VARICELLA	Rash
(chicken pox)	Soreness at the injection site
	Anaphylactic reaction

▷ **Principal Uses**

As a Single Drug Product: Uses currently included in FDA-approved labeling: Prevention of chicken pox.

Other (unlabeled) generally accepted uses: (1) Prevention of herpes zoster (in people more than 55 years old) who have previously had chicken pox.

How This Drug Works: By stimulating the immune system, the vaccine prepares the body to fight any exposure to the wild-type virus.

Available Dosage Forms and Strengths

Vaccine: single-dose vials with a final dose of 1350 PFU per 0.5 ml.

How to Store

This product must be kept frozen prior to use.

▷ **Recommended Dosage Ranges** (Actual dose and schedule must be determined for each patient individually.)

Infants and Children 1 to 12 Years Old: Not indicated in infants. Children 1 year old or older are given 0.5 ml injected under the skin.

12 to 55 Years of Age: Same as the children's dose, providing the patient has not had chicken pox.

Over 55 Years of Age: Not studied.

Author's Note: The Centers for Disease Control (CDC) Immunization Practices Committee has recommended that all children 12- to 18-months-old should be given varicella vaccine if they have not previously contracted chicken pox. The vaccine is also recommended by the committee for children 19 months to 13 years old. Finally, adults or adolescents who have not had chicken pox and are at risk for exposure may also be given the vaccine.

Conditions Requiring Dosing Adjustments

Liver Function: Not a consideration.

Kidney Function: Not a consideration.

▷ **Dosing Instructions:** This vaccine is to be injected under the skin. It may be given with measles, mumps and rubella vaccine. If you forget to get vaccinated: Get the vaccine and talk with your pediatrician about vaccine schedules. It's always better to PREVENT a disease or condition than to have to treat it.

Usual Duration of Benefit: Exposure to chicken pox 5 years after vaccination may result in 20% of patients developing mild disease. More experience is needed before the question of repeat vaccination is answered. Immunity may last 10 years.

Typical Treatment Goals and Measurements (Outcomes and Markers)

Immune response/protection from varicella (chicken pox): The general goal is to challenge the immune system of the person receiving the vaccination enough to elicit an immune response that will protect the person from the virus itself. For example, my generation was "expected" to get many of the childhood diseases. Subsequently, measles, mumps and varicella vaccines were created, and possible mortality and morbidity may be avoided in those who received the "shots." The varicella vaccine is important as it probably protects adults from shingles later in life. Clinical markers include gpELISA of greater than 0.3 and avoidance of varicella infection despite subsequent exposure.

Possible Advantages of This Drug

Prevention of chicken pox and avoidance of shingles later in life.

Currently a Drug of Choice
For prevention of chicken pox. Some company-based information can be obtained by calling 1-800-Merck-RX or 1-800-637-2579.

▷ **This Drug Should Not Be Taken If**
- you are allergic to any component of the vaccine (even gelatin).
- you have a history of anaphylactic reaction to neomycin.
- you have a history of blood diseases or leukemia or have AIDS.
- you are taking medicines that suppress the immune system.
- you have tuberculosis that has not been treated.
- you are allergic to eggs, gelatin or any other vaccine component.
- you are pregnant (avoid pregnancy for 3 months after vaccine).
- you have an active infection.

▷ **Inform Your Physician Before Taking This Drug If**
- you are planning pregnancy in the near future.
- you have a condition that may require steroids.
- you have had blood or plasma transfusions (vaccination should be delayed for 5 months).
- you take salicylates (aspirin, others) on a regular basis. This should NOT be done for 6 weeks following vaccination, as it is a risk for Reye's syndrome.
- you live with someone who has a depressed immune system (such as an AIDS patient). Because this vaccine is a live-virus vaccine, you may be infectious to them.

Possible Side Effects (natural, expected and unavoidable drug actions)
Pain at the injection site, fever—infrequent to frequent.

▷ **Possible Adverse Effects** (unusual, unexpected and infrequent reactions)
If any of the following develop, consult your physician promptly for guidance.
Mild Adverse Effects
Allergic reactions: skin rash.
Varicellalike rash—infrequent.
Headache, irritability, fatigue and loss of appetite—rare to infrequent.
Increased sensitivity to light (photophobia)—case reports.
Chills, stiff neck and joint pain—infrequent.
Nausea, vomiting—rare.
Serious Adverse Effects
Allergic reactions: anaphylactic reaction—case reports.
Idiosyncratic reactions: none reported.
Febrile seizures—case reports.
Thrombocytopenic purpura—case reports.
Herpes zoster—possible.
Pneumonitis—case report and of questionable causation.
May be possible for a recently vaccinated person to transmit varicella to a susceptible contact—one case report.

▷ **Possible Effects on Sexual Function:** None reported.

Possible Delayed Adverse Effects: None reported.

▷ **Adverse Effects That May Mimic Natural Diseases or Disorders**
Rash may resemble chicken pox.

Natural Diseases or Disorders That May Be Activated by This Drug
None reported.

Possible Effects on Laboratory Tests
 None reported.

CAUTION
 Do not give aspirin or other salicylates to patients who have recently received the vaccine. The risk of Reye's syndrome is associated with such aspirin use.

Precautions for Use
 By Infants and Children: Safety and effectiveness for use by those under 12 months of age have not been established.
 By Those Over 60 Years of Age: Not studied.

▷ **Advisability of Use During Pregnancy**
 Pregnancy Category: C. See Pregnancy Risk Categories at the back of this book.
 Animal studies: Have not been conducted with this vaccine.
 Human studies: Information from adequate studies of pregnant women is not available.
  The manufacturer says that the vaccine should not be given to pregnant women, and pregnancy should be avoided for 3 months following vaccination.

Advisability of Use If Breast-Feeding
 Presence of this drug in breast milk: Expected.
 Avoid drug or refrain from nursing.

Habit-Forming Potential: None.

Effects of Overdose: Not defined.

Possible Effects of Long-Term Use: Not intended for long-term use.

Suggested Periodic Examinations While Taking This Drug (at physician's discretion)
 None suggested.

▷ **While Taking This Drug, Observe the Following**
 Foods: No restrictions.
 Herbal Medicines or Minerals: Some patients use echinacea to attempt to boost their immune systems. Unfortunately, use of echinacea is not recommended in people with damaged immune systems. This herb may also actually weaken any immune system if it is used too often or for too long a time. Mistletoe has also not been studied and can not be recommended.
 Beverages: No restrictions.
▷ *Alcohol:* No interactions expected.
 Tobacco Smoking: No interactions expected. I advise everyone to quit smoking.
▷ *Other Drugs*
  Varicella vaccine *taken concurrently* with
  • acyclovir (Zovirax) may result in a blunted immune benefit from the vaccine.
  • aspirin or any salicylates (various) may result in Reye's syndrome—DO NOT take aspirin for 6 weeks after vaccination.
  • chemotherapy (various) may lead to infection risk by the vaccine.
  • corticosteroids (see Drug Classes) may result in extreme reactions.
  • etanercept (Enbrel) may blunt immune response to varicella vaccine.
  • hepatitis B immune globulin may blunt immune response to varicella vaccine.
  • immune globulins (such as rabies or tetanus immune globulin) may blunt beneficial response to the vaccine.
  • immunosuppressant medicines (such as cyclosporine [Sandimmune],

sirolimus [Rapamune] or tacrolimus [Prograf]) may result in blunted beneficial vaccine response as well as unexpected reactions, sometimes extreme reactions.

- infliximab (Remicade) may increase risk of varicella infection from varicella vaccine itself.
- leflunomide (Arava) may blunt immune response to varicella vaccine. Rapid elimination procedure for leflunomide may be needed.
- mesalamine (Asacol) may result in risk of Reye's syndrome—DO NOT take salicylates for 6 weeks after vaccination.
- olsalazine (Dipentum) may result in risk of Reye's syndrome—DO NOT take salicylates for 6 weeks after vaccination.

▷ *Driving, Hazardous Activities:* This drug may cause soreness at the injection site. Restrict activities as necessary.

Aviation Note: The use of this drug *is probably not a disqualification* for piloting. Consult a designated Aviation Medical Examiner.

Exposure to Sun: No restrictions.

Occurrence of Unrelated Illness: This vaccination should not be given in the presence of any other active infection.

Special Storage Instructions: This vaccine must be stored frozen.

Author's Note: There is now a Vaccine Adverse Event Reporting System (VAERS). The toll-free number is 1-800-822-7967.

VENLAFAXINE (ven la FAX een)

Introduced: 1993   **Class:** Antidepressant   **Prescription:** USA: Yes
Controlled Drug: USA: No; Canada: No   **Available as Generic:** USA: No
Brand Names: Effexor, Effexor XR

BENEFITS versus RISKS	
Possible Benefits	*Possible Risks*
EFFECTIVE TREATMENT OF DEPRESSION	INCREASED BLOOD PRESSURE
	Seizures
BETTER SIDE-EFFECT PROFILE THAN TRICYCLIC ANTIDEPRESSANTS	Constipation
	Increased heart rate
	Increased serum lipids
RAPID ONSET OF EFFECT	
EXCELLENT REMISSION RATE IN MAJOR DEPRESSION	
HELPS PREVENT RELAPSE AND RECURRENCE OF DEPRESSION	
EFFECTIVE TREATMENT OF ANXIETY	
TREATS GENERALIZED ANXIETY DISORDER	
Second line treatment of children who have both depression and ADHD (XR form)	
May decrease hot flashes in cancer survivors and after menopause	

▷ **Principal Uses**

As a Single Drug Product: Uses currently included in FDA-approved labeling: (1) Treatment of depression; (2) treatment of generalized anxiety disorder; (3) prevention of relapse and recurrence of depression.

Other (unlabeled) generally accepted uses: (1) May be useful in obsessive-compulsive disorder; (2) may treat chronic fatigue syndrome; (3) may have a role in easing hot flashes in cancer survivors and after menopause; (4) second line treatment in children who have both depression and ADHD.

How This Drug Works: This bicyclic (second-generation) antidepressant inhibits the return (reuptake) of nerve transmitters (serotonin, norepinephrine and dopamine) and helps return normal mood and thinking.

Available Dosage Forms and Strengths

Tablets — 25 mg, 37.5 mg, 50 mg, 75 mg, 100 mg

Tablets, extended release — 37.5 mg, 75 mg, 100 mg, 150 mg (100 and 150 mg in Canada)

▷ **Recommended Dosage Ranges** (Actual dose and schedule must be determined for each patient individually.)

Infants and Children: Safety and efficacy for those under 18 years of age are not established.

18 to 60 Years of Age: For depression and generalized anxiety disorder: Start with 75 mg per day, as 25-mg doses three times daily taken with food. If needed and tolerated, the dose may be increased at 4-day intervals up to a maximum of 225 mg per day. Some hospitalized patients have been given a maximum of 375 mg per day. The XR form is started at 37.5 milligrams per day. Dose increases of 75 mg/day can be made at intervals of at least 4 days. Daily maximum is 225 mg per day. In general, conversion from immediate release to venlafaxine XR can be done using the total immediate release daily dose and converting that to the nearest equal dose of the XR form.

For reducing hot flashes in cancer survivors: 12.5 mg twice daily.

Over 60 Years of Age: Low starting doses and slow increases are indicated. Natural declines in kidney function may lead to drug accumulation at higher doses. May worsen constipation.

Conditions Requiring Dosing Adjustments

Liver Function: Total daily dose must be reduced by 50% for patients with moderate liver compromise. Further dose decreases and individualized dosing is needed in liver cirrhosis.

Kidney Function: Patients with compromised kidneys (creatinine clearance of 10 to 70 ml/min) should take 75% of the usual daily dose.

▷ **Dosing Instructions:** Best to take this medicine with food. The XR form should NOT be crushed or chewed. If you forget a dose: Take the missed dose as soon as you remember it, unless it's nearly time for your next dose—if that is the case, skip the missed dose and take the next dose right on schedule. DO NOT double up on doses. Because this medicine must reach an equilibrium (or steady state) in the brain, it is very important to take it exactly as prescribed to get the best results in helping depression. Talk with your doctor if you find yourself missing doses.

Usual Duration of Use: Regular use for 2 weeks usually determines benefits in treating depression. Decreasing hot flashes in cancer survivors may take several weeks. Long-term use requires follow-up by your doctor.

Typical Treatment Goals and Measurements (Outcomes and Markers)

Depression: The general goal: to at least help lessen the degree and severity of depression, letting patients return to their daily lives. Specific measures of depression involve testing or inventories (such as Hamilton Depression) and can be valuable in helping check benefits from this medicine.

Possible Advantages of This Drug

Effective treatment of depression with fewer side effects than other currently available agents. Starts to have a therapeutic effect more rapidly than other available agents. One study of 1,108 patients with major depression found a 45% remission rate. Works on both serotonin and norepinephrine nerve transmitters (neurotransmitters).

▷ **This Drug Should Not Be Taken If**
- you had an allergic reaction to any form of it previously.
- you are taking a monoamine oxidase (MAO) inhibitor (see Drug Classes).

▷ **Inform Your Physician Before Taking This Drug If**
- you have a history of high blood pressure.
- you've recently had a heart attack.
- you have a history of abnormally increased lipids (hyperlipidemia).
- you are planning pregnancy.
- you have a history of seizures.
- you have a history of suicide attempts or think about suicide.
- you have trouble sleeping.
- you have a history of hypomania or mania.
- you are unsure how much to take or how often to take this medicine.

Possible Side Effects (natural, expected and unavoidable drug actions)

Constipation and headache. Sleepiness, weight loss, dry mouth. Small increases in cholesterol (2–3 mg/dl).

▷ **Possible Adverse Effects** (unusual, unexpected and infrequent reactions)

If any of the following develop, consult your physician promptly for guidance.

Mild Adverse Effects

Allergic reactions: Possible.

Palpitations or fast heart rate—rare.

Nausea and vomiting—infrequent.

Dizziness (may disappear without treatment), fatigue and headache—infrequent to frequent.

Anxiety, somnolence or insomnia (may stop on its own).

Blurred vision—possible.

Spontaneous and easy bruising (ecchymosis)—case report.

Sweating—possible

Serious Adverse Effects

Allergic reactions: Possible.

Idiosyncratic reactions: one case report of lowered white blood cells (agranulocytosis).

Liver toxicity—case report.

SIADH and very low sodium—case reports.

Increased blood pressure—case reports.

Serotonin syndrome—case reports.

Seizures—very rare during premarketing studies.

▷ **Possible Effects on Sexual Function:** Delayed orgasm, abnormal ejaculation, priapism, impotence and erectile failure—all rare.

Possible Delayed Adverse Effects: None reported.

▷ **Adverse Effects That May Mimic Natural Diseases or Disorders**
None reported.

Natural Diseases or Disorders That May Be Activated by This Drug
None reported.

Possible Effects on Laboratory Tests
Serum cholesterol: increased slightly.

CAUTION
1. This drug should not be taken with MAO inhibitors (see Glossary). If you have recently stopped an MAO inhibitor, 14 days should pass before venlafaxine is started.

▷ **Advisability of Use During Pregnancy**
Pregnancy Category: C. See Pregnancy Risk Categories at the back of this book.
Animal studies: There was an increase in stillborn rats at 10 times the usual human dose.
Human studies: Adequate studies of pregnant women are not available.
Ask your doctor for guidance.

Advisability of Use If Breast-Feeding
Presence of this drug in breast milk: Unknown.
Monitor nursing infant closely, and discontinue drug or nursing if adverse effects develop.

Habit-Forming Potential: None.

Effects of Overdose: Nausea, vomiting, constipation, seizure potential.

Possible Effects of Long-Term Use: None noted.

Suggested Periodic Examinations While Taking This Drug (at physician's discretion)
Blood pressure checks.

▷ **While Taking This Drug, Observe the Following**
Foods: No restrictions.
Herbal Medicines or Minerals: Since venlafaxine and St. John's wort may act to increase serotonin, the combination is not advised (St. John's wort may also cause fast heart rate). Since part of the way ginseng and ginkgo work may be as an MAO inhibitor, do not combine ginseng or ginkgo with venlafaxine. Ma huang, yohimbe, Indian snakeroot and kava kava are also best avoided while taking this medicine. Talk to your doctor BEFORE combining any herbals with this medicine.
Nutritional Support: No special support indicated.
Beverages: Since venlafaxine is metabolized in the liver and grapefruit juice has been shown to inhibit the removal (metabolism) of some other medications, caution is advised. Water is the best liquid to take this medicine with.
▷ *Alcohol:* May increase somnolence if combined.
Tobacco Smoking: No interactions expected. I advise everyone to quit smoking.
Marijuana Smoking: Additive effect on somnolence.
▷ *Other Drugs*
Venlafaxine taken concurrently with
• beta blockers (see Drug Classes) may result in larger than expected phar-

macological effects from the beta blockers; because these agents are metabolized in the liver and venlafaxine may block this metabolism, caution is advised.

- calcium channel blockers (see Drug Classes) may result in toxicity; because these agents are metabolized in the liver and venlafaxine may block this metabolism, caution is advised.
- cimetidine (Tagamet) may lead to venlafaxine toxicity.
- dextromethorphan (the DM in many cough and cold preparations) may result in dextromethorphan or venlafaxine toxicity. Caution is advised.
- dofetilide (Tikosyn) may result in dofetilide toxicity.
- MAO inhibitors (see Drug Classes) may lead to undesirable side effects—DO NOT COMBINE.
- quinidine (Quinaglute, others) may result in venlafaxine toxicity.
- ritonavir (Norvir) may lead to venlafaxine toxicity.
- drugs with sedative properties will increase those effects.
- paroxetine (Paxil—a SSRI) or SNRIs can lead to a serotonin syndrome if a sufficient time does not pass between stopping a first medicine and starting an alternative therapy. The time required (washout) may vary patient to patient, but the generally accepted time is two weeks.
- sibutramine (Meridia) increases toxicity risk (serotonin syndrome)—DO NOT COMBINE.
- sumatriptan (Imitrex), naratriptan (Amerge), rizatriptan (Maxalt) or zolmitriptan (Zomig) may lead to incoordination and weakness—DO NOT COMBINE.
- tramadol (Ultram) may increase the risk of seizures.
- tricyclic antidepressants (see Drug Classes) may result in toxicity; because these agents are metabolized in the liver and venlafaxine may block this metabolism, caution is advised.
- warfarin (Coumadin) may result in bleeding; more frequent INR (prothrombin time or protime) testing is needed. Ongoing warfarin doses should be adjusted to laboratory results.
- zolpidem (Ambien) may increase risk of hallucinations—DO NOT COMBINE.

▷ *Driving, Hazardous Activities:* This drug may cause somnolence. Restrict activities as necessary.

Aviation Note: The use of this drug *is a disqualification* for piloting. Consult a designated Aviation Medical Examiner.

Exposure to Sun: No restrictions.

Exposure to Heat: No restrictions.

Discontinuation: If this medicine is to be stopped, the dose should be slowly lowered over 2–3 weeks on your doctor's advice. Tapering over this time helps your body best adjust to not having this medicine, minimizing risk of undesirable discontinuation symptoms.

VERAPAMIL (ver AP a mil)

Introduced: 1967   **Class:** Anti-anginal, antiarrhythmic, antihypertensive, calcium channel blocker   **Prescription:** USA: Yes   **Controlled Drug:** USA: No; Canada: No   **Available as Generic:** USA: Yes (verapamil SR); Canada: Yes

Brand Names: ❦Alti-Verapamil, ❦Apo-Verap, Calan, Calan SR, ❦Chronovera, Covera-HS, ❦Dom-Verapamil SR, ❦Gen-Verapamil, Isoptin, Isoptin SR, ❦Med-Verapamil, ❦Novo-Veramil, ❦Nu-Verap, ❦PMS-Verapamil, Tarka [CD], Verelan, Verelan PM

Controversies in Medicine: Medicines in this class have had many conflicting reports. The FDA has held hearings on the calcium channel blocker (CCB) class. Amlodipine got the first FDA approval to treat high blood pressure or angina in people with congestive heart failure. Early research at New York University found that nifedipine is a cause of reversible male infertility. CCBs are currently second-line agents for high blood pressure according to the JNC VI (see Glossary).

BENEFITS versus RISKS

Possible Benefits	*Possible Risks*
EFFECTIVE PREVENTION OF BOTH MAJOR TYPES OF ANGINA	Congestive heart failure
	Low blood pressure (infrequent)
EFFECTIVE CONTROL OF HEART RATE IN CHRONIC ATRIAL FIBRILLATION AND FLUTTER	Heart rhythm disturbance
	Fluid retention
	Constipation
EFFECTIVE PREVENTION OF PAROXYSMAL ATRIAL TACHYCARDIA (PAT)	Liver damage without jaundice
	Swelling of male breast tissue
EFFECTIVE TREATMENT OF HYPERTENSION	

▷ **Principal Uses**

As a Single Drug Product: Uses currently included in FDA-approved labeling: Used to treat (1) angina pectoris due to coronary artery spasm (Prinzmetal's variant angina) that occurs spontaneously and is not associated with exertion; (2) classical angina of effort (due to atherosclerotic disease of the coronary arteries) in individuals who have not responded to or cannot tolerate the nitrates and beta-blocker drugs customarily used to treat this disorder; (3) abnormally rapid heart rate due to chronic atrial fibrillation or flutter; (4) recurrent paroxysmal atrial or supraventricular tachycardia; (5) primary hypertension.

Other (unlabeled) generally accepted uses: (1) May help decrease keloid formation; (2) prevents abnormal heart rhythms that occur after surgery; (3) relieves symptoms of and may help reverse hypertrophic cardiomyopathy; (4) may help decrease the severity or occurrence of cluster headaches; (5) helps control symptoms of panic attacks; (6) can be of use in post-ischemic-acute-kidney failure; (7) may stop the progression of abnormal buildup on the inside of blood vessels (atherosclerosis); (8) may help decrease severity and occurrence of nocturnal leg cramps; (9) can help stuttering; (10) may have a role in treating Tourette's syndrome.

As a Combination Drug Product [CD]: This drug is available in combination (Tarka brand) with an ACE inhibitor (trandolapril). The combination offers benefits of two different mechanisms of action in the same medicine in treating high blood pressure.

How This Drug Works: By blocking passage of calcium through certain cell walls (which is necessary for the function of nerve and muscle tissue), this drug slows the spread of electrical activity through the heart and inhibits the contraction of coronary arteries and peripheral arterioles. As a result of these combined effects, this drug

- prevents spontaneous coronary artery spasm (Prinzmetal's type of angina).
- reduces heart rate and contraction force during exertion, thus lowering the oxygen requirement of the heart muscle; this reduces the occurrence of effort-induced angina (classical angina pectoris).
- reduces degree of contraction of peripheral arterial walls, resulting in relaxation and lowering of blood pressure. This further reduces the workload of the heart during exertion and contributes to the prevention of angina.
- slows the rate of electrical impulses through the heart and thereby prevents excessively rapid heart action (tachycardia).

Available Dosage Forms and Strengths

Caplets, sustained-release — 120 mg, 180 mg, 240 mg
Capsules, sustained-release — 360 mg
Injection — 5 mg/2 ml
Tablets — 40 mg, 80 mg, 120 mg
Tablets, combination (Tarka) — 1 mg trandolapril/240 mg verapamil,
2 mg trandolapril/180 mg verapamil,
2 mg trandolapril/ 240 mg verapamil,
4 mg trandolapril/240 mg verapamil
Tablets, extended-release — 180 mg, 240 mg
Tablets, sustained-release — 120 mg, 180 mg, 240 mg
Tablets, timed-release (Verelan PM) — 100 mg, 200 mg, 300 mg

▷ **Usual Adult Dosage Ranges:** Hypertension: Initially 80 mg three times daily. The dose may be increased gradually at 1- to 7-day intervals as needed and tolerated. The usual maintenance dose is from 240 to 360 mg daily in three or four divided doses. The prolonged-action (sustained-release) dose forms permit once-a-day dosing. The total daily dose should not exceed 360 mg.

Once-a-day treatment may be initiated with one prolonged-action capsule of 120 mg or one tablet of 180 mg.

The Covera HS form is given as one 180 mg extended-release tablet at bedtime. If adequate response is not obtained, the dose may be increased to 240 mg at bedtime. Dose may be subsequently increased as needed and tolerated to a maximum of 480 mg. The lowest effect or trough effect would be best evaluated just before bedtime.

The VereZlan PM form is designed to be taken at bedtime. Dosing generally starts at 100 mg at bedtime.

Tarka form: Talk to your doctor.

Note: Actual dose and schedule must be determined for each patient individually.

Conditions Requiring Dosing Adjustments

Liver Function: Blood levels should be obtained to guide dosing. In liver disease, dose should be decreased to 20–50% of usual doses at the usual times. This drug is also a rare cause of liver damage. Electrocardiogram changes may provide an early indication of increasing blood levels.

Kidney Function: In severe kidney compromise, the dose should be decreased by 50–75%.

Heart (Myocardial) Dysfunction: Intravenous doses (0.0001 mg/kg/minute) are started and adjusted (titrated) against heart rate. Also adjusted if you are taking digoxin or a beta blocker.

▷ **Dosing Instructions:** Preferably taken with meals and with food at bedtime. The regular tablet may be crushed for administration. The prolonged-action dose forms (capsules and tablets) should be swallowed whole and not altered. Verelan capsules may be taken without regard to food intake. The Verelan PM form IS NOT a sleeping pill. The PM is meant to stand for bedtime dosing. If you forget a dose: Take the missed dose as soon as you remember it, unless it's nearly time for your next dose—if that is the case, skip the missed dose and take the next dose right on schedule. DO NOT double up on doses. Talk with your doctor if you find yourself missing doses.

Usual Duration of Use: Use on a regular schedule for 2 to 4 weeks usually determines effectiveness in reducing the frequency and severity of angina. Reduction of elevated blood pressure may be apparent within the first 1 to 2 weeks. For long-term use (months to years), the smallest effective dose should be used. Periodic physician evaluation is needed.

Typical Treatment Goals and Measurements (Outcomes and Markers)

Blood pressure: The most recent treatment guidelines (JNC VI) actually define optimal blood pressure (BP) as less than 120/80 and high normal as 139/89. The American Diabetes Association has chosen a target of 130/80 as the blood pressure goal for people living with diabetes. Most clinicians try to achieve a BP that achieves the best balance of lower cardiovascular risk while avoiding the problem of too low a blood pressure. The goal and time frame (see peak benefits above) should be discussed with you when the prescription is written.

Abnormal heartbeats: The general goal is to return the heart to a normal rhythm or at least to markedly reduce the occurrence of abnormal heartbeats. In life-threatening arrhythmias, the goal is to abort the abnormal beats and return the pattern to normal. Success at ongoing suppression may involve ambulatory checks of heart rate and rhythm for a day (such as in Holter monitoring). This kind of testing involves placement of adhesive backed temporary electrodes on the skin in several positions around the heart. A small heart rate and rhythm (EKG or ECG) recording device is carried around via a shoulder strap and records what the heart is doing over 24 hours. Once the recording is made, a scanning machine reviews the record, tallies abnormal heart beats or rhythms and gives a close and extended look at how the heart is reacting or benefiting from the medicines that the patient is taking. Repeat measurements can be made if doses are changed to check the success at keeping the heart in normal sinus rhythm!

Possible Advantages of This Drug

No adverse effects on blood levels of glucose, potassium or uric acid. Does not increase blood cholesterol or triglyceride levels. Does not impair capacity for exercise. The 360-mg strength of Verelan allows once-daily dosing for those patients who require more than 240 mg daily. The company has noted that there is no increase in side effects when comparing the 240-mg capsules to the new 360-mg ones.

The Verelan PM and the Covera HS forms are specifically made to reach their peak levels in the body in the morning. The thinking here is that since heart attacks most often happen in the morning, they may actually be related to early morning increases in heart rate and blood pressure. These medicines seek to avoid low medicine blood levels at a time when it appears they are needed most.

Currently a "Drug of Choice"

For treating (with once-daily forms) people who have trouble remembering to take their medicines (nonadherent patients).

▷ **This Drug Should Not Be Taken If**
- you have had an allergic reaction to it previously.
- you have active liver disease.
- you have a "sick sinus" syndrome (and do not have an artificial pacemaker).
- you have a fast heart rate (ventricular tachycardia) arising in the ventricles.
- you have atrial fibrillation or flutter.
- you have been told that you have a second- or third-degree heart block or congestive heart failure.
- you have low blood pressure (systolic pressure below 90).

▷ **Inform Your Physician Before Taking This Drug If**
- you have had an unfavorable response to any calcium channel blocker.
- you are currently taking any other drugs, especially digitalis or a beta-blocker drug (see Drug Classes).
- you have had a recent stroke or heart attack.
- you have a history of congestive heart failure, angina or heart rhythm disorders.
- you have aortic stenosis (ask your specialist).
- you have poor circulation to your extremities or gangrene.
- you have impaired liver or kidney function.
- you have a history of drug-induced liver damage.

Possible Side Effects (natural, expected and unavoidable drug actions)

Low blood pressure, fluid retention—rare. Change in how well platelets work (antiplatelet effect)—may be significant if combined with aspirin. Constipation (up to 42%).

▷ **Possible Adverse Effects** (unusual, unexpected and infrequent reactions)

If any of the following develop, consult your physician promptly for guidance.

Mild Adverse Effects

Allergic reactions: skin rash, hives, itching, aching joints.

Flushing—infrequent.

Headache—frequent.

Dizziness, fatigue—infrequent.

Nausea, indigestion, constipation—rare to infrequent.

Abnormal growth of the gums—infrequent to frequent.

Sensation of numbness or coldness in the extremities—case reports.

Hair color change—case report.

Cough—rare.

Serious Adverse Effects

Allergic reactions: skin rash (Stevens-Johnson syndrome)—possible.

Serious disturbances of heart rate and/or rhythm, congestive heart failure—rare.

Drug-induced liver damage without jaundice—case reports.

Antiplatelet effect and extended time to form blood clots—possible.

Lung problems (pulmonary edema).

Excessive lowering of blood pressure—case reports.

Unmasking of parkinsonism or movement disorders—rare.

Low blood sugar—possible.

▷ **Possible Effects on Sexual Function:** Altered timing and pattern of menstruation.

Male breast enlargement and tenderness (gynecomastia)—case reports.

Impotence—frequent.

Possible Effects on Laboratory Tests

Blood total cholesterol and HDL cholesterol levels: no effect in some; decreased in others.

Blood LDL cholesterol or triglyceride level: no effect.

Glucose tolerance test (GTT): decreased.

Liver function tests: increased enzymes (ALT/GPT, AST/GOT), increased bilirubin (case reports).

CAUTION

1. Be sure to inform all physicians and other health care professionals who provide medical care for you that you take this drug. Note the use of this drug on your card of personal identification.
2. You may use nitroglycerin and other nitrate drugs as needed to relieve acute episodes of angina pain. If angina attacks become more frequent or intense, call your doctor promptly.
3. If this drug is used concurrently with a beta-blocker drug, you may develop excessively low blood pressure.
4. This drug may cause swelling of the feet and ankles. This may not be indicative of either heart or kidney dysfunction.

Precautions for Use

By Infants and Children: Safety and effectiveness for those under 12 years of age are not established.

By Those Over 60 Years of Age: You may be more susceptible to weakness, dizziness, fainting and falling. Take necessary precautions to prevent injury. Report promptly any changes in your pattern of thirst and urination.

▷ **Advisability of Use During Pregnancy**

Pregnancy Category: C. See Pregnancy Risk Categories at the back of this book.

Animal studies: Toxic effects on the embryo and retarded growth of the fetus (but no birth defects) reported in rat studies.

Human studies: Adequate studies of pregnant women are not available.

Avoid this drug during the first 3 months. Use during the final 6 months only if clearly needed. Ask your doctor for help.

Advisability of Use If Breast-Feeding

Presence of this drug in breast milk: Yes.

Discuss the benefits and risks of nursing your infant. Most clinicians find breast milk drug levels to be insignificant. Monitor infant for adverse effects.

Habit-Forming Potential: None. A withdrawal syndrome is possible (increased frequency and severity of angina). If the medicine must be stopped, it should be slowly decreased—NOT stopped abruptly.

Effects of Overdose: Flushed and warm skin, sweating, light-headedness, irritability, rapid heart rate, low blood pressure, loss of consciousness.

Possible Effects of Long-Term Use: None reported.

Suggested Periodic Examinations While Taking This Drug (at physician's discretion)

Evaluations of heart function, including electrocardiograms.

Liver and kidney function tests, with long-term use.

▷ **While Taking This Drug, Observe the Following**

Foods: DO NOT take this medicine with grapefruit or grapefruit juice. Avoid excessive salt intake.

Herbal Medicines or Minerals: Ginseng may increase blood pressure, blunting the benefits of this medicine. Hawthorn, saw palmetto, ma huang, goldenseal, yohimbe and licorice may also cause increased blood pressure. Garlic and calcium may work to lower blood pressure. The combination may work to require lower verapamil doses. St. John's wort may work to lower calcium channel blocker levels (because it increases P-glycoprotein in the gut). This combination may also increase sun sensitivity. Eleuthero root and ephedra should be avoided by people living with hypertension.

Indian snakeroot has a German Commission E monograph indication for hypertension—talk to your doctor. Discuss any plans for herbal medicines or minerals with your doctor.

Beverages: Caffeine levels will be increased if caffeine-containing beverages are consumed while you are on verapamil. DO NOT take this medicine with grapefruit or grapefruit juice. May be taken with milk.

▷ *Alcohol:* Use with caution until combined effects have been determined. Alcohol may exaggerate the drop in blood pressure and change the elimination of alcohol (experienced by some patients). This may lead to an exaggerated effect of alcohol.

Tobacco Smoking: Nicotine can reduce the effectiveness of this drug. Avoid all forms of tobacco.

Marijuana Smoking: Possible reduced effectiveness of this drug; mild to moderate increase in angina; possible changes in electrocardiogram, confusing interpretation.

▷ *Other Drugs*

Verapamil may ***increase*** the effects of

- buspirone (Buspar).
- carbamazepine (Tegretol) and cause carbamazepine toxicity.
- digitoxin and digoxin (Lanoxin) and cause digitalis toxicity.
- lovastatin (Mevacor), simvastatin (Zocor) and other HMG CoA reductase inhibitors that use cytochrome P 450 3A4 for removal.
- neuromuscular blocking agents (such as pancuronium—Pavulon or vecuronium—Norcuron) may prolong muscle weakness.
- sirolimus (Rapamune).
- tacrolimus (Prograf).
- tretinoin (Vesanoid).
- tricyclic antidepressants (see Drug Classes).
- vincristine (Oncovin).

Verapamil ***taken concurrently*** with

- amiodarone (Cordarone) may result in cardiac arrest.
- aspirin (various) may result in excessive verapamil levels and excessive lowering of blood pressure.

- beta blockers (see Drug Classes) may affect heart rate and rhythm adversely. Careful monitoring by your physician is necessary if these drugs are taken concurrently.
- calcium supplements (various) may blunt the therapeutic benefits of verapamil—separate calcium and verapamil dosing by 2 hours.
- cilostazol (Pletal) may result in cilostazol toxicity. Lower cilostazol doses are prudent.
- colesevelam (Welchol) will decrease the therapeutic blood level of verapamil.
- cyclosporine (Sandimmune) may result in cyclosporine toxicity and renal compromise.
- dantrolene will cause elevated blood potassium and depression of the heart.
- dofetilide (Tikosyn) may result in dofetilide toxicity. Checks of dofetilide levels and dosing adjustments to levels are prudent.
- disopyramide (Norpace) can cause congestive heart failure.
- flecainide (Tambocor) may have additive heart effects (excessively low heart rate or cardiogenic shock).
- lithium (Lithobid, others) may result in lithium toxicity and mania.
- midazolam (Versed) may result in midazolam toxicity. Lower doses (by 50%) and careful patient monitoring are critical.
- NSAIDs (see Drug Classes) may blunt the therapeutic effect of verapamil on blood pressure.
- NSAIDs (see Drug Classes) may blunt the therapeutic effect of verapamil on blood pressure.
- oral hypoglycemic agents (see Oral Antidiabetic Drugs in Drug Classes) may lead to excessively low blood sugar.
- phenytoin (Dilantin) may result in decreased effectiveness of verapamil.
- prazosin (Minipres, others) may increase risk of orthostatic hypotension.
- quinidine (Quinaglute, others) can result in quinidine toxicity.
- rifampin (Rifadin, others) will decrease the therapeutic benefits of verapamil.
- sulfinpyrazone increases the removal of verapamil and lessens its therapeutic effects.
- terazosin (Hytrin) can lead to excessive decreases in blood pressure.
- theophylline (Theo-Dur, others) can lead to theophylline toxicity.
- warfarin (Coumadin) or other oral anticoagulants may increase risk of stomach or intestinal (GI) hemorrhage. More frequent INR tests are indicated.

The following drugs may *increase* the effects of verapamil:
- cimetidine (Tagamet) and other histamine (H_2) blocking drugs (see Drug Classes).
- clarithromycin (Biaxin).
- quinupristin/dalfopristin (Synercid).
- ritonavir (Norvir) and perhaps other protease inhibitors (see Drug Classes).
- tricyclic antidepressants (see Drug Classes).

▷ *Driving, Hazardous Activities:* Usually no restrictions. This drug may cause dizziness. Restrict activities as necessary.

Aviation Note: Coronary artery disease *is a disqualification* for piloting. Consult a designated Aviation Medical Examiner.

Exposure to Sun: Use caution until sensitivity has been determined. This drug may cause photosensitivity (see Glossary).

Exposure to Heat: Caution is advised. Hot environments can exaggerate the blood-pressure-lowering effects of this drug. Observe for light-headedness or weakness.

Heavy Exercise or Exertion: This drug may improve your ability to be more active without resulting angina pain. Use caution and avoid excessive exercise that could impair heart function in the absence of warning pain.

Discontinuation: Do not stop this drug abruptly. Consult your physician regarding gradual withdrawal to prevent the development of rebound angina.

WARFARIN (WAR far in)

Introduced: 1941   **Class:** Anticoagulant, coumarins   **Prescription:** USA: Yes   **Controlled Drug:** USA: No; Canada: No   **Available as Generic:** USA: Yes; Canada: Yes

Brand Names: Athrombin-K, Carfin, Coumadin, PanWarfarin, Sofarin, ♣ Warnerin

---

BENEFITS versus RISKS

Possible Benefits	*Possible Risks*
EFFECTIVE PREVENTION OF BOTH ARTERIAL AND VENOUS THROMBOSIS	NARROW TREATMENT RANGE Dose-related bleeding Skin and soft tissue hemorrhage with tissue death
EFFECTIVE PREVENTION OF EMBOLIZATION IN THROMBOEMBOLIC DISORDERS	
HELPS PREVENT RECURRENCE OF HEART ATTACK	
HELPS PREVENT STROKES IN PATIENTS WITH ATRIAL FIBRILLATION	
TREATS ACUTE CORONARY SYNDROME	
HELPS PREVENT BLOOD CLOTS AFTER MITRAL VALVE REPLACEMENT	
May have a role in helping to prevent cancer	

▷ **Principal Uses**

As a Single Drug Product: Uses currently included in FDA-approved labeling: Used in (1) acute thrombosis (clot) or thrombophlebitis of the deep veins; (2) acute pulmonary embolism, resulting from blood clots that originate anywhere in the body; (3) atrial fibrillation, to prevent clotting of blood inside the heart that could result in embolization of small clots to any part of the body; (4) acute myocardial infarction (heart attack), to prevent clotting and embolization and therefore a recurrence of heart attack; (5)

mitral valve replacement; (6) helping prevent blood clots in the lungs (pulmonary embolism) that may start after hip replacement surgery.

Other (unlabeled) generally accepted uses: (1) Helps prevent embolization from the heart in people with artificial heart valves; (2) may help patients with low blood platelets caused by heparin; (3) one case report of benefits in treatment-resistant migraines; (4) A study of 854 patients (after suffering a first blood clot) who were then treated with warfarin appeared to have a lower risk of newly diagnosed cancer. This possible chemoprotective effect must be further evaluated.

How This Drug Works: The coumarin anticoagulants interfere with the production of four essential blood-clotting factors by blocking the action of vitamin K. This leads to a deficiency of these clotting factors in circulating blood and inhibits blood-clotting mechanisms. Mechanism in possibly decreasing cancer risk is not known.

Available Dosage Forms and Strengths

Injection — 5 mg

Tablets — 1 mg, 2 mg, 2.5 mg, 3 mg, 4 mg, 5 mg, 6 mg, 7.5 mg, 10 mg

Tablets (Canada) — 25 mg

▷ **Usual Adult Dosage Ranges:** Initially an induction dose of 2 to 5 mg daily is used. A large loading dose is inappropriate and may be hazardous—hence an induction dose is used in the aforementioned range and then the ongoing dose is decided based on INR (prothrombin time or protime) results and the condition being treated. Defined ranges exist for treating or preventing problems with various diagnoses. The usual ongoing maintenance dose range is 2 to 10 mg daily, adjusted to maintain the prothrombin time (protime) to 1.2 to 2 times the control value which corresponds to an International Normalized Ratio (INR) of 2.0 to 3.0 for most indications (1.5 to 5.0 is a possible INR range). **Note: Actual dose and schedule must be determined for each patient individually.**

Conditions Requiring Dosing Adjustments

Liver Function: Blood testing (prothrombin times) should be obtained to guide dosing. This drug is contraindicated in patients with liver disease.

Kidney Function: This drug should be used with caution in renal compromise, as warfarin may cause microscopic kidney stones.

▷ **Dosing Instructions:** The tablet may be crushed and is preferably taken when the stomach is empty and at the same time each day to ensure uniform results. If you forget a dose: Take the missed dose as soon as you remember it. If you don't remember until the next day, skip the missed dose and take the next dose right on schedule. Let your doctor know you missed a dose. Be honest if you find yourself missing doses, there are timers and beeper-based systems that can be very helpful.

Usual Duration of Use: Use on a regular schedule for 3 to 5 days usually determines effectiveness in providing significant anticoagulation. An additional 10 to 14 days is required to determine the optimal maintenance dose for each person. INR ranges vary according to the condition warranting use of warfarin in the first place. The appropriate duration of therapy is controversial and should be discussed with your doctor according to the condition being treated. Ongoing use (months to years) requires physician supervision. Patient self-testing (INR) monitors are now available.

Typical Treatment Goals and Measurements (Outcomes and Markers)

Anticoagulation: The goal of anticoagulation is to prevent further extention of an existing clot or to prevent a clot in patients who are at risk for getting a blood clot. Additionally, a balance must be struck between thinning the blood enough to avoid an undesirable blood clot and thinning it so much that bleeding occurs. The INR (a ratio involving a prothrombin time test and standardization to make results "the same" lab to lab) is used to check to what degree the blood has been made less likely to clot by warfarin.

While you are taking this medicine you will have blood drawn on a regular basis to make sure that your blood is in the right range. Many patients refer to anticoagulation as being "thin" enough and to warfarin as a blood thinner. The key, however, is to make the blood less likely to form abnormal clots, yet have it retain enough of an ability to clot to keep you from bleeding. For example, the Antithrombotic Therapy in Acute Coronary Syndrome (ACTACS) study reported that when INR is adjusted to a range of between 2 and 3, the frequency of bleeding complications was about the same (not statistically different) for aspirin alone (162.5 mg) or aspirin plus warfarin in people with chest pain (ischemic pain) due to unstable angina or non-Q-wave heart attack (myocardial infarction).

▷ **This Drug Should Not Be Taken If**
- you have had an allergic reaction to it previously.
- you have an active peptic ulcer or active ulcerative colitis.
- you are pregnant, and are experiencing eclampsia or a threatened abortion.
- you have had recent anesthesia (lumbar block) to the spine.
- you've had a spinal tap (lumbar puncture).
- you have arterial aneurysm.
- you have malignant hypertension, low blood platelets.
- you have low blood platelets.
- you have infective pericarditis or endocarditis.
- you have liver disease.
- you have esophageal varices (ask your doctor).
- you have had a recent stroke.

▷ **Inform Your Physician Before Taking This Drug If**
- you are now taking any other drugs, either prescription drugs or over-the-counter drug products.
- you are planning pregnancy.
- you have a history of a bleeding disorder.
- you have congestive heart failure.
- you have high blood pressure.
- you have abnormally heavy or prolonged menstrual bleeding.
- you have diabetes.
- you are using an indwelling catheter.
- you have impaired liver or kidney function.
- you will have surgery or dental extraction.

Possible Side Effects (natural, expected and unavoidable drug actions)

Minor episodes of bleeding may occur even though dose and INR or prothrombin times are well within the recommended range.

▷ **Possible Adverse Effects** (unusual, unexpected and infrequent reactions)

If any of the following develop, consult your physician promptly for guidance.

Mild Adverse Effects

Allergic reactions: skin rash, hives.

Loss of scalp hair (alopecia)—case reports.

Loss of appetite, nausea, vomiting, cramping, diarrhea—case reports.

Serious Adverse Effects

Allergic reactions: drug fever (see Glossary).

Idiosyncratic reactions: bleeding into skin and soft tissues, causing gangrene of breast, toes and localized areas of necrosis anywhere—rare.

Hereditary warfarin resistance—rare.

Abnormal bleeding from nose, gastrointestinal tract (one case of esophageal ulcer), lungs, urinary tract, uterus or other sites—possible and dose-related.

Pericardial tamponade—case reports.

Hemolytic anemia—rare.

Sudden nerve damage (femoral neuropathy)—case reports.

Kidney problems (tubulointerstitial nephritis)—case reports.

Liver toxicity (viral hepatitis-like syndrome)—case report.

▷ **Possible Effects on Sexual Function:** None reported.

▷ **Adverse Effects That May Mimic Natural Diseases or Disorders**

Drug-induced fever may suggest infection.

Natural Diseases or Disorders That May Be Activated by This Drug

Bleeding from "silent" peptic ulcer, intestinal or bladder polyp or tumor.

Possible Effects on Laboratory Tests

Complete blood cell counts: decreased red cells, hemoglobin and white cells.

Bleeding time: increased.

INR (prothrombin time): increased (desirable when in therapeutic range).

Blood uric acid level: increased (in men).

Liver function tests: increased liver enzymes (ALT/GPT, AST/GOT and alkaline phosphatase).

CAUTION

1. Always carry a personal identification card that includes a statement that *you are taking an anticoagulant drug. A medicine alert bracelet is also prudent.*
2. While taking this drug, always consult your physician *before* starting any new drug, changing the dose schedule of any drug or stopping any drug.
3. Data from the Agency for Health Care Policy and Research have shown that expanded use of warfarin could cut in half the 80,000 strokes that occur every year in patients who have atrial fibrillation.
4. **If** you start taking the brand, it is prudent to keep taking the brand. Conversely, if you have your anticoagulation adjusted using the generic form, it is prudent to continue the generic. Changing from one form to the other may result in differences in degree of anticoagulation.
5. **If** you choose to use acetaminophen while taking this medicine, talk to your doctor about adjusting the warfarin and INR testing.
6. Hereditary or acquired warfarin resistance is possible.
7. Some herbal medicines can lead to additive bleeding problems. Avoid garlic, ginkgo, ginseng and echinacea (amongst others—see below) prior to any surgery and while you are taking this medicine.
8. Checks of INR are MANDATORY while you are taking this medicine.

Home monitors can be extremely helpful by increasing access to INR tests. They are available from CoaguCheck (1-800-852-8766) and Pro-Time (1-800-631-5945).

Precautions for Use

By Those Over 60 Years of Age: Small starting doses are mandatory. Watch regularly for excessive drug effects: prolonged bleeding from shaving cuts, bleeding gums, bloody urine, rectal bleeding, excessive bruising. Some study data reveal that the beneficial effects of this medicine are not as widely known as needed and it is underprescribed for those over 60.

▷ **Advisability of Use During Pregnancy**

Pregnancy Category: X. See Pregnancy Risk Categories at the back of this book.
Animal studies: Fetal hemorrhage and death due to this drug have been reported in mice.
Human studies: Information from studies of pregnant women indicates fetal defects and fetal hemorrhage due to this drug. The manufacturers state that this drug is contraindicated during entire pregnancy.

Advisability of Use If Breast-Feeding

Presence of this drug in breast milk: Yes, but in inactive forms.
Breast-feeding appears to be safe. Checking the infant for warfarin effects is prudent.

Habit-Forming Potential: None.

Effects of Overdose: Episodes of bleeding, from minor surface bleeding (nose, gums, small lacerations) to major internal bleeding (vomiting blood, bloody urine or stool).

Possible Effects of Long-Term Use: None reported.

Suggested Periodic Examinations While Taking This Drug (at physician's discretion)

Regular determinations of INR (prothrombin time or protime) are essential to safe dose and proper control.
Urine analysis for blood.

▷ **While Taking This Drug, Observe the Following**

Foods: A larger intake than usual of foods rich in vitamin K may reduce the effectiveness of this drug and make larger doses necessary. Foods rich in vitamin K include asparagus, bacon, beef liver, cabbage, fish, cauliflower and green leafy vegetables. Vitamin C in high doses has some conflicting reports of warfarin resistance. Vitamin E (high dose) may increase risk of bleeding.
Herbal Medicines or Minerals: Because many herbal products are extracts from plants with a variety of active compounds in addition to those listed on the label—and since many compounds can have activity as anticoagulants—herbal medicines in general SHOULD NOT be combined with warfarin.
Specifically, angelica root, anise, borage seed oil, devil's claw, papain, garlic, ginseng, ginger, ginkgo, horse chestnut, alfalfa, red clover, clove oil, feverfew, passionflower herb, salvia root (danshen), willow bark, cinchona bark, turmeric and garlic may also change clotting, so combining those herbals with these medicines cannot be recommended. Dong quai appears to have a true pharmacodynamic interaction with warfarin (potentiation), and since it is as yet uncharacterized, these medicines should not be com-

bined. Boldo-Fenugreek caused more than a 50% increase in INR in one case report. Co-enzyme Q10 (ubiquinone) and green tea may decrease warfarin benefits. TALK TO YOUR DOCTOR BEFORE taking any herbal medicine with warfarin—but again—-this combination is not advisable.

Beverages: No restrictions. May be taken with milk.

▷ *Alcohol:* Limit alcohol to one drink daily. Note: Heavy users of alcohol with liver damage may be very sensitive to anticoagulants and require smaller than usual doses.

Tobacco Smoking: Heavy smokers may require relatively larger doses of this drug. I advise everyone to quit smoking.

▷ *Other Drugs*

Warfarin may ***increase*** the effects of
- oral hypoglycemic agents (see Oral Antidiabetic Drugs in Drug Classes).
- phenytoin (Dilantin) or fosphenytoin (Cerebyx).

Warfarin may ***decrease*** the effects of
- cyclosporine (Sandimmune, others).
- phenytoin (Dilantin) or fosphenytoin (Cerebyx).

The following drugs may ***increase*** the effects of warfarin:
- abciximab (Reopro).
- acarbose (Precose).
- acetaminophen (Tylenol, others—especially if more than 2,275 mg per week is taken).
- allopurinol (Zyloprim).
- alteplase (Activase) and is contraindicated if the prothrombin time is more than 15 seconds.
- amiodarone (Cordarone).
- amprenavir (Agenerase).
- androgens (see Drug Classes).
- argatroban (Acova).
- aspirin and some other NSAIDs (see Drug Classes).
- azithromycin (Zithromax).
- bismuth subsalicylate (Pepto-Bismol).
- some calcium channel blockers (various) have been associated with an increased risk of stomach and intestine (gastrointestinal) hemorrhage. This risk may be exacerbated by warfarin use.
- carbamazepine (Tegretol).
- cephalosporins (see Drug Classes).
- chloral hydrate (Noctec).
- chloramphenicol (Chloromycetin).
- cimetidine (Tagamet).
- ciprofloxacin and other quinolone antibiotics (see Drug Classes).
- cisapride (Propulsid).
- clarithromycin (Biaxin).
- clofibrate (Atromid-S).
- clopidogrel (Plavix).
- cloxacillin (various).
- cotrimoxazole (Bactrim).
- COX II inhibitors (celecoxib and rofecoxib).
- dextrothyroxine.
- dirithromycin and other macrolide antibiotics (see Drug Classes).

- disopyramide (Norpace).
- disulfiram (Antabuse).
- enoxaparin (Lovenox) and other low molecular weight heparins (see Drug Classes).
- eptifibatide (Integrelin).
- erythromycin (various).
- felbamate (Felbatol).
- fluconazole (Diflucan).
- fluoxetine (Prozac).
- fluvastatin (Lescol) and perhaps similar drugs.
- fluvoxamine (Luvox).
- fosphenytoin (Cerebyx) or phenytoin (Dilantin).
- gemfibrozil (Lopid).
- glucagon.
- heparin (various).
- HMG CoA-reductase inhibitors (see Drug Profiles).
- influenza vaccine (various).
- isoniazid (INH).
- itraconazole (Sporanox).
- ketoconazole (Nizoral).
- mesna (Mesnex).
- methyltestosterone (any 17-alkylated androgen).
- metronidazole (Flagyl).
- miconazole (Monistat).
- minocycline.
- nonsteroidal anti-inflammatory drugs (see Drug Classes).
- omeprazole (Prilosec).
- orlistat (Xenical).
- paroxetine (Paxil).
- pravastatin (Pravachol).
- propafenone (Rythmol).
- propranolol (Inderal).
- propoxyphene (various).
- quinidine (Quinaglute).
- quetiapine (Seroquel).
- raloxifene (Evista)—more frequent INR checks are prudent.
- ranitidine (Zantac).
- ritonavir (Norvir) and perhaps other protease inhibitors (see Drug Classes).
- salicylates (aspirin, etc.).
- sertraline (Zoloft).
- simvastatin (Zocor).
- streptokinase.
- sulfinpyrazone (Anturane).
- sulfonamides (see Drug Classes).
- tamoxifen (Nolvadex).
- tamsulosin (Flomax).
- terbinafine (Lamisil).
- testosterone (various).
- tetracyclines (see Drug Classes).

- thyroid hormones (various).
- thrombolytic drugs (such as alteplase).
- tramadol (Ultram).
- trastuzumab (Herceptin).
- tricyclic antidepressants (see Drug Classes).
- vancomycin (Vancoled).
- vitamin E (higher doses).
- zafirlukast (Accolate).
- zileuton (Zyflo).
- zotepine (Nipolept).

The following drugs may *decrease* the effects of warfarin:

- antithyroid agents (various) by decreasing prior high rates of clotting factor metabolism.
- azathioprine (Imuran).
- barbiturates (see Drug Classes).
- birth control pills (oral contraceptives).
- carbamazepine (Tegretol).
- chlordiazepoxide (Librium).
- cholestyramine (Questran).
- estrogens (various).
- ethchlorvynol (Placidyl).
- glutethimide (Doriden).
- griseofulvin (Gris-PEG).
- phenobarbital (various).
- phytonadione (vitamin K).
- primidone (Mysoline).
- rifampin (Rifadin).
- spironolactone.
- sucralfate (Carafate).
- telmisartan (Micardis)—slight decrease.
- thiazide diuretics (see Drug Classes).
- vitamin K.

▷ *Driving, Hazardous Activities:* No restrictions.

Aviation Note: The use of this drug *is a disqualification* for piloting. Consult a designated Aviation Medical Examiner.

Exposure to Sun: No restrictions.

Discontinuation: Do not stop this drug abruptly unless abnormal bleeding occurs. Ask your physician for guidance regarding gradual reduction in dose over a period of 3 to 4 weeks.

ZALCITABINE (zal SIT a been)

Other Names: Dideoxycytidine, DDC

Introduced: 1987   **Class:** Antiviral, anti-AIDS   **Prescription:** USA: Yes
Controlled Drug: USA: No; Canada: No   **Available as Generic:** USA: No
Brand Name: Hivid

BENEFITS versus RISKS

Possible Benefits	*Possible Risks*
DELAYED PROGRESSION OF DISEASE IN HIV-INFECTED PATIENTS	DRUG-INDUCED PERIPHERAL NEURITIS
PART OF REASONABLY EFFECTIVE COMBINATION REGIMENS	DRUG-INDUCED PANCREATITIS
	LACTIC ACIDOSIS
	HEPATOMEGALY
	LIVER FAILURE
	Drug-induced esophageal ulcers or arthritis
	Drug-induced cardiomyopathy/ congestive heart failure

▷ **Principal Uses**

As a Single Drug Product: Uses currently included in FDA-approved labeling: (1) This drug is approved for use as part of combination therapy of HIV infection.

Author's Note: Adherence or taking medicines for HIV exactly on time and in the right amount is ABSOLUTELY critical to getting the best possible results or outcomes. The new antiretroviral therapy guidelines (from NIAID) take into account how easily the medicine treating HIV can fit into a patient's life.

Other (unlabeled) generally accepted uses: None.

How This Drug Works: Combines with phosphorous in cells (is phosphorylated) to zalcitabine triphosphate. This active triphosphate form interferes with essential HIV enzyme systems, and prevents the growth and reproduction of HIV particles within infected cells, thus limiting the severity and extent of HIV infection.

Available Dosage Forms and Strengths

Tablets — 0.375 mg, 0.75 mg

▷ **Recommended Dosage Ranges** (Actual dose and schedule must be determined for each patient individually.)

Infants and Children: Under investigation.

12 to 60 Years of Age: In combination therapy: one 0.75-mg tablet orally every 8 hours in combination with other antiretroviral medicines. The initial dose does not need to be reduced unless the patient has a body mass of less than 30 kg (66 lb).

Conditions Requiring Dosing Adjustments

Liver Function: Liver toxicity more likely in people with a prior history of alcohol abuse or liver damage. Patients should be watched closely and dose reduced or drug interrupted if toxicity occurs. Those with liver function enzymes more than five times the upper limit of the normal range should stop the drug.

Kidney Function: Patients with moderate kidney failure can take 0.75 mg of zalcitabine every 12 hours. In severe kidney failure, the patient can take 0.75 mg every 24 hours.

▷ **Dosing Instructions:** When combination therapy is being given, dose adjustments must be based on the toxicity profiles for each drug. For example, if peripheral neuropathy or severe oral ulcers occur, the zalcitabine dose should be decreased to 0.375 mg every 8 hours. If the patient experiences anemia or granulocytopenia, and zidovudine is being used, dose should be decreased or interrupted. If the zalcitabine is interrupted or stopped, the zidovudine dose should be changed from 200 mg every 8 hours to 100 mg every 4 hours. If zalcitabine is stopped, salvage therapy or appropriate sequencing strategies must be used.

The largest peak concentration, the time that it takes for the peak to be achieved and the amount absorbed are all changed if this drug is taken with food. It is better to take this medication on an empty stomach. If you forget a dose: Take the missed dose as soon as you remember it, unless it's nearly time for your next dose—if that is the case, skip the missed dose and take the next dose right on schedule. DO NOT double up on doses. Talk with your doctor if you find yourself missing doses. IT IS ABSOLUTELY CRITICAL to take HIV medicines exactly as prescribed. There are beeper-based systems that can be of great help.

Usual Duration of Use: Use on a regular schedule for several months usually determines effectiveness in slowing the progression of AIDS (VIRAL BURDEN NADIR). Long-term use (months to years) requires periodic physician evaluation of response (viral load and CD4) and dose adjustment. It is not unusual for medicines to be changed over the course of treatment

Typical Treatment Goals and Measurements (Outcomes and Markers)

HIV: Goals for HIV treatment presently are maximum suppression of viral replication, maximum lowering of the amount of virus in your body (viral load or burden), and maximum patient survival. The loftier goal of eradication of HIV from the body does not appear possible given the medicines presently available. Markers of successful therapy include undetectable viral load, increased CD4 cells, absence of indicator or opportunistic infections (OIs) and in the case of the HIV-positive patient, failure of the infection to progress to AIDS.

Possible Advantages of This Drug

Does not cause serious depression of bone marrow function (production of blood cells).

▷ **This Drug Should Not Be Taken If**
- you have had an allergic reaction to it previously.
- you have had pancreatitis recently.
- you have severe myelosuppression (ask your doctor).

▷ **Inform Your Physician Before Taking This Drug If**
- you have had allergic reactions to any drugs in the past.
- you are taking any other drugs currently.
- you have a history of pancreatitis or peripheral neuritis.
- you have a history of severe myelosuppression (ask your doctor).
- you have a history of esophageal ulcers.
- you have congestive heart failure or cardiac muscle damage (cardiac myopathy).
- you have a history of or existing signs or symptoms of peripheral nerve damage.
- you have a history of alcoholism.
- you have impaired liver or kidney function.

Possible Side Effects (natural, expected and unavoidable drug actions)

Mild and infrequent decreases in red blood cell, white blood cell and platelet counts.

▷ **Possible Adverse Effects** (unusual, unexpected and infrequent reactions)

If any of the following develop, consult your physician promptly for guidance.

Mild Adverse Effects

Allergic reactions: skin rash and itching.

Fever, joint pains—infrequent.

Ringing in the ears—case reports.

Mouth sores, nausea, vomiting, diarrhea, stomach pain—infrequent.

Serious Adverse Effects

Allergic reactions: anaphylaxis—rare.

Drug-induced peripheral neuritis (see Glossary), usually occurring after 7 to 18 weeks of treatment. This is more frequent and severe with high doses and less frequent and mild with low doses.

Drug-induced cardiomyopathy/congestive heart failure—infrequent.

Drug-induced pancreatitis (may happen in the first 6 months of treatment)—rare.

Electrolyte changes (lowered phosphorous, sodium, magnesium or calcium)—rare to infrequent.

Ototoxicity and hearing loss—rare.

Lowered white blood cell counts—infrequent.

Worsening of preexisting liver disease or hepatotoxicity—rare.

▷ **Possible Effects on Sexual Function:** None reported.

▷ **Adverse Effects That May Mimic Natural Diseases or Disorders**

Increased liver enzymes may resemble infectious hepatitis.

Possible Effects on Laboratory Tests

Complete blood cell counts: decreased red cells, white cells and platelets (infrequent and mild).

Blood amylase level: increased (infrequent).

Blood glucose level: increased.

Liver function tests: increased (SGOT, SGPT and LDH).

CD4: increased.

Viral burden: decreased.

CAUTION

1. This drug does not cure HIV infection.
2. This drug should not be taken with lamivudine because both medicines are cytidine analogs and need to use the same enzymes to become active (phosphorylated) in the cells of the body.
3. Call your doctor right away if stomach pain with nausea and vomiting occurs; this could indicate the onset of pancreatitis. It may be necessary to discontinue this drug.
4. Combination treatment is now a standard of care.
5. Pain, numbness, tingling or burning in the hands or feet should prompt a call to your doctor; this could indicate the onset of peripheral neuritis. Drug may need to be stopped.
6. Best to avoid all other drugs known to cause pancreatitis or peripheral neuritis; ask your physician for guidance.

Precautions for Use

By Infants and Children: Safety and effectiveness for use by this age group have not been established. Children may also be at risk for developing drug-induced pancreatitis and peripheral neuritis; monitor closely for significant symptoms.

By Those Over 60 Years of Age: Reduced kidney function may require dose reduction.

▷ **Advisability of Use During Pregnancy**

Pregnancy Category: C. See Pregnancy Risk Categories at the back of this book.

Animal studies: This drug has been shown to be teratogenic in mice at doses of 1,365 and 2,730 times of the maximum recommended human dose (MRHD). Increased embryolethality was observed in mice with doses of 2,730 times the MRHD.

Human studies: Information from adequate studies of pregnant women is not available.

The manufacturer recommends that fertile women should not receive zalcitabine unless they are using effective contraception during therapy. Consult your physician for specific guidance.

Advisability of Use If Breast-Feeding

Presence of this drug in breast milk: Unknown.

Avoid drug or refrain from nursing.

Note: HIV has been found in human breast milk. Breast-feeding may result in transmission of HIV infection to the nursing infant.

Habit-Forming Potential: None.

Effects of Overdose: Drowsiness, nausea, vomiting, stomach pain, diarrhea, liver toxicity, hand and foot pain (neuropathy).

Possible Effects of Long-Term Use: Peripheral neuritis (see Glossary).

Suggested Periodic Examinations While Taking This Drug (at physician's discretion)

Complete blood cell counts before starting treatment and weekly thereafter until tolerance is established.

Neurologic exam/peripheral neuritis check.

Blood amylase levels, fractionated for salivary gland and pancreatic origin.

Triglyceride levels should be tested at baseline (before therapy is started) and periodically during therapy.

Assessment of CD4 counts and viral load. These tell of pending failure and reason to change to other agents.

▷ **While Taking This Drug, Observe the Following**

Foods: Best taken on an empty stomach.

Herbal Medicines or Minerals: Some patients use echinacea to attempt to boost their immune systems. Unfortunately, use of echinacea is not recommended in people with damaged immune systems. This herb may also actually weaken any immune system if it is used too often or for too long a time.

Beverages: No restrictions.

▷ *Alcohol:* No interactions expected.

Tobacco Smoking: No interactions expected. I advise everyone to quit smoking.

▷ *Other Drugs*

Zalcitabine may ***increase*** the effects of

• zidovudine (Retrovir) and enhance its antiviral effect against HIV—serious patient reactions to either of these medicines should be reported to the FDA.

Zalcitabine *taken concurrently* with

- antacids (various) may blunt zalcitabine effectiveness.
- cimetidine (Tagamet) may result in toxic zalcitabine levels.
- didanosine (Videx) may result in additive neurotoxicity.
- metoclopramide (Reglan) may result in lowered blood levels of zalcitabine and reduced therapeutic benefits.
- other drugs that cause neurotoxicity or pancreatitis may lead to addictive toxicity—these combinations are best avoided.
- pentamidine (Nebupent) may lead to increased risk of pancreatitis.
- probenecid (Benemid) may lead to zalcitabine toxicity.

▷ *Driving, Hazardous Activities:* This drug may cause pain and weakness in the extremities. Restrict activities as necessary.

Aviation Note: The use of this drug *is a disqualification* for piloting. Consult a designated Aviation Medical Examiner.

Exposure to Sun: No restrictions.

Discontinuation: Do not stop this drug without your physician's knowledge and guidance.

ZALEPLON (ZAH la plon)

Introduced: 1999   **Class:** Hypnotic, nonbenzodiazepine   **Prescription:** USA: Yes   **Controlled Drug:** USA: C-IV*; Canada: Prescription   **Available as Generic:** USA: No

Brand Name: Sonata, ❧Starnoc

BENEFITS versus RISKS

Possible Benefits	*Possible Risks*
GIVES SHORT-TERM RELIEF OF INSOMNIA WITH MINIMAL SLEEP DISRUPTION (REM)	Habit-forming potential with prolonged use
REDUCES SLEEP LATENCY	
MAY BE TAKEN AT BEDTIME OR LATER (AS LONG AS FOUR HOURS OF TIME IN BED ARE LEFT)	
SHORT HALF-LIFE (AVOIDS HANGOVER EFFECT)	

▷ **Principal Uses**

As a Single Drug Product: Uses currently included in FDA-approved labeling: Treatment of insomnia in adults for up to 5 weeks (new and longer period of approved use).

Other (unlabeled) generally accepted uses: None at present.

How This Drug Works: This drug attaches (binds) to a specific receptor (GABA-BZ subunit modulation) and reduces the time it takes to fall asleep.

*See Schedules of Controlled Drugs at the back of this book.

Available Dosage Forms and Strengths

Tablets — 5 mg, 10 mg

▷ **Recommended Dosage Ranges** (Actual dose and schedule must be determined for each patient individually.)

Infants and Children: Safety and efficacy for those under 18 years of age are not established.

18 to 60 Years of Age: 10 mg is taken immediately before bedtime. Patients should be reevaluated after taking this drug for 7–10 days. Maximum length of use was 28 days in clinical studies. Patients of low body weight should be given 5 mg as a starting dose. Dose may be increased slowly to a maximum of 20 mg as needed and tolerated.

Over 60 Years of Age: Therapy should be started with 5 mg taken at bedtime. The dose may be cautiously increased to 10 mg at bedtime.

Conditions Requiring Dosing Adjustments

Liver Function: The dose should be reduced by 50% in mild to moderate liver compromise.

Kidney Function: No changes thought to be needed in mild compromise. This medicine HAS NOT been studied in severe kidney insufficiency.

▷ **Dosing Instructions:** The tablet may be crushed. Best taken on an empty stomach (taking it with a high-fat meal delays absorption). Do not stop this drug abruptly if taken more than 7 days. If you forget a dose: Take the missed dose as soon as you remember it, as long as you will be in bed for another four hours.

Usual Duration of Use: Use on a regular schedule for 2 nights usually determines effectiveness in treating insomnia. Your physician should assess the benefit of this drug after 7 to 10 days. New recommended maximum length of use is 5 weeks.

Typical Treatment Goals and Measurements (Outcomes and Markers)

Insomnia: The general goal is to decrease the amount of time it takes between the time you go to bed and the time you fall asleep (shortened sleep latency). Additionally, the number of times that you wake up is expected to decrease, enabling a full night of sleep. How alert you feel in the morning is also a consideration. Many other hypnotics with longer half-lives also have significant effects the next morning ("hangover" effects).

Possible Advantages of This Drug

Low occurrence of adverse effects. Short half-life. No difference between a dummy pill (placebo) and this medicine was seen when patients were checked for next-day sleepiness. Now approved for up to 5 weeks of insomnia treatment.

▷ **This Drug Should Not Be Taken If**

• you had an allergic reaction to it previously.
• you have severe liver compromise.

▷ **Inform Your Physician Before Taking This Drug If**

• you have abnormal liver or kidney function.
• you are pregnant or planning pregnancy or are breast-feeding your infant.
• you have a history of alcoholism or drug abuse.
• you have a serious lung problem (respiratory impairment).
• you have a history of serious depression or mental disorder.

- you are elderly or are debilitated.
- you are unsure how much to take or how often to take this medicine.

Possible Side Effects (natural, expected and unavoidable drug actions)
   Sleepiness.

▷ **Possible Adverse Effects** (unusual, unexpected and infrequent reactions)
   If any of the following develop, consult your physician promptly for guidance.
   Mild Adverse Effects
   Allergic reactions: Itching and rash.
   Drowsiness and dizziness—possible and dose related.
   Psychomotor impairment—possible and dose related.
   Blurred vision—dose related—rare.
   Rebound insomnia—possible, dose-dependent and appears to resolve by the second night.
   Lowered white blood cell counts—rare and transitory and of questionable causation.
   Nausea, anorexia or indigestion—infrequent.
   Muscle aches (myalgia)—infrequent.
   Increased liver enzymes—rare and transient and of questionable causality.
   Serious Adverse Effects
   Allergic reactions: not defined.
   Abnormal thoughts or hallucinations—very rare.

▷ **Possible Effects on Sexual Function:** Dysmenorrhea—very rare.

Possible Effects on Laboratory Tests
   Liver function tests: possibly increased SGOT, SGPT and CPK.

CAUTION
   1. This drug works quickly. It is best to take it just before bedtime.
   2. Do not drink alcohol while taking this drug.
   3. Withdrawal (see Glossary) may occur, even if this drug was only taken for a week or two. Ask your doctor for advice before stopping zaleplon.
   4. You may experience trouble going to sleep for 1 or 2 nights after stopping this drug (rebound insomnia). This effect is usually short-term.
   5. Sleep disturbances may be a symptom of underlying psychological problems. Tell your doctor if unusual behaviors or odd thoughts occur.
   6. Drugs that depress the central nervous system may produce additive effects with this drug. Ask your doctor or pharmacist before combining other prescription or nonprescription drugs with zaleplon.

Precautions for Use
   By Infants and Children: Safety and effectiveness for those under 18 years of age are not established.
   By Those Over 60 Years of Age: The starting dose should be decreased to 5 mg. Since this drug works quickly, it is best taken immediately before going to bed. You may be at increased risk for falls if the drug remains in your system in the morning. Watch for lethargy, unsteadiness, nightmares and paradoxical agitation and anger.

▷ **Advisability of Use During Pregnancy**
   Pregnancy Category: C. See Pregnancy Risk Categories at the back of this book.
   Animal studies: In rats, there was increased stillbirth and postnatal death as well as slower growth and development in offspring of females treated

with 7 mg per kg per day during the later part of pregnancy and throughout lactation.

Human studies: Adequate studies of pregnant women are not available.
Use during pregnancy is not recommended.

Advisability of Use If Breast-Feeding
Presence of this drug in breast milk: Yes, in small amounts.
Avoid drug or refrain from nursing.

Habit-Forming Potential: This drug may cause dependence (see Glossary).

Effects of Overdose: One case of 100 mg taken in combination with a benzodiazepine reported that the patient recovered without ill effects. Supportive
and symptomatic care is recommended.

Possible Effects of Long-Term Use: Psychological and/or physical dependence.

Suggested Periodic Examinations While Taking This Drug (at physician's discretion)
Liver function tests.

▷ **While Taking This Drug, Observe the Following**
Foods: This drug is best taken on an empty stomach because food delays
absorption.

Herbal Medicines or Minerals: Kava kava and valerian may exacerbate central
nervous system depression (avoid this combination). Kola nut, Siberian
ginseng, mate, ephedra and ma huang may blunt the benefits of this medicine. While St. John's wort is indicated for anxiety, it is also thought to
increase (induce) cytochrome P450 enzymes and could tend to blunt zaleplon effectiveness.

Beverages: Avoid caffeine-containing beverages: coffee, tea, cola, chocolate.

▷ *Alcohol:* This drug should not be combined with alcohol.

Tobacco Smoking: Nicotine is a stimulant and should be avoided. I advise
everyone to quit smoking.

Marijuana Smoking: May cause additive drowsiness.

▷ *Other Drugs*
Zaleplon *taken concurrently* with
- cimetidine (Tagamet, others) may increase zaleplon effects (inhibits aldehyde oxidase and CYP 3A4—both methods that the body uses to eliminate
this drug). A starting dose of 5 mg and careful patient follow up are needed
if these medicines are combined.
- medicines that inhibit both aldehyde oxidase (primary removal mechanism) and CYP 3A4 will inhibit removal of zaleplon and may lead to zaleplon toxicity.
- medicines that induce both aldehyde oxidase (primary removal mechanism)
and CYP 3A4 will blunt benefits of zaleplon by decreasing blood levels.
- rifampin (Rifater, others) may decrease zaleplon benefits.
- ritonavir (Norvir) and perhaps other protease inhibitors (see Drug Classes)
may lead to toxicity.

Zaleplon may *increase* the effects of
- chlorpromazine (Thorazine).
- narcotics or other CNS-depressant drugs (see Drug Classes for Opioids,
Phenothiazines, Antihistamines and Benzodiazepines).

▷ *Driving, Hazardous Activities:* This drug may cause drowsiness and impair
coordination. Restrict activities as necessary.

Aviation Note: The use of this drug ***is a disqualification*** for piloting. Consult a designated Aviation Medical Examiner.

Discontinuation: This drug should not be stopped abruptly, even after a week of use. Ask your doctor for help regarding an appropriate withdrawal schedule.

ZIDOVUDINE (zi DOH vyoo deen)

Other Names: AZT, azidothymidine, compound S, ZDV

Introduced: 1987   **Class:** Antiviral, anti-HIV   **Prescription:** USA: Yes
Controlled Drug: USA: No; Canada: No   **Available as Generic:** USA: No; Canada: No

Brand Name: Retrovir, Combivir [CD], Trizivir [CD]

BENEFITS versus RISKS	
Possible Benefits	*Possible Risks*
DELAYED PROGRESSION OF DISEASE IN HIV-INFECTED PATIENTS WHEN COMBINATION TREATMENT IS USED	SERIOUS BONE MARROW DEPRESSION
REDUCED INCIDENCE OF INFECTIONS (OPPORTUNISTIC) WITH COMBINATION THERAPY	Brain toxicity
COMBIVIR and TRIZIVIR FORMS ENCOURAGES COMPLIANCE BY COMBINING 3 MEDICINES IN ONE PILL	Lip, mouth and tongue sores
REDUCED POSSIBILITY OF TRANSMISSION OF HIV FROM MOTHER TO FETUS (Zidovudine)	

▷ **Principal Uses**

As a Single Drug Product: Uses currently included in FDA-approved labeling: (1) Used to treat selected patients who have acquired immunodeficiency syndrome (AIDS)—this drug is not a cure for HIV; (2) approved to help prevent transmission of HIV from mother to infant; (3) approved for combination therapy with other agents; (4) approved for children 3 months or older who have laboratory values that indicate HIV infection or HIV immunosuppression; (5) approved for use in HIV-positive patients who are as yet asymptomatic.

Author's Note: Adherence or taking medicines for HIV exactly on time and in the right amount is ABSOLUTELY critical to getting the best possible results or outcomes. The new antiretroviral therapy guidelines (from NIAID) take into account how easily the medicine treating HIV can fit into a patient's life. One researcher has questioned whether zidovudine may have the decreasing benefits of other HIV medicines. Further research is needed.

Other (unlabeled) generally accepted uses: (1) Used to treat Kaposi's sarcoma; (2) helps remove hairy leukoplakia in the mouth; (3) used to treat heart dysfunction in people with HIV; (4) may prevent HIV in health care workers exposed to the AIDS virus (combined with other HIV medicines); (5) appears to increase AIDS-related low platelet counts; (6) may have a role treating adult T-cell leukemia or lymphoma with interferon alpha.

As a Combination Drug Product [CD]: This drug is available in combination (Combivir—lamivudine and zidovudine; Trizivir—abacavir, lamivudine and zidovudine). The combinations offer two different and three different medicines in the same pills.

How This Drug Works: By interfering with essential enzyme systems, this drug is thought to prevent the growth and reproduction of HIV particles within tissue cells, thus limiting the severity and extent of HIV infection.

Available Dosage Forms and Strengths

> Capsules — 100 mg
> Injection — 10 mg/ml
> Syrup — 50 mg/5 ml
> Tablet (Combivir) — lamivudine 150 mg
> — zidovudine 300 mg
> Tablet (Trizivir) — abacavir 300 mg
> — lamivudine 150 mg
> — zidovudine 300 mg

▷ **Usual Adult Dosage Ranges:** *HIV infection:* The product information insert for zidovudine recommends 600 mg daily, divided into equal doses in combination with other antiretroviral agents. Further, 500 mg as 100 mg every 4 hours while awake or 600 mg daily divided into equal doses is suggested. Combivir form—one tablet twice daily. Trizivir form—one tablet twice daily in people weighing more than 40 kg.

Prevention of maternal–fetal transmission in pregnancy: Once the mother has passed 14 weeks of pregnancy—100 mg by mouth five times per day until the start of labor. During labor, AZT is given intravenously (2 mg per kg of body mass), followed by 1 mg per kg of body mass per hour. This dose is continued until the umbilical cord is clamped. The infant then receives 1.5 mg per kg of body mass every 6 hours. The CDC recommends combination therapy for pregnant women.

Note: Actual dose and administration schedule must be determined for each patient individually.

Conditions Requiring Dosing Adjustments

Liver Function: Dose decreased by 50% or the dosing interval doubled in significant liver disease. Drug can be a rare cause of liver damage, and patients should be followed closely.

Kidney Function: Specific guidelines for dose adjustments in patients with compromised kidneys are not available. This drug should be used with caution in kidney compromise.

Granulocytopenia: If counts of this type of white blood cell are less than 750/ml cubed or if there is a decrease in number of this kind of cell of more than 50% of what a patient starts with, this medicine may need to be stopped until the bone marrow recovers.

Anemia: If the hemoglobin drops more than 25% from the starting point or is less than 7.5 g per deciliter, zidovudine may have to be stopped. Occurrence increases with higher doses and/or lower CD4 counts. Erythropoietin may help reduce the need for blood transfusions.

▷ **Dosing Instructions:** Preferably taken on an empty stomach, but may be taken with or following food. Take exactly as prescribed. Zidovudine capsule may be opened and the contents mixed with food just prior to taking it. Best to take the capsule with at least 120 ml of water, and patients should then NOT lie down for an hour. If you forget a dose: Take the missed dose as soon as you remember it, unless it's nearly time for your next dose—if that is the case, skip the missed dose and take the next dose right on schedule. DO NOT double dose. Talk with your doctor if you find yourself missing doses. IT IS ABSOLUTELY CRITICAL to take HIV medicines exactly as prescribed. There are beeper-based systems that can be a great help in complicated medication schedules.

Usual Duration of Use: Use on a regular schedule for 10 to 12 weeks usually determines effectiveness in improving the course of symptomatic AIDS infection. Long-term use requires periodic physician evaluation of response (viral load and CD4) and dose adjustment. It is not uncommon for antiretrovirals to be changed during HIV treatment.

Typical Treatment Goals and Measurements (Outcomes and Markers)

HIV: Goals for HIV treatment presently are maximum suppression of viral replication, maximum lowering of the amount of virus in your body (viral load or burden), and maximum patient survival. The loftier goal of eradication of HIV from the body does not appear possible given the medicines presently available. Markers of successful therapy include undetectable viral load, increased CD4 cells, absence of indicator or opportunistic infections (OIs) and in the case of the HIV-positive patient, failure of the infection to progress to AIDS.

▷ **This Drug (These Drugs) Should Not Be Taken If**
- you have had a serious allergic reaction to it previously.
- you have a serious degree of uncorrected bone marrow depression.

▷ **Inform Your Physician Before Taking This Drug (These Drugs) If**
- you have a history of either folic acid or vitamin B_{12} deficiency.
- you have impaired liver or kidney function.
- you take other drugs that can have a bad effect on the bone marrow (are myelosuppressive).

Possible Side Effects (natural, expected and unavoidable drug actions)
None reported.

▷ **Possible Adverse Effects** (unusual, unexpected and infrequent reactions)
If any of the following develop, consult your physician promptly for guidance.

Mild Adverse Effects
Allergic reactions: skin rash, hives, itching.
Headache, weakness, drowsiness, dizziness, nervousness, insomnia—infrequent.
Nausea, diarrhea, vomiting, altered taste, lip sores, swollen mouth or tongue—infrequent (incidence higher with combination forms).
Paresthesias, muscle aches, fever, sweating—infrequent.

Serious Adverse Effects
Allergic reactions: one case report of toxic epidermolysis for zidovudine. **A severe and life-threatening hypersensitivity reaction (3–5%) has been reported with abacavir.**

Confusion, loss of speech, twitching, tremors, seizures (representing brain toxicity)—infrequent.

Eye problems (macular edema)—case reports.

Muscle toxicity (myopathy)—infrequent.

Mania or seizures—rare.

Muscle toxicity of the heart (cardiomyopathy)—case reports.

Bone marrow depression (see Glossary): fatigue, weakness, fever, sore throat, abnormal bleeding or bruising.

Anemia occurs most commonly after 4 to 6 weeks of treatment; abnormally low white blood cell counts occur after 6 to 8 weeks of treatment—infrequent.

Esophageal ulcers (patients should take this medicine with at least 120 ml of water and not lie down for an hour)—possible.

Liver toxicity—infrequent.

Increased blood sugar (Trizivir form)—may be frequent.

Increased triglycerides (Trizivir form)—frequent (up to 25% in some populations).

▷ **Possible Effects on Sexual Function:** None reported.

Possible Delayed Adverse Effects: Significant anemia and deficient white blood cell counts may develop after this drug has been discontinued. Myopathy, increased triglycerides, blood sugar increases.

▷ **Adverse Effects That May Mimic Natural Diseases or Disorders**

Seizures may suggest the possibility of epilepsy.

Possible Effects on Laboratory Tests

Complete blood cell counts: decreased red cells, hemoglobin, white cells and platelets

Triglycerides (Trizivir form)—frequent increases

Blood glucose (sugar) (Trizivir form)—may be increased frequently.

CAUTION

1. These drugs are not a cure for AIDS; nor do they protect completely against other infections or complications. Follow your doctor's instructions. Take all medications exactly as prescribed.
2. These drugs do not reduce the risk of transmitting AIDS to others through sexual contact or contamination of the blood. The use of an effective condom is mandatory. Needles for drug administration should not be shared.
3. Triglyceride and blood sugar increases should be followed with combination forms.
4. Follow-up viral burden and CD4 tests are critical. Medicines that have failed MUST be changed (salvage therapy).

Precautions for Use

By Infants and Children: Zidovudine syrup is used in HIV-infected pediatric patients who are greater than 3 months old. The usual dose is 180 mg per square meter.

By Those Over 60 Years of Age: Impaired kidney function will require dose reduction.

▷ **Advisability of Use During Pregnancy**

Pregnancy Category: C. See Pregnancy Risk Categories at the back of this book.

Animal studies: Rat studies reveal no birth defects.

Human studies: Adequate studies of pregnant women are not available.

Consult your physician for specific guidance. This medicine has been shown to dramatically reduce the transference of HIV from mother to infant. If the decision is made to use this medicine in pregnancy, cases should be reported to 1-800-722-9292, extension 39437.

Advisability of Use If Breast-Feeding

Presence of this drug in breast milk: Unknown.

Breast-feeding may pass the HIV to the infant. DO NOT BREAST-FEED.

Habit-Forming Potential: None.

Effects of Overdose: Nausea, vomiting, diarrhea, bone marrow depression.

Possible Effects of Long-Term Use: Serious anemia and loss of white blood cells. Muscle toxicity (myopathy).

Suggested Periodic Examinations While Taking This Drug (at physician's discretion)

Complete blood cell counts before starting treatment and weekly thereafter until tolerance is established.

Continual monitoring for bone marrow depression is necessary during entire course of treatment.

Periodic CD4 counts or measurements of viral load are indicators that treatment is failing and demand change of antiretroviral therapy.

▷ **While Taking This Drug, Observe the Following**

Foods: No restrictions.

Herbal Medicines or Minerals: Some patients use echinacea to attempt to boost their immune systems. Unfortunately, use of echinacea is not recommended in people with damaged immune systems. This herb may also actually weaken any immune system if it is used too often or for too long a time. Use of mistletoe is also not recommended.

Beverages: No restrictions. May be taken with milk.

▷ *Alcohol:* No interactions expected with zidovudine or Combivir, but the Trizivir form contains abacavir. Abacavir blood levels are significantly increased when combined with alcohol and this combination should be avoided.

Tobacco Smoking: No interactions expected. I advise everyone to quit smoking.

▷ *Other Drugs*

The following drugs may ***increase*** the effects of zidovudine and enhance its toxicity:

- acetaminophen (Tylenol, others) although reports have NOT been consistent.
- acyclovir (Zovirax).
- amphotericin B (Fungizone).
- aspirin.
- benzodiazepines (see Drug Classes).
- cidefovir (Vistide) which is given with probenecid, may lead to increased zidovudine levels because of the probenecid.
- cimetidine (Tagamet).
- cotrimoxazole (various).
- fluconazole (Diflucan).
- ganciclovir (Cytovene).
- indomethacin (Indocin).
- interferon alpha, beta-1-A and natural.
- methadone (Dolophine).

- morphine (various).
- probenecid (Benemid).
- sulfonamides (see Drug Classes).

Zidovudine *taken concurrently* with

- dapsone may suppress bone marrow and increase risk of blood (hematologic) toxicity; more frequent complete blood counts are warranted.
- didanosine may result in increased risk of myelosuppression.
- doxorubicin (various) and other chemotherapy increases risk of bone marrow depression.
- filgrastim (Neupogen) may help maintain the white blood cell count.
- flucytosine (Ancobon) may suppress bone marrow and increase risk of blood (hematologic) toxicity; more frequent complete blood counts are warranted.
- fosphenytoin (Cerebyx) or phenytoin (Dilantin) may change blood levels of all drugs. Phenytoin levels and more, frequent complete blood counts are warranted.
- ganciclovir (Cytovene) may suppress bone marrow and increase risk of blood (hematologic) toxicity; more frequent complete blood counts are warranted.
- nimodipine (Nimotop) can increase toxicity to nerves.
- other nucleoside analogs for HIV may lower the ability of other HIV treatment requiring phosphorylation to become active.
- pyrazinamide (Rifater, others) may lower concentrations of pyrazinamide and increase risk of progression of tuberculosis. Pyrazinamide levels and dosing adjustments are prudent.
- rifabutin (Mycobutin) and rifampin (Rifadin) can lead to decreased zidovudine blood levels. Zidovudine levels may need to be increased if these medicines are combined.
- ritonavir (Norvir) may lower zidovudine levels.
- stavudine (D4T) may lessen effectiveness, as both agents are cell cycle specific.
- trimexate may cause additive hematological toxicity.
- valproic acid (Depakene) increases zidovudine blood levels. Lower doses of zidovudine and change from fixed dosage forms may be needed if valproic acid is required.

▷ *Driving, Hazardous Activities:* This drug may cause dizziness or fainting. Restrict activities as necessary.

Aviation Note: The use of this drug *is a disqualification* for piloting. Consult a designated Aviation Medical Examiner.

Exposure to Sun: No restrictions.

Discontinuation: Do not stop this drug without your physician's knowledge and guidance.

ZIPRASIDONE (ZIH praise ih dohn)

Introduced: 2001   **Class:** Antipsychotic   agent   **Prescription:** USA: Yes   **Controlled Drug:** USA: No; Canada: No   **Available as Generic:** USA: No; Canada: No

Brand Name: Geodon

```
┌──────────────────────────────────────────────────────────────┐
│                    BENEFITS versus RISKS                       │
│        Possible Benefits              Possible Risks           │
│  TREATMENT OF SCHIZOPHRENIA      PROLONGATION OF THE QT         │
│  DECREASED SIDE EFFECTS            INTERVAL                     │
│    COMPARED TO OTHER             ABNORMAL HEART RHYTHMS         │
│    AVAILABLE DRUGS               Abnormal lowering of blood pressure │
│  EFFECTIVE TREATMENT OF            on standing (postural hypotension) │
│    CERTAIN PSYCHOTIC DISORDERS   Involuntary movement disorder  │
│  LESS WEIGHT THAN OTHER          Neuroleptic malignant syndrome │
│    AVAILABLE MEDICINES FOR         (possible)                  │
│    SCHIZOPHRENIA                                               │
│  TWICE A DAY DOSING                                            │
│  LOW OCCURRENCE OF MOVEMENT                                    │
│    (EXTRAPYRAMIDAL) DISORDERS                                  │
└──────────────────────────────────────────────────────────────┘
```

▷ **Principal Uses**

As a Single Drug Product: Uses currently included in FDA-approved labeling: (1) Manages adult schizophrenia; (2) helps sudden (acute) episodes of schizoaffective disorder in adults.

Other (unlabeled) generally accepted uses: (1) None at present.

How This Drug Works: Goes to work at serotonin (also known as 5HT-2A) and dopamine D2 (D2 agonist) sites. This medicine also is active at 5HT-1A type sites which might account for greater protection against movement (extrapyramidal) disorders all of which help restore more normal thinking and mood.

Available Dosage Forms and Strengths

Capsules — 20 mg, 40 mg, 60 mg, 80 mg

▷ **Recommended Dosage Ranges** (Actual dose and schedule must be determined for each patient individually.)

Infants and Children: Safety and efficacy for those less than 18 years of age are not established.

18 to 60 Years of Age: Starting dose is 20 mg. Dose can be increased as needed and tolerated after as little as 2 days, but preferably after several weeks up to a dose of 80 mg twice a day. The lowest effective dose should be used. Doses greater than 80 mg per day are not recommended.

Over 60 Years of Age: No specific dosing changes thought to be needed. Additionally, no changes thought to be needed in mild to moderate kidney problems (CrCl of 60 down to 10 ml/min) which encompasses the "usual" age-related decline in kidney function. Because older patients may be more susceptible to sudden decreases in blood pressure (orthostatic hypotension), careful attention must be paid to blood pressure and development of adverse effects in this population.

Author's Note: Information in this profile will be broadened as more information becomes available and if broadened inclusion in the guide is warranted.

ZOLPIDEM (ZOL pi dem)

Introduced: 1993   **Class:** Hypnotic, imidazopyridine   **Prescription:** USA: Yes   **Controlled Drug:** USA: C-IV*; Canada: Prescription   **Available as Generic:** USA: No
Brand Name: Ambien

BENEFITS versus RISKS	
Possible Benefits	*Possible Risks*
GIVES SHORT-TERM RELIEF OF INSOMNIA WITH MINIMAL SLEEP DISRUPTION (REM)	Habit-forming potential with prolonged use

▷ **Principal Uses**
  As a Single Drug Product: Uses currently included in FDA-approved labeling: Short-term treatment of insomnia in adults.
    Other (unlabeled) generally accepted uses: (1) Long-term (more than 1 year) treatment of insomnia has been accomplished successfully in limited trials; (2) use in treating insomnia resulting from some antidepressants (SSRIs—see Drug Classes) has been investigated.
How This Drug Works: This drug attaches (binds) to a specific receptor (omega-1) and reduces the time it takes to fall asleep and increases total sleep time while producing a pattern and benefit of sleep that is similar to normal sleep patterns.
Available Dosage Forms and Strengths
    Tablets — 5 mg, 10 mg
▷ **Recommended Dosage Ranges** (Actual dose and schedule must be determined for each patient individually.)
  Infants and Children: Safety and efficacy for those under 18 years of age are not established.
  18 to 60 Years of Age: 10 mg is taken immediately before bedtime. Patients should be reevaluated after taking this drug for 7–10 days.
  Over 60 Years of Age: Therapy should be started with 5 mg taken at bedtime. The dose may be cautiously increased to 10 mg at bedtime. In general, any given dose will lead to about 50% higher peak concentrations. Confusion and falls are more likely in this population.
Conditions Requiring Dosing Adjustments
  Liver Function: The dose should be reduced by 50% in liver compromise.
  Kidney Function: No changes thought to be needed.
▷ **Dosing Instructions:** The tablet may be crushed. Best taken on an empty stomach. Do not stop this drug abruptly if taken more than 7 days. If you forget a dose: Because this medicine is taken when you can't sleep, a specific schedule is usually not required. Some patients take this medicine just before going to sleep, while others take it only if they can't sleep. DO NOT double up on doses.
Usual Duration of Use: Use on a regular schedule for 2 nights usually determines effectiveness in treating insomnia. Your physician should assess the benefit of this drug after a week to 10 days.

*See Schedules of Controlled Drugs at the back of this book.

Typical Treatment Goals and Measurements (Outcomes and Markers)

Insomnia: The general goal is to decrease the amount of time it takes between the time you go to bed and the time you fall asleep (sleep latency). Additionally, the number of times that you wake up is expected to decrease, enabling a full night of sleep. How alert you feel in the morning is also a consideration as many other hypnotics with longer half-lives also have significant effects the next morning ("hangover" effects). Two scales often used are the Stanford Sleepiness Scale (SSS) and the Saint Mary Hospital Sleep Questionnaire (SMHSQ).

Possible Advantages of This Drug

Low occurrence of adverse effects. May produce less of an undesirable effect on normal sleep patterns (sleep architecture).

Author's Note: The National Institute of Mental Health has an information page on anxiety. It can be found on the World Wide Web (www. nimh.nih.gov/anxiety).

Currently a Drug of Choice

For short-term management of insomnia in adults.

▷ **This Drug Should Not Be Taken If**

- you had an allergic reaction to it previously.

▷ **Inform Your Physician Before Taking This Drug If**

- you have abnormal liver or kidney function.
- you are pregnant or planning pregnancy.
- you have a history of alcoholism or drug abuse.
- you have a serious lung problem (respiratory impairment).
- you have a history of serious depression or mental disorder.
- you are unsure how much to take or how often to take this medicine.

Possible Side Effects (natural, expected and unavoidable drug actions)

Drowsiness.

▷ **Possible Adverse Effects** (unusual, unexpected and infrequent reactions)

If any of the following develop, consult your physician promptly for guidance.

Mild Adverse Effects

Allergic reactions: skin rash.

Drowsiness and dizziness—rare.

Central nervous system reactions (confusion, nightmares), sleep walking (somnambulism)—case reports.

Nausea and diarrhea—infrequent.

Elevation of liver function tests—rare.

Muscle tremors—infrequent.

Blurred vision—infrequent.

Serious Adverse Effects

Allergic reactions: not defined.

Abnormal thoughts or hallucinations—case reports.

Paradoxical aggression, agitation or suicidal thoughts—rare.

▷ **Possible Effects on Sexual Function:** None reported.

Possible Effects on Laboratory Tests

Liver function tests: increased SGOT, SGPT and CPK.

CAUTION

1. This drug works quickly. It is best to take it just before bedtime.

2. Do **not** drink alcohol while taking this drug
3. This medicine does not work to resolve anxiety. Your doctor should talk to you about NOT using it excessively if anxiety is a root cause of your sleep problem.
4. Withdrawal (see Glossary) may occur, even if this drug was only taken for a week or two. Ask your doctor for advice before stopping zolpidem.
5. You may experience trouble going to sleep for 1 or 2 nights after stopping this drug (rebound insomnia). This effect is usually short-term.
6. Sleep disturbances may be a symptom of underlying psychological problems. Tell your doctor if unusual behaviors or odd thoughts occur.
7. Drugs that depress the central nervous system may produce additive effects with this drug. Ask your doctor or pharmacist before combining other prescription or nonprescription drugs with zolpidem.

Precautions for Use

By Infants and Children: Safety and effectiveness for those under 18 years of age are not established.

By Those Over 60 Years of Age: The starting dose should be decreased to 5 mg. Since this drug works quickly, it is best taken immediately before going to bed. You may be at increased risk for falls if the drug remains in your system in the morning. Watch for lethargy, unsteadiness, nightmares and paradoxical agitation and anger.

▷ **Advisability of Use During Pregnancy**

Pregnancy Category: B. See Pregnancy Risk Categories at the back of this book.

Animal studies: In rats, abnormal skull bone formation was reported. In rabbits, abnormal bone formation was found.

Human studies: Adequate studies of pregnant women are not available.

Use during pregnancy is not advisable. Ask your doctor for guidance.

Advisability of Use If Breast-Feeding

Presence of this drug in breast milk: Yes.

Avoid drug or refrain from nursing.

Habit-Forming Potential: This drug may cause dependence (see Glossary).

Effects of Overdose: Marked change from lethargy to coma. Cardiovascular and respiratory compromise was also reported. The drug flumazenil may help reverse symptoms.

Possible Effects of Long-Term Use: Psychological and/or physical dependence.

Suggested Periodic Examinations While Taking This Drug (at physician's discretion)

Liver function tests.

▷ **While Taking This Drug, Observe the Following**

Foods: This drug should not be taken with food (food slows the time to beneficial effects).

Herbal Medicines or Minerals: Kava kava and valerian may exacerbate central nervous system depression (avoid this combination). Kola nut, Siberian ginseng, mate, ephedra and ma huang may blunt the benefits of this medicine. While St. John's wort is indicated for anxiety, it is also thought to increase (induce) cytochrome P450 enzymes and could tend to blunt zolpidem effectiveness.

Beverages: Avoid caffeine-containing beverages: coffee, tea, cola, chocolate.

▷ *Alcohol:* This drug should not be combined with alcohol.

Tobacco Smoking: Nicotine is a stimulant and should be avoided. I advise everyone to quit smoking.

Marijuana Smoking: : May cause additive drowsiness.

▷ *Other Drugs*

Zolpidem *taken concurrently* with

- azole antifungals (ketoconazole, fluconazole, others) may lead to zolpidem toxicity.
- bupropion (Wellbutrin) may increase risk of hallucinations.
- desipramine (Norpramin) may increase risk of hallucinations.
- fluoxetine (Prozac, SARAFEM) may increase risk of hallucinations.
- rifampin (Rifater, others) may decrease zolpidem benefits.
- ritonavir (Norvir) and perhaps other protease inhibitors (see Drug Classes) may lead to zolpidem toxicity.
- sertraline (Zoloft or venlafaxine (Effexor) may increase risk of hallucinations.

Zolpidem may *increase* the effects of

- chlorpromazine (Thorazine).
- narcotics or other CNS-depressant drugs (see Drug Classes for Opioids, Phenothiazines, Antihistamines and Benzodiazepines).

▷ *Driving, Hazardous Activities:* This drug may cause drowsiness and impair coordination. Restrict activities as necessary.

Aviation Note: The use of this drug *is a disqualification* for piloting. Consult a designated Aviation Medical Examiner.

Discontinuation: This drug should not be stopped abruptly, even after a week of use. Ask your doctor for help regarding an appropriate withdrawal schedule.

Author's Note: This marks the end of the medicine profiles in this edition. Your Guide continues with 17 helpful tables and a glossary of medical terms!

THE LEADING EDGE

This section is designed to help you become more fully aware of medicines that show promise for a variety of reasons. Some are novel applications or are now FDA-approvable. "The Leading Edge" can also explain new information about concepts in how medicines are packaged for better delivery into the body.

A few interesting medicines or therapeutic products still in early clinical trials are included as "stars on the horizon." It is impossible to predict which medicines or delivery systems will achieve final FDA approval or will be used in specific medicines, but many successful ones will be covered in subsequent editions of this book.

Finally, many medicines or delivery systems that could be covered in a given year may be omitted simply because of space limitations. The author will select those that in his opinion offer the most potential benefit to his readers.

ALZHEIMER'S VACCINE (ALLS high murs)

Novel Approach

We've heard about the two medicines (tacrine [Cognex] and donepezil [Aricept]) that can help control Alzheimer's disease. These both work to inhibit acetyl cholinesterase. Some original research has resulted in a new approach—a vaccine that appears to work in mice. The senior medical advisor to the Alzheimer's Association called the study a landmark. The original research appeared in the July 1999 issue of *Nature* and showed that the vaccine excited the immune system and kept sticky deposits called amyloid plaques from being deposited in the brain. The company who will be making the vaccine, Elan, started human studies. I'll update you in future editions and on my web site at www.medicineinfo.com.

ANGIOGENESIS INHIBITORS (ANN jee oh jen ih sis)

Stars on the Horizon

Progress has stopped after clinical trials of these medicines did not pan out. This class of medicines is an example of something that appeared to have great promise, but did not stand up to rigorous scientific research.

ANTI-IGE (An TIE Eye jee EE)

Novel Approach

I've often said that it's always better to prevent a disease or condition than to have to treat it. Asthma is a really good example. Researchers at the National Jewish Medical and Research Center found that anti-IgE injections, given once every two weeks or as infrequently as once a month, worked to stop allergies to a wide variety of pollen, dust and molds. The injections appear to work both in adults and children without major side effects. One study found that 40% of those receiving the injections required no other treatment. Further research is needed, and approval may be granted in a year or two.

ATHEROSCLEROSIS VACCINE (ATH er oh skler oh sis)

Novel Approach

We've all heard that high levels of "bad" cholesterol are harmful. There are numerous profiles in this book outlining medicines (HMG-CoA reductase inhibitors) that block formation of or otherwise work to lower harmful cholesterol. A vaccine is being tested against CETP (cholesterol ester transfer protein) by a company named Avant. The hope of the vaccine is that it may improve the ratio of good (HDL) to bad (LDL) cholesterol.

B LYMPHOCYTE STIMULANT (bee LYMFF oh site)

Star on the Horizon

A human protein has been discovered that works to trigger one of the most important infection-fighting cells in the body. The protein is called B lymphocyte stimulant or BlyS, and it actually causes the body to make more of a specific kind of white blood cell, called B lymphocyte. These cells play a critical role in HIV/AIDS, lymphoma and leukemia. Human trials continue.

CERVICAL CANCER VACCINE (SIR vi kal) (KAN sir)

Novel Approach

It may be possible to prevent cervical cancer with a vaccine. The vaccine will be directed against the human papilloma virus (HPV). While you may not have heard about this previously, this virus is the most common sexually transmitted disease in the United States. The vaccine will help those vaccinated avoid the virus—and avoid one cause of cervical cancer.

ETORICOXIB (EE tor ah kox ib)

Star on the Horizon
Many aspects of pain therapy have progressed because of pain guidelines from the Joint Commission on Accreditation of Health Care Organizations. COX II inhibitors have recently come under questions of increased risk of blood clots/cardiovascular risk. A new COX II inhibitor called etoricoxib is now being studied. This medicine appears to be even more selective than previously available "coxibs."

GENETIC THERAPY (JA neh tik therapy)

Stars on the Horizon
Many aspects of genetic therapy are being researched, but a most promising approach uses specific genetic probes to treat congestive heart failure (CHF). CHF affects more than 2 million people in the U.S. Early research by a company called Collateral Therapeutics continues to show promise for a one-time, nonsurgical treatment that may reverse CHF! Other companies, such as Glaxo, are exploring use of gene therapy to reverse high cholesterol.

GLIAL CELL LINE-DERIVED NEUROTROPHIC FACTOR (GDNF) (GLEE ahll)

Star on the Horizon
Still another aspect of genetic therapy seeks to reverse Parkinson's disease. A company called Cell Genesys has used its adeno-associated viral (AAV) gene delivery system to actually stimulate nerve growth in mice. The goal of survival without L-dopa for a year was achieved, and the company is now actively investigating collaboration for further development of Parkinson's gene therapy.

HDL (HIGH-DENSITY LIPOPROTEIN) THERAPY

Star on the Horizon
HDL or good cholesterol has long been known to help keep cholesterol and fat from depositing on the inside of blood vessels (atherosclerosis). Does your HDL (whatever level) work? Could HDL or an HDL-like treatment help unclog blood vessels? A company called Esperion Therapeutics is working on HDL therapy. Their first product is called Apo A Milano and is progressing through clinical trials. The concept involves use of an intravenous medicine to pull cholesterol off the blood vessels! Visit www.esperion.com and my website at www.medicine info.com for more information.

HUMAN GENOME (JEE nohm)

Star on the Horizon
Many medicines today address the symptoms of a disease or condition (such as high blood pressure) rather than addressing the cause. In what I consider to be the

most incredible effort at understanding how our bodies work in health and in illness, a project to map the entire group of human genes reached completion. It was projected that this effort would take more than five years, but the map was finished early. The potential for developing medicines that actually correct the underlying CAUSE of a disease or condition is suddenly very, very real. A medicine called STI571 listed below is one of the first candidates using a new treatment called pharmacogenomics. Interestingly, some 20 diseases cause more than 80% of deaths around the world and about 200–300 genes are responsible for these diseases. One prevalent example might be found in the fact that about every three weeks we in essence get a new heart from the same genes, if it would be possible to eliminate a "bad" gene from a gene pair, it might be possible to reverse some heart disease!

IC-351 (HYDROXYLASE) (hi DROX ul ace)

Star on the Horizon
Sildenafil (Viagra) has been one of the most widely publicized medicines ever to be approved by the FDA. A new medicine for impotence is progressing through clinical trials, which activates the same blood flow system as the existing medicine. IC-351 may have an advantage in that it may cause fewer possible side effects.

INSULIN, ORAL (IN sue lyn)

Medication Delivery
Would you prefer a shot (injection) or a spray? I think we all know the answer to this. A new insulin delivery system promises to replace an insulin shot with a sprayer that is actually sprayed into the mouth. I saw the data at the 2001 American Diabetes Association meeting. I've reviewed the available data and it looks like the insulin is absorbed into the blood and offers similar efficacy to the less desirable needle. Generex Biotechnology (www.generex.com) has progressed their product through clinical trials and its Oralin product via the Rapidmist device is currently in Phase III (the last phase before approval). Blood sugar control without a shot may soon be here.

FLU NASAL SPRAY (Vaccine)

Once again—another stall. The FDA panel who reviewed the application for FluMist said that they needed to finish their safety data studies so that more safety data could be presented. As of this writing, the FDA is expected to follow the advisory panel recommendation and ask the company to finish its safety analysis. Perhaps for the 2002–2003 flu season, a spray in the nose will finally replace the shot.

NESIRITIDE (NEH sear ih tyde)

Star on the Horizon
Congestive heart failure has been treated with the same medicines for more than a decade. A company called Scios has received a unanimous recommenda-

tion from an expert FDA panel for FDA approval of nesiritide (Natrecor). Historically, nitroglycerin has been used to try to reverse congestive heart failure. Nesiritide is a heart hormone that could represent the first new weapon in treating congestive heart failure in more than 10 years.

ORAL HEPARIN (HEP ere in)

Star on the Horizon

Historically, heparin (an effective anticoagulant or blood thinner) has required intravenous dosing. The first research on taking heparin and low molecular weight heparin by mouth (orally) has been started by Emisphere in conjunction with DuPont Pharmaceuticals. An oral liquid dosage form may be available.

PAIN TREATMENT IMPLANT

Novel Application

Dr. Stewart (Skip) Grossman is leading a team of researchers at Johns Hopkins University looking into actually implanting a pain medicine under the skin. Dr. Grossman originally envisioned use of the medicine in countries where clocks and time are less widely used concepts. It appears, however, that Dr. Grossman's team has identified a way to bring long-lasting relief (the insert may provide a reliable amount of medicine for up to a month) to chronic pain patients. The clear benefit here is that a reliable level of pain medicine could be regularly delivered while having a minimal impact on a patient's life. Even pain patients can have problems trying to remember to take a pill!

PARATHORMONE (PARA thor moan)

Star on the Horizon

A modified hormone called parathyroid hormone or parathormone has shown great promise in helping decrease bone fractures. This injection is being studied in women with osteoporosis and reduced fractures by 65% in early trials. This hormone works by stimulating new growth of bone (osteoblast action) and is a new approach versus the antiresorptive (osteoclast) approach of medicines like alendronate (Fosamax). I expect clinical trials will progress. The brand name is projected to be Forteo.

PROSTATE CANCER VACCINE (PRAH state)

Star on the Horizon

A vaccine to help prevent prostate cancer is in the works. A phase I/II study showed that a vaccine named GVAX stabilized disease in 71% of patients and was also safe and well tolerated. It is expected that the company researching this vaccine (Cell Genesys) will move forward with further testing.

TELOMERASE (TELL om er ace)

Star on the Horizon

Work has continued on this new enzyme that appears to have a role in aging and may also be part of the cancer mystery. Much research needs to be done to see where this enzyme fits in.

VASOPEPTIDE INHIBITORS (VAY soh pep tyde)

Stars on the Horizon

Work has moved forward on this new class of medicines for high blood pressure. They appear to inhibit both the angiotensin converting enzyme (ACE) system as well as neural endopeptidases. I expect that a medicine called omapatrilat (Vanlev) from Bristol-Myers Squibb will receive expedited review by the FDA. A major study of the Bristol drug (OVERTURE or omapatrilat versus enalapril) will be completed in 2002.

ZOLEDRONATE (ZOH lead roh nate)

Star on the Horizon

Osteoporosis treatment has undergone major benefits from alendronate which itself has recently benefited from a once a week dosing schedule. Adherence is a critical issue in the US with nearly half of the people who live with an asymptomatic chronic condition stopping their medicines after about a year. A new medicine called zoledronic acid or zoledronate belongs to the same chemical family as alendronate. In Madrid at the 1st joint meeting of the International Bone and Mineral Society and the European Calcified Tissue Society an abstract detailed information about this ONCE A YEAR injection to treat osteoporosis. Early data showed that bone mineral density increased in both the spine and the hip!

DRUG CLASSES

Throughout the drug profiles, I often refer you to various drug classes. Use this section to protect yourself and your family. Medicines in the same class often share important characteristics in their chemistry, how they work in the body and even the problems or side effects that they may cause. Any drug (or all drugs) in a given class can be expected to behave in a similar way. This knowledge helps you prevent interactions or unanticipated or hazardous adverse effects.

Each Drug Class is named, followed by an alphabetic listing of the generic names of the drugs in the class. Following each generic name (and enclosed in parentheses) is the widely recognized brand name(s) of that particular drug. A complete listing is not possible. If your medicine is not present, call your doctor or pharmacist to get the generic name of the drug that concerns you. The generic name listings are sufficiently complete to serve the scope of this book.

ACE (Angiotensin-Converting Enzyme) Inhibitors

benazepril (Lotensin)
captopril (Capoten)
cilazapril (investigational)
enalapril (Vasotec)
enalapril/felodipine (Lexxel)
fosinopril (Monopril)
lisinopril (Prinivil, Zestril
lisinopril/hctz (Prinzide, Zestoretic)
moexipril (Univasc)

moexipril/hydrochlorothiazide
  (Uniretic)
perindopril (Aceon)
quinapril (Accupril)
ramipril (Altace)
spirapril (Renormax)
trandolapril (Mavik)
trandolapril/verapamil (Tarka)

Adrenocortical Steroids (Cortisonelike Drugs)

amcinonide (Cyclocort)

beclomethasone (Beclovent, Vanceril)

betamethasone (Celestone)

budesonide (Pulmicort)

cortisone (Cortone)

dexamethasone (Decadron)

fludrocortisone (Florinef)

flunisolide (AeroBid, Nasarel)

fluorometholone (FML)

fluticasone (Flonase)

halcinonide (Halog)

halobetasol (Ultravate)

hydrocortisone (Cortef)

medrysone (HMS Ophthalmic Suspension)

methylprednisolone (Medrol)

mometasone (Elocon)

paramethasone (Haldrone)

prednisolone (Delta-Cortef)

prednisone (Deltasone)

rimexalone (Vexol)

triamcinolone (Aristocort, Azmacort)

Alpha-Glucosidase Inhibitors

acarbose (Precose)

miglitol (Glyset)

Amebicides (Anti-Infectives)

chloroquine (Aralen)

emetine

iodoquinol (Yodoxin)

metronidazole (Flagyl)

paromomycin (Humatin)

Aminoglycosides (Anti-Infectives)

amikacin (Amikin)

gentamicin (Garamycin)

kanamycin (Kantrex)

neomycin (Mycifradin, Neobiotic)

paromomycin (Humatin)

tobramycin (Tobicin)

Amphetaminelike Drugs

amphetamine

benzphetamine (Didrex)

dextroamphetamine (Dexedrine)

diethylpropion (Tenuate, Tepanil)

methamphetamine (Desoxyn)

methylphenidate (Ritalin)

phendimetrazine (Adipost, Anorex, Plegine)

phenmetrazine (Preludin)

phentermine (Adipex-P, Fastin)

phentermine resin complex (Ionamin)

phenylpropanolamine (Dexatrim)

Analgesics (Pain relievers)

Acetaminophen (Datril, Tylenol)

acetaminophen/propoxyphene (Darvocet-N 100)

aspirin

capsaicin (Zostrix)

COX II inhibitors (rofecoxib-Vioxx, celecoxib-Celebrex, etoricoxib, parecoxib)

Fentanyl (Duragesic)

Gabapentin (Neurontin)

lidocaine/prilocaine cream (Emla)

morphine (Kadian, MS-Contin)

oxycodone (Oxycontin)

propoxyphene (Darvon)

tramadol (Ultram)

zinconotide (investigational)

See also Nonsteroidal Anti-Inflammatory Drugs (NSAIDs) and Opioid Drugs

Androgens (Male Sex Hormones)

fluoxymesterone (Halotestin)
methyltestosterone (Android,
    Metandren, Oreton)

testosterone (Androderm, Andriol,
    AndroGel, Depotest, Testoderm,
    Testone)

Angiotensin-II-Receptor Antagonists

candesartan (Atacand)
candesartan/hctz (Atacand HCT)
eprosartan (Teveten)
irbesartan (Avapro)
irbesartan/HCTZ (Avalide)

losartan (Cozaar)
losartan/hctz (Hyzaar)
telmisartan (Micardis)
valsartan (Diovan)
valsartan/hctz (Diovan HCT)

Anorexiants (Appetite Suppressants)

mazindol (Mazanor, Sanorex)
sibutramine (Meridia)

See also Amphetaminelike Drugs

Anti-Acne Drugs

adapalene (Differin)
azelaic acid (Azelex)
benzoyl peroxide (Epi-Clear, others)
erythromycin (Eryderm)
isotretinoin (Accutane)

sodium sulfacetamide 10% lotion
    (Klaron)
tetracycline (Achromycin V)
tretinoin (Retin-A)

Anti-AIDS/HIV Drugs (Anti-Retrovirals)

abacavir (Ziagen)
abacavir/lamivudine/zidovudine
    (Trizivir)
amprenavir (Agenerase or VX-1478)
delavirdine (Rescriptor)
didanosine (DDI, Videx)
efavirenz (Sustiva)
hydroxyurea (Droxia)
indinavir (Crixivan)
integrase (Zintevir) (investigational)
lamivudine (3TC, Epivir)
lopinavir/ritonvair (Kaletra)

nelfinavir (Viracept)
nevirapine (Viramune)
ritonavir (Norvir)
saquinavir (Invirase)
stavudine (D4T, Zerit)
T-20 (investigational)
T-1249 (investigational)
zalcitabine (dideoxycytidine, DDC,
    Hivid)
zidovudine (AZT, Retrovir)
232632 (azantavir-Investigational)

Antialcoholism Drugs

disulfiram (Antabuse)

naltrexone (Trexan, ReVia)

Anti-Alzheimer's Drugs

donepezil (Aricept)
galantamine (newly approved in the
    U.S. as Reminyl)
gingko biloba (herbal preparation-
    standardization pending by USP)

metrifonate (Bilarcil)
rivastigmine (Exelon)
tacrine (Cognex)
vitamin E (various brands)

Anti-Anginal Drugs

bepridil (Vascor)
diltiazem (Cardizem)
nicardipine (Cardene)
nifedipine (Adalat, Procardia)

nitrates (see class below)
verapamil (Calan, Isoptin)
See also Beta Blockers

Antianxiety Drugs

buspirone (Buspar)
chlormezanone (Trancopal)
hydroxyzine (Atarax, Vistaril)
lorazepam (Ativan)

meprobamate (Equanil, Miltown)
paroxetine (Paxil)—generalized and
   adult social anxiety disorder
See also Benzodiazepines

Antiarrhythmic Drugs (Heart Rhythm Regulators)

Class or Group One

disopyramide (Norpace)
flecainide (Tambocor)
mexiletine (Mexitil)
procainamide (Procan SR, Pronestyl)

quinidine (Quinaglute, Quinidex,
   Quinora)
propafenone (Rythmol)
tocainide (Tonocard)

Class or Group Two

acebutolol (Sectral)
propranolol (Inderal)

sotalol (Betapace)

Class or Group Three

amiodarone (Cordarone)
dofetilide (Tikosyn)

ibutilide (Corvert)
sotalol (Betapace)

Class or Group Four

diltiazem (Cardizem)

verapamil (Calan, Isoptin)

Miscellaneous

adenosine (Adenocard)

digoxin (Lanoxin)

Antiarthritics

aspirin
azathioprine (Imuran; rheumatoid only)
chloroquine (Aralen; rheumatoid only)
COX-II inhibitor family
etanercept (Enbrel)
infliximab (Remicade)

leflunomide (Arava)
penicillamine (Cuprimine)
See also Nonsteroidal Anti-
   Inflammatory Drugs (NSAIDs)
   and Adrenocorticosteroids

Antiasthmatic Drugs

Anti-Inflammatory Agents, Corticosteroids

beclomethasone (Beclovent, Vanceril)
flunisolide (AeroBid)
fluticasone (Flovent)

fluticasone/salmeterol (Advair Diskus)
triamcinolone (Azmacort)

Anti-Leukotrienes

montelukast (Singulair)

zafirlukast (Accolate)

zileuton (Zyflo)

Bronchodilators

albuterol (Proventil, Ventolin)

aminophylline (Phyllocontin)

bitolterol (Tornalate)

dyphylline (Lufyllin)

ephedrine (Efed II)

epinephrine (Adrenalin, Bronkaid Mist, Primatene Mist)

formoterol (Foradil)

ipratropium

isoetharine (Bronkosol, Dey-Lute)

isoproterenol (Isuprel)

metaproterenol (Alupent, Metaprel)

oxtriphylline (Choledyl)

pirbuterol (Maxair)

salmeterol (Serevent) (see combination form above)

terbutaline (Brethaire, Brethine, Bricanyl)

theophylline (Bronkodyl, Elixophyllin, Slo-Phyllin, others)

Combination Agents

fluticasone/salmeterol (Advair Diskus)

Mast-Cell-Stabilizing Agents

cromolyn sodium (Gastrocrom, Intal)

nedocromil (Tilade)

Preventive Agents

cromolyn (Intal)

nedocromil (Tilade)

Xanthines

theophylline (Slo-bid, Theo-Dur)

Anti-Attention-Deficit-Hyperactivity-Disorder Drugs

clonidine (Catapres)

methylphenidate (Ritalin)

pemoline (Cylert)

Anti-Benign-Prostatic-Hyperplasia Drugs

doxazosin (Cardura)

finasteride (Proscar)

prazosin (Minipres)

saw palmetto (various)—herbal product

tamsulosin (Flomax)

terazosin (Hytrin)

Antibiotics

See specific antibiotic class (Cephalosporins, Penicillins, Tetracyclines, etc.)

Topical, Anti-Infectives

mupirocin (Bactroban)

Anticancer Drugs (Antineoplastics or Chemotherapy)

capecitabine (Zeloda)

chlorambucil (Leukeran)

cyclophosphamide (Cytoxan)

flutamide (Eulexin)

hydroxyurea (Hydrea)

liposomally encapsulated doxorubicin (Evacet) (investigational)

mercaptopurine (Purinethol)

methotrexate (Rheumatrex)

tamoxifen (Nolvadex)

Signal Transduction Inhibitor

imatinib STI571 (Gleevec)

Anti-Canker-Sore Drugs

amlexanox (Apthasol)

Anticholesterol Drugs

See Cholesterol-Reducing Drugs
See HMG-CoA Reductase Inhibitors

See "The Leading Edge" section of this
  book

Anticholinergic Drugs (Atropinelike Drugs)

atropine
belladonna
hyoscyamine
scopolamine
See also the specific drug class:

Antidepressant Drugs, Tricyclic
Antihistamines, some
Anti-Parkinsonism Drugs, some
Antispasmodics, Synthetic, some
Muscle Relaxants, some

Anticoagulant Drugs

anisindione (Miradon)
dicumarol
low-molecular-weight heparins
  (ardeparin-Normiflo, dalteparin-
  Fragmin, enoxaparin-Lovenox,
  tinzaparin-Innohep)

warfarin (Coumadin and generic)

Anticonvulsant Drugs (Antiepileptic Drugs)

acetazolamide (Diamox)
carbamazepine (Tegretol)
clonazepam (Klonopin)
clorazepate (Tranxene)
diazepam (Valium)
ethosuximide (Zarontin)
ethotoin (Peganone)
felbamate (Felbatol)
gabapentin (Neurontin)
lamotrigine (Lamictal)
levetiracetam (Keppra)
mephenytoin (Mesantoin)

methsuximide (Celontin)
oxcarbamazepine (Trileptal)
paramethadione (Paradione)
phenacemide (Phenurone)
phenobarbital (Luminal)
phensuximide (Milontin)
phenytoin (Dilantin)
primidone (Mysoline)
topiramate (Topamax)
trimethadione (Tridione)
valproic acid (Depakene)
zonisamide (Zonegran)

Anti-Cystic-Fibrosis Agents (Recombinant DNase)

dornase alfa (Pulmozyme)

Antidepressant Drugs

Bicyclic Antidepressants

fluoxetine (Prozac, Prozac Weekly)   venlafaxine (Effexor)

Tetracyclic Antidepressants

maprotiline (Ludiomil)   mirtazapine (Remeron)

Tricyclic Antidepressants

amitriptyline (Elavil, Endep)
amoxapine (Asendin)
clomipramine (Anafranil)
desipramine (Norpramin, Pertofranc)
doxepin (Adapin, Sinequan)
imipramine (Tofranil)
nortriptyline (Aventyl, Pamelor)
protriptyline (Vivactil)
trimipramine (Surmontil)
Other Antidepressants

bupropion (Wellbutrin, Wellbutrin SR)
fluvoxamine (Luvox)
Hypericum (St. John's wort)
nefazodone (Serzone)
paroxetine (Paxil)
sertraline (Zoloft)
trazodone (Desyrel)
See also Monoamine Oxidase (MAO)
    Inhibitors

Antidiabetic Drugs

Oral

See Alpha-Glucosidase Inhibitors,
    Biguanides, D-phenylalanine
    derivatives, Meglitinides,
    Sulfonylureas and
    Thiazolindinediones

Injectable

insulin

Mouth (Oral) Spray

insulin (Oralin—investigational)

Antidiarrheal Drugs

loperamide

Antiemetic Drugs (Anti-Motion-Sickness, Antinausea Drugs)

chlorpromazine (Thorazine)
cyclizine (Marezine)
dimenhydrinate (Dramamine)
diphenhydramine (Benadryl)
ginger (various)
granisetron (Kytril)
hydroxyzine (Atarax, Vistaril)

meclizine (Antivert, Bonine)
ondansetron (Zofran)
prochlorperazine (Compazine)
promethazine (Phenergan)
scopolamine (Transderm Scop)
trimethobenzamide (Tigan)

Antiepileptic Drugs

See Anticonvulsant Drugs

Antifungal Drugs (Anti-Infectives)

amphotericin B (Fungizone)
butenafine (Mentax)
caspofungin (Cancidas)
fluconazole (Diflucan)
flucytosine (Ancobon)
griseofulvin (Fulvicin, Grifulvin,
   Grisactin)
itraconazole (Sporanox)

ketoconazole (Nizoral)
lipid-associated amphotericin B
   (Abelcet)
miconazole (Monistat)
nystatin (Mycostatin)
terbinafine (Lamisil)
tioconazole (Vagistat-1)

Antiglaucoma Drugs

acetazolamide (Diamox)
betaxolol (Betoptic)
bimatoprost (Lumigan)
brimonidine (Alphagan)
brinzolamide (Azopt)
dipivefrin (Propine)
dorzolamide (Trusopt)
dorzolamide and timolol (Cosopt)
epinephrine (Glaucon)

latanoprost (Xalatan)
levobetaxolol (Betaxon)
levobunolol (Betagan)
metipranolol (Optipranolol)
pilocarpine (Pilocar)
timolol (Betimol, Timoptic,
   Timoptic-XE)
travaprost (Travatan)

Antigout Drugs

allopurinol (Zyloprim)
colchicine
diclofenac (Cataflam, Voltaren)
fenoprofen (Nalfon)
ibuprofen (Advil, Motrin, Nuprin, Rufin)
indomethacin (Indocin)
ketoprofen (Orudis)

mefenamic acid (Ponstel)
naproxen (Anaprox, Naprosyn)
oxaprozin (Daypro)
piroxicam (Feldene)
probenecid (Benemid)
sulfinpyrazone (Anturane)
sulindac (Clinoril)

Antihistamines

astemizole (Hismanal) (now
   removed from the market)
azatadine (Optimine)
azelastine (Astelin)
brompheniramine (Dimetane, others)
carbinoxamine (Clistin, Rondec)
cetirizine (Zyrtec)
chlorpheniramine (Chlor-Trimeton, Teldrin)
clemastine (Tavist)
cyclizine (Marezine)
cyproheptadine (Periactin)
dimenhydrinate (Dramamine)

diphenhydramine (Benadryl)
doxylamine (Unisom)
hydroxyzine (Atarax)
loratadine (Claritin, Claritin Extra)
meclizine (Antivert, Bonine)
orphenadrine (Norflex)
pheniramine (component of Triaminic)
promethazine (Phenergan, others)
pyrilamine (component of Triaminic)
tripelennamine (Pyribenzamine, PBZ)
triprolidine (component of Actifed and
   Sudahist)

Nonsedating or Minimally Sedating

astemizole (Hismanal) (now removed from
   the market)
cetirizine (Zyrtec)

fexofenadine (Allegra)
loratadine (Claritin)

Antihypertensive Drugs

amlodipine/benazepril (Lotrel)
bisoprolol/hydrochlorothiazide (Ziac)
carvedilol (Coreg)
clonidine (Catapres)
doxazosin (Cardura)
enalapril/felodipine (Lexxel)
guanabenz (Wytensin)
guanadrel (Hylorel)
guanethidine (Ismelin)
guanfacine (Tenex)
hydralazine (Apresoline)

hydrochlorothiazide/benazepril
   (Lotensin)
methyldopa (Aldomet)
minoxidil (Loniten)
prazosin (Minipres)
reserpine (Serpasil)
terazosin (Hytrin)
See also ACE Inhibitors, Angiotensin-
   II-Receptor Antagonists, Beta
   Blockers, Calcium Blockers and
   Diuretics

Anti-Impotence Drugs

alprostadil injection (Caverject)
apomorphine (Uprima)

IC-151 hydroxylase (investigational)
sildenafil (Viagra)

Anti-Infective Drugs

See the specific anti-infective drug
   classes:
Amebicides
Aminoglycosides
Antifungal Drugs
Antileprosy Drugs
Antimalarial Drugs
Antituberculosis Drugs

Antiviral Drugs
Cephalosporins
Fluoroquinolones
Macrolide Antibiotics
Oxazolidinones
Penicillins
Sulfonamides
Tetracyclines

Miscellaneous Anti-Infective Drugs

atovaquone (Mepron)
chloramphenicol (Chloromycetin)
clindamycin (Cleocin)
colistin (Coly-Mycin S)
furazolidone (Furoxone)
lincomycin (Lincocin)
linezolid (Zyvox)

nalidixic acid (NegGram)
nitrofurantoin (Furadantin,
   Macrodantin)
novobiocin (Albamycin)
pentamidine (Pentam-300)
trimethoprim (Proloprim, Trimpex)
vancomycin (Vancocin)

Antileprosy Drugs (Anti-Infectives)

clofazimine (Lamprene)

dapsone

Antimalarial Drugs (Anti-Infectives)

chloroquine (Aralen)
doxycycline (Vibramycin)
hydroxychloroquine (Plaquenil)
mefloquine (Lariam)
primaquine

pyrimethamine (Daraprim)
quinacrine (Atabrine)
quinine
sulfadoxine (Fansidar)

Antimigraine Drugs

almotriptan (Axert)
atenolol (Tenormin)
ergotamine (Ergostat)
methysergide (Sansert)
metoprolol (Lopressor)
nadolol (Corgard)
naratriptan (Amerge)

nifedipine (Procardia)
propranolol (Inderal)
rizatriptan (Maxalt, Maxalt MLT)
sumatriptan (Imitrex)
timolol (Blocadren)
verapamil (Calan, Isoptin)
zolmatriptan (Zomig)

Anti-Motion-Sickness/Antinausea Drugs

See Antiemetic Drugs

Anti-Myasthenics

neostigmine

Antimycobacterial Agents

rifabutin (Mycobutin)

Anti-Osteoporotics

alendronate (Fosamax)
antiestrogens (SERM)
calcitonin (Miacalcin)
calcium (various brands)
estrogen (various brands)
parathormone PTH (investigational)
pravastatin (Pravachol—one study
    reported improvement—not an
    FDA-approved use)

raloxifene (Evista)
risedronate (Actonel)
synthetic conjugated estrogens
tiludronate (Skelid)
zoledronic acid (Zoledronate—
    investigational)

Anti-Parkinsonism Drugs

amantadine (Symmetrel)
benztropine (Cogentin)
bromocriptine (Parlodel)
diphenhydramine (Benadryl)
levodopa (Dopar, Larodopa)
levodopa/bensarazide (Prolopa)
levodopa/carbidopa (Sinemet, Sinemet CR)
pergolide (Permax)

prampexole (Myrapex)
ropinirole (Requip)
selegiline (Eldepryl)
tolcapone (Tasmar)
trihexyphenidyl (Artane)
vitamin E (various)
Catechol O-Methyl Tranferase (COMT) Drugs
tolcapone (Tasmar)

Antiplatelet Drugs (Platelet Aggregation Inhibitors)

aspirin
aspirin/dipyridamole (Aggrenox)
clopidogrel (Plavix)
dipyridamole (Persantine)

sulfinpyrazone (Anturane)
ticlopidine (Ticlid)
tirofiban (Aggrastat)

Antipsoriatic Drugs

acitretin (Soriatane)
etretinate

methotrexate

Antipsychotic Drugs (Neuroleptics, Major Tranquilizers)

chlorprothixene (Taractan)
clozapine (Clozaril)
haloperidol (Haldol)
loxapine (Loxitane)
molindone (Moban)
olanzapine (Zyprexa)
pimozide (Orap)

quetiapine (Seroquel)
risperidone (Risperdal)
thiothixene (Navane)
ziprasidone (Geodon)
See also Phenothiazines and
  Thienobenzodiazepines

Antipyretic Drugs (Fever-Reducing Drugs)

acetaminophen
aspirin
See also COX II inhibitors

See also Nonsteroidal Anti-
  Inflammatory Drugs (NSAIDs)

Anti-Sickle-Cell-Anemia Drugs

hydroxyurea (Droxia, Hydrea)

Antispasmodics, Synthetic

anisotropine (Valpin)
clidinium (Quarzan)
glycopyrrolate (Robinul)
hexocyclium (Tral)
isopropamide (Darbid)

mepenzolate (Cantil)
methantheline (Banthine)
methscopolamine (Pamine)
propantheline (Pro-Banthine)
tridihexethyl (Pathilon)

Antituberculosis Drugs

aminosalicylate sodium (Sodium P.A.S.)
capreomycin (Capastat)
cycloserine (Seromycin)
ethambutol (Myambutol)
ethionamide (Trecator-SC)
isoniazid (Laniazid, Nydrazid)

pyrazinamide
rifabutin (Mycobutin)
rifampin (Rifadin, Rimactane, Rifater)
rifapentine (Priftin)
streptomycin

Antitussive Drugs (Cough Suppressants)

benzonatate (Tessalon)
codeine (various brands)
dextromethorphan (Hold DM, Suppress)
diphenhydramine (Benylin)

hydrocodone (Hycodan)
hydromorphone (Dilaudid)
promethazine (Phenergan)

Antiulcer Drugs

Antacids

various brands

Antibiotics

amoxicillin
clarithromycin
metronidazole

tetracycline
See Histamine (H2) Blockers
See Proton Pump Inhibitors

Miscellaneous Antiulcer Drugs

amoxicillin/clarithromycin/
  lansoprazole (Prevpac)
bismuth subsalicylate (Pepto-Bismol, others)

misoprostol (Cytotec)
ranitidine bismuth citrate (Tritec)
sucralfate (Carafate)

Antiviral Drugs (Anti-Infectives)

Abacavir (Ziagen)
Abacavir, lamivudine, zidovudine
  (Trizivir)
acyclovir (Zovirax)
amantadine (Symmetrel)
amprenavir (Agenerase)
cidofovir (Vistide)
didanosine (Videx)
docosanol (Abreva)
efavirenz (Sustiva)
famciclovir (Famvir)
foscarnet (Foscavir)
ganciclovir (Cytovene)
indinavir (Crixivan)
lamivudine (Epivir,
Epivir HBV)

lopinavir/ritonavir (Kaletra)
nelfinavir (Viracept)
nevirapine (Viramune)
oseltamivir (Tamiflu)
penciclovir (Denavir)
ribavirin (Virazole)
rimantadine (Flumadine)
ritonavir (Norvir)
saquinavir (Invirase)
stavudine (Zerit)
valacyclovir (Valtrex)
vidarabine (Vira A)
zalcitabine (Hivid)
zanamivir (Relenza)
zidovudine (Retrovir)
232632 azantavir (investigational)

Appetite Suppressants

See Anorexiants

Atropinelike Drugs

See Anticholinergic Drugs

Barbiturates

amobarbital (Amytal)
aprobarbital (Alurate)
butabarbital (Butisol)
mephobarbital (Mebaral)
metharbital (Gemonil)

pentobarbital (Nembutal)
phenobarbital (Luminal, Solfoton)
secobarbital (Seconal)
talbutal (Lotusate)

Benzodiazepines

alprazolam (Xanax)
bromazepam (Lectopam)
chlordiazepoxide (Libritabs, Librium)
clonazepam (Klonopin)
clorazepate (Tranxene)
diazepam (Valium, Vazepam)
estazolam (Prosom)
flurazepam (Dalmane)
halazepam (Paxipam)

ketazolam (Loftran)
lorazepam (Ativan)
midazolam (Versed)
nitrazepam (Mogadon)
oxazepam (Serax)
prazepam (Centrax)
quazepam (Doral)
temazepam (Restoril)
triazolam (Halcion)

Beta Blockers (Beta-Adrenergic-Blocking Drugs)

acebutolol (Sectral)
atenolol (Tenormin)
betaxolol (Kerlone)
bisoprolol (Zebeta)
bisoprolol/hydrochlorothiazide (Ziac)
carteolol (Cartrol)
carvedilol (Coreg)

labetalol (Normodyne, Trandate)
metoprolol (Lopressor)
nadolol (Corgard)
penbutolol (Levatol)
pindolol (Visken)
propranolol (Inderal)
timolol (Blocadren)

Biguanides (Oral Antidiabetic Drugs)

metformin (Glucophage)

Bisphosphonates

alendronate (Fosamax)
risedronate (Actonel)

tiludronate (Skelid)
zoledronate (investigational)

Blood Flow Agents

cilostazol (Pletal)
ginkgo biloba (various)

pentoxifylline (Trental)

Bowel Anti-Inflammatory Drugs (Inflammatory Bowel Disease Suppressants)

azathioprine (Imuran)
infliximab (Avakine)
mesalamine (Rowasa, Asacol)

metronidazole (Flagyl)
olsalazine (Dipentum)
sulfasalazine (Azulfidine)

Bronchodilators

See Antiasthmatic Drugs

Calcium Blockers (Calcium-Channel-Blocking Drugs)

amlodipine (Norvasc)
bepridil (Vascor)
diltiazem (Cardizem, Tiazac)
felodipine (Plendil)
isradipine (DynaCirc)
mibefradil (Posicor) (removed by the
   company)

nicardipine (Cardene, Cardene SR)
nifedipine (Adalat CC, Procardia XL)
nimodipine (Nimotop)
nisoldipine (Sular)
verapamil (Calan, Isoptin, Verelan)

Cephalosporins (Anti-Infectives)

cefaclor (Ceclor)
cefadroxil (Duricef, Ultracef)
cefamandole (Mandol)
cefatrizine (Cefaperos)
cefazolin (Ancef, Kefzol, Zolicef)
cefdinir (Omnicef)
cefepime (Maxipime)
cefixime (Suprax)
cefmetazole (Zefazone)
cefonicid (Monocid)
cefoperazone (Cefobid)
ceforanide (Precef)
cefotaxime (Claforan)
cefotetan (Cefotan)

cefoxitin (Mefoxin)
cefpodoxime (Vantin)
cefprozil (Cefzil)
ceftazidime (Fortaz, Tazidime, Tazicef)
ceftibuten (Cedax)
ceftizoxime (Cefizox)
ceftriaxone (Rocephin)
cefuroxime (Ceftin, Kefurox, Zinacef)
cephalexin (Keflex, Keftab)
cephalothin (Keflin)
cephapirin (Cefadyl)
cephradine (Anspor, Velosef)
loracarbef (Cefobid)
moxalactam (Moxam)

Cholesterol-Reducing Drugs

atorvastatin (Lipitor)
cerivastatin (Baycol) (Removed form
   the market)
cholestyramine (Questran, Prevalite)
clofibrate (Atromid-S)
colesevelam (Welchol)
colestipol (Colestid)
dextrothyroxine (Choloxin)

fenofibrate (Tricor)
fluvastatin (Lescol)
gemfibrozil (Lopid)
lovastatin (Mevacor)
niacin (Nicobid, Slo-Niacin, others)
pravastatin (Pravachol)
simvastatin (Zocor)

Cortisonelike Drugs

See Adrenocortical Steroids

Cough Suppressants

See Antitussive Drugs

COX II Inhibitors

celecoxib (Celebrex)
etoricoxib (investigational; please see
   The Leading Edge section)

parecoxib (investigational and
   pending in the FDA)
rofecoxib (Vioxx)

Decongestants

ephedrine (Efedron, Ephedrol)
naphazoline (Naphcon, Vasocon)
oxymetazoline (Afrin, Duration, others)
phenylephrine (Neo-Synephrine,
    others)
phenylpropanolamine (Propadrine,
    Propagest, others)

pseudoephedrine (Afrinol, Sudafed,
    others)
tetrahydrozoline (Tyzine, Visine,
    others)
xylometazoline (Otrivin)

Digitalis Preparations

deslanoside (Cedilanid-D)
digitoxin (Crystodigin)

digoxin (Lanoxicaps, Lanoxin)

Disease-Modifying Antirheumatic Drugs (DMARDs)

etanercept (Enbrel)
leflunomide (Arava)

methotrexate (Rheumatrex)

Diuretics

acetazolamide (Diamox)
amiloride (Midamor)
bumetanide (Bumex)
chlorthalidone (Hygroton)
ethacrynic acid (Edecrin)
furosemide (Lasix)

indapamide (Lozol)
metolazone (Diulo, Zaroxolyn)
spironolactone (Aldactone)
triamterene (Dyrenium)
See also Thiazide Diuretics

D-phenylalanine derivative oral hypoglycemics

nateglinide (Starlix)

Ergot Derivatives

bromocriptine (Parlodel)
ergotamine (Bellergal)

methysergide (Sansert)
pergolide (Permax)

Estrogens (Female Sex Hormones)

chlorotrianisene (Tace)
diethylstilbestrol (DES, Stilphostrol)
estradiol (Estrace, Estraderm, others)
estrogens, conjugated (Premarin,
    Prempro)
estrogens, esterified (Estratab, Menest)

estrone (Theelin, others)
estropipate (Ogen)
ethinyl estradiol (Estinyl)
quinestrol (Estrovis)
plant-derived synthetic conjugated
    estrogens (Cenestin)

Female Sex Hormones

See Estrogens and Progestins

Fever-Reducing Drugs
See Antipyretic Drugs

5-Alpha-Reductase Inhibitors
finasteride (Proscar)

Fluoroquinolones (Anti-Infectives)

balofloxacin (pending)
ciprofloxacin (Cipro)
fleroxacin (Quinodis [Germany])
gatiloxacin (Tequin)
grepafloxacin (Raxar)
levofloxacin (Levaquin)

lomefloxacin (Maxaquin)
moxifloxacin (Avelox)
norfloxacin (Noroxin)
ofloxacin (Floxin)
sparfloxacin (Zagam)
trovafloxacin (Trovan)

Gastrointestinal Drugs

Miscellaneous

cisapride (Propulsid)
infliximab (Avakine)

metoclopramide (Reglan)

Ulcer Preventatives

misoprostol (Cytotec)

Hair Growth Stimulants

finasteride (Proscar, Propecia)

minoxidil (Rogaine)

Heart Rhythm Regulators
See Antiarrhythmic Drugs

Hematopoietic Agents
filgrastim (Neupogen)

HMG-CoA reductase inhibitors

atorvastatin (Lipitor)
cerivastatin (Baycol) (removed from
  the US market)
fluvastatin (Lescol)

lovastatin (Mevacor)
pravastatin (Pravachol)
simvastatin (Zocor)

Hormones

Miscellaneous

nafarelin (Synarel)
See also Androgens for male sex
  hormones

See also Estrogens and Progestins for
  female sex hormones

H2 Blockers (Histamine [H2] Blocking Drugs)

cimetidine (Tagamet, Tagamet HB 200)

famotidine (Pepcid, Pepcid AC, Pepcid Complete)

nizatidine (Axid, Axid AR)

ranitidine (Zantac, Zantac 75)

Hypnotic Drugs (Sedatives/Sleep Inducers)

acetylcarbromal (Paxarel)

chloral hydrate (Aquachloral, Noctec)

estazolam (Prosom)

ethchlorvynol (Placidyl)

ethinamate (Valmid)

flurazepam (Dalmane)

glutethimide (Doriden)

methyprylon (Noludar)

paraldehyde (Paral)

propiomazine (Largon)

quazepam (Doral)

temazepam (Restoril)

triazolam (Halcion)

zaleplon (Sonata)

zolpidem (Ambien)

See also Barbiturates

Immunosuppressants

azathioprine (Imuran)

chlorambucil (Leukeran)

cyclophosphamide (Cytoxan)

cyclosporine (Sandimmune)

hydroxychloroquine (Plaquenil)

leflunomide (Arava)

serolimus (Rapamune)

tacrolimus (Prograf)

Macrolide Antibiotics (Anti-Infectives)

azithromycin (Zithromax)

clarithromycin (Biaxin)

dirithromycin (Dynabac)

erythromycin (E-Mycin, Ilosone, Erythrocin, E.E.S.)

troleandomycin (TAO)

Male Sex Hormones

See Androgens

Mast-Cell-Stabilizing Agents

See Antiasthmatic Drugs

Meglitinides

repaglinide (Prandin)

Monoamine Oxidase (MAO) Inhibitor Drugs (Type A: Antidepressants)

isocarboxazid (Marplan)

phenelzine (Nardil)

tranylcypromine (Parnate)

Muscarinic Receptor Antagonists (Anti-Incontinence)

tolteradine (Detrol)

Muscle Relaxants (Skeletal Muscle Relaxants)

baclofen (Lioresal)
carisoprodol (Rela, Soma, others)
chlorphenesin carbamate (Maolate)
chlorzoxazone (Paraflex, Parafon Forte)
cyclobenzaprine (Flexeril)
dantrolene (Dantrium)

diazepam (Valium)
meprobamate (Equanil, Miltown, others)
metaxalone (Skelaxin)
methocarbamol (Robaxin, others)
orphenadrine (Norflex, others)

Neuramidase inhibitors

oseltamivir (Tamiflu)

zanamivir (Relenza)

Nitrates

amyl nitrate (amyl nitrate generic,
    Vaporole, others)
erythrityl tetranitrate (Cardilate)
isosorbide dinitrate (Isordil,
    Sorbitrate, others)

isosorbide mononitrate (Ismo, Imdur)
nitroglycerin (Nitrostat, Nitrolingual,
    Nitrogard, Nitrong, others)
pentaerythritol tetranitrate (Duotrate,
    Peritrate)

Nonnucleoside Reverse Transcriptase Inhibitors

delavirdine (Rescriptor)
efavirenz (Sustiva)

nevirapine (Viramune)

Nonsteroidal Anti-Inflammatory Drugs (NSAIDs)
(Aspirin Substitutes)

Acetic Acids

bromfenac sodium (Duract)
diclofenac potassium (Cataflam)
diclofenac sodium (Voltaren)
etodolac (Lodine)
indomethacin (Indochron E-R,
    Indocin, Indocin SR)
ketorolac (Toradol)

meloxicam (Mobic)
nabumetone (Relafen)
sulindac (Clinoril)
tolmetin (Tolectin, Tolectin DS)
Fenamates
meclofenamate (Meclomen)
mefenamic acid (Ponstel)

Oxicams

piroxicam (Feldene)

Propionic Acids

diflunisal (Dolobid)
fenoprofen (Nalfon)
flurbiprofen (Ansaid)
ibuprofen
ketoprofen (Orudis, Oruvail)
naproxen (Naprosyn)

naproxen sodium (Aleve, Anaprox,
    Anaprox DS)
oxaprozin (Daypro)
oxyphenbutazone (Oxalid)
suprofen (Profenal)

Opioid Antagonists

naltrexone (ReVia)

Opioid Drugs (Narcotics)

alfentanil (Alfenta)
codeine
fentanyl (Actiq, Sublimaze, Duragesic)
hydrocodone (Hycodan)
hydromorphone (Dilaudid)
levorphanol (Levo-Dromoran)
meperidine (Demerol)

methadone (Dolophine)
morphine (Astramorph, Duramorph, MS Contin, Roxanol)
oxycodone (OxyContin, Roxicodone)
oxymorphone (Numorphan)
propoxyphene (Darvon)
sufentanil (Sufenta)

Pain Syndrome Modifiers (also adjuvants)

carbamazepine (Tegretol)
gabapentin (Neurontin)
phenytoin (Dilantin)

samarium-EDTMP (Quadramet)
strontium-89 (Metastron)

Penicillins (Anti-Infectives)

amoxicillin (Amoxil, Larotid, Polymox, Trimox, others)
amoxicillin/clavulanate (Augmentin)
ampicillin (Omnipen, Polycillin, Principen, Totacillin)
ampicillin/sulbactam (Unasyn)
bacampicillin (Spectrobid)
carbenicillin (Geocillin, Geopen, Pyopen)
cloxacillin (Cloxapen, Tegopen)
dicloxacillin (Dynapen, Pathocil, Veracillin)

methicillin (Staphcillin)
mezlocillin (Mezlin)
nafcillin (Nafcil, Unipen)
oxacillin (Prostaphlin)
penicillin G (Pentids, others)
penicillin V (Pen Vee K, V-Cillin K, Veetids, others)
piperacillin (Pipracil)
ticarcillin (Ticar)
ticarcillin/clavulanate (Timentin)

Phenothiazines (Antipsychotic Drugs)

acetophenazine (Tindal)
chlorpromazine (Thorazine)
fluphenazine (Permitil, Prolixin)
mesoridazine (Serentil)
perphenazine (Trilafon)
prochlorperazine (Compazine)

promazine (Sparine)
thioridazine (Mellaril)
trifluoperazine (Stelazine)
triflupromazine (Vesprin)
ziprasidone (Geodon)

Potassium Replacement Products

K-Dur

Potassium chloride (various)

Progestins (Female Sex Hormones)

ethynodiol

hydroxyprogesterone (Duralutin, Gesterol L.A., others)

medroxyprogesterone (Amen, Curretab, Prempro, Premphase, Provera)

megestrol (Megace)

norethindrone (Micronor, Norlutate, Norlutin)

norgestrel (Ovrette)

progesterone (Gesterol 50, Progestaject)

Protease Inhibitors

amprenavir (VX-1478) Agenerase

BMS-232632 azantavir (investigational)

indinavir (Crixivan)

lopinavir/ritonvair (Kaletra)

nelfinavir (Viracept)

ritonavir (Norvir)

saquinavir (Fortovase, Invirase)

Proton Pump Inhibitors (H/K ATPase Inhibitors)

esomeprazole (Nexium)

lansoprazole (Prevacid, Prevpac)

omeprazole (Prilosec)

pantoprazole (Protonix)

rabeprazole (Aciphex)

Radiopharmaceuticals

samarium-EDTMP (Quadramet)

strontium-89 (Metastron)

Salicylates

aspirin

choline salicylate (Arthropan)

magnesium salicylate (Doan's, Magan, Mobidin)

salsalate (Amigesic, Disalcid, Salsitab)

sodium salicylate

sodium thiosalicylate (Rexolate, Tusal)

Sedatives/Sleep Inducers

See Hypnotic Drugs

Selective Serotonin Reuptake Inhibitors (SSRIs)

citalopram (Celexa)

fluoxetine (Prozac)

fluvoxamine (Luvox)

nefazodone (Serzone)

paroxetine (Paxil)

sertraline (Zoloft)

trazodone (Desyrel)

venlafaxine (Effexor)

Selective Estrogen Receptor Modulators (SERMs)

raloxifene (Evista)

tamoxifen (Nolvadex)

Smoking Cessation Adjuncts
bupropion (Zyban)
nicotine (Nicorette, various patch
   brands such as Nicotrol)

Sulfonamides (Anti-Infectives)
multiple sulfonamides (Triple Sulfa No. 2)
sulfacytine (Renoquid)
sulfadiazine
sulfamethizole (Thiosulfil)
sulfamethoxazole (Gantanol)

sulfasalazine (Azulfidine)
sulfisoxazole (Gantrisin)
COX Two Inhibitor
celecoxib (Celebrex)

Sulfonylureas (Oral Antidiabetic Drugs)
acetohexamide (Dymelor)
chlorpropamide (Diabinese)
glimepiride (Amaryl)
glipizide (Glucotrol)

glyburide (DiaBeta, Micronase)
tolazamide (Ronase, Tolamide, Tolinase)
tolbutamide (Orinase)

Tetracyclines (Anti-Infectives)
demeclocycline (Declomycin)
doxycycline (Doryx, Doxychel,
   Vibramycin)
methacycline (Rondomycin)

minocycline (Minocin)
oxytetracycline (Terramycin)
tetracycline (Achromycin V, Panmycin,
   Sumycin)

Thiazide Diuretics
bendroflumethiazide (Naturetin)
benzthiazide (Aquatag, Exna, Marazide)
chlorothiazide (Diuril)
cyclothiazide (Anhydron)
hydrochlorothiazide (Esidrix,
   HydroDiuril, Oretic)

hydroflumethiazide (Diucardin, Saluron)
methyclothiazide (Enduron, Aquatensen)
polythiazide (Renese)
trichlormethiazide (Metahydrin, Naqua)

Thiazolidinediones
pioglitazone (Actos)
rosiglitazone (Avandia)

troglitazone (Rezulin)—
   no longer available in the US

Thienobenzodiazepines
olanzapine (Zyprexa)

Thyroid Hormones
levothyroxine (Synthroid)

liothyronine (Cytomel)

Tranquilizers, Major

See Antipsychotic Drugs

Tranquilizers, Minor

See Antianxiety Drugs

Vaccines (Immune Modulators)

influenza vaccine (Fluogen, Flu-Shield,
   Fluzone, FluMist)
Lyme disease vaccine (LYMErix)

pneumococcal vaccine (Prevnar)
varicella virus vaccine (Varivax)

Vasodilators (Peripheral Vasodilators)

cyclandelate (Cyclospasmol)
ethaverine (Ethaquin, Isovex)
isoxsuprine (Vasodilan)

nylidrin (Arlidin)
papaverine (Cerespan, Pavabid)

Weight Loss Agents (Miscellaneous)

Orlistat (Xenical)

Xanthines (Bronchodilators)

aminophylline (Phyllocontin,
   Truphylline)
dyphylline (Dilor, Lufyllin)

oxtriphylline (Choledyl)
theophylline (Bronkodyl, Slo-Phyllin,
   Theolair, others)

A GLOSSARY
OF
DRUG-RELATED TERMS

Glossary

addiction This is generally recognized as intense drug dependence, with uncontrollable drug-seeking behavior, *tolerance* for pleasure-giving effects, and *withdrawal* if the drug is withheld. This is *physical dependence*—where the drug is incorporated into the fundamental biochemistry of the brain. Some clinicians characterize this as a loss of control (centrality) of drug use—with continued drug use by those addicted even though it proves to be harmful. (See the terms dependence and tolerance for accounts of physical and psychological dependence.)

adherence (prior term: compliance. European term: concordance) How appropriately a patient takes their medicine according to the way it was prescribed. For example: If a medicine is to be taken three times a day and the patient actually takes it three times a day—they are perfectly adherent to their medicine (100 % adherent).

adverse effect or reaction An abnormal, unexpected, infrequent and often unpredictable injurious response to a drug. This does not include a pharmacological action, even though some may be undesirable and unintended. (See side effect.) Adverse reactions are those due to drug *allergy*, individual *idiosyncrasy*, and *toxic* effects of drugs on tissues (see allergy [drug], idiosyncrasy and toxicity).

allergy (drug) An abnormal drug response that happens after antibodies* are made to the drug itself. People with history of hay fever, asthma, hives or eczema are more likely to develop drug allergies. Allergies can develop slowly, or they can appear suddenly and require lifesaving medical attention.

alternative delivery system (ADS) A term describing a variety of health care forms other than the established fee-for-service model, such as HMOs, PPOs and others.

analgesic A drug used to relieve pain. There are three types:
- simple nonnarcotics, which block production of chemicals that cause or worsen pain (prostaglandins, etc.)—examples are acetaminophen, aspirin, nonsteroidal anti-inflammatory drugs (Motrin, Advil, etc.) and the new COX II inhibitors
- narcotic analgesics or opioids, which relieve pain by blunting pain perception in the brain—examples are morphine, codeine and hydrocodone (natural derivatives of opium) and meperidine or pentazocine (synthetic drug products)

*Antibodies are proteins that combine with foreign substances. Protective antibodies destory bacteria and neutralize toxins. Injurious antibodies react with foreign substances such as drugs to cause release of histamine, a chemical causing allergic reactions.

- local anesthetics, which relieve pain by making sensory nerve endings insensitive to pain—such as phenazopyridine (Pyridium)

anaphylactic (anaphylactoid) reaction Signs and symptoms that indicate an extreme hypersensitivity to a drug. Anaphylactic reactions often involve several body systems. Mild symptoms include itching, hives, congestion, nausea, cramping or diarrhea. Sometimes these precede severe problems, such as choking, shortness of breath and loss of consciousness (usually referred to as anaphylactic shock). Anaphylactic reactions can happen after a very small dose; they may develop suddenly and can be rapidly fatal. They are true medical emergencies. Any adverse effect appearing within 20 minutes after taking a drug should be considered an early sign of anaphylactic reaction. Get medical attention immediately! (See allergy [drug] and hypersensitivity.)

antihypertensive A drug used to lower high blood pressure. *Hypertension* describes blood pressure above a normal range. It is not nervous or emotional tension. Currently, the National Heart, Lung and Blood Institute or NHLBI describes three stages of hypertension. Optimal is 120/80 for those without diabetes and 130/80 for those living with diabetes. Stage one hypertension begins at 149/89. There are also categories a, b and c within those numerical ranges which seek to stratify risk factors onto blood pressure ranges. Medicines to treat hypertension fall into several major groups:

- drugs that increase urine production (the diuretics)
- drugs that relax blood vessel walls
- drugs that reduce sympathetic nervous system activity

  Some clinicians classify antihypertensives based on their site or mechanism of action—For example, ACE inhibitors which inhibit angiotensin converting enzyme or ARBs—antihypertensives that act as angiotensin two (AT1 subtype) receptor blockers. Please note—although high blood pressure often does not have any symptoms, you MUST treat it for life. Take your medicine EXACTLY as prescribed.

antipyretic A drug that lowers body temperature. It reduces fever by working on the hypothalamus of the brain. This leads to dilation of blood vessels (capillary beds) in the skin and brings heated blood to the skin surface for cooling. Sweat glands arc also stimulated to cool the body through evaporation. An antipyretic may also be a pain reliever (analgesic, such as acetaminophen) or analgesic and anti-inflammatory (aspirin).

aplastic anemia Also known as pancytopenia, where production of the three types of blood cells is seriously impaired. Aplastic anemia can occur from unknown causes, but about half of reported cases are caused by drugs or chemicals. A delay of one to six months may occur between the use of a drug and anemia. Symptoms include lower red blood cells (anemia), resulting in fatigue and pallor; deficiency of white blood cells (leukopenia), predisposing to infections; and low blood platelets (thrombocytopenia), which can cause spontaneous bruising or bleeding. Treatment is difficult. Even with the best of care, half the cases may be fatal. Aplastic anemia is rare, but anyone taking a drug that can cause it should have periodic complete blood cell counts. For a listing of causative drugs, see Table 5, Section Six.

Bad Med Syndrome (BMS) The decreased quality of life, decrease in expected beneficial drug results, loss of time from work, unnecessary stays in the hospital or additional treatment resulting from medicines themselves or from the improper use of medicines. Improper use includes drug interactions resulting from inappropriate medicine combinations; too low a dose (subtherapeutic dosing); too high a dose (overdose); as well as taking the medicine "every once in a while" when it was prescribed for ongoing use.

No one intends to cause Bad Med Syndrome (BMS), yet patients, pharmacists, physicians, other health care providers and many organizations all contribute to it. I believe it will take a team effort to solve it.

bioavailability How fast and how much active drug is absorbed into the blood. Two types of measurements—blood levels after it was taken and how long the drug stays in the blood—show how much drug is available to work and for how long. The two major factors that govern bioavailability are (1) the chemical and physical characteristics of the dose and (2) how well the digestive system of the person taking it works. A drug that falls apart quickly in a normal stomach or small intestine produces blood levels quite promptly. Such a drug product has good bioavailability. Drugs such as metoclopramide or cisapride that slow the gastrointestinal system may act to actually increase the amount of drug that gets into the body.

bioequivalence The ability of a drug product to cause its intended therapeutic effect is related to bioavailability. When a drug is made by several manufacturers, it is critical to pick the one that has the bioavailability needed to work. While the drug in medicines from different firms may be the same chemical, don't assume that they are equally available.

Bioavailability depends mostly on physical characteristics of how a drug is made. These determine how well a drug falls apart and releases its active drug component(s). Drug products that have the same drug but are combined with different inert additives, coated with different substances or enclosed in different capsules may or may not have the same bioavailability. Those that do are termed bioequivalent and can be relied upon to give the same result.

If you consider having your prescription filled with a generic, ask your physician and pharmacist for help. This requires professional judgment in each case. In some cases, reasonable differences in bioavailability are acceptable. For serious illnesses, or when blood levels must be kept in a narrow range, it is essential to use the drug product that has been shown to have reliable bioavailability. This has been a major area of controversy for blood thinners (anticoagulants) and medicines used to control seizures.

blood platelets The smallest of the blood cells made by bone marrow. Platelets are normally present in very large numbers. They are the basis of normal blood clotting and prevent excessive bruising or bleeding if you are injured. Platelets preserve smaller blood vessel walls. If there is damage, platelets seal small holes in vessel walls. Some drugs and chemicals may lower the platelet count. Many slow formation; other drugs hasten destruction. If the platelet count gets too low, blood begins to leak through the walls of smaller vessels. This shows as scattered bruises in the skin of the thighs or legs and is called purpura. Bleeding happens anywhere, internally as well as into the tissues immediately beneath the skin. For a listing of causative drugs, see Table 5, Section Six.

body mass index (BMI) A calculation used to measure the relative degree of a patient's obesity. This measurement is used in deciding the appropriateness of using sibutramine (Meridia). BMI is calculated using weight in kilograms divided by height in meters squared. If the BMI is greater than 30 kg per square meter or is 27 kg per square meter with other risk factors such as diabetes, sibutramine is approved for use in weight loss considering those additional factors.

bone marrow depression A decrease in the ability of bone marrow to make blood cells. This can be an adverse reaction to drugs or chemicals. Bone marrow makes most of the body's blood cells: red blood cells (erythrocytes), white blood cells (leukocytes) and platelets (thrombocytes). Each type of cell has one or more functions, critical to life and health.

Drugs that depress bone marrow may impair all types of blood cells right away or only one type selectively. Blood tests can show drug effects on bone marrow. If fewer red blood cells are made, anemia results, causing weakness, cold intolerance and shortness of breath. Low white blood cells lowers resistance to infection (fever, sore throat or pneumonia). If platelets fall to very low levels, the blood loses its ability to clot quickly. Bruising or prolonged bleeding may happen. Any of these symptoms require immediate studies of blood and bone marrow. For a listing of causative drugs, see Table 5, Section Six.

brand name The registered trade name given to a drug by its manufacturer. Each company creates a trade name to distinguish its brand of the generic drug from its competitors'. A brand name designates a proprietary drug—one that is protected by patent or copyright. Generally, brand names are shorter, easier to pronounce and more readily remembered than their generic counterparts.

capitation A system where a set amount of money is used to cover the cost of health care for a given person. For instance, a health plan or hospital is paid monthly on a negotiated per-person rate and the plan or hospital provides all health services for the people in the plan.

cause-and-effect relationship An association between a drug and a biological event—most commonly a side effect or an adverse effect. Important factors are when the drug was given, the use of multiple drugs and their possible interactions, the effects of the disease being treated, the physiological and psychological patient factors and the influences of unrecognized disorders or malfunctions.

The majority of adverse drug reactions occur sporadically, unpredictably and infrequently in the general population. A *definite* cause-and-effect relationship between drug and reaction is shown when (1) the adverse effect immediately follows dosing of the drug or (2) the adverse effect disappears after the drug is stopped (dechallenge) and reappears when the drug is used again (rechallenge) or (3) the adverse effects are clearly the expected and predictable toxic consequences of drug overdose.

There is also a large gray area of "probable," "possible" and "coincidental" associations. Clarification of cause-and-effect relationships requires observation over a long period of time, followed by sophisticated statistical analysis. Some news stories are based on suggestive but incomplete data. Though early warning is in the public interest, these stories should make clear whether the presumed relationship is based on definitive criteria or is inferred. It is critical to avoid losing valuable medicines because of poorly designed studies that find their way to the news.

The most competent techniques for evaluating cause-and-effect relationships of adverse drug reactions have been devised by the Division of Tissue Reactions to Drugs, a research unit of the Armed Forces Institute of Pathology:

No association	5.0%
Coincidental	14.5%
Possible	33.0%
Probable	30.0%
Causative	17.5%

It is significant that expert evaluation of 2,800 drug-related cases concluded that only 47.5% could be substantiated as causative or probably causative.

contraindication A condition or disease that precludes the use of a drug. Some contraindications are absolute, meaning that the drug should NEVER be used in a particular situation. Other contraindications are relative, meaning that using the drug requires expert consideration of all factors.

coordinated performance measurement for the management of adult diabetes A term used to describe a great new consensus reached by the American Medical Association (AMA), the Joint Commission on Accreditation of Healthcare Organizations (JCAHO) and The National Committee on Quality Assurance (NCQA). This body of information was released in April of 2001 and seeks to look at how typical measures, markers or preventive measures used in diabetes (such as lipid management, hemoglobin A1c and flu shots should be approached to get the best frequency of testing and avoidance of disease progression or incidental or at risk infections.

covered lives A term used by health maintenance organizations to indicate how many people have enrolled in their plan. From the HMO's point of view, a minimum number of covered lives is needed to support a certain number of family practice physicians, specialists and so on. Understanding their logic helps explain why some HMOs have one specialist while others have several.

COX-II Inhibitor A medicine that inhibits the action of cyclooxygenase or COX type two. While type one COX can have some protective functions in the body, COX-II is an enzyme that works to make compounds that lead to swelling (inflammation). If COX-II is blocked, inflammation is prevented or relieved.

creatinine clearance A measure of how well the kidneys are eliminating waste, toxins and impurities from the body. A low creatinine clearance (such as 20 ml per minute or ml/min) means poorer kidney function; a high creatinine clearance (such as 120 ml/min) means better kidney function. People who have low creatinine clearances often receive lower initial doses and smaller increases of medicines that are removed by the kidneys.

critical or clinical pathway An assortment of coordinated measures taken by a health care organization to effectively group care of specific diseases or conditions. All diagnostic tests, treatments, discharge plans and other factors are carefully studied, and practice is aimed at giving the best patient results in the most cost-effective manner.

dependence A term identifying *psychological dependence* (or *habituation*) and *physical dependence* (or *addiction*). In addition, functional dependence—the need to use a drug continuously in order to sustain a particular body function—is included.

Psychological dependence is a form of neurotic behavior—an "emotional" dependence. This characterizes itself as an obsession to satisfy a particular desire. Psychological dependence is also seen in many more socially acceptable patterns such as entertainment, sports and collecting. Unfortunately, we often see an increasing reliance on medicines to cope with everyday problems: pills for frustration, nervous stomach, tension headache and insomnia. This compulsive abuse shows little or no tendency to increase the dose (see tolerance) and minor or nonexistent physical symptoms if the medicine is taken away (withdrawn). Some clinicians include psychological dependence in their definition of addiction.

Physical dependence, which is true addiction, includes two elements: tolerance and withdrawal. Addicting drugs provide relief from anguish and pain, but can also cause a physiological tolerance requiring increased doses or repeated use to remain effective. These two features foster its becoming a functioning component in brain biochemistry. (Thus some authorities prefer the term chemical dependence.) Sudden removal of the drug causes a major upheaval in body chemistry, provoking a withdrawal syndrome—intense mental and physical pain—that is the hallmark of addiction. True addiction is rare, and fear of addiction, even with potent narcotics, should never stand in the way of effective pain control.

Functional dependence differs from both psychological and physical dependence. It occurs when a drug relieves a distressing condition and provides a sense of well-being. Drugs that cause functional dependence are often used for symptom relief. The most familiar example of functional dependence is the "laxative habit." Some types of constipation are made worse by the wrong laxative, and natural bowel function fades as the colon becomes more and more dependent on the laxative drug.

disease management An approach to prevention and treatment of a specific condition that checks how often it happens in a population, organizes resources and allocates money to reach the best balance of dollars spent and results achieved.

disulfiramlike (Antabuse-like) reaction Symptoms resulting from the interaction of alcohol and a drug causing the "Antabuse effect." Symptoms include intense facial flushing, severe throbbing headache, shortness of breath, chest pains, nausea, repeated vomiting, sweating and weakness. If a large enough amount of alcohol is present, the reaction may progress to blurred vision, vertigo, marked drop in blood pressure and loss of consciousness. Severe reactions may lead to convulsions and death. The reaction can last from 30 minutes to several hours, depending upon the amount of alcohol in the body. As the symptoms subside, the person is exhausted and often sleeps for several hours.

diuretic A drug that increases urine volume. Diuretics work in several ways to accomplish this. Diuretics are used to (1) remove excess water from the body (as in congestive heart failure and some types of liver and kidney disease) and (2) treat hypertension by promoting excretion of sodium from the body.

divided doses The total daily dose of a medicine is split into smaller individual doses over the course of a day.

DMARD A Disease-Modifying Antirheumatic Drug. These medicines represent a true breakthrough in rheumatoid arthritis (RA) because they actually attack the cause of RA. For example, leflunomide (Arava) works to shut down T-cells destroying tissue, and etanercept (Enbrel) works to bind tumor necrosis factor (TNF) so that it can't harm joints.

dosage forms and strengths This information category in the individual Drug Profiles (Section Two) uses several abbreviations to designate measurements of weight and volume:

mcg	= microgram	=	1,000,000th of a gram (weight)
mg	= milligram	=	1,000th of a gram (weight)
ml	= milliliter	=	1,000th of a liter (volume)
gm	= gram	=	1,000 milligrams (weight)

There are approximately 65 mg in 1 grain.
There are approximately 5 ml in 1 teaspoon.
There are approximately 15 ml in 1 tablespoon.
There are approximately 30 ml in 1 ounce.
One milliliter of water weighs 1 g.
There are approximately 454 g in 1 pound.

drug, drug product Terms used interchangeably to describe a medicine (in any form) used in medical practice. The term *drug* refers to the single chemical that provokes a specific response when put in a biological system—the "active" ingredient. A *drug product* is the dosage form—tablet, capsule, elixir, etc.—that has the active drug mixed with inactive ingredients to provide convenient dosing. Drug products that have one active ingredient are called single-entity drugs. Drug products with two or more active ingredients are called combination drugs ([CD] in the brand names in the Drug Profiles, Section Two).

drug class A group of drugs that are similar in chemistry, method of action, and use. Because of their common characteristics, many drugs in a class will cause the same side effects and have similar potential for related adverse reactions and interactions. Variations among members within a drug class can occur. This can let choices be made if certain benefits are desired or particular side effects are to be minimized. Examples: Antihistamines and phenothiazines (see Drug Classes, Section Four).

drug family A group of drugs that are similar in chemistry, method of action and purpose. In *The Essential Guide*, drug families are identified by entries such as the Minimally Sedating Antihistamine Family. This allows you to easily compare the drugs meeting the criteria for listing in the book.

drug fever Increased body temperature caused by a medicine. Drugs can cause fever by allergic reactions, tissue damage, acceleration of tissue metabolism, constriction of skin blood vessels and direct action on the brain. The most common form of drug fever is allergic. It may be the only allergic symptom, or it may include skin rash, hives, joint swelling and pain, enlarged lymph glands, hemolytic anemia or hepatitis. The fever usually appears about 7 to 10 days after starting the drug and varies from low-grade to alarmingly high levels. It may be sustained or intermittent, but it usually lasts for as long as the drug is taken. Although many drugs can cause fever, the following are more commonly responsible:

allopurinol
antihistamines
atropinelike drugs
barbiturates
coumarin anticoagulants
hydralazine
iodides
isoniazid
methyldopa
nadolol
novobiocin
para-aminosalicylic acid
penicilin
pentazocine
phenytoin
procainamide
propylthiouracil
quinidine
rifampin
sulfonamindes

evidence-based medicine An important concept in therapeutics that impacts which medicines are used and how they are used. This involves combining recent best research (evidence) with knowledge of how disease happens (pathophysiology), patient preferences and clinical expertise in order to come up with the best individualized medicine for any given patient. Fortunately, development and use of evidence-based medicine skills is now being integrated into US medical schools.

extension effect An unwanted but predictable drug response that is a result of mild to moderate overdose. It is an exaggeration of the drug's pharmacological action; it can be thought of as a mild form of dose-related toxicity (see overdosage and toxicity).

Example: The continued "hangover" of mental sluggishness that persists in the morning is a common extension effect of a long-acting sleep-inducing drug (a hypnotic such as Dalmane) taken the night before.

FDA-approvable A stage in the Food and Drug Administration's review and approval process. A medicine is considered FDA-approvable once the panel that reviewed the supporting data submitted to the FDA finds that data acceptable. In general, at this point only final details need to be resolved before the drug becomes FDA-approved and is made available for general use.

FDA-review status A description of chemical types and review status has been developed by the FDA. Chemical types are divided into:

1. New molecular entity
2. New ester, new salt form or other covalent derivative
3. New formulation
4. New combination
5. New manufacturer
6. New indication
7. Drug already marketed, but without an approved NDA

The review process is divided into:

Fast track: Critical review for a new treatment for a life threatening condition (such as a new HIV/AIDS drug)

Priority review: Significant improvement compared to marketed products, in the treatment, diagnosis, or prevention of a disease.

Standard review: The drug appears to have therapeutic qualities similar to those of one or more already marketed drugs.

fructosamine A new term in diabetes which is also known as Glycated protein. Fructosamine is used in conjunction with glycosylated hemoglobin (hemoglobin A1C) to check to see how well blood sugar has been controlled. Unlike A1C, fructosamine gives a picture of glucose control for prior weeks versus months. There is a home glucose meter that tests fructosamine.

generic name The official, common or public name used to describe an active drug. Generic names are coined by committees of drug experts and are approved by governmental agencies for national and international use. Many drug products are marketed only under a generic name. The drugs most commonly prescribed as generics are listed below, ranked in descending order of new or refill prescriptions issued.

amoxicillin	cephalexin
hydrocodone/acetaminophen	acetaminophen/codeine
furosemide	propoxyphene-N/acetaminophen
albuterol aerosol	triamterene/HCTZ
trimethoprim/Sulfa	ibuprofen

genetic diversity This is actually a descriptive term used to identify ways in which a given person's genetic makeup differs from the expected sequences of the human genome. Snippets of nuclear material are analyzed, and once variant sequences are identified, in time we may be able to remove them and restore people to health.

genetic therapy Perhaps the most promising area of therapy in medicine today. Healthy genetic material is isolated and inserted into appropriate but diseased cells. For example, normal lung genes are given to a person with cystic fibrosis. Still very experimental, it may someday allow people suffering with genetically based diseases or conditions to receive therapy that changes the affected genes and actually *cures* those conditions. The latest approaches are working on causing the heart to grow new blood vessels and actually reversing congestive heart failure by the AC-6 gene. One of the true break-throughs in medicine for this edition was the complete identification of the human genome by a private US company. There are some 3 billion base pairs, and an estimated 40,000 genes in the human genome. Some 20 dis-eases cause more than 80% of deaths around the world. About 200–300 genes are responsible for these diseases. Considering that about every three weeks we in essence get a new heart from the same set of genes, if controlling the genes becomes a reality—-we can possibly knock out heart disease!

habituation A form of drug dependence based upon strong psychological gratifi-cation. Ongoing use of mood-altering drugs or those relieving minor discom-forts results from compulsive need to feel pleasure and satisfaction or to escape emotional distress. If these drugs are abruptly stopped, a withdrawal does not result. Thus habituation is a *psychological dependence.* (See depend-ence for more on psychological and physical dependence.)

hemolytic anemia Lower red blood cells and hemoglobin caused by premature destruction (hemolysis) of red blood cells. One way that this happens is from a genetic lowering of glucose-6-phosphate dehydrogenase (G6PD), a needed enzyme. If patients with this condition are given antimalarial drugs or sulfa drugs, red cells will be destroyed. One type of drug-induced hemolytic ane-mia is a form of allergy. Many widely used drugs (such as quinidine and lev-odopa) can cause hemolytic destruction of red cells as an allergic reaction. Hemolytic anemia can occur abruptly or silently. The acute form lasts about 7 days and shows as fever, pallor, weakness, dark-colored urine and varying degrees of jaundice. If drug-induced hemolytic anemia is mild, there may be no symptoms (see idiosyncrasy and allergy [drug]). For drugs that may cause this, see Table 5, Section Six.

hepatitislike reaction Some drugs may cause liver damage similar to viral hep-atitis. Symptoms of drug-induced hepatitis and viral hepatitis are often so similar that only laboratory tests can tell the difference. Hepatitis from drugs may be allergy, or it may be a toxic adverse effect. Serious liver reactions usu-ally lead to jaundice (see jaundice). For drugs that can cause this, see Table 8, Section Six.

HMO Abbreviation for Health Maintenance Organization—a health care system that provides a broad spectrum of medical therapies and services by a collec-tive group of people in a common organization.

hospitalist A relatively new term used to denote a physician who specializes in working in a hospital as opposed to a doctor who primarily has an office-based practice. The intent here is to create a group of doctors who are very familiar with critical paths, streamlining and other hospital methods to make length of stay as appropriate as possible.

hypersensitivity Over-responsiveness to drugs. Used in this sense, it means that the response is appropriate but the degree of response is exaggerated. More widely used today to identify allergy. To have *hypersensitivity* to a drug is to be allergic to it (see allergy [drug]). Some people develop cross-hypersensi-tivity. This means that allergy to one drug will also lead to a reaction to other closely related drugs.

Example: A *hypersensitive* patient had seasonal hay fever and asthma since child-hood. His *allergy* to penicillin developed after his third treatment. The *hypersen-sitivity* was a diffuse, measleslike rash. When he was later given a cephalosporin antibiotic (chemically related to penicillins), he developed the same rash.

hypnotic A drug used to cause sleep. Classes include antihistamines, barbiturates, benzodiazepines and several unrelated compounds. In the past 15 years, benzodiazepines have largely replaced barbiturates. In general, they are safer and have lower dependence potential. Tolerance to the hypnotic effect can happen after several weeks of continual use, so hypnotics should be used for short periods of time.

hypoglycemia Sugar (glucose) in blood below the normal range. Since the brain only runs on sugar, the brain can be seriously impaired by too low a sugar level. Early warnings include headache, mild drunkenness feeling, hunger and an inability to think clearly. If blood sugar falls further, nervousness and confusion develop. Weakness, numbness, trembling, sweating and rapid heartbeat follow. If blood sugar drops further, impaired speech and unconsciousness, with or without convulsions, will follow. Treatment for any low blood sugar (hypoglycemia) is important. If you take a drug that can cause hypoglycemia it is prudent to know the symptoms and what to do if hypoglycemia occurs.

hypothermia When internal body temperature falls below 98.6 degrees F or 37 degrees C. By definition, hypothermia is a body temperature of less than 95 degrees F or 35 degrees C. The elderly and debilitated are more prone to hypothermia. Most cases are initiated by room temperatures below 65 degrees F or 18.3 degrees C. This can develop suddenly, can mimic a stroke and has a mortality rate of 50%. Some drugs, such as phenothiazines, barbiturates and benzodiazepines, may make hypothermia more likely.

idiosyncrasy An abnormal drug response that happens in people with a defect in body chemistry (often hereditary) that produces an effect totally unrelated to the drug's normal action. This is not a form of allergy. Some defects responsible for idiosyncratic drug reactions are well understood; others are not.

Example: Some 100 million people (including 10% of African-Americans) have a low glucose-6-phosphate dehydrogenase (G6PD) in red blood cells. The cells then disintegrate when exposed to sulfonamides (Gantrisin, Kynex), nitrofurantoin (Furadantin, Macrodantin), probenecid (Benemid), quinine and quinidine. This can lead to a serious anemia.

immunosuppressive A drug that suppresses the immune system. Immunosuppression may be an intended drug effect, such as cyclosporine preventing the rejection of a transplanted kidney. In other cases, it is an unwanted side effect, as in the long-term use of cortisonelike drugs (to control asthma) suppressing the immune system. Chronic disorders thought to be auto-immune—such as rheumatoid arthritis, ulcerative colitis and systemic lupus erythematosus—may be eased by immunosuppressive medicines.

INR This is a term used in blood thinning or anticoagulation. It stands for International Normalized Ratio. The intent of the INR is to remove the problem of testing variation in reagents from laboratory to laboratory in coagulation results. The INR helps make a coagulation test (protime number and then calculated ratio) mean the same thing for a patient being tested in New York or Omaha. The sequence happens like this: Blood is drawn from the patient, and a prothrombin time or protime test is done. The protime number is then put into a calculation that standardizes the result. The end of the math is an INR, a ratio that tells a clinician to what degree the ability of the blood to clot (coagulate) has been changed by warfarin or a clotting factor problem.

interaction A change in a drug that results when a second drug (altering the action of the first) is given to the same person. Some interactions can enhance the effect of either drug, giving a response similar to overdose.

Other interactions may reduce drug effectiveness and cause inadequate response. A third interaction can produce an unrelated toxic response with no increase or decrease in the interacting drugs. Many interactions can be anticipated, and appropriate adjustments in dose can be made to prevent or minimize fluctuations in drug response.

jaundice A yellowing in the color of skin (and the white portion of the eyes) that occurs when bile accumulates in blood because of impaired liver function. Jaundice can happen from a wide variety of diseases or may be an adverse reaction to a drug. Jaundice due to a drug is always a serious adverse effect. If you take a medicine that can cause jaundice, watch closely for any change in urine or feces color. Dark discoloration of urine or pale (lack of color) stools may be early indication of developing jaundice. If this happens, call your doctor promptly. Lab tests can clarify the nature of the jaundice. Table 8, Section Six lists causative drugs.

JNC VI A national committee of experts that meets to try to establish a framework of medicines used to treat high blood pressure. The committee reviews the currently available drugs and attempts to organize possible treatments into a logical approach for lowering high blood pressure and prolonging lives.

low dose medications A group of medicines which have been found to be effective in some patients in doses that are lower than the doses recommended by the manufacturer. This area of therapeutics is controversial and results from the gap between valid and valuable research publication and the time it takes for a manufacturer to send needed data to the FDA, the FDA review and approval for changes to the approved labeling of the medicine. Some of the controversy also revolves around varying opinion as to required outcomes from treatment from medicines.

low molecular weight heparins A group of blood thinning (anticoagulant) medicines used to prevent abnormal blood clots (venous thromboembolisms or VTEs). New recommendations from the Sixth American College of Chest Physicians may lead to increased use of these medicines versus unfractionated heparins to prevent these clots (VTEs) in high risk patients.

lupus erythematosus (LE) A serious disease, seen in two forms: one limited to skin (discoid LE) and the other involving several body systems (systemic LE). Both forms occur mostly in young women. About 5% of cases of discoid form convert to the systemic form. Systemic LE is an immune disorder that can be chronic, with progressive inflammation destroying connective tissue of the skin, blood vessels, joints, brain, heart muscle, lungs and kidneys. Altered proteins in the blood lead to antibody formation that attacks the person's own organs or tissues. Low white blood cells and platelets often occur. The course of systemic LE is usually quite protracted and unpredictable. There is no cure, but acceptable management may be achieved in some cases by judicious use of cortisonelike drugs.

Several drugs can start a form of systemic LE quite similar to that which occurs spontaneously. Symptoms may appear as early as two weeks or as late as years after starting the drug. Initial symptoms are usually low-grade fever, skin rashes of various kinds, aching muscles and multiple joint pains. Chest pains (pleurisy) are fairly common. Enlargement of the lymph glands occurs less frequently. Symptoms usually subside if the drug is stopped, but laboratory evidence of the reaction may persist for many months.

medication map (MM) A new concept in medicines pioneered by Dr. Rybacki. One of the flaws in current drug information is that it is provided for individual medicines when patients actually often take medicines during the same day and in combination as well. Patients are not given a schedule that organizes their medicines into a framework that works well with their usual day. The medication map seeks to organize any and all of the medicines a patient takes into a clear schedule using the best possible times, combinations and results or outcomes data. A medication map helps avoid drug-drug, drug-food and drug activity interactions, and gives the patient the best possible quality of life.

national cholesterol education program (NCEP) A program of the National Institutes of Health that works to standardize the approach to cholesterol laboratory values, treatments and patient care using evidence-based medicine principles. The new guidelines ATP III (Adult Treatment) were released in 2001 and will probably help save thousands of lives when they are successfully implemented.

neuroleptic malignant syndrome (NMS) A rare, serious, sometimes fatal idiosyncratic reaction to neuroleptic (antipsychotic) drugs. Symptoms include hyperthermia (temperatures of 102 to 104 degrees F), marked muscle rigidity and coma. Rapid heart rate and breathing, profuse sweating, tremors and seizures can also occur. Two-thirds of cases happen in men, one-third in women. Mortality rate is 15 to 20%.

The following drugs may cause this reaction:

amantadine (Symmetrel)
amitripyline+perphenazine
(Triavil)
amoxapine (Asendin)
bromocriptine (Parlodel)
carbamazepine (Tegretol)
chlorpromazine (Thorazine)
chlorprothixine (Taractan)
clomipramine (Anafranil)
clozapine (Clozaril)
cyclobenzaprine
doxepin (Asendin)
fluoxetine (Prozac)
fluphenazine (Permitil, Prolixin)
fluvoxamine (Luvox)
haloperidol (Haldol)
imipramine (Tofranil, etc.)

levoda + carbidopa (Sinemet)
lithium (Lithobid)
loxapine (Loxitane)
metoclopramide (Reglan, Octamide)
molindone (Moban)
oral contraceptives (combination)
paroxetine (Paxil)
perphenazine (Etrafon, Trilafon)
pimozide (Orap)
prochlorperzine (Compazine)
risperidone (Risperdal)
sertraline (Zoloft)
thioridazine (Mellaril)
thiothixene (Navane)
trifluoperazine (Stelazine)
trimeprazine (Temaril)
zotepine (Nipolept)

orthostatic hypotension A type of low blood pressure related to body position or posture (also called postural hypotension). People who get orthostatic hypotension may have normal blood pressure lying down, but on sitting upright or standing will feel light-headed, dizzy and as if they are going to faint. These symptoms come from inadequate blood flow (oxygen supply) to the brain.

Many drugs may cause orthostatic hypotension. Tell your doctor if you have this effect so that changes can be made. If this situation isn't corrected, severe falls or injury may result. It is prudent to avoid sudden standing, prolonged standing, vigorous exercise and exposure to hot environments. Alcoholic beverages should be used cautiously until combined effects with the drug in use have been determined.

outcomes research A concept in health care evaluation that considers the benefits (gauged by a variety of measures) of using a particular drug versus another. This may lead to the cheapest drug not being the drug of choice, because the outcomes from therapy don't stand up over time or may result in significant treatment failure.

overdose The meaning of this term is not limited to doses exceeding the normal range recommended by a manufacturer. The "best" dose of many drugs varies greatly from person to person. An average dose for most people can be an overdose for some and an underdose for others. Factors such as age, body size, nutritional status and liver and kidney function have significant great impact on dosing.

Drugs with narrow safety margins often give signs of overdose if removal of the daily dose is delayed. Massive overdose—as in accidental ingestion of drugs by children or with suicides—is referred to as poisoning.

over-the-counter (OTC) drugs Medicines that can be bought without prescriptions. Many people do not look upon OTC medicines as drugs. It is important to remember that OTC medicines can have a variety of actions. OTC drugs may react with one another and can also react with prescription medicines. Serious problems can arise when (1) the patient fails to tell the doctor about OTC drug(s) he or she is taking ("because they really aren't drugs") and (2) the doctor fails to specify that his or her question about which drugs are being taken includes all OTC drugs and herbal meds as well. During any treatment, patients need to talk with their doctor or pharmacist about any OTC drug that he or she wishes to take. The major classes of OTC drugs for internal use include:

allergy medicines (antihistamines)	menstrual aids
antacids	motion sickness remedies
antiworm medicines	pain relievers
aspirin and aspirin combinations	salt substitutes
aspirin substitutes	sedatives and tranquilizers
asthma aids	sleeping pills
cold medicines (decongestants)	smoking cessation products
cough medicines	stimulants (caffeine)
diarrhea remedies	sugar substitutes (saccharin)
digestion aids	tonics
diuretics	vaginal yeast infection medicines
heartburn medicines	vitamins
iron laxatives	weight-reduction aids
laxatives	

paradoxical reaction A drug response that does not follow the known pharmacology of a drug. These effects are due to individual sensitivity and can occur at any age. They are seen more commonly in children and the elderly.

Example: An 80-year-old man was sent to a nursing home after his wife died. He had trouble adjusting to his new environment and was agitated and irritable. He was given diazepam (Valium) to relax him, starting with small doses. On the second day he became confused. The dose of diazepam was increased. On the third day he began to wander, talked incessantly and was angry when attempts were made to help him. Suspecting a paradoxical reaction, his health care provider stopped the diazepam. All behavioral disturbances subsided in three days.

Parkinson-like disorders (parkinsonism) A group of symptoms resembling Parkinson's disease. The typical features of parkinsonism include a fixed, emotionless facial expression (masklike in appearance); trembling hands, arms or legs; and stiffness of extremities that produces rigid posture and gait. Parkinsonism is a fairly common adverse effect that occurs in about 15% of patients who take large doses of phenothiazines or use them over an extended period. If found early, the Parkinson-like features will lessen or disappear with lower doses or different medicines. In some cases, Parkinson-like changes may become permanent.

peripheral neuritis (peripheral neuropathy) A group of symptoms that results from injury to nerve tissue in the extremities. A variety of drugs or chemicals can cause this. The sensation of numbness and tingling usually starts in the toes and fingers and is accompanied by altered sensation to touch. Vague discomfort from aching sensations to burning pain is also seen. Severe forms of peripheral neuritis may include loss of muscular strength and coordination. Isoniazid can cause this condition.

If vitamin B6 (pyridoxine) is not given with isoniazid, peripheral neuritis may occur. Vitamin B6 can be both preventive and curative in this form of drug-induced peripheral neuritis.

Since peripheral neuritis can also be a late complication of many viral infections, care must be taken to avoid assigning a cause-and-effect relationship to a drug that is not responsible for the nerve injury (see cause-and-effect relationship). See Table 10, Section Six, for further discussion of drug-induced nerve damage.

Peyronie's disease A permanent deformity of the penis caused by dense fibrous (scarlike) tissue within in the penile vessels that become engorged with blood during an erection. During sexual arousal, inelastic fibrous tissue causes painful downward bowing of the penis that hampers or precludes intercourse. This condition has been caused by phenytoin (Dilantin, etc.) and with most members of the beta-blocker drugs (see Drug Classes, Section Four). For a listing of causative drugs, see Table 11, Section Six.

pharmacoeconomics The discipline within pharmacology that studies the issues of costs versus benefits, utilizing a variety of measures: material and personnel costs, treatment outcomes, quality of patient life, etc. Study results are used in deciding where and how health care resources should be utilized.

pharmacogenomics The use of knowledge of the human genome, actions of genes and the way that certain genes are active or inactive in a disease to design medicines. This new area also takes into account the concept of individualizing an approach to patients based on THEIR specific genes. The first medicine to result from pharmacogenomics is imatinib or Gleevec (see new drug profile). This medicine is a signal transduction inhibitor that works to turn off a gene that is active in leukemia and a rare kind of stomach tumor.

pharmacology The medical science relating to development and use of drugs as well as their composition and action in animals and humans. Used in its broadest sense, pharmacology embraces related sciences of medicinal chemistry, experimental therapeutics and toxicology.

photosensitivity A drug-induced skin change resulting in a rash or exaggerated sunburn on exposure to the sun or ultraviolet lamps. The reaction is confined to uncovered areas of skin, giving a clue to the nature of its cause. For a list of causative drugs, see Table 2, Section Six.

porphyria Hereditary disorders where excessive amounts of respiratory pigments known as porphyrins are made. (One porphyrin is part of hemoglobin in red blood cells.) Two forms of porphyria—acute intermittent porphyria and cutaneous porphyria—can be activated by drugs. Acute intermittent porphyria involves nervous system damage. An attack can include fever, rapid heart rate, vomiting, pain in the abdomen and legs, hallucinations, seizures, paralysis and coma. Some examples of causative drugs include: barbiturates, "sulfa" drugs, chlordiazepoxide (Librium), chlorpropamide (Diabinese), methyldopa (Aldomet) and phenytoin (Dilantin).

Cutaneous porphyria involves skin and liver damage. Symptoms include red and blistered skin, followed by crusting, scarring and excessive hair growth. Repeated liver damage can lead to cirrhosis. This form of porphyria can be caused by chloroquine, estrogen, oral contraceptives and excessive iron.

priapism Prolonged, painful erection of the penis usually on sexual arousal. It is caused by obstruction to drainage of blood through the veins at the root of the penis. Erection may last for 30 minutes to a few hours and then subside, or it may persist for up to 30 hours and require surgical drainage. More than half priapism from drugs results in permanent impotence. Sickle cell anemia may predispose to priapism, and those with this disorder should avoid all drugs that may cause priapism.

Drugs reported to induce priapism include:

anabolic steroids (male hormonelike
   drugs: Anadrol, Anavar, Android,
   Halotestin, Metandren, Oreton,
   Testred, Winstrol
chlorpromazine (Thorazine)
cocaine
guanethidine (Ismelin)
heparin

levodopa (Sinemet)
molindone (Moban)
prazosin (Minipres)
prochlorperzine (Compazine)
trazodone (Desyrel)
trifluoperazine (Stelazine)
warfarin (Coumadin)

prostatism The difficulties that happen with an enlarged prostate. As the prostate enlarges, it constricts the urethra (outflow passage) and impedes urination. This causes a lower size and force of the urinary stream, hesitancy, interruption and incomplete bladder emptying. Atropine and drugs with atropinelike effects can impair the bladder's ability to compensate for the prostate gland, intensifying all of the above symptoms.

QT interval medicines This new term is used to describe drugs that can have an effect on part of the heart beat (QT interval) and pose a complicated benefit to risk decision in people with heart rhythm problems or who are at increased risk for heart rhythm problems (such as the elderly, people with existing heart disease, women, those with low magnesium or potassium and others). These medicines have led to such concern that the FDA will now require all new drugs to be tested for QT interval prolongation.

Raynaud's phenomenon Intermittent episodes of reduced blood flow to fingers or toes, with resulting paleness, discomfort, numbness and tingling. Stress or exposure to cold can cause attack. It can occur as part of a systemic disorder (lupus erythematosus, scleroderma), or it can occur without apparent cause (Raynaud's disease). Beta-adrenergic blockers and products that contain ergotamine can lead to Raynaud-like symptoms in predisposed people.

Reye (Reye's) syndrome A sudden, often fatal, childhood illness where the brain swells and the liver degenerates. It usually develops during a viral infection (flu), measles or chicken pox. Cases have been seen with lupus (SLE). Symptoms include fever, headache, delirium, loss of consciousness and seizures. It is one of the 10 major causes of death in children ages 1 to 10 years. Those younger than 18 may be affected. The syndrome may be due to combined effects of viral infection and chemical toxins in a genetically predisposed child. Drugs that have been used prior to symptoms include salicylates (aspirin) and drugs to control nausea and vomiting. This is why salicylates (aspirin and aspirinlike medicines) should be avoided in children with flu-like infections, chicken pox or measles. Some clinicians question use of any NSAID. Remember to look for salicylates in combination cold or flu products and inflammatory bowel drugs. Valproic acid (a seizure medicine) can cause a Reye-like syndrome. Acetaminophen appears to be the medicine of choice in those less than 18 with fever from a sudden viral illness.

secondary effect A complication of drug use that does not occur as part of the drug's primary pharmacological activity. Secondary effects are unwanted consequences and are adverse effects.

Example: Cramping of leg muscles can be a secondary effect of diuretic (urine-producing) drug treatment for high blood pressure. Excessive loss of potassium renders the muscle vulnerable to painful spasm during exercise.

SIADH A Syndrome of Inappropriate Antidiuretic Hormone excretion. This may be caused by medicines and is repeatedly cited where appropriate in the text. Since antidiuretic hormone (ADH) works to control the amount of water that the body retains, excessive ADH causes the body to retain water. This can be very serious, as the excessive water dilutes minerals such as sodium, which is critical for life.

side effect A normal, expected and predictable response to a drug. Side effects are part of a drug's pharmacological activity and are unavoidable. Most side effects are undesirable. The majority cause minor annoyance and inconvenience; a few can be hazardous.

superinfection (suprainfection) A second infection superimposed on an initial infection. The superinfection is caused by organisms not killed by the drug(s) used to treat the original (primary) infection. This kind of infection usually happens during or following use of a broad-spectrum antibiotic. The disturbance of the normal balance of bacteria permits overgrowth of organisms usually found in numbers too small to cause disease. The superinfection may also require treatment, using those drugs that are effective against the offending organism.

Example: A woman is given an antibiotic for a sinus infection. This medicine changes the bacteria usually present in her vagina, allowing yeast to grow. The yeast infection must then be treated with a second medicine.

tardive dyskinesia A drug-induced nervous system disorder with involuntary and bizarre movements of eyelids, jaws, lips, tongue, neck and fingers. It can happen after use of potent drugs for mental illness. It may occur in any age group but is more common in the middle-aged and especially in chronically ill older women. Once it starts, it may be irreversible. To date, there is no way of identifying who may develop this reaction. The abnormal movement (dyskinesia) is not associated with decline in mental function.

tolerance A situation where the body adapts to a medicine and reacts to it less vigorously over time. Tolerance can be beneficial or harmful in treatment.

Example: Beneficial tolerance happens when someone with hay fever finds that drowsiness from their antihistamine gradually disappears after 4 or 5 days of continuous use. Harmful tolerance occurs when the patient with "shingles" (herpes zoster) finds that the usual dose of pain medicine no longer works to relieve pain.

toxicity Capacity of a drug to impair body functions or damage tissues. Most drug toxicity is related to total dose: the larger the dose, the greater the toxic effects. Some drugs are toxic in normal doses. Toxic effects due to overdose are often a harmful extension of normal pharmacological actions and may be predictable and preventable.

Treat to Goal An important yet widely underused concept. One of the features in this edition of the Guide is the concept of treatment goals, measurements and outcomes. Treating to goal means that when a particular medicine is considered, results and timeframes to achieve those goals are set and communicated to the patient. If goals are NOT achieved, medication doses can often be increased (if not at maximum), new medicines can be added or different non-pharmacological approaches may be tried in order to reach the goal. A good example is treatment of high cholesterol (hyperlipidemia). It is not enough to find elevated cholesterol, start a medicine (such as an HMG-CoA reductase inhibitor or statin) and forget about it. The treatment goal of the medicine (such as getting the LDL to less than 130 mg/dl or HDL to more than 40 mg/dl) should be explained, the medicine started, and then cholesterol rechecked in a reasonable interval (such as three months). If the goal is achieved, and the treatment well tolerated—the medicine should be continued. If the goal is not reached and a medicine such as Pravachol (Pravastatin) is being used, it is reasonable (depending on the starting dose) to increase the dose and then recheck the cholesterol in three months. The process then continues until the National Cholesterol Education Program (NCEP) target or the target chosen by your doctor is reached.

trough-to-peak ratio (T/P) A concept used to check dosing of medicines for high blood pressure. The T/P ratio is calculated by dividing the blood pressure level immediately before the next drug dose (trough) by the largest blood pressure drop during the time between doses. A result greater than 50% means that the effect of the medicine over the entire time between doses is ideal.

tyramine A chemical present in many common foods and beverages that raises blood pressure. Normally, enzymes in the body neutralize tyramine (monoamine oxidase [MAO] type A). If the action of MAO type A is blocked, substances such as tyramine can cause alarming and dangerous increases in blood pressure.

Several drugs can block monoamine oxidase type A. They are called monoamine oxidase (MAO) type A inhibitors (see Drug Classes, Section Four). If you take one of these drugs and your diet includes foods or beverages high in tyramine, sudden increases in blood pressure may happen. Talk with your doctor or pharmacist about an appropriate diet and before combining any other medicine with an MAO inhibitor.

The following foods and beverages have been reported to contain varying amounts of tyramine. Unless their tyramine content is known to be insignificant, they should be avoided altogether while taking an MAO type A inhibitor drug.

FOODS	BEVERAGES
Aged cheeses of all kinds*	Beer (unpasteurized)
Avocado	Chianti wine
Banana skins	Sherry wine
Bean curd	Vermouth
Bologna	
"Bovril" extract	
Broad bean pods	

Chicken liver (unless fresh
  and used at once)
Chocolate
Figs, canned
Fish, canned
Fish, dried and salted
Herring, pickled
Liver, if not very fresh
"Marmite" extract
Meat extracts
Meat tenderizers
Pepperoni
Raisins
Raspberries
Salami
Shrimp paste
Sour cream
Soy sauce
Yeast extracts

Note: *Any* high-protein food that is aged or has undergone breakdown by putrefaction probably contains tyramine and could produce a hypertensive crisis in anyone taking MAO type A inhibitor drugs.

viral load or viral burden A term used in reference to AIDS patients to describe the amount of HIV virus present in the body at any given time. The amount of virus relates to how well drug therapy is working, and can be a reason to change drugs if the load increases.

WHO Pain Ladder A therapeutic scheme using increasing strengths and combinations of pain medicines (analgesics) that includes NSAIDs, opiates and adjuvant drugs to control pain as specified by the World Health Organization (WHO). It is not an absolute treatment scheme, but it should be used to organize the approach to effective pain prevention.

WOMAC A widely used approach to measure the health status of osteoarthritis patients. This scale is the Western Ontario and McMaster University index or WOMAC. What it does is work to check (assess) the therapeutic scheme using increasing strengths and combinations of pain medicines (analgesics) that include NSAIDs, opiates and adjuvant drugs to control pain as specified by the World Health Organization (WHO). It is not an absolute assessment scheme, but used correctly, organizes patient information into a rational approach to checking how compromised the patient is before the medicine is added and then allows an objective follow-up check on how well the medicine is working.

TABLES OF DRUG INFORMATION

TABLE 1

Drugs That May Adversely Affect the Fetus and Newborn Infant

In 1961, a decision was made to use thalidomide to try to make pregnancy less stressful. Despite these laudable intensions, this became the thalidomide disaster of 1961 because this medicine (and many others) causes birth defects or even fetal death if used during pregnancy (possible teratogens or embryocidal medicines). This does NOT mean that the medicines are "bad" medicines. For example, extremely effective medicines such as the HMG-CoA inhibitors for lowering cholesterol should NEVER be taken during pregnancy (Category X). Thalidomide itself has seen a resurrection because it fights an important body chemical called Tumor Necrosis Factor or TNF. It still should NEVER be used in pregnancy, but now has a valuable role treating erythema nodosum leprosum (ENL).

Our understanding of how drugs can affect the fetus or newborn infant continues to grow, and the list of the drugs that can cause significant harm to the unborn and newborn child has gotten larger and larger. In many cases, it is not possible to clearly separate adverse effects due to the mother's disease or disorder from those that may be caused by medicines. Based on current knowledge, it is strongly recommended that only those drugs that confer clear and essential benefits should be used during pregnancy. Some medicines also have pregnancy registries sponsored by the company that makes the product. Where possible, I have included the 800 numbers for these as I consider them to be a good idea if the decision is made to use a medicine in pregnancy. Talk to your doctor for more information.

Drugs that *probably* cause adverse effects when taken during the *first* trimester

aminopterin	finasteride	misoprostol
anticonvulsants*	fluorouracil	opioid analgesics*
antithyroid drugs	HMG-CoA reductase	progestins*
cytarabine	inhibitors*	quinine
danazol	iodides	streptomycin
diethylstilbestrol	isotretinoin	testosterone
ethanol (large amounts	kanamycin	thalidomide
and for long periods)	mercaptopurine	warfarin
etretinate	methotrexate	

Drugs that *possibly* cause adverse effects when taken during the *first* trimester

angiotensin-converting	lithium	oral contraceptives
enzyme inhibitors*	mebendazole	piperazine
busulfan	monoamine oxidase	rifampin
chlorambucil	(MAO) inhibitors*	tetracyclines*
estrogens*		

Drugs that *probably* cause adverse effects when taken during the *second* and *third* trimesters

amiodarone	chloramphenicol	iodides
androgens*	estrogens*	kanamycin
angiotensin-converting	ethanol (large amounts	lithium
enzyme inhibitors*	and for long periods)	nonsteroidal anti-
antithyroid drugs	finasteride	inflammatory drugs*
aspirin	HMG-CoA reductase	opioid analgesics*
benzodiazepines*	inhibitors*	phenothiazines*

*See Drug Class, Section Four

1229

Drugs that *probably* cause adverse effects when taken during the *second* and *third* trimesters (cont.)

progestins*
rifampin
streptomycin
sulfonamides*

sulfonylureas*
tetracyclines*
thalidomide
thiazide diuretics*

tricyclic antidepressants*
warfarin

Drugs that *possibly* cause adverse effects when taken during the *second* and *third* trimesters

acetazolamide
clemastine
diphenhydramine

ethacrynic acid
fluoroquinolones*
haloperidol

hydroxyzine
promethazine

TABLE 2

Drugs That May Increase Sensitivity to the Sun (Photosensitivity)

Some drugs can sensitize skin to ultraviolet light. This can cause the skin to react with a rash or exaggerated burn on exposure to sun or ultraviolet lamps. If you are taking any of the following drugs, ask your doctor for help about sun exposure and sunblocks.

acetazolamide
acetohexamide
alprazolam
amantadine
amiloride
aminobenzoic acid
amiodarone
amitriptyline
amoxapine
barbiturates
bendroflumethiazide
benzocaine
benzophenones
benzoyl peroxide
benzthiazide
captopril
carbamazepine
chlordiazepoxide
chloroquine
chlorothiazide
chlorpromazine
chlorpropamide
chlortetracycline
chlorthalidone
ciprofloxacin
clindamycin
clofazimine
clofibrate
clomipramine
cyproheptadine
dacarbazine
dapsone
demeclocycline

desipramine
desoximetasone
diethylstilbestrol
diflunisal
diltiazem
diphenhydramine
disopyramide
doxepin
doxycycline
enoxacin
estrogen
etretinate
flucytosine
fluorescein
fluorouracil
fluphenazine
flutamide
furosemide
glipizide
glyburide
gold preparations
griseofulvin
haloperidol
hexachlorophene
hydrochlorothiazide
hydroflumethiazide
ibuprofen
imipramine
indomethacin
isotretinoin
ketoprofen
lincomycin
lomefloxacin

maprotiline
mesoridazine
methacycline
methotrexate
methyclothiazide
methyldopa
metolazone
minocycline
minoxidil
nabumetone
nalidixic acid
naproxen
nifedipine
norfloxacin
nortriptyline
ofloxacin
oral contraceptives
oxyphenbutazone
oxytetracycline
para-aminobenzoic acid
perphenazine
phenelzine
phenobarbital
phenylbutazone
phenytoin
piroxicam
polythiazide
prochlorperazine
promazine
promethazine
protriptyline
pyrazinamide
quinidine

*See Drug Class, Section Four

Drugs That May Increase Photosensitivity to the Sun (Cont.)

quinine
St. John's wort
sulfonamides
sulindac
tetracycline
thiabendazole
thioridazine
thiothixene
tolazamide

tolbutamide
tranylcypromine
trazodone
tretinoin
triamterene
trichlormethiazide
trifluoperazine
triflupromazine
trimeprazine

trimethoprim
trimipramine
triprolidine
vinblastine

TABLE 3

Drugs That May Adversely Affect Behavior

Medicines can alter mood and emotional stability. They can also cause unpredictable patterns of thinking or behavior. These responses are relatively infrequent, but the nature and degree of mental disturbance can be alarming as well as dangerous for both patient and family.

Such paradoxical responses are often of an idiosyncratic nature, and someone with a history of a serious mental or emotional disorder is more likely to experience bizarre reactions. In some cases, it may be hard to separate the disorder being treated from an effect of one (or more) medicines the patient may be taking. If in doubt, it is best to talk with your doctor.

Drugs reported to impair *concentration* and/or *memory*

acyclovir
anticonvulsants
antihistamines*
anti-parkinsonism drugs*

barbiturates*
benzodiazepines*
isoniazid
monoamine oxidase

(MAO) inhibitors*
phenytoin
primidone
scopolamine

Drugs reported to cause *confusion, delirium,* or *disorientation*

acetazolamide
acyclovir
amantadine
aminophylline
amphetamines
amphotericin B
anticholinergics
antidepressants*
antihistamines*
antipsychotics
atropinelike drugs*
barbiturates*
benzodiazepines*
beta adrenergic blockers
    (some)
bromides
carbamazepine
chloroquine
cimetidine
clonidine
cortisonelike drugs*
cycloserine

dantrolene
digitalis
digitoxin
digoxin
disulfiram
diuretics
ethchlorvynol
ethinamate
fenfluramine
fluoroquinolone
    antibiotics*
glutethimide
histamine (H2) receptor
    antagonists
interferons
isoniazid
lamotrigine
levodopa
lidocaine
liposomal amphotericin B
lisinopril
melatonin

meprobamate
mesalamine
methyldopa
metoclopramide
narcotic pain relievers
    (analgesics)
NSAIDs*
para-aminosalicylic acid
phenelzine
phenothiazines*
phenytoin
piperazine
primidone
propranolol
quinidine
reserpine
scopolamine
tacrine
theophylline
tricyclic antidepressants
zolpidem

*See Drug Class, Section Four

Drugs reported to cause *paranoid thinking*

acyclovir
amphetaminelike
    medicines
anticholinergic drugs
benzodiazepines
bromides

cocaine
cortisonelike drugs*
cycloserine
diphenhydramine
disopyramide
disulfiram

isoniazid
levodopa
propafenone
propranolol
tricyclic antidepressants

Drugs reported to cause *schizophreniclike behavior*

amphetamines*
anabolic steroids
cimetidine (case reports
    and in elderly or
    debilitated)

ciprofloxacin (case
    reports and
    idiosyncratic)
ephedrine

fenfluramine
phenmetrazine
phenylpropanolamine

Drugs reported to cause *maniclike behavior*

antidepressants*
clarithromycin (case
    reports)
cortisonelike drugs*
levodopa

metoclopramide (case
    reports)
monoamine oxidase
    (MAO) inhibitors*
selective serotonin

reuptake inhibitors
    (SSRIs) (when drug
    is stopped)

Some medicines have mood-altering *side effects,* although they are prescribed for altogether unrelated conditions. Emotional and behavioral secondary effects will be quite unpredictable and vary enormously from person to person. However, the following experiences have been seen with sufficient frequency to establish recognizable patterns.

Drugs reported to cause *nervousness* (anxiety and irritability)

amantadine
amphetaminelike drugs*
    (appetite suppressants)
anabolic steroids
antihistamines*
caffeine
chlorphenesin
cimetidine (case reports in
    elderly)
cocaine
cortisonelike drugs*

ephedrine
epinephrine
isoproterenol
levodopa
liothyronine (in excessive
    dosage)
methylphenidate
methysergide
monoamine oxidase
    (MAO) inhibitors*
nylidrin

oral contraceptives
selective serotonin
    reuptake inhibitors
    (SSRIs)
theophylline
thyroid (in excessive
    dosage)
thyroxine (in excessive
    dosage)

Drugs reported to cause *emotional depression*

amantadine
amphetamines* (on
    withdrawal)
baclofen
benzodiazepines*
beta adrenergic blockers
    (some)
calcium channel blockers
    (case reports)
carbamazepine
chloramphenicol

cimetidine
clonidine
clotrimazole
cortisonelike drugs*
cycloserine
digitalis
digitoxin
digoxin
diphenoxylate
estrogens
ethionamide

fenfluramine (on
    withdrawal)
fluoroquinolone antibiotics
fluphenazine
guanethidine
haloperidol
HMG-CoA reductase
    inhibitors (case reports)
hydrocortisone
indomethacin
isoniazid

*See Drug Class, Section Four

Drugs reported to cause *emotional depression* (cont.)

isotretinoin
levodopa
methsuximide
methyldopa
methysergide
metoclopramide (case
  reports)
metoprolol
oral contraceptives

phenylbutazone
procainamide
progesterones
propranolol
raloxifene
reserpine
sulfonamides*
thiazide diuretics (may
  start after weeks to

months)
tretinoin
vinblastine (possibly dose-
  related)
vitamin D (in excessive
  dosage)

Drugs reported to cause *euphoria*

amantadine
aminophylline
amphetamines
antihistamines* (some)
antispasmodics, synthetic*
aspirin
barbiturates*
benzphetamine
cephalosporins (increased
  risk with kidney disease)
chloral hydrate
clorazepate

codeine
cortisonelike drugs*
diethylpropion
diphenoxylate
dronabinol
ethosuximide
flurazepam
ginseng (sign of abuse)
haloperidol
levodopa
meprobamate
methysergide

monoamine oxidase
  (MAO) inhibitors*
morphine
opioids
pargyline
pentazocine
phenmetrazine
propoxyphene
scopolamine
tybamate

Drugs reported to cause *excitement*

acetazolamide
amantadine
amphetaminelike drugs*
antidepressants*
antihistamines*
atropinelike drugs*
barbiturates* (paradoxical
  response)
benzodiazepines*
  (paradoxical response)
cortisonelike drugs
cycloserine

diethylpropion
digitalis
ephedrine
epinephrine
ethinamate (paradoxical
  response)
ethionamide
glutethimide (paradoxical
  response)
isoniazid
isoproterenol
levodopa

meperidine and MAO
  inhibitor drugs*
methyldopa and MAO
  inhibitor drugs*
methyprylon (paradoxical
  response)
nalidixic acid
orphenadrine
quinine
scopolamine

TABLE 4
Drugs That May Adversely Affect Vision

A significant percentage of all adverse drug effects involve visual changes or eye damage. Some effects, such as blurring of vision or double vision, may occur shortly after starting a drug. More subtle and serious effects, such as cataract development or damage to the retina or optic nerve, may not happen until a drug has been in use for a long time. Some changes are irreversible. If you are taking a drug that can affect the eye, promptly report any eye discomfort or change in vision.

*See Drug Class, Section Four

Drugs reported to cause *blurring of vision*

acetazolamide
antiarthritic/anti-
  inflammatory drugs
antidepressants*
antihistamines*
atropinelike drugs*
chlorthalidone

ciprofloxacin
cortisonelike drugs*
diethylstilbestrol
etretinate
fenfluramine
norfloxacin
oral contraceptives

phenytoin
sildenafil
sulfonamides*
tetracyclines*
thiazide diuretics*

Drugs reported to cause *double vision*

antidepressants*
antidiabetic drugs*
antihistamines*
aspirin
barbiturates*
benzodiazepines*
bromides
carbamazepine
carisoprodol
chloroquine
chlorprothixene
ciprofloxacin
clomiphene
colchicine
colistin
cortisonelike drugs*

digitalis
digitoxin
digoxin
ethionamide
ethosuximide
etretinate
guanethidine
hydroxychloroquine
indomethacin
isoniazid
levodopa
mephenesin
methocarbamol
methsuximide
morphine
nalidixic acid

nitrofurantoin
norfloxacin
oral contraceptives
orphenadrine
oxyphenbutazone
pentazocine
phenothiazines*
phensuximide
phenylbutazone
phenytoin
primidone
propranolol
quinidine
sedatives/sleep inducers*
thiothixene
tranquilizers*

Drugs reported to cause *farsightedness*

ergot
penicillamine

sulfonamides* (possibly)
tolbutamide (possibly)

Drugs reported to cause *nearsightedness*

acetazolamide
aspirin
carbachol
chlorthalidone
codeine
cortisonelike drugs*

ethosuximide
methsuximide
morphine
oral contraceptives
penicillamine
phenothiazines*

phensuximide
spironolactone
sulfonamides*
tetracyclines*
thiazide diuretics*

Drugs reported to *alter color vision*

acetaminophen
amodiaquine
amyl nitrite
aspirin
atropine
barbiturates*
belladonna
chloramphenicol
chloroquine
chlorpromazine
chlortetracycline
ciprofloxacin
cortisonelike drugs*

digitalis
digitoxin
digoxin
disulfiram
epinephrine
ergotamine
erythromycin
ethchlorvynol
ethionamide
fluphenazine
furosemide
hydroxychloroquine
indomethacin

isocarboxazid
isoniazid
mefenamic acid
mesoridazine
methysergide
nalidixic acid
norfloxacin
oral contraceptives
oxyphenbutazone
paramethadione
pargyline
penicillamine
pentylenetetrazol

*See Drug Class, Section Four

Drugs reported to *alter color vision* (cont.)

perphenazine
phenacetin
phenylbutazone
primidone
prochlorperazine
promazine
promethazine

quinacrine
quinidine
quinine
reserpine
sildenafil
sodium salicylate
streptomycin

sulfonamides*
thioridazine
tranylcypromine
trifluoperazine
triflupromazine
trimeprazine
trimethadione

Drugs reported to cause *sensitivity to light* (photophobia)

antidiabetic drugs*
atropinelike drugs*
bromides
chloroquine
ciprofloxacin
clomiphene
digitoxin
doxepin
ethambutol

ethionamide
ethosuximide
etretinate
hydroxychloroquine
mephenytoin
methsuximide
monoamine oxidase
(MAO) inhibitors*
nalidixic acid

norfloxacin
oral contraceptives
paramethadione
phenothiazines*
quinidine
quinine
sildenafil
tetracyclines*
trimethadione

Drugs reported to cause *halos around lights*

amyl nitrite
chloroquine
cortisonelike drugs*
digitalis
digitoxin

digoxin
hydrochloroquine
nitroglycerin
norfloxacin
oral contraceptives

paramethadione
phenothiazines*
quinacrine
trimethadione

Drugs reported to cause *visual hallucinations*

amantadine
amphetaminelike drugs*
amyl nitrite
antihistamines*
aspirin
atropinelike drugs*
barbiturates*
benzodiazepines*
bromides
carbamazepine
cephalexin
cephaloglycin
chloroquine
cycloserine

digitalis
digoxin
disulfiram
ephedrine
furosemide
gabapentin
griseofulvin
haloperidol
hydroxychloroquine
indomethacin
isosorbide
levodopa
nialamide
oxyphenbutazone

pargyline
pentazocine
phenothiazines*
phenylbutazone
phenytoin
primidone
propranolol
quinine
sedatives/sleep inducers*
sulfonamides*
tetracyclines*
tricyclic antidepressants*
tripelennamine

Drugs reported to impair the use of *contact lenses*

brompheniramine
carbinoxamine
chlorpheniramine
cyclizine
cyproheptadine

dexbrompheniramine
dexchlorpheniramine
dimethindene
diphenhydramine
furosemide

oral contraceptives
terfenadine
tripelennamine

*See Drug Class, Section Four

Drugs reported to cause *cataracts* or *lens deposits*

allopurinol
busulfan
chlorpromazine
chlorprothixene
cortisonelike drugs*
fluphenazine
mesoridazine

methotrimeprazine
perphenazine
phenmetrazine
pilocarpine
prochlorperazine
promazine
promethazine

thioridazine
thiothixene
trifluoperazine
triflupromazine
trimeprazine

TABLE 5

Drugs That May Cause Blood Cell Dysfunction or Damage

All blood cells come from and mature in the bone marrow: red blood cells (erythrocytes), white blood cells (leukocytes) and blood platelets (thrombocytes). There are three kinds of white blood cells: granulocytes, monocytes (macrophages) and lymphocytes. Drugs that affect formation or development of blood cells can (1) act on any stage of cell production; (2) impair one cell type or line; (3) influence all cell lines. Some medicines can damage mature cells in the bloodstream.

Drugs that cause inevitable (dose-dependent) *aplastic anemia* (see Glossary)

actinomycin D
azathioprine
busulfan
carboplatin
carmustine
chlorambucil
cisplatin
cyclophosphamide

cytarabine
doxorubicin
epirubicin
etoposide
fluorouracil
hydroxyurea
lomustine
melphalan

mercaptopurine
methotrexate
mitomycin
mitoxantrone
plicamycin
procarbazine
thioguanine
thiotepa

Drugs that may cause idiosyncratic (dose-independent) *aplastic anemia*

amodiaquine
benoxaprofen
carbimazole
chloramphenicol
chlorpromazine
gold
indomethacin

mepacrine
oxyphenbutazone
penicillamine
phenylbutazone
phenytoin
piroxicam
prothiaden

pyrimethamine
sulfonamides*
sulindac
thiouracils
trimethoprim/
    sulfamethoxazole

Drugs that may impair red blood cell production (only)

azathioprine
carbamazepine
chloramphenicol
chlorpropamide
dapsone
fenoprofen
gold
halothane

isoniazid
methyldopa
penicillin
pentachlorophenol
phenobarbital
phenylbutazone
phenytoin
pyrimethamine

sulfasalazine
sulfathiazol
sulfonamides*
sulfonylureas*
thiamphenicol
tolbutamide
trimethoprim/
    sulfamethoxazole

*See Drug Class, Section Four

Drugs that may significantly *reduce granulocyte cell counts* (various mechanisms)

acetaminophen
acetazolamide
allopurinol
amitriptyline
amodiaquine
benzodiazepines*
captopril
carbamazepine
carbimazole
cephalosporins*
chloramphenicol
chloroquine
chlorothiazide
chlorpromazine
chlorpropamide
chlorthalidone
cimetidine
clindamycin
dapsone
desipramine
disopyramide

ethacrynic acid
gentamicin
gold
hydralazine
hydrochlorothiazide
imipramine
indomethacin
isoniazid
levamisole
meprobamate
methimazole
methyldopa
oxyphenbutazone
penicillamine
penicillins*
pentazocine
phenacetin
phenothiazines*
phenylbutazone
phenytoin
procainamide

propranolol
propylthiouracil
pyrimethamine
quinidine
quinine
ranitidine
rifampin
sodium aminosalicylate
streptomycin
sulfadoxine
sulfadoxine/
  pyrimethamine
sulfonamides*
tetracyclines*
tocainide
tolbutamide
trimethoprim/
  sulfamethoxazole
vancomycin

Drugs that may significantly *reduce blood platelet counts*

acetazolamide
actinomycin
allopurinol
alpha-interferon
amiodarone
ampicillin
aspirin
carbamazepine
carbenicillin
cephalosporins*
chenodeoxycholic acid
chloroquine
chlorothiazide
chlorpheniramine
chlorpropamide
chlorthalidone
cimetidine
cyclophosphamide
danazol
desferrioxamine

diazepam
diazoxide
diclofenac
digoxin
diltiazem
furosemide
gentamicin
gold
hydrochlorothiazide
imipramine
isoniazid
isotretinoin
levamisole
meprobamate
methyldopa
mianserin
minoxidil
morphine
nitrofurantoin
oxprenolol

oxyphenbutazone
penicillamine
penicillin
phenylbutazone
phenytoin
piroxicam
procainamide
quinidine
quinine
ranitidine
rifampin
sodium aminosalicylate
sulfasalazine
sulfonamides*
thioguanine
trimethoprim/
  sulfamethoxazole
valproate
vancomycin

Drugs that cause *hemolytic anemia* due to glucose-6-phosphate dehydrogenase (G6PD) deficiency of red blood cells

acetanilid
dapsone
methylene blue
nalidixic acid
naphthalene
niridazole

nitrofurantoin
pamaquine
phenazopyridine
phenylhydrazine
primaquine
sulfacetamide

sulfamethoxazole
sulfanilamide
sulfapyridine
thiazolsulfone
toluidine blue

*See Drug Class, Section Four

Drugs that may cause *hemolytic anemia* by other mechanisms

antimony	methotrexate	quinidine
chlorpropamide	para-aminosalicylic acid	quinine
cisplatin	penicillamine	rifampin
mephenesin	phenazopyridine	sulfasalazine

Drugs that may cause *megaloblastic anemia*

acyclovir	metformin	primidone
alcohol	methotrexate	pyrimethamine
aminopterin	neomycin	sulfasalazine
azathioprine	nitrofurantoin	tetracycline
colchicine	nitrous oxide	thioguanine
cycloserine	oral contraceptives	triamterene
cytarabine	para-aminosalicylic acid	trimethoprim
floxuridine	pentamidine	vinblastine
fluorouracil	phenformin	vitamin A
hydroxyurea	phenobarbital	vitamin C (large doses)
mercaptopurine	phenytoin	zidovudine

Drugs that may cause *sideroblastic anemia*

alcohol	isoniazid	pyrazinamide
chloramphenicol	penicillamine	
cycloserine	phenacetin	

TABLE 6

Drugs That May Cause Heart Dysfunction or Damage

Drugs may damage either heart structure or function. Heart problems themselves often decide the nature of adverse drug effects. Some are direct pharmacological actions of a drug on heart tissues, and others are caused indirectly by altering chemical balances that diminish how well the heart works (as with potassium or magnesium loss from diuretics).

Drugs that may cause or contribute to *abnormal heart rhythms* (arrhythmias)

aminophylline	digitoxin	gatifloxacin
amiodarone	digoxin	grepafloxacin (no longer on the US market)
amitriptyline	diltiazem	
antiarrhythmic drugs*	disopyramide	halofantrene
arsenic trioxide	diuretics*	haloperidol
astemizole (no longer on the US market)	dofetilide	ibutilide
	doxepin	indapamide
bepridil	droperidol	isoproterenol
beta adrenergic blockers*	encainide	isradipine
beta-adrenergic bronchodilators*	erythromycin (intravenous)	ketanserin
		levofloxacin
carbamazepine	fentolterol	levomethadyl
chlorpromazine	felbamate	lidocaine
cimetidine	flecainide	maprotiline
cisapride (use is now limited)	fluoxetine	methyldopa
	foscarnet	mesoridazine
clarithromycin	fosphenytoin	mexiletine

*See Drug Class, Section Four

Drugs that may cause or contribute to *abnormal heart rhythms* (cont.)

milrinone
moexipril/hctz
moxifloxacin
naratriptan
nicardipine
octreotide
pentamidine
phenothiazines*
pimozide
prenylamine
procainamide
quetiapine
quinidine

ranitidine
risperidone
salmeterol
sertraline
sotalol
sparfloxacin
sumatriptan
tacrolimus
tamoxifen
terbutaline
terfenadine (no longer
    on the US market)
theophylline

thiazide diuretics*
thioridazine
tizanidine
trazodone
tricyclic antidepressants
    (such as Elavil,
    Sinequan, Tofranil)*
venlafaxine
verapamil
ziprasidone
zolmitriptan

Drugs that may *depress heart function* (reduce pumping efficiency)

beta adrenergic blockers*
cocaine
daunorubicin
diltiazem

disopyramide
doxorubicin
epinephrine
flecainide

fluorouracil
isoproterenol
nifedipine
verapamil

Drugs that may *reduce coronary artery blood flow* (reduce oxygen supply to heart muscle)

amphetamines*
beta adrenergic blockers*
    (abrupt withdrawal)
cocaine

ergotamine
fluorouracil
nifedipine
oral contraceptives

ritodrine
vasopressin
vinblastine
vincristine

Drugs that may *impair healing of heart muscle* following heart attack (myocardial infarction)

adrenocortical steroids*
nonsteroidal anti-inflammatory drugs (NSAIDs)*

Drugs that may cause *heart valve damage*

dexfenfluramine (Redux)
ergotamine
fen-phen (fenfluramine-phenteramine)

methysergide
minocycline (blue-black
    pigmentation)

Drugs that may cause *pericardial disease*

actinomycin D
anthracyclines
bleomycin
cisplatin
cyclophosphamide

cytarabine
fluorouracil
hydralazine
methysergide
minoxidil

phenylbutazone
practolol
procainamide
sulfasalazine

TABLE 7

Drugs That May Cause Lung Dysfunction or Damage

Lung damage from medicines may be difficult to distinguish from natural diseases or disorders that involve lung function or structure. Type A reactions are those due to known pharmacological drug actions; Type B are unexpected and unpredictable allergic or idiosyncratic reactions.

*See Drug Class, Section Four

Drugs that may adversely affect *blood vessels of the lung*

Drugs that may cause thromboembolism

chlorpromazine	oral contraceptives
estrogens*	(high-estrogen type)

Drugs that may cause pulmonary hypertension

amphetamines*	oral contraceptives	the label, but effect has
dexfenfluramine (Redux)	sibutramine (Meridia)	NOT been reported)
fenfluramine	(carries a warning on	tryptophan

Drugs that may cause vasculitis (blood vessel damage) with or without hemorrhage

aminoglutethimide	febarbamate	phenytoin
amphotericin	nitrofurantoin	
cocaine	penicillamine	

Drugs that may cause adult respiratory distress syndrome (ARDS)

bleomycin	heroin	naloxone
codeine	hydrochlorothiazide	ritodrine
cyclophosphamide	methadone	terbutaline
dextropropoxyphene	mitomycin	vinblastine

Drugs that may adversely affect the *bronchial tubes*

Drugs that may cause bronchoconstriction (asthma)

acetaminophen	griseofulvin	nonsteroidal anti-
aspirin	maprotiline	inflammatory drugs*
beta adrenergic blockers*	methacholine	penicillins*
carbachol	methoxypsoralen	pilocarpine
cephalosporins*	metoclopramide	propafenone
chloramphenicol	morphine	pyridostigmine
deanol	neomycin	streptomycin
demeclocycline	neostigmine	tartrazine (coloring
erythromycin	nitrofurantoin	agent)

Drugs that may cause bronchiolitis (with permanent obstruction of small bronchioles)

penicillamine	sulfasalazine

Drugs that may *damage lung tissues*

Drugs that may cause acute allergic-type pneumonitis

ampicillin	methotrexate	penicillamine
bleomycin	metronidazole	penicillin
cephalexin	mitomycin	phenylbutazone
chlorpropamide	nalidixic acid	phenytoin
gold	nitrofurantoin	procarbazine
imipramine	nomifensine	sulfonamides*
mephenesin	nonsteroidal anti-	tetracycline
mercaptopurine	inflammatory drugs*	vinblastine
metformin	para-aminosalicylic acid	

*See Drug Class, Section Four

Drugs that may cause chronic pneumonitis and/or fibrosis (scarring)

amiodarone	chlorambucil	mercaptopurine
azathioprine	cyclophosphamide	methysergide
BCNU	ergotamine	nitrofurantoin
bleomycin	gold	pentolinium
bromocriptine	hexamethonium	practolol
busulfan	lomustine	sulfasalazine
carmustine	mecamylamine	tocainide
CCNU	melphalan	tolfenamic acid

Drugs that may *damage the pleura*

bromocriptine	methysergide	practolol

TABLE 8

Drugs That May Cause Liver Dysfunction or Damage

The liver often changes drugs into forms easily removed from the body. Medicines can hurt liver structure or function. Reactions range from mild and transient changes in liver function tests to complete liver failure and death. Many drugs may affect the liver in more than one way. Careful liver monitoring is required.

Drugs that may *cause acute dose-dependent liver damage* (resembling acute viral hepatitis)

acetaminophen (overdose)	salicylates (doses over
amiodarone	2 g daily)
niacin	6-mercaptopurine

Drugs that may cause *acute dose-independent liver* damage (resembling acute viral hepatitis)

acebutolol	indomethacin	phenytoin
allopurinol	isoniazid	piroxicam
atenolol	ketoconazole	probenecid
carbamazepine	labetalol	pyrazinamide
cimetidine	maprotiline	quinidine
cocaine	metoprolol	quinine
dantrolene	mianserin	ranitidine
diclofenac	naproxen	rifampin
diltiazem	nifedipine	sulfonamides*
disulfiram	para-aminosalicylic acid	sulindac
enflurane	penicillins*	tricyclic antidepressants*
ethambutol	phenelzine	trovafloxacin
ethionamide	phenindione	valproic acid
halothane	phenobarbital	verapamil
ibuprofen	phenylbutazone	

Drugs that may cause *acute fatty infiltration of the liver*

adrenocortical steroids*	phenothiazines*	tetracyclines*
antithyroid drugs	phenytoin	valproic acid
isoniazid	salicylates*	
methotrexate	sulfonamides*	

*See Drug Class, Section Four

Drugs that may cause *cholestatic jaundice*

acetaminophen
actinomycin D
amitriptyline
amoxicillin/clavulanate
azathioprine
captopril (case reports)
carbamazepine
carbimazole
cephalosporins*
chlordiazepoxide
chlorpromazine
chlorpropamide
cimetidine
cloxacillin
cyclophosphamide
cyclosporine
danazol
desipramine
diazepam
diclofenac
disopyramide
enalapril

erythromycin (estolate)
estradiol
flecainide
flurazepam
flutamide
glyburide
gold
griseofulvin
haloperidol
imipramine
indomethacin
ketoconazole
mercaptopurine
methyltestosterone
nafcillin
niacin
nifedipine
nitrofurantoin
nonsteroidal anti-
    inflammatory drugs*
norethandrolone
oral contraceptives

oxacillin
penicillamine
phenothiazines*
phenytoin
piroxicam
propoxyphene
propylthiouracil
rifampin
sulfonamides*
sulindac
tamoxifen
thiabendazole
tolazamide
tolbutamide
tricyclic antidepressants*
trimethoprim/sulfamethox
    azole
troleandomycin
verapamil
zidovudine

Drugs that may cause *liver granulomas* (chronic inflammatory nodules)

allopurinol
aspirin
carbamazepine
chlorpromazine
chlorpropamide
diltiazem
disopyramide

gold
hydralazine
isoniazid
methyldopa
nitrofurantoin
penicillin
phenylbutazone

phenytoin
procainamide
quinidine
ranitidine
sulfonamides*
tolbutamide

Drugs that may cause *chronic liver disease*

Drugs that may cause active chronic hepatitis

acetaminophen (chronic
    use, large doses)
dantrolene

isoniazid
methyldopa
nitrofurantoin

salicylates (aspirin)
trazodone

Drugs that may cause liver cirrhosis or fibrosis (scarring)

methotrexate
methyldopa

nicotinic acid
vitamin A

Drugs that may cause chronic cholestasis (resembling primary biliary cirrhosis)

chlorpromazine/valproic
    acid (combination)
chlorpropamide/erythro-
    mycin (combination)

imipramine
phenothiazines*
phenytoin
thiabendazole

tolbutamide

Drugs that may cause *liver tumors* (benign and malignant)

anabolic steroids
androgens (C17
    substituted kinds)

danazol
oral contraceptives
testosterone

thorotrast

*See Drug Class, Section Four

Drugs that may cause damage to liver blood vessels

adriamycin	sporine (combination)	mitomycin
anabolic steroids	dacarbazine	oral contraceptives
azathioprine	herbal teas, some	thioguanine
carmustine	mercaptopurine	vincristine
cyclophosphamide/cyclo-	methotrexate	vitamin A (excessive doses)

Drugs that can cause *idiosyncratic liver damage*

acebutolol (case reports)	dacarbazine	troglitazone
amoxicillin/clavulanate	procainamide	trovafloxacin
carbamazepine	propylthiouracil	valproic acid
chlorpromazine	sulfonamides	

TABLE 9

Drugs That May Cause Kidney Dysfunction or Damage

The kidneys perform two major drug functions: (1) alteration of the drug to help remove it; (2) elimination of the drug from the body in the urine. As with effects on the liver, many drugs can harm the kidneys in several ways. Careful monitoring is prudent when taking any of the drugs listed below.

Drugs that may primarily *impair kidney function* (without damage)

amphotericin	demeclocycline	nifedipine
angiotensin-converting	diuretics/NSAIDs* (avoid	nitroprusside
enzyme inhibitors*	this combination)	nonsteroidal anti-
(with renal artery	glyburide	inflammatory drugs
stenosis; with congestive	isofosfamide	(NSAIDs)*
heart failure)	lithium/tricyclic	rifampin
beta adrenergic blockers*	antidepressants* (avoid	vinblastine
ceftazidime	this combination)	
colchicine	methoxyflurane	

Drugs that may cause *acute kidney failure* (due to kidney damage)

Drugs that may damage the kidney filtration unit (the nephron)

acetaminophen	cisplatin	oral contraceptives
(excessive dosage)	cyclosporine	penicillamine
allopurinol	enalapril	phenytoin
aminoglycoside	ergometrine	quinidine
antibiotics*	hydralazine	rifampin
amphotericin	methy-CCNU	streptokinase
bismuth thiosulfate	metronidazole	sulfonamides*
carbamazepine	mitomycin	thiazide diuretics*

*See Drug Class, Section Four

Drugs that may cause *acute interstitial nephritis*

allopurinol
amoxicillin
ampicillin
aspirin
azathioprine
aztreonam
captopril
carbamazepine
carbenicillin
cefaclor
cefoxitin
cephalexin
cephalothin
cephapirin
cephradine
cimetidine
ciprofloxacin
clofibrate
cloxacillin
diazepam

diclofenac
diflunisal
fenoprofen
foscarnet
furosemide
gentamicin
glafenine
ibuprofen
indomethacin
ketoprofen
mefenamate
methicillin
methyldopa
mezlocillin
minocycline
nafcillin
naproxen
oxacillin
penicillamine
penicillin

phenindione
phenobarbital
phenylbutazone
phenytoin
piroxicam
pirprofen
pyrazinamide
rifampin
sodium valproate
sulfamethoxazole
sulfinpyrazone
sulfonamides*
sulindac
thiazide diuretics*
tolmetin
trimethoprim
vancomycin
warfarin

Drugs that may cause *muscle destruction* and associated *acute kidney failure*

adrenocortical steroids*
alcohol
amphetamines*
amphotericin
aristolochic acid
  (prompted removal
  of several herbal
  products from the

market by the FDA)
carbenoxolone
chlorthalidone
clofibrate
cocaine
cytarabine
fenofibrate
haloperidol

halothane
heroin
lovastatin
opioid analgesics*
pentamidine
phenothiazines*
streptokinase
suxamethonium

Drugs that may cause kidney damage resembling *glomerulonephritis or nephrosis*

captopril
fenoprofen
gold
ketoprofen

lithium
mesalamine
penicillamine
phenytoin

practolol
probenecid
quinidine

Drugs that may cause *chronic interstitial nephritis and papillary necrosis* (analgesic kidney damage)

acetaminophen
aspirin

phenacetin
(All with long-term use)

Drugs that may cause or contribute to urinary tract crystal or stone formation

acetazolamide
acyclovir
cytotoxic drugs
dihydroxyadenine
magnesium trisilicate
mercaptopurine
methotrexate

methoxyflurane
phenylbutazone
probenecid
salicylates*
sulfonamides*
thiazide diuretics*
triamterene

uricosuric drugs
vitamin A
vitamin C
vitamin D
warfarin
zoxazolamine

*See Drug Class, Section Four

TABLE 10

Drugs That May Cause Nerve Dysfunction or Damage

Medicines may affect any part of the nervous system from the brain to peripheral nerves. The extent of benefits or problems varies widely from person to person.

Drugs that may cause *significant headache*

albuterol	inhibitors	perhexiline
amyl nitrate	hydralazine	propranolol
bepridil	ibuprofen	ranitidine
bromocriptinc	indomcthacin	scrtralinc
caffeine	labetalol	sibutramine
cilostazol	liposomal amphotericin B	sildenafil
clonidine	lithium	stavudine
cocaine	lomefloxacin	sulindac
delavirdine	mesalamine	terbutaline
ergotamine (prolonged use)	naproxen	tetracyclines*
etretinate	nifedipine	theophylline
felodipine	nisoldipine	tolmetin
fluticasone	nitrofurantoin	trimethoprim/sulfamethox
fluvoxamine	nitroglycerin	azole
HMG-CoA reductase	oral contraceptives	valacyclovir

Drugs that may cause *seizures* (convulsions)

acyclovir	cisapride	nalidixic acid
alprostadil	cocaine	ofloxacin
amantadine	cycloserine	oxacillin
amitriptyline	disopyramide	paclitaxel
ampicillin	enoxacin	penicillins* (synthetic)
atenolol	ether	phenothiazines*
baclofen	gabapentin	pyrimethamine
bromocriptine	halothane	tacrine
bupropion	indomethacin	terbutaline
carbamazepine (exacer-	isoniazid	theophylline
bation of absence)	lidocaine	ticarcillin
carbenicillin	lithium	tramadol
cephalosporins*	mefenamic acid	tricyclic antidepressants*
chloroquine	metronidazole (high doses)	venlafaxine
cimetidine	morphine (high-dose	vincristine
ciprofloxacin	intravenous)	

Drugs that may cause *stroke*

amitriptyline	nicotine	sumatriptan
anabolic steroids	oral contraceptives	trazodone
cocaine	phenylpropanolamine	

Drugs that may cause features of *parkinsonism*

amitriptyline	diltiazem	lithium
amodiaquine	diphenhydramine	methyldopa
chloroquine	droperidol	metoclopramide
chlorprothixene	fluoxetine	phenothiazines*
clozapine	haloperidol	reserpine
desipramine	imipramine	thiothixene
diazoxide	levodopa	trifluperidol

*See Drug Class, Section Four

Drugs that may cause *acute dystonias* (acute involuntary movement syndromes—AIMS)

carbamazepine	haloperidol	phenytoin
chlorzoxazone	metoclopramide	propranolol
fluoxetine	phenothiazines*	tricyclic antidepressants*

Drugs that may cause *tardive dyskinesia* (see Glossary)

haloperidol	phenothiazines*	thiothixene

Drugs that may cause *neuroleptic malignant syndrome* (NMS)

See this term in the Glossary for a list of causative drugs.

Drugs that may cause *peripheral neuropathy* (see Glossary)

amiodarone	emetine	penicillamine
amitriptyline	ergotamine	penicillin
amphetamines*	ethambutol	perhexiline
amphotericin	ethanol	phenelzine
anticoagulants*	glutethimide	phenylbutazone
carbutamide	gold	phenytoin
chlorambucil	hydralazine	podophyllin
chloramphenicol	imipramine	procarbazine
chloroquine	indomethacin	propranolol
chlorpropamide	isoniazid	propylthiouracil
cimetidine	lamotrigine	ritonavir
cisplatin	losartan	stavudine
clioquinol	methaqualone	streptomycin
clofibrate	methimazole	sulfonamides*
colchicine	methysergide	sulfoxone
colistin	metronidazole	thalidomide
cytarabine	nalidixic acid	tolbutamide
dapsone	nelfinavir	vinblastine
didanosine	nitrofurantoin	vincristine
disopyramide	nitrofurazone	
disulfiram	paclitaxel	

Drugs that may cause a *myasthenia gravis* syndrome

aminoglycoside antibiotics*	codeine	of existing MG)
amitriptyline	erythromycin (exacerbation of existing MG)	penicillamine
azithromycin (exacerbation of existing MG)	lithium	phenytoin
	morphine	polymixin B
beta adrenergic blockers*	norfloxacin (exacerbation	procainamide
		tetracycline
		trihexyphenidyl

TABLE 11

Drugs That May Adversely Affect Sexuality

Many commonly used drugs can cause obvious or subtle changes on one or more aspects of sexual expression. Patients may be unaware that sexual changes can be related to medicines and are often reluctant to talk about them. Sexual dysfunction

*See Drug Class, Section Four

may also be a result of the disorder being treated or an undetected problem. Diabetes, kidney failure, hypertension, depression, and alcoholism may reduce libido and cause failure of erection. Many drugs used to treat these conditions may worsen subclinical sexual dysfunction. This requires the closest cooperation between therapist and patient in order to correctly assess possible cause-and-effect relationships and change therapy appropriately.

Possible Drug Effects on Male Sexuality

1. Increased libido
  androgens (replacement therapy in deficiency states)
  baclofen (Lioresal)
  bupropion (Wellbutrin)
  chlordiazepoxide (Librium) (antianxiety effect)
  diazepam (Valium) (antianxiety effect)
  haloperidol (Haldol)
  levodopa (Larodopa, Sinemet) (may be an indirect effect due to improved sense of well-being)
  sildenafil (Viagra) (may be an effect of confidence from the drug)

2. Decreased libido
  amphetamines
  antihistamines
  barbiturates
  chlordiazepoxide (Librium), sedative effect
  chlorpromazine (Thorazine), 10% to 20% of users
  cimetidine (Tagamet)
  clofibrate (Atromid-S)
  clonidine (Catapres), 10% to 20% of users
  danazol (Danocrine)
  diazepam (Valium), sedative effect
  disulfiram (Antabuse)
  estrogens (therapy for prostatic cancer)
  fenfluramine (Pondimin)
  finasteride (Propecia, Proscar)
  heroin
  licorice
  medroxyprogesterone (Provera)
  methyldopa (Aldomet), 10% to 15% of users
  metoclopramide (Reglan), 80% of users
  perhexiline (Pexid)
  prazosin (Minipres), 15% of users
  propranolol (Inderal), rarely
  reserpine (Serpasil, Ser-Ap-Es)
  spironolactone (Aldactone)
  tricyclic antidepressants

3. Impaired erection (impotence)
  amitriptyline
  amphetamines
  angiotensin-converting enzyme (ACE) inhibitors
  anticholinergics
  antihistamines
  baclofen (Lioresal)
  barbiturates (when abused)
  beta blockers*
  captopril

*See Drug Class, Section Four

chlordiazepoxide (Librium) (in high dosage)
chlorpromazine (Thorazine)
cimetidine (Tagamet)
citalopram (Celexa)
clofibrate (Atromid-S)
clonidine (Catapres)
cocaine
diazepam (Valium) (in high dosage)
digitalis and its glycosides
disopyramide (Norpace)
disulfiram (Antabuse), uncertain
estrogens (therapy for prostatic cancer)
ethacrynic acid (Edecrin)
ethionamide (Trecator-SC)
fenfluramine (Pondimin)
Finasteride (Proscar)
furosemide (Lasix)
gabapentin (Neurontin)
guanethidine (Ismelin)
haloperidol (Haldol)
heroin
hydrochlorothiazide (ESPECIALLY if combined with a beta blocker)
hydroxyprogesterone (therapy for prostatic cancer)
indomethacin
itraconazole
licorice
lisinopril
lithium (Lithonate)
losartan (Cozaar)
marijuana
mesoridazine (Serentil)
methantheline (Banthine)
methyldopa (Aldomet)
metoclopramide (Reglan)
mirtazapine (Remeron)
monoamine oxidase (MAO) type A inhibitors*
perhexiline (Pexid)
pravastatin
prazosin (Minipres), infrequently
reserpine (Serpasil, Ser-Ap-Es)
simvastatin
spironolactone (Aldactone)
telmisartan (Micardis)
thiazide diuretics
thioridazine (Mellaril)
tricyclic antidepressants
venlafaxine (Effexor)

4. Impaired ejaculation
   anticholinergics
   barbiturates (when abused)
   chlorpromazine (Thorazine)
   clonidine (Catapres)
   cocaine
   estrogens (therapy for prostatic cancer)
   guanethidine (Ismelin)

*See Drug Class, Section Four

heroin
mesoridazine (Serentil)
methyldopa (Aldomet)
monoamine oxidase (MAO) type A inhibitors*
phenoxybenzamine (Dibenzyline)
phentolamine (Regitine)
reserpine (Serpasil, Ser-Ap-Es)
thiazide diuretics*
thioridazine (Mellaril)
tricyclic antidepressants*

5. Decreased testosterone
adrenocorticotropic hormone (ACTH)
barbiturates
digoxin (Lanoxin)
haloperidol (Haldol)—increased testosterone with low dosage, decreased
   testosterone with high dosage
lithium (Lithonate)
marijuana
medroxyprogesterone (Provera)
monoamine oxidase (MAO) type A inhibitors*
spironolactone (Aldactone)

6. Impaired spermatogenesis (reduced fertility)
adrenocorticosteroids (prednisone, etc.)
androgens (moderate to high dosage, extended use)
antimalarials
aspirin (abusive, chronic use)
chlorambucil (Leukeran)
cimetidine (Tagamet)
colchicine
cotrimoxazole (Bactrim, Septra)
cyclophosphamide (Cytoxan)
estrogens (therapy for prostatic cancer)
marijuana
medroxyprogesterone (Provera)
methotrexate
metoclopramide (Reglan)
monoamine oxidase (MAO) type A inhibitors
niridazole (Ambilhar)
nitrofurantoin (Furadantin)
spironolactone (Aldactone)
sulfasalazine (Azulfidine)
testosterone (moderate to high dosage, extended use)
vitamin C (doses of 1 g or more)

7. Testicular disorders
Swelling
—tricyclic antidepressants
Inflammation
—oxyphenbutazone (Tandearil)
Atrophy
—androgens (moderate to high dosage, extended use)
—chlorpromazine (Thorazine)
—cyclophosphamide (Cytoxan) (in prepubescent boys)
—spironolactone (Aldactone)

*See Drug Class, Section Four

8. Penile disorders
   Priapism (see Glossary)
   —alfentanil
   —anabolic steroids (male hormonelike drugs)
   —chlorpromazine (Thorazine)
   —clozapine (Clozaril)
   —cocaine
   —fluphenazine (Prolixin)
   —guanethidine (Ismelin)
   —haloperidol (Haldol)
   —heparin
   —hydralazine (Apresoline)
   —levodopa (Sinemet)
   —mesoridazine (Serentil)
   —molindone (Moban)
   —phenelzine (Nardil)
   —phenytoin (Dilantin)
   —prazosin (Minipres)
   —prochlorperazine (Compazine)
   —risperidone (Risperdal)
   —tamoxifen (Nolvadex)
   —thioridazine (Mellaril)
   —trazodone (Desyrel)
   —trifluoperazine (Stelazine)
   —warfarin (Coumadin)
   Peyronie's disease (see Glossary)
   —beta blockers*
   —phenytoin (Dilantin, etc.)

9. Gynecomastia (excessive development of the male breast)
   anabolic steroids
   androgens (partial conversion to estrogen)
   busulfan (Myleran)
   captopril
   carmustine (BiCNU)
   chlormadinone
   chlorpromazine (Thorazine)
   chlortetracycline (Aureomycin)
   cimetidine (Tagamet)
   clonidine (Catapres), infrequently
   diazepam
   diethylstilbestrol (DES)
   digitalis and its glycosides
   diltiazem
   enalapril
   estrogens (therapy for prostatic cancer)
   ethionamide (Trecator-SC)
   finasteride (Propecia, Proscar)
   fluphenazine
   griseofulvin (Fulvicin, etc.)
   haloperidol (Haldol)
   heroin
   human chorionic gonadotropin
   indinavir (Crixivan)
   isoniazid (INH, Nydrazid)
   marijuana
   mestranol

*See Drug Class, Section Four

methyldopa (Aldomet)
metoclopramide (Reglan)
nifedipine
omeprazole (Prilosec)
penicillamine
phenelzine (Nardil)
phenothiazines
reserpine (Serpasil, Ser-Ap-Es)
spironolactone (Aldactone)
thioridazine (Mellaril)
tricyclic antidepressants (TCAs)
verapamil
vincristine (Oncovin)

10. Feminization (loss of libido, impotence, gynecomastia, testicular atrophy)
conjugated estrogens (Premarin, etc.)

11. Precocious puberty
anabolic steroids
androgens
isoniazid (INH)

Possible Drug Effects on Female Sexuality

1. Increased libido
androgens
chlordiazepoxide (Librium) (antianxiety effect)
diazepam (Valium) (antianxiety effect)
mazindol (Sanorex)
oral contraceptives (freedom from fear of pregnancy)

2. Decreased libido
See list of drug effects on male sexuality. Some of these may have potential for
reducing libido in the female. The literature is sparse on this subject.

3. Impaired arousal and orgasm
anticholinergics
clonidine (Catapres)
methyldopa (Aldomet)
monoamine oxidase (MAO) inhibitors*
tricyclic antidepressants*

4. Breast enlargement
penicillamine
tricyclic antidepressants*

5. Galactorrhea (spontaneous flow of milk)
amphetamine
chlorpromazine (Thorazine)
cimetidine (Tagamet)
haloperidol (Haldol)
heroin
methyldopa (Aldomet)
metoclopramide (Reglan)
oral contraceptives
phenothiazines
reserpine (Serpasil, Ser-Ap-Es)
sulpiride (Equilid)
tricyclic antidepressants*

*See Drug Class, Section Four

6. Ovarian failure (reduced fertility)
  anesthetic gases (operating room staff)
  cyclophosphamide (Cytoxan)
  cytostatic drugs
  danazol (Danocrine)
  medroxyprogesterone (Provera)

7. Altered menstruation (menstrual disorders)
  adrenocorticosteroids (prednisone, etc.)
  androgens
  barbiturates (when abused)
  chlorambucil (Leukeran)
  chlorpromazine (Thorazine)
  cyclophosphamide (Cytoxan)
  danazol (Danocrine)
  estrogens
  ethionamide (Trecator-SC)
  haloperidol (Haldol)
  heroin
  isoniazid (INH, Nydrazid)
  marijuana
  medroxyprogesterone (Provera)
  metoclopramide (Reglan)
  oral contraceptives
  phenothiazines
  progestins
  radioisotopes
  rifampin (Rifadin, Rifamate, Rimactane)
  spironolactone (Aldactone)
  testosterone
  thioridazine (Mellaril)
  vitamin A (in excessive dosage)

8. Virilization (acne, hirsutism, lowering of voice, enlargement of clitoris)
  anabolic drugs
  androgens
  haloperidol (Haldol)
  oral contraceptives (lowering of voice)

9. Precocious puberty
  estrogens (in hair lotions)
  isoniazid (INH, Nydrazid)

TABLE 12

Drugs That May Interact with Alcohol

Alcohol may interact with a wide variety of drugs. The most important problem happens when the depressant action on the brain of sedatives, sleep-inducing drugs, tranquilizers and narcotic drugs is intensified by alcohol. Alcohol may also reduce drug benefits or lead to toxic effects. Some drugs may increase the intoxicating effects of alcohol, further impairing mental alertness, judgment, coordination and reaction time.

The intensity and significance can vary greatly from one person to another and from one occasion to another. This is because many factors influence what happens when drugs and alcohol interact. Factors include variations in sensitivity to drugs, the chemistry and quantity of the drug, type and amount of alcohol consumed, and the sequence in which drugs and alcohol are taken. If you need to use any of the drugs in the following table, ask your doctor for help about alcohol use.

Drugs with which it is advisable to avoid alcohol completely

Drug name or class	Possible interaction with alcohol
amphetamine	excessive rise in blood pressure with alcoholic beverages containing tyramine**
antidepressants	excessive sedation, increased intoxication
barbiturates*	excessive sedation
bromides	confusion, delirium, increased intoxication
calcium carbimide	disulfiramlike reaction**
carbamazepine	excessive sedation
chlorprothixene	excessive sedation
chlorzoxazone	excessive sedation
disulfiram	disulfiram reaction**
ergotamine	reduced effectiveness of ergotamine
fenfluramine	excessive stimulation of nervous system with some beers and wines
furazolidone	disulfiramlike reaction**
haloperidol	excessive sedation
MAO inhibitors*	excessive rise in blood pressure with alcoholic beverages containing tyramine**
meperidine	excessive sedation
meprobamate	excessive sedation
methotrexate	increased liver toxicity and excessive sedation
metronidazole	disulfiramlike reaction**
narcotic drugs	excessive sedation
oxyphenbutazone	increased stomach irritation and/or bleeding
pentazocine	excessive sedation
pethidine	excessive sedation
phenothiazines*	excessive sedation
phenylbutazone	increased stomach irritation and/or bleeding
procarbazine	disulfiramlike reaction**
propoxyphene	excessive sedation
reserpine	excessive sedation, orthostatic hypotension**
sleep-inducing drugs (hypnotics) —carbromal —chloral hydrate —ethchlorvynol —ethinamate —flurazepam —glutethimide —methaqualone —methyprylon —temazepam —triazolam	excessive sedation
thiothixene	excessive sedation
tricyclic antidepressants*	excessive sedation, increased intoxication
trimethobenzamide	excessive sedation

*See Drug Class, Section Four
**See Glossary

Drugs with which alcohol should be used only in small amounts (use cautiously until combined effects have been determined)

Drug name or class	Possible interaction with alcohol
acetaminophen (Tylenol, etc.)	increased liver toxicity
antiarthritic/anti-inflammatory drugs	increased stomach irritation and/or bleeding
anticoagulants (coumarins)*	increased anticoagulant effect
antidiabetic drugs (sulfonylureas)*	increased antidiabetic effect, excessive hypoglycemia**
antihistamines*	excessive sedation
antihypertensives*	excessive orthostatic hypotension**
aspirin (large doses or continuous use)	increased stomach irritation and/or bleeding
benzodiazepines*	excessive sedation
carisoprodol	increased alcoholic intoxication
diethylpropion	excessive nervous system stimulation with alcoholic beverages containing tyramine**
dihydroergotoxine	excessive lowering of blood pressure
diphenoxylate	excessive sedation
dipyridamole	excessive lowering of blood pressure
diuretics*	excessive orthostatic hypotension**
ethionamide	confusion, delirium, psychotic behavior
fenoprofen	increased stomach irritation and/or bleeding
griseofulvin	flushing and rapid heart action
ibuprofen	increased stomach irritation and/or bleeding
indomethacin	increased stomach irritation and/or bleeding
insulin	excessive hypoglycemia**
iron	excessive absorption of iron
isoniazid	decreased effectiveness of isoniazid, increased incidence of hepatitis
lithium	increased confusion and delirium (avoid all alcohol if any indication of lithium overdosage)
methocarbamol	excessive sedation
methotrimeprazine	excessive sedation
methylphenidate	excessive nervous system stimulation with alcoholic beverages containing tyramine**
metoprolol	excessive orthostatic hypotension**
nalidixic acid	increased alcoholic intoxication
naproxen	increased stomach irritation and/or bleeding
nicotinic acid	possible orthostatic hypotension**
nitrates* (vasodilators)	possible orthostatic hypotension**
nylidrin	increased stomach irritation
orphenadrine	excessive sedation
phenelzine	increased alcoholic intoxication
phenoxybenzamine	possible orthostatic hypotension**

*See Drug Class, Section Four
**See Glossary

phentermine	excessive nervous system stimulation with alcoholic beverages containing tyramine**
phenytoin	decreased effect of phenytoin
pilocarpine	prolongation of alcohol effect
prazosin	excessive lowering of blood pressure
primidone	excessive sedation
propranolol	excessive orthostatic hypotension**
sulfonamides*	increased alcoholic intoxication
sulindac	increased stomach irritation and/or bleeding
tolmetin	increased stomach irritation and/or bleeding
tranquilizers (mild) —chlordiazepoxide —clorazepate —diazepam —hydroxyzine —meprobamate —oxazepam —phenaglycodol —tybamate	excessive sedation
tranylcypromine	increased alcoholic intoxication

Drugs capable of producing a disulfiramlike reaction** when used concurrently with alcohol

antidiabetic drugs (sulfonylureas)*
calcium carbimide
chloral hydrate
chloramphenicol
disulfiram
furazolidone
metronidazole
nifuroxime
nitrofurantoin
procarbazine
quinacrine
sulfonamides*
tinidazole
tolazoline

*See Drug Class, Section Four
**See Glossary

TABLE 13

High-Potassium Foods

Drugs that cause loss of potassium are often used to treat conditions that also require a reduced intake of sodium. The high-potassium foods listed below have been selected for compatibility with a sodium-restricted diet (500 to 1,000 mg of sodium daily). Water pills (diuretics) may also cause loss of magnesium. Make sure magnesium is tested if you take a diuretic and discuss the results with your doctor.

Beverages

orange juice	skim milk	tomato juice
prune juice	tea	whole milk

Breads and Cereals

brown rice	muffins	waffles
cornbread	oatmeal	
griddle cakes	shredded wheat	

Fruits

apricot	fig	orange
avocado	honeydew melon	papaya
banana	mango	prune

Meats

beef	haddock	rockfish
chicken	halibut	salmon
codfish	liver	turkey
flounder	pork	veal

Vegetables

baked beans	parsnips	tomato
lima beans	radishes	white potato
mushrooms	squash	
navy beans	sweet potato	

TABLE 14
Your Personal Drug Profile

I have spoken to countless patients who were sure that they knew how much of their medicines to take, and when to take them, only to learn that they were not only taking the wrong dose, but had also been taking a second medicine too many or too few times a day. Knowing as much as possible about your body and your medicines can save your life. Please take the time to fill out this profile with the latest information. **Medicine never does you any good if you forget to take it. Take control of that chronic disease or condition by finding the goals and taking the medicine.** Also make time to copy the Medication Map and have your doctor or pharmacist fill it in and discuss it with you. Make sure you work with your doctor to fit your medicines into your life.

Name: _____

Age: _____

Weight in kilograms (pounds divided by 2.2): _____

Height in inches: _____

Prescription drug allergies: _____

_____

Non-prescription drug allergies: _____

_____

Food allergies: _____

_____

My kidneys* are: normal_____

mildly_____   moderately_____   severely_____   compromised.

My liver* is: normal_____

mildly_____   moderately_____   severely_____   compromised.

Conditions or diseases that I have or have had: _____

_____

Prescription and nonprescription medications I take regularly:_____

_____

Prescription and nonprescription medications I take periodically:_____

_____

*Make certain your dose is decreased if the drug is eliminated by an organ (such as the liver or kidneys) with which you have a problem. To determine which organs are involved, refer to the drug profile, and in particular the "Conditions Requiring Adjustments" section, for each medication you are taking.

I find it very difficult_____ to remember to take medicines.

I find it very easy_____ to remember to take medicines.

I become constipated rarely_____ occasionally_____ never_____.

Urination is usually easy_____ rather difficult_____ difficult_____.

The phone number of the nearest Poison Control Center is_____.

I sleep well_____ OK_____ poorly_____ little_____ on most nights.

I have_____ have never_____ had blood problems in the past.

I am considering becoming_____ might be_____ am_____ pregnant.

I want the medications that offer the best balance of price and outcomes for my specific medical history and present conditions.

TABLE 15

The Medication Map

Getting four new prescriptions often means that you will get four brief patient package inserts or papers stapled to the pharmacy bag when you pick up your prescriptions. Rarely does anyone take the time to understand YOUR INDIVIDUAL day and select medicines based on how your day REALLY works or help you fit the medicines into the way that you actually live. I believe that this is a critical cause of drug interactions, irrational drug combinations and taking the medicine incorrectly. It also dooms to failure what otherwise might be brilliant use of medicines.

This reality contributes to the more than 100 billion dollars spent EACH YEAR and leads to the more than 100,000 deaths caused by the medicine itself. I can't begin to count the number of times I've found that medicines prescribed three times a day were actually only taken twice a day or less. The cure can easily become the disease.

Use the map below to talk with your doctor or pharmacist to schedule your prescription, nonprescription or herbal medicines as you really plan or are able to take them. Make sure the timing and combinations are OK! Important questions to ask include:

Have all of these medicines been checked for drug interactions?

Do I really need to take all of these medicines at this time?

Are there newer medicines that might have fewer possible side effects or that might treat the conditions or diseases being treated more effectively (get better results or outcomes)?

Are there medicines that only need to be taken twice or once daily that could be substituted for one or more of those I take now?

Can food react with any of the medicines I take?

Midnight	Medicine and dose planned:	
1 A.M.	Medicine and dose planned:	
2 A.M.	Medicine and dose planned:	
3 A.M.	Medicine and dose planned:	
4 A.M.	Medicine and dose planned:	
5 A.M.	Medicine and dose planned:	
6 A.M.	Medicine and dose planned:	
7 A.M.	Medicine and dose planned:	*Morning Meal Time is:*
8 A.M.	Medicine and dose planned:	
9 A.M.	Medicine and dose planned:	
10 A.M.	Medicine and dose planned:	
11 A.M.	Medicine and dose planned:	
12 noon	Medicine and dose planned:	*Lunch or Brunch Time:*
1 P.M.	Medicine and dose planned:	
2 P.M.	Medicine and dose planned:	
3 P.M.	Medicine and dose planned:	
4 P.M.	Medicine and dose planned:	
5 P.M.	Medicine and dose planned:	
6 P.M.	Medicine and dose planned:	*Evening Meal Time:*
7 P.M.	Medicine and dose planned:	
8 P.M.	Medicine and dose planned:	
9 P.M.	Medicine and dose planned:	*Snack Time (if any):*
10 P.M.	Medicine and dose planned:	
11 P.M.	Medicine and dose planned:	

TABLE 16

Medicines Removed from the Market

Once again, either the FDA or the companies that make medicines have seen fit to remove some medicines from the market. As in the 2000 edition, I've included prior removals for continuity. While removals could be seen as disconcerting, it also shows that the Phase Four (reporting after a drug is FDA-approved) system sometimes works. This also means that more than ever, you need to be a partner in your health care! Talk to your doctor right away if you suspect you are having a reaction to one of your medicines. It is literally impossible for the FDA to check EVERY medicine against one that is pending approval for possible drug interactions or side effects. Encourage your doctor to report serious new adverse effects to the company that makes the drug or to the FDA (FDA MedWatch can be reached at 1-800-332-1088).

The information in this table will be updated for each subsequent *Essential Guide* edition. The listings will give the general category to which the medicine belongs, the generic name and at least one brand name and the reason for removal. While the web address and location give a rough idea of the date of removal, beginning with the 2002 edition, removals will have the FDA MedWatch removal report date with each new listing.

Antibiotics

grepafloxacin (Raxar)   Reason removed: Risks of adverse effects (abnormal heart rhythms or arrhythmias) outweighed the benefits.

Sparfloxacin (Zagam)   Reason removed: Drug interactions, safety profile.

Antidiabetic Drugs (Diabetes Treatments)

troglitazone (Rezulin)   Reason removed: Negative publicity regarding liver damage and death precluded effective use of the product. The FDA requested and the company voluntarily removed the medicine.

Antipsoriatic Drugs (Psoriasis Treatments)

etretinate (Tegison)   Reason removed: Newer medicines available.

Cholesterol Reducing Drugs

probucol (Lorelco)   Reason removed: More effective medicines available.

cerivastatin (Baycol)   Reason removed: Reports of sometimes fatal muscle damage (rhabdomyolysis)
FDA MedWatch report date 8/9/01: www.fda.gov/medwatch/safety/2001safety01.html#bayco2

Gastrointestinal Medicines (GERD, heartburn)

cisapride (Propulsid)   Reason removed: Serious cardiovascular side effects and drug interactions with multiple drugs.
More information can be found at www.fda.gov/medwatch/safety/2000/safety00.htm#propul

Herbal Medicines (Various indications and there have been a variety of herbs and herbal products)

Aristolochic Acid (Akebia   Reason removed: aristolochic acid has been found
Trifoliata Caulis-Mu Tong   to be a potent carcinogen and has been associated

and Asarum Sieboldii
Herba cum Radix-Xi Xin)

with several kidney failure cases. More
information can be found at www.fda.gov/medwatch/
satety/2001/safety01.htm#aristo

High Blood Pressure Medicines (antihypertensives)

mibefradil (Posicor)

Reason removed: Serious drug interactions with
multiple drugs.
More information is at www.fda.gov/bbs/topice/
answers/ans00876.html

Immunosuppressant

cyclosporine
(Gegraf form only)

Reason removed: Found NOT to be bioequivalent to
Neoral when mixed with apple juice.
More information is at www.fda.gov

Irritable Bowel Syndrome Treatment

alosetron (Lotronex)

Reason removed: Voluntarily withdrawn because of
serious bowel impactions, ischemic colitis cases and
deaths. More information is available from the FDA
at www.fda.gov

Minimally Sedating Antihistamines

astemizole (Hismanal)

Reason removed: Voluntarily withdrawn because
of serious drug interactions with multiple drugs.
More information is available at: http://www.fda.gov/
bbs/topics/answers/ans00961.html

terfenadine (Seldane)

Reason removed: Voluntarily withdrawn because of
serious drug interactions with multiple drugs. Find
more info at: www.fda.gov/bbs/topics/answers/
ans00843.html

Vaccines

Rotavirus vaccine
(RotaShield)

Reason removed: Withdrawn because it can cause
the bowel to collapse or telescope onto itself
(intussusception). Find out more at www.fda.gov

Weight Loss Agents (Anorexiants)

dexfenfluramine (Redux)
fenfluramine (Pondimin)

Reason removed: Possible heart valve damage.
Reason removed: Possible heart valve damage.
Questions and answers about this can be found at
www.fda.gov/cder/news/fenphenqa2.htm

TABLE 17
Helpful, Balanced, and Objective Web Sites

There has been an explosion of information available on the Internet. Unfortunately,
like information found elsewhere, all of it is NOT reliable. From my own activities in
research, and from my experience with MY web site, I'm please to augment this new
table that tells you about web sites that I've found to offer balanced, objective and scientifically rigorous information. I've also added three sites that have been highly rated
in a survey by the Rowin Group. Happy surfing, and ALWAYS TALK TO YOUR
HEALTH CARE PROVIDER BEFORE YOU CHANGE ANY THERAPY.

To find information on taking your medicines (adherence, compliance or concordance)

www.4woman.gov
www.acog.org
www.nwhn.org
www.fda.gov/womens/tttc.html
www.health.gov/healthypeople
www.medicineinfo.com
www.medscape.com
www.aarp.org
www.talkaboutrx.org
www.americanheart.org/CAP/
www.onelife.americanheart.org

To find information on AIDS

www.amfar.org
www.cdc.org
www.Hopkins-aids.edu

To find information on Anxiety

www.nimh.nih.gov/anxiety

To find information on Arthritis

www.arthritis.org

To find information on Bacteria that have become resistant to treatment

www.fda.gov/oc/opacom/hottopics/anti_resist.html

To find information on Cancer

www.cancer.org
www.fda.gov/cder/cancer
www.cancertrails.nci.nih.gov
www.fda.gov/bs/topics/NEWS/2001/NEW00766.html
www.cancer.med.upenn.edu

To find information on Counterfeit Medicines

www.fda.gov/medwatch/safety/2001/sero_faked.html
www.amgen.com/news/news01/release01510.html
www.gene.com/gene/products/nutropin_aq/product_update.html

To find information on How to Stop Smoking (Cessation)

www.lungusa.org

To find information on Cholesterol Reducing Drugs

www.americanheart.org
www.onelife.americanheart.org
www.americanheart.org/getwiththeguidelines.html
www.acc.org
www.nhlbi.nih.gov

To find highly rated Consumer-Oriented web sites (breast cancer treatment, heartburn/ulcer treatment and high cholesterol treatment)

www.nolvadex.com
www.prevacid.com
www.zocor.com

To find information on Diabetes

www.diabetes.org

To find information on Health Care Policy and Research

www.ahcpr.gov

To find information on the Heart and Heart Health

www.americanheart.org
www.clevelandclinic.org
www.//sln.fi.edu/biosci/heart.html
www.med.yale.edu/library/heartbk/

To find information on Hospital Accreditation

www.jcaho.org

To find High Blood Pressure Medicines (Antihypertensives)

www.americanheart.org
www.cdc.gov
www.acc.org
www.nhlbi.nih.gov
www.ash-us.org

To find the FDA

www.fda.gov

To find out about Herbal Supplements and Disease/Structure Function Claims and Prudent Steps Regarding Herbals

http://vm.cfsan.fda.gov/;sllrd/fr000106.html
www.talkaboutrx.org

To find information on Menopause

www.acog.org
www.americanheart.org
www.asrm.org
www.menopause.org
www.4woman.gov

To find out about Nutrition

www.americanheart.org
www.eatright.org

To find out about Osteoporosis

www.nof.org
www.asbmr.org
www.iscd.org

To find information about Pain and Pain Guidelines

www.ahcpr.gov
www.jcaho.org/standard/pm_hap.html
www.painandhealth.org
www.backincontrol.net

To find information on Pediatrics

www.aap.org
www.tchin.org

To find information on Reproductive Health/Contraception

www.acog.org
www.amwa.org
www.nwhn.org
www.plannedparenthood.org
www.americanheart.org (as contraception impacts cardiovascular system)

To find information on Strokes

www.apacure.com
www.strokes.org

To find information on Transplantation

www.otf.org

To find information on Health Around the World

www.cdc.gov

To find information on Weight Control

www.americanheart.org/heart_and_stroke_A_Z_guide/obesity.html
www.eatright.org
www.naaso.org

Sources

The following sources were consulted in the compilation and revision of this book:

Abramowicz, M., ed. *The Choice of Antibacterial Drugs: The Medical Letter on Drugs and Therapeutics.* 1999. New Rochelle, NY: The Medical Letter.

Abramowicz, M., ed. *Drug Interactions: The Medical Letter on Drugs and Therapeutics.* Vol. 41 (issue 1056), July 2, 1999. New Rochelle, NY: The Medical Letter.

Abramowicz, M., ed. *Drugs of Choice: The Medical Letter on Drugs and Therapeutics.* 1997. New Rochelle, NY: The Medical Letter.

Abramowicz, M., ed. *Drugs of Choice: The Medical Letter on Drugs and Therapeutics.* 1999. New Rochelle, NY: The Medical Letter.

Abramowicz, M., ed. *Rofecoxib for Osteoarthritis Pain: The Medical Letter on Drugs and Therapeutics.* Vol. 41 (issue 1056), July 2, 1999. New Rochelle, NY: The Medical Letter.

Abramowicz, M., ed. *Some Drugs That Cause Psychiatric Symptoms: The Medical Letter on Drugs and Therapeutics.* 1998. New Rochelle, NY: The Medical Letter.

Ackerman, B.H., and N. Kasbekar. Disturbances of Taste and Smell Induced by Drugs. *Pharmacotherapy* 17(3):482–496. 1997.

Adrogue, H.J., and Madias, N.E. Hyponatremia. *The New England Journal of Medicine* 342(21):1581–1589. 2000.

Advances in Osteoporosis. 1996, 1997.

AIDS Clinical Care. 1997, 1998, 1999, 2000. Boston: Massachusetts Medical Society.

American Botanical Society. *The Complete German Commission E Monographs Therapeutic Guide to Herbal Medicines.* 1st ed. 1998. Austin, Texas: American Botanical Council and Integrative Medicine Communications.

American Heart Association. *2001 Heart and Stroke Statistical Update.* Dallas, Texas: American Heart Association, 2000.

American Heart Association. *Get With the Guidelines.* On www.americanheart.org. Dallas, Texas: American Heart Association, 2001.

American Journal of Clinical Nutrition. Harper, A.E., ed. Physiologically Active Food Components: Their Role in Optimizing Health and Aging. June 2000. Weston, MA.

American Journal of Hospice and Palliative Care. Enk, R., ed. 1998. Weston, MA.

American Medical Association (AMA), Joint Commission on Accreditation of Healthcare Organizations (JCAHO) and the National Committee for Quality Assurance (NCQA). *Coordinated Performance Measurement for the Management of Adult Diabetes.* April 2001, pages 1–42. 2001.

American Pharmaceutical Association Special Report: A Review of the Sixth Report of the Joint National Committee on Prevention, Detection, Evaluation and Treatment of High Blood Pressure. 1998. Washington, DC: American Pharmaceutical Association.

Anderson, A.S., et al. Current Management of Chronic Heart Failure. *Postgraduate Medicine.* 109(3):35–61. March, 2001.

Annals of Pharmacotherapy. 1996–1998. Cincinnati, OH: Harvey Whitney Books.

Aparasu, R.R. and Flinginger, S.E. Inappropriate Medication Prescribing for the Elderly by Office-Based Physicians. *Annals of Pharmacotherapy.* 31:823–836. July/August, 1997.

Adult Treatment Panel 3 (ATP III). Third Report of the National Cholesterol Education Program (NCEP) Expert Panel on Detection, Evaluation and Treatment of High Blood Cholesterol in Adults. June, 2001. The National Institutes of Health.

Baron, J.A., et al. Calcium Supplements for the Prevention of Colorectal Adenomas. *New England Journal of Medicine.* 340:101–107. January 14, 1999.

Bartlett, J., et al. *The Hopkins HIV Report.* Volume 13, Number 3 (Updated Guidelines for Managing HIV in Pregnancy From the USPHS Task Force and Update from the 8th CROI: Adverse Effects of HAART and Structured Treatment Interruption, Number 4. The Johns Hopkins University AIDS Service, Division of Infectious Diseases. 2001.

Bartlett, J. *The Johns Hopkins Hospital 1996 Guide to Medical Care of Patients with HIV Infection.* Baltimore: Williams and Wilkins.

Bartlett, J. *Medical Management of HIV Infection: 1998 Edition.* Baltimore: Port City Press.

Bartlett, J. and Gallant, J.E. 2000–2001 *Medical Management of HIV Infection.* Baltimore: Port City Press.

Bates, D., et al. Effect of Computerized Physician Order Entry and a Team Intervention on Prevention of Serious Medication Errors. *Journal of the American Medical Association.* 280(15):1311–1316. October 21, 1998.

Beard, S.L. HMG-CoA Reductase Inhibitors: Assessing Differences in Drug Interactions and Safety Profiles. *Journal of the American Pharmaceutical Association Sept/Oct 2000.* 40(5):637–644. 2000.

Beckman, S.E., et al., Consumer Use of St. John's Wort: A Survey on Effectiveness, Safety and Tolerability. *Pharmacotherapy 2000.* 20(5):568–574. 2000.

Berchou, R.C. and Scheife, R.T. Contemporary Issues in the Pharmacotherapy of Parkinson's Disease. *Pharmacotherapy the Journal of Human Pharmacology and Drug Therapy.* Vol. 20, No. 1 Part 2, January, 2000.

Berger, K., et al. Light-to-Moderate Alcohol Consumption and the Risk of Stroke Among U.S. Male Physicians. *The New England Journal of Medicine.* 341(21):1557. November 18, 1999.

Berkow, R., ed. *The Merck Manual.* 15th ed. 1996. Rahway, NJ: Merck Sharp and Dohme Research Laboratories.

Bonnick, S.L. *The Osteoporosis Handbook.* 1994. Dallas: Taylor Publishing.

Borenstein, D. *Back in Control A Conventional and Complimentary Prescription for Eliminating Back Pain.* M. Evans, New York. 2001.

Burke, L.E. and Ockene, I.S. *Compliance in Healthcare and Research.* The American Heart Association. Futura Publishing Company, Armonk, NY. 2000.

Boullata, J.I. and Nace, A.M. Safety Issues with Herbal Medicine. *Pharmacotherapy The Journal of Human Pharmacology and Drug Therapy.* 20(3):257–269. 2000.

Briggs, G.G., Bodendorfer, T.W., Freeman, R.K., and S.J. Yaffee. *Drugs in Pregnancy and Lactation.* 1983. Baltimore: Williams and Wilkins.

Brooke, M.H. *A Clinician's View of Neuromuscular Diseases.* 2nd ed. 1986. Baltimore: Williams and Wilkins.

Business Wire: June 28, 2001. Roche and Trimeris Correct Previous Announcement on Complete Enrollment in T-20 Phase III Clinical Trial. Nutley, NJ and Durham, NC.

Cabana, M.D., et al. Why Don't Physicians Follow Clinical Practice Guidelines? A Framework for Improvement. *Journal of the American Medical Association,* 282:1458–1465.

Canadian Pharmaceutical Association, St. Paul's Hospital British Columbia Center of Excellence for HIV-AIDS. 1997, 1998. Vancouver, BC: Canadian Pharmaceutical Association.

Cape, R. *Aging: Its Complex Management.* 1978. Hagerstown, MD: Harper and Row.

Caring for the Dying. 1996. American Board of Internal Medicine.

Carnahan, R.M., et al. Ziprasidone, a New Atypical Antipsychotic Drug. *Pharmacotherapy* 2001;21(6):717–730. 2001.

Cheng, J.W.M., et al. Patient-Reported Adherence to Guidelines of the Sixth Joint National Committee on Prevention, Detection, Evaluation and Treatment of High Blood Pressure. *Pharmacotherapy* 2001;21(7):828–841. 2001.

Classen, D.C., et al. Adverse Drug Events in Hospitalized Patients. *Journal of the American Medical Association.* 277:301–306. 1997.

Clin-Alert. 1996–1997. Medford, NJ: Clin-Alert.

Clinisphere. Facts and Comparisons 2.0. 1999. St. Louis: Facts and Comparisons.

Compendium of Pharmaceuticals and Specialties. 26th ed. 1991. Ottawa: Canadian Pharmaceutical Association.

Conroy, W.E., et al. Lipid Screening in Adults. Working to prevent coronary artery disease. *Postgraduate Medicine.* 107(4):229–235. April, 2000.

Cooper, S.M. Improving Outcomes in Osteoarthritis. *Postgraduate Medicine.* 105(6):29–38. 1999.

Crouse, J.R., et al. A Randomized Trial Comparing the Effect of Casein With That of Soy Protein Containing Varying Amounts of Isoflavones on Plasma Concentrations of Lipids and Lipoproteins. *Arch Int. Med* 159:2070–2076. September 27, 1999.

Cumming, R.G., et al. Use of Inhaled Corticosteroids and the Risk of Cataracts. *New England Journal of Medicine.* 337(1):8–14. 1997.

Cupp, M.J. Herbal Remedies: Adverse Effects and Drug Interactions. *American Family Physician.* 59(5):1239–1244. 1999.

Daniels, J.B., ed. *Infectious Disease in Clinical Practice.* 1997. Baltimore: Williams and Wilkins.

Davis, E.A. and Pathak, D.S. Psychometric Evaluation of Four HIV Disease-Specific Quality-of-Life Instruments. *Annals of Pharmacotherapy.* 159:546–552. May, 2001.

Depression in Primary Care. Volume 1: Detection and Diagnosis. 1993. Washington, DC: U.S. Department of Health and Human Services.

DiGregorio, J.G., et al. *Handbook of Pain Management.* 1991. Westchester, NY: Medical Surveillance.

Drug Information Journal. 1996–1998.

Drug Interactions Newsletter. 1997. Spokane, WA: Applied Therapeutics.

DrugLink. 1998. St. Louis: J.B. Lippincott, Facts and Comparisons.

Drug Newsletter. 1998. St. Louis: J.B. Lippincott, Facts and Comparisons.

Drugs and Therapy Perspectives. 1996–1997.

Drug Therapy: Physicians Prescribing Update. 1992. Lawrenceville, NJ: Excerpta Medica.

Dukes, M.N.G., ed. *Meyler's Side Effects of Drugs.* 11th ed. 1988. Amsterdam: Excerpta Medica.

Eastell, R., et al. Treatment of Postmenopausal Osteoporosis. *New England Journal of Medicine.* 338(11):736–746. 1998.

Electronic Library of Medicine. 1996. Boston: Little, Brown.

Epstein, F.H., et al. Acute-Phase Proteins and Other Systemic Responses to Inflammation. *New England Journal of Medicine.* 340(6):448–454. February 11, 1999.

Erramouspe, J. and Heyneman, A. Treatment and Prevention of Otitis Media. *The Annals of Pharmacotherapy.* 34:1452. 2001.

Farrell, B., and B. Farrell, eds. *Pain in the Elderly.* 1996. International Association for the Study of Pain Press.

Favus, M., ed. *Primer on the Metabolic Bone Diseases and Disorders of Mineral Metabolism.* 3rd ed. 1996. Philadelphia, New York: Lippincott-Raven.

FDA Drug Bulletin. 1996–1997. Rockville, MD: Department of Health and Human Services, Food and Drug Administration.

FDA News Digest. July 16, 2001. Guidance on Levothyroxine Sodium Products. Rockville, MD: Department of Health and Human Services, Food and Drug Administration.

Fitzgerald, G.A. and Patrono, C. The Coxibs, Selective Inhibitors of Cyclooxygenase-2. *The New England Journal of Medicine.* August 9, 2000. Vol 345(6). Content.nejm.org/cgi/content/short/345/6/433.

Frackiewicz, Edyta J., *Endometriosis: An Overview of the Disease and Its Treatment. Journal of the American Pharmaceutical Association.* Vol. 40, No. 5, September/October 2000.

Frackiewicz, Edyta J. and N. Cutler. *Women's Health Care During the Perimenopause. Journal of the American Pharmaceutical Association.* Vol. 40, No. 6. November/December 2000.

Francis, G. S., ed. *The Cleveland Clinic Heart Advisor.* 3(4):3. 2000.

Fraunfelder, F. T. *Drug-Induced Ocular Side Effects and Drug Interactions.* 3rd ed. 1989. Philadelphia: Lea and Febiger.

Generali, M. S., ed., et al. *Clini-Alert Reporting on Adverse Clinical Events.* 38(7):1–8. 2000.

Ghandi, S. K., et al. The Pathogenesis of Acute Pulmonary Edema Associated with Hypertension. *The New England Journal of Medicine.* 344(1):17–22. January 4, 2001.

Gleason, P. P., et al. Medical Outcomes and Antimicrobial Costs With the Use of the American Thoracic Society Guidelines for Outpatients With Community Acquired Pneumonia. *Journal of the American Medical Association.* 278(1):32–39. 1997.

Goldman, S. A., et al. Minimizing the Risks of Drug Interactions. *Patient Care.* March 30, 1999:26–68.

Goodman, L. S., and A. Gilman, eds. *The Pharmacological Basis of Therapeutics.* 9th ed. 1996. New York: Macmillan.

Graham, A. S. Cytochrome P450 Drug Interactions. *The Rx Consultant.* 8(2):1–8. 1999.

Graham, I. M., et al. Plasma Homocysteine as a Risk Factor for Vascular Disease. *Journal of the American Medical Association.* 277(22):1775–1781. 1997.

Graumlich, J. F., MD. Preventing gastrointestinal complications of NSAIDS Risk factors, recent advances, and latest strategies. *Postgraduate Medicine* 109(5):117–128. May 2001.

Gray, S. L., et al. Medication Adherence in Elderly Patients Receiving Home Health Services Following Hospital Discharge. The Annals of Pharmacotherapy. 35(5): 539–545. May 2001.

Greenland, P. Beating High Blood Pressure with Low-Sodium DASH. *The New England Journal of Medicine.* 344(1): 53–55. January 4, 2001.

Griffiths, M. C., ed. *USAN* 1989. Rockville, MD: United States Pharmacopeial Convention.

Griffiths, M. C., ed. *The USP Dictionary of Drug Names.* 1988. Rockville, MD: United States Pharmacopeial Convention.

Guay, DRP. Cefdinir: An expanded Spectrum Oral Cephalosporin. *The Annals of Pharmacotherapy 2000.* 34:1469–1477. 2000.

Hambrecht, M. D., et al. Effect of Exercise on Coronary Endothelial Function in Patients With Coronary Artery Disease. *The New England Journal of Medicine.* 342(7):454–460. 2000.

Handbook of Clinical Drug Data. 1993. Hamilton, IL: Drug Intelligence Publications.

Handbook of Nonprescription Drugs. 11th ed. 1996. Washington, DC: American Pharmaceutical Association.

Hanlon, J. T., et al. Inappropriate Drug Use Among Community-Dwelling Elderly. *Pharmacotherapy 2000.* 20(5):575–582. 2000.

Hansten, P. D. *Drug Interactions.* 6th ed. 1992. Philadelphia: Lea and Febiger.

Hansten, P. D. and Horn, J. R. *The Top 100 Drug Interactions. A Guide to Patient Management.* 2001. Edmonds: H&H Publications.

Hart, S. Influence of B-Blockers on Mortality in Chronic Heart Failure. *The Annals of Pharmacotherapy.* 34:1440–1451. 2001.

Hasketh, P. L., ed. *The Journal of Oncology.* 1998. Cedar Knolls, NJ: National Medical Information Network.

Hayden, F, et al. Inhaled Zanamivir for the Prevention of Influenza in Families. *The New England Journal of Medicine.* 343(18):1282–1289. 2000.

Heck, A. M., et al. Orlistat, a New Lipase Inhibitor for the Management of Obesity. *Pharmacotherapy the Journal of Human Pharmacology and Drug Therapy.* 20(3):270–279. 2000.

Hecht, H. S., et al. Electron Beam Tomography and National Cholesterol Education Program Guidelines in Asymptomatic Women. *Journal of the American College of Cardiology.* 37(6): 1506–1511. 2001.

Heinonen, O.P., Slone, D., and S. Shapiro. *Birth Defects and Drugs in Pregnancy.* 1977. Littleton, MA: PSG Publishing.

Herrerias, C.T., et al. The Child with ADHD. Using the AAP Clinical Practice Guideline. *American Family Physician.* 63(9):1803–1812. 2001.

Hilleman, D.E. and Bauman, J.L. Role of Antiarrhythmic Therapy in Patients at Risk for Sudden Cardiac Death: An Evidence-Based Review. *Pharmacotherapy 2001.* 21(5):556–574. 2001.

Hollister, L.E. *Clinical Pharmacology of Psychotherapeutic Drugs.* 2nd ed. 1983. New York: Churchill Livingstone.

Houston Miller, N., et al. The Multilevel Compliance Challenge: Recommendations for a Call to Action. *Circulation* 95:1085–1090. The American Heart Association 1997.

Hussar, D.A. New Drugs of 2000. *Journal of the American Pharmaceutical Association.*41(2):229–280. The American Pharmaceutical Association. March/April 2001.

The Hospice Journal. 1998. New York: The Haworth Press.

Influenza and Pneumococcal Vaccination Levels Among Adults Aged Greater Than or Equal to 65. *Morbidity and Mortality Weekly Report.* 47:797–802. October 2, 1998.

International Drug Therapy Newsletter. 1997. Baltimore: Ayd Medical Communications.

Janne, P.A., and Mayer, R.J. Chemoprevention of Colorectal Cancer. *New England Journal of Medicine.* 342(26):1960–1968. 2000.

Jefferson, J.W., and J.H. Greist. *Primer of Lithium Therapy.* 1977. Baltimore: Williams and Wilkins.

Jellin, J.M., et al. Pharmacist's Letter. 17(1):1–6. 2001.

Johnson, M.D., et al. Clinically Significant Drug Interactions: What You Need to Know Before Writing Prescriptions. *Postgraduate Medicine.* 105(2):193–222. 1999.

Jorenby, D.E., Ph.D., et al. A Controlled Trial of Sustained-Release Bupropion, a Nicotine Patch, or Both for Smoking Cessation. *New England Journal of Medicine.* 340(9):685–691. 1999.

Journal of Acquired Immune Deficiency Syndromes. 1999. Hagerstown, MD: Lippincott-Raven.

Journal of the American Medical Association. 1997–1999.

Journal of Bone and Mineral Research. 1996–2000. Malden, MA: Blackwell Science, Inc.

Journal of the National Cancer Institute. 1999. Cary, NC: Oxford University Press.

Journal Watch. 1996–2000. Waltham, MA: The Massachusetts Medical Society.

Journal Watch: Women's Health. 1996–2000. Waltham, MA: The Massachusetts Medical Society.

Kaplan, N.M. *Management of Hypertension.* 6th ed. 1995. Durant, OK: Essential Medical Information Systems.

Kelly, William N. Can the Frequency and Risks of Fatal Adverse Drug Events Be Determined? *Pharmacotherapy.* 21(5). May 2001.

Klippel, J.H., ed. Systemic Lupus Erythematosus Demographics, Prognosis and Outcome. *Journal of Rheumatol Suppl* 48:67–71. 1997.

Koda-Kimbal (Lloyd Yee Young). *Applied Therapeutics: The Clinical Use of Drugs.* 6th ed. 1995. Vancouver, WA: Applied Therapeutics.

Koller, W.C., ed. *Handbook of Parkinson's Disease.* 1987. New York: Marcel Dekker.

Kolodny, R.C., Masters, W.H., and V.E. Johnson. *Textbook of Sexual Medicine.* 1979. Boston: Little, Brown.

Kovacs, J.A., and Masur, H. Prophylaxis Against Opportunistic Infections in Patients with Human Immunodeficiency Virus Infection. *NEJM.* 342(19):1416–1429. May 11, 2000.

Lambing, C.L. Osteoporosis prevention, detection, and Treatment. A mandate for primary care physicians. *Postgraduate Medicine.* 107(7):37–56. June, 2000.

Lawrence, R.A. *Breast-Feeding.* 1980. St. Louis: Mosby.

Leon, A.C., et al., Prospective Study of Fluoxetine Treatment of Suicidal Behavior in Affectively Ill Subjects. *American Journal of Psychiatry.* 156:195–201. 1999.

Lieberman, M.L. *The Sexual Pharmacy.* 1988. New York: New American Library.

Long, J.W. *Clinical Management of Prescription Drugs.* 1984. Philadelphia: Harper and Row.

Long, J.W. *The Essential Guide to Chronic Illness*. 1997. New York: HarperCollins.

Love, N., et al. Symposium: A New Era in Breast Cancer. *Postgraduate Medicine*. 105(6): 43–103. 1999.

Lowy, F.D. Staphylococcus Aureus Infections. *New England Journal of Medicine*. 339 (8):520–532. August 20, 1998.

Maddin, S., ed. *Current Dermatologic Therapy*. 1982. Philadelphia: W.B. Saunders.

Marcus, A.O. Lipid Disorders in Patients with Type 2 Diabetes Meeting the Challenges of Early, Aggressive Treatment. *Postgraduate Medicine*. 110(1):111–123. 2001.

Martin, W.R., Fuller, R.E. Suspected Chromium Picolinate-Induced Rhabdomyolysis. *Pharmacotherapy*. 18(4):860–862. 1998.

Mayeuz, R., and Sano, M. Treatment of Alzheimer's Disease. *The New England Journal of Medicine*. 341(22):1670–1679. November 25, 1999.

Mayo Clinic Proceedings. 1996–2000.

McEvoy, G.K., ed. *American Hospital Formulary Service: Drug Information 1997*. Bethesda, MD: American Society of Hospital Pharmacists.

Medical Letter on Drugs and Therapeutics. 1998, 1999, 2000. New Rochelle, NY: The Medical Letter.

Mehta, S.R., M.D., et al. The Clopidogrel in Unstable angina to prevent Recurrent Events (CURE) trial programme. Rationale, design and baseline characteristics including a meta-analysis of the effects of thienopyridines in vascular disease CURE study investigators. *European Heart Journal (2000)*. 21,2022–2041. 2000.

Melmon, K.L., and Morrelli, H.F. *Clinical Pharmacology*. 2nd ed. 1978. New York: Macmillan.

Michelson, M.D., et al. Bone Mineral Density in Women with Depression. *New England Journal of Medicine*. 335(16):1176–1181. 1996.

Micromedex: Drugdex. 1999, 2000. Englewood, CO: Computerized Clinical Information System.

Milgrom, H., et al. Treatment of Allergic Asthma with Monoclonal Anti-IgE Antibody. *The New England Journal of Medicine*. 341(26): 1964–1972. December 23, 1999.

Modi, P., et al. *The Evolving Role of Oral Insulin Spray (RapidMist) in the Treatment of Diabetes*. 5th International Congress of Immunology. Madrid, India February 2001.

Modi, P., et al. *The Role of Oral Insulin Combined with Metformin in the Treatment of Diabetes*. American Association National Meeting. Philadelphia, PA, USA June 2001.

Mohler, S.R. *Medication and Flying: A Pilot's Guide*. 1982. Boston: Boston Publishing.

Mossad, S.B. Prophylactic and Symptomatic Treatment of Influenza Current and Developing Options. *Postgraduate Medicine* 109. 97–105. January 2001.

Mongthuong, TT, et al. Role of Coenzyme Q10 in Chronic Heart Failure, Angina, and Hypertension. *Pharmacotherapy* 2001;21(7):797–806.

Montserrat, V.L. et al. Cost-Effectiveness Results from the US Carvedilol Heart Failure Trials Program. *The Annals of Pharmacotherapy;*35:846–851. 2001.

Morbidity and Mortality Weekly Report (MMWR): Prevention and Control of Influenza. Vol. 48 No. RR-4 April 30, 1999. Washington, DC: U.S. Department of Health and Human Services.

Morbidity and Mortality Weekly Report (MMWR): Report of the NIH Panel to Define Principles of Therapy of HIV Infection and Guidelines for the Use of Antiretroviral Agents in HIV-Infected Adults and Adolescents. April 24, 1998. Washington, DC: U.S. Department of Health and Human Services, CDC Atlanta, Georgia.

Mosca, L., et al. Guide to Preventive Cardiology for Women. *Circulation*. 1999;99:2480–2484. 1999.

Mossad, S.B. Prophylactic and Symptomatic Treatment of Influenza Current and Developing Options. *Postgraduate Medicine* 109. 97–105. January 2001.

Mosher, M. *Clinical Management of Hypertension*. Fourth Edition. 1999. Caddo, OK: Professional Communications, Inc.

Mukherjee, D., Nissen, S.E. and Topol, E.J. Risk of Cardiovascular Events Associated With Selective COX-2 Inhibitors. *Journal of the American Medical Association*. 286(8); August 22/29, 2001. accessed from www.jama.ama-assn.org/issues/v286n8/rfull/jsc10193.html.

Murphy, J. E. *Clinical Pharmacokinetics.* 1993. Bethesda, MD: American Society of Hospital Pharmacists.

Nallamothu, M., Fendrick, M. Rubenfire, et al. Lowering Elevated Homocysteine Levels Could Result in Substantial Clinical Benefits at a Reasonable Cost. *Archives of Internal Medicine* 160. 3406–3412. December 11, 2000.

National Center For Health Statistics, CDC. *Leading Causes of Death.* 2001. www.cdc.gov/nchs/fastats/icod.htm.

National Institutes of Health's (NIH, NHLBI) Guidelines for Diagnosis and Management of Asthma. 1997.

Nephropathy, urinary tract cancer from herbal products containing aristolochic acid. FDA. www.cfsan.fd.gov/;sldms/ds-bot3.html. Pharmacy Today. Page 5, June 2001.

Nerhood, RC. Making a Decision about ERT/HRT. *Postgraduate Medicine.* 109 (3):167–178. 2001.

New England Journal of Medicine. 1997–2001.

Nielsen, J.W., MD, et al. Optimal Antidepressant Dosing. Practical framework for selection, titration, and duration of therapy. *Postgraduate Medicine.* 108 (5):111–115. Oct. 2000.

Olin, B. R., ed. *Facts and Comparisons.* 1997, 1998, 2000. St. Louis: J. B. Lippincott, Facts and Comparisons.

Olin, B. R., ed. 1992. *Patient Drug Facts.* St. Louis: J. B. Lippincott, Facts and Comparisons.

O'Laughlin, J., et al. The Role of Community Pharmacists in Health Education and Disease Prevention: A Survey of Their Interests and Needs in Relation to Cardiovascular Disease. *Preventive Medicine.* 28:324–331. 1999.

Pain Forum: Official Journal of the American Pain Society. 1997, 1998, 2000. Secaucus, NJ: Churchill Livingstone.

Palacioz, K. P. et al. Drug-Induced Long QT Interval. *Detail-Document 170401 Therapeutic Resource Center. Pharmacist's Letter/Prescriber's Letter 2001.*

Penzak, et al. Depression in patients with HIV infection. *American Journal of Health System Pharm.* 57:376–389. Feb 15, 2000.

Perazella, M. A. COX-2 Inhibitors and the Kidney. Hospital Practice, March 15, 2001.

Pharmacotherapy: The Journal of Human Pharmacology and Drug Therapy. 1997–2001.

Physicians' Desk Reference. Electronic Library 2000.1, version 5.1 AT. Montvale, NJ: Medical Economics.

Physician's GenRX. 1996. Version 96.1a. St. Louis, MO: Mosby.

Physician's Therapeutics and Drug Alert. 1998–2001.

Postgraduate Medicine: The Journal of Applied Medicine for the Primary Care Physician. 1998–2000.

Practice Guideline for the Treatment of Patients With Alzheimer's Disease and Other Dementias of Late Life. 1997. Washington, DC: American Psychiatric Association.

Pratt, D. S., and Kaplan, M. M. Evaluation of Abnormal Liver-Enzyme Results in Asymptomatic Patients. *New England Journal of Medicine.* 342(17):1266–1271. April 27, 2000.

Principles of Analgesic Use in the Treatment of Acute Pain and Cancer Pain. 3rd ed. 1996. Glenview, IL: American Pain Society.

Principles of Analgesic Use in the Treatment of Acute Pain and Cancer Pain. 4th ed. 1999. Glenview, IL: American Pain Society.

Qtdrugs.org. International Registry for Drug-Induced Arrhythmias "drugs to avoid in patients with congenital Long QT syndrome." June 2001.

Quality Improvement Guidelines for the Treatment of Acute Pain and Cancer Pain. 1995. Glenview, IL: American Pain Society Quality of Care Committee.

Quintiliani, R., MD, et al. Optimizing Antiinfective Transition Therapy In Community-Acquired Pneumonia. *Pharmacotherapy.*21(7)Part two: 1-108S. July 2001.

Raj, P. P. *Practical Management of Pain.* 1986. Chicago: Year Book Medical Publishers.

Rakel, R. E., ed. *Conn's Current Therapy* 1992. Philadelphia: W. B. Saunders.

Rational Drug Therapy and Pharmacology for Physicians. 1990. Bethesda, MD: American Society for Pharmacology and Experimental Therapeutics.

The Diabetes Control and Complication Trial. Retinopathy and Nephropathy in Patients with Type 1 Diabetes Four Years After a Trial of Intensive Therapy. *The New England Journal of Medicine.* 342(6): 381–389. February 10, 2000.

Reynolds, J.E.F., ed. *Martindale: The Extra Pharmacopoeia.* 29th ed. 1997. London: The Pharmaceutical Press.

Rogers, C.S., and J.D. McCue, eds. *Managing Chronic Disease.* 1987. Oradell, NJ: Medical Economics Books.

Romanelli, F., et al., Human Immunodeficiency Virus Drug Resistance Testing: State of the Art in Genotypic and Phenotypic Testing of Antiretrovirals. *Pharmacotherapy 2000;* 20(2):151–157.

Russo, R.L. and D'Aprille, M. Role of Antimicrobial Therapy in Acute Exacerbations of Chronic Obstructive Pulmonary Disease. *The Annals of Pharmacotherapy.* 35, 576–580. May 2001.

Rybacki, J.J. Letter to the editor. *Journal of the American Medical Association.* 277(17):1351. 1997.

Rybacki, J.J. "What was the CURE trial?" Good News and New Medicines. 3(2):page 3 on www.medicineinfo.com. April 2001.

Sacks, F.M., et al. Effects on Blood Pressure of Reduced Dietary Sodium and the Dietary Approaches to Stop Hypertension (DASH) Diet. *The New England Journal of Medicine.* 344(1): 3–10. January 4, 2001.

Sanford, J., et al. *The Sanford Guide to HIV/AIDS Therapy.* 5th ed. 1996. Antimicrobial Therapy, Inc. Vienna, VA: Lippincott-Raven.

Sauer, G.C. *Manual of Skin Diseases.* 5th ed. 1985. Philadelphia: J.B. Lippincott.

Scan Newsletter. 1996–1998. Norwich, NY: Society for Clinical Densitometry.

Schardein, J.L. *Drugs as Teratogens.* 1976. Cleveland: CRC Press.

Scheife, R.T., et al. Low Molecular Weight Heparins for Venous Thromboembolism: Making an Evidence-based Treatment Choice. *Pharmacotherapy.* 21(6), Part 2. June 2001.

Scheife, R.T., et al. New Strides in Asthma. *Pharmacotherapy.* 21(3), Part 2. March 2001.

Scientific American Medicine. 1999. CD-ROM. New York: Enigma Information Systems.

Second Scientific Forum on Quality of Care and Outcomes Research in Cardiovascular Disease and Stroke. April 2000. The American Heart Association Councils on Clinical Cardiology, Cardiovascular Nursing, Cardiovascular Disease in the Young, Cardio-Thoracic and Vascular Surgery, Epidemiology and Prevention, High Blood Pressure Research and the American College of Cardiology. Abstracts. Washington, DC.

Semla, T.P., et al. *Geriatric Dosage Handbook.* 1993. Cleveland: Lexi-comp.

Shavelle, D. M., et al. Exercise Testing and Electron Beam Computed Tomography in the Evaluation of Coronary Artery Disease. *Journal of the American College of Cardiology.* 36(1). 2000.

Shepard, J.E. Effects of Estrogen on Cognition, Mood, and Degenerative Brain Diseases. *Journal of the American Pharmaceutical Association* 41(2): 221–228. March/April 2001.

Shepard, T.H. *Catalog of Teratogenic Agents.* 6th ed. 1989. Baltimore: Johns Hopkins University Press.

Sickle Cell Disease: Screening, Diagnosis, Management and Counseling in Newborns and Infants. 1993. Washington, DC: U.S. Department of Health and Human Services.

Simpson, S.H., et al. Economic Impact of Community Pharmacist Intervention in Cholesterol Risk Management: An Evaluation of the Study of Cardiovascular Risk Intervention by Pharmacists. *Pharmacotherapy.* 21(5):627–635. Mar 1, 2001.

Skaehill, P.A. Tacrolimus in Dermatologic Disorders. *The Annals of Pharmacotherapy.* 35:582–588. May 2001.

Sleeper, R., et al. Psychotropic Drugs and Falls: New Evidence Pertaining to Serotonin Reuptake Inhibitors. *Pharmacotherapy 2000.* 20(3):308–317. 2000.

Smith, L.H., and Thier, S.O. *Pathophysiology: The Biological Principles of Disease.* 2nd ed. 1985. Philadelphia: W.B. Saunders.

Song, J.C., et al. Pharmacologic, Pharmacokinetic and Therapeutic Differences Among Angiotensin II Receptor Antagonists. *Pharmacotherapy The Journal of Human Pharmacology and Drug Therapy.* 20(2):130–39. 2000.

Sorensen, S.J., and S.R. Abel. Comparison of the Ocular Beta-Blockers. *Annals of Pharmacotherapy.* 30:43–54. 1997.

Sotiriou, C.G. and Cheng, J. Beneficial Effects of Statins in Coronary Artery Disease—Beyond Lowering Cholesterol. *The Annals of Pharmacotherapy.* 34:1432–1439. 2000.

Spanheimer, R.G. Reducing Cardiovascular Risk in Diabetes: Which Factors to Modify First? *Postgraduate Medicine.* 109(4):26–36. 2001.

Spath, P.L., ed. *Clinical Paths, Tools for Outcomes Management.* 1994. Chicago: The American Hospital Association

Speight, T.M., and N.H.G. Holford, eds. *Avery's Drug Treatment.* 4th ed. 1997. Auckland, NZ: Adis International.

Spinler, S.A. New Recommendations from the 1999 American College of Cardiology/American Heart Association Acute Myocardial Infarction Guidelines. *The Annals of Pharmacotherapy.* 35:589–588. May 2001.

Struckman, D.R. and Rivey, M.P. Combined Therapy with an Angiotensin II Receptor Blocker and an Angiotensin-Converting Enzyme Inhibitor in Heart Failure. *The Annals of Pharmacotherapy.* 35:242–248. 2001.

Sumpton, J.E. and Moulin, D.E. Treatment of Neuropathic Pain with Venlafaxine. *The Annals of Pharmacotherapy.* 35(5): 557–559. May 2001.

Swash, M., and Schwartz, M.S. *Neuromuscular Diseases.* 2nd ed. 1988. Berlin: Springer-Verlag.

Swenson, C.N., and Fundak, G. Observational cohort study of switching warfarin sodium products in a managed care organization. *Am Jrn Health Syst. Pharm.* 57:452–455. Mar 1, 2000.

Szefler, S., et al. (The Childhood Asthma Research Group) Long-term Effects of Budesonide or Nedocromil in Children with Asthma. *The New England Journal of Medicine.* 343 (15): 1054–1069.

Tatro, D.S., ed. *Drug Interaction Facts.* 1997. St. Louis: J.B. Lippincott, Facts and Comparisons.

Temple, M.E., and Nahata, M.C. Treatment of Pediatric Hypertension. *Pharmacotherapy.* 20(2):140–150. 2000.

Thordsen, D.J., and Welty, T.E., eds. *Clinical Abstracts: Current Therapeutic Findings.* 1998. Cincinnati, OH: Harvey Whitney Books.

Tran M.T., et al. Role of Coenzyme Q10 in Chronic Heart Failure, Angina, and Hypertension. *Pharmacotherapy 2001;* 21(7)797–806. 2001.

Tsuyuki, R.T. and Bungard, T.J. Poor Adherence with Hypolipidemic Drugs: A Lost Opportunity. *Pharmacotherapy.* 21(5)576–582. Mar 1, 2001.

Tuchmann-Duplessis, H. *Drug Effects on the Fetus.* 1975. Sydney, Australia: ADIS Press.

Tyler, V.E. *The Honest Herbal: A Sensible Guide to the Use of Herbs and Related Remedies.* 3rd ed. 1993. New York: Pharmaceutical Products Press, Haworth Press, Inc.

United States Pharmacopeial Convention (USP) Dispensing Information 1997. Vol. 1: Drug Information for the Health Care Provider. 12th ed. Rockville, MD: United States Pharmacopeial Convention.

Utian, W.H. *Menopause in Modern Perspective.* 1980. New York: Appleton-Century-Crofts.

Wallach, J.B. *Interpretation of Diagnostic Tests.* 6th ed. 1996. Boston: Little, Brown.

Watanabe, M.D. Antipsychotics The Treatment of Schizophrenia. *The Rx Consultant.* X(5):1–7. 2001.

Weimerskirch, P.R., and Ernst, M.E. Newer Dopamine Agonists in the Treatment of Restless Legs Syndrome. *The Annals of Pharmacotherapy.* 35:627–635. May 2001.

Ward, M.W., and Holimon, T.D. Calcium Treatment for Premenstrual Syndrome. *The Annals of Pharmacotherapy.* 33:1356–1358. 1999.

Wenzel, R.P. and Edmond, M.B. Managing Antibiotic Resistance. *New England Journal of Medicine.* 343(26): 1961–1963. December 28, 2000.

Willhite, L.A., and O'Connell, B. Urogenital Atrophy: Prevention and Treatment. *Pharmacotherapy;* 21(4):464–480.

Wolf, M.M., et al. Gastrointestinal Toxicity of Nonsteroidal Anti-Inflammatory Drugs. *New England Journal of Medicine.* June 17, 1999:1888–1899.

Wood, A.J.J., and Ito, S. Drug Therapy for Breast-Feeding Women. *New England Journal of Medicine.* 343(2):118–126. July 13, 2000.

Wood, A.J.J., et al. Diuretic Therapy. *New England Journal of Medicine.* 339(6):387–395. August 6, 1998.

Wood, M.J., and Cox J.L. HRT to Prevent Cardiovascular Disease. What studies show, how to advise patients. *Postgraduate Medicine.* 108 (3):59–72. Sept 1, 2000.

Worley, R.J., ed. Menopause. *Clinical Obstetrics and Gynecology.* 24(1):163–164. 1981.

www.backincontrol.net: Back Pain resource.

www.cdc.gov/ncidod/flu/fluvac.htm Vaccine Information Influenza Vaccine. July, 2001.

www.fda.gov/cder/approval?index.htm: The Food And Drug Administration. June, 2001.

www.fda.gov/cder/orange/docket/pdf: The Food And Drug Administration: CDERNEW6 June, 2001.

www.fdanewsdigest@oc.FDA.GOC (FDA News Digest): The Food And Drug Administration. July, August, 2001.

www.fda.gov/medwatch: The Food And Drug Administration: MedWatch various dates including 8/6/01, 2001.

www.medanews.com: MedAdNews. 20(5) May 2001.

www.naturaldatabase.com: The Pharmacist's Letter/Prescriber's Letter. August, 2001.

www.nlm.nih.gov/medlineplus/news/fullstory 2647.html: Herbal Medicines Pose Risk During Surgery: Report. July 11, 2001.

Yiu-Chung Chan, et al. Atypical Antipsychotics in Older Adults. *Pharmacotherapy.* 19:811–822. 1999.

Yki-Jarvinen, H., et al. Bedtime Insulin Plus Metformin Prevents Weight Gain and Reduces Frequency of Hypoglycemia in Type 2 Diabetes. *Annals of Internal Medicine.* 130:389–396. 1999.

Young, D.S. *Effects of Drugs on Clinical Laboratory Tests.* 1991 supplement. Washington, DC: AACC Press.

Young, L.L., ed. *Nonprescription Products: Formulations and Features '96–97.* Washington, DC: American Pharmaceutical Association.

Zametkin, A.J., and Ernst, M. Problems in the Management of Attention-Deficit-Hyperactivity Disorder. *New England Journal of Medicine.* 340(1):40–46. January 1999.

Index

This index contains all the brand and generic drug names included in Section Two.

Brand names of drugs appear in italic type and are capitalized.

Each brand name is followed by its generic name. The generic name is the name under which you'll find the drug profile in Section Two.

The symbol [CD] indicates that the brand name represents a combination drug that contains other generic drug components; see the Drug Profile for details on other components present. To be fully familiar with any combination drug [CD], it is necessary to read the Drug Profile of each component.

The symbol ✽ before the brand name of a combination drug indicates that the brand name is used in both the United States and Canada, but that the ingredients in the combination product in each country differ. The Canadian drug is marked with the symbol ✽ to distinguish it from the American drug with the same name.

A generic name with no page designation indicates an active component of a combination drug for which there is no Profile in Section Two. It is included to alert you to its presence, should you wish to consult your physician regarding its significance.

About the Author

JAMES J. RYBACKI, Pharm.D., was born in Oneonta, New York. He received his prepharmacy education at Creighton University and his Doctor of Pharmacy degree from the University of Nebraska Medical Center, College of Pharmacy, in Omaha. Dr. Rybacki has nearly three decades of hospital and clinical experience which include early efforts in gas-liquid chromatography research characterizing human drug metabolites, and data collection for the College of American Pathologists to establish normal values for laboratory studies. He is a member of the clinical faculty at the University of Maryland School of Pharmacy and has provided clinical rounding and hospital experience for Pharm.D. and bachelor students. He presently teaches a Drug Information rotation for Pharm.D. students at The Clearwater Group. He is board certified in pain management at the Diplomat level by the American Academy of Pain Management, and he provides ongoing clinical pain management and medicine information consulting nationwide. He lectures for the Department of Family Medicine at the Georgetown University School of Medicine. He is a member of The National Council of Hospice Professionals. Dr. Rybacki is actively involved in the postmarketing monitoring of medicines via The Drug Surveillance Network, a nationwide association of clinical pharmacists, and he is an approved External New Drug Application reviewer for the Canadian Drug Ministry. He lives in Maryland.

Dr. Rybacki's efforts in drug information and clinical pharmacy include many years of active practice, including infectious disease, pharmacokinetic, nutrition support, pain management and pharmacological consultations. Through an Occupational Health Unit, he has offered independent pain management and pharmacological consultations nationwide. He has also advised the World Health Organization's Expert Committee regarding revisions as well as the selection of drugs to be listed in the next edition of *The Use of Essential Drugs* and is an assistant editor for the Drugdex drug information system. His past role as a Vice President Clinical Services bought him added expertise in overseeing occupational health, physical medicines, laboratory services, imaging, cardiology, respiratory therapy, cancer programs and continuing medical education. He served as conference coordinator for the first and second annual Dorchester General Hospital Pain conferences and as seminar coordinator for the eastern shore of Maryland for the "Take Control" physician and public pain education programs with Johns Hopkins.

Dr. Rybacki is now president of The Clearwater Group and the lead clinical consultant of the Medicine Information Institute—both headquartered in Easton, Maryland. He provides drug information support and clinical pharmacy services to physician groups, consumers and employers; holds seminars and continuing education meetings on infectious disease, adherence, osteoporosis, pain management, Women's Health and therapeutics; provides information support to insurance companies and HMOs; on-site hospital consulting on JCAHCO Pain standards, optimizing use of medicines and other programs, produces educational tapes and television programming on medicines; designs clinical programs; and conducts independent pharmacological evaluations. He is actively involved in the Compliance Action Program (CAP) of the American Heart Association on a national level, and is actively designing research involving how, why and how to enhance the way people take their medicines and decrease risk factors for cardiovascular disease. You can find out more about the CAP program on the web at www.americanheart.org/cap. Dr. Rybacki is also working with the American Heart Association to involve pharmacists and pharmacy associations, pharmacies as information and management sites and pharmacy chains in checking adherence. He is a strong advocate of a multilevel/multidisciplinary approach and is designing projects to involve pharmacists/physicians/PAs/nurses/nurse practitioners/cardiac rehab programs at the practice site itself in communicating risk factor reduction and medication adherence importance. He is also working to further a new hospital-based Secondary Prevention program (after a heart attack) called Get With The Guidelines (GWTG). Visit www.americanheart.org and www.medicineinfo.com for more details.

He was selected for full membership in the American College of Clinical Pharmacy, is a Certified Clinical Densitometrist (CCD) through the Society for Clinical Densitometry and became a Fellow to the American College of Forensic Examiners in 1997. He is a lifetime member of Who's Who in Global Business. Dr. Rybacki is director of clinical research, therapeutics and outcomes at the Medicine Information Institute—an interdisciplinary consulting group. Dr. Rybacki has been a frequent guest on Comcast's *Family Talk* live television program as well as their new *Real Life* TV. He is now the writer and host of a new television/radio program and video tape series called Medicines and Your Family with Dr. Jim Rybacki. This program will be taped to be broadcast in both a half an hour interview format as well as in short-segment on the web and radio. Catch Dr. Jim on the web, on the radio and on TV!

Current goals include creation of a special report on heart medications as well as phase two and four research on medicines among other projects. An active national speaker, Dr. Rybacki participates in numerous medical speakers bureaus, including Merck Pain management, Miles, Dupont Pharma and Glaxo. He has been a member of the Bristol-Myers Squibb Distinguished Speakers in HIV faculty since 1994 and lectures across the country. He has jointly authored several articles in professional journals on use of medicines in infectious diseases, critical care, therapeutics and cost containment and adherence. *The Essential Guide to Prescription Drugs*, first published in 1977, was co-authored by Dr. Rybacki since 1994, before he assumed full authorship in 1996. "The Medicine Man," a nationwide live radio show, was developed, written, produced and hosted by Dr. Rybacki in 1995. He is the original writer and host of the American Pharmaceutical Association's *The Pharmacist Minute* radio program, sponsored by a grant from Johnson and Johnson Merck (Pepcid AC®). Dr. Rybacki believes that the new art of prescribing medicines lies in setting and communicating goals and time frames and the importance of adherence for medicines, while achieving cost containment without sacrifice of clinical outcomes. He has created a popular site on the World Wide Web at www.medicineinfo.com.

Controlled Drug Schedules

Schedule I: These medicines have a high abuse and dependence potential. Typically, the only use for these drugs is for research purposes. Examples include LSD and heroin. A prescription cannot be legally written for these drugs for medicinal use.

Schedule II: These medicines have therapeutic uses and the highest abuse and dependence potential for drugs with medicinal purposes. Examples include analgesics such as morphine (MS Contin) and meperidine (Demerol). A written prescription is required and refills are not allowed.

Schedule III: Medicines in this schedule have an abuse and dependence potential that is less than those in schedule II, but greater than those in schedule IV. These medicines have clear medicinal uses and include such medicines as codeine, or paregoric in combination. A common name is Tylenol Number 3 with codeine. A telephone prescription is permitted for medications in this class; however, it must be converted to a written form by a pharmacist. Prescriptions for these medicines may be refilled, but only five times in 6 months.

Schedule IV: This schedule contains medicines with less abuse and dependence potential than those in schedule III. Examples of medicines in this schedule include diazepam (Valium) and chlordiazepoxide (Librium). Prescriptions for these medicines may be refilled, but only five times in 6 months.

Schedule V: These medicines have the lowest abuse and dependence potential. Medicines in this class include diphenoxylate (Lomotil) and loperamide (Imodium). Drugs in this class that require a prescription are handled the same as any nonscheduled prescription medicine. Some drugs in this class do not require a prescription, and can be sold only with the approval of a pharmacist. The buyer may be required to sign a logbook when the drug is dispensed. Examples include codeine and hydrocodone in combination with other active nonnarcotic drugs, sold in preparations that have limited quantities of codeine or hydrocodone for control of diarrhea or cough.

Pregnancy Risk Categories

Definitions of FDA Pregnancy Categories

Category A: Adequate and well-controlled studies in pregnant women are negative for fetal abnormalities. Risk to the fetus is remote.

Category B: Animal reproduction studies are negative for fetal abnormalities, and data from adequate and well-controlled studies in pregnant women are not available.
OR:
Animal reproduction studies are positive for fetal abnormalities. Adequate and well-controlled studies in pregnant women are negative for fetal abnormalities, and fail to show a risk to the fetus.

Category C: Animal reproduction studies are positive for fetal abnormalities. Information from adequate and well-controlled studies in pregnant women is not available.
OR:
Information from animal reproduction studies and from adequate and well-controlled studies in pregnant women is not available.

Category D: Studies in pregnant women and/or premarketing (investigational) or postmarketing uses show positive evidence of human fetal risk. The drug is only used in serious disease or in life-threatening situations where safer medicines will not work or cannot be used. These situations may make the medicine acceptable despite its risks.

Category X: Animal reproduction studies and/or human pregnancy studies are positive for fetal abnormalities.
OR:
Studies in pregnant women and/or premarketing (investigational) or postmarketing (Phase Four) experience show **positive** evidence of human fetal risk.
AND:
Potential fetal risks outweigh possible benefits of the drug. These medicines should never be used in pregnancy.

The FDA is currently evaluating these pregnancy categories, and may opt to modify them.